ESSENTIALS OF Clinical Psychopharmacology

THIRD EDITION

ESSENTIALS OF
Clinical Psychopharmacology

THIRD EDITION

EDITED BY

Alan F. Schatzberg, M.D.
Charles B. Nemeroff, M.D., Ph.D.

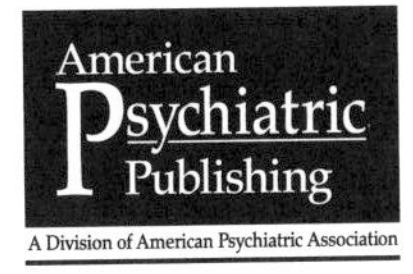

Washington, DC
London, England

Note: The authors have worked to ensure that all information in this book is accurate at the time of publication and consistent with general psychiatric and medical standards, and that information concerning drug dosages, schedules, and routes of administration is accurate at the time of publication and consistent with standards set by the U.S. Food and Drug Administration and the general medical community. As medical research and practice continue to advance, however, therapeutic standards may change. Moreover, specific situations may require a specific therapeutic response not included in this book. For these reasons and because human and mechanical errors sometimes occur, we recommend that readers follow the advice of physicians directly involved in their care or the care of a member of their family.

Books published by American Psychiatric Publishing (APP) represent the findings, conclusions, and views of the individual authors and do not necessarily represent the policies and opinions of APP or the American Psychiatric Association.

Manufactured in the United States of America on acid-free paper
17 16 15 14 13 5 4 3 2 1
Third Edition

American Psychiatric Publishing,
a Division of American Psychiatric Association
1000 Wilson Boulevard
Arlington, VA 22209-3901
www.appi.org

Typeset in Adobe's Bembo and Futura.

Library of Congress Cataloging-in-Publication Data

Essentials of clinical psychopharmacology / edited by Alan F. Schatzberg, Charles B. Nemeroff. — 3rd ed.

p. ; cm.

Includes bibliographical references and index.

ISBN 978-1-58562-419-5 (pbk. : alk. paper)

I. Schatzberg, Alan F. II. Nemeroff, Charles B.

[DNLM: 1. Mental Disorders—drug therapy. 2. Psychopharmacology. 3. Psychotropic Drugs. WM 402]

616.89′18—dc23

2012034906

British Library Cataloguing in Publication Data

A CIP record is available from the British Library.

Contents

Antipsychotics

Contributors

Elias Aboujaoude, M.D.
Associate Clinical Professor, Department of Psychiatry and Behavioral Sciences, Stanford University School of Medicine, Stanford, California

Donna Ames, M.D.
Professor in Residence, Department of Psychiatry and Behavioral Sciences, David Geffen School of Medicine, University of California Los Angeles; Program Leader, Psychosocial Rehabilitation and Recovery Center, Greater Los Angeles VA Medical Center, Los Angeles, California

Jacob S. Ballon, M.D.
Assistant Professor of Clinical Psychiatry, Department of Psychiatry, College of Physicians and Surgeons, Columbia University, and New York State Psychiatric Institute, New York, New York

Pierre Blier, M.D., Ph.D.
Professor, Departments of Psychiatry and Cellular/Molecular Medicine, University of Ottawa; Research Director, Mood Disorders Research Unit, University of Ottawa Institute of Mental Health Research, Ottawa, Ontario, Canada

David R. Block, M.D.
Staff Psychiatrist, Student Health Services, San Francisco State University, San Francisco, California

Charles L. Bowden, M.D.
Clinical Professor of Psychiatry and Pharmacology, Nancy U. Karren Endowed Chair of Psychiatry, Department of Psychiatry, University of Texas Health Science Center, San Antonio, Texas

Frank W. Brown, M.D.
Associate Professor of Psychiatry and Behavioral Sciences, Emory University School of Medicine, and Chief Medical Officer, Wesley Woods Geriatric Hospital, Emory HealthCare, Atlanta, Georgia

Mary F. Brunette, M.D.
Associate Professor of Psychiatry, Department of Psychiatry, Dartmouth Psychiatric Research Center, Dartmouth Medical School, Hanover, New Hampshire

Peter F. Buckley, M.D.
Dean, Medical College of Georgia, Georgia Health Sciences University, Augusta, Georgia

Matthew Byerly, M.D.
Associate Professor, University of Texas Southwestern Medical Center, Dallas, Texas

Joseph R. Calabrese, M.D.
Director, Mood Disorders Program, University Hospitals of Cleveland, and Professor of Psychiatry, Case Western Reserve University School of Medicine, Cleveland, Ohio

Carla M. Canuso, M.D.
Senior Director, External Innovation, Neuroscience Therapeutic Area, Janssen Pharmaceutical Research & Development LLC, Titusville, New Jersey

Linda L. Carpenter, M.D.
Professor, Department of Psychiatry and Human Behavior, Warren Alpert Medical School of Brown University, Providence, Rhode Island

Leslie L. Citrome, M.D., M.P.H.
Clinical Professor of Psychiatry and Behavioral Sciences, New York Medical College, Valhalla, New York

Anita H. Clayton, M.D.
David C. Wilson Professor, Department of Psychiatry and Neurobehavioral Sciences, and Professor of Clinical Obstetrics and Gynecology, University of Virginia, Charlottesville, Virginia

Yvonne I. Cole, Ph.D.
Research Coordinator, Department of Psychiatry, Columbia University College of Physicians and Surgeons, New York, New York

James W. Cornish, M.D.
Associate Professor, Department of Psychiatry, University of Pennsylvania and Philadelphia Veterans Affairs Medical Center, Philadelphia, Pennsylvania

Daniella David, M.D.
Chief of Psychiatry, Bruce W. Carter Department of Veterans Affairs Medical Center; Professor of Clinical Psychiatry, Department of Psychiatry and Behavioral Sciences, University of Miami Miller School of Medicine, Miami, Florida

Jonathan R. T. Davidson, M.D.
Emeritus Professor, Department of Psychiatry and Behavioral Sciences, Duke University Medical Center, Durham, North Carolina

Karon Dawkins, M.D.
Associate Professor of Psychiatry and Director of General Psychiatry Residency Training, School of Medicine, University of North Carolina at Chapel Hill, Chapel Hill, North Carolina

Charles DeBattista, D.M.H., M.D.
Professor, Department of Psychiatry and Behavioral Sciences, Stanford University School of Medicine, Stanford, California

William C. Dement, M.D., Ph.D.
Lowell W. and Josephine Q. Berry Professor, Department of Psychiatry and Behavioral Sciences, Stanford University School of Medicine, Stanford, Palo Alto, California

Jamie M. Dupuy, M.D.
Instructor in Psychiatry, Harvard Medical School; Attending Psychiatrist, Harvard Vanguard Medical Associates, Boston, Massachusetts

Adriana E. Foster, M.D.
Associate Professor, Department of Psychiatry and Health Behavior, Medical College of Georgia, Georgia Health Sciences University, Augusta, Georgia

Marlene P. Freeman, M.D.
Associate Professor of Psychiatry, Harvard Medical School; Director of Clinical Services, Center for Women's Mental Health, Perinatal and Reproductive Psychiatry Clinical Research Program, Massachusetts General Hospital, Boston, Massachusetts

Oliver Freudenreich, M.D.
Associate Professor, Department of Psychiatry, Massachusetts General Hospital, Harvard Medical School, Boston, Massachusetts

Mark A. Frye, M.D.
Consultant, Professor, and Chair, Department of Psychiatry and Psychology, and Director, Mayo Clinic Depression Center, Mayo Clinic, Rochester, Minnesota

Keming Gao, M.D., Ph.D.
Director, Mood and Anxiety Clinic, Assistant Professor of Psychiatry, University Hospitals Case Medical Center, Case Western Reserve University School of Medicine, Cleveland, Ohio

Alan J. Gelenberg, M.D.
Shively-Tan Professor and Chair, Department of Psychiatry, Penn State College of Medicine, Hershey, Pennsylvania

Elizabeth H. Gillespie, D.O.
Consulting Psychiatrist, Johns Hopkins University Counseling Center, Baltimore, Maryland

Ira D. Glick, M.D.
Professor Emeritus of Psychiatry and Behavioral Sciences, Stanford University School of Medicine, Stanford, California

Donald C. Goff, M.D.
Director, Nathan S. Kline Institute for Psychiatric Research, Orangeburg, New York

Robert N. Golden, M.D.
Dean, School of Medicine and Public Health, and Vice Chancellor for Medical Affairs, University of Wisconsin–Madison, Madison, Wisconsin

Alan I. Green, M.D.
Raymond Sobel Professor of Psychiatry and Chairman, Department of Psychiatry, Dartmouth Medical School, Hanover, New Hampshire

Philip D. Harvey, Ph.D.
Professor and Chief, Division of Psychology, Department of Psychiatry and Behavioral Sciences, University of Miami Miller School of Medicine, Miami, Florida

Joseph Henry, M.D.
Assistant Professor of Clinical Psychiatry, Department of Psychiatry and Behavioral Sciences, University of Miami Miller School of Medicine, Miami, Florida

Michele Hill, M.R.C.Psych.
Research Fellow, Schizophrenia Program, Massachusetts General Hospital, Boston, Massachusetts

Ned H. Kalin, M.D.
Hedberg Professor and Chair, Department of Psychiatry; and Director, HealthEmotions Research Institute, University of Wisconsin School of Medicine and Public Health, Madison, Wisconsin

Paul E. Keck Jr., M.D.
President–CEO, Lindner Center of HOPE, Mason, Ohio; Lindner Professor of Psychiatry and Behavioral Neuroscience and Executive Vice Chair, University of Cincinnati College of Medicine, Cincinnati, Ohio

David E. Kemp, M.D., M.S.
Director, Mood and Metabolic Clinic, Assistant Professor of Psychiatry, University Hospitals Case Medical Center, Case Western Reserve University School of Medicine, Cleveland, Ohio

Terence A. Ketter, M.D.
Professor of Psychiatry and Behavioral Sciences and Chief, Bipolar Disorders Clinic, Stanford University School of Medicine, Stanford, California

Lorrin M. Koran, M.D.
Professor of Psychiatry, Emeritus, Department of Psychiatry and Behavioral Sciences, Stanford University School of Medicine, Stanford, California

K. Ranga Rama Krishnan, M.D.
Professor and Chairman, Department of Psychiatry and Behavioral Sciences, Duke University Medical Center, Durham, North Carolina; Dean, Duke–NUS Graduate Medical School Singapore

Jeffrey A. Lieberman, M.D.
Chairman, Department of Psychiatry, College of Physicians and Surgeons, Columbia University; Director, New York State Psychiatric Institute; Director, Lieber Center for Schizophrenia Research; Psychiatrist-in-Chief, New York Presbyterian Hospital and Columbia University Medical Center, New York, New York

Stephen R. Marder, M.D.
Professor and Director, Section on Psychosis, Semel Institute of Neuroscience and Human Behavior, University of California at Los Angeles; Director, Desert Pacific Mental Illness Research, Education, and Clinical Center, West Los Angeles Veterans Administration Medical Center, Los Angeles, California

Susan L. McElroy, M.D.
Chief Research Officer, Lindner Center of HOPE, Mason, Ohio; Professor of Psychiatry and Behavioral Neuroscience, University of Cincinnati College of Medicine, Cincinnati, Ohio

Laura F. McNicholas, M.D., Ph.D.
Clinical Associate Professor, Department of Psychiatry, University of Pennsylvania, Philadelphia, Pennsylvania, and Philadelphia Veterans Affairs Medical Center, Philadelphia, Pennsylvania

Emmanuel Mignot, M.D., Ph.D.
Craig Reynolds Professor of Sleep Medicine and Professor of Psychiatry and Behavioral Sciences, Stanford University School of Medicine, Palo Alto, California; Director, Stanford Center for Sleep Sciences and Medicine, Palo Alto, California

Kazuo Mishima, M.D., Ph.D.
Director, National Institute of Mental Health, National Center of Neurology and Psychiatry, Kodaira, Tokyo, Japan

Katherine Marshall Moore, M.D.
Consultant, Department of Psychiatry and Psychology, Mayo Clinic, Rochester, Minnesota

Henry A. Nasrallah, M.D.
Professor of Psychiatry and Neuroscience, Department of Psychiatry, University of Cincinnati College of Medicine, Cincinnati, Ohio

J. Craig Nelson, M.D.
Leon J. Epstein Professor of Psychiatry, Director of Geriatric Psychiatry, University of California San Francisco

Charles B. Nemeroff, M.D., Ph.D.
Leonard M. Miller Professor and Chairman, Department of Psychiatry and Behavioral Sciences, University of Miami Miller School of Medicine, Miami, Florida

John W. Newcomer, M.D.
Leonard M. Miller Professor of Psychiatry and Behavioral Sciences, Leonard M. Miller School of Medicine, University of Miami, Miami, Florida

D. Jeffrey Newport, M.D.
Associate Professor, Department of Psychiatry and Behavioral Sciences, Emory University School of Medicine, Atlanta, Georgia

Linda Nicholas, M.D.
Professor of Psychiatry, School of Medicine, University of North Carolina at Chapel Hill, Chapel Hill, North Carolina

Seiji Nishino, M.D., Ph.D.
Professor of Psychiatry and Behavioral Sciences, Stanford University School of Medicine, Stanford, California; Director, Sleep and Circadian Neurobiology Laboratory, Stanford Sleep Research Center, Palo Alto, California

Sandhaya Norris, M.D.
Physician, Mood Disorders Research Unit, University of Ottawa Institute of Mental Health Research, Ottawa, Ontario, Canada

Charles P. O'Brien, M.D., Ph.D.
Kenneth Appel Professor, Department of Psychiatry, University of Pennsylvania and Philadelphia Veterans Affairs Medical Center, Philadelphia, Pennsylvania

Eric D. Peselow, M.D.
Adjunct Professor of Psychiatry and Behavioral Sciences, New York Medical College, Valhalla, New York

Steven R. Pliszka, M.D.
Professor and Chief, Division of Child and Adolescent Psychiatry, Department of Psychiatry, The University of Texas Health Science Center at San Antonio

Robert M. Post, M.D.
Adjunct Professor of Psychiatry, George Washington University, Washington, DC; Head, Bipolar Collaborative Network, Bethesda, Maryland

Michelle M. Primeau, M.D.
Clinical Instructor, Department of Psychiatry, Stanford University, Stanford, California

B. Ashok Raj, M.D.
Physician Researcher, University of South Florida College of Medicine, Tampa, Florida

Mark Hyman Rapaport, M.D.
Chairman, Department of Psychiatry and Behavioral Sciences, Emory University School of Medicine, and Chief of Psychiatric Services, Emory Healthcare System, Atlanta, Georgia

Karl Rickels, M.D.
Stuart and Emily B.H. Mudd Professor of Behavior and Reproduction in Psychiatry, Department of Psychiatry, University of Pennsylvania, Philadelphia, Pennsylvania

Donald S. Robinson, M.D.
Consultant, Worldwide Drug Development, Shelburne, Vermont

Patrick H. Roseboom, Ph.D.
Associate Scientist in Psychiatry and Lecturer in Pharmacology, University of Wisconsin School of Medicine and Public Health, Madison, Wisconsin

Jerrold F. Rosenbaum, M.D.
Chief of Psychiatry, Massachusetts General Hospital; Stanley Cobb Professor of Psychiatry, Harvard Medical School, Boston, Massachusetts

Noriaki Sakai, D.V.M., Ph.D.
Visiting Scholar, Department of Psychiatry and Behavioral Sciences, Stanford University School of Medicine, Palo Alto, California

Erika F. H. Saunders, M.D.
Assistant Professor of Psychiatry, Penn State College of Medicine, Hershey, Pennsylvania

Alan F. Schatzberg, M.D.
Kenneth T. Norris Jr. Professor, Department of Psychiatry and Behavioral Sciences, Stanford University School of Medicine, Stanford, California

S. Charles Schulz, M.D.
Professor and Head, Department of Psychiatry, University of Minnesota School of Medicine, Minneapolis, Minnesota

Zafar A. Sharif, M.D.
Associate Clinical Professor of Psychiatry, Columbia University, New York, New York; Director, Department of Psychiatry, Harlem Hospital Center, New York, New York

Jonathan Shaywitz, M.D.
Director, Anxiety Disorders Program, Department of Psychiatry and Health Behavior, Cedars-Sinai Medical Center, Los Angeles, California

David V. Sheehan, M.D., M.B.A.
Distinguished University Health Professor Emeritus, University of South Florida College of Medicine, Tampa, Florida

George M. Simpson, M.D.
Professor of Research Psychiatry, Department of Psychiatry and Behavioral Sciences, USC Keck School of Medicine, Los Angeles, California

Justin B. Smith, M.D.
Chief Resident, Department of Psychiatry and Neurobehavioral Sciences, University of Virginia School of Medicine, Charlottesville, Virginia

Joseph K. Stanilla, M.D.
Assistant Professor of Psychiatry, Jefferson Medical College of Thomas Jefferson University, Philadelphia, Pennsylvania

Zachary N. Stowe, M.D.
Professor in Psychiatry, Pediatrics, and Obstetrics & Gynecology, University of Arkansas for Medical Sciences, Little Rock, Arkansas

Martin T. Strassnig, M.D.
Assistant Professor of Psychiatry and Behavioral Sciences, and Medical Director, Mood Disorders and ECT Program, Leonard M. Miller School of Medicine, University of Miami, Miami, Florida

Rajiv Tandon, M.D.
Professor of Psychiatry, University of Florida College of Medicine, Gainesville, Florida

Michael E. Thase, M.D.
Professor, Department of Psychiatry, University of Pennsylvania School of Medicine (Philadelphia) and Philadelphia Veterans Affairs Medical Center; Adjunct Professor, University of Pittsburgh Medical Center, Pittsburgh, Pennsylvania

Marc L. van der Loos, M.D., Ph.D.
Department of Psychiatry, Isala Klinieken, Location Sophia, Zwolle, The Netherlands

Scott Van Sant, M.D.
Assistant Professor, Department of Psychiatry and Health Behavior, Georgia Health Sciences University, Augusta, Georgia

Karen Dineen Wagner, M.D., Ph.D.
Marie B. Gale Centennial Professor and Vice Chair, Department of Psychiatry and Behavioral Sciences, and Director, Division of Child and Adolescent Psychiatry, University of Texas Medical Branch, Galveston, Texas

Po W. Wang, M.D.
Clinical Associate Professor, Department of Psychiatry and Behavioral Sciences, Stanford University School of Medicine, Stanford, California

Curtis W. Wittmann, M.D.
Instructor in Psychiatry, Harvard Medical School; Associate Director, Acute Psychiatric Service, Massachusetts General Hospital, Boston, Massachusetts

Joanne D. Wojcik, Ph.D., P.M.H.C.N.S.-B.C.
Instructor in Psychiatry and Associate Director, Commonwealth Research Center, Beth Israel Deaconess Medical Center, Harvard Medical School, Boston, Massachusetts

Tsung-Ung W. Woo, M.D., Ph.D.
Assistant Professor of Psychiatry, Harvard Medical School, Boston, Massachusetts; Director, Laboratory for Cellular Neuropathology, McLean Hospital, Belmont, Massachusetts

Kimberly A. Yonkers, M.D.
Professor, Departments of Psychiatry, Obstetrics, Gynecology and Reproductive Sciences, Yale School of Medicine, New Haven, Connecticut

Daniel Zigman, M.D.
Physician, Mood Disorders Research Unit, University of Ottawa Institute of Mental Health Research, Ottawa, Ontario, Canada

Disclosure of Interests

The contributors have declared all forms of support received within the 12 months prior to manuscript submittal that may represent a competing interest in relation to their work published in this volume, as follows:

Pierre Blier, M.D., Ph.D. *Consultant:* AstraZeneca, Bristol-Myers Squibb, Eli Lilly, Janssen Pharmaceuticals, Lundbeck, Merck, Pfizer, Servier, and Takeda; *Lecture Honoraria:* Janssen Pharmaceuticals, Lundbeck, and Pfizer; *Grant Support:* AstraZeneca, Bristol-Myers Squibb, Janssen Pharmaceuticals, Labopharm, Lundbeck, Merck, Pfizer, and Servier; *Contract Employee:* Steelbeach Productions.

Joseph R. Calabrese, M.D. *Federal Funding:* U.S. Department of Defense, Health Resources and Services Administration, and National Institute of Mental Health; *Research Support:* Abbott, AstraZeneca, Bristol-Myers Squibb, Cephalon, Cleveland Foundation, Eli Lilly, GlaxoSmithKline, Janssen, National Alliance for Research on Schizophrenia and Depression, Repligen, Stanley Medical Research Institute, Takeda, and Wyeth; *Consultant/Advisory Board:* Abbott, AstraZeneca, Bristol-Myers Squibb, Dainippon Sumitomo, EPI-Q, Forest, France Foundation, GlaxoSmithKline, Janssen, Johnson & Johnson, Lundbeck, Merck, Neurosearch, OrthoMcNeil, Otsuka, Pfizer, Repligen, Schering-Plough, Servier, Solvay, Supernus, Synosia, Takeda, and Wyeth; *CME Lecture Support:* AstraZeneca, Bristol-Myers Squibb, France Foundation, GlaxoSmithKline, Janssen, Johnson & Johnson, Merck, Sanofi-Aventis, Schering-Plough, Pfizer, Solvay, and Wyeth.

Carla M. Canuso, M.D. *Employed by:* Janssen Pharmaceutical Research & Development LLC; *Stock:* Johnson & Johnson.

Linda L. Carpenter, M.D. *Grant/Research Support:* National Alliance for Research on Schizophrenia and Depression (2006–2009), National Institute of Mental Health (2005–2012), Pfizer (2006), UCB Pharma (2006–2009), Sepracor (2007–2009), Cyberonics (2007–2010), U.S. Department of Defense (2006–2009), Medtronic (2009–2012), Neuronetics (2009–2012), NeoSync (2011–2012); *Consultant/Advisory Board:* Abbott (2006, 2010, 2011, 2012),

Bristol-Myers Squibb (2005), Cyberonics (2006, 2007, 2008), Johnson & Johnson (2012), Medtronic (2005), Takeda Lundbeck (2011), Novartis (2006, 2007, 2008), Pfizer (2006), Wyeth (2006, 2007, 2008, 2009), Sepracor (2005), AstraZeneca (2008), Neuronetics (2007, 2009, 2010, 2011) (Note: No financial compensation received from Neuronetics since 2009; consultancy in 2010 and thereafter on volunteer basis only); *Honoraria for CME:* No commercial entity support since 2008; all CME presentations supported by hosting academic institutions and American Psychiatric Association (none since 2009); *Full-Time Employee:* Butler Hospital, Providence, RI.

Leslie L. Citrome, M.D., M.P.H. *Consultant/Honoraria/Clinical Research Support:* Alexza, Alkermes, AstraZeneca, Avanir, Bristol-Myers Squibb, Eli Lilly, Genentech, Janssen, Lundbeck, Merck, Novartis, Noven, Otsuka, Pfizer, Shire, Sunovion, and Valeant.

Anita H. Clayton, M.D. *Grant/Research Support:* Pfizer; *Consultant/Advisory Board:* AstraZeneca, Bristol-Myers Squibb, PGxHealth, Pfizer, and Sanofi-Aventis.

Jonathan R. T. Davidson, M.D. *Advisor:* CeNeRx BioPharma; *Data and Safety Monitoring Board:* University of California at San Diego; *Royalties and Licence Fees:* Connor-Davidson Resilience Scale, Multi-Health Systems Inc. (for Davidson Trauma Scale), Social Phobia Inventory, Guilford Publications, and McFarland Publishing.

Mark A. Frye, M.D. *Grant Support:* Mayo Foundation, Myriad Genetics, National Alliance for Research on Schizophrenia and Depression, National Institute on Alcohol Abuse and Alcoholism, National Institute of Mental Health, and Pfizer.

Keming Gao, M.D., Ph.D. *Grant/Research Support:* AstraZeneca, National Alliance for Research on Schizophrenia and Depression.

Alan J. Gelenberg, M.D. *Grant/Research Support:* Eli Lilly, GlaxoSmithKline; *Consultant:* AstraZeneca, Best Practice, Dey Pharma, Eli Lilly, eResearch Technology (ERT), GlaxoSmithKline, Jazz Pharmaceuticals, Lundbeck, Myriad Genetics, PGxHealth, Takeda, Wyeth, and ZARS Pharma; *Stock Holdings:* Healthcare Technology Systems.

Ira D. Glick, M.D. *Consultant/Honoraria/Clinical Research Support:* AstraZeneca, Bristol-Myers Squibb/Otsuka, Eli Lilly, GlaxoSmithKline, Janssen, Lundbeck, National Institute of Mental Health, Organon, Pfizer, Shire, Solvay, and Vanda.

Donald C. Goff, M.D. *Consultant/Advisory Board:* Abbott Laboratories, Biovail, Bristol-Myers Squibb, Cypress, Dainippon Sumitomo, Eli Lilly, Endo Pharmaceuticals, Hoffman-La Roche, Indevus Pharmaceuticals, H. Lundbeck, Schering-Plough, Solvay, and Takeda; *Data and Safety Monitoring Board:* Otsuka; *Research Support:* GlaxoSmithKline, Janssen, Novartis, and Pfizer.

Robert N. Golden, M.D. *Associate Editor: Psychosomatic Medicine; Board of Directors:* The Shapiro Foundation.

Alan I. Green, M.D. *Research Support:* AstraZeneca, Eli Lilly, and Janssen; *Data and Safety Monitoring Board:* Eli Lilly (no personal compensation); *Pending Patents:* Treatment for Substance Abuse.

Philip D. Harvey, Ph.D. *Consultant:* Abbott Laboratories, Bristol-Myers Squibb, Cypress Bioscience, EnVivo Pharmaceuticals, Genentech, Johnson & Johnson, Merck, Shire Pharmaceuticals, and Sunovion Pharmaceuticals.

Ned H. Kalin, M.D. *Scientific Advisory Board:* AstraZeneca, Bristol-Myers Squibb, CeNeRx BioPharma, Centocor Ortho Biotech, CME Outfitters, Corcept Therapeutics, Double Helix, Elsevier, Eli Lilly, Letters and Sciences, Medivation, Neuronetics, Otsuka American Pharmaceuticals, Sanofi-Aventis, Wyeth Pharmaceuticals; *Research Grants:* National Institute of Mental Health, Stanley Medical Research Institute; *Editor: Psychoneuroendocrinology* (Elsevier); *Stock/Equity Holdings:* CeNeRx BioPharma, Corcept Therapeutics; *Owner:* Promoter Neurosciences LLC; *Patents:* U.S. Patent Nos. 7,071,323 and 7,531,356—Kalin NH, Roseboom PH, Landry CF, Nanda SA: Promoter sequences for corticotropin-releasing factor CRF2alpha and method of identifying agents that alter the activity of the promoter sequences; U.S. Patent No. 7,087,385—Kalin NH, Roseboom PH, Nanda SA: Promoter sequences for urocortin 2 and the use thereof; U.S. Patent No. 7,122,650—Roseboom PH, Kalin NH, Nanda SA: Promoter sequences for corticotropin-releasing factor binding protein and use thereof.

Paul E. Keck Jr., M.D. *Employers:* University of Cincinnati College of Medicine and Lindner Center of HOPE; *Research Sponsorship:* Alkermes, AstraZeneca, Cephalon, GlaxoSmithKline, Eli Lilly, Jazz Pharmaceuticals, Marriott Foundation, National Institute of Mental Health, Orexigen, Pfizer, and Shire; *Consultant (2010):* Sepracor and Medco; *CME Presentation Support (2010):* CME Neuroscience; *Patents:* Co-inventor on U.S. Patent No. 6,387,956—Shapira NA, Goldsmith TD, Keck PE Jr. (University of Cincinnati): Methods of treating obsessive-compulsive spectrum disorder comprises the step of administering an effective amount of tramadol to an individual. Filed March 25, 1999; approved May 14, 2002. (Dr. Keck has received no financial gain from this patent.)

David E. Kemp, M.D., M.S. *Consultant:* Bristol-Myers Squibb; *Speakers Bureau:* AstraZeneca and Pfizer; *Other:* Spouse holds shares in Abbott.

Terence A. Ketter, M.D. *Grant/Research Support:* AstraZeneca, Cephalon, Eli Lilly, Pfizer, and Sunovion; *Consultant:* Merck; *Lecture Honoraria:* AstraZeneca and GlaxoSmithKline; *Publishing Royalties:* American Psychiatric Publishing; *Other:* Spouse is an employee of and owns stock in Johnson & Johnson.

K. Ranga Rama Krishnan, M.D. *Indirect Stock Ownership and Scientific Advisory Board:* CeNeRx BioPharma; *Stock Ownership:* Orexigen, Sonexa Therapeutics, and Corcept.

Stephen R. Marder, M.D. *Consultant/Advisory Board:* Abbott, Amgen, Boehringer, Genentech, Otsuka, Roche, Shire, and Targacept; *Research Support:* Novartis, PsychoGenics, and Sunovion.

Susan L. McElroy, M.D. *Employers:* University of Cincinnati College of Medicine and Lindner Center of HOPE; *Consultant/Scientific Advisory Board:* Alkermes, Eli Lilly, and Shire; *Research Sponsorship:* Agency for Healthcare Research and Quality, Alkermes, AstraZeneca, Bristol-Myers Squibb, Cephalon, Eli Lilly, Forest Labs, GlaxoSmithKline, Jazz Pharmaceuticals, Marriott Foundation, National Institute of Mental Health, Orexigen Therapeutics, Pfizer, Shire, and Takeda; *Patents:* Inventor on U.S. Patent No. 6,323,236 B2 (Use of Sulfamate Derivatives for Treating Impulse Control Disorders), and, along with the patent's assignee (University of Cincinnati, Cincinnati, OH), has received payments from Johnson & Johnson Pharmaceutical Research & Development LLC, which has exclusive rights under the patent.

J. Craig Nelson, M.D. *Lecture Honoraria:* Biovail, Eli Lilly Global, Lundbeck, Otsuka Asia, and Schering-Plough/Merck (Asia); *Consultant:* Bristol-Myers Squibb, Corcept, Covidien, Eli Lilly, Forest, Lundbeck, Medtronic, Merck, Orexigen, Otsuka, and Pfizer; *Advisory Board:* Bristol-Myers Squibb, Dey Pharma, Eli Lilly, Labopharm, and Otsuka; *Research Support:* Health Resources and Services Administration and National Institute of Mental Health; *Stock Ownership:* Atossa Genetics.

Charles B. Nemeroff, M.D., Ph.D. *Consultant:* Takeda, Xhale; *Research/Grant Support:* Agency for Healthcare Research and Quality, National Institutes of Health; *Stock Holdings:* CeNeRx BioPharma, Corcept Therapeutics, NovaDel Pharma, PharmaNeuroBoost, Revaax Pharma, Xhale; *Other Financial Interests:* CeNeRx BioPharma, PharmaNeuroBoost; *Scientific Advisory Board:* American Foundation for Suicide Prevention (AFSP), Anxiety Disorders Association of America, CeNeRx BioPharma, National Alliance for Research on Schizophrenia and Depression, NovaDel Pharma, PharmaNeuroBoost; *Board of Directors:* AFSP, NovaDel Pharma; *Patents:* U.S. Patent No. 6,375,990B1—Method and devices for transdermal delivery of lithium; U.S. Patent No. 7,148,027B2—Method of assessing antidepressant drug therapy via transport inhibition of monoamine neurotransmitters by ex vivo assay.

John W. Newcomer, M.D. *Grant Support:* National Alliance for Research on Schizophrenia and Depression, National Institute of Mental Health, Bristol-Myers Squibb, Pfizer, Wyeth; *Consultant:* AstraZeneca, Bristol-Myers Squibb, Biovail; *Litigation Consultant:* H. Lundbeck, Janssen Pharmaceutica, Obecure, Otsuka Pharmaceuticals, Pfizer, Sepracor, Solvay Pharma, Vanda Pharmaceutica, Wyeth Pharmaceuticals; *Data and Safety Monitoring Board:* Dainippon Sumitomo Pharma America, Organon Pharmaceuticals, Schering-Plough/Merck, Vivus; *Product Development Royalties:* Jones & Bartlett Publishing.

D. Jeffrey Newport, M.D. *Research Support:* Eli Lilly, GlaxoSmithKline, Janssen, National Alliance for Research on Schizophrenia and Depression, National Institutes of Health, and Wyeth; *Speakers Honoraria:* AstraZeneca, Eli Lilly, GlaxoSmithKline, and Pfizer.

Eric D. Peselow, M.D. *Consultant/Honoraria/Clinical Research Support:* Forest and Pfizer.

Steven R. Pliszka, M.D. *Expert Witness:* Eli Lilly; *Research Grants:* Ortho-McNeil-Janssen, Shire; *Consultant:* Therazance (one time).

Robert M. Post, M.D. *Consultant:* AstraZeneca, Bristol-Myers Squibb, GlaxoSmithKline, and PureTech Ventures; *Speakers Honoraria:* AstraZeneca, Bristol-Myers Squibb, GlaxoSmithKline, Janssen-Cilag, Novartis, and PureTech Ventures.

Mark Hyman Rapaport, M.D. *Consultant:* National Institute on Drug Abuse and National Institute of Mental Health; *Unpaid Science Advisory Board:* National Center for Complementary and Alternative Medicine and Pax Pharmaceutical.

Patrick H. Roseboom, Ph.D. *Research Grant:* Stanley Medical Research Institute; *Co-Owner and Part-Time Employee:* Promoter Neurosciences LLC; *Patents:* U.S. Patent Nos. 7,071,323 and 7,531,356—Kalin NH, Roseboom PH, Landry CF, Nanda SA: Promoter sequences for corticotropin-releasing factor CRF2alpha and method of identifying agents that alter the activity of the promoter sequences; U.S. Patent No. 7,087,385—Kalin NH, Roseboom PH, Nanda SA: Promoter sequences for urocortin 2 and the use thereof; U.S. Patent No. 7,122,650—Roseboom PH, Kalin NH, Nanda SA: Promoter sequences for corticotropin-releasing factor binding protein and use thereof.

Alan F. Schatzberg, M.D. *Consultant:* BrainCells, CeNeRx BioPharma, CNS Response, Eli Lilly, Forest Labs, GlaxoSmithKline, Jazz Pharmaceuticals, Lundbeck, Merck, Neuronetics, NovaDel Pharma, Novartis, Pathway Diagnostics, Pfizer, PharmaNeuroBoost, Quintiles, Sanofi-Aventis, Sunovion, Synosia, Takeda, Xytis, and Wyeth; *Honoraria:* Merck, Pfizer, and Roche; *Equity Holdings:* Amnestix, BrainCells, CeNeRx BioPharma, Corcept (co-founder), Delpor, Forest Labs, Merck, Neurocrine, NovaDel Pharma, Pfizer, PharmaNeuroBoost, Somaxon, and Synosia; *Intellectual Property:* Named inventor on pharmacogenetic use patents on prediction of antidepressant response and glucocorticoid antagonists in psychiatry.

S. Charles Schulz, M.D. *Advisory Board:* Biovail, Bristol-Myers Squibb, Eli Lilly; *Grant Support:* AstraZeneca, Otsuka, Rules-Based Medicine Inc.

David V. Sheehan, M.D., M.B.A. *Lectures/Presentations/Publications:* Abbott Laboratories, Angelini-Labopharm, AstraZeneca, Boehringer Ingelheim Pharmaceuticals, Boots Pharmaceuticals, Bristol-Myers Squibb, Burroughs Wellcome, Charter Hospitals, Ciba Geigy, Dista Products, Eli Lilly, Excerpta Medica Asia, Glaxo Pharmaceuticals, GlaxoSmithKline, Harvard University, Hikma Pharmaceuticals, Hospital Corporation of America, Humana, Janssen Pharmaceutica, Kali-Duphar, Kennedy Krieger Institute LLC, Labopharm, McNeil Pharmaceuticals, Mead Johnson, Merck Sharp & Dohme, Organon, Novo Nordisk, Parke-Davis, Pfizer, Pharmacia & Upjohn, Quadrant HealthCom, Rhone-Poulenc Rorer Pharmaceuticals, Rhone Laboratories, Roerig, Sandoz Pharmaceuticals, Schering, SmithKlineBeecham, Solvay Pharmaceuticals, TAP Pharmaceuticals, Tampa General Hospital/University Psychiatry Center, The Upjohn Company, United BioSource Corporation, Warner Chilcott, Wyeth-Ayerst Laboratories; *Stock Shareholder:* Medical Outcome Systems; *Grant/Research Support:* Abbott Laboratories, American Medical Association, Anclote Foundation, AstraZeneca, Bristol-Myers Squibb, Burroughs Wellcome, Cephalon, Eisai America, Eli Lilly, Forest Laboratories, GlaxoSmithKline, Institute of Clinical Research (ICR), Janssen Pharmaceutica Products, Jazz Pharmaceuticals, Kali Duphar Laboratories, Mead Johnson, Medicinova, Merck Sharp & Dohme, National Institute of Drug Abuse, National Institutes of Health, Novartis Pharmaceuticals, Parke-Davis, Pfizer, Quintiles, Sandoz Pharmaceuticals, Sanofi-Aventis, Sanofi-Synthelabo Recherche, SmithKlineBeecham Pharmaceuticals, Tampa General Hospital/University Psychiatry Center, TAP Pharmaceuticals, The Upjohn Company, Warner Chilcott, Worldwide Clinical Trials, and Wyeth-Ayerst; *Consultant:* Angelini-Labopharm, Applied Health Outcomes/Xcenda, INC Research, International Society for CNS Drug Development, National Anxiety Foundation, NovaDel Pharma, Pfizer, PharmaNeuroBoost, and Sagene.

Zachary N. Stowe, M.D. *Grant/Research Support:* GlaxoSmithKline, National Institutes of Health, and Wyeth; *Advisory Board:* Bristol-Myers Squibb, GlaxoSmithKline, and Wyeth; *Speakers Honoraria:* Eli Lilly, GlaxoSmithKline, Pfizer, and Wyeth.

Martin T. Strassnig, M.D. *Research Grant:* Pfizer Global Investigator-Initiated Research Program.

Michael E. Thase, M.D. *Consultant:* AstraZeneca, Bristol-Myers Squibb, Dey Pharma, Eli Lilly, Forest Pharmaceuticals, Gerson Lehman Group, GlaxoSmithKline, Guidepoint Global, H. Lundbeck A/S, MedAvante, Merck, Neuronetics, Novartis, Otsuka, Ortho-McNeil Pharmaceuticals, PamLab, Pfizer, Schering-Plough, Shire US, Supernus Pharmaceuticals, Takeda (Lundbeck), and Transcept Pharmaceuticals; *Speakers Bureau:* AstraZeneca, Bristol-Myers Squibb, Eli Lilly, Merck, and Pfizer; *Grant Support:* Eli Lilly, GlaxoSmithKline, National Institute of Mental Health, Agency for Healthcare Research and Quality, and Sepracor; *Royalties:* American Psychiatric Publishing, Guilford Publications, Herald House, Oxford University Press, and W.W. Norton; *Equity Holdings:* MedAvante; *Other:* Spouse is employed as the Group Scientific Director for Embryon (formerly Advogent), which does business with Bristol-Myers Squibb and Pfizer/Wyeth.

Marc L. van der Loos, M.D., Ph.D. *Advisory Board:* Bristol-Myers Squibb; *Speakers Bureau:* AstraZeneca; *Research Support:* Employer (Isala Klinieken Zwolle) was compensated by GlaxoSmithKline for time spent on research.

Karen Dineen Wagner, M.D., Ph.D. *Honoraria:* American Academy of Child Adolescent Psychiatry, American Psychiatric Association, CME LLC, CMP Medica, Contemporary Forums, Doctors Hospital at Renaissance, Physicians Postgraduate Press, Quantia Communications, and UMB Medica.

Kimberly A. Yonkers, M.D. *Study Medication:* Pfizer (for a National Institute of Mental Health trial); *Investigator-Initiated Trial Support:* Eli Lilly; *Royalties:* Up To Date.

The following authors have no competing interests to report:

Elias Aboujaoude, M.D.
David R. Block, M.D.
Charles L. Bowden, M.D.
Frank W. Brown, M.D.
Mary F. Brunette, M.D.
Yvonne I. Cole, Ph.D.
James W. Cornish, M.D.
Daniella David, M.D.
Jamie M. Dupuy, M.D.
Elizabeth H. Gillespie, D.O.
Joseph Henry, M.D.
Michele Hill, M.R.C.Psych.
Lorrin M. Koran, M.D.
Katherine Marshall Moore, M.D.
Sandhaya Norris, M.D.
Michelle M. Primeau, M.D.
Karl Rickels, M.D.
Donald S. Robinson, M.D.
Jerrold F. Rosenbaum, M.D.
Noriaki Sakai, D.V.M., Ph.D.
Erika F. H. Saunders, M.D.
George M. Simpson, M.D.
Justin B. Smith, M.D.
Joseph K. Stanilla, M.D.
Curtis W. Wittmann, M.D.
Joanne D. Wojcik, Ph.D., P.M.H.C.N.S.-B.C.
Tsung-Ung W. Woo, M.D., Ph.D.
Daniel Zigman, M.D.

Preface

Psychopharmacology has developed as a medical discipline over the past six decades. The discoveries of the earlier effective antidepressants, antipsychotics, and mood stabilizers were frequently based on serendipitous observations. Repeated demonstration of efficacy of these agents then served as an impetus for considerable research into the neurobiological bases of their therapeutic effects and of emotion and cognition themselves, as well as the biological basis of the major psychiatric disorders. Moreover, the emergence of an entire new multidisciplinary field, neuropsychopharmacology, which has led to newer specific agents to alter maladaptive central nervous system processes or activity, was another by-product of these early endeavors.

The remarkable proliferation of knowledge in this area—coupled with the absence of any comparable, currently available text—led us to edit the first edition of *The American Psychiatric Press Textbook of Psychopharmacology* (Schatzberg and Nemeroff 1995). The response to that edition was overwhelmingly positive. In the second edition of the *Textbook* (Schatzberg and Nemeroff 1998), we expanded considerably on the earlier text, covering a number of areas in much greater detail, adding several new chapters, and updating all of the previous material. For the third and fourth editions of *The American Psychiatric Publishing Textbook of Psychopharmacology* (Schatzberg and Nemeroff 2004, 2009), we broadened the scope of the text to encompass the ever-growing volume of new knowledge. New authors were invited to contribute, and new topics—including pharmacogenetics, research methodology, brain imaging, and neurostimulatory devices—were addressed.

For some potential readers, the textbooks seemed to provide far more material than a busy clinician needed for day-to-day practice. Thus, after the second edition of the *Textbook*, we developed a distilled "essentials" version—*Essentials of Clinical Psychopharmacology*—that focused on core information of greatest relevance to the practicing clinician. We have organized this synopsis, now in its third edition, around two major parts of the *Textbook:*

- The first part, "Classes of Psychiatric Treatments: Animal and Human Pharmacology," systematically reviews medications within each drug class, presenting key information on preclinical and clinical pharmacology, pharmacokinetics, approved indications, drug interactions, side effects, and other prescribing factors. This section is pharmacopoeia-like. New chapters or chapter sections on recently introduced medications have been added to each successive edition of the *Textbook*, and this material—with further updates—is included in the *Essentials*.

- The second part, "Psychopharmacological Treatment," outlines state-of-the-art pharmacotherapeutic approaches for the major psychiatric disorders as well as for specific patient populations. This section incorporates the latest research and treatment advances, providing the clinician with detailed information on selecting, prescribing, and monitoring medication treatment.

Because of the time gap between publication of the fourth edition of the *Textbook* and this third edition of the *Essentials*, we have thoroughly updated the material and references in the chapters. Thus, the *Essentials* is much more than a pared-down version of the *Textbook*. With all content brought up to date as well as condensed, this book serves as a current-state transition from the fourth edition to the anticipated fifth edition of *The American Psychiatric Publishing Textbook of Psychopharmacology*.

References

Schatzberg AF, Nemeroff CB (eds): The American Psychiatric Press Textbook of Psychopharmacology. Washington, DC, American Psychiatric Press, 1995

Schatzberg AF, Nemeroff CB (eds): The American Psychiatric Press Textbook of Psychopharmacology, 2nd Edition. Washington, DC, American Psychiatric Press, 1998

Schatzberg AF, Nemeroff CB (eds): Essentials of Clinical Psychopharmacology. Washington, DC, American Psychiatric Publishing, 2001

Schatzberg AF, Nemeroff CB (eds): The American Psychiatric Publishing Textbook of Psychopharmacology, 3rd Edition. Washington, DC, American Psychiatric Publishing, 2004

Schatzberg AF, Nemeroff CB (eds): Essentials of Clinical Psychopharmacology, 2nd Edition. Washington, DC, American Psychiatric Publishing, 2006

Schatzberg AF, Nemeroff CB (eds): The American Psychiatric Publishing Textbook of Psychopharmacology, 4th Edition. Washington, DC, American Psychiatric Publishing, 2009

Schatzberg AF, Nemeroff CB (eds): Essentials of Clinical Psychopharmacology, 3rd Edition. Washington, DC, American Psychiatric Publishing, 2013

Acknowledgments

This book would not have been possible without the superb work of the chapter authors in editing and updating their material.

In addition, we wish to thank Editorial Director John McDuffie and his staff at American Psychiatric Publishing. In particular, we appreciate the major efforts of Tina Coltri-Marshall, Publications Coordinator/Project Editor; Bessie Jones, Acquisitions Coordinator; Greg Kuny, Managing Editor; Rebecca Richters, Senior Editor; Tammy J. Cordova, Graphic Design Manager; and Judy Castagna, Assistant Director of Production Services.

Finally, we extend our thanks to Marlene Crane and Adrienne Bronfeld at Stanford University and Carmen Alsina at the University of Miami for their invaluable assistance.

Alan F. Schatzberg, M.D.
Charles B. Nemeroff, M.D., Ph.D.

PART I

Classes of Psychiatric Treatments: Animal and Human Pharmacology

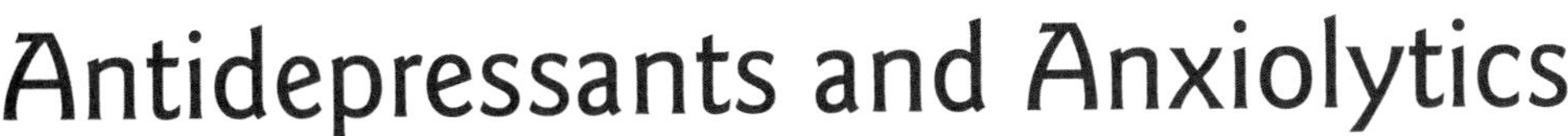

Antidepressants and Anxiolytics

CHAPTER 1

Tricyclic and Tetracyclic Drugs

J. Craig Nelson, M.D.

The tricyclic antidepressant agents hold an important place in the history of treatments for depression. They were the first class of antidepressant compounds to be widely used in depression and remained the first-line treatment for more than 30 years. The observation of their activity led to theories of drug action involving norepinephrine and serotonin. Indeed, this "psychopharmacological bridge" suggested that alterations of these neurotransmitters might cause depression (Bunney and Davis 1965; Prange 1965; Schildkraut 1965). The tricyclics were extensively studied, and through this study the field developed several principles for the management of depressive illness. For example, in addition to understanding the need for adequate dose and duration during acute treatment, the importance of continuation treatment was described. The adverse events associated with these agents required that psychiatrists become familiar with a variety of syndromes, such as anticholinergic delirium, delayed cardiac conduction, and orthostatic hypotension. The observation that tricyclic plasma concentrations varied widely stimulated interest in understanding the relationships of clinical activity and drug concentrations and the metabolism of tricyclic drugs. The field was introduced to the concepts of genetic polymorphisms in the cytochrome P450 (CYP) enzyme system. Finally, our knowledge of how these drugs worked became the basis for the discovery of new drugs such as the selective serotonin reuptake inhibitors (SSRIs).

History and Discovery

In 1957, Roland Kuhn, a Swiss psychiatrist, investigated the clinical effects of imipramine in human subjects in part to determine if its sedative properties would be useful (Kuhn 1958, 1970). He found that imipramine was not useful for calming agitated patients; however, he observed that it did appear to ameliorate symptoms in depressed patients.

After imipramine was introduced, several other antidepressant compounds were developed and marketed. These compounds had a basic tricyclic or tetracyclic structure and shared many of the secondary effects for which the tricyclics came to be known.

Structure-Activity Relations

Tricyclic and tetracyclic compounds are categorized on the basis of their chemical structure (Figure 1–1). The tricyclics have a central three-ring structure, hence the name. The tertiary-amine tricyclics, such as amitriptyline and imipramine, have two methyl groups at the end of the side chain. These compounds can be demethylated to secondary amines, such as desipramine and nortriptyline. The tetracyclic compound maprotiline (Ludiomil) has a four-ring central structure. Five tertiary amines have been marketed in the United States—amitriptyline (Elavil), clomipramine (Anafranil), doxepin (Sinequan), imipramine (Tofranil), and trimipramine (Surmontil). The three secondary-amine compounds are desipramine (Norpramin, Pertofrane), nortriptyline (Aventyl, Pamelor), and protriptyline (Vivactil). All of these compounds, in addition to amoxapine (Asendin) and maprotiline (Ludiomil), have been approved for use in major depression with the exception of clomipramine (Anafranil), which in the United States is approved for use only in obsessive-compulsive disorder (OCD).

The nature of the side chain appears to be important for the tricyclics' function. The tertiary tricyclic agents—amitriptyline, imipramine, and clomipramine—are more potent in blocking the serotonin transporter. The secondary tricyclics are much more potent in blocking the norepinephrine transporter (Table 1–1) (Bolden-Watson and Richelson 1993; Tatsumi et al. 1997).

The structure of amoxapine differs from the structures of the other tricyclics. With a central three-ring structure and a side chain that differ from those of the tricyclics, amoxapine is structurally more similar to the antipsychotic loxapine, from which it is derived.

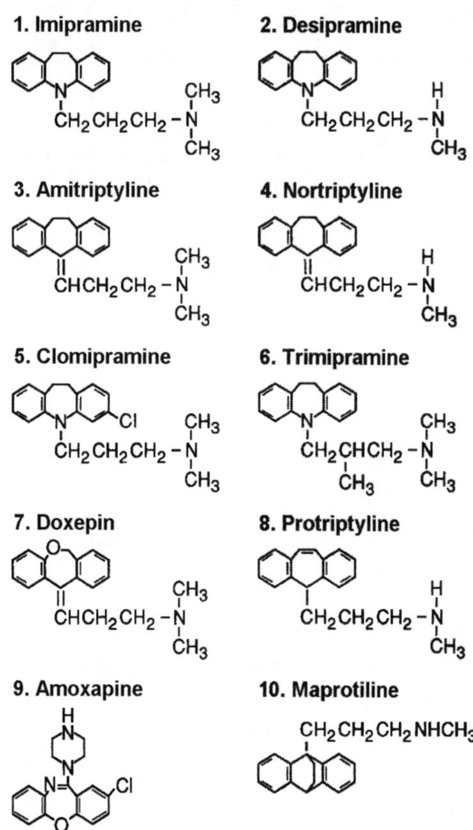

FIGURE 1–1. Drugs marketed in the United States as tricyclics (1–9) and a tetracyclic (10).

Source. Reprinted from Potter WZ, Manji HK, Rudorfer MV: "Tricyclics and Tetracyclics," in *The American Psychiatric Press Textbook of Psychopharmacology*, Second Edition. Edited by Schatzberg AF, Nemeroff CB. Washington, DC, American Psychiatric Press, 1998, p. 200. Copyright 1998, American Psychiatric Press, Inc. Used with permission.

Similar to the secondary tricyclics, it is a potent norepinephrine reuptake inhibitor. Unlike all of the other compounds in this group, amoxapine, and particularly its metabolite 7-hydroxyamoxapine, blocks postsynaptic dopamine receptors (Coupet et al. 1979). As a result, it is the only compound in the group that has antipsychotic activity in addition to antidepressant effects.

Maprotiline also differs from the others

TABLE 1–1. Affinity of tricyclics and tetracyclics for neurotransmitter transporters and specific receptors (expressed as equilibrium dissociation constants)

	Potency uptake blockade			Receptor binding affinity					
Drug	**5-HT**	**NE**	**DA**	α_1	α_2	H_1	M_1	5-HT_{1A}	5-HT_2
Amitriptyline	4.3	35	3,250	27	940	1.1	18	450	18
Amoxapine	58.0	16	4,310	50	2,600	25	1,000	220	1.0
Clomipramine	0.28	38	2,190	38	3,200	31	37	7,000	27
Desipramine	17.6	0.83	3,190	130	7,200	110	198	6,400	350
Doxepin	68.0	29.5	12,100	24	1,100	0.24	80	276	27
Imipramine	1.4	37	8,500	90	3,200	11	90	5,800	150
Maprotiline	5,800.0	11.1	1,000	90	9,400	2	570	12,000	120
Nortriptyline	18.0	4.37	1,140	60	2,500	10	150	294	41
Protriptyline	19.6	1.41	2,100	130	6,600	25	25	3,800	67
Trimipramine	149.0	2,450	3,780	24	680	0.27	58	8,400	32
Reference									
Pentolamine				15					
Yohimbine					1.6				
D-Chlorpheniramine						15			
Atropine							2.4		
Serotonin								0.72	
Ketanserin									2.5

Note. Affinity and potency = equilibrium dissociation constants in molarity. $\alpha_1 = \alpha_1$-adrenergic; $\alpha_2 = \alpha_2$-adrenergic; DA = dopamine; 5-HT = serotonin; 5-HT_{1A} = serotonin$_{1A}$; 5-HT_2 = serotonin$_2$; H_1 = histamine$_1$; M_1 = muscarinic$_1$; NE = norepinephrine.

Source. Uptake potency data adapted from Tatsumi et al. 1997. Receptor affinity data adapted from Richelson and Nelson 1984.

in this group. Although maprotiline is tetracyclic, its side chain is identical to that in desipramine, nortriptyline, and protriptyline. As would be predicted from this similarity, maprotiline is most potent in blocking the norepinephrine transporter (Randrup and Braestrup 1977).

Pharmacological Profile

Reuptake Blockade

Early in the history of the tricyclic and tetracyclic antidepressants, the ability of these compounds to block the transporter site for norepinephrine was described (Axelrod et al. 1961) (see Table 1–1). The tertiary amines have greater affinity for the serotonin transporter, whereas the secondary amines are relatively more potent at the norepinephrine transporter. During the administration of amitriptyline, imipramine, or clomipramine, these tertiary amines are demethylated to secondary amines; thus, both serotonergic and noradrenergic effects occur. In addition, because dopamine is inactivated by norepinephrine transporters in the frontal cortex (Bymaster et al. 2002), norepinephrine reuptake inhibitors would be expected to increase dopamine concentrations in that region.

Receptor Sensitivity Changes

The initial reuptake blockade described above is followed by a sequence of events (Blier et al. 1987; Charney et al. 1991; Tremblay and Blier 2006). The tertiary tricyclic compounds inhibit the uptake of serotonin, and serotonin levels rise. As the result of inhibitory feedback from the presynaptic somatodendritic serotonin$_{1A}$ (5-HT$_{1A}$) autoreceptor, the firing rate of the presynaptic serotonin neuron falls, and concentrations of 5-hydroxyindoleacetic acid (5-HIAA), the major metabolite of serotonin, decline rapidly. During a 10- to 14-day period, the presynaptic autoreceptor is desensitized, and at this point, the tonic firing rate returns to its pretreatment rate. With both a normal firing rate and reuptake blockade, serotonin transmission is enhanced. The tricyclic agents also sensitize or upregulate postsynaptic 5-HT$_{1A}$ receptors (de Montigny and Aghajanian 1978). These changes further enhance the effects of serotonin.

The tricyclics also downregulate the 5-HT$_2$ receptors (G.M. Goodwin et al. 1984; Peroutka and Snyder 1980). In preclinical experiments, when the 5-HT$_2$ receptor was blocked by an antagonist, the effects of serotonin were enhanced (Lakoski and Aghajanian 1985; Marek et al. 2003). Some of the tricyclics—particularly amoxapine and doxepin, and to some extent amitriptyline—have 5-HT$_2$ antagonist properties relatively comparable to their reuptake potency (see Table 1–1) (Tatsumi et al. 1997).

The sequence of events with chronic dosing in the noradrenergic system is more complicated (Tremblay and Blier 2006). As in the serotonergic system, reuptake inhibition results in a rapid decline in norepinephrine turnover, as reflected by a fall in concentrations of 3-methoxy-4-hydroxyphenylglycol (MHPG), a metabolite of norepinephrine, and attenuation of the firing rate of the noradrenergic neuron. This effect appears to be mediated by the presynaptic somatodendritic α_2-adrenergic autoreceptor, which provides inhibitory feedback to the presynaptic neuron. In contrast to the serotonergic system, the firing rate of noradrenergic neurons remains inhibited with chronic treatment (Szabo and Blier 2001), suggesting that somatodendritic α_2 receptors do not desensitize. Norepinephrine concentrations do increase at postsynaptic sites such as the hippocampus and frontal cortex. This may indicate desensitization of terminal α_2 autoreceptors.

With chronic treatment, the postsynaptic β-adrenergic receptor is downregulated or decreased in density (Sulser et al. 1978).

Current evidence suggests that β-adrenergic receptor downregulation is likely a compensatory change. Overall, chronic administration of a noradrenergic reuptake inhibitor appears to override the downregulation of the postsynaptic β-receptor, resulting in enhanced noradrenergic transmission. This effect is manifested as enhanced formation of the second messenger cyclic adenosine monophosphate (cAMP) (Duman et al. 1997) and is reflected clinically by a persistent increase in heart rate (Roose et al. 1998; Rosenstein and Nelson 1991).

Secondary Effects

The tricyclic and tetracyclic compounds also have a variety of other actions mediated by other receptors (Cusack et al. 1994; Richelson and Nelson 1984) (see Table 1–1). For example, these compounds block muscarinic receptors, producing anticholinergic effects. Although these anticholinergic effects have generally been thought to mediate adverse effects, a double-blind, randomized crossover study in 19 subjects with major depression found that the anticholinergic drug scopolamine had a beneficial effect on depressive and anxious symptoms (Furey and Drevets 2006). The tricyclics also block histamine$_1$ (H_1) receptors and α_1- and α_2-adrenergic receptors, resulting in a variety of other effects (as discussed in the next section). Tricyclics act on fast sodium channels, which explains their adverse cardiac effects; however, these same actions may contribute to the beneficial effects of tricyclics on pain (Priest and Kaczorowski 2007). The potency of secondary effects of the tricyclics and tetracyclics varies considerably. Among the tricyclics, amitriptyline is the most anticholinergic and desipramine the least anticholinergic. Doxepin is the most potent H_1 antagonist among the tricyclics, but mirtazapine is even more potent. The consequences of these secondary effects are discussed below.

Pharmacokinetics and Disposition

Absorption

Absorption of the tricyclic and tetracyclic drugs occurs in the small intestine and is rapid and reasonably complete. Peak levels are reached within 2–8 hours following ingestion. Exceptions include protriptyline (peak levels reached between 6 and 12 hours after ingestion) and maprotiline (peak levels not reached until 8 hours or longer). Although peak levels may have implications for side effects, peak levels are relatively unimportant with respect to efficacy because the antidepressant action of these drugs occurs over several weeks.

Volume of Distribution

The tricyclic and tetracyclic compounds are basic lipophilic amines and are concentrated in a variety of tissues throughout the body. As a result, they have a high volume of distribution. For example, concentrations of these drugs in cardiac tissue exceed concentrations in plasma.

Plasma Protein Binding

The tricyclic and tetracyclic compounds are extensively bound to plasma proteins (e.g., 90% or greater) because of their lipid solubility. Exceptions are the hydroxy metabolites, which have lower plasma protein binding than the parent compounds.

First-Pass Metabolism

Following absorption, the tricyclics are taken up in the circulation but pass first through the liver, and metabolism of the drug begins—the so-called first-pass effect. As a result, the amount of the compound that enters the systemic circulation is reduced.

Hepatic Metabolism

Hepatic metabolism is the principal method of clearance for the tricyclic and tetracyclic compounds. Only a small portion of drug is eliminated by the kidneys. Rates of hepatic metabolism vary widely from person to person, resulting in dramatic differences in steady-state plasma concentrations. Elimination half-lives for most of the tricyclic and tetracyclic compounds average about 24 hours or longer; thus, the drugs can be given once a day (Table 1–2). Amoxapine has a shorter half-life than the other tricyclics and is an exception.

Hepatic metabolism of the tricyclics and tetracyclics occurs along two principal metabolic pathways. *Demethylation of the side chain* converts the tertiary amines to secondary amines. The other pathway in hepatic metabolism is *hydroxylation of the ring structure*, which produces hydroxy metabolites. In some cases, the levels of the metabolite are substantial. The concentration of 10-hydroxynortriptyline usually exceeds that of the parent compound (Bertilsson et al. 1979). Usually 2-hydroxydesipramine is present at levels approximately 40%–50% of those present in the parent compound, but these ratios are quite variable, depending on the rate of hydroxylation (Bock et al. 1983; Potter et al. 1979). Hydroxyimipramine and hydroxyamitriptyline are present at very low concentrations and are clinically unimportant. The hydroxy metabolites are then conjugated and excreted. The conjugated metabolites are not active.

Hydroxynortriptyline and hydroxydesipramine both block the norepinephrine transporter (Bertilsson et al. 1979; Potter et al. 1979). Both have antidepressant activity (Nelson et al. 1988b; Nordin et al. 1987). The norepinephrine reuptake potency of hydroxydesipramine is comparable to that of the parent compound. There are two isomers of hydroxynortriptyline, *E*- and *Z*-10-hydroxynortriptyline. *E*-10-hydroxynortriptyline is present at levels four times higher than those of the *Z* isomer and is about 50% as potent as nortriptyline in blocking norepinephrine uptake.

The principal metabolic pathway for amoxapine is hydroxylation, during which 7-hydroxyamoxapine and 8-hydroxyamoxapine are produced (Coupet et al. 1979). These compounds differ: 7-hydroxyamoxapine has high-potency antipsychotic properties but a short half-life; 8-hydroxyamoxapine is metabolized more slowly and appears to contribute to the drug's antidepressant action.

The CYP2D6 pathway appears responsible for hydroxylation of desipramine and nortriptyline (Brosen et al. 1991). In fact, desipramine has been considered the prototypic substrate for CYP2D6 because it has no other major metabolic pathways. Demethylation of the tertiary-amine compounds involves a number of CYP isoenzymes, including 1A2, 3A4, and 2C19. These hepatic isoenzymes are under the control of specific genes, and the gene loci have been identified for several of these isoenzymes, including CYP2D6. Approximately 5%–10% of Caucasians are homozygous for the recessive autosomal 2D6 trait, resulting in deficient hydroxylation of desipramine and nortriptyline (Brosen et al. 1985; Evans et al. 1980). These individuals are termed *poor metabolizers*, whereas those with adequate 2D6 enzyme are referred to as *extensive metabolizers*. Approximately 20% of individuals of Asian descent have a genetic polymorphism resulting in deficient CYP2C19 metabolism.

The variability in plasma concentrations that results from these metabolic differences is substantial. For example, in a sample of 83 inpatients who were given a fixed dose of 2.5 mg/kg of desipramine, we observed steady-state plasma concentrations ranging from 20 ng/mL to 934 ng/mL (Nelson 1984).

Steady-State Concentrations

Steady state, an important pharmacological concept. is the point on a fixed dose at which plasma concentrations of the drug reach a plateau. Steady state is achieved after five half-lives. If blood level monitoring is employed, a

TABLE 1–2. Dosage, clearance, and apparent therapeutic plasma concentrations of tricyclics and tetracyclics

	Plasma		Therapeutic	
Drug	**Half-life (hours)**	**Clearance (L/hour)**	**Dosage range (mg/day)**	**Plasma level (ng/mL)**
Tertiary tricyclics				
Amitriptyline	5–45	20–70	150–300	
Clomipramine	15–60	20–120	150–300	>150[a]
Doxepin	10–25	40–60	150–300	
Imipramine	5–30	30–100	150–300	>200[a]
Trimipramine	15–40	40–105		
Secondary tricyclics				
Desipramine	10–30	80–170	75–300	>125
Nortriptyline	20–55	15–80	50–150	50–150
Protriptyline	55–200	5–25	15–60	
Tetracyclics				
Amoxapine	5–10	225–275	150–300	
Maprotiline	25–50	15–35	100–225	

[a]Total concentration of the parent compound and the desmethyl metabolite.

Source. Adapted from Nelson JC: "Tricyclic and Tetracyclic Drugs," in *Comprehensive Textbook of Psychiatry/VII*, 7th Edition. Edited by Kaplan HI, Sadock BJ. Baltimore, MD, Lippincott Williams & Wilkins, 2000, p. 2494. Copyright 2000, Lippincott Williams & Wilkins. Used with permission.

sample is drawn before the next dose is given, usually in the morning, after the patient's level has reached steady state. Steady-state drug concentrations should remain relatively stable as long as the dose is constant, the patient is compliant, and no interactive drugs are added. If only one sample is drawn, the clinician needs to remember that even if the laboratory error is low, there will be moderate biological variability (±10%–15%). Single blood levels are better viewed as estimates than as precise measures.

When the drug concentration is measured, the total of both the free and bound drug is reported. Drug concentrations in the cerebrospinal fluid are proportional to the free levels. The *free concentration* is dependent on dose and hepatic clearance but is not affected by plasma protein binding (Greenblatt et al. 1998). Factors that affect plasma proteins—malnutrition, inflammation—may lead to changes in the bound fraction, but the absolute free concentration is unaffected.

Linear Kinetics

Most of the tricyclics have linear kinetics; that is, concentration increases in proportion to dose within the therapeutic range. There are exceptions. Desipramine, for example, appears to have nonlinear kinetics in the usual dose range (Nelson and Jatlow 1987). In cases of overdose, nonlinear changes are more likely to occur, and the clinician cannot assume that usual rates of drug elimination will be maintained.

Effects of Aging

Many changes in the pharmacodynamics and pharmacokinetics of drug treatment occur with aging, yet some may be relatively unimportant (Greenblatt et al. 1998). The ratio of fat to lean body mass increases, and cardiac output and hepatic blood flow decrease. There may be further changes associated with medical illness. But the clinical importance of these changes is usually relatively minor because of the dramatic variability of hepatic metabolism. The activity of the CYP3A4 pathway does slow with age (von Moltke et al. 1995), and concentrations of the tertiary amines are increased somewhat in older individuals (Abernathy et al. 1985). Alternatively, most studies of nortriptyline (Katz et al. 1989; Young et al. 1984) and desipramine (Abernathy et al. 1985; Nelson et al. 1985, 1995) indicate that ratios of blood level to dosage of these drugs are relatively unaffected by aging, suggesting that the 2D6 isoenzyme is not similarly affected. Renal clearance of the hydroxy metabolites does decrease with age (Nelson et al. 1988a; Young et al. 1984). As a result, concentrations of hydroxynortriptyline may be substantially elevated in older patients.

In children, the clearance of tricyclic compounds is increased. Half-lives of imipramine are shorter and ratios of desmethylimipramine to imipramine are higher, consistent with more rapid metabolism (Geller 1991; Rapoport and Potter 1981). Alternatively, a study of desipramine in children found that the clearance of both desipramine and hydroxydesipramine was increased so that hydroxy metabolite–parent compound ratios were not elevated (Wilens et al. 1992).

Relationship of Plasma Concentration to Clinical Action

Plasma Concentration and Response

Marked interindividual variability of tricyclic plasma concentrations was described by Hammer and Sjöqvist in 1967. This finding suggested that drug level monitoring might ensure that therapeutic blood levels are achieved and might help to avoid toxic levels. In carefully selected inpatients with endogenous or melancholic major depression, treatment with adequate levels of imipramine or desipramine resulted in robust response rates of about 85% (Glassman et al. 1977; Nelson et al. 1982). But similar relationships have proven difficult to demonstrate in depressed outpatients. In outpatients, drug-placebo differences are often small, and the effect of drug treatment is harder to detect. Depressed outpatients may be more heterogeneous and include individuals who are not responsive to any drug treatment. It is logical to conclude that blood level relationships determined in severely depressed inpatients might be used as a guide for treatment of outpatients, but this assumption has not been empirically validated.

A task force of the American Psychiatric Association (1985) that reviewed these studies concluded that relationships between plasma level and response had been demonstrated for imipramine, desipramine, and nortriptyline (see Table 1–2). The data relating blood levels and response in depression are limited or conflicting for the other tricyclic and tetracyclic compounds.

Plasma Concentration and Toxicity

Blood level monitoring may help to avoid toxicity. The risk of delirium is substantially increased at amitriptyline plasma concentrations above 450 ng/mL and is moderately increased at concentrations above 300 ng/mL (Livingston et al. 1983; Preskorn and Simpson 1982). But amitriptyline is the most anticholinergic tricyclic and is most likely to produce delirium. The risk of first-degree atrioventricular block is also increased with plasma concentrations of imipramine greater than 350 ng/mL (Preskorn and Irwin 1982). The risk of seizures also increases at higher doses and, presumably, higher blood levels, although a clear plasma level threshold for seizures has not been demonstrated. Following overdose, tricyclic blood levels greater than 1,000 ng/mL can be achieved, and the risks of delirium, stupor, cardiac abnormalities, and seizures are all substantially increased (Preskorn and Irwin 1982; Rudorfer and Young 1980; Spiker et al. 1975). The value of blood level monitoring to avoid serious adverse effects has been hard to demonstrate because rates of serious toxicity are low so that large samples are required to demonstrate any increase in risk at higher blood levels.

If blood level monitoring is undertaken, the clinician needs to remember that many factors—such as laboratory variability, blood sampling errors, missed doses, and biological variability— can affect drug concentrations. For this reason, the clinician should not view the concentration reported as a precise measure. Yet because concentrations vary across such a wide range, it may be very helpful to know if the level is low (e.g., 25–75 ng/mL), moderate (e.g., 100–300 ng/mL), or high (e.g., 300–1,000 ng/mL).

Prospective Dosing Techniques

The demonstrated relationship between timed drug concentrations after a single tricyclic dose and the steady-state level achieved suggests the possibility of using plasma levels obtained early in treatment to rapidly adjust the dose. A clinical study using desipramine found that treatment could be initiated at full dose once the dose needed to reach a therapeutic level was determined from a 24-hour blood level following a test dose (Nelson et al. 1987). However, the practical application of this method was limited. Most laboratories are not prepared to determine drug concentrations accurately at very low levels (as needed following a test dose) and are unable to report results quickly. A more practical and clinically feasible method is to start the drug at a low or moderate fixed dose, obtain a blood sample after 5–7 days on that dose, and then make further adjustments based on that level. There are exceptions. Elderly depressed patients often require gradual dosing in order to assess tolerance. In patients with panic attacks, lower starting doses are employed to avoid exacerbation of panic attacks.

Mechanism of Action

Observations that the tricyclic agents blocked uptake of monoamines at the norepinephrine and serotonin transporters occurred early in their history (Axelrod et al. 1961). This drug effect was quickly advanced as a possible mechanism of action. The observation that reserpine, which depletes presynaptic catecholamines, might induce depression in vulnerable individuals supported this hypothesis (F. K. Goodwin and Bunney 1971). Confirmation that norepinephrine and serotonin do in fact mediate the action of these antidepressants was provided by subsequent challenge studies in depressed patients. For example, administration of a tryptophan-free diet rapidly depletes serotonin and causes relapse in depressed patients who have been successfully treated with a serotonin reuptake inhibitor but not a norepinephrine reuptake inhibitor (Delgado et al. 1990). Alternatively, administration of α-methyl-*p*-tyrosine (AMPT), which interrupts the synthesis of catecholamines, caused relapse in patients who were being successfully treated with noradrenergic agents but not those receiving serotonergic drugs (Delgado et al. 1993). These studies provide supporting evidence that serotonin and norepinephrine mediate antidepressant effects, but they do not necessarily imply that alterations in these neurotransmitter systems are central to the etiology of depression.

More recent research into the mechanism of action of the tricyclics and other antidepressant drugs has shifted to include consideration of factors affecting postsynaptic signal transduction (Manji et al. 1995). These factors include coupling of G proteins to the adrenergic receptor or to adenylyl cyclase and the activity of membrane phospholipases and protein kinases. Other novel targets, including glucocorticoid receptors (Barden 1996), neurotrophic factors (Duman et al. 1997), and gene expression (Lesch and Manji 1992; Nibuya et al. 1996; Schwaninger et al. 1995), have been explored.

Indications and Efficacy

Major Depression

The efficacy of the tricyclic and tetracyclic compounds in major depression is well established. The evidence for their effectiveness has been reviewed previously (Agency for Health Care Policy and Research 1993; Davis and Glassman 1989). Imipramine is the most extensively studied tricyclic antidepressant, in part because new drugs were often compared with it. In 30 of 44 placebo-controlled studies, imipramine was more effective than placebo. If data from these studies are combined, 65% of 1,334 patients *completing* treatment with imipramine were substantially improved, whereas 30% of those on placebo improved. *Intention-to-treat* response rates for placebo-controlled studies of imipramine in outpatients were 51% for imipramine and 30% for placebo (Agency for Health Care Policy and Research 1993). The other tricyclic and tetracyclic antidepressants appeared comparable to imipramine in efficacy.

The tricyclic compounds are also effective when used for maintenance treatment. The Pittsburgh group found that imipramine, at full dose, effectively maintained nearly 80% of the depressed patients for a 3-year period compared with 10% of those on placebo (Frank et al. 1990). In this study, maintenance psychotherapy had an intermediate effect, with about 30% of the patients remaining well. In practice, clinicians may encounter patients with chronic depression, with residual symptoms, or with comorbid medical and psychiatric disorders. For such patients, the effects of maintenance treatment are less robust.

The U.S. Food and Drug Administration (FDA) has approved all of the tricyclic and tetracyclic compounds discussed in this chapter for the treatment of depression with the exception of clomipramine. In Europe, clomipramine is also used for depression; in fact, it is regarded by many as the most potent antidepressant.

Melancholia and Severe Depression

The efficacy of the tricyclic compounds appears to vary in different subtypes of depression. The early studies of tricyclic compounds were frequently conducted in hospitalized patients with severe or endogenous depression, and in these patients the tricyclics were found to be effective. In fact, these agents may be especially effective in this group. Two studies of imipramine and desipramine found rates of response of about 85% in severely depressed hospitalized patients who did not have a refractory history, did not have prominent personality disorder, received an adequate plasma concentration of the drug, and completed treatment (Glassman et al. 1977; Nelson et al. 1982).

When the SSRIs were introduced, it was suggested that they might be less effective than the tricyclic antidepressants in treating severe or melancholic depression. In a large meta-analysis of more than 100 comparison studies, Anderson (2000) found that tricyclic antidepressants and SSRIs had comparable efficacy. In a separate meta-analysis of 25 inpatient studies (Anderson 1998), the advantage of the tricyclics appeared limited to those with dual action, namely amitriptyline and clomipramine. In outpatients, the designation of melancholia does not appear to predict an advantage for tricyclic antidepressants versus SSRIs (Anderson and Tomenson 1994; Montgomery 1989).

Anxious Depression

Anxious depression is not recognized in DSM-IV-TR (American Psychiatric Association

2000) as a subtype of depression; nevertheless, it has been frequently studied. Doxepin, amoxapine, and maprotiline have received FDA approval for use in patients with depression and symptoms of anxiety. Direct comparison studies, however, have found little indication that one tricyclic is better than another for treatment of anxious depression. Depressed patients who are anxious may respond less well than less anxious patients to amitriptyline (Kupfer and Spiker 1981), imipramine (Roose et al. 1986), and desipramine (Nelson et al. 1994). Yet these drugs are still more effective than placebo in anxious depressed patients, and it is not established that another drug class is more effective in these patients.

Atypical Depression

A series of studies by the Columbia University group examined the efficacy of imipramine in depressed patients with atypical features (Liebowitz et al. 1984, 1988). Imipramine was more effective than placebo but significantly less effective than the monoamine oxidase inhibitor (MAOI) phenelzine. Other investigators have reported the value of switching from a tricyclic to an MAOI in tricyclic-refractory depressed patients with atypical features (McGrath et al. 1987; Thase et al. 1992). In fact, the validity and utility of atypical depression were in large part supported by this observed difference.

Psychotic Depression

In 1975, Glassman et al. observed that imipramine was less effective in patients with major depression who had delusions. Subsequently, Chan et al. (1987) reviewed several studies involving more than 1,000 patients and found that antidepressants—usually tricyclics—given alone were effective in approximately two-thirds of the nonpsychotic patients but only about one-third of those with psychotic features. Several open studies reviewed elsewhere (Nelson 1987) and one prospective study (Spiker et al. 1985) found that the tricyclics, when combined with an antipsychotic, are effective in psychotic depression.

Anton and Burch (1990) suggested that because of its antipsychotic effects, amoxapine might be effective for psychotic depression. In a double-blind study, these researchers demonstrated that amoxapine was comparable in efficacy to the combination of perphenazine and amitriptyline in treating psychotic depression (Anton and Burch 1990).

Bipolar Depression

Forty years ago, it was suggested that the MAOI antidepressants might be more effective than the tricyclics in treating bipolar depression (Himmelhoch et al. 1972). Later, Himmelhoch et al. (1991) demonstrated in a double-blind study that tranylcypromine was more effective than imipramine for bipolar depression. In addition, tricyclics are more likely than other agents to induce mania (Weir and Goodwin 1987). As a result, the tricyclics are not recommended for monotherapy of bipolar depression.

Chronic Major Depression and Dysthymia

Imipramine appears to be effective in treating chronic depression and dysthymia and to be relatively comparable to sertraline in efficacy (Keller et al. 1998; Kocsis et al. 1988; Thase et al. 1996). Imipramine and desipramine have both been studied in controlled trials and have been found to be more effective than placebo both for acute treatment and for maintenance treatment (Miller et al. 2001).

Late-Life Depression

Gerson et al. (1988) reviewed the studies of tricyclic antidepressants reported prior to 1986. They found 13 placebo-controlled trials but noted several methodological problems. Although tricyclics were effective, overall response rates in older patients appeared to be lower than rates in nonelderly patients (Agency for Health Care Policy and Research 1993). Katz et al. (1990) performed one of the first placebo-controlled trials of nortriptyline in the treatment of patients older than 80 years living in a residential care facility. Nortriptyline was more effective than placebo. The doses employed and levels achieved were similar to those in younger subjects. This study remains the only study to date showing an advantage for an antidepressant over placebo in depressed nursing home patients.

Depression in Children

In children and adolescents, the tricyclic antidepressants have not demonstrated superiority over placebo (Ryan 1992).

Obsessive-Compulsive Disorder

Unlike depression, which responds to a variety of antidepressant agents, OCD appears to require treatment with a serotonergic agent. Clomipramine, the most serotonergic of the tricyclics, is approved by the FDA for use in OCD, and its efficacy in this disorder is well established (Greist et al. 1995). Studies comparing its effectiveness with noradrenergic agents such as desipramine found that clomipramine was substantially superior (Leonard et al. 1989). Although the SSRIs are effective in treating OCD, there is a suggestion that clomipramine may be superior (Greist et al. 1995). Whether this suggested superiority is due to the dual mechanism of clomipramine or to other factors is unclear.

Panic Disorder

None of the tricyclic or tetracyclic drugs is approved for use in panic disorder. Yet imipramine was the first drug described for use in this disorder (Klein 1964). The efficacy of both tertiary and secondary tricyclics has been demonstrated in controlled trials (Jobson et al. 1978; Munjack et al. 1988; Zitrin et al. 1980). In treating this disorder, the drug is initiated at a low dose to avoid exacerbation of panic symptoms.

Attention-Deficit/Hyperactivity Disorder

The efficacy of the stimulant drugs in treating attention-deficit/hyperactivity disorder (ADHD) is well established. The tricyclics, especially desipramine, also appear to be of value. In one study, desipramine, given at dosages greater than 4 mg/kg for 3–4 weeks, was effective in two-thirds of the children, whereas placebo was effective in only 10% (Biederman et al. 1989). Desipramine was also found to be more effective than placebo in adults with ADHD (Wilens et al. 1996). One of the advantages of desipramine is its low potential for abuse. Unfortunately, five cases of sudden death were reported in the early 1990s in children being treated with desipramine (Riddle et al. 1991, 1993). All were under the age of 12 years. As a result, desipramine is now contraindicated in children younger than 12 years (discussed in greater detail below; see section "Side Effects and Toxicology"). Given that tricyclics as a group share the same adverse cardiac effects, there is reason to be concerned that other tricyclics might also have safety issues in young children (see also Chapter 40, "Treatment of Child and Adolescent Disorders").

Pain Syndromes

The tricyclics and maprotiline have been widely used in various chronic pain syndromes. In a review of the literature, O'Malley et al. (1999) identified 56 controlled studies involving tricyclic antidepressant therapy for various pain syndromes, including headache (21 studies), fibromyalgia (18 studies), functional gastrointestinal syndromes (11 studies), idiopathic pain (8 studies), and tinnitus (2 studies), and Salerno et al. (2002) identified 7 more placebo-controlled trials of tricyclics or maprotiline used for chronic back pain. These agents were quite effective; the mean effect size (0.87) and the drug-placebo difference in response rates (32%) in the pain trials are more robust than those usually observed in placebo-controlled studies in depression. The analgesic effects of these compounds were not simply the result of their antidepressant effects.

The mechanism of these agents' analgesic effects appears to differ from that of their antidepressant effects. The antinociceptive actions of the antidepressants result from actions on descending norepinephrine and serotonin pathways in the spinal cord (Yoshimura and Furue 2006). In animals, norepinephrine reuptake inhibitors and combined norepinephrine–serotonin reuptake inhibitors appear to be more potent than SSRIs (Mochizucki 2004). In humans, there is some evidence that the combined-action agents amitriptyline and clomipramine are more effective than the SSRI fluoxetine (Max et al. 1992) or the norepinephrine-selective agents maprotiline (Eberhard et al. 1988) and nortriptyline (Panerai et al. 1990). In humans, antidepressant dosing and timing of effects for pain differ from those observed in depression. For example, usual dosages of amitriptyline required for pain management (≤75 mg/day) are lower than those required to treat depression (15–300 mg/day), and response occurs more quickly, usually within the first 1 or 2 weeks.

Other Indications

Imipramine has been used for treatment of nocturnal enuresis in children with FDA approval, and controlled trials indicate efficacy (Rapoport et al. 1980). The dose of imipramine is usually 25–50 mg at bedtime. Amitriptyline and nortriptyline also appear to be useful, although they are not approved for use in this disorder. The mechanism of action is unclear but may in part be anticholinergic. It is not clear, however, that the risk of cardiac problems would be substantially less with tricyclics other than desipramine in children younger than 12 years, although the low doses required may reduce this risk.

Tricyclic antidepressant drugs have been extensively studied in patients with schizophrenia. However, in the absence of a major depressive syndrome, these agents appear to be of limited value (Siris et al. 1978).

Side Effects and Toxicology

Distinguishing side effects during tricyclic treatment from the somatic symptoms of depression can be complicated. During treatment, patients may attribute somatic symptoms to drug side effects even if the symptoms were preexisting. One study found that the strongest predictor of overall somatic symptom severity was the severity of the depression at the time of assessment (Nelson et al. 1984).

Another general factor contributing to side effects is the patient's vulnerability. For example, one of the best predictors of orthostatic hypotension during treatment is the presence of orthostatic hypotension prior to treatment (Glassman et al. 1979). Seizures are most likely in a patient with a history of seizures (Rosenstein et al. 1993). Cardiac conduction problems are most likely to occur in patients with preexisting conduction delay (Roose et al. 1987a).

Antidepressant drugs do have effects on a variety of organs and can produce adverse effects. The in vitro potency or affinity of antidepressant compounds for various receptor sites (see Table 1–1) is one measure for comparing the likelihood that various agents will produce specific side effects. A related issue is how the in vitro potency of a secondary effect relates to the potency of the primary action of the drug. If the secondary effect is more potent, it will occur at concentrations below the therapeutic level of the drug. For example, orthostatic hypotension often occurs at plasma concentrations below the usual therapeutic threshold. Alternatively, the proarrhythmic and proconvulsant effects of the tricyclic antidepressants become more frequent at elevated blood levels or those encountered in overdose.

Central Nervous System Effects

The principal action of the tricyclic and tetracyclic agents in the central nervous system is to reduce the symptoms of depression. Nondepressed subjects given imipramine may feel sleepy, quieter, light-headed, clumsy, and tired. These effects are generally unpleasant (DiMascio et al. 1964).

The anticholinergic and antihistaminic effects of the tricyclics and tetracyclics can produce confusion or delirium. The incidence of delirium is dose dependent and increases at blood levels above 300 ng/mL (Livingston et al. 1983; Preskorn and Simpson 1982). The risk of delirium appears to be higher for the more anticholinergic agents, such as amitriptyline. Patients with concurrent dementia are particularly vulnerable to the development of delirium, and the more anticholinergic tricyclics should be avoided in these patients. Intramuscular or intravenous physostigmine can be used to reverse or reduce the symptoms of delirium, but physostigmine's short duration of action makes the continued use of this agent difficult.

Seizures can occur with all of the tricyclic and tetracyclic agents and are dosage- and blood level–related (Rosenstein et al. 1993). For clomipramine, the risk for seizures is reported to be 0.5% at dosages up to 250 mg/day. At dosages above 250 mg/day, the seizure risk increases to 1.67% (new drug application data on file with the FDA). The seizure risk for the older compounds was not as well established at the time of marketing. At moderate dosages, seizure rates were below 1%; however, at high dosages, the risk may exceed 1% (Jick et al. 1983; Peck et al. 1983). The risk of seizures is substantially increased following overdose (Spiker et al. 1975). The risk of convulsions is increased in patients with predisposing factors such as a prior history of seizures, brain injury, or presence of antipsychotics. The mechanism by which tricyclics produce seizures is not well understood.

A fine, rapid tremor can occur with use of tricyclic agents. Because tremors are dose dependent, tend to occur at higher blood levels, and are not typical depressive symptoms, development of a tremor may be a clinical indicator of an elevated blood level (Nelson et al. 1984).

Because the 7-hydroxy metabolite of amoxapine has antipsychotic properties, administration of amoxapine carries the potential risk of neuroleptic malignant syndrome and tardive dyskinesia. Although these adverse events are rare, the seriousness of the risk and the availability of alternatives suggest that use of amoxapine should be reserved for patients whose clinical condition warrants the use of an agent with antipsychotic properties.

Anticholinergic Effects

The tricyclics block muscarinic receptors and can cause a variety of anticholinergic side effects, such as dry mouth, constipation, blurred vision, and urinary hesitancy. These effects can precipitate an ocular crisis in patients with narrow-angle glaucoma. The tricyclic and tetracyclic compounds vary substantially in their muscarinic potency (see Table 1–1). Amitriptyline is the most potent, and desipramine is the least anticholinergic. Amoxapine and maprotiline also have minimal anticholinergic effects. Anticholinergic effects can contribute to tachycardia, but tachycardia also occurs as a result of stimulation of β-adrenergic receptors in the heart. Thus, tachycardia also occurs in patients receiving desipramine, which is minimally anticholinergic (Rosenstein and Nelson 1991).

Although anticholinergic effects are annoying, they are usually not serious. They can, however, become severe. An ocular crisis in patients with narrow-angle glaucoma is an acute condition associated with severe pain. Urinary retention can be associated with stretch injuries to the bladder. Constipation can progress to severe obstipation. (Paralytic ileus has been described but is rare.) In these conditions, medication must be discontinued and appropriate supportive measures instituted. Elderly patients are at greatest risk for severe adverse consequences.

The frequency of severe anticholinergic adverse reactions is increased by concomitant antipsychotic administration. Use of nortriptyline or desipramine, either of which is less anticholinergic, can help to reduce the likelihood of these problems.

Anticholinergic effects may benefit from other interventions. Bethanechol (Urecholine) at a dosage of 25 mg three or four times a day may be helpful in patients with urinary hesitancy. The regular use of stool softeners helps to manage constipation. Patients with narrow-angle glaucoma who are receiving pilocarpine eyedrops regularly can be treated with a tricyclic, as can those who have had an iridectomy. Tricyclic agents do not affect patients with chronic open-angle glaucoma.

Antihistaminic Effects

Several of the tricyclic compounds and maprotiline have clinically significant antihistaminic effects. Doxepin, the most potent H_1 antagonist among the tricyclics, is more potent than diphenhydramine but less potent than mirtazapine. Central H_1 receptor blockade can contribute to sedation and delirium and also appears to be related to the increased appetite and associated weight gain that patients may develop with chronic treatment. Because of their sedating effects, the tricyclic antidepressants, especially amitriptyline, have been used as hypnotics. Given their cardiac effects and lethality in overdose, this practice should be discouraged.

Cardiovascular Effects

Orthostatic hypotension is one of the most common reasons for discontinuation of tricyclic antidepressant treatment (Glassman et al. 1979). It can occur with all of the tricyclics but appears to be less pronounced with nortriptyline (Roose et al. 1981; Thayssen et al. 1981). The α_1-adrenergic blockade associated with the tricyclics contributes to orthostatic hypotension; however, it is the postural reflex that is primarily affected. Resting supine blood pressure may be unaffected or can even be elevated (Walsh et al. 1992). Orthostatic hypotension is most likely to occur or is most severe in patients who have preexisting orthostatic hypotension (Glassman et al. 1979). It is also aggravated by concurrent antihypertensive medications, especially volume-depleting diuretic agents. The elderly are more likely to have preexisting hypotension and are also more vulnerable to the consequences of orthostatic hypotension, such as falls and hip fractures.

Orthostatic hypotension often occurs at low blood levels. Gradual dosage adjustment may allow accommodation to the subjective experience of light-headedness, but the actual orthostatic blood pressure changes do not accommodate within a reasonable period of time (e.g., 4 weeks) (Roose et al. 1998). As a consequence, patients who experience serious symptomatic orthostatic hypotension may not be treatable with a tricyclic antidepressant. Fludrocortisone (Florinef) has been used to raise blood pressure, but in this author's experience it is not very effective. If patients are receiving antihypertensives, it may be possible and helpful to reduce the dose of these agents.

Desipramine has been reported to raise supine blood pressure in younger patients, although it is not clear this effect is limited to that age group (Walsh et al. 1992). This effect may be similar to that reported for venlafaxine.

Tachycardia occurs with all the tricyclics, not just the more anticholinergic agents. Both supine and postural pulse changes can occur, and the standing pulse can be markedly elevated. A study of nortriptyline, dosed to a therapeutic plasma concentration, found a mean pulse rise of 11% (8 beats per minute) (Roose et al. 1998). Patients do not accommodate to the pulse rise, which can persist for months. Tachycardia is more prominent in younger patients, who appear more sensitive to sympathomimetic effects, and is one of the most common reasons for drug discontinuation in adolescents. A persistent pulse rise in older patients, however, increases cardiac work and may be clinically significant in patients with ischemic heart disease.

The effect of tricyclic antidepressants on cardiac conduction has been a subject of great interest. Cardiac arrhythmia is the principal cause of death following overdose (Spiker et al. 1975). Apparently, through inhibition of Na^+/K^+-ATPase, the tricyclics stabilize electrically excitable membranes and delay conduction, particularly His ventricular conduction. Consequently, the tricyclics have type I antiarrhythmic qualities or quinidine-like effects.

At therapeutic blood levels, the tricyclics can have beneficial effects on ventricular excitability. In patients with preexisting conduction delay, however, the tricyclic antidepressants can cause heart block (Glassman and Bigger 1981; Roose et al. 1987b). A pretreatment QTc interval of 450 milliseconds or greater indicates that conduction is already delayed and that the patient is not a candidate for tricyclic antidepressant treatment. High drug plasma levels (e.g., imipramine plasma concentrations >350 ng/mL) increase the risk of first-degree atrioventricular heart block (Preskorn and Irwin 1982). The tricyclic antidepressants do not reduce cardiac contractility or cardiac output (Roose et al. 1987a).

Glassman et al. (1993), noting that the type I antiarrhythmic drugs given following myocardial infarction actually increased the risk of sudden death, suggested that the tricyclics may pose similar risks. The risk of sudden death is also increased when heart rate variability is reduced, and the tricyclics reduce heart rate variability (Roose et al. 1998).

As mentioned earlier (see subsection "Attention-Deficit/Hyperactivity Disorder"), sudden death has been reported in five children under the age of 12 years who were receiving desipramine (Riddle et al. 1991, 1993). It was suggested that the immature conduction system in some children might render them more vulnerable to the cardiac effects of desipramine. Subsequently, no cardiac abnormalities were observed in a study of 71 children with 24-hour cardiac monitoring (Biederman et al. 1993). These findings suggest that cardiac events in children are not dose dependent and that electrocardiogram monitoring is not likely to identify those at risk.

Hepatic Effects

Acute hepatitis has been associated with administration of imipramine (Horst et al. 1980; Moskovitz et al. 1982; Weaver et al. 1977) and desipramine (Powell et al. 1968; Price and Nelson 1983). Mild increases of liver enzymes (less than three times normal) are not uncommon and usually can be monitored safely over a period of days or weeks. Enzyme changes do not appear to be related to drug concentrations (Price et al. 1984). Acute hepatitis is relatively uncommon but can occur. The etiology is not well established but in some cases appears to be a hypersensitivity reaction. It is characterized by very high enzyme levels (e.g., aspartate aminotransferase [AST] levels >800), which develop within days. The enzyme pattern can be either hepatocellular or cholestatic. Enzyme changes may precede clinical symptoms, especially in the hepatocellular form. If a random blood test indicates mildly elevated liver enzymes, enzyme levels can be followed for a few days. Because of the rapid rise in liver enzyme levels in acute hepatitis, that condition will become evident quickly and will be easily distinguished from mild, persistent enzyme level elevations.

Acute hepatitis is a dangerous and potentially fatal condition. The antidepressant must be discontinued and should not be introduced again because the next reaction may be more severe.

Other Side Effects

Increased sweating can occur with the tricyclic compounds and occasionally can be marked. Another side effect for which the mechanism is unclear is carbohydrate craving. This effect, when coupled with antihistaminic effects, can lead to significant weight gain. Weight gain appears to be greater with the tertiary compounds. Sexual dysfunction has been described with the tricyclics but appears to be less common than with the SSRIs. This side effect appears to be associated with the more serotonergic compounds such as clomipramine. Tricyclic antidepressants can cause allergic skin rashes, which are sometimes associated with photosensitivity reactions. Various blood dyscrasias also have been reported; fortunately, these are very rare.

Overdose

Because antidepressants are used for depressed patients who are at risk for overdose, the lethality of antidepressant drugs in overdose is of great concern. A tricyclic overdose of 10 times the total daily dose can be fatal (Gram 1990; Rudorfer and Robins 1982). Death most commonly occurs as a result of cardiac arrhythmia. However, seizures and central nervous system depression can occur. Although the use of tricyclics in depression has declined, amitriptyline remains widely used for other disorders, such as pain. The total number of deaths associated with amitriptyline is comparable to that for all other tricyclics and tetracyclics combined. All of the tricyclic and tetracyclic compounds are dangerous in overdose. Differences among these drugs are relatively minor in comparison with the improved safety of the second-generation antidepressant agents.

Teratogenicity

The long history of tricyclic use without observation of birth defects argues for the safety of these agents. Of course, the patient must be informed of the possible risks and benefits of taking the drug and the risks of discontinuing treatment before making a decision. The risk of recurrence is particularly high for patients with a prior history of depression during or following pregnancy.

If tricyclics are continued during pregnancy, dosage adjustment may be required because of metabolic changes (Altshuler and Hendrick 1996). Drug withdrawal following delivery can occur in the infant and is characterized by tachypnea, cyanosis, irritability, and poor sucking reflex. Drugs in this class should be discontinued 1 week prior to delivery if possible. The tricyclics are excreted in breast milk at concentrations similar to those in plasma, but the actual quantity delivered is very small, so that drug levels in the infant are usually undetectable (Rudorfer and Potter 1997; also see Chapter 41, "Psychopharmacology During Pregnancy and Lactation").

Drug-Drug Interactions

Both pharmacodynamic and pharmacokinetic drug interactions should be considered.

Pharmacodynamic Interactions

Serious pharmacodynamic interactions can occur between the tricyclics and the MAOI drugs. The most dangerous sequence is to give a large dose of a tricyclic to a patient who is already taking an MAOI. This can result in a sudden increase in catecholamines and a potentially fatal hypertensive reaction. These two compounds have been used together to treat patients with refractory depression (Goldberg and Thornton 1978; Schuckit et al. 1971). Treatment is begun with lower doses, and either the two compounds are started together or the tricyclic is started first.

The most common pharmacodynamic interaction involving tricyclics occurs when they are added to other sedating agents, resulting in increased sedation. By blocking the transporters, the tricyclics block the uptake and thus interfere with the action of guanethidine. Desipramine and the other tricyclics reduce the effect of clonidine.

Quinidine is an example of a drug with a potential dynamic and kinetic interaction with tricyclics. Because the tricyclics have quinidine-like effects, the effects of tricyclics and quinidine on cardiac conduction are potentially additive. In addition, quinidine is a potent CYP2D6 isoenzyme inhibitor that can raise tricyclic levels, further adding to the problem.

Pharmacokinetic Interactions

A number of drugs can block the metabolic pathways of the tricyclics, resulting in higher and potentially toxic levels. Desipramine has been of particular interest because it is metabolized via the CYP2D6 isoenzyme and there are no major alternative pathways. Inhibition of CYP2D6 can result in very high desipramine plasma levels, and toxicity can occur (Preskorn et al. 1990). Quinidine, mentioned above, is a very potent CYP2D6 inhibitor. Fluoxetine and paroxetine, duloxetine, bupropion, and some antipsychotics also inhibit CYP2D6. Fluoxetine and paroxetine at usual doses raise desipramine levels, on average, three- to fourfold in extensive metabolizers (Preskorn et al. 1994). CYP2D6 inhibitors would be expected to block nortriptyline metabolism, but the magnitude of this interaction has not been well studied.

Because the tertiary tricyclics are metabolized by several pathways (CYP1A2, 3A4, 2C19), a selective inhibitor of one pathway would be likely to have less of an effect on these compounds. Methylphenidate appears to inhibit demethylation of imipramine to desipramine. At this point, numerous drug interactions have been described, although many are of doubtful clinical significance (for comprehensive reviews, see Nemeroff et al. 1996; Pollock 1997).

Enzyme induction can also occur. The result of this interaction may render the drug acted upon ineffective. Unlike enzyme inhibition, which occurs quickly, enzyme induction requires synthesis of new enzyme, and the effect may take 2–3 weeks to develop. Barbiturates and carbamazepine are potent inducers of CYP3A4. Induction with phenytoin appears to be less dramatic. Although CYP2D6 is a noninducible isoenzyme, phenobarbital reduces the availability of desipramine substantially. Apparently when CYP3A4 is induced, it becomes an important metabolic pathway for desipramine and the other tricyclics. In this author's experience, it can be difficult to attain an effective blood level of desipramine in the presence of a barbiturate.

Nicotine induces the CYP1A2 pathway and may lower concentrations of the tertiary tricyclics, but the secondary tricyclics (e.g., desipramine, nortriptyline) appear to be less affected.

Acute ingestion of alcohol can reduce first-pass metabolism, resulting in higher tricyclic levels. Because tricyclic overdose is often associated with alcohol ingestion, this is an important consideration. Alternatively, chronic use of alcohol appears to induce hepatic isoenzymes and may lower tricyclic levels (Shoaf and Linnoila 1991).

The tricyclics themselves appear to be weak enzyme inhibitors, and few clinically significant interactions have been described. The tertiary tricyclics compete with warfarin for some metabolic enzymes (e.g., CYP1A2) and may raise warfarin levels.

Conclusion

The tricyclic drugs were the mainstay of treatment for depression for three decades. Although the second-generation antidepressants appear to be better tolerated, no new agent has been shown to be more effective than the tricyclics, and if anything, there has been concern that the new agents may be less effective. The tricyclics were "dirty" drugs; that is, they had multiple actions. Although their side effects have been emphasized, these multiple actions may have contributed to their efficacy. Not only does amitriptyline block uptake of 5-HT, but its metabolite blocks uptake of norepinephrine, and in addition, amitriptyline is a 5-HT_2 antagonist. The principal drawback of this class of agents is the risk of serious cardiac adverse effects. They can aggravate arrhythmia in patients with preexisting conduction delay. They also may increase the risk of sudden death in children and in patients with ischemic heart disease. Moreover, a week's supply of medication taken in overdose could be fatal. Because of these adverse effects, it is unlikely that there will be a resurgence of interest in the tricyclics. Nevertheless, the efficacy of these agents across a range of disorders, including pain, suggests the possible advantage of antidepressant drugs with multiple actions.

References

Abernathy DR, Greenblatt DJ, Shader RI: Imipramine and desipramine disposition in the elderly. J Pharmacol Exp Ther 232:183–188, 1985

Agency for Health Care Policy and Research: Clinical Practice Guideline: Depression in Primary Care: Treatment of Major Depression, Vol 2. Rockville, MD, U.S. Government Printing Office, 1993

Altshuler LL, Hendrick VC: Pregnancy and psychotropic medication: changes in blood levels. J Clin Psychopharmacol 16:78–80, 1996

American Psychiatric Association: Diagnostic and Statistical Manual of Mental Disorders, 4th Edition, Text Revision. Washington, DC, American Psychiatric Association, 2000

American Psychiatric Association Task Force: Tricyclic antidepressants—blood level measurements and clinical outcome: an APA Task Force report. Task Force on the Use of Laboratory Tests in Psychiatry. Am J Psychiatry 142:155–162, 1985

Anderson I: SSRIs versus tricyclics antidepressants in depressed inpatients: a meta-analysis of efficacy and tolerability. Depress Anxiety 7 (suppl 1): 11–17, 1998

Anderson I: Selective serotonin reuptake inhibitors versus tricyclics antidepressant: a meta-analysis of efficacy and tolerability. J Affect Disord 58:19–36, 2000

Anderson I, Tomenson B: A meta-analysis of the efficacy of selective serotonin reuptake inhibitors compared to tricyclic antidepressants in depression (abstract). Neuropsychopharmacology 10 (suppl):106, 1994

Anton RF, Burch EA: Amoxapine versus amitriptyline combined with perphenazine in the treatment of psychotic depression. Am J Psychiatry 147:1203–1208, 1990

Axelrod J, Whitby LG, Herting G: Effect of psychotropic drugs on the uptake of H3-norepinephrine by tissues. Science 133:383–384, 1961

Barden N: Modulation of glucocorticoid receptor gene expression by antidepressant drugs. Pharmacopsychiatry 29:12–22, 1996

Bertilsson L, Mellstrom B, Sjöqvist P: Pronounced inhibition of noradrenaline uptake by 10-hydroxy metabolites of nortriptyline. Life Sci 25:1285–1292, 1979

Biederman J, Baldessarini RJ, Wright V, et al: A double-blind placebo-controlled study of desipramine in the treatment of ADD, I: efficacy. J Am Acad Child Adolesc Psychiatry 32:805–813, 1989

Biederman J, Baldessarini RJ, Goldblatt A, et al: A naturalistic study of 24-hour electrocardiographic recording and echocardiographic findings in children and adolescents treated with desipramine. J Am Acad Child Adolesc Psychiatry 32:805–813, 1993

Blier P, de Montigny C, Chaput Y: Modification of the serotonin system by antidepressant treatments: implications for the therapeutic response in major depression. J Clin Psychopharmacol 7:24S–35S, 1987

Bock J, Nelson JC, Gray S, et al: Desipramine hydroxylation: variability and effect of antipsychotic drugs. Clin Pharmacol Ther 33:190–197, 1983

Bolden-Watson C, Richelson E: Blockade of newly developed antidepressants of biogenic amine uptake into rat brain synaptosomes. Life Sci 52:1023–1029, 1993

Brosen K, Otton SV, Gram LF: Sparteine oxidation polymorphism in Denmark. Acta Pharmacol Toxicol 57:357–360, 1985

Brosen K, Zeugin T, Myer UA: Role of P450IID6, the target of the sparteine/debrisoquin oxidation polymorphism, in the metabolism of imipramine. Clin Pharmacol Ther 49:609–617, 1991

Bunney WE, Davis JM: Norepinephrine in depressive reactions: a review. Arch Gen Psychiatry 13:483–494, 1965

Bymaster FP, Katner JS, Nelson DL, et al: Atomoxetine increases extracellular levels of norepinephrine and dopamine in prefrontal cortex of rat: a potential mechanism for efficacy in attention deficit/hyperactivity disorder. Neuropsychopharmacology 27:699–711, 2002

Chan CH, Janicak PG, Davis JM: Response of psychotic and nonpsychotic depressed patients to tricyclic antidepressants. J Clin Psychiatry 48:197–200, 1987

Charney DS, Delgado PL, Price LH, et al: The receptor sensitivity hypothesis of antidepressant action: a review of antidepressant effects on serotonin function, in The Role of Serotonin in Psychiatric Disorders. Edited by Brown SL, van Praag HM. New York, Brunner/Mazel, 1991, pp 29–56

Coupet I, Rauh CE, Szucs-Myers VA, et al: 2-Chloro-11(piperazinyl)[b,f][1,4]oxazepine (amoxapine), an antidepressant with antipsychotics properties—a possible role for 7-hydroxyamoxapine. Biochem Pharmacol 28:2514–2515, 1979

Cusack B, Nelson A, Richelson E: Binding of antidepressants to human brain receptors: focus on newer generation compounds. Psychopharmacology 114:559–565, 1994

Davis JM, Glassman AH: Antidepressant drugs, in Comprehensive Textbook of Psychiatry. Edited by Kaplan HI, Sadock BJ. Baltimore, MD, Williams & Wilkins, 1989, pp 1627–1655

Delgado PL, Charney DS, Price LH, et al: Serotonin function and the mechanism of antidepressant action. Reversal of antidepressant-induced remission by rapid depletion of plasma tryptophan. Arch Gen Psychiatry 47:411–418, 1990

Delgado PL, Miller HL, Salomon RM, et al: Monoamines and the mechanism of antidepressant action: effects of catecholamine depletion on mood of patients treated with antidepressants. Psychopharmacol Bull 29:389–396, 1993

de Montigny C, Aghajanian GK: Tricyclic antidepressants: long-term treatment increases responsivity of rat forebrain neurons to serotonin. Science 202:1303–1306, 1978

DiMascio A, Heninger G, Klerman GL: Psychopharmacology of imipramine and desipramine: a comparative study of their effects in normal males. Psychopharmacologia 5:361–371, 1964

Duman RS, Heninger GR, Nestler EJ: A molecular and cellular theory of depression. Arch Gen Psychiatry 54:597–606, 1997

Eberhard G, von Knorring L, Nilsson HL, et al: A double-blind randomized study of clomipramine versus maprotiline in patients with idiopathic pain syndromes. Neuropsychobiology 19:25–34, 1988

Evans DAP, Mahgoub A, Sloan TP, et al: A family and population study of the genetic polymorphism of debrisoquin oxidation in a white British population. J Med Genet 17:102–105, 1980

Frank E, Kupfer DJ, Perel JM, et al: Three-year outcomes for maintenance therapies in recurrent depression. Arch Gen Psychiatry 47:1093–1099, 1990

Furey ML, Drevets WC: Antidepressant efficacy of the antimuscarinic drug scopolamine: a randomized, placebo-controlled clinical trial. Arch Gen Psychiatry 63:1121–1129, 2006

Geller B: Psychopharmacology of children and adolescents: pharmacokinetics and relationships of plasma/serum levels to response. Psychopharmacol Bull 27:401–409, 1991

Gerson SC, Plotkin DA, Jarvik LF: Antidepressant drug studies, 1964 to 1986: empirical evidence for aging patients. J Clin Psychopharmacol 8:311–322, 1988

Glassman AH, Bigger JT: Cardiovascular effects of therapeutic doses of tricyclic antidepressants. Arch Gen Psychiatry 38:815–820, 1981

Glassman AH, Kantor S, Shostak M: Depression, delusions, and drug response. Am J Psychiatry 132:716–719, 1975

Glassman AH, Perel JM, Shostak M, et al: Clinical implications of imipramine plasma levels for depressive illness. Arch Gen Psychiatry 34:197–204, 1977

Glassman AH, Bigger JT Jr, Giardina EV, et al: Clinical characteristics of imipramine induced orthostatic hypotension. Lancet 1(8114):468–472, 1979

Glassman AH, Roose SP, Bigger JT Jr: The safety of tricyclic antidepressants in cardiac patients: risk/benefit reconsidered. JAMA 269:2673–2675, 1993

Goldberg RS, Thornton WE: Combined tricyclic-MAOI therapy for refractory depression: a review, with guidelines for appropriate usage. J Clin Pharmacol 18:143–147, 1978

Goodwin FK, Bunney WE Jr: Depressions following reserpine: a reevaluation. Semin Psychiatry 3:435–448, 1971

Goodwin GM, Green AR, Johnson P: 5-HT2 receptor characteristics in frontal cortex and 5-HT2 receptor mediated head-twitch behavior following antidepressant treatment to mice. Br J Pharmacol 83:235–242, 1984

Gram LF: Inadequate dosing and Pharmacokinetic variability as confounding factors in assessment of efficacy of antidepressants. Clin Neuropharmacol 13 (suppl):S35–S44, 1990

Greenblatt DJ, Moltke LL, Shader RI: Pharmacokinetics of psychotropic drugs, in Geriatric Psychopharmacology. Edited by Nelson JC. New York, Marcel Dekker, 1998, pp 27–41

Greist JH, Jefferson JW, Kobak KA, et al: Efficacy and tolerability of serotonin transport inhibitors in obsessive-compulsive disorder: a meta-analysis. Arch Gen Psychiatry 52:53–60, 1995

Hammer W, Sjöqvist F: Plasma levels of monomethylated tricyclic antidepressants during treatment with imipramine-like compounds. Life Sci 6:1895–1903, 1967

Himmelhoch JM, Detre T, Kupfer DJ, et al: Treatment of previously intractable depressions with tranylcypromine and lithium. J Nerv Ment Dis 155:216–220, 1972

Himmelhoch JM, Thase ME, Mallinger AG, et al: Tranylcypromine versus imipramine in anergic bipolar depression. Am J Psychiatry 148:910–916, 1991

Horst DA, Grace ND, Le Compte PM: Prolonged cholestasis and progressive hepatic fibrosis following imipramine therapy. Gastroenterology 79:550–554, 1980

Jick H, Dinan BJ, Hunter JR, et al: Tricyclic antidepressants and convulsions. J Clin Psychopharmacol 3:182–185, 1983

Jobson K, Linnoila M, Gillam J, et al: Successful treatment of severe anxiety attacks with tricyclic antidepressants: a possible mechanism of action. Am J Psychiatry 135:863–864, 1978

Katz IR, Simpson GM, Jethanandani V, et al: Steady state pharmacokinetics of nortriptyline in the frail elderly. Neuropsychopharmacology 2:229–236, 1989

Katz IR, Simpson GM, Curlik SM, et al: Pharmacologic treatment of major depression for elderly patients in residential care settings. J Clin Psychiatry 51 (7, suppl):41–47, 1990

Keller MB, Gelenberg AJ, Hirschfeld RMA, et al: The treatment of chronic depression: a double-blind, randomized trial of sertraline and imipramine. J Clin Psychiatry 59(pt 2):598–607, 1998

Klein DF: Delineation of two drug responsive anxiety syndromes. Psychopharmacologia 5:397–408, 1964

Kocsis JH, Frances AJ, Voss CB, et al: Imipramine treatment for chronic depression. Arch Gen Psychiatry 45:253–257, 1988

Kuhn R: The treatment of depressive states with G22355 (imipramine hydrochloride). Am J Psychiatry 115:459–464, 1958

Kuhn R: The imipramine story, in Discoveries in Biological Psychiatry. Edited by Ayd FJ, Blackwell B. Philadelphia, PA, JB Lippincott, 1970, pp 205–217

Kupfer DJ, Spiker DG: Refractory depression: prediction of nonresponse by clinical indicators. J Clin Psychiatry 42:307–312, 1981

Lakoski JM, Aghajanian GK: Effects of ketanserin on neuronal responses to serotonin in the prefrontal cortex, lateral geniculate and dorsal raphe nucleus. Neuropharmacology 24:265–273, 1985

Leonard HL, Swedo S, Rapoport JL, et al: Treatment of obsessive compulsive disorder in children and adolescents with clomipramine and desipramine: a double-blind crossover comparison. Arch Gen Psychiatry 46:1088–1092, 1989

Lesch KP, Manji HK: Signal-transducing G proteins and antidepressant drugs: evidence for modulation of alpha subunit gene expression in rat brain. Biol Psychiatry 32:549–579, 1992

Liebowitz MR, Quitkin FM, Stewart JW, et al: Phenelzine vs imipramine in atypical depression. Arch Gen Psychiatry 41:669–677, 1984

Liebowitz MR, Quitkin FM, Stewart JW, et al: Antidepressant specificity in atypical depression. Arch Gen Psychiatry 45:129–137, 1988

Livingston RL, Zucker DK, Isenberg K, et al: Tricyclic antidepressants and delirium. J Clin Psychiatry 44:173–176, 1983

Manji HK, Potter WZ, Lenox RH: Signal transduction pathways: molecular targets for lithium's actions. Arch Gen Psychiatry 52:531–543, 1995

Marek GJ, Carpenter LL, McDougle CJ, et al: Synergistic action of 5-HT2A antagonists and selective serotonin reuptake inhibitors in neuropsychiatric disorders Neuropsychopharmacology 28:402–412, 2003

Max MB, Lynch SA, Muir J, et al: Effects of desipramine, amitriptyline, and fluoxetine on pain in diabetic neuropathy. N Engl J Med 326:1250–1256, 1992

McGrath PJ, Stewart JW, Harrison W, et al: Treatment of tricyclic refractory depression with a monoamine oxidase inhibitor antidepressant. Psychopharmacol Bull 23:169–172, 1987

Miller NL, Kocsis JH, Leon AC, et al: Maintenance desipramine for dysthymia: a placebo-controlled study. J Affect Disord 64:231–237, 2001

Mochizucki D: Serotonin and noradrenaline reuptake inhibitors in animal models of pain. Hum Psychopharmacol 19 (suppl 1):S15–S19, 2004

Montgomery SA: The efficacy of fluoxetine as an antidepressant in the short and long term. Int Clin Psychopharmacol 4 (suppl):113–119, 1989

Moskovitz R, DeVane CL, Harris R, et al: Toxic hepatitis and single daily dosage imipramine therapy. J Clin Psychiatry 43:165–166, 1982

Munjack DJ, Usigli R, Zulueta A, et al: Nortriptyline in the treatment of panic disorder and agoraphobia with panic attacks. J Clin Psychopharmacol 8:204–207, 1988

Nelson JC: Use of desipramine in depressed inpatients. J Clin Psychiatry 45:10–15, 1984

Nelson JC: The use of antipsychotic drugs in the treatment of depression, in Treating Resistant Depression. Edited by Zohar J, Belmaker RH. New York, PMA Publishing, 1987, pp 131–146

Nelson JC, Jatlow PI: Nonlinear desipramine kinetics: prevalence and importance. Clin Pharmacol Ther 41:666–670, 1987

Nelson JC, Jatlow P, Quinlan DM, et al: Desipramine plasma concentrations and antidepressant response. Arch Gen Psychiatry 39:1419–1422, 1982

Nelson JC, Jatlow PI, Quinlan DM: Subjective complaints during desipramine treatment: relative importance of plasma drug concentrations and the severity of depression. Arch Gen Psychiatry 41:55–59, 1984

Nelson JC, Jatlow P, Mazure C: Desipramine plasma levels and response in elderly melancholics. J Clin Psychopharmacol 5:217–220, 1985

Nelson JC, Jatlow PI, Mazure C: Rapid desipramine dose adjustment using 24-hour levels. J Clin Psychopharmacol 7:72–77, 1987

Nelson JC, Mazure C, Attilasoy E, et al: Hydroxydesipramine in the elderly. J Clin Psychopharmacol 8:428–433, 1988a

Nelson JC, Mazure C, Jatlow PI: Antidepressant activity of 2-hydroxy-desipramine. Clin Pharmacol Ther 44:283–288, 1988b

Nelson JC, Mazure CM, Jatlow PI: Characteristics of desipramine refractory depression. J Clin Psychiatry 55:12–19, 1994

Nelson JC, Mazure CM, Jatlow PI: Desipramine treatment of major depression in patients over 75 years of age. J Clin Psychopharmacol 15:99–105, 1995

Nemeroff CB, DeVane CL, Pollock BG: Newer antidepressants and the cytochrome P450 system. Am J Psychiatry 153:311–320, 1996

Nibuya M, Nestler EJ, Duman RS: Chronic antidepressant administration increases the expression of cAMP response element-binding protein (CREB) in rat hippocampus. J Neurosci 16:2365–2372, 1996

Nordin C, Bertilsson L, Siwers B: Clinical and biochemical effects during treatment of depression with nortriptyline—the role of 10-hydroxynortriptyline. Clin Pharmacol Ther 42:10–19, 1987

O'Malley PG, Jackson JL, Santoro J, et al: Antidepressant therapy for unexplained symptoms and symptom syndromes. J Fam Pract 48:980–990, 1999

Panerai AE, Monza G, Movilia P, et al: A randomized, within-patient, cross-over, placebo-controlled trial on the efficacy and tolerability of the tricyclic antidepressants chlorimipramine and nortriptyline in central pain. Acta Neurol Scand 82:34–38, 1990

Peck AW, Stern WC, Watkinson C: Incidence of seizures during treatment with tricyclic antidepressant drugs and bupropion. J Clin Psychiatry 44 (5, pt 2):197–201, 1983

Peroutka SJ, Snyder SH: Long term antidepressant treatment decreases spiroperidol-labeled serotonin receptor binding. Science 210:88–90, 1980

Pollock BG: Drug interactions, in Geriatric Psychopharmacology. Edited by Nelson JC. New York, Marcel Dekker, 1997, pp 43–60

Potter WZ, Calil NM, Manian AA, et al: Hydroxylated metabolites of tricyclic antidepressants: preclinical assessment of activity. Biol Psychiatry 14:601–613, 1979

Powell WJ, Koch-Weser J, Williams RA: Lethal hepatic necrosis after therapy with imipramine and desipramine. JAMA 206:1791–1792, 1968

Prange AI: The pharmacology and biochemistry of depression. Dis Nerv Syst 25:217–221, 1965

Preskorn SH, Irwin HA: Toxicity of tricyclic antidepressants: kinetics, mechanism, intervention: a review. J Clin Psychiatry 43:151–156, 1982

Preskorn SH, Simpson S: Tricyclic antidepressant–induced delirium and plasma drug concentration. Am J Psychiatry 139:822–823, 1982

Preskorn SH, Beber JH, Faul JC, et al: Serious adverse effects of combining fluoxetine and tricyclic antidepressants. Am J Psychiatry 147:532, 1990

Preskorn SH, Alderman J, Chung M, et al: Pharmacokinetics of desipramine co-administered with sertraline or fluoxetine. J Clin Psychopharmacol 14:90–98, 1994

Price LH, Nelson JC: Desipramine associated hepatitis. J Clin Psychopharmacology 3:243–246, 1983

Price LH, Nelson JC, Jatlow P: Effects of desipramine on clinical liver function tests. Am J Psychiatry 414:798–800, 1984

Priest BT, Kaczorowski GJ: Blocking sodium channels to treat neuropathic pain. Expert Opin Ther Targets 11:291–306, 2007

Randrup A, Braestrup C: Uptake inhibition of biogenic amines by newer antidepressant drugs: relevance to the dopamine hypothesis of depression. Psychopharmacology (Berl) 53:309–314, 1977

Rapoport J, Potter WZ: Tricyclic antidepressants: use in pediatric psychopharmacology, in Pharmacokinetics: Youth and Age. Edited by Raskin A, Robinson D. Amsterdam, The Netherlands, Elsevier, 1981, pp 105–123

Rapoport JL, Mikkelson EJ, Zavadil AP, et al: Childhood enuresis, II: psychopathology, tricyclic concentrations in plasma and anti-enuretic effect. Arch Gen Psychiatry 37:1146–1152, 1980

Richelson E, Nelson A: Antagonism by antidepressants of neurotransmitter receptors of normal human brain in vitro. J Pharmacol Exp Ther 230:94–102, 1984

Riddle MA, Nelson JC, Kleinman CS, et al: Sudden death in children receiving Norpramin: a review of three reported cases and commentary. J Am Acad Child Adolesc Psychiatry 30:104–108, 1991

Riddle MA, Geller B, Ryan N: Another sudden death in a child treated with desipramine. J Am Acad Child Adolesc Psychiatry 32:792–797, 1993

Roose SP, Glassman AH, Siris SG, et al: Comparison of imipramine and nortriptyline-induced orthostatic hypotension: a meaningful difference. J Clin Psychopharmacol 1:316–319, 1981

Roose SP, Glassman AH, Walsh BT, et al: Tricyclic nonresponders, phenomenology and treatment. Am J Psychiatry 143:345–348, 1986

Roose SP, Glassman AH, Giardina EG, et al: Cardiovascular effects of imipramine and bupropion in depressed patients with congestive heart failure. J Clin Psychopharmacol 7:247–251, 1987a

Roose SP, Glassman AH, Giardina EG, et al: Tricyclic antidepressants in depressed patients with cardiac conduction disease. Arch Gen Psychiatry 44:273–275, 1987b

Roose S, Laghrissi-Thode F, Kennedy JS, et al: A comparison of paroxetine and nortriptyline in depressed patients with ischemic heart disease. JAMA 279:287–291, 1998

Rosenstein DL, Nelson JC: Heart rate during desipramine treatment as an indicator of $beta_1$-adrenergic function. Society of Biological Psychiatry Scientific Program. Biol Psychiatry 29:132A, 1991

Rosenstein DL, Nelson JC, Jacobs JC: Seizures associated with antidepressants: a review. J Clin Psychiatry 54:289–299, 1993

Rudorfer MV, Potter WZ: The role of metabolites of antidepressant in the treatment of depression. CNS Drugs 7:273–312, 1997

Rudorfer MV, Robins E: Amitriptyline overdose: clinical effects of tricyclic antidepressant plasma levels. J Clin Psychiatry 43:457–460, 1982

Rudorfer MV, Young RC: Desipramine: cardiovascular effects and plasma levels. Am J Psychiatry 137:984–986, 1980

Ryan ND: The pharmacologic treatment of child and adolescent depression. Psychiatric Clin North Am 15:29–40, 1992

Salerno SM, Browning R, Jackson JL: The effect of antidepressant treatment on chronic back pain. Arch Intern Med 162:19–24, 2002

Schildkraut JJ: The catecholamine hypothesis of affective disorders: a review of supporting evidence. Am J Psychiatry 122:509–522, 1965

Schuckit M, Robins E, Feighner J: Tricyclic antidepressants and monoamine oxidase inhibitors: combination therapy in the treatment of depression. Arch Gen Psychiatry 24:509–514, 1971

Schwaninger M, Schofl C, Blume R, et al: Inhibition by antidepressant drugs of cyclic AMP response element-binding protein/cyclic AMP response element-directed gene transcription. Mol Pharmacol 47:1112–1118, 1995

Shoaf SE, Linnoila M: Interaction of ethanol and smoking on the pharmacokinetics and pharmacodynamics of psychotropic medications. Psychopharmacol Bull 27:577–594, 1991

Siris SG, van Kammen DP, Docherty JP: Use of antidepressant drugs in schizophrenia. Arch Gen Psychiatry 35:1368–1377, 1978

Spiker DG, Weiss JC, Chang S, et al: Tricyclic antidepressant overdose: clinical presentation and plasma levels. Clin Pharmacol Ther 18:539–546, 1975

Spiker DG, Weiss JC, Dealy RS, et al: The pharmacologic treatment of delusional depression. Am J Psychiatry 142:430–436, 1985

Sulser F, Vetulani J, Mobley PL: Mode of action of antidepressant drugs. Biochem Pharmacol 27:257–261, 1978

Szabo ST, Blier P: Effect of the selective noradrenergic reuptake inhibitor reboxetine on the firing activity of noradrenaline and serotonin neurons. Eur J Neurosci 13:2077–2087, 2001

Tatsumi M, Groshan K, Blakely RD, et al: Pharmacological profile of antidepressants and related compounds at human monoamine transporters. Eur J Pharmacol 340:249–258, 1997

Thase ME, Malinger AG, McKnight D, et al: Treatment of imipramine-resistant recurrent depression, IV: a double-blind crossover study of tranylcypromine for anergic bipolar depression. Am J Psychiatry 149:195–198, 1992

Thase ME, Fava M, Halbreich U, et al: A placebo-controlled, randomized clinical trial comparing sertraline and imipramine for the treatment of dysthymia. Arch Gen Psychiatry 53:777–784, 1996

Thayssen P, Bjerre M, Kragh-Sorenson P, et al: Cardiovascular effects of imipramine and nortriptyline in elderly patients. Psychopharmacology 74:360–364, 1981

Tremblay P, Blier P: Catecholaminergic strategies for the treatment of major depression. Curr Drug Targets 7:149–158, 2006

von Moltke LL, Greenblatt DJ, Harmatz JS, et al: Psychotropic drug metabolism in old age: principles and problems of assessment, in Psychopharmacology: The Fourth Generation of Progress. Edited by Bloom FE, Kupfer DJ. New York, Raven, 1995, pp 1461–1469

Walsh T, Hadigan CM, Wong LM: Increased pulse and blood pressure associated with desipramine treatment of bulimia nervosa. J Clin Psychopharmacol 12:163–168, 1992

Weaver GA, Pavinoc D, Davis JS: Hepatic sensitivity to imipramine. Dig Dis 22:551–553, 1977

Weir TA, Goodwin FK: Can antidepressants cause mania and worsen the course of affective illness? Am J Psychiatry 144:1403–1411, 1987

Wilens TE, Biederman J, Baldessarini RJ, et al: Developmental changes in serum concentrations of desipramine and 2-hydroxydesipramine during treatment with desipramine. J Am Acad Child Adolesc Psychiatry 31:691–698, 1992

Wilens TE, Biederman J, Prince J, et al: Six week, double-blind, placebo-controlled study of desipramine for adult attention deficit hyperactivity disorder. Am J Psychiatry 153:1147–1153, 1996

Yoshimura M, Furue H: Mechanisms for the antinociceptive actions of the descending noradrenergic and serotonergic systems in the spinal cord. J Pharmacol Sci 101:107–117, 2006

Young RC, Alexopoulos GS, Shamoian CA, et al: Plasma 10-hydroxy-nortriptyline in elderly depressed patients. Clin Pharmacol Ther 35:540–544, 1984

Zitrin CM, Klein DF, Woerner MG: Treatment of agoraphobia with group exposure in vivo and imipramine. Arch Gen Psychiatry 37:63–72, 1980

CHAPTER 2

Fluoxetine

Jerrold F. Rosenbaum, M.D.

The introduction of fluoxetine as the first selective serotonin reuptake inhibitor (SSRI) approved in the United States, initially for the treatment of depression, represents an important advance in psychopharmacology and has been the catalyst for much subsequent basic and clinical research. Considerable evidence has demonstrated that fluoxetine, like other SSRIs, has a broad spectrum of clinical indications. There is a consensus, however, that the commercial success of fluoxetine (and subsequently marketed SSRIs) derived from its advantageous safety profile, which propelled SSRIs to dominance in the antidepressant drug market. Fluoxetine, under the brand name Prozac, became a cultural icon—a symbol of the growth in antidepressant prescribing and depression recognition. Consequently, it also became a focus of controversies about rare events attributed to side effects, such as violent acts and suicide, and a symbol of the medicalization of mental health concerns. Fluoxetine was also the first of the SSRI blockbuster drugs to become available in generic form; ironically, with decreased cost came decreased market share, likely reflecting the reduction in marketing and availability of office samples. Although SSRIs, as a class, share several common features, individual agents, such as fluoxetine, also have unique characteristics.

History and Discovery

Serotonin (5-HT) is an indoleamine with wide distribution in plants, animals, and humans. Pioneering histochemistry by Falck et al. (1962) found that 5-HT was localized within specific neuronal pathways and cell bodies. These originate principally from two discrete nuclei, the medial and dorsal raphe. Across animal species, 5-HT innervation is widespread. Although regional variations exist, several limbic structures manifest especially high levels of 5-HT (Amin et al. 1954).

However, the 5-HT levels in the central nervous system (CNS) represent only a small fraction of the 5-HT levels in the body (Bradley 1989). Because 5-HT does not cross the blood-brain barrier, it must be synthesized locally. 5-HT is released into the synapse from the cytoplasmic and vesicular reservoirs (Elks et al. 1979). Following its release, 5-HT is principally inactivated by reuptake into nerve terminals through a sodium/potassium (Na^+/K^+) adenosine triphosphatase (ATPase)–dependent carrier (Shaskan and Snyder 1970). The transmitter is subsequently subject to either degradation by monoamine oxidase (MAO) or vesicular restorage. Abnormalities in central 5-HT function have been hypothesized to underlie disturbances in mood, anxiety, satiety, cognition, aggression, and sexual drives, to highlight a few. As described by Fuller (1985), there are several loci at which therapeutic drugs might alter 5-HT neurotransmission. The explosion of knowledge regarding the serotonergic system can largely be traced to the development of compounds, such as fluoxetine, that block the reuptake of this neurotransmitter.

Structure-Activity Relations

Drugs that inhibit 5-HT reuptake vary in their selectivity. Despite the tendency to lump the contemporary SSRIs into the same class designation, significant structural and activity differences exist. Their chemical structures help illustrate this diversity. In contrast to paroxetine and sertraline, which exist as single isomers, fluoxetine, like citalopram, is a racemate. The family of SSRIs manifests diverse structural and activity relations. Such data are in vitro and thus subject to methodological variability (Thomas et al. 1987). Fluoxetine is less potent than paroxetine in vitro and less selective for 5-HT reuptake inhibition, relative to norepinephrine, than citalopram. However, note that in vitro potency does not necessarily equate with in vivo dosing experience, clinical efficacy, or adverse-event profile.

Although the tricyclic antidepressants (TCAs), like the SSRIs, antagonize 5-HT receptors (Dempsey et al. 2005; Eisensamer et al. 2003), they also exhibit inhibitory activity at other receptor targets mediating their adverse-event profile (Hall and Ogren 1981; Snyder and Yamamura 1977; U'Prichard et al. 1978). These include histaminergic, α_1-adrenergic, and muscarinic receptors. For fluoxetine, the median inhibitory concentration (IC_{50}) at histaminergic and adrenergic sites is in the micromolar range and thus unlikely to be of clinical significance. Activity at the muscarinic receptor is negligible for fluoxetine. Stauderman et al. (1992) reported that fluoxetine and paroxetine inhibit the binding of ^{3}H-nitrendipine to L-type calcium channels; however, this was at concentrations that were probably in excess of those achieved during in vivo treatment of depression.

In summary, in vitro radioligand-binding techniques showed that fluoxetine had a lower probability of many of the troublesome side effects associated with TCAs and was relatively selective in its 5-HT reuptake inhibition.

Pharmacological Profile

Serotonin

The action of any SSRI extends beyond the inhibition of 5-HT reuptake. At least 14 different 5-HT receptor subtypes reside at pre- and postsynaptic locations (Fuller 1996). Serotonin$_{1A}$ (5-HT$_{1A}$) binding sites include both somatodendritic and presynaptic autoreceptors (which inhibit 5-HT firing) and postsynaptic receptors. The latter are predominantly hippocampal, and their sensitivity is increased after chronic antidepressant exposure (Aghajanian et al. 1988; Elena Castro et al. 2003).

After chronic administration, many antidepressants downregulate or reduce the density of serotonin$_2$ (5-HT$_2$) binding sites in rat frontal cortex (Peroutka and Snyder 1980). Some, but not all, SSRIs have been associated with this effect (Fraser et al. 1988), and fluoxetine has been demonstrated to normalize 5-HT$_{1A}$ density in rats

(Sodero et al. 2006). SSRIs, as a drug class, have been reported to normalize both 5-HT_{1A} and 5-HT_2 receptor density among patients with depression (Leonard 1992).

The mechanisms by which fluoxetine and other SSRIs interact with the human serotonin transporter (SERT) are not fully understood. Some evidence suggests that fluoxetine's effect on SERT is partially based on SERT promoter polymorphism; it can lead to increased or decreased SERT expression, depending on an individual's genotype (Little et al. 2006). Further studies have shown that SERT may also be inhibited at the posttranslational stage, likely through multiple binding sites on the SERT molecule itself (Henry et al. 2006; Iceta et al. 2007).

Fluoxetine transiently inhibits dorsal raphe firing, decreases terminal autoreceptor function, and ultimately increases net 5-HT synaptic transmission within CA3 pyramidal cells in the hippocampus (Blier et al. 1988). Electrophysiological studies indicate that most antidepressants enhance net 5-HT transmission after chronic administration (Blier et al. 1990), albeit at different loci: the TCAs via enhanced sensitivity of postsynaptic 5-HT_{1A} receptors, and the SSRIs (and MAO inhibitors [MAOIs]) via reduced sensitivity of somatodendritic (5-HT_{1A}) and terminal (serotonin$_{1D}$ [5-HT_{1D}]) autoreceptors. SSRIs and TCAs also exert an inhibitory effect on 5-HT_3 receptors in a noncompetitive fashion (Eisensamer et al. 2003). These observations of different mechanisms may help to explain why certain depressive symptoms that do not respond to one class of antidepressant will respond to another class and may also explain the enhanced response reported when combinations of antidepressant agents are used.

Norepinephrine

Chronic administration of most somatic treatments for depression downregulates or reduces the density of β-adrenergic binding sites in the brain (Bergstrom and Kellar 1979). These treatments include traditional norepinephrine-specific and mixed uptake inhibitors (Charney et al. 1981). However, results with the SSRIs have been less consistent (Johnson 1991). Despite its in vitro 5-HT selectivity, fluoxetine has been observed, with autoradiography, to induce β-adrenergic receptor downregulation. It has also been shown in at least one study to increase extracellular norepinephrine concentrations in rat prefrontal cortex after acute systemic administration; this effect was not observed with other SSRIs tested (Bymaster et al. 2002). Fluoxetine has also been demonstrated to potentiate the noradrenergic effects of bupropion (Li et al. 2002).

Most studies with SSRIs have not shown a consistent change in β-adrenergic binding or β-adrenergic-stimulated cyclic adenosine monophosphate (cAMP) production. However, Baron et al. (1988) reported that fluoxetine, when it was coadministered with desipramine, augmented the reduction in cortical β-adrenergic receptors expected with desipramine alone. In contrast, investigations with fluvoxamine, paroxetine, and citalopram have not yielded consistent results. In general, the greater the 5-HT selectivity of a compound, the less in vitro evidence for β-adrenergic downregulation has been seen. Thus, β-adrenergic downregulation may not be essential for clinical efficacy.

Current data do not support a significant effect on α-adrenergic receptor affinity or density by the SSRIs. Studies using radiolabeling to investigate fluoxetine (Wong et al. 1985) have shown relative inactivity at this site. Fluoxetine has been reported to reduce desipramine-induced release of growth hormone after 4 weeks of treatment (O'Flynn et al. 1991). This effect suggests a possible indirect activity at the α_2-adrenergic receptor.

In summary, although relative differences in adrenoreceptor affinity exist across the SSRI class, and fluoxetine may have more adrenergic activity than some of the other SSRIs, the clinical significance of these differences appears to be negligible.

Dopamine

Animal studies provide evidence that the serotonergic system may exert tonic inhibition on the central dopaminergic system. Serotonin has also been shown to decrease the generation of dopaminergic cells from mesencephalic precursors in rats, an effect mediated by 5-HT_4 and 5-HT_7 receptors found on glial cells (Parga et al. 2007). Thus, fluoxetine might diminish dopaminergic transmission, consistent with anecdotes of extrapyramidal side effects (EPS) occurring during fluoxetine therapy (Bouchard et al. 1989). 5-HT agonists, however, also exert a facilitatory influence on dopamine release (Benloucif and Galloway 1991), which can be antagonized by the 5-HT_1 blocker pindolol, and evidence suggests that SSRIs may actually sensitize mesolimbic dopamine receptors (Arnt et al. 1984a, 1984b). Furthermore, repeated administration of fluoxetine, citalopram, or paroxetine to rats increased spontaneous dopaminergic neuronal activity (Sekine et al. 2007), and chronic fluoxetine treatment also increased brain-derived neurotrophic factor (BDNF) expression within rat dopaminergic regions (Molteni et al. 2006).

Summary of Neurotransmitter Effects

In summary, fluoxetine enhances central 5-HT transmission through increased output and/or increased postsynaptic receptor sensitivity (Blier et al. 1987). Fluoxetine's overall effects on the noradrenergic and dopaminergic systems are less straightforward and are also less likely to play a role in the drug's antidepressant effects. However, such changes alone, in any of the neurotransmitter systems, do not guarantee a clinically meaningful response (Charney et al. 1984). A change in baseline 5-HT function or a "permissive" set of interactions with other collocated neurotransmitter receptors is likely involved in the highly individualized responses in patients with depression.

Pharmacokinetics and Disposition

Considerable pharmacokinetic variability exists within the SSRI class (Leonard 1992). Of particular note, discussion of drug half-life must also include consideration of the presence or absence of active metabolites. Fluoxetine is extensively metabolized by the liver's cytochrome P450 (CYP) system to its active metabolite, norfluoxetine. Fluoxetine is a potent CYP2D6 inhibitor, and norfluoxetine has a moderate inhibitory effect on CYP3A4 (Hemeryck and Belpaire 2002). The elimination half-life of norfluoxetine (4–16 days) is significantly longer than that of fluoxetine (4–6 days); in fact, norfluoxetine's half-life is the longest of any of the SSRIs or their active metabolites. Half-life is not significantly affected by hemodialysis or renal impairment (Aronoff et al. 1984).

The relatively long half-life of fluoxetine confers greater protection from the discontinuation syndrome that is associated with abrupt discontinuation or noncompliance related to interruption of treatment than more rapidly cleared SSRIs. Conversely, more prolonged vigilance for drug-drug interactions following discontinuation is required for fluoxetine; for example, a 5-week washout from fluoxetine is recommended before initiating an MAOI (Ciraulo and Shader 1990; Lane and Baldwin 1997). Variability in drug half-life is associated with a range in time to steady-state plasma concentrations, which does not clearly predict or correlate with onset of antidepressant activity.

Mechanism of Action

In the absence of pharmacological manipulation, the reuptake of 5-HT into the presynaptic nerve terminal typically leads to its inactivation. Fluoxetine, through blockade of the reuptake process, acutely enhances serotonergic neurotransmission by permitting 5-HT to act for an extended period of time at synaptic binding sites. A net result is an acute increase in synaptic 5-HT. One difference separating SSRIs from direct-acting agonists is that SSRIs are dependent on neuronal release of 5-HT for their action—that is, SSRIs can be considered augmenters of basal physiological signals, but they are not direct stimulators of postsynaptic receptor function, and they are dependent on presynaptic neuronal integrity. These pharmacodynamic features might explain SSRI nonresponse. If the release of 5-HT from presynaptic neuronal storage sites is substantially compromised, and in turn, if net synaptic 5-HT concentration is negligible, a clinically meaningful response to an SSRI would not be expected.

Serotonin receptors also include a family of presynaptic autoreceptors that suppresses the further release of 5-HT, thus limiting the degree of postsynaptic receptor stimulation that can be achieved. De Montigny et al. (1989) investigated the mechanism of action of several SSRIs and suggested that the enhanced efficacy of serotonergic synaptic transmission is not the result of increased postsynaptic sensitivity. Rather, longer-term SSRI treatment induced a desensitization of somatodendritic and terminal 5-HT autoreceptors. This desensitization would permit 5-HT neurons to reestablish a normal rate of firing, despite sustained reuptake blockade. These neurons could then release a greater amount of 5-HT (per impulse) into the synaptic cleft. This modification reportedly occurs over a time course that is compatible with the antidepressant response.

Indications and Efficacy

The U.S. Food and Drug Administration (FDA)–labeled indications for fluoxetine are major depressive disorder, obsessive-compulsive disorder (OCD), panic disorder, bulimia nervosa, and premenstrual dysphoric disorder (PMDD). We will review these as well as some other disorders for which fluoxetine is commonly used.

Major Depressive Disorder

Placebo-controlled, double-blind trials have established the superiority of fluoxetine over placebo (Kasper et al. 1992). Statistically significant reductions from baseline in the Hamilton Rating Scale for Depression (Ham-D; Hamilton 1960) score have been seen as early as the second week of treatment; however, the rate and quality of response to any SSRI are highly individualized (range, 10–42 days). Overall, the efficacy of fluoxetine has been found to be comparable to or slightly better than that of the conventional TCAs (Cipriani et al. 2005; Wernicke et al. 1987) and comparable to that of venlafaxine (Nemeroff et al. 2007; Schatzberg and Roose 2006). Notwithstanding, in a survey of 439 clinicians, about one-quarter indicated that they believed SSRIs to be the most efficacious antidepressant class, despite a lack of clear empirical evidence (Petersen et al. 2002). Within the class of SSRIs, there is no clear and consistent evidence for superior effectiveness of one agent over another in primary care settings (Kroenke et al. 2001).

In general, the range for dose titration with most SSRIs is relatively narrow, and higher dosages are more often associated with increased adverse events (Altamura et al. 1988; Amin et al. 1989). Schweizer et al. (1990) reported that in a study of 108 subjects treated with 20 mg of fluoxetine for 3 weeks and then randomly assigned to either 20 mg or 60 mg for another 5 weeks, both groups did equally well after 8 weeks.

However, early implementation of high-dose therapy may be appropriate in some circumstances. Conversion of nonresponders by prescribing at the higher end of the dose range has been described with fluoxetine (Fava et al. 1992). Unfortunately, plasma-level studies have contributed little to the understanding of the dose-response relationship. Most studies have failed to confirm any relationship between clinical response and plasma concentration with fluoxetine (Kelly et al. 1989). This suggests that synaptic concentrations and/or pharmacodynamic effects are not accurately reflected by plasma levels.

Continued efficacy of fluoxetine during maintenance therapy has been established in several trials (Danion 1989; Dufour 1987; Ferrey et al. 1989; Montgomery et al. 1988; Reimherr et al. 1998). One trial reported a recurrence in 54 of 94 placebo subjects (57%) versus 23 of 88 fluoxetine-maintained subjects (26%) ($P<0.0001$) who had at least 4.5 months of recovery before randomization (Montgomery et al. 1988). Study participants were required to have had at least two previous episodes.

Although fluoxetine is perceived as "activating," considerable evidence supports its utility in depression with anxious features. Montgomery (1989a) conducted a meta-analysis of several fluoxetine trials that indicated efficacy in depression featuring anxiety and psychomotor agitation. Similar findings have been reported by Jouvent et al. (1989) and Beasley et al. (1991).

In an attempt to improve compliance with long-term antidepressant treatment, a once-weekly formulation of fluoxetine was developed and approved. Although the concept appears reasonable and the preparation, a once-weekly enteric-coated 90-mg tablet, is safe and efficacious for continuation treatment (Schmidt et al. 2000), this formulation has not attracted widespread use, which suggests that a once-daily formulation may be convenient enough for most patients.

Obsessive-Compulsive Disorder

Clomipramine, a potent inhibitor of both 5-HT and norepinephrine reuptake, was observed more than 30 years ago to reduce obsessive-compulsive symptoms (Renynghe de Voxurie 1968). The superior benefit of this potent serotonergic TCA over desipramine represents a cornerstone in the 5-HT hypothesis of OCD (Benkelfat et al. 1989). Fluoxetine has been shown to be effective in OCD independent of a patient's comorbid mood status (Jenike et al. 1989). Patients who have OCD may require higher doses of medication and longer treatment periods than do patients with depression to determine response. Currently, clomipramine and the SSRIs are considered to be the first-line agents for treatment of OCD (Kaplan and Hollander 2003).

Because OCD is a chronic disorder, prolonged fluoxetine therapy may be necessary. In patients whose symptoms have been minimally or only moderately reduced with SSRI treatment, numerous augmentation strategies have been proposed and include tryptophan, fenfluramine, lithium, buspirone, trazodone, or a neuroleptic (see Goodman et al. 1992). In addition, fluoxetine has shown efficacy in children and adolescents with OCD (Geller et al. 2001). In so-called OCD spectrum disorders, such as skin picking (Bloch et al. 2001) and body dysmorphic disorder (Phillips et al. 2002), controlled trials also indicate efficacy for fluoxetine.

Panic Disorder

SSRIs are the drugs of choice in the prevention of panic attacks and in the treatment of panic disorder. Positive results from double-blind, placebo-controlled trials in patients with panic disorder are available for fluoxetine (Michelson et al. 2001). In general, patients with panic disorder need a low initial dose of fluoxetine (e.g., 10 mg); however, often usual antidepressant dosing for optimal response (e.g., 20–80 mg) is required. The initial low dose serves to minimize early side effects in anxious patients who are particularly sensitive to somatic symptoms of anxiety, and it sets the stage for long-term compliance. The recurrent and chronic nature of panic disorder requires individual medication regimens that may include multiple agents as well as variable dosages.

Eating Disorders

Manipulation of central 5-HT results in significantly altered feeding behaviors (e.g., an increased satiety response) (Carruba et al. 1986). Blundell (1986) reported that pharmacological enhancement of 5-HT reduced meal size, rate of eating, and body weight. The predominant locus of this 5-HT effect is likely within the hypothalamus and may be mediated through gene expression of neuropeptide Y (NPY) and pro-opiomelanocortin (POMC) (Myung et al. 2005). In general, the ability of an antidepressant to diminish appetite and, in turn, to reduce weight is related to its ability to block 5-HT uptake (Angel et al. 1988).

Bulimia Nervosa

Agents with at least some degree of 5-HT uptake inhibition have been useful in bulimia nervosa (see Brewerton et al. 1990). Clinical trials with fluoxetine have found a positive treatment effect on binge eating and purging behaviors (Goldstein et al. 1995). In a large placebo-controlled trial, Enas et al. (1989) studied dosing of 20 mg versus 60 mg of fluoxetine in 382 female outpatients with bulimia. A clinical benefit was observed in binge frequency, purging, mood, and carbohydrate craving. In a smaller study of 91 female patients in a primary care setting, women assigned to fluoxetine kept more physician appointments, exhibited greater reductions in binge eating and vomiting, and had a greater improvement in psychological symptoms than those assigned to placebo (Walsh et al. 2004). Continued treatment with fluoxetine is associated with improvement and decreased risk of relapse (Romano et al. 2002).

Anorexia Nervosa

Pharmacological trials with SSRIs in patients with anorexia nervosa have been relatively sparse. Kaye et al. (1991) suggested that fluoxetine may help maintain body weight in patients with anorexia nervosa who have gained weight. This group also completed a similar study with fluoxetine under controlled conditions, suggesting some benefit for fluoxetine in improving outcome and preventing relapse (Kaye et al. 2001). On the other hand, Walsh et al. (2006) found no benefit for continued treatment with fluoxetine after weight restoration in a randomized, double-blind, placebo-controlled trial of 93 patients. Efficacy of SSRIs has been linked to the food obsessions of many patients with eating disorders.

Premenstrual Dysphoric Disorder

Several randomized, blinded, placebo-controlled trials that used various diagnostic criteria and outcome measures have established the efficacy and tolerability of fluoxetine in the treatment of PMDD (Menkes et al. 1993; Pearlstein et al. 1997; Steiner et al. 1995; Su et al. 1993, 1997; Wood et al. 1992). In the largest study, 313 women with DSM-III-R-defined late luteal phase dysphoric disorder (American Psychiatric Association 1987) received 20 mg of fluoxetine, 60 mg of fluoxetine, or placebo daily for six menstrual cycles after a two-cycle placebo washout period (Steiner et al. 1995). One hundred eighty women completed the study. Both doses of fluoxetine were superior to placebo, beginning at the first menstrual cycle and continuing throughout the six cycles. More patients treated with 60 mg of fluoxetine discontinued because of adverse events than did patients treated with 20 mg of fluoxetine or placebo. More patients treated with placebo discontinued because of lack of response than did patients treated with either fluoxetine dose. In a subsequent study of 34 women, fluoxetine was significantly superior to bupropion and placebo in treating PMDD (Pearlstein et al. 1997).

Anger and Aggression

Diminished serotonergic activity has been implicated in the personality features of impulsivity, anger, hostility, and aggression (Coccaro et al. 1989). These clinical attributes best associate with DSM-IV (American Psychiatric Association 1994) Cluster B personality disorders. Fluoxetine reduced impulsivity in small groups of patients with borderline personality disorder (Cornelius et al.

1991; Norden 1989). Fluoxetine significantly reduced anger attacks in patients with and without depression (Fava et al. 1991, 1993, 1996; Rubey et al. 1996; Salzman et al. 1995).

Posttraumatic Stress Disorder

Fluoxetine significantly reduced symptoms of posttraumatic stress disorder (PTSD), compared with placebo, in 64 patients (veterans and nonveterans), as measured by the Clinician-Administered PTSD Scale (CAPS) (Van der Kolk et al. 1994). It also showed efficacy by week 6 in a large double-blind, placebo-controlled trial (Martenyi et al. 2002).

Premature Ejaculation

SSRIs, including fluoxetine, are effective in the treatment of premature ejaculation, although increased latency to ejaculation is highest with paroxetine (Waldinger et al. 1998). In a 1-year follow-up study, patients treated with fluoxetine (20 mg/day or less) in combination with sexual behavior therapy reported significant improvement in ejaculation latency (Graziottin et al. 1996). Another study demonstrated efficacy from a weekly fluoxetine dose of 90 mg (Manasia et al. 2003). Clear-cut dosing recommendations have not been clarified, however, and titration (upward or downward) may be necessary.

Pain Syndromes

Fluoxetine has shown efficacy in reducing pain associated with diabetic neuropathy (Max et al. 1992). Fluoxetine (20 mg/day) improved scores on measures of pain and discomfort in subjects with fibromyalgia, compared with subjects on placebo (Arnold et al. 2002; Goldenberg et al. 1996). The effect of fluoxetine combined with amitriptyline was superior to the effect of either agent used alone. Fluoxetine reduced the number of attacks in patients with migraine headaches (Saper et al. 1994). More recent work has demonstrated that antidepressants that also affect the norepinephrine system (i.e., serotonin-norepinephrine reuptake inhibitors [SNRIs]) are more effective than the SSRIs in treating neuropathic pain (Mochizucki 2004; Pedersen et al. 2005). In fact, the SNRI duloxetine has received FDA approval for the treatment of neuropathic pain.

Alcohol Abuse and Dependence

A substantial amount of evidence supports a 5-HT dysfunction in alcohol abuse and dependence. Animal studies have shown that increased 5-HT levels reduce alcohol consumption (Farren 1995). For example, Murphy et al. (1988) reported beneficial effects with fluoxetine and fluvoxamine in reducing alcohol intake in a rat model.

Although results are not consistent, some clinical trials with SSRIs have reported reduced alcohol consumption in patients with and without depression, in contrast to patients treated with TCAs, which have less robust efficacy (Cornelius et al. 1997; Lejoyeux 1996). A precise mechanism for the role of SSRIs in the treatment of alcohol dependence is not understood. To date, the beneficial effect, if any, appears to be independent of antidepressant activity (Naranjo et al. 1986, 1990). More work is needed to determine the specific patient subpopulations that might benefit most from SSRIs (see Gorelick 1989).

From a risk-benefit assessment, it is reassuring that fluoxetine does not appear to potentiate the effects of ethanol (Lemberger et al. 1985) and does not carry a high risk of fatal poisoning when taken in combination with alcohol (Koski et al. 2005). SSRIs may help selected patients with alcohol dependence in recovery when these drugs are used as part of a multifaceted treatment program.

Obesity

SSRIs have been extensively investigated for an effect on food consumption. This interest stems from evidence that perturbation of 5-HT receptors modifies animal feeding behavior (Garattini et al. 1986). This modification appears to be independent of a local gastrointestinal effect (e.g., the perception of nausea). 5-HT innervation to the hypothalamus influences satiety and may selectively affect carbohydrate consumption (Wurtman et al. 1981). In one large trial, 458 patients were treated for 52 weeks with fluoxetine (60 mg/day) or placebo (Goldstein et al. 1994). Weight loss was significantly greater in the fluoxetine-treated group at 28 weeks, but not at 52 weeks. Long-term benefits may be better sustained when fluoxetine is combined with behavior modification (Marcus et al. 1990).

The broad involvement of the serotonergic system in modulating behavior and cognition supports the wide potential utility of SSRIs.

Other Medical Conditions

Fluoxetine has been evaluated and observed to be efficacious in a variety of medical conditions, including poststroke depression, fibromyalgia, chronic pain, and depression in cancer patients. It has also proved useful in some patients with chronic fatigue syndrome.

Side Effects and Toxicology

Safety and a favorable side-effect profile, as well as the lack of multiple receptor affinity that mediates adverse events associated with TCAs, distinguish fluoxetine and other SSRIs from TCAs. Medications in the SSRI class generally have similar side-effect profiles.

For most patients, SSRIs are better tolerated than TCAs, based on the number of early trial discontinuations attributable to an adverse event (see Boyer and Feighner 1991). In general, for three-arm trials, the incidence of early discontinuation due to an adverse event was 5%–10% for placebo, 10%–20% for SSRIs, and 30%–35% for TCAs. The SSRIs, presumably by enhancement of 5-HT within the CNS, may induce agitation, anxiety, sleep disturbance, tremor, sexual dysfunction (primarily anorgasmia), or headache. Baseline clinical features do not appear to predispose patients to these adverse events (Montgomery 1989b). Although CNS adverse events may occur with SSRIs, Kerr et al. (1991) suggested that these drugs have a more favorable profile of behavioral toxicity overall than do conventional TCAs.

Because the enteric nervous system is richly innervated by 5-HT, adverse events may include altered gastrointestinal motility and nausea. Certain autonomic adverse events, including dry mouth, sweating, and weight change, also occur.

Fluoxetine decreases rapid eye movement (REM) and increases non–rapid eye movement (NREM) sleep at dose ranges of 5–40 mg/kg in rodent models (Gao et al. 1992). This is a common property of many antidepressant medications. Of interest, fluoxetine induces higher rates of sedation as dosages are increased.

As was discussed earlier in this chapter (see section "Summary of Neurotransmitter Effects"), fluoxetine is unlikely to alter dopamine function; nonetheless, some side effects, such as hyperprolactinemia, extrapyramidal symptoms, sexual and cognitive dysfunction, galactorrhea, mammary hypertrophy, and gynecomastia, have been attributed to SSRI effects on the dopaminergic system (Damsa et al. 2004). Anecdotal reports of EPS (Meltzer et al. 1979) associated with SSRIs are not more frequent than those reported historically with TCAs (Fann et al. 1976; Zubenko et al. 1987), MAOIs (Teusink et al. 1984), or trazodone (Papini et al. 1982). Very rare events, including arthralgia, lymphadenopathy, syndrome of inappropriate antidiuretic hormone (SIADH) secretion, agranulocytosis, and hypoglycemia, have been reported during clinical trials or postmarketing surveillance; however, causality typically is uncertain.

One additional rare and life-threatening event associated with all SSRIs (and more prominently, their interaction with MAOIs or other 5-HT enhancers) is the central 5-HT syndrome. This phenomenon appears to represent an overactivation of central 5-HT receptors and may manifest with features such as abdominal pain, diarrhea, sweating, fever, tachycardia, elevated blood pressure, altered mental state (e.g., delirium), myoclonus, increased motor activity, irritability, hostility, and mood change. Severe manifestations of this syndrome can induce hyperpyrexia, cardiovascular shock, or death. When switching from an SSRI to an MAOI, drug half-life (and that of any active metabolite, where applicable) should serve as a guide to the length of the washout period. A standard recommendation is to wait at least five times the half-life of the SSRI or its metabolite, whichever is longer, before administering the next serotonergic agent (for a review, see Lane and Baldwin 1997). For fluoxetine, this means a minimum 5-week washout period.

Tolerance to an adverse event may change with dose and/or length of exposure; higher doses are typically associated with higher rates of adverse events (Bressa et al. 1989). Many events, such as activation, are transient, usually beginning early in the course of therapy and then remitting (Beasley et al. 1991). Comparisons between A.M. and P.M. administration did not identify differences in efficacy (Usher et al. 1991). Individual patient differences suggest the need for some flexibility in dosing schedules. TCAs behave like type IA antiarrhythmics; therefore, in a dose-dependent fashion, they may retard His-Purkinje conduction. SSRIs are essentially devoid of this property. In clinical trials, the incidence of increased heart rate or conduction disturbance has been very low with fluoxetine (Fisch 1985). For a review of the relative side-effect profiles of TCAs and SSRIs, see Brambilla et al. (2005).

Specific Issues

Suicidality

Evidence implicating 5-HT in suicide or violence is compelling. Reduced cerebrospinal fluid (CSF) 5-hydroxyindoleacetic acid (5-HIAA) concentrations correlate highly with completed suicides in patients with depression (Edman et al. 1986; Ninan et al. 1984). In vitro binding assays have shown an increased density (B_{max}) of 5-HT_2 receptors in individuals with depression and suicidal tendencies (Pandey et al. 1990). Both observations are consistent with a relative state of 5-HT depletion among subjects with suicidal tendencies. The American College of Neuropsychopharmacology (1992) reviewed evidence showing that antidepressants result in substantial improvement or remission of suicidal ideation and impulses in the vast majority of patients; SSRIs were thought to potentially "carry a lower risk for suicide than older tricyclic antidepressants" (p. 181) when taken in overdose. Furthermore, the task force stated that no evidence indicated that SSRIs triggered emergent suicidal ideation above base rates associated with depression. In addition, Warshaw and Keller (1996) determined that fluoxetine use did not increase the rate of suicide in a group of 654 patients with anxiety disorders. In a large retrospective review of patients receiving one or more of 10 antidepressants (including fluoxetine), Jick et al. (1995) concluded that the risk for suicide was similar among all agents.

Concern about suicidality surged in 2003 after the industry alerted the FDA that there might be an increased risk of suicide-related adverse events in children being treated with paroxetine. The FDA's review of available data found that approximately 4% of children taking SSRI medications reported or exhibited suicidal thinking or behavior (including suicide attempts), twice the rate of those taking placebo. No completed suicides occurred among nearly 2,200 children treated with SSRIs, however.

The FDA's review was followed by a number of other studies examining this issue, including a meta-analysis of 24 pediatric trials of nine antidepressant drugs by Hammad et al. (2006). These authors found a modestly increased risk of suicidality (risk ratio = 1.66) for SSRIs in depression trials (95% confidence interval = 1.02–2.68). This risk must be balanced against the benefit—in the form of general improvement in mood and overall functioning—experienced by most depressed patients when they are placed on antidepressant therapy. In most cases, the therapeutic benefit of SSRIs will outweigh the risk of increased suicidal thoughts or behaviors (Bridge et al. 2007).

Black Box Warning

On March 22, 2004, the FDA issued a public health advisory warning of the risk of worsened depression and suicidality in children and adolescents being treated with antidepressant medications. This was followed by placement of a black box warning on the packaging of all antidepressant medications, revised in 2006 to include adults through age 25 years (for the full text of the 2007 revision, see www.fda.gov/cder/drug/antidepressants/antidepressants_label_change_2007.pdf).

Pregnancy and Lactation

Given the widespread use of SSRIs and the high prevalence of mood disorders during the childbearing years, it is likely that these agents are being used during pregnancy and breast-feeding. Published information about the use and safety of SSRIs in this special population is greatest for fluoxetine. Goldstein et al. (1997) evaluated the outcomes of 796 prospectively identified pregnancies with confirmed first-trimester exposure to fluoxetine. Historical reports of newborn surveys were used for comparison. Abnormalities were observed in 5% of the fluoxetine-exposed newborns, which was consistent with historical controls.

Pregnancy outcomes and follow-up cognitive and behavioral assessments of 135 children exposed in utero to a TCA or fluoxetine (55 infants) were compared with those in a control group of infant-mother pairs (Nulman et al. 1997). The incidence of major malformations and perinatal complications was similar among the three groups. No statistically significant differences in mean global intelligence quotient (IQ) scores or language development were found in the children of mothers who received a TCA or fluoxetine or control mothers. There were also no differences among the groups on several behavioral assessments. The results of children exposed during the first trimester were not different from those of children exposed throughout the pregnancy. Prospectively derived data are not available for paroxetine, sertraline, fluvoxamine, or citalopram.

Fluoxetine is secreted into breast milk (Hendrick et al. 2001). The implications of this minimal exposure are unclear, but one naturalistic study (Taddio et al. 1996) and two case reports (Burch and Wells 1992; Isenberg 1990), with a total of 13 infants, noted no adverse effects in these infants during the short-term study periods. One case report did describe adverse events in a breastfed infant whose mother was taking fluoxetine (Lester et al. 1993).

SSRI Discontinuation Syndrome

Discontinuation symptoms have been described with several classes of antidepressants, including TCAs and MAOIs. SSRI discontinuation symptoms have been reported most frequently with paroxetine (short elimination half-life and no active metabolite) and least frequently with fluoxetine (long elimination half-lives of parent compound and active metabolite) (Haddad 1997; Stahl et al. 1997). SSRIs are not drugs of abuse; when these agents are discontinued, patients show neither the characteristic abstinence syndrome of CNS-depressant withdrawal nor drug-seeking behavior. The most common physical symptoms are dizziness, nausea and vomiting, fatigue, lethargy, flulike symptoms (e.g., aches and chills), and sensory and sleep disturbances. The psychological symptoms most commonly reported are anxiety, irritability, and crying spells. For most patients, the discontinuation symptoms are different from the adverse effects that they may have experienced while taking an SSRI. Discontinuation symptoms most often emerge within 1–3 days (Schatzberg et al. 1997).

Until recently, most information about SSRI discontinuation syndrome came from case reports or retrospective analyses. Rosenbaum et al. (1998) compared the effects of a 5- to 8-day abrupt discontinuation period from fluoxetine, paroxetine, or sertraline in three groups of patients with depression receiving maintenance therapy. Patients from the paroxetine and sertraline groups had a significant increase in adverse events, whereas patients in the fluoxetine group experienced no increase in adverse events.

In a more extended evaluation, the effects of abrupt discontinuation of fluoxetine were studied in 195 patients with depression (Zajecka et al. 1998). Patients whose depression remitted while they were taking fluoxetine were randomly assigned to continue fluoxetine (20 mg/day) or to discontinue abruptly to placebo, and they were monitored for 6 weeks. Reports of adverse events were similar for both groups.

In summary, SSRIs with short half-lives (paroxetine and fluvoxamine) and related drugs, such as venlafaxine, should be tapered. Fluoxetine does not require tapering because of its extended half-life.

Overdose

A major advantage of SSRIs, relative to other antidepressants, has been their superior therapeutic index (Cooper 1988; Pedersen et al. 1982). The number of deaths per 1 million prescriptions, across several SSRIs (0–6), is substantially lower than that for conventional TCAs (8–53) or MAOIs (0–61) (Leonard 1992).

Borys et al. (1992) reported on 234 cases of fluoxetine overdose (serum level = 232–1,390 ng/mL) obtained in a prospective multicenter study. Fluoxetine was the sole ingestant in 87 cases; in the remaining 147 cases, it was taken in combination with alcohol and/or other drugs. Common symptoms included tachycardia, sedation, tremor, nausea, and emesis. The authors concluded that the emergent symptoms were minor and of short duration; thus, aggressive supportive care "is the only intervention necessary" (Borys et al. 1992, p. 115).

Drug-Drug Interactions

Although the potential for significant interactions exists, SSRIs are unlikely to be associated with many of the conventional problems seen with the earlier antidepressants. These problems include the cumulative CNS-depressant effects with alcohol, anticholinergic agents, or antihistaminic compounds. The structural differences among SSRIs offer a basis for some intraclass differences. Lithium concentrations are generally unaffected.

One potential for clinically relevant antidepressant pharmacokinetic interactions is based on the drug effect on the cytochrome P450 family of enzymes (Brosen and Gram 1989). For example, SSRIs are both substrates for and inhibitors of oxidation via cytochrome P450 2D6. Crewe et al. (1992) ranked the potency of 2D6 inhibition for serotonergic antidepressants, revealing the most clinically relevant effects on 2D6 for paroxetine and fluoxetine and less relevant effects for sertraline, fluvoxamine, citalopram, clomipramine, and amitriptyline.

Through inhibition of 2D6, fluoxetine may elevate the concentration of concomitantly administered drugs that rely on this enzyme for metabolism. This has particular clinical relevance when the second agent has a narrow therapeutic index. Examples of such agents include flecainide, quinidine, carbamazepine, propafenone, TCAs, and several antipsychotics (Rudorfer and Potter 1989). The clinical consequence of such an interaction may either enhance or impair efficacy and/or heighten the adverse-event profile.

The data with respect to fluoxetine's inhibition of other cytochrome P450 enzymes, such as 3A3/4, 2C9, and 2C19, are less consistent, but the potential for such interaction exists.

Conclusion

Fluoxetine has been shown to be a safe and effective drug that has proved to be better tolerated than TCAs and to have a superior safety profile in overdose for patients with comorbid medical illness. Evidence suggests a broad utilitarian role for fluoxetine across a spectrum of psychopathology.

References

Aghajanian JK, Sprouse JS, Rasmussen K: Electrophysiology of central serotonin receptor subtypes, in The Serotonin Receptors. Edited by Sanders-Bush E. Clifton, NJ, Humana Press, 1988, pp 225–252

Altamura AC, Montgomery SA, Wernicke JF: The evidence for 20 mg a day of fluoxetine as the optimal dose in the treatment of depression. Br J Psychiatry 153:109–112, 1988

American College of Neuropsychopharmacology: Suicidal behavior and psychotropic medication (consensus statement). Neuropsychopharmacology 8:177–183, 1992

American Psychiatric Association: Diagnostic and Statistical Manual of Mental Disorders, 3rd Edition, Revised. Washington, DC, American Psychiatric Association, 1987

American Psychiatric Association: Diagnostic and Statistical Manual of Mental Disorders, 4th Edition. Washington, DC, American Psychiatric Association, 1994

Amin AH, Crawford TBB, Gaddum JH: The distribution of substance P and 5-hydroxytryptamine in the central nervous system of the dog. J Physiol (Lond) 126:596–618, 1954

Amin M, Lehmann H, Mirmiran J: A double blind, placebo-controlled, dose-finding study with sertraline. Psychopharmacol Bull 25:164–167, 1989

Angel I, Taranger MA, Claustrey Y, et al: Anorectic activities of serotonin uptake inhibitors: correlation with their potencies at inhibiting serotonin uptake in vivo and with 3H-mazindol binding in vitro. Life Sci 43:651–658, 1988

Arnold LM, Hess EV, Hudson JI, et al: A randomized, placebo-controlled, double-blind, flexible-dose study of fluoxetine in the treatment of women with fibromyalgia. Am J Med 112:191–197, 2002

Arnt J, Hyttel J, Overo FK: Prolonged treatment with the specific 5-HT uptake inhibitor citalopram: effect on dopaminergic and serotonergic functions. Pol J Pharmacol Pharm 36:221–230, 1984a

Arnt J, Overo KF, Hyttel J, et al: Changes in rat dopamine and serotonin function in vivo after prolonged administration of the specific 5-HT uptake inhibitor citalopram. Psychopharmacology (Berl) 84:457–465, 1984b

Aronoff GR, Bergstrom RF, Pottratz ST, et al: Fluoxetine kinetics and protein binding in normal and impaired renal function. Clin Pharmacol Ther 36:138–144, 1984

Baron BM, Ogden AM, Siegel BW, et al: Rapid down-regulation of β-adrenoceptors by coadministration of desipramine and fluoxetine. Eur J Pharmacol 154:125–134, 1988

Beasley CM, Sayler ME, Bosomworth JC, et al: High-dose fluoxetine: efficacy and activating-sedating effects in agitated and retarded depression. J Clin Psychopharmacol 11:166–174, 1991

Benkelfat C, Murphy DL, Zohar J, et al: Clomipramine in obsessive-compulsive disorder: further evidence for a serotonergic mechanism of action. Arch Gen Psychiatry 46:23–28, 1989

Benloucif S, Galloway MP: Facilitation of dopamine release in vivo by serotonin agonists: studied with microdialysis. Eur J Pharmacol 200:1–8, 1991

Bergstrom DA, Kellar JK: Adrenergic and serotonergic receptor binding in rat brain after chronic desmethyl imipramine treatment. J Pharmacol Exp Ther 209:256–261, 1979

Blier P, de Montigny C, Chaput Y: Modifications of the serotonin system by antidepressant treatments: implications for the therapeutic response in major depression. J Clin Psychopharmacol 7 (suppl):24S–35S, 1987

Blier P, Chaput Y, de Montigny C: Long-term 5-HT reuptake blockade, but not monoamine oxidase inhibition, decreases the function of terminal 5-HT autoreceptors: an electrophysiological study in the rat brain. Naunyn Schmiedebergs Arch Pharmacol 337:246–254, 1988

Blier P, de Montigny C, Chaput Y: A role for the serotonin system in the mechanism of action of antidepressants. J Clin Psychiatry 51 (suppl 4): 14–20, 1990

Bloch MR, Elliott M, Thompson H, et al: Fluoxetine in pathologic skin-picking: open-label and double-blind results. Psychosomatics 42:314–319, 2001

Blundell JE: Serotonin manipulations and the structure of feeding behaviour. Appetite 7 (suppl): 39–56, 1986

Borys DJ, Setzer SC, Ling LJ, et al: Acute fluoxetine overdose: a report of 234 cases. Am J Emerg Med 10:115–120, 1992

Bouchard RH, Pourcher E, Vincent P: Fluoxetine and extrapyramidal side effects. Am J Psychiatry 146:1352–1353, 1989

Boyer WF, Feighner JP: The efficacy of selective serotonin uptake inhibitors in depression, in Selective Serotonin Uptake Inhibitors. Edited by Feighner JP, Boyer WF. Chichester, UK, Wiley, 1991, pp 89–108

Bradley PB: Introduction to Neuropharmacology. Boston, MA, Wright, 1989

Brambilla P, Cipriani A, Hotopf M, et al: Side-effect profile of fluoxetine in comparison with other SSRIs, tricyclic and newer antidepressants: a meta-analysis of clinical trial data. Pharmacopsychiatry 38:69–77, 2005

Bressa GM, Brugnoli R, Pancheri P: A double-blind study of fluoxetine and imipramine in major depression. Int Clin Psychopharmacol 4 (suppl 1): 69–73, 1989

Brewerton TD, Brandt HA, Lessem MD, et al: Serotonin in eating disorders, in Serotonin in Major Psychiatric Disorders. Edited by Coccaro EF, Murphy DL. Washington, DC, American Psychiatric Press, 1990, pp 153–184

Bridge JA, Iyengar S, Salary CB, et al: Clinical response and risk for reported suicidal ideation and suicide attempts in pediatric antidepressant treatment: a meta-analysis of randomized controlled trials. JAMA 297:1683–1696, 2007

Brosen K, Gram LF: Clinical significance of the sparteine/debrisoquine oxidation polymorphism. Eur J Clin Pharmacol 36:537–547, 1989

Burch KJ, Wells BG: Fluoxetine/norfluoxetine concentrations in human milk. Pediatrics 89:676–677, 1992

Bymaster FP, Zhang W, Carter PA, et al: Fluoxetine, but not other selective serotonin uptake inhibitors, increases norepinephrine and dopamine extracellular levels in prefrontal cortex. Psychopharmacology (Berl) 160:353–361, 2002

Carruba MO, Mantegazza P, Memo M, et al: Peripheral and central mechanisms of action of serotoninergic anorectic drugs. Appetite 7 (suppl): 105–113, 1986

Charney DS, Menkes DB, Heninger GR: Receptor sensitivity and the mechanism of action of antidepressant treatment. Arch Gen Psychiatry 38:1160–1180, 1981

Charney DS, Heninger GR, Sternberg DE: Serotonin function and mechanism of action of antidepressant treatment. Arch Gen Psychiatry 41:359–365, 1984

Cipriani A, Brambilla P, Furukawa T, et al: Fluoxetine versus other types of pharmacotherapy for depression. Cochrane Database Syst Rev (4):CD004185, 2005

Ciraulo DA, Shader RI: Fluoxetine drug-drug interactions, I: antidepressants and antipsychotics. J Clin Psychopharmacol 10:48–50, 1990

Coccaro EF, Siever LJ, Klar HM, et al: Serotonergic studies in patients with affective and personality disorders: correlates with suicidal and impulsive aggressive behavior. Arch Gen Psychiatry 46:587–599, 1989

Cooper GL: The safety of fluoxetine—an update. Br J Psychiatry 153:77–86, 1988

Cornelius JR, Soloff PH, Perel JM, et al: A preliminary trial of fluoxetine in refractory borderline patients. J Clin Psychopharmacol 11:116–120, 1991

Cornelius JR, Salloum IM, Ehler JG, et al: Fluoxetine in depressed alcoholics: a double-blind, placebo-controlled trial. Arch Gen Psychiatry 54:700–705, 1997

Crewe HK, Lennard MS, Tucker GT, et al: The effect of selective serotonin reuptake inhibitors on the cytochrome P4502D6 (CYP2D6) activity in human liver microsomes. Br J Clin Pharmacol 34:262–265, 1992

Damsa C, Bumb A, Bianchi-Demicheli F, et al: "Dopamine-dependent" side effects of selective serotonin reuptake inhibitors: a clinical review. J Clin Psychiatry 65:1064–1068, 2004

Danion JM: The effectiveness of fluoxetine in acute studies and long-term treatment, in Psychiatry Today: VIII World Congress of Psychiatry Abstracts. Edited by Stefanis CN, Soldatos CR, Rabavilas AD. New York, Elsevier, 1989, p 334

de Montigny C, Chaput Y, Blier P: Long-term tricyclic and electroconvulsive treatment increases responsiveness of dorsal hippocampus 5-HT1A receptors: an electrophysiological study. Soc Neurosci Abstracts 15:854, 1989

Dempsey CM, Mackenzie SM, Gargus A, et al: Serotonin (5-HT), fluoxetine, imipramine and dopamine target distinct 5-HT receptor signaling to modulate Caenorhabditis elegans egg-laying behavior. Genetics 169:1425–1436, 2005

Dufour H: Fluoxetine: long-term treatment and prophylaxis in depression. Paper presented at the International Fluoxetine Symposium, Tyrol, Austria, October 13–17, 1987

Edman G, Åsberg M, Levander S, et al: Skin conductance habituation and cerebrospinal fluid 5-hydroxyindoleacetic acid in suicidal patients. Arch Gen Psychiatry 43:586–592, 1986

Eisensamer B, Rammes G, Gimpl G, et al: Antidepressants are functional antagonists at the serotonin type 3 (5-HT3) receptor. Mol Psychiatry 8:994–1007, 2003

Elena Castro M, Diaz A, del Olmo E, et al: Chronic fluoxetine induces opposite changes in G protein coupling at pre and postsynaptic 5-HT1A receptors in rat brain. Neuropharmacology 44:93–101, 2003

Elks ML, Youngblood WW, Kizer JS: Serotonin synthesis and release in brain slices, independence of tryptophan. Brain Res 172:471–486, 1979

Enas GG, Pope HJ, Levine LR: Fluoxetine and bulimia nervosa: double-blind study, in 1989 New Research Program and Abstracts, American Psychiatric Association 142nd Annual Meeting, San Francisco, CA, May 6–11, 1989. Washington, DC, American Psychiatric Association, 1989, p 204

Falck B, Hillarp N-A, Thieme G, et al: Fluorescence of catecholamines and related compounds condensed with formaldehyde. J Histochem Cytochem 10:348–354, 1962

Fann WE, Sullivan JL, Richman BW: Dyskinesias associated with tricyclic antidepressants. Br J Psychiatry 128:490–493, 1976

Farren CK: Serotonin and alcoholism: clinical and experimental research. Journal of Serotonin Research 2:9–26, 1995

Fava M, Rosenbaum JF, McCarthy M, et al: Anger attacks in depressed outpatients and their response to fluoxetine. Psychopharmacol Bull 27:275–280, 1991

Fava M, Rosenbaum JF, Cohen L, et al: High dose fluoxetine in the treatment of depressed patients not responsive to a standard dose of fluoxetine. J Affect Disord 25:229–234, 1992

Fava M, Rosenbaum JF, Pava JA, et al: Anger attacks in unipolar depression, I: clinical correlates and response to fluoxetine treatment. Am J Psychiatry 150:1158–1163, 1993

Fava M, Alpert J, Nierenberg AA, et al: Fluoxetine treatment of anger attacks: a replication study. Ann Clin Psychiatry 8:7–10, 1996

Ferrey G, Gailledrau J, Beuzen JN: The interest of fluoxetine in prevention of depressive recurrences, in Psychiatry Today: VIII World Congress of Psychiatry Abstracts. Edited by Stefanis CN, Soldatos CR, Rabavilas AD. New York, Elsevier, 1989, p 99

Fisch C: Effect of fluoxetine on the electrocardiogram. J Clin Psychiatry 46:42–44, 1985

Fraser A, Offord SJ, Lucki I: Regulation of serotonin receptors and responsiveness in the brain, in The Serotonin Receptors. Edited by Sanders-Bush E. Clifton, NJ, Humana Press, 1988, pp 319–362

Fuller RW: Drugs altering serotonin synthesis and metabolism, in Neuropharmacology of Serotonin. Edited by Green AR. New York, Oxford University Press, 1985, pp 1–20

Fuller RW: Mechanisms and functions of serotonin neuronal systems: opportunities for neuropeptide interactions. Ann N Y Acad Sci 780:176–184, 1996

Gao B, Duncan WC Jr, Wehr ATA: Fluoxetine decreases brain temperature and REM sleep in Syrian hamsters. Psychopharmacology (Berl) 106:321–329, 1992

Garattini S, Mennini T, Bendotti C, et al: Neurochemical mechanism of action of drugs which modify feeding via the serotonergic system. Appetite 7 (suppl):15–38, 1986

Geller DA, Hoog SL, Heiligenstein JH, et al: Fluoxetine treatment for obsessive-compulsive disorder in children and adolescents: a placebo-controlled clinical trial. J Am Acad Child Adolesc Psychiatry 40:773–779, 2001

Goldenberg D, Mayskiy M, Mossey C, et al: A randomized, double-blind crossover trial of fluoxetine and amitriptyline in the treatment of fibromyalgia. Arthritis Rheum 39:1852–1859, 1996

Goldstein DJ, Rampey AH, Enas GG, et al: Fluoxetine: a randomized clinical trial in the treatment of obesity. Int J Obes Relat Metab Disord 18:129–135, 1994

Goldstein DJ, Wilson MG, Thompson VL, et al: Long-term fluoxetine treatment of bulimia nervosa. Br J Psychiatry 166:660–666, 1995

Goldstein DJ, Corbin LA, Sundell KL: Effects of first-trimester fluoxetine exposure on the newborn. Obstet Gen 89 (5, pt 1): 713–718, 1997

Goodman WK, McDougle CJ, Price LH: Pharmacotherapy of obsessive-compulsive disorder. J Clin Psychiatry 53 (suppl 4):29–37, 1992

Gorelick DA: Serotonin uptake blockers and the treatment of alcoholism. Recent Dev Alcohol 7:267–281, 1989

Graziottin A, Montorsi F, Guazzoni G, et al: Combined fluoxetine and sexual behavioral therapy for premature ejaculation: one-year follow-up analysis of results, complications and success predictors (abstract). J Urol 155 (5, suppl): 497A, 1996

Haddad P: Newer antidepressants and the discontinuation syndrome. J Clin Psychiatry 58 (suppl 7): 17–21, 1997

Hall H, Ogren SO: Effects of antidepressant drugs on different receptors in rat brain. Eur J Pharmacol 70:393–407, 1981

Hamilton M: A rating scale for depression. J Neurol Neurosurg Psychiatry 23:56–62, 1960

Hammad TA, Laughren T, Racoosin J: Suicidality in pediatric patients treated with antidepressant drugs. Arch Gen Psychiatry 63:332–339, 2006

Hemeryck A, Belpaire FM: Selective serotonin reuptake inhibitors and cytochrome P-450 mediated drug-drug interactions: an update. Curr Drug Metab 3:13–37, 2002

Hendrick V, Stowe ZN, Altshuler LL, et al: Fluoxetine and norfluoxetine concentrations in nursing infants and breast milk. Biol Psychiatry 50:775–782, 2001

Henry LK, Field JR, Adkins EM, et al: Tyr-95 and Ile-172 in transmembrane segments 1 and 3 of human serotonin transporters interact to establish high affinity recognition of antidepressants. J Biol Chem 281:2012–2023, 2006

Iceta R, Mesonero JE, Alcalde AI: Effect of long-term fluoxetine treatment on the human serotonin transporter in Caco-2 cells. Life Sci 80:1517–1524, 2007

Isenberg KE: Excretion of fluoxetine in human breast milk (letter). J Clin Psychiatry 51:169, 1990

Jenike MA, Buttolph L, Baer L, et al: Open trial of fluoxetine in obsessive-compulsive disorder. Am J Psychiatry 146:909–911, 1989

Jick SS, Dean AD, Jick H: Antidepressants and suicide. BMJ 310:215–218, 1995

Johnson AM: The comparative pharmacological properties of selective serotonin reuptake inhibitors in animals, in Selective Serotonin Uptake Inhibitors. Edited by Feighner JP, Boyer WF. Chichester, UK, Wiley, 1991, pp 37–70

Jouvent R, Baruch P, Ammar S, et al: Fluoxetine efficacy in depressives with impulsivity vs blunted affect, in Psychiatry Today: VIII World Congress of Psychiatry Abstracts. Edited by Stefanis CN, Soldatos CR, Rabavilas AD. New York, Elsevier, 1989, p 398

Kaplan A, Hollander E: A review of pharmacologic treatments for obsessive-compulsive disorder. Psychiatr Serv 54:1111–1118, 2003

Kasper S, Fuger J, Moller H-J: Comparative efficacy of antidepressants. Drugs 43 (suppl 2):11–23, 1992

Kaye WH, Weltzin TE, Hsu LK, et al: An open trial of fluoxetine in patients with anorexia nervosa. J Clin Psychiatry 52:464–471, 1991

Kaye WH, Nagat T, Weltzin TE, et al: Double-blind, placebo controlled administration of fluoxetine in restricting- and restricting-purging-type anorexia nervosa. Biol Psychiatry 49:644–652, 2001

Kelly MW, Perry J, Holstad SG, et al: Serum fluoxetine and norfluoxetine concentrations and antidepressant response. Ther Drug Monit 11:165–170, 1989

Kerr JS, Sherwood N, Hindmarch I: The comparative psychopharmacology of 5-HT reuptake inhibitors. Hum Psychopharmacol 6:313–317, 1991

Koski A, Vuori E, Ojanpera I: Newer antidepressants: evaluation of fatal toxicity index and interaction with alcohol based on Finnish postmortem data. Int J Legal Med 119:344–348, 2005

Kroenke K, West SL, Swindle R, et al: Similar effectiveness of paroxetine, fluoxetine, and sertraline in primary care: a randomized trial. JAMA 286:2947–2955, 2001

Lane R, Baldwin D: Selective serotonin reuptake inhibitor-induced serotonin syndrome: review. J Clin Psychopharmacol 17:208–221, 1997

Lejoyeux M: Use of serotonin (5-hydroxytryptamine) reuptake inhibitors in the treatment of alcoholism. Alcohol 31 (suppl 1):69–75, 1996

Lemberger L, Rowe H, Bergstrom RF, et al: Effect of fluoxetine on psychomotor performance, physiologic response and kinetics of ethanol. Clin Pharmacol Ther 37:658–664, 1985

Leonard BE: Pharmacological differences of serotonin reuptake inhibitors and possible clinical relevance. Drugs 43 (suppl 2):3–10, 1992

Lester BM, Cucca J, Andreozzi BA, et al: Possible association between fluoxetine hydrochloride and colic in an infant. J Am Acad Child Adolesc Psychiatry 32:1253–1255, 1993

Li SX, Perry KW, Wong DT: Influence of fluoxetine on the ability of bupropion to modulate extracellular dopamine and norepinephrine concentrations in three mesocorticolimbic areas of rats. Neuropharmacology 42:181–190, 2002

Little KY, Zhang L, Cook E: Fluoxetine-induced alterations in human platelet serotonin transporter expression: serotonin transporter polymorphism effects. J Psychiatry Neurosci 31: 333–339, 2006

Manasia P, Pomerol J, Ribe N, et al: Comparison of the efficacy and safety of 90 mg versus 20 mg fluoxetine in the treatment of premature ejaculation. J Urol 170:164–165, 2003

Marcus MD, Wing RR, Ewing L, et al: Double-blind, placebo-controlled trial of fluoxetine plus behavior modification in the treatment of obese binge eaters and non-binge eaters. Am J Psychiatry 147:876–881, 1990

Martenyi F, Brown EB, Zhang H, et al: Fluoxetine versus placebo in posttraumatic stress disorder. J Clin Psychiatry 63:199–206, 2002

Max MB, Lynch SA, Muir J, et al: Effects of desipramine, amitriptyline, and fluoxetine on pain in diabetic neuropathy. N Engl J Med 326:1250–1256, 1992

Meltzer HY, Young M, Metz J, et al: Extrapyramidal side effects and increased serum prolactin following fluoxetine, a new antidepressant. J Neural Transm 45:165–175, 1979

Menkes DB, Taghavi E, Mason PA, et al: Fluoxetine's spectrum of action in premenstrual syndrome. Int Clin Psychopharmacol 8:95–102, 1993

Michelson D, Allgulander C, Dantendorfer K, et al: Efficacy of usual antidepressant dosing regimens of fluoxetine in panic disorder: randomized placebo-controlled trial. Br J Psychiatry 179:514–518, 2001

Mochizucki D: Serotonin and noradrenaline reuptake inhibitors in animal models of pain. Hum Psychopharmacol 19 (suppl 1): S15–S19, 2004

Molteni R, Calabrese F, Bedogni F, et al: Chronic treatment with fluoxetine upregulates cellular BDNF mRNA expression in rat dopaminergic regions. Int J Neuropsychopharmacol 9:307–317, 2006

Montgomery SA, Dufour H, Brion S, et al: The prophylactic efficacy of fluoxetine in unipolar depression. Br J Psychiatry 153:69–76, 1988

Montgomery SA: Fluoxetine in the treatment of anxiety, agitation and suicidal thoughts, in Psychiatry Today: VIII World Congress of Psychiatry Abstracts. Edited by Stefanis CN, Soldatos CR, Rabavilas AD. New York, Elsevier, 1989a, p 335

Montgomery SA: New antidepressants and 5-HT uptake inhibitors. Acta Psychiatr Scand 80 (suppl 350):107–116, 1989b

Murphy JM, Waller MB, Gatto GJ, et al: Effects of fluoxetine on the intragastric self-administration of ethanol in the alcohol preferring P line of rats. Alcohol 5:283–286, 1988

Myung CS, Kim BT, Choi SH, et al: Role of neuropeptide Y and proopiomelanocortin in fluoxetine-induced anorexia. Arch Pharm Res 28:716–721, 2005

Naranjo CA, Sellers EM, Lawrin MO: Modulation of ethanol intake by serotonin uptake inhibitors. J Clin Psychiatry 47 (suppl 4):16–22, 1986

Naranjo CA, Kadlec KE, Sanhueza P, et al: Fluoxetine differentially alters alcohol intake and other consummatory behaviors in problem drinkers. Clin Pharmacol Ther 47:490–498, 1990

Nemeroff CB, Thase ME; EPIC 014 Study Group: A double-blind, placebo-controlled comparison of venlafaxine and fluoxetine treatment in depressed outpatients. J Psychiatr Res 41:351–359, 2007

Ninan PT, van-Kammen DP, Scheinin M, et al: CSF 5-hydroxyindoleactic acid levels in suicidal schizophrenic patients. Am J Psychiatry 141: 566–569, 1984

Norden MJ: Fluoxetine in borderline personality disorder. Prog Neuropsychopharmacol Biol Psychiatry 13:885–893, 1989

Nulman I, Rovet J, Stewart DE, et al: Neurodevelopment of children exposed in utero to antidepressant drugs. N Engl J Med 336:258–262, 1997

O'Flynn K, O'Keane V, Lucey JV, et al: Effect of fluoxetine on noradrenergic mediated growth hormone release: a double-blind, placebo-controlled study. Biol Psychiatry 30:377–382, 1991

Pandey GN, Pandey SC, Janicak PG, et al: Platelet serotonin-2 receptor binding sites in depression and suicide. Biol Psychiatry 28:215–222, 1990

Papini M, Martinetti MJ, Pasquinelli A: Trazodone symptomatic extrapyramidal disorders of infancy and childhood. Ital J Neurol Sci 3:161–162, 1982

Parga J, Rodriguez-Pallares J, Munoz A, et al: Serotonin decreases generation of dopaminergic neurons from mesencephalic precursors via serotonin type 7 and type 4 receptors. Dev Neurobiol 67:10–22, 2007

Pearlstein TB, Stone AB, Lund SA, et al: Comparison of fluoxetine, bupropion, and placebo in the treatment of premenstrual dysphoric disorder. J Clin Psychopharmacol 17:261–266, 1997

Pedersen LH, Nielsen AN, Blackburn-Munro G: Anti-nociception is selectively enhanced by parallel inhibition of multiple subtypes of monoamine transporters in rat models of persistent and neuropathic pain. Psychopharmacology (Berl) 182:551–561, 2005

Pedersen OL, Kragh-Sorenson P, Bjerre M, et al: Citalopram, a selective serotonin reuptake inhibitor: clinical antidepressive and long-term effect—a phase II study. Psychopharmacology (Berl) 77:199–204, 1982

Peroutka SJ, Snyder SH: Long-term antidepressant treatment decreases spiroperidol-labelled serotonin receptor binding. Science 210:88–90, 1980

Petersen T, Dording C, Neault NB, et al: A survey of prescribing practices in the treatment of depression. Prog Neuropsychopharmacol Biol Psychiatry 26:177–187, 2002

Phillips KA, Albertini RS, Rasmussen SA: A randomized placebo-controlled trial of fluoxetine in body dysmorphic disorder. Arch Gen Psychiatry 59:381–388, 2002

Reimherr FW, Amsterdam JD, Quitkin FM, et al: Optimal length of continuation therapy in depression: a prospective assessment during long-term fluoxetine treatment. Am J Psychiatry 155:1247–1253, 1998

Renynghe de Voxurie GE: Anafranil (G34586) in obsessive neurosis. Acta Neurol Belg 68:787–792, 1968

Romano SJ, Halmi KA, Sarkar NP, et al: A placebo-controlled study of fluoxetine in continued treatment of bulimia nervosa after successful acute fluoxetine treatment. Am J Psychiatry 159:96–102, 2002

Rosenbaum JF, Fava M, Hoog SL, et al: Selective serotonin reuptake inhibitor discontinuation syndrome: a randomized clinical trial. Biol Psychiatry 44:77–87, 1998

Rubey RN, Johnson MR, Emmanuel N, et al: Fluoxetine in the treatment of anger: an open clinical trial. J Clin Psychiatry 57:398–401, 1996

Rudorfer MV, Potter WZ: Combined fluoxetine and tricyclic antidepressants. Am J Psychiatry 146:562–564, 1989

Salzman C, Wolfson AN, Schatzberg A, et al: Effect of fluoxetine on anger in symptomatic volunteers with borderline personality disorder. J Clin Psychopharmacol 15:23–29, 1995

Saper JR, Silberstein SD, Lake AE III, et al: Double-blind trial of fluoxetine: chronic daily headache and migraine. Headache 34:497–502, 1994

Schatzberg A, Roose S: A double-blind, placebo-controlled study of venlafaxine and fluoxetine in geriatric outpatients with major depression. Am J Geriatr Psychiatry 14:361–370, 2006

Schatzberg AF, Haddad P, Kaplan EM, et al: Serotonin reuptake discontinuation syndrome: a hypothetical definition (discontinuation consensus panel). J Clin Psychiatry 58 (suppl 7):5–10, 1997

Schmidt ME, Fava M, Robinson JM, et al: The efficacy and safety of a new enteric-coated formulation of fluoxetine given once weekly during the continuation treatment of major depressive disorder. J Clin Psychiatry 61:851–857, 2000

Schweizer E, Rickels K, Amsterdam JD, et al: What constitutes an adequate antidepressant trial for fluoxetine? J Clin Psychiatry 51:8–11, 1990

Sekine Y, Suzuki K, Ramachandran PV, et al: Acute and repeated administration of fluoxetine, citalopram, and paroxetine significantly alters the activity of midbrain dopamine neurons in rats: an in vivo electrophysiological study. Synapse 61:72–77, 2007

Shaskan EG, Snyder SH: Kinetics of serotonin accumulation into slices from rat brain: relationship to catecholamine uptake. J Pharmacol Exp Ther 175:404–418, 1970

Snyder SH, Yamamura HI: Antidepressants and the muscarinic acetylcholine receptor. Arch Gen Psychiatry 34:236–239, 1977

Sodero AO, Orsingher OA, Ramirez OA: Altered serotonergic function of dorsal raphe nucleus in perinatally protein-deprived rats: effects of fluoxetine administration. Eur J Pharmacol 532:230–235, 2006

Stahl MMS, Lindquist M, Pettersson M, et al: Withdrawal reactions with selective serotonin reuptake inhibitors as reported to the WHO system. Eur J Clin Pharmacol 53:163–169, 1997

Stauderman KA, Gandhi DC, Jones DJ: Fluoxetine-induced inhibition of synaptosomal [3H] 5-HT release: possible calcium-channel inhibition. Life Sci 50:2125–2138, 1992

Steiner M, Steinberg S, Stewart D, et al: Fluoxetine in the treatment of premenstrual dysphoria. N Engl J Med 332:1529–1534, 1995

Su T-P, Danaceau M, Schmidt PJ, et al: Fluoxetine in the treatment of patients with premenstrual syndrome. Biol Psychiatry 33:159A–160A, 1993

Su T-P, Schmidt PJ, Danaceau MA, et al: Fluoxetine in the treatment of premenstrual dysphoria. Neuropsychopharmacology 16:346–356, 1997

Taddio A, Ito S, Koren G: Excretion of fluoxetine and its metabolite, norfluoxetine, in human breast milk. J Clin Pharmacol 36:42–47, 1996

Teusink JP, Alexopoulos GS, Shamoian CA: Parkinsonian side effects induced by a monoamine oxidase inhibitor. Am J Psychiatry 141:118–119, 1984

Thomas DR, Nelson DR, Johnson AM: Biochemical effects of the antidepressant paroxetine, a specific 5-hydroxytryptamine uptake inhibitor. Psychopharmacology (Berl) 93:193–200, 1987

U'Prichard DC, Greenberg DA, Sheehan PB, et al: Tricyclic antidepressants: therapeutic properties and affinity for alpha-noradrenergic receptor binding sites in the brain. Science 199:197–198, 1978

Usher RW, Beasley CM, Bosomworth JC: Efficacy and safety of morning versus evening fluoxetine administration. J Clin Psychiatry 52:134–136, 1991

Van der Kolk BA, Dreyfuss D, Michaels M, et al: Fluoxetine in posttraumatic stress disorder. J Clin Psychiatry 55:517–522, 1994

Waldinger MD, Hengeveld MW, Zwinderman AH, et al: Effect of SSRI antidepressants on ejaculation: a double-blind, randomized, placebo-controlled study with fluoxetine, fluvoxamine, paroxetine and sertraline. J Clin Psychopharmacology 18:274–281, 1998

Walsh BT, Fairburn CG, Mickley D, et al: Treatment of bulimia nervosa in a primary care setting. Am J Psychiatry 161:556–561, 2004

Walsh BT, Kaplan AS, Attia E, et al: Fluoxetine after weight restoration in anorexia nervosa: a randomized controlled trial. JAMA 295:2605–2612, 2006

Warshaw MG, Keller MB: The relationship between fluoxetine use and suicidal behavior in 654 subjects with anxiety disorders. J Clin Psychiatry 57:158–166, 1996

Wernicke JF, Bremner JD, Bosomworth J, et al: The efficacy and safety of fluoxetine in the long-term treatment of depression. Paper presented at the International Fluoxetine Symposium, Tyrol, Austria, October 13–17, 1987

Wong DT, Reid LR, Bymaster FP, et al: Chronic effects of fluoxetine, a selective inhibitor of serotonin uptake, on neurotransmitter receptors. J Neural Transm 64:251–269, 1985

Wood SH, Mortola JF, Chan Y-F, et al: Treatment of premenstrual syndrome with fluoxetine: a double-blind placebo-controlled crossover study. Obstet Gen 80:339–344, 1992

Wurtman JJ, Wurtman RJ, Growdon JH, et al: Carbohydrate craving in obese people: suppression by treatments affecting serotonergic transmission. Int J Eat Disord 1:2–15, 1981

Zajecka J, Fawcett J, Amsterdam J, et al: Safety of abrupt discontinuation of fluoxetine: a randomized, placebo-controlled study. J Clin Psychiatry 18:193–197, 1998

Zubenko GS, Cohen BM, Lipinski JF: Antidepressant-related akathisia. J Clin Psychopharmacol 7:254–257, 1987

CHAPTER 3

Sertraline

Linda L. Carpenter, M.D.

Kimberly A. Yonkers, M.D.

Alan F. Schatzberg, M.D.

David R. Block, M.D.

History and Discovery

Research has implicated dysregulation of serotonin (5-HT) in mood and anxiety disorders. Researchers thus identified compounds that are selective in blocking neurotransmitter reuptake and yet have little agonist and antagonist activity at receptors thought to be associated with adverse effects. Sertraline [(+)-*cis*-(1S,4S)-4-(3,4-dichlorophenyl)-1,2,3,4-tetrahydro-*N*-methyl-1-naphthylamine], a naphthylamino compound that is structurally different from monoamine oxidase inhibitors (MAOIs) and tricyclic antidepressants (TCAs), is one of this class of drugs (Guthrie 1991; Heym and Koe 1988).

For the 12 months ending June 2006, it was estimated that sales of sertraline (under the brand name Zoloft) in the United States exceeded $3 billion (Rancourt 2006). In August 2006, a generic formulation of sertraline became available in the United States, and within the first 2 weeks of its availability, the substitution rate exceeded 77% (Block 2006).

Structure–Activity Relations

Sertraline hydrochloride specifically blocks the reuptake of 5-HT in the soma and terminal regions of serotonergic neurons. The ability of sertraline to inhibit 5-HT reuptake is approximately 20-fold higher than its capacity to inhibit uptake of either norepinephrine or dopamine (Heym and Koe 1988). However, sertraline is more potent at blocking dopamine receptor uptake than are other selective serotonin reuptake inhibitors (SSRIs) and TCAs (Hiemke and Härtter 2000; Richelson 1994).

Serotonin neurons in the midbrain raphe nuclei have inhibitory autoreceptors in both the soma (serotonin$_{1A}$ [5-HT$_{1A}$] receptors) and terminal area (serotonin$_{1B}$ [5-HT$_{1B}$] receptors) that are stimulated by the acute increase in 5-HT. The immediate effect of serotonin transporter (5-HTT) blockade is to increase the amount of 5-HT in axosomatic synapses and to decrease neuronal firing (Blier 2001; Blier et al. 1990; Heym and Koe 1988). Over several weeks, these autoreceptors are desensitized and firing rates increase.

Unlike the older TCAs, sertraline has little appreciable antagonistic effect on histamine$_1$ (H_1), muscarinic, or dopamine$_2$ (D_2) receptors and thus is associated with few difficulties with severe constipation, drowsiness, and dry mouth (Hiemke and Härtter 2000; Richelson 1994). The antagonism of α_1-adrenoreceptors by sertraline is at least 10-fold more than that of other SSRIs (Hiemke and Härtter 2000), although this antagonism does not translate into clinically meaningful hypotension or reflex tachycardia. However, there is a report suggesting that sertraline decreases sympathetic nervous system activity, a property consistent with α receptor blockade (Shores et al. 2001). It is also possible that the decrease in sympathetic response is related to stimulation of the 5-HT_{1A} receptors noted above.

Sertraline is metabolized to desmethylsertraline (see section "Pharmacokinetics and Distribution" below). This compound is approximately one-tenth as active in blocking the reuptake of 5-HT; it also lacks antidepressant activity in animal models (Heym and Koe 1988).

Pharmacological Profile

Among the various antidepressant agents that block the 5-HTT, sertraline is second only to paroxetine in potency for 5-HT reuptake blockade, as demonstrated in animal models (Hiemke and Härtter 2000; Owens et al. 2001; Richelson 1994). The selectivity of sertraline over norepinephrine follows that of escitalopram (Hiemke and Härtter 2000; Owens et al. 2001), although other work suggests greater selectivity for fluvoxamine than for sertraline (Richelson 1994). The relative selectivity for the 5-HTT, compared with the dopamine transporter (DAT), is lowest for sertraline (Owens et al. 2001).

Sertraline exhibits inhibitory activity on several cytochrome P450 (CYP) enzymes. The ability of the compound to slightly elevate dextromethorphan and desipramine supports modest inhibition of CYP2D6 (Hiemke and Härtter 2000; Ozdemir et al. 1998; Preskorn 1996). It has little appreciable inhibition of CYP1A2, even when used at higher doses (Ozdemir et al. 1998). A very mild elevation of CYP2C9/10 substrates has been found in several studies (Preskorn 1996). Sertraline has complex effects on the CYP3A3/4 enzyme system: it initially shows slight inhibition, but it also induces this system, albeit modestly, over time (Preskorn 1996).

Pharmacokinetics and Distribution

Sertraline is absorbed slowly via the gastrointestinal tract, with peak plasma levels occurring between 6 and 8 hours after ingestion (Warrington 1991). The delay may be the result of enterohepatic circulation (Hiemke and Härtter 2000; van Harten 1993). When sertraline is taken with food, the peak level decreases to about 5.5 hours (Pfizer 2001). The medication is more than 95% protein bound; however, because it binds weakly to α_1-glycoproteins, it does not cause substantial displacement of other protein-bound drugs (Preskorn 1996).

The volume of distribution (V_d) of sertraline is large, exceeding 20 L/kg. The distribution is larger in young females than in young males (Warrington 1991). In animal models, the concentration of sertraline is 40 times higher in brain than in plasma (Hiemke and Härtter 2000).

The elimination half-life of sertraline is 26–32 hours, and steady-state levels are achieved after 7 days. Sertraline shows linear pharmacokinetics within a range of 50–200 mg/day (Warrington 1991) and does not appear to inhibit or induce its own metabolism.

Peak plasma levels are somewhat lower in young males, compared with females and older males (Pfizer 2001; Ronfeld et al. 1997; Warrington 1991), and the elimination rate constant is higher in young males than in females or older males (0.031/hour in young males; 0.022/hour in young females and 0.019/hour in older males and females). Maximal plasma concentrations of sertraline may be significantly reduced following gastric bypass procedure (Roerig et al. 2011).

In children between the ages of 6 and 17 years, weight-corrected metabolism is more rapid. The maximum concentration and area under the curve (AUC) are 22% lower than in adults. Despite this relatively greater metabolism, the smaller body mass of most children suggests that lower dosages of sertraline should be used in pediatric populations (Pfizer 2001).

Sertraline is metabolized in the liver via oxidative metabolism; the concentration of the primary metabolite, desmethylsertraline, is up to threefold higher than that of the parent compound (Hiemke et al. 1991; Ronfeld et al. 1997; Warrington 1991). Desmethylsertraline levels are also lower in young males than in females and elderly males. The peak concentration (t_{max}) of desmethylsertraline is attained more quickly in young females than in young males (6 hours in young females vs. 9 hours in young males, 8 hours in older females, and 14 hours in older males) (Warrington 1991). The half-life of desmethylsertraline is 1.6–2.0 times that of the parent compound (Warrington 1991).

Whereas desmethylsertraline is the major metabolite of sertraline, other minor metabolites include a ketone and an alcohol compound (Warrington 1991). Less than 0.2% of an oral dose of sertraline is excreted unchanged in urine, whereas approximately 50% is found in feces. The enzymes involved in metabolism of sertraline to desmethylsertraline remain unclear (Greenblatt et al. 1999). Although six different CYP enzymes have the capacity to catalyze this reaction, none accounts for more than 25% of sertraline's clearance. The contribution of each CYP enzyme is dependent on not only the protein's activity on the substrate, as evidenced through in vitro models, but also the abundance of the enzyme. Given these properties, one computer model identified 2C9 as the greatest contributor (~23%) to sertraline demethylation, with 3A4 and 2C19 each contributing about 15%, 2D6 adding 5%, and 2B6 contributing 2% to the process (Greenblatt et al. 1999; Lee et al. 1999). These percentages can vary across individuals, depending on the amount of enzyme that is available or enzyme inhibition that occurs. Because multiple CYP enzymes are involved in sertraline's metabolism, concurrent use of medications with specific CYP inhibition is unlikely to substantially impair the process (Greenblatt et al. 1999). However, increased CYP2B activity was seen in mice as a consequence of sertraline coadministration with bupropion (Molnari et al. 2011).

Patients with liver disease experience decreased sertraline metabolism (Hiemke and Härtter 2000). For individuals with mild liver impairment, the half-life of drug may be increased threefold (Pfizer 2001), and concentrations are likely to be greater in patients with severe impairment. Although renal impairment does not appreciably influence the metabolism of sertraline (Hiemke and Härtter 2000), hemodialysis patients with severe end-stage renal disease do not appear to tolerate sertraline 25 mg/day without risk of significant toxicity (Chander et al. 2011).

Mechanism of Action

The means by which all antidepressants exert their therapeutic action are largely unknown, although some of the properties noted above have been related to hypothetical mechanisms (Blier 2001; Blier et al. 1990). As previously noted, the immediate effect of sertraline is to decrease neuronal firing rates. This is followed by normalization and an increase in firing rates, as autoreceptors are desensitized. As activity in the presynaptic neuron increases, noradrenergic neurons are stimulated by postsynaptic 5-HT receptors located on noradrenergic nerve terminals, leading to eventual downregulation of β-adrenergic receptors, a property caused by many, but not all, antidepressant agents (Frazer and Scott 1994; Guthrie 1991).

Not inconsistent with the above are findings suggesting that SSRI treatment decreases production of 5-HT_{1B} messenger RNA (mRNA), the message for a regulatory autoreceptor on dorsal raphe neurons that controls the amount of 5-HT released with each impulse (Anthony et al. 2000). Again, the decrease in mRNA production coincides temporally with the time frame for SSRI therapeutic effects. In addition to inhibition of 5-HT reuptake, preclinical research has shown that sertraline inhibits hippocampal presynaptic sodium channels to control neurotransmitter release (Aldana and Sitges 2012), and sertraline's ability to increase extracellular dopamine concentration in nucleus accumbens and striatum differentiated it from other SSRIs (Kitaichi et al. 2010).

Indications and Efficacy

Sertraline is currently approved by the U.S. Food and Drug Administration (FDA) for use in the treatment of major depressive disorder (MDD), obsessive-compulsive disorder (OCD) and pediatric OCD, posttraumatic stress disorder (PTSD), panic disorder, premenstrual dysphoric disorder (PMDD), and social anxiety disorder. Some of the pivotal studies using this compound for these indications are reviewed below.

Major Depressive Disorder

The efficacy of sertraline in the treatment of MDD was established by a number of placebo-controlled trials for acute-phase therapy (Fabre et al. 1995; Opie et al. 1997; Reimherr et al. 1990). In a multicenter trial, 369 patients were randomly assigned to a fixed dose of sertraline (50 mg, 100 mg, or 200 mg daily) or placebo for 6 weeks (Fabre et al. 1995). Patients at all dosages of sertraline showed approximately equivalent improvement, which was greater than placebo for most measures.

Sertraline was compared with amitriptyline and placebo in a multicenter trial of 448 patients (Reimherr et al. 1990). Sertraline was dosed flexibly up to 200 mg daily, and amitriptyline was administered at dosages as high as 150 mg/day. Both active treatments were superior to placebo, as indicated by Hamilton Rating Scale for Depression (Ham-D) and Clinical Global Impressions (CGI) Scale scores; similarly, response rates (rates at which patients attained a 50% decrease in the Ham-D or a CGI Scale score of 1 or 2) were higher with the active treatment compared with placebo.

In a multicenter study of 235 men and 400 women with either chronic MDD (enduring at least 2 years) or MDD superimposed on dysthymic disorder, subjects were randomly assigned to 12 weeks of either sertraline or imipramine in a 2-to-1 ratio (Kornstein et al. 2000). Treatment was double-blinded, and the study medication was titrated to a flexible maximum daily dose of 200 mg sertraline or 300 mg imipramine. Response to both drugs was similar, but sertraline was better tolerated. Results revealed that many who benefited had not achieved response until after 8 weeks of treatment, underscoring the need for extended sertraline trials in patients with chronic depression (Keller et al. 1998a). Another interesting finding from this study is that men and women had differential response rates to sertraline and imipramine (Kornstein et al. 2000). Remission and response outcomes were combined in an intent-to-treat analysis that showed that 57% of women but only 46% of men benefited from sertraline. Among men, response was somewhat better for imipramine compared with sertraline (62% and 45%, respectively). Response rates were more rapid for men assigned to imipramine and for women assigned to sertraline. Premenopausal women were more likely to respond to sertraline, whereas postmenopausal women were equally likely to respond to either agent.

Sertraline has been shown to be effective for maintenance-phase treatment, both in patients with MDD (Doogan and Caillard 1992) and in patients with chronic MDD (defined as a major depressive episode enduring at least 2 years or co-occurring with dysthymic disorder) (Keller et al. 1998b). The Doogan and Caillard (1992) study followed 300 patients throughout 44 weeks of double-blind, placebo-controlled maintenance therapy and found that 13% of sertraline-treated patients, compared with 46% of placebo-treated patients, experienced a relapse.

The utility of sertraline in preventing illness recurrence among chronic MDD patients who responded to acute antidepressant therapy ($n = 161$) was examined in the Keller et al. (1998b) study, which involved random assignment to 52 weeks of maintenance treatment with either placebo or sertraline. More than 60% of the sample were female and had a current episode duration that exceeded 8 years. Sertraline significantly outperformed placebo for all outcome measures; 6% of sertraline-treated patients and 23% of placebo-treated patients experienced depressive episode recurrence, and clinically significant depressive symptom re-emergence was observed in 26% of sertraline-treatment patients versus 50% on placebo.

Sertraline can be used to treat MDD in special populations. In addition to the above trials, several studies found sertraline to be at least as effective as TCAs in treating younger adults (Cohn et al. 1990; Lydiard et al. 1997; Moller et al. 1998) and elderly patients (Bondareff et al. 2000; Finkel et al. 1999; Forlenza et al. 2001) with MDD. Sertraline has been shown to be as beneficial as nortriptyline in women with postpartum major depression (Wisner et al. 2006). Furthermore, sertraline may also confer a prophylactic advantage in women at high risk for developing postpartum episodes of major depression (Wisner et al. 2004), and sertraline is one of three antidepressants judged to be evidence-based choices for MDD in women who are breast-feeding (Lanza di Scalea and Wisner 2009). Several trials have shown roughly equivalent response between sertraline and other SSRIs (Aguglia et al. 1993; Franchini et al. 1997; Nemeroff et al. 1996; Newhouse et al. 2000; Stahl 2000), but a recent Cochrane Database review and meta-analysis of all randomized controlled trials of sertraline against an active antidepressant comparator revealed that sertraline was superior for treatment of MDD, in terms of both efficacy and acceptability (Cipriani et al. 2010).

Obsessive-Compulsive Disorder

Several multicenter trials found benefit for sertraline over placebo in the acute- and maintenance-phase treatment of OCD in adults. One study failed to show superiority of sertraline over placebo, perhaps because of the limited sample size ($n = 19$) or the treatment-resistant characteristics of the cohort (Jenike et al. 1990). Larger-scale studies with diverse patients had differing results. By week 3 of a 12-week flexible-dose study in 167 patients (Kronig et al. 1999), sertraline (mean 165 mg/day) differentiated from placebo. At study endpoint, 41% of patients receiving sertraline and 23% of those receiving placebo had achieved a CGI–Improvement scale (CGI-I) score of 1 or 2.

A fixed-dose study (Greist et al. 1995) also found superior results with three different daily dosages (50, 100, or 200 mg) of sertraline, compared with placebo, over 1 year of treatment in a multisite trial. OCD patients ($n = 325$) were randomly assigned to 12 weeks of double-blind treatment after a 1-week washout period. Responders (40% of sertraline-treated patients and 26% of placebo-treated patients) were offered enrollment in an additional 40 weeks of continuation treatment. Over the 52 weeks of the study, sertraline-treated subjects demonstrated significantly greater improvement than did subjects given placebo.

Some evidence suggests that higher daily dosages of sertraline may be helpful for patients who fail to respond at standard dosages. In one study, 66 patients with OCD who failed to respond to sertraline therapy at dosages of 200 mg/day after 16 weeks of treatment were randomly assigned to continue on the same dose for an additional 12 weeks or to increase their dosage to 250–400 mg/day (Ninan et al. 2006). At the end of the trial, those receiving higher dosages had greater improvement in Yale-Brown Obsessive Compulsive Scale (Y-BOCS) scores, although responder rates between the two groups were similar.

Other studies supporting the utility of sertraline in OCD include head-to-head comparison studies with other antidepressants (Bergeron et al. 2002; Bisserbe et al. 1995; Hoehn-Saric et al. 2000). In a comparison of lower-dose sertraline with cognitive-behavioral group therapy, both treatments were shown to be efficacious, though OCD patients treated with group therapy had greater reduction in symptoms (Sousa and Isolan 2006).

Pediatric Obsessive-Compulsive Disorder

Sertraline is approved for use in children for the treatment of OCD. In a 12-week double-blind, placebo-controlled, parallel-group multicenter trial in 187 pediatric subjects (107 children ages 6–12 years, and 80 adolescents ages 13–17 years), March et al. (1998) found that subjects treated with sertraline (mean endpoint dosage 167 mg/day) showed significant improvement on the Y-BOCS, National Institute of Mental Health–Global Obsessive-Compulsive Scale (NIMH-GOCS), and CGI-I, compared with subjects receiving placebo. There were few dropouts related to adverse events, and the authors concluded that sertraline is a safe, well-tolerated treatment in this age group. A subsequent study in children and adolescents treated with sertraline (50–200 mg/day) over 12 months found that many responders to acute treatment can achieve full or partial remission status with longer-term treatment (Wagner et al. 2003).

Posttraumatic Stress Disorder

The efficacy of sertraline for the treatment of PTSD is supported by two large acute-phase, double-blind, placebo-controlled multicenter studies (Brady et al. 2000; Davidson et al. 2001), a long-term treatment study (Londborg et al. 2001), and a relapse prevention trial (Davidson et al. 2001). In one acute-phase trial (Davidson et al. 2001), 208 civilian patients were randomly assigned to either sertraline or placebo for 12 weeks of treatment. Observed symptom reductions with active treatment were about 50% for reexperiencing/intrusion, just under 50% for avoidance/numbing, and 40% for arousal. The probability of response, defined as a CGI Scale score of 1 or 2 and a minimal 30% decrease in the Clinician-Administered PTSD Scale—Part 2 (CAPS-2), was 0.65 in sertraline-treated patients and 0.38 in placebo-treated patients at the 12-week endpoint. Approximately 40% of each group had comorbid MDD, with mean baseline 21-item Ham-D scores around 21. Of interest, there were no significant differences among groups in depression symptom severity. An acute-phase study by Brady et al. (2000) yielded similarly positive results. In a pediatric sample with PTSD, 10 weeks of treatment with sertraline 50–200 mg/day appeared generally safe but did not produce outcomes superior to those with placebo (Robb et al. 2010).

While the overall acute-phase efficacy of sertraline for PTSD was significant for women in the large controlled studies reviewed above (Brady et al. 2000; Davidson et al. 2001), sertraline failed to differentiate from placebo in men. Some research suggests that treatment efficacy may vary by gender and by type of traumas experienced. Other research has shown no significant gender differences in efficacy of sertraline among patients with combat-related PTSD (Friedman et al. 2007). Reasons for the sex differences in efficacy findings are not clear, although one possible explanation is that women are more likely to experience sexual or physical trauma and childhood abuse than men. It is possible that the nature of the trauma itself (age at exposure, chronicity, contextual factors) may alter the biology of the disorder and its responsiveness to medication (Stein et al. 2006). Recent data suggest that certain serotonin transporter genotypes may be associated with better outcomes (Mushtaq et al. 2011).

Findings from a U.S. Department of Veterans Affairs (VA) medical center study failed to show that sertraline was superior to placebo in patients with predominantly combat-related PTSD (Friedman et al. 2007), but a subsequent trial in Iranian combat veterans (n=70) did show robust efficacy of sertraline when compared with placebo (Panahi et al. 2011).

The long-term benefit of sertraline for PTSD was demonstrated in a continuation study in which patients who had completed 12 weeks of double-blind, placebo-controlled acute-phase treatment for PTSD with sertraline (Brady et al. 2000) were enrolled in a 24-week open-label follow-up study (Londborg et al. 2001). It was observed that about 20%–25% of the total improvement in PTSD symptoms occurred during the continuation phase (weeks 12–36). The greatest improvement over time was among patients who were originally considered "nonresponders" in the acute phase, leading the authors to conclude that as many as one-third of PTSD patients may require longer treatment to achieve a clinically significant response. Davidson et al. (2001) also examined the durability of sertraline response and efficacy in preventing PTSD relapse in a 28-week double-blind continuation study (n=96). Sertraline was found to be superior to placebo on three primary outcome measures: full syndrome relapse (sertraline vs. placebo, 5.3% and 26.1%, respectively), relapse or discontinuation due to clinical deterioration (sertraline vs. placebo, 15.8% and 45.7%, respectively), and acute exacerbation (sertraline vs. placebo, 15.8% and 52.2%, respectively). Relative risk of relapse (RR) after discontinuing sertraline was 6.35.

Panic Disorder

Sertraline has also proven effective in the treatment of panic disorder, as demonstrated by several studies. In a 12-week randomized, placebo-controlled, flexible-dose multicenter trial in outpatients with panic disorder (with and without agoraphobia) but without depression (Pohl et al. 1998), sertraline was superior to placebo on a number of efficacy measures. One hundred sixty-eight patients meeting diagnostic criteria for panic disorder without depression were randomly assigned to receive sertraline or placebo after a 2-week single-blind lead-in. The mean sertraline dosage at endpoint was 126 mg/day (SD=62 mg/day), and the reduction in frequency of panic attacks was significantly greater for the sertraline group (77% vs. 51% for the placebo group), with significantly fewer panic symptom episodes occurring in that group. Similar results supporting sertraline's efficacy for panic disorder were reported by Pollack et al. (1998), who randomly assigned 178 patients to sertraline or placebo.

A fixed-dose study that employed 50 mg, 100 mg, or 200 mg of sertraline or placebo for 12 weeks (Londborg et al. 1998) demonstrated sertraline's superiority over placebo in numerous trial outcomes, including number of panic attacks and limited-symptom attacks, severity of anticipatory anxiety, dimensional anxiety measures, and global measures of improvement. Pooled sertraline data indicated a 65% reduction in the number of panic attacks, compared with a 39% decrease in the placebo group. Effect sizes, reflecting the magnitude of difference between the two treatments, for the three different sertraline doses tested were 0.58 (50 mg), 0.41 (100 mg), and 0.60 (200 mg), but response rates did not differ significantly among dose groups. In the above panic studies, the authors reported a low incidence of attrition secondary to sertraline adverse events, concluding that sertraline is a safe, as well as effective, treatment for patients with panic disorder. The beneficial effect of sertraline for panic disorder may be further enhanced when used in combination with self-administered cognitive-behavior therapy (Koszycki et al. 2010).

Premenstrual Dysphoric Disorder

In one of the first multicenter trials to test the efficacy of an antidepressant agent for PMDD, sertraline was compared with placebo (Yonkers et al. 1997). Either placebo or sertraline, administered flexibly and daily, was given to 243 women. After three menstrual cycles of treatment, total daily rating scores had decreased by 32% and 11% in the sertraline- and placebo-treated groups, respectively. Both emotional and physical symptom clusters improved by 32% with sertraline treatment, a reduction nearly threefold higher than that seen with placebo. At the endpoint, CGI-I scores of 1 or 2 were achieved by 62% and 34% of those assigned to sertraline and placebo, respectively.

In a second multicenter trial, it was shown that sertraline treatment could be commenced halfway through the menstrual cycle (i.e., at ovulation) and still be more effective than placebo (Halbreich et al. 2002). In this three-cycle flexible-dose study, 281 women were randomly assigned to receive daily doses of 50–100 mg of sertraline or placebo. The responder rates in this study, after three cycles of luteal-phase treatment, were 50% and 26% for sertraline and placebo, respectively. As with the daily treatment study, functional improvement paralleled symptomatic improvement. Only 8% of the women taking sertraline and 1% of the women receiving placebo discontinued the study because of side effects. The efficacy of this platform of drug administration for women with PMDD has the potential to revolutionize treatment approaches because many women with PMDD prefer to avoid taking medication during nonsymptomatic periods.

A secondary analysis of data from three large federally sponsored trials ($n=447$) indicated that women with premenstrual syndrome (PMS) showed positive responses to sertraline, similar to outcomes observed in women with PMDD (Freeman et al. 2011). Examination of symptom-based subtypes in that analysis revealed that predominantly psychological symptoms or mixed psychological/physical symptoms predicted better response to sertraline than predominantly physical symptoms.

Social Anxiety Disorder

Several studies have established the efficacy of sertraline in the treatment of social anxiety disorder (also known as social phobia). In one of the earliest studies, sertraline treatment (at flexible doses of 50–100 mg/day) showed a statistically significant improvement compared with placebo, as measured by the Liebowitz Social Anxiety Scale (LSAS) (Katzelnick et al. 1995). A large double-blind, placebo-controlled study followed more than 200 Canadian outpatients with generalized social phobia for 20 weeks, measuring response on CGI-I scores and mean reductions on the social phobia subscale of the Marks Fear Questionnaire and the Brief Social Phobia scale (Van Ameringen et al. 2001). Fifty-three percent of patients treated with sertraline, compared with only 29% of patients receiving placebo, were either much or very much improved by the study's end, as measured by CGI-I scores. When subjects who responded to sertraline were randomly assigned to continue sertraline or switch to placebo for an additional 24 weeks, the relative risk of relapse for those who were randomly assigned to placebo was greater than 10 (Walker et al. 2000).

Liebowitz et al. (2003) demonstrated that sertraline produced a significant reduction in LSAS scores and resulted in a greater proportion of responders after 12 weeks of treatment (at dosages up to 200 mg/day) compared with placebo. In a placebo-controlled study that compared sertraline, exposure therapy, and combined treatment and involved more than 380 Norwegian patients with generalized social phobia, sertraline alone or in combination with exposure therapy yielded statistically significant improvements in CGI social phobia scores, whereas exposure therapy alone did not (Blomhoff et al. 2001). While not FDA approved in the pediatric population, sertraline has been well tolerated and has shown efficacy in childhood social anxiety disorder (Compton et al. 2001).

Off-Label Use and Special Populations

Sertraline has also been studied for off-label use in the treatment of a variety of disorders. Sertraline has been used to treat mood symptoms associated with a number of neurological conditions, including depression associated with Parkinson's disease (Antonini et al. 2006; Hauser and Zesiewicz 1997; Meara and Hobson 1998) and depression-linked fatigue in multiple sclerosis (Mohr et al. 2003). A study in children and adolescents with epilepsy and depression demonstrated sertraline's efficacy in treating depressive symptoms while maintaining good seizure control (Thome-Souza et al. 2007). A 10-week study of sertraline in patients with chronic tension headaches showed a decline in analgesic medication use, suggesting sertraline may be a good alternative for patients who cannot tolerate the adverse events associated with TCAs (Singh and Misra 2002). Sertraline has been also used to improve pathological crying and pseudobulbar-type affects (Benedek and Peterson 1995; Mukand et al. 1996; Okun et al. 2001; Peterson et al. 1996).

Following initial results suggesting a possible role for sertraline in Alzheimer's dementia (Lyketsos et al. 2000; Magai et al. 2000), more recent studies have failed to show superiority in comparison with placebo at 12, 13, and 24 weeks (Banerjee et al. 2011; Rosenberg et al. 2010; Weintraub et al. 2010). However, sertraline does appear to improve subsyndromal depressive symptoms and cognitive function in elderly patients without dementia (Rocca et al. 2005).

Sertraline has also demonstrated some success in the treatment of depression in patients with schizophrenia (Addington et al. 2002; Kirli and Caliskan 1998; Mulholland et al. 2003) and in the treatment of generalized anxiety disorder (GAD). Two randomized GAD trials showed that sertraline had superiority over placebo (Allgulander et al. 2004; Brawman-Mintzer et al. 2006) and efficacy similar to that of paroxetine (Ball et al. 2005).

Trials of sertraline for impulse-control disorders have yielded mixed results; positive outcomes were observed in a trichotillomania sample (Dougherty et al. 2006), but there was no therapeutic effect demonstrated for gambling disorders (Saiz-Ruiz et al. 2005). One study in depressed patients showed that sertraline increased adaptive traits associated with psychopathic personality (social charm and interpersonal and physical boldness) and reduced maladaptive traits associated with psychopathy (dysregulated impulsivity and externalization), independent of its antidepressant effects (Dunlop et al. 2011). A number of studies have highlighted the effective use of sertraline in treating aggressive behaviors (Buck 1995; Feder 1999), specifically in patients with personality disorders (Kavoussi et al. 1994) and patients with Huntington's disease (Ranen et al. 1996). Results from some investigations suggest a role for sertraline in the treatment of various eating disorders, including anorexia nervosa (Santonastaso et al. 2001), bulimia nervosa (Milano et al. 2004), binge-eating disorder (Leombruni et al. 2006; McElroy et al. 2000), and night-eating syndrome (O'Reardon et al. 2006).

In a placebo-controlled trial (Rynn et al. 2001), sertraline was both effective and safe in children with GAD. It has also been used successfully in the treatment of children and adolescents with major depression and dysthymic disorder (Ambrosini et al. 1999; Nixon et al. 2001). Patients with pervasive developmental disorder have also benefited from sertraline, according to at least two reports (Hellings et al. 1996; McDougle et al. 1998).

Numerous studies have examined the potential for sertraline to benefit patients with substance use disorders. An acute-phase trial of sertraline in alcohol dependence did not suggest benefit over placebo (Kranzler et al. 2006), but subsequent analyses and follow-up data suggested potential benefit for alcohol-dependent patients with certain genotypes (Kranzler et al. 2012). The combination of sertraline plus naltrexone may be particularly useful for treating depression symptoms and maintaining sobriety in individuals with co-occurring depression and alcohol dependence (Pettinati et al. 2010). Most studies of sertraline for dependence on other substances of abuse such as methamphetamine (Shoptaw et al. 2006), opiates (Carpenter et al. 2004), and cocaine (Winhusen et al. 2005) do not suggest any benefit in helping curb substance abuse. However, a recent trial did find that delay in time to relapse of cocaine use was a benefit for cocaine-dependent patients with depressive symptoms (Oliveto et al. 2012).

Sertraline is one of the few antidepressants shown to be safe for the treatment of depression in patients with cardiovascular disease. In a well-publicized study by the Sertraline Antidepressant Heart Attack Randomized Trial (SADHART) Group, 369 patients with a recent myocardial infarction or hospitalization for unstable angina who also met criteria for a current major depressive episode were randomly assigned to sertraline (at flexible dosages of 50–200 mg/day) or placebo for 24 weeks (Glassman et al. 2002). There were no significant treatment-emergent effects of sertraline on cardiac measures (including change from baseline left ventricular ejection fraction [LVEF], runs of ventricular premature complexes, or prolonged QTc intervals). For the entire sample, sertraline was superior to placebo in improving rates of response when defined by CGI ratings, but not when defined by Ham-D scores (Glassman et al. 2002). A separate analysis of the SADHART data showed a trend for sertraline-treated patients to have fewer psychiatric or cardiovascular hospitalizations during the treatment period (O'Connor et al. 2005) and indicated that sertraline was most beneficial for those patients whose depressive episodes predated the acute cardiac syndrome, those who had a past history of MDD, and those whose episodes were more severe (Glassman et al. 2006). However, although sertraline's safety was again demonstrated in a study of 469 SADHART patients with chronic heart failure (CHF), in this sample there was no evidence of antidepressant superiority of sertraline over placebo (O'Connor et al. 2010). Compared with nonremitters, CHF patients who achieved remission from depression had fewer cardiovascular events at pretreatment baseline and went on to have better cardiovascular outcomes over a 5-year period (Jiang et al. 2011).

Other data relevant to cardiac health include a sertraline trial in nondepressed patients with chronic ischemic heart failure, where the drug appeared to decrease ventricular extrasystoles (Leftheriotis et al. 2010). While the potential mechanism of cardiovascular benefit is not entirely clear, sertraline may decrease platelet adherence, thus decreasing the likelihood of recurrent myocardial events (McFarlane et al. 2001; Shapiro et al. 1999). A review of the literature relevant to abnormal bleeding associated with sertraline and other SSRIs suggested increased risk for gastrointestinal bleeding may be caused by SSRI-induced increase in gastric acid secretion, whereas a protective effect against ischemic heart disease may be attributable to SSRI effects on platelet reactivity, endothelial reactivity, and inflammatory markers (Andrade et al. 2010). Of note, examination of pretreatment inflammatory markers in a sample ($n=122$) with coronary heart disease (CHD) and comorbid depression did not suggest that elevated baseline inflammatory markers predict inferior response to sertraline (Bot et al. 2011), but depressed CHD patients with comorbid obstructive sleep apnea/hypopnea syndrome had inferior outcomes with sertraline (Roest et al. 2011). Other studies demonstrate that sertraline can improve quality of life in depressed patients with acute coronary syndrome (Swenson et al. 2003) and stroke (Murray et al. 2005). Sertraline alone and sertraline in combination with coping skills training showed efficacy in treating noncardiac chest pain, including associated symptoms of catastrophizing and anxiety (Keefe et al. 2011).

Sertraline has been studied in patients with cancer and depression. A 12-week open-label, flexible-dose trial during chemotherapy showed positive effects of treatment for patients with depressed mood (Torta et al. 2008), but in a controlled trial of almost 200 patients with advanced disease but without major depression, sertraline had no mood benefit over placebo (Stockler et al. 2007).

There has been some research into the potential benefit of sertraline in addressing nonpsychiatric symptoms. Several studies have used sertraline to treat premature ejaculation (Arafa and Shamloul 2006; Biri et al. 1998). Sertraline has proven useful in preventing dialysis-induced hypotension, a condition that can be exacerbated by other antidepressive agents (Perazella 2001). Sertraline has also been used to treat pruritus associated with cholestatic liver disease (Mayo et al. 2007) and severe refractory tinnitus (Zoger at al. 2006).

Another proposed off-label use for sertraline is the alleviation of hot flashes associated with menopause (Aedo et al. 2011; Gordon et al. 2006; Grady et al. 2007) or with tamoxifen treatment for breast cancer (Kimmick et al. 2006) in women, as well as in men following medical castration for advanced prostate cancer (Roth and Scher 1998). One study suggested that positive response to sertraline for hot flashes is related to activity level, education, and menopausal status (Kerwin et al. 2007). Sertraline did prove superior to placebo in a study that examined its potential for controlling hot flashes in women with or at high risk of breast cancer, for whom hormone therapy was not recommended (Wu et al. 2009).

Side Effects and Toxicology

Sertraline has been demonstrated to have a low incidence of anticholinergic, sedative, or cardiovascular effects because of its low affinity for adrenergic, cholinergic, histaminergic, or benzodiazepine receptors. However, sertraline was associated with a number of adverse effects in premarketing evaluation, the most common of which included gastrointestinal disturbance (nausea, 27%; diarrhea/loose stools, 21%), sleep disturbance (insomnia, 22%; somnolence, 14%), headache (26%), dry mouth (15%), and sexual dysfunction (ejaculation failure, 14%; decreased libido, 6%). Other side effects reported by subjects, described as frequent (i.e., they occurred in at least 1 of 100 subjects) in premarketing pooled data from clinical trials, include impotence, palpitations, chest pain, hypertonia, hypoesthesia, increased appetite, back pain, asthenia, malaise, weight gain, myalgia, yawning, rhinitis, and tinnitus (Pfizer 2001).

Sertraline and other SSRIs have been associated with instances of hyponatremia, as well as with the syndrome of inappropriate antidiuretic hormone (SIADH) secretion (see Bouman et al. 1997; Bradley et al. 1996; Catalano et al. 1996; Goldstein et al. 1996; Kessler and Samuels 1996). Bradley et al. (1996), in a review of the literature, noted that the average age of patients experiencing

SIADH is over 70 years, suggesting that the elderly may be more vulnerable to age-related changes in water balance, which may make them more susceptible to developing SIADH with an SSRI.

Extrapyramidal side effects (EPS), including dyskinesias, dystonias, and akathisia, have also been seen with sertraline use, although they are infrequent (Altshuler and Szuba 1994; Lambert et al. 1998; Madhusoodanan and Brenner 1997; Opler 1994). Hamilton and Opler (1992) suggested that the underlying mechanism of SSRI-induced akathisia is serotonergic inhibition of the nigrostriatal dopamine pathway, which can be associated with parkinsonism (Leo et al. 1995; Pina Latorre et al. 2001). Madhusoodanan and Brenner (1997), in a case report of choreiform dyskinesia and EPS associated with sertraline therapy, proposed that 5-HT-driven antagonism of dopaminergic transmission in the nigrostriatal pathway, as well as in the ventral tegmental area (VTA), might be responsible.

Sexual side effects are a well-known side effect of SSRIs, including sertraline. A Cochrane Database review noted that while there is currently limited evidence available, some trials suggest that the addition of sildenafil or bupropion can reduce antidepressant-induced erectile dysfunction in men (Rudkin et al. 2004).

Other adverse events associated with sertraline are rare and include seizures (Raju et al. 2000; Saraf and Schrader 1999), stuttering (Brewerton et al. 1996; Christensen et al. 1996; McCall 1994), altered platelet function and bleeding time (Calhoun and Calhoun 1996; Mendelson 2001), and galactorrhea (Bronzo and Stahl 1993; Lesaca 1996). Urinary hesitancy and retention have been reported in a few cases in women (Lowenstein et al. 2007).

As with all other antidepressants, sertraline carries an FDA black box warning regarding increased risk of suicidality in children and adolescents. Interestingly, one study of suicidal thinking and behavior in more than 700 seniors with late-life depression showed no increase in suicidality with sertraline versus placebo (Nelson et al. 2007).

Sertraline has also been associated with a discontinuation syndrome. Leiter et al. (1995) described two cases in which patients experienced alterations in mood, cognition, energy, gait, and equilibrium, in addition to gastrointestinal symptoms, headaches, and paresthesias. Elsewhere there have been reports of insomnia, impaired short-term memory, myalgias, dyspnea, and chills without fevers (Louie et al. 1994). In a systematic 28-week study involving panic disorder patients (Rapaport et al. 2001), abrupt discontinuation of sertraline was primarily associated only with insomnia (15.7% of patients randomly assigned to placebo vs. 4.3% continuing on sertraline) and dizziness (4.3% of patients continuing to take sertraline and 16.4% switched to placebo). There was no statistically significant clinical deterioration in headache or in general malaise.

Drug-Drug Interactions

Sertraline has a number of potential drug-drug interactions. Because the drug is tightly bound to plasma proteins, caution should be employed when sertraline is used in combination with pharmaceuticals possessing similar characteristics, such as warfarin, and prothrombin time should be monitored when sertraline and warfarin are used concurrently (Pfizer 2001). The potential for serotonin syndrome may be increased when sertraline is combined with other SSRIs, serotonin–norepinephrine reuptake inhibitors, or triptans used for the acute treatment of migraines. Coadministration of sertraline with MAOIs is contraindicated because of the significant risk of serotonin syndrome with this combination.

The degree of sertraline's inhibition of the cytochrome P450 system, most significantly CYP2D6, is relatively minor in comparison with other SSRIs, such as fluoxetine and paroxetine (Preskorn et al. 2007), although mouse data have shown a mild pharmacokinetic drug-drug interaction between bupropion and sertraline resulting in a small elevation in bupropion metabolism (Molnari et al. 2011). Because TCAs are substrates of CYP2D6, drug levels and dosages need to be closely monitored when TCAs are used in combination with sertraline.

Conclusion

Controlled clinical trials support the efficacy of sertraline in the treatment of a variety of psychiatric conditions, including depressive and anxiety disorders. Uncontrolled studies suggest an expanded role for sertraline in a variety of other conditions. The safety profile is superior to that of the older antidepressant agents, thus increasing the potential target population of patients in whom sertraline treatment can be beneficial.

References

Addington DD, Azorin JM, Falloon IR, et al: Clinical issues related to depression in schizophrenia: an international survey of psychiatrists. Acta Psychiatr Scand 105:189–195, 2002

Aedo S, Cavada G, Campodonico I, et al: Sertraline improves the somatic and psychological symptoms of the climacteric syndrome. Climacteric 14:590–595, 2011

Aguglia E, Casacchia M, Cassano G, et al: Double-blind study of the efficacy and safety of sertraline versus fluoxetine in major depression. Int Clin Psychopharmacol 8:197–202, 1993

Aldana BI, Sitges M: Sertraline inhibits pre-synaptic Na+ channel-mediated responses in hippocampus-isolated nerve endings. J Neurochem 121:197–205, 2012

Allgulander C, Dahl AA, Austin C, et al: Efficacy of sertraline in a 12-week trial for generalized anxiety disorder. Am J Psychiatry 161:1642–1649, 2004

Altshuler LL, Szuba MP: Course of psychiatric disorders in pregnancy: dilemmas in pharmacologic management. Neurol Clin 12:613–635, 1994

Ambrosini P, Wagner K, Biederman J, et al: Multicenter open-label sertraline study in adolescent outpatients with major depression. J Am Acad Child Adolesc Psychiatry 38:566–572, 1999

Andrade C, Sandarsh S, Chethan KB, et al: Serotonin reuptake inhibitor antidepressants and abnormal bleeding: a review for clinicians and a reconsideration of mechanisms. J Clin Psychiatry 71:1565–1575, 2010

Anthony J, Sexton T, Neumaier J: Antidepressant-induced regulation of 5-HT 1B mRNA in rat dorsal raphe nucleus reverses rapidly after drug discontinuation. J Neurosci Res 61:82–87, 2000

Antonini A, Tesei S, Zecchinelli A, et al: Randomized study of sertraline and low-dose amitriptyline in patients with Parkinson's disease and depression: effect on quality of life. Mov Disord 21:1119–1122, 2006

Arafa M, Shamloul R: Efficacy of sertraline hydrochloride in treatment of premature ejaculation: a placebo-controlled study using a validated questionnaire. Int J Impot Res 18:534–538, 2006

Ball SG, Kuhn A, Wall D, et al: Selective serotonin reuptake inhibitor treatment for generalized anxiety disorder: a double-blind, prospective comparison between paroxetine and sertraline. J Clin Psychiatry 66:94–99, 2005

Banerjee S, Hellier J, Dewey M, et al: Sertraline or mirtazapine for depression in dementia (HTA-SADD): a randomised, multicentre, double-blind, placebo-controlled trial. Lancet 378:403–411, 2011

Benedek D, Peterson K: Sertraline for treatment of pathological crying. Am J Psychiatry 152:953–954, 1995

Bergeron R, Ravindran A, Chaput Y, et al: Sertraline and fluoxetine treatment of obsessive-compulsive disorder: results of a double-blind, 6-month treatment study. J Clin Psychopharmacol 22:148–154, 2002

Biri H, Isen K, Sinik Z, et al: Sertraline in the treatment of premature ejaculation: a double-blind placebo controlled study. Int Urol Nephrol 30:611–615, 1998

Bisserbe J, Lane R, Flament M: A double-blind comparison of sertraline and clomipramine in outpatients with obsessive-compulsive disorder. Eur Psychiatry 12:82–93, 1995

Blier P: Pharmacology of rapid-onset antidepressant treatment strategies. J Clin Psychiatry 62:12–17, 2001

Blier P, de Montigny C, Chaput Y: A role for the serotonin system in the mechanism of action of antidepressant treatments: preclinical evidence. J Clin Psychiatry 51 (4, suppl):14–20, 1990

Block J: Zoloft erosion outpaces recent generic launches. "The Pink Sheet" Daily. September 5, 2006. Available at: www.thepinksheetdaily.com. Accessed November 2007.

Blomhoff S, Haug TT, Hellstrom K, et al: Randomised controlled general practice trial of sertraline, exposure therapy and combined treatment in generalized social phobia. Br J Psychiatry 179:23–30, 2001

Bondareff W, Alpert M, Friedhoff A, et al: Comparison of sertraline and nortriptyline in the treatment of major depressive disorder in late life. Am J Psychiatry 157:729–736, 2000

Bot M, Carney RM, Freedland KE, et al: Inflammation and treatment response to sertraline in patients with coronary heart disease and comorbid major depression. J Psychosom Res 71:13–17, 2011

Bouman W, Johnson H, Trescoli-Serrano C, et al: Recurrent hyponatremia associated with sertraline and lofepramine. Am J Psychiatry 154:580, 1997

Bradley M, Foote E, Lee E, et al: Sertraline-associated syndrome of inappropriate antidiuretic hormone: case report and review of the literature. Pharmacotherapy 16:680–683, 1996

Brady K, Pearlstein T, Asnis G, et al: Efficacy and safety of sertraline treatment of posttraumatic stress disorder. JAMA 283:1837–1844, 2000

Brawman-Mintzer O, Knapp RG, Rynn M, et al: Sertraline treatment for generalized anxiety disorder: a randomized, double-blind, placebo-controlled study. J Clin Psychiatry 67:874–881, 2006

Brewerton T, Markowitz J, Keller S, et al: Stuttering with sertraline. J Clin Psychiatry 57:90–91, 1996

Bronzo M, Stahl S: Galactorrhea induced by sertraline (letter). Am J Psychiatry 150:1269–1270, 1993

Buck O: Sertraline for reduction of violent behavior. Am J Psychiatry 152:953, 1995

Calhoun J, Calhoun D: Prolonged bleeding time in a patient treated with sertraline. Am J Psychiatry 153:443, 1996

Carpenter KM, Brooks AC, Vosburg SK, et al: The effect of sertraline and environmental context on treating depression and illicit substance use among methadone maintained opiate dependent patients: a controlled clinical trial. Drug Alcohol Depend 74:123–134, 2004

Catalano G, Kanfer S, Catalano M, et al: The role of sertraline in a patient with recurrent hyponatremia. Gen Hosp Psychiatry 18:278–283, 1996

Chander WP, Singh N, Mukhiya GK: Serotonin syndrome in maintenance haemodialysis patients following sertraline treatment for depression. J Indian Med Assoc 109:36–37, 2011

Christensen R, Byerly M, McElroy R: A case of sertraline-induced stuttering. J Clin Psychopharmacol 16:92–93, 1996

Cipriani A, La Ferla T, Furukawa TA, et al: Sertraline versus other antidepressive agents for depression. Cochrane Database Syst Rev 4: CD006117, 2010

Cohn CK, Shrivastava R, Mendels J, et al: Double-blind, multicenter comparison of sertraline and amitriptyline in elderly depressed patients. J Clin Psychiatry 51 (12, suppl B):28–33, 1990

Compton S, Grant P, Chrisman A, et al: Sertraline in children and adolescents with social anxiety disorder: an open trial. J Am Acad Child Adolesc Psychiatry 40:564–571, 2001

Davidson J, Rothbaum B, van der Kolk B, et al: Multicenter, double-blind comparison of sertraline and placebo in the treatment of posttraumatic stress disorder. Arch Gen Psychiatry 58:485–492, 2001

Doogan DP, Caillard V: Sertraline in the prevention of depression. Br J Psychiatry 160:217–222, 1992

Dougherty DD, Loh R, Jenike MA, et al: Single modality versus dual modality treatment for trichotillomania: sertraline, behavioral therapy, or both? J Clin Psychiatry 67:1086–1092, 2006

Dunlop BW, DeFife JA, Marx L, et al: The effects of sertraline on psychopathic traits. Int Clin Psychopharmacol 26:329–337, 2011

Fabre L, Abuzzahab F, Amin M, et al: Sertraline safety and efficacy in major depression: a double-blind fixed dose comparison with placebo. Biol Psychiatry 38:592–602, 1995

Feder R: Treatment of intermittent explosive disorder with sertraline in 3 patients. J Clin Psychiatry 60:195–196, 1999

Finkel S, Richter E, Clary C, et al: Comparative efficacy of sertraline vs. fluoxetine in patients age 70 or over with major depression. Am J Geriatr Psychiatry 7:221–227, 1999

Forlenza O, Almeida O, Stoppe A, et al: Antidepressant efficacy and safety of low-dose sertraline and standard-dose imipramine for the treatment of depression in older adults: results from a double-blind, randomized, controlled clinical trial. Int Psychogeriatr 13:75–84, 2001

Franchini L, Gasperini M, Perez J, et al: A double-blind study of long-term treatment with sertraline or fluvoxamine for prevention of highly recurrent unipolar depression. J Clin Psychiatry 58:104–107, 1997

Frazer A, Scott PA: Onset of action of antidepressant treatments: neuropharmacological aspects. Int Acad Biomed Drug Res 9:1–7, 1994

Freeman EW, Sammel MD, Lin H, et al: Clinical subtypes of premenstrual syndrome and responses to sertraline treatment. Obstet Gynecol 118:1293–1300, 2011

Friedman MJ, Marmar CR, Baker DG, et al: Randomized, double-blind comparison of sertraline and placebo for posttraumatic stress disorder in a Department of Veterans Affairs setting. J Clin Psychiatry 68:711–720, 2007

Glassman A, O'Connor C, Califf R, et al: Sertraline treatment of major depression in patients with acute MI or unstable angina. JAMA 6:701–709, 2002

Glassman AH, Bigger JT, Gaffney M, et al: Onset of major depression associated with acute coronary syndromes: relationship of onset, major depressive disorder history, and episode severity to sertraline benefit. Arch Gen Psychiatry 63:283–288, 2006

Goldstein L, Barker M, Segall F, et al: Seizure and transient SIADH associated with sertraline (letter). Am J Psychiatry 153:732, 1996

Gordon PR, Kerwin JP, Boesen KG, et al: Sertraline to treat hot flashes: a randomized controlled, double-blind, crossover trial in a general population. Menopause 13:568–575, 2006

Grady D, Cohen B, Tice J, et al: Ineffectiveness of sertraline for treatment of menopausal hot flashes: a randomized controlled trial. Obstet Gynecol 109:823–840, 2007

Greenblatt D, von Moltke L, Harmatz J, et al: Human cytochromes mediating sertraline biotransformation: seeking attribution. J Clin Psychopharmacol 19:489–493, 1999

Greist J, Jefferson J, Kobak K, et al: A 1 year double-blind placebo-controlled fixed dose study of sertraline in the treatment of obsessive-compulsive disorder. Int Clin Psychopharmacol 10:57–65, 1995

Guthrie S: Sertraline: a new specific serotonin reuptake blocker. DICP 25:952–961, 1991

Halbreich U, Bergeron R, Yonkers K, et al: Efficacy of intermittent, luteal phase sertraline treatment of premenstrual dysphoric disorder. Obstet Gynecol 100:1219–1229, 2002

Hamilton M, Opler L: Akathisia, suicidality, and fluoxetine. J Clin Psychiatry 53:401–406, 1992

Hauser R, Zesiewicz T: Sertraline for the treatment of depression in Parkinson's disease. Mov Disord 12:756–759, 1997

Hellings J, Kelley L, Gabrielli W, et al: Sertraline response in adults with mental retardation and autistic disorder. J Clin Psychiatry 57:333–336, 1996

Heym J, Koe BK: Pharmacology of sertraline: a review. J Clin Psychiatry 49:40–45, 1988

Hiemke C, Härtter S: Pharmacokinetics of selective serotonin reuptake inhibitors. Pharmacol Ther 85:11–28, 2000

Hiemke C, Jussofie A, Juptner M: Evidence that 3-alpha-hydroxy-5-alpha-pregnan-20-one is a physiologically relevant modulator of GABA-ergic neurotransmission. Psychoneuroendocrinology 16:517–523, 1991

Hoehn-Saric R, Ninan P, Black D, et al: Multicenter double-blind comparison of sertraline and desipramine for concurrent obsessive-compulsive and major depressive disorders. Arch Gen Psychiatry 57:76–82, 2000

Jenike M, Baer L, Summergrad P, et al: Sertraline in obsessive-compulsive disorder: a double-blind comparison with placebo. Am J Psychiatry 147:923–928, 1990

Jiang W, Krishnan R, Kuchibhatla M, et al. Characteristics of depression remission and its relation with cardiovascular outcome among patients with chronic heart failure (from the SAD HART-CHF Study). Am J Cardiol 107:545–551, 2011

Katzelnick DJ, Kobak KA, Greist JH, et al: Sertraline for social phobia: a double-blind, placebo-controlled crossover study. Am J Psychiatry 152:1368–1371, 1995

Kavoussi R, Liu J, Coccaro E: An open trial of sertraline in personality disordered patients with impulsive aggression. J Clin Psychiatry 55:137–141, 1994

Keefe FJ, Shelby RA, Somers TJ, et al: Effects of coping skills training and sertraline in patients with non-cardiac chest pain: a randomized controlled study. Pain 152:730–741, 2011

Keller MB, Gelenberg AJ, Hirschfeld RM, et al: The treatment of chronic depression, part 2: a double-blind, randomized trial of sertraline and imipramine. J Clin Psychiatry 59:598–607, 1998a

Keller MB, Kocsis JH, Thase ME, et al: Maintenance phase efficacy of sertraline for chronic depression: a randomized controlled trial. JAMA 280:1665–1672, 1998b

Kerwin JP, Gordon PR, Senf JH: The variable response of women with menopausal hot flashes when treated with sertraline. Menopause 14: 841–845, 2007

Kessler J, Samuels S: Sertraline and hyponatremia (letter). N Engl J Med 335:524, 1996

Kimmick GG, Lovato J, McQuellon R, et al: Randomized, double-blind, placebo-controlled, crossover study of sertraline (Zoloft) for the treatment of hot flashes in women with early stage breast cancer taking tamoxifen. Breast J 12:114–122, 2006

Kirli S, Caliskan M: A comparative study of sertraline versus imipramine in postpsychotic depressive disorder of schizophrenia. Schizophr Res 33:103–111, 1998

Kitaichi Y, Inoue T, Nakagowa S, et al: Sertraline increases extracellular levels not only of serotonin, but also of dopamine in the nucleus accumbens and striatum of rats. Eur J Pharmacol 647:90–96, 2010

Kornstein S, Schatzberg A, Thase M, et al: Gender differences in treatment response to sertraline versus imipramine in chronic depression. Am J Psychiatry 157:1445–1452, 2000

Koszycki D, Taljaard M, Segal Z, et al: A randomized trial of sertraline, self-administered cognitive behavior therapy, and their combination for panic disorder. Psychol Med 41:373-383, 2010

Kranzler HR, Mueller T, Cornelius J, et al: Sertraline treatment of co-occurring alcohol dependence and major depression. J Clin Psychopharmacol 26:13–20, 2006

Kranzler HR, Armeli S, Tennen H: Post-treatment outcomes in a double-blind, randomized trial of sertraline for alcohol dependence. Alcohol Clin Exp Res 36:739–744, 2012

Kronig M, Apter J, Asnis G, et al: Placebo-controlled, multicenter study of sertraline treatment for obsessive-compulsive disorder. J Clin Psychopharmacol 19:172–176, 1999

Lambert M, Trutia C, Petty F, et al: Extrapyramidal adverse effects associated with sertraline. Prog Neuropsychopharmacol Biol Psychiatry 22:741–748, 1998

Lanza di Scalea T, Wisner KL: Antidepressant medication use during breastfeeding. Clin Obstet Gynecol 52:483–497, 2009

Lee A, Chan W, Harralson A, et al: The effects of grapefruit juice on sertraline metabolism: an in vitro and in vivo study. Clin Ther 21:1890–1899, 1999

Leftheriotis D, Flevari P, Ikonomidis I, et al: The role of the selective serotonin re-uptake inhibitor sertraline in nondepressive patients with chronic ischemic heart failure: a preliminary study. Pacing Clin Electrophysiol 33:1217–1223, 2010

Leiter F, Nierenberg A, Sanders K, et al: Discontinuation reactions following sertraline. Biol Psychiatry 38:694–695, 1995

Leo R, Lichter D, Hershey L: Parkinsonism associated with fluoxetine and cimetidine: a case report. J Geriatr Psychiatry Neurol 8:231–233, 1995

Leombruni P, Piero A, Brustolin A, et al: A 12 to 24 weeks pilot study of sertraline treatment in obese women binge eaters. Hum Psychopharmacol 21:181–188, 2006

Lesaca T: Sertraline and galactorrhea. J Clin Psychopharmacol 16:333–334, 1996

Liebowitz MR, DeMartinis NA, Weihs K, et al: Efficacy of sertraline in severe generalized social anxiety disorder: results of a double-blind, placebo-controlled study. J Clin Psychiatry 64:785–792, 2003

Londborg P, Wolkow R, Smith W, et al: Sertraline in the treatment of panic disorder. Br J Psychiatry 173:54–60, 1998

Londborg P, Hegel M, Goldstein S, et al: Sertraline treatment of posttraumatic stress disorder: results of 24 weeks of open-label continuation treatment. J Clin Psychiatry 62:325–331, 2001

Louie AK, Lannon RA, Ajari LJ: Withdrawal reaction after sertraline discontinuation. Am J Psychiatry 151:450–451, 1994

Lowenstein L, Mueller ER, Sharma S, et al: Urinary hesitancy and retention during treatment with sertraline. Int Urogynecol J Pelvic Floor Dysfunct 18:827–829, 2007

Lydiard RB, Stahl S, Hertzman M, et al: A double-blind, placebo-controlled study comparing the effects of sertraline versus amitriptyline in the treatment of major depression. J Clin Psychiatry 58:484–491, 1997

Lyketsos C, Sheppard J, Steele C, et al: Randomized, placebo-controlled, double-blind clinical trial of sertraline in the treatment of depression complicating Alzheimer's disease: initial results from the Depression in Alzheimer's Disease study. Am J Psychiatry 157:1686–1689, 2000

Madhusoodanan S, Brenner R: Reversible choreiform dyskinesia and extrapyramidal symptoms associated with sertraline therapy. J Clin Psychopharmacol 17:138–139, 1997

Magai C, Kennedy G, Cohen C, et al: A controlled clinical trial of sertraline in the treatment of depression in nursing home patients with late-stage Alzheimer's disease. Am J Geriatr Psychiatry 8:66–74, 2000

March J, Biederman J, Wolkow R, et al: Sertraline in children and adolescents with obsessive-compulsive disorder: a multicenter randomized controlled trial. JAMA 280:1752–1756, 1998

Mayo MJ, Handem I, Saldana S, et al: Sertraline as a first-line treatment for cholestatic pruritus. Hepatology 45:666–674, 2007

McCall W: Sertraline induced stuttering. J Clin Psychiatry 55:316, 1994

McDougle C, Brodkin E, Naylor S, et al: Sertraline in adults with pervasive developmental disorders: a prospective open-label investigation. J Clin Psychopharmacol 18:62–66, 1998

McElroy S, Casuto L, Nelson E, et al: Placebo-controlled trial of sertraline in the treatment of binge eating disorder. Am J Psychiatry 157:1004–1006, 2000

McFarlane A, Kamath M, Fallen E, et al: Effect of sertraline on the recovery rate of cardiac autonomic function in depressed patients after acute myocardial infarction. Am Heart J 142:617–623, 2001

Meara J, Hobson P: Depression, anxiety and hallucinations in Parkinson's disease. Elder Care 10 (suppl 4–5), 1998

Mendelson S: Platelet function and sertraline. Am J Psychiatry 158:823–824, 2001

Milano W, Petrella C, Sabatino C, et al: Treatment of bulimia nervosa with sertraline: a randomized control trial. Adv Ther 21:232–237, 2004

Mohr DC, Hart SL, Goldberg A: Effects of treatment for depression on fatigue in multiple sclerosis. Psychosom Med 65:542–547, 2003

Moller J, Gallinat J, Hegerl U, et al: Double-blind, multicenter comparative study of sertraline and amitriptyline in hospitalized patients with major depression. Pharmacopsychiatry 31:170–177, 1998

Molnari JC, Hassan HE, Myers AL: Effects of sertraline on the pharmacokinetics of bupropion and its major metabolite, hydroxybupropion, in mice. Eur J Drug Metab Pharmacokinet 37:57–63, 2011

Mukand J, Kaplan M, Senno R, et al: Pathological crying and laughing: treatment with sertraline. Arch Phys Med Rehabil 77:1309–1311, 1996

Mulholland C, Lynch G, King DJ, et al: A double-blind, placebo-controlled trial of sertraline for depressive symptoms in patients with stable, chronic schizophrenia. J Psychopharmacol 17: 107–112, 2003

Murray V, von Arbin M, Bartfai A, et al: Double-blind comparison of sertraline and placebo in stroke patients with minor depression and less severe major depression. J Clin Psychiatry 66:708–716, 2005

Mushtaq D, Ali A, Margoob MA, et al: Association between serotonin transporter gene promoter-region polymorphism and 4- and 12-week treatment response to sertraline in posttraumatic stress disorder. J Affect Disord 136:955–962, 2011

Nelson JC, Delucchi K, Schneider L: Suicidal thinking and behavior during treatment with sertraline in late-life depression. Am J Geriatr Psychiatry 15:573–580, 2007

Nemeroff CB, DeVane CL, Pollock BJ: Newer antidepressants and the cytochrome P450 system. Am J Psychiatry 153:311–320, 1996

Newhouse P, Krishnan K, Doraiswamy P, et al: A double-blind comparison of sertraline and fluoxetine in depressed elderly outpatients. J Clin Psychiatry 61:559–568, 2000

Ninan PT, Koran LM, Kiev A, et al: High-dose sertraline strategy for non-responders to acute treatment for obsessive-compulsive disorder: a multicenter double-blind trial. J Clin Psychiatry 67:15–22, 2006

Nixon M, Milin R, Simeon J, et al: Sertraline effects in adolescent major depression and dysthymia: a six month open trial. J Child Adolesc Psychopharmacol 11:131–142, 2001

Okun M, Riestra A, Nadeau S: Treatment of ballism and pseudobulbar affect with sertraline. Arch Neurol 58:1682–1684, 2001

Oliveto A, Poling J, Mancino MJ et al: Sertraline delays relapse in recently abstinent cocaine-dependent patients with depressive symptoms. Addiction 107:131–141, 2012

Opie J, Gunn K, Katz E: A double-blind placebo-controlled multicenter study of sertraline in the acute and continuation treatment of major depression. Psychiatry 12:34–41, 1997

Opler L: Sertraline and akathisia. Am J Psychiatry 151:620–621, 1994

O'Connor CM, Glassman AH, Harrison DJ: Pharmacoeconomic analysis of sertraline treatment of depression in patients with unstable angina or a recent myocardial infarction. J Clin Psychiatry 66:346–352, 2005

O'Connor CM, Jiang W, Kuchibhatla M, et al: Safety and efficacy of sertraline for depression in patients with heart failure: results of the SADHART-CHF (Sertraline Against Depression and Heart Disease in Chronic Heart Failure) trial. J Am Coll Cardiol 56:692–699, 2010

O'Reardon JP, Allison KC, Martino NS, et al: A randomized, placebo-controlled trial of sertraline in the treatment of night eating syndrome. Am J Psychiatry 163:893–898, 2006

Owens MJ, Knight DL, Nemeroff CB: Second-generation SSRIs: human monoamine transporter binding profile of escitalopram and R-fluoxetine. Soc Biol Psychiatry 50:345–350, 2001

Ozdemir V, Naranjo C, Herrmann N, et al: The extent and determinants of changes in CYP2D6 and CYP1A2 activities with therapeutic doses of sertraline. J Clin Psychopharmacol 18:55–61, 1998

Panahi Y, Moghaddam BR, Sahebkar A, et al: A randomized, double-blind, placebo-controlled trial on the efficacy and tolerability of sertraline in Iranian veterans with post-traumatic stress disorder. Psychol Med 41:2159–2166, 2011

Perazella MA: Pharmacologic options available to treat symptomatic intradialytic hypotension. Am J Kidney Dis 38 (4, suppl 4):S26–S36, 2001

Peterson K, Armstrong S, Moseley J: Pathologic crying responsive to treatment with sertraline (letter). J Clin Psychopharmacol 16:333, 1996

Pettinati HM, Oslin SW, Kampman KM, et al: A double-blind, placebo-controlled trial combining sertraline and naltrexone for treating co-occurring depression and alcohol dependence. Am J Psychiatry 167:668–675, 2010

Pfizer: Zoloft (sertraline hydrochloride) tablets and oral concentrate (package insert), 2001

Pina Latorre M, Modrego P, Rodilla F, et al: Parkinsonism and Parkinson's disease associated with long-term administration of sertraline. J Clin Pharm Ther 26:111–112, 2001

Pohl R, Wolkow R, Clary C: Sertraline in the treatment of panic disorder: a double-blind multicenter trial. Am J Psychiatry 155:1189–1195, 1998

Pollack M, Otto M, Worthington J, et al: Sertraline in the treatment of panic disorder: a flexible-dose multicenter trial. Arch Gen Psychiatry 55:1010–1016, 1998

Preskorn S: Effects of antidepressants on the cytochrome P450 system. Am J Psychiatry 153: 1655–1670, 1996

Preskorn SH, Shah R, Neff M, et al: The potential for clinically significant drug-drug interactions involving the CYP 2D6 system: effects with fluoxetine and paroxetine versus sertraline. J Psychiatr Pract 13:5–12, 2007

Raju G, Kumar T, Khanna S: Seizures associated with sertraline. Can J Psychiatry 45:491, 2000

Rancourt J: Teva Launches First Generic Zoloft. "The Pink Sheet" Daily. August 14, 2006. Available at: www.thepinksheetdaily.com. Accessed November 2007.

Ranen N, Lipsey J, Treisman G, et al: Sertraline in the treatment of severe aggressiveness in Huntington's disease. J Neuropsychiatry Clin Neurosci 8:338–340, 1996

Rapaport M, Wolkow R, Rubin A, et al: Sertraline treatment of panic disorder: results of a long-term study. Acta Psychiatr Scand 104:289–298, 2001

Reimherr FW, Chouinard G, Cohn CK, et al: Antidepressant efficacy of sertraline: a double-blind, placebo- and amitriptyline-controlled multicenter comparison study in outpatients with major depression. J Clin Psychiatry 51 (12, suppl B):18–27, 1990

Richelson E: Pharmacology of antidepressants—characteristics of the ideal drug. Mayo Clin Proc 69:1069–1081, 1994

Robb AS, Cueva JE, Sporn J, et al: Sertraline treatment of children and adolescents with posttraumatic stress disorder: a double-blind, placebo-controlled trial. J Child Adolesc Psychopharmacol 20:463–471, 2010

Rocca P, Calvarese P, Faggiano F, et al: Citalopram versus sertraline in late-life nonmajor clinically significant depression: a 1-year follow-up clinical trial. J Clin Psychiatry 66:360–369, 2005

Roerig JL, Steffen K, Zimmerman C, et al: Preliminary comparison of sertraline levels in postbariatric surgery patients versus matched nonsurgical cohort. Surg Obes Relat Dis 8:62–66, 2011

Roest AM, Carney RM, Stein PK, et al.: Obstructive sleep apnea/hypopnea syndrome and poor response to sertraline in patients with coronary heart disease. J Clin Psychiatry 73:31–36, 2011

Ronfeld RA, Tremaine LM, Wilner KD: Pharmacokinetics of sertraline and its N-demethyl metabolite in elderly and young male and female volunteers. Clin Pharmacokinet 32 (suppl 1): 22–30, 1997

Rosenberg PB, Drye LT, Martin BK, et al: Sertraline for the treatment of depression in Alzheimer's disease. Am J Geriatr Psychiatry 18:136–145, 2010

Roth A, Scher H: Sertraline relieves hot flashes secondary to medical castration as treatment of advanced prostate cancer. Psychooncology 7:129–132, 1998

Rudkin L, Taylor MJ, Hawton K: Strategies for managing sexual dysfunction induced by antidepressant medication. Cochrane Database Syst Rev (4):CD003382, 2004

Rynn M, Siqueland L, Rickels K: Placebo-controlled trial of sertraline in the treatment of children with generalized anxiety disorder. Am J Psychiatry 158:2008–2014, 2001

Saiz-Ruiz J, Blanco C, Ibáñez A, et al: Sertraline treatment of pathological gambling: a pilot study. J Clin Psychiatry 66:28–33, 2005

Santonastaso P, Friederici S, Favaro A: Sertraline in the treatment of restricting anorexia nervosa: an open controlled trial. J Child Adolesc Psychopharmacol 11:143–150, 2001

Saraf M, Schrader G: Seizure associated with sertraline. Aust N Z J Psychiatry 33:944–945, 1999

Shapiro P, Lesperance F, Frasure-Smith N, et al: An open-label preliminary trial of sertraline for treatment of major depression after acute myocardial infarction (the SADHAT Trial). Am Heart J 137:1100–1106, 1999

Shoptaw S, Huber A, Peck J, et al: Randomized, placebo-controlled trial of sertraline and contingency management for the treatment of methamphetamine dependence. Drug Alcohol Depend 85:12–18, 2006

Shores M, Pascualy M, Lewis N, et al: Short-term sertraline treatment suppresses sympathetic nervous system activity in healthy human subjects. Psychoneuroendocrinology 26:433–439, 2001

Singh NN, Misra S: Sertraline in chronic tension-type headache. J Assoc Physicians India 50:873–878, 2002

Sousa MB, Isolan LR: A randomized clinical trial of cognitive-behavioral group therapy and sertraline in the treatment of obsessive-compulsive disorder. J Clin Psychiatry 67:1133–1139, 2006

Stahl S: Placebo-controlled comparison of the selective serotonin reuptake inhibitors citalopram and sertraline. Biol Psychiatry 48:894–901, 2000

Stein DJ, van der Kolk BA, Austin C, et al: Efficacy of sertraline in posttraumatic stress disorder secondary to interpersonal trauma or childhood abuse. Ann Clin Psychiatry 18:243–249, 2006

Stockler MR, O'Connell R, Nowak AK, et al: Effect of sertraline on symptoms and survival in patients with advanced cancer, but without major depression: a placebo-controlled double-blind randomized trial. Lancet Oncol 8:603–612, 2007

Swenson JR, O'Connor CM, Barton D, et al: Influence of depression and effect of treatment with sertraline on quality of life after hospitalization for acute coronary syndrome. Am J Cardiol 92:1271–1276, 2003

Thome-Souza MS, Kuczynski E, Valente KD: Sertraline and fluoxetine: safe treatments for children and adolescents with epilepsy and depression. Epilepsy Behav 10:417–425, 2007

Torta R, Siri I, Caldera P: Sertraline effectiveness and safety in depressed oncological patients. Support Care Cancer 16:83–91, 2008

Van Ameringen M, Lane R, Walker J, et al: Sertraline treatment of generalized social phobia: a 20 week, double-blind, placebo-controlled study. Am J Psychiatry 158:275–281, 2001

van Harten J: Clinical pharmacokinetics of selective serotonin reuptake inhibitors. Clin Pharmacokinet 24:203–220, 1993

Wagner KD, Cook EH, Chung H, et al: Remission status after long-term sertraline treatment of pediatric obsessive-compulsive disorder. J Child Adolesc Psychopharmacol 13 (suppl 1):S53–S60, 2003

Walker JR, Van Ameringen MA, Swinson R, et al: Prevention of relapse in generalized social phobia: results of a 24-week study in responders to 20 weeks of sertraline treatment. J Clin Psychopharmacol 20:636–644, 2000

Warrington SJ: Clinical implications of the pharmacology of sertraline. Int Clin Psychopharmacol 6:11–21, 1991

Weintraub D, Rosenberg PB, Drye LT, et al: Sertraline for the treatment of depression in Alzheimer's disease: week 24 outcomes. Am J Geriatr Psychiatry 18:332–340, 2010

Winhusen TM, Somoza EC, Harrer JM, et al: A placebo-controlled screening trial of tiagabine, sertraline and donepezil as cocaine dependence treatments. Addiction 100 (suppl 1):68–77, 2005

Wisner KL, Perel JM, Peindl KS, et al: Prevention of postpartum depression: a pilot randomized clinical trial. Am J Psychiatry 161:1290–1292, 2004

Wisner KL, Hanusa BH, Perel JM, et al: Postpartum depression: a randomized trial of sertraline versus nortriptyline. J Clin Psychopharmacol 26:353–360, 2006

Wu MF, Hilsenbeck SG, Tham YL, et al: The efficacy of sertraline for controlling hot flashes in women with or at high risk of developing breast cancer. Breast Cancer Res Treat 118:369–375, 2009

Yonkers KA, Halbriech U, Freeman E, et al: Symptomatic improvement of premenstrual dysphoric disorder with sertraline treatment. JAMA 278:983–988, 1997

Zoger S, Svedlund J, Holgers KM: The effects of sertraline on severe tinnitus suffering—a randomized, double-blind, placebo-controlled study. J Clin Psychopharmacol 26:32–39, 2006

Chapter 4

Paroxetine

Michelle M. Primeau, M.D.

Joseph Henry, M.D.

Charles B. Nemeroff, M.D., Ph.D.

Paroxetine (Paxil) is classified as one of the selective serotonin reuptake inhibitors (SSRIs) because of its potent inhibition of presynaptic serotonin (5-HT) uptake. It is also a relatively potent norepinephrine reuptake inhibitor, particularly at higher doses. Paroxetine has been granted U.S. Food and Drug Administration (FDA) approval for the treatment of depression, panic disorder, obsessive-compulsive disorder (OCD), social anxiety disorder, generalized anxiety disorder (GAD), posttraumatic stress disorder (PTSD), premenstrual dysphoric disorder (PMDD), and child and adolescent OCD. Paroxetine also has demonstrated efficacy in postmenopausal hot flashes and child and adolescent social anxiety disorder.

Paroxetine is available in 10-, 20-, 30-, and 40-mg tablets and in suspension form. A controlled-release (CR) formulation is available in 12.5-, 25-, and 37.5-mg tablets. It exhibits equal or better efficacy than the paroxetine immediate-release (IR) formulation, as well as clear advantages in tolerability (Golden et al. 2002).

Structure-Activity Relations and Pharmacological Profile

Paroxetine is the most potent inhibitor of the serotonin transporter (5-HTT) among the SSRIs (Frazer 2001); 85%–100% of 5-HTT binding sites are occupied following 20- to 40-mg daily doses of paroxetine (Kent et al. 2002; Meyer et al. 2001), and transporter binding is maintained for up to 14 days after 4 weeks of treatment (Magnussen et al. 1982; Thomas et al. 1987).

Paroxetine is the most potent inhibitor of the norepinephrine transporter (NET) among drugs classified as SSRIs. Despite its relatively high affinity for the NET, paroxetine has an even higher affinity for the 5-HTT (Finley 1994). In an 8-week high-dose forced-titration protocol comparing paroxetine CR dosages of 12.5 and 75 mg/day with venlafaxine extended release (XR) dosages of 75–375 mg/day, both paroxetine and venlafaxine produced dose-dependent inhibition of 5-HTT and NET (Owens et al. 2008); at 8 weeks, maximal 5-HTT inhibition for paroxetine and venlafaxine, respectively, was 90% and 85%, and maximal NET inhibition was 33% and 61%. Substantial NET antagonism occurs at paroxetine IR dosages of 40 mg/day and higher (Gilmor et al. 2002).

Paroxetine has no appreciable affinity for the dopamine transporter (DAT) or for dopamine$_1$ (D_1), dopamine$_2$ (D_2), serotonin$_{1A}$ (5-HT$_{1A}$), serotonin$_{2A}$ (5-HT$_{2A}$), α_1- and α_2-adrenergic, and histamine$_1$ (H_1) receptors (Hyttel 1994; Owens et al. 1997). It is distinguished from sertraline by its high affinity for the NET and low affinity for the DAT. Sertraline, by contrast, has a relatively high affinity for the DAT but no affinity for the NET (Tulloch and Johnson 1992). The affinity of paroxetine for the muscarinic cholinergic receptor is similar to that of desipramine, though paroxetine is used at lower dosages than desipramine and is therefore less anticholinergic than this tricyclic agent. However, this property may account for paroxetine's mild anticholinergic side effects, including dry mouth, blurry vision, and constipation (Owens et al. 1997).

Pharmacokinetics and Disposition

Paroxetine is well absorbed from the alimentary tract, and absorption is not affected by the presence or absence of food (Kaye et al. 1989). Paroxetine is highly lipophilic and is readily distributed into peripheral tissues, with a high volume of distribution and 95% protein binding (Kaye et al. 1989). Oral bioavailability is affected by extensive first-pass metabolism (Lane 1996). With serial dosing, bioavailability increases as the hepatic metabolic system becomes saturated and a larger proportion of the parent compound enters systemic circulation (Kaye et al. 1989). Following oral dosing, steady-state concentrations of paroxetine exhibit wide intersubject variability (Sindrup et al. 1992a); however, there appears to be no relationship between paroxetine levels and clinical response or adverse outcomes (Tasker et al. 1989).

The rate-limiting step in the metabolism of paroxetine is the P450 (CYP) 2D6 enzyme system (Crewe et al. 1992; Sindrup et al. 1992a). Genetic studies have demonstrated up to 40 polymorphisms of the 2D6 enzyme, which in part may explain the differences in pharmacokinetic parameters observed among individuals (Lane 1996). Individual probands can be categorized as poor, intermediate, extensive, or ultrarapid metabolizers, denoting that they have very high, high, low, or very low serum paroxetine concentrations, respectively (Charlier et al. 2003). Patients with negligible or diminished CYP2D6 activity are thought to use alternative enzyme systems (Gunasekara et al. 1998; Lane 1996).

Paroxetine is the most potent inhibitor of the CYP2D6 enzyme system among the SSRIs (Crewe et al. 1992; Nemeroff et al. 1996), and its inhibition of 2D6 can continue for up to 5 days after discontinuation (Liston et al. 2002). As both a substrate and an inhibitor of its own metabolism, paroxetine has a nonlinear pharmacokinetic profile, such that higher doses produce disproportionately greater plasma drug concentrations as the enzyme becomes saturated (Preskorn 1993). With paroxetine IR, peak plasma concentration is attained in approximately 5 hours, and plasma steady-state concentration is achieved within 4–14 days (Kaye et al. 1989). The terminal half-life ($t_{1/2}$) of the parent compound is approximately 1 day and increases at higher doses, consequent to autoinhibition of CYP2D6 (Preskorn 1993). The pharmacokinetic properties of paroxetine appear to be affected by age. Bayer et al. (1989) reported a threefold increase in maximum plasma concentration in elderly subjects, compared with younger subjects, following a single dose of paroxetine. Furthermore, $t_{1/2}$ in the elderly subgroup was extended by nearly 100%.

In individuals with renal impairment, both half-life and maximum plasma levels of paroxetine have been shown to increase relative to the extent of renal disease (Doyle et al. 1989). In patients with severe liver disease, there are considerable elevations in the steady-state concentration and the $t_{1/2}$ of paroxetine (Dalhoff et al. 1991). Patients with substantial renal or hepatic impairment should be treated initially with lower doses of paroxetine to avoid potential side effects.

Paroxetine CR is designed to slow absorption and delay the release of paroxetine until after the tablet has passed through the stomach. With this formulation, 20% of the drug is excreted unchanged from the gastrointestinal tract, such that 20% higher doses of paroxetine CR are necessary to achieve the same bioavailability (DeVane 2003). Dissolution after single dosing takes 4–5 hours; otherwise paroxetine CR displays the same pharmacokinetic parameters with regard to $t_{1/2}$ and nonlinearity as the IR formulation.

Paroxetine mesylate is a generic formulation available in European countries. Although no studies have compared this formulation's efficacy or bioequivalence against that of paroxetine hydrochloride, case reports have indicated problems of decreased efficacy and poor tolerability in patients switched from paroxetine hydrochloride to paroxetine mesylate (Borgherini 2003).

Pharmacogenomics

Paroxetine's primary mode of action is likely mediated by its binding to the 5-HTT. A well-known polymorphism (5-HT transporter gene–linked polymorphic region [5-HTTLPR]) has been located in the promoter region of the gene (SLC6A4) that encodes 5-HTT. This polymorphism may be a pharmacogenetic marker for antidepressant efficacy. The 5-HTTLPR polymorphism was first reported as two alleles, referred to as "long" (L) and "short" (S); a third allele (Lg) has also been identified but has not been studied in relation to SSRI response to any great extent. There exists some evidence that cells with the S allele express 50% less 5-HTT than cells with the L allele, resulting in reduced efficacy of SSRI medications, including paroxetine (Lotrich et al. 2008; Zanardi et al. 2000). The S allele may influence tolerability of paroxetine as well (Murphy et al. 2004). Because patients with the S allele have less expression of 5-HTT, they require a higher serum paroxetine concentration to achieve an effect (Lotrich et al. 2008). It may be that patients with major depressive disorder who are L/L homozygotes have greater 5-HTT occupancy and improved clinical response (Ruhe et al. 2009b).

Another possible genetic marker for antidepressant efficacy is the 102 T/C single-nucleotide polymorphism (SNP) in the serotonin$_{2A}$ (5-HT$_{2A}$) gene (*5HTR2A*). Survival analysis has shown a more or less linear relationship between the number of C alleles and the odds of patients discontinuing paroxetine therapy due to untoward effects (Murphy et al. 2003).

Mechanism of Action

Paroxetine and all of the other SSRIs cause immediate elevations in extracellular 5-HT concentrations in serotonergic synapses, resulting from the decreased 5-HT clearance associated with 5-HTT inhibition (Wagstaff et al. 2002). Paroxetine initially causes a paradoxical *decrease* in 5-HT neurotransmission, likely due to activation of a negative feedback system mediated by increased 5-HT binding to the 5-HT$_{1A}$ autoreceptor and subsequent diminution in serotonergic neural activity (Blier et al. 1990). After 2 weeks of paroxetine treatment, the 5-HT$_{1A}$ autoreceptors are desensitized, and there is an associated increase in serotonergic neurotransmission (Chaput et al. 1991). The delayed changes in 5-HT$_{1A}$ receptor sensitivity and 5-HT neurotransmission seen after chronic daily paroxetine administration are temporally associated with clinical improvement, hinting at a possible mechanistic link.

Pindolol, a nonselective β-adrenergic receptor antagonist/5-HT_{1A} antagonist, has been studied as a novel approach to accelerate the therapeutic response to SSRIs, as well as to convert SSRI nonresponders to responders. It was hypothesized that blockade of the presynaptic 5-HT_{1A} autoreceptor might prevent the initial reduction in serotonergic transmission, leading to a more rapid and robust clinical response (Perez et al. 1999).

This hypothesis was supported by results from open studies as well as by multiple double-blind, placebo-controlled trials indicating that the addition of pindolol (2.5–5 mg three times a day) to paroxetine in the early phase of treatment for major depression might increase the rapidity of clinical improvement (Artigas et al. 1994; Blier and Bergeron 1995). However, data on augmentation of clinical efficacy with pindolol were not compelling, especially in individuals with depression refractory to paroxetine monotherapy (Bordet et al. 1998; Perez et al. 1999; Tome et al. 1997; Zanardi et al. 1997). In another study, paroxetine with pindolol augmentation was found to be most efficacious in patients with depression who were drug naive and patients who had bipolar depression (Geretsegger et al. 2008). It may be that the doses of pindolol previously studied were inadequate to obtain a response (Martinez et al. 2000).

Paroxetine has also been shown to have an effect on the hypothalamic-pituitary-adrenal (HPA) axis. It is well established that many individuals with depression have HPA axis hyperactivity and hypersecretion of corticotropin-releasing factor (CRF) from the hypothalamic and extrahypothalamic circuits (Heim and Nemeroff 1999). Early life stress is associated with hyperactivity of the HPA axis and increased CRF messenger RNA (mRNA) expression (Nemeroff 1996; Newport et al. 2002). In adult animals, these effects are reversed by chronic—but not acute—paroxetine treatment.

Indications and Efficacy

Depression

Comparison With Other Agents

The efficacy of paroxetine in major depression has been established in several randomized, placebo-controlled studies, as well as in studies comparing the effects of paroxetine with those of other antidepressants, including tricyclic antidepressants (TCAs), serotonin-norepinephrine reuptake inhibitors (SNRIs), and other SSRIs. Many studies have compared paroxetine with other SSRIs; however, many of these studies were sponsored by the pharmaceutical industry and therefore must be evaluated with caution. The earliest placebo-controlled trials used 10–50 mg of paroxetine and were 6 weeks in duration. Outcome variables used were typically the Hamilton Rating Scale for Depression (Ham-D), the Montgomery-Åsberg Depression Rating Scale (MADRS), and the Clinical Global Impressions (CGI) Scale to assess improvement.

Recently there has been some debate regarding the use of such scales in the assessment of medication efficacy, as well as concerns that there exists a publication bias toward positive results. A minority of authors have suggested using "hard measures" of treatment effectiveness—namely, suicide attempts, treatment switching, hospital admission, job loss, or dropout from the trial (Barbui et al. 2008)—although such endpoints are not currently acceptable to the FDA. Barbui et al. (2008) undertook a systematic review of paroxetine, evaluating both published and unpublished data according to one specific "hard measure"—treatment discontinuation—by looking at the number of patients who left a study early for any reason. The authors found that when this measure was used as a primary outcome, paroxetine was not effective, whereas when rate of response (defined as ≥50% reduction in Ham-D score) was used, paroxetine was superior to placebo (Barbui et al. 2008).

Tricyclic and tetracyclic antidepressants. A meta-analysis by Montgomery (2001) compared the efficacy and tolerability of paroxetine with those of TCAs, including amitriptyline, imipramine, clomipramine, doxepin, and nortriptyline, as well as the tetracyclics mianserin and maprotiline. The data demonstrated no overall significant difference in antidepressant response rates between paroxetine and TCAs or tetracyclics. Paroxetine was better tolerated, had lower rates of discontinuation attributed to adverse events, and had a greater effect on concomitant anxiety.

Other SSRIs. Many studies have found paroxetine and fluoxetine to be equally effective in the treatment of major depression and associated anxiety (Chouinard et al. 1999; De Wilde et al. 1993; Fava et al. 1998, 2000; Tignol 1993). Similar results have been obtained from trials comparing paroxetine with sertraline or escitalopram. Equivalent efficacy has been demonstrated in comparisons of paroxetine against either sertraline or escitalopram; however, these studies tend to also show a greater dropout rate in paroxetine groups, likely due to adverse medication effects (Aberg-Wistedt et al. 2000; Baldwin et al. 2006; Zanardi et al. 1996).

Other agents. Paroxetine has also been compared with a variety of other agents in the treatment of depression. Nefazodone and paroxetine were shown to possess similar efficacy and tolerability (Baldwin et al. 1996), and mirtazapine and paroxetine were found to be equivalent in terms of efficacy and tolerability (Benkert et al. 2000).

In the meta-analysis of the venlafaxine worldwide database, the SNRI venlafaxine showed a slight statistically significant advantage in efficacy over SSRIs as a class, although no such difference was demonstrated between venlafaxine and paroxetine (Nemeroff et al. 2003). A comparison between venlafaxine XR and paroxetine in the maintenance treatment of depression found higher rates of remission with venlafaxine (Shelton et al. 2005). In patients with treatment-resistant depression (defined as failure to respond to two prior adequate treatments from different classes of medication in the current depressive episode), venlafaxine (200–300 mg/day) was shown to be superior to paroxetine (30–40 mg/day) in bringing about remission (Poirier and Boyer 1999). By contrast, a recent study in Chinese patients with treatment-resistant depression showed no significant differences among paroxetine, mirtazapine, and venlafaxine XR (Fang et al. 2010). Similarly, a study comparing paroxetine with the SNRI duloxetine (40–80 mg/day) revealed a higher probability of remission with duloxetine 80 mg/day than with paroxetine (Goldstein et al. 2004). However, in evaluating studies comparing paroxetine with SNRI agents, it is important to consider the dosages used for paroxetine, as paroxetine 20 mg/day is too low to exhibit any NET blockade.

Paroxetine has also been compared with investigational agents such as substance P (NK_1) receptor antagonists. In the Merck-sponsored NK_1 receptor antagonist trials in major depression, paroxetine 20 mg/day was superior to both placebo and the novel agent (Cutler et al. 2000).

Depression in the Elderly

Following successful treatment for depression, elderly patients are more likely than nonelderly patients to experience early relapses (Zis et al. 1980). SSRIs are currently the treatment of choice in this population because of their demonstrated efficacy and their relative safety over TCAs and monoamine oxidase inhibitors (MAOIs). While paroxetine, clomipramine, and amitriptyline are equally effective in geriatric patients (Geretsegger et al. 1995; Guillibert et al. 1989; Hutchinson et al. 1992), paroxetine and fluoxetine have both been shown to elicit improved depression response rates and improved cognitive functioning, and they are equally well tolerated (Geretsegger et al. 1994; Gunasekara et al. 1998; Schöne and Ludwig 1993). Paroxetine and bupropion sustained release (SR) also have been shown to be equally effective in this population and to have low discontinuation rates (Weihs et al. 2000). Paroxetine CR at daily dosages of 12.5 mg and 25 mg was found to be well tolerated by elderly patients and superior to placebo; at the higher dosage, patients showed numerically larger decreases in total Ham-D scores, and a greater number of patients achieved remission (Ham-D ≤7) (Rapaport et al. 2009).

For maintenance treatment in elderly (≥65 years old) patients with depression, paroxetine and nortriptyline are similarly effective in preventing relapse (Bump et al. 2001). In a maintenance study comparing continuation of combined treatment consisting of either interpersonal therapy (IPT) plus paroxetine or IPT plus placebo, patients who continued on paroxetine were significantly less likely to experience a recurrence, whereas therapy alone was not successful in preventing relapse (Reynolds et al. 2006).

One issue of concern in treating the elderly with paroxetine is the potential risk of anticholinergic side effects, leading to delirium. Fluoxetine has minimal anticholinergic activity, and in a study comparing the effects of fluoxetine and paroxetine in depressed elderly patients without dementia, both medications produced marked improvement in cognitive functioning and mood symptoms and were well tolerated (Cassano et al. 2002).

Long-Term Treatment

Given that it is now well recognized that unipolar depression is a chronic and recurrent disorder, the prevention of recurrence should be a primary aim. Studies have demonstrated the effectiveness of paroxetine in maintaining remission over an extended period without adverse effects (Duboff 1993), particularly when compared with placebo (Montgomery and Dunbar 1993). However, studies comparing paroxetine with escitalopram report that although both medications produce improvement in measures of depression, escitalopram appears to be more efficacious and to have better tolerability (Baldwin et al. 2006; Boulenger et al. 2006; Kasper et al. 2009).

The paroxetine dosages used in the long-term phases were typically the same ones used in the acute studies (20–40 mg/day). Thus, for maintenance therapy for depression, the recommended dose of paroxetine is the dose that was effective during the acute phase.

In most patients with an acute major depressive episode, an initial daily dosage of 20 mg is sufficient for the duration of the illness episode, at least when response (defined as ≥50% reduction in symptoms) is used as an endpoint (Dunner and Dunbar 1992). One study demonstrated that in patients with major depression, dosage escalation of 20 mg/day and subsequent increased plasma levels were not associated with improved clinical outcomes (Ruhe et al. 2009a). However, to improve the likelihood of remission, we recommend increasing the dosage in 10-mg increments each week—up to 50 mg/day or more of the IR form and up to 75 mg/day of the CR form (Nemeroff 1993). Elderly patients and those with renal or hepatic dysfunction should be initiated at a lower dosage, with gradual dose titration to therapeutic effect while monitoring for side effects.

Bipolar Depression

Paroxetine has demonstrated efficacy and safety in treating patients with bipolar depression, an often treatment-refractory disorder. In one study in lithium-treated patients, augmentation with paroxetine was shown to be superior to augmentation with amitriptyline (Bauer et al. 1999); in another study, paroxetine and imipramine were equally efficacious and superior to placebo as augmentation agents (Nemeroff et al. 2001). However, a more recent study evaluating antidepressant augmentation of a mood stabilizer showed no differences in efficacy among paroxetine, bupropion SR, and placebo (Sachs et al. 2007). Paroxetine was not associated with an increased rate of switch into mania or hypomania in any of these studies.

Depression Associated With Medical Illness

Paroxetine has been found to be efficacious in treating depression comorbid with several medical disorders, including rheumatoid arthritis, irritable bowel syndrome, cardiovascular disease, and Parkinson disease (Bird and Broggini 2000; Masand et al. 2001; Richard et al. 2012; Roose et al. 1998). Paroxetine also was demonstrated to be efficacious in the prevention of interferon-α-induced depression in patients with malignant melanoma (Musselman et al. 2001; see Figure 4–1).

Child and Adolescent Depression

In 2003, the FDA released a statement regarding a possible increased risk of suicidal thinking and suicide attempts in children and adolescents 18 years of age and younger treated with paroxetine for major depressive disorder (U.S. Food and Drug Administration 2003). The statement was based on data from three well-controlled unpublished studies, each showing no benefit for paroxetine above placebo in the treatment of pediatric depression. The data also revealed an increased rate of suicidal ideation and suicide attempts with paroxetine treatment versus placebo (3.4% vs. 1.2%). Published data on paroxetine have shown limited efficacy as well (Emslie et al. 2006; Keller et al. 2001).

Differences in pharmacokinetics in children and adults may explain the observed age-related discrepancy in efficacy and suicide risk. In children, an increase in dosage from 10 to 20 mg results in a sixfold increase in serum paroxetine levels (Findling et al. 1999). This dramatic increase in child serum levels could potentially cause activation, akathisia, or disinhibition, explaining suicidal thoughts or acts (Brent 2004), and the effect is even greater in children who are slow metabolizers at CYP2D6 (roughly 10% of the Caucasian population) (Riddle 2004). Additionally, paroxetine has a relatively short half-life (11 hours vs. 5 days with fluoxetine), and limited treatment adherence—not uncommon in children and teens—could lead to SSRI discontinuation syndrome and dysphoria (Brent 2004).

Recent studies utilizing animal models have confirmed these observations. In a rat model, depressive symptoms appear with an increase in locus coeruleus (LC) activity, and effective antidepressant treatment decreases LC activity; however, in younger rats, administration of paroxetine initially increases LC activity, which then declines with prolonged administration (West et al. 2010). Furthermore, increased LC activity is also associated with low or decreasing serum paroxetine levels, further supporting the hypothesis that poor adherence to or faster metabolism of medication may contribute to the risk of suicidality (West et al. 2010).

The FDA's black box warning concerning antidepressant use and suicidality risk in children and adolescents has led to a decline in SSRI prescribing for the under-18 age group (Nemeroff et al. 2007). The Centers for Disease Control and Prevention (2007) reported that suicide rates in American children and adolescents increased 18% in 2004, after 10 years of steady decline. A recent cohort study of 20,906 adolescents (ages 10–18 years) prescribed SSRIs in British Columbia demonstrated a risk of suicidal behavior (attempted or completed suicide) five times higher than that in the general population; however, the authors noted that this increased rate likely reflects the risk associated with a diagnosis of depression (Schneeweiss et al. 2010a). Most of the suicidal events occurred during the first 6 months of SSRI treatment. Interestingly, the authors found no significant difference in risk of suicidal behavior among the specific SSRIs (fluoxetine, citalopram, fluvoxamine, paroxetine, and sertraline) evaluated (Schneeweiss et al. 2010a).

Obsessive-Compulsive Disorder

Currently, the SSRIs fluvoxamine, fluoxetine, sertraline, and paroxetine are FDA approved for the treatment of OCD in adults. Although two meta-analyses assessing the efficacy and tolerability of the TCA clomipramine and SSRIs in OCD seemed to favor clomipramine in terms of overall effectiveness (Greist et al. 1995; Piccinelli et al. 1995), the only placebo-controlled multicenter study to compare clomipramine directly against an SSRI (paroxetine) revealed equal efficacy and greater tolerability for paroxetine (Zohar and Judge 1996).

In addition to its proven efficacy in adult OCD, paroxetine has been FDA approved for pediatric OCD. In a randomized, double-blind, placebo-controlled multicenter trial (Geller et al. 2004), paroxetine was found to be an effective and generally well-tolerated treatment for OCD in children and adolescents. Patients with comorbid major depressive disorder were excluded from this study, and only one incident of treatment-emergent suicidal behavior or ideation was reported.

In adults, daily doses of ≥60 mg of paroxetine are usually required to optimally treat OCD. Although patients characteristically respond to treatment within 3–4 weeks, clinical improvement may not be discernible until 10–12 weeks; therefore, a standard trial of up to 12 weeks should be conducted before an alternative medication is considered (Rasmussen et al. 1993).

Panic Disorder

Paroxetine was the first SSRI to be granted FDA approval for the treatment of panic disorder. Paroxetine and clomipramine have been shown to be equally efficacious in the treatment of panic attacks, and a faster onset of action was noted with paroxetine (Lecrubier et al. 1997). The long-term efficacy and tolerability of paroxetine have also been demonstrated in patients with panic disorder (Lecrubier and Judge 1997; Nardi et al. 2012). The combination of cognitive-behavioral therapy (CBT) and paroxetine is more effective in the treatment of panic disorder than CBT alone (Bakker et al. 1999; Oehrberg et al. 1995).

In general, patients with panic disorder should initially be treated with a low dose of paroxetine (e.g., 10 mg/day), with gradual increases in dose, as clinically indicated. The data that led to FDA approval indicated that 40 mg/day is the minimum effective dosage for this condition; however, clinical experience indicates that lower dosages may be sufficient in some patients and higher dosages may be required in other patients (Ballenger et al. 1998). The standard duration of treatment ranges from 6 to 12 months; however, rates of relapse appear to be greater than those for major depressive disorder, indicating that panic disorder may require an indefinite course of treatment (Hirschfeld 1996).

Social Anxiety Disorder

Paroxetine, sertraline, fluvoxamine CR, and venlafaxine XR are the only medications with FDA approval for the treatment of social anxiety disorder, which is also known as social phobia. The efficacy of paroxetine in the treatment of social anxiety disorder was first suggested by the results of open clinical trials (Mancini and van Amerigen 1996; Stein et al. 1996) and was later confirmed by findings from double-blind, placebo-controlled studies (Baldwin et al. 1999; Stein et al. 1998). Paroxetine and venlafaxine XR have been shown to be similarly effective and superior to placebo in the treatment of social anxiety disorder (Liebowitz et al. 2005).

In children and adolescents (ages 8–17 years) with social anxiety disorder, paroxetine was found to be superior to placebo (Wagner et al. 2004). It is important to note that a total of five patients in the paroxetine group ($n=163$), versus none in the placebo group ($n=156$), exhibited suicidal threats or gestures.

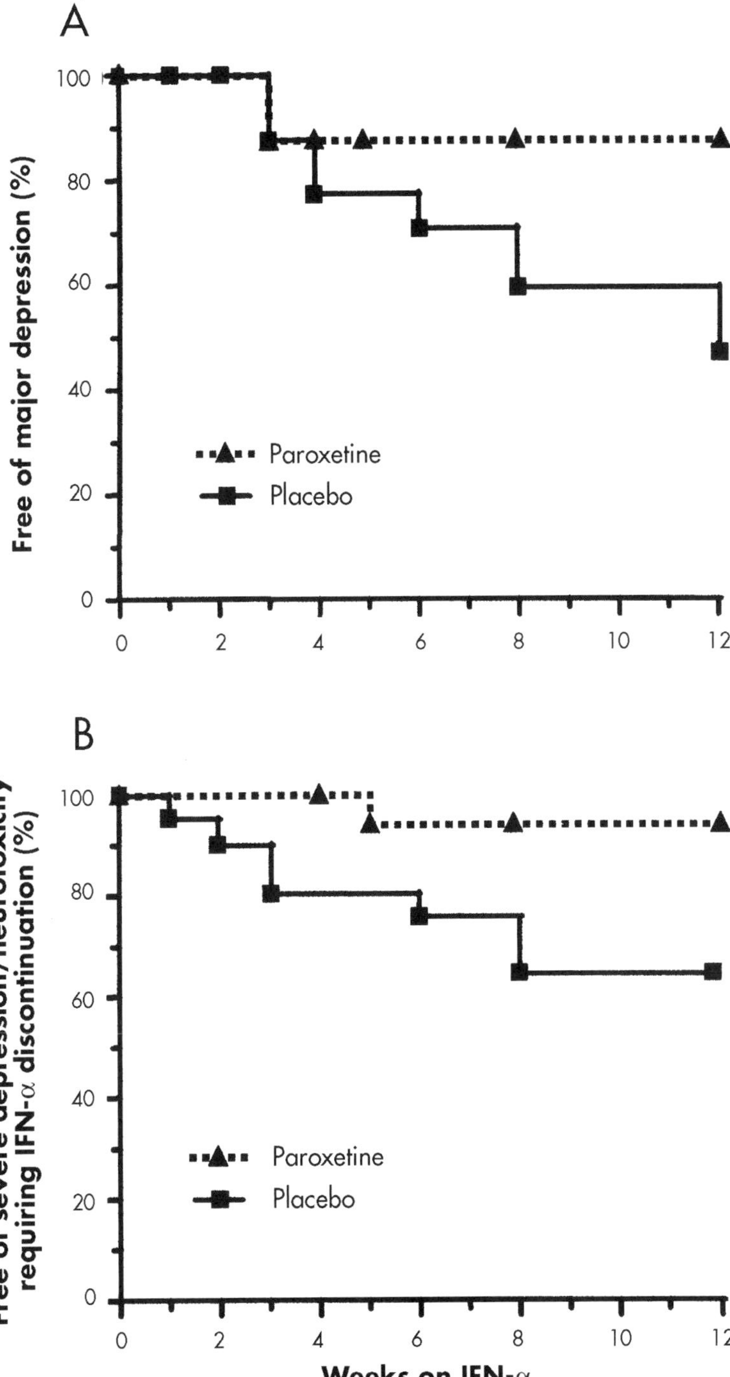

FIGURE 4–1. Paroxetine effect on interferon-α (IFN-α)–induced depression.

Kaplan-Meier analysis of the percentage of patients in the placebo and paroxetine groups who were free of major depression (**A**) and of severe depression, requiring the discontinuation of IFN-α (**B**).

Source. Musselman et al. 2001.

It appears that the optimal daily dose of paroxetine for the treatment of social anxiety disorder is 20–40 mg, with no additional benefit seen for 60 mg (Lydiard and Bobes 2000). In patients who respond to paroxetine, it is also advisable to continue treatment to prevent relapse (Stein et al. 2002).

Generalized Anxiety Disorder

Venlafaxine XR, escitalopram, duloxetine, and paroxetine have all been approved by the FDA for treatment of GAD. The first published study supporting the use of paroxetine in GAD compared it with both imipramine and 2′-chlorodesmethyldiazepam, a benzodiazepine (Rocca et al. 1997). Not surprisingly, patients receiving the benzodiazepine showed the earliest improvement in symptoms; however, both paroxetine and imipramine showed significant reductions in Ham-A total score, exceeding that of the benzodiazepine by week 4 of the 8-week trial. Subsequent studies further confirmed the efficacy of paroxetine in treatment of GAD (Bielski et al. 2005; Pollack et al. 2001; Rickels et al. 2003).

Long-term treatment of GAD with paroxetine may be necessary (Stocchi et al. 2003). Clinical experience and investigative research indicate that the usual effective paroxetine dosage for treating GAD is 20 mg/day (Paxil 2001).

Posttraumatic Stress Disorder

Among the SSRIs, sertraline and paroxetine have FDA approval for the treatment of PTSD. Compared with placebo, paroxetine (20–40 mg/day) has been shown to produce significant improvements in the three main cluster groups of reexperiencing, avoiding/numbing, and hyperarousal and to reduce disability and depression (Marshall et al. 1998, 2001). Patients with comorbid major depression (40%) respond just as favorably as subjects without depression. Similar findings have been replicated by other groups (Tucker et al. 2001, 2004), in combination with prolonged exposure therapy (Schneier et al. 2012), and with long-term treatment (Bremner et al. 2003; Kim et al. 2008).

Premenstrual Dysphoric Disorder

Fluoxetine, sertraline, and paroxetine are FDA approved for the treatment of PMDD. The somatic features of PMDD—bloating, weight gain, breast tenderness, poor concentration, and disturbed sleep and appetite—manifest in the luteal phase of ovulation and disappear upon menstruation. These symptoms are cyclical, predictably appearing prior to each menses (Dimmock et al. 2000). The psychological symptoms of PMDD are more severe and prominent and include irritability, dysphoria, tension, and mood lability. Paroxetine has been shown to be significantly more effective than the tetracyclic maprotiline, a norepinephrine reuptake inhibitor, in reducing both psychological and somatic symptoms of PMDD (Eriksson et al. 1995). Two small open trials reported positive findings with paroxetine treatment (Sunblad et al. 1997; Yonkers et al. 1996), and a double-blind, placebo-controlled study demonstrated that paroxetine CR (25 mg/day) was both well tolerated and effective in the treatment of PMDD (Cohen et al. 2004).

PMDD can be successfully managed with intermittent luteal-phase dosing, in which the medication is started 14 days prior to the estimated next menses and continued until the onset of menstruation (Steiner et al. 2005). It has been shown that paroxetine improves irritability within 14 hours of taking the first dose (Landen et al. 2009). Both luteal- and continuous-phase dosing of paroxetine (either the CR or the IR formulation) are superior to placebo in treating the psychological symptoms of PMDD, but not the somatic symptoms (food craving, breast tenderness) (Steiner et al. 2005, 2008). Somatic symptoms may be better addressed with continuous treatment (Landen et al. 2007; Wu et al. 2008); however, with intermittent dosing, patients experience fewer adverse effects (Steiner et al. 2008).

Menopausal Vasomotor Symptoms

In addition to its proven efficacy in PMDD, paroxetine has been found to be efficacious in treating perimenopausal hot flashes (Soares et al. 2008; Stearns et al. 2003), possibly via a paroxetine-induced increase in brain-derived neurotrophic factor (BDNF) plasma levels (Cubeddu et al. 2010).

Earlier studies also demonstrated paroxetine (20 mg/day) to be effective in the treatment of postmenopausal hot flashes in breast cancer survivors with chemotherapy-induced ovarian failure (Stearns et al. 2000, 2005; Weitzner et al. 2002). This finding has important implications in women with estrogen receptor–positive breast cancer who are taking tamoxifen to decrease the risk of breast cancer relapse. Tamoxifen is a prodrug that requires CYP2D6 metabolism to create the more active metabolite endoxifen; however, as a potent inhibitor of CYP2D6, paroxetine blocks the conversion of tamoxifen to endoxifen (Kelly et al. 2010). An increased risk of death from breast cancer has been observed in women taking tamoxifen and paroxetine (Kelly et al. 2010).

Side Effects and Toxicology

The popularity of SSRIs, as a class, in the treatment of psychiatric disorders is owed not to their superiority in efficacy over their predecessors but rather to their overall tolerability and safety. The most commonly cited adverse experiences in patients treated with paroxetine are, in order of frequency, nausea, headache, somnolence, dry mouth, asthenia, sweating, constipation, dizziness, and tremor (Boyer and Blumhardt 1992).

According to the worldwide preregistration clinical trial database, anticholinergic side effects, tremor, dizziness, postural hypotension, and somnolence were more common in comparison drugs (generally TCAs) (Jenner 1992). The most common side effect associated with early termination for paroxetine was nausea. Clinical experience demonstrates that this effect can be mitigated with a conservative starting dose and administration with food, as well as with the use of the CR form of the compound (Golden et al. 2002). Furthermore, patients reported that nausea diminishes markedly with prolonged administration (Jenner 1992). As noted earlier, elderly patients do not appear to be more susceptible to the side effects of paroxetine, and cognitive function remains intact or improves during treatment (Cassano et al. 2002; Nebes et al. 1999).

Sexual Side Effects

All SSRIs and SNRIs have been associated with male and female sexual dysfunction. In a comparison study of 200 subjects who were treated with paroxetine, fluoxetine, fluvoxamine, or sertraline, paroxetine treatment was associated with higher rates of anorgasmia in women and ejaculation difficulty or impotence in men (Montejo-Gonzalez et al. 1997). In a large cross-sectional observational study (Clayton et al. 2002), paroxetine was associated with the highest rates of sexual dysfunction among the antidepressants evaluated (mirtazapine, venlafaxine, sertraline, citalopram, fluoxetine, nefazodone, and bupropion).

On the other hand, the sexual side effects of paroxetine have been capitalized on in the application to the treatment of premature ejaculation. Paroxetine produces a greater delay in time to ejaculation compared with fluoxetine, fluvoxamine, sertraline, dapoxetine (a short-acting SSRI awaiting FDA approval for the treatment of premature ejaculation), and mirtazapine (Safarinejad 2006; Waldinger et al. 1998, 2003).

Sexual side effects emerge in a dose-dependent fashion and do not appear to diminish with prolonged administration; however, the effect is reversible, with most patients returning to normal functioning within 1 month of discontinuing the medication (Tanrikut et al. 2010). Strategies to lessen the impact of psychotropic medications on sexual function include reducing the dosage, changing to a different antidepressant with less sexual side-effect liability, and adding an agent (e.g., sildenafil, yohimbine, buspirone, cyproheptadine, amantadine, methylphenidate, bupropion) to reverse the sexual side effects (Rosen et al. 1999). Ephedrine, an α- and β-adrenergic agonist previously shown to enhance genital blood flow in women, has been evaluated in women experiencing SSRI-induced sexual dysfunction from paroxetine, sertraline, or fluoxetine (Meston 2004). Both ephedrine and placebo improved self-reported scores of desire and orgasm intensity compared with baseline, although women taking sertraline and paroxetine fared better than did women taking fluoxetine, a finding the authors attributed to differences in the mechanism of action of these SSRIs (Ahrold and Meston 2009).

Suicidality

As previously discussed (see "Childhood and Adolescent Depression" subsection earlier in this chapter), in 2004 the FDA ordered pharmaceutical companies to place a black box warning on all antidepressants, stating that suicidal behavior might increase in children and adolescents taking these medications. Concerns about a link between antidepressant usage and suicidal ideation led FDA regulators to request that antidepressant manufacturers examine their databases for similar findings in adult. GlaxoSmithKline (Paxil/Seroxat) conducted a meta-analysis of its clinical data comparing suicidality with paroxetine versus placebo. Among depressed patients taking paroxetine, 0.32% (11 of 3,455) attempted suicide, compared with 0.05% (1 of 1,978) of depressed patients taking placebo, an odds ratio of 6.7 (GlaxoSmithKline 2006). Cases of completed suicide in both samples were exceedingly rare, with one reported in the paroxetine sample versus none reported with placebo. GlaxoSmithKline further examined the data to identify clinical features of those patients who developed suicidal behaviors (Kraus et al. 2010). Common features among these patients included some improvement in depressive symptoms, younger age (<30 years old), psychosocial stressor preceding the attempt, and no identified suicidality at the prior study visit (Kraus et al. 2010).

Another analysis of both published and unpublished data on paroxetine in the treatment of depression evaluated suicidality as a secondary outcome (Barbui et al. 2008), finding an odds ratio of 2.55, with a number needed to harm of 142. The authors noted that whereas suicidality is exceedingly rare, the data are also variably recorded, making it more difficult to track this outcome through retrospective reports (Barbui et al. 2008). A cohort study of 287,543 adult residents of British Columbia ages 18 years and older who were receiving antidepressants (Schneeweiss et al. 2010b) found no significant difference in suicidality risk between individual SSRIs (fluoxetine, citalopram, fluvoxamine, paroxetine, and sertraline). As in the study of children and adolescents mentioned earlier (Schneeweiss et al. 2010a), most of the suicidal events that occurred did so during the first 6 months of treatment (Schneeweiss et al. 2010b).

These findings are limited by the fact that suicidal ideation and self-harming behaviors were not the main outcome measures in the pooled studies. Procedures to assess suicidality have not, until recently, been standardized and are based largely on unsolicited and unstructured reports and observations. Also, depression is a risk factor for suicidal behavior, and suicide is a potential complication of the disease. Transient suicidal thinking must be considered in the context of the overall risk-benefit analysis of paroxetine in the treatment of adults with major depressive disorder.

Nevertheless, in late 2006, an FDA advisory panel extended the black box warning to cover young adults up to their mid-20s (U.S. Food and Drug Administration 2007). They reported that in patients 18–24 years of age, antidepressant use was associated with four cases of suicidal ideation per 1,000 patients treated, whereas drug therapy for patients older than 30 years was unequivocally protective against suicidality.

Clinicians should inform their patients about the possible risks and should monitor depressed patients closely once paroxetine or any other antidepressants are prescribed, particularly during the early phase of treatment. The FDA advisory committee has made it clear that the black box warning should not dissuade physicians from prescribing antidepressants to patients in need (U.S. Food and Drug Administration 2007).

Medical Safety

Paroxetine treatment in clinical trials has not been associated with any significant abnormalities in standard laboratory tests, including hematological indices and chemistry panels, electroencephalogram (EEG), or electrocardiogram (ECG). One possible concern regarding paroxetine had been the potential for decreasing heart rate variability (HRV), which is a significant risk factor for myocardial infarction and cardiovascular mortality (Carney et al. 2005). Other norepinephrine reuptake–inhibiting antidepressants have been shown to cause decreases in this electrophysiological variable (Rechlin 1994), and depressed patients have been shown to exhibit lower HRV than nondepressed persons (Gorman and Sloan 2000); however, paroxetine does not exhibit this effect.

Paroxetine and other SSRIs have been implicated in the precipitation of the syndrome of inappropriate antidiuretic hormone (SIADH), particularly in elderly individuals; symptoms resolve upon discontinuation of the medication (Strachan and Shepherd 1998). One study demonstrated that hyponatremia (defined as plasma sodium levels <135 mEq/L) occurred in 12% (9 of 75) of subjects, typically within the first 10 days of paroxetine treatment (Fabian et al. 2004). Risk factors for developing hyponatremia were low body mass index (BMI) and low starting plasma sodium levels.

Discontinuation Syndrome

With abrupt discontinuation or treatment interruption, patients may develop what has become known as the SSRI discontinuation syndrome. Symptoms occur as early as the second day after a missed dose and may persist for several days. Postmarketing data reported the occurrence of withdrawal-related events to be greater in paroxetine-treated patients than in patients treated with sertraline, fluvoxamine, or fluoxetine and to have a mean duration of 10.2 days (Price et al. 1996); similar results were reported by other groups (Michelson et al. 2000; Montgomery et al. 2004; Rosenbaum et al. 1998). Shorter treatment interruptions (3–5 days), similar to what a patient would experience if he or she missed just a few doses, demonstrate that whereas paroxetine-treated patients develop significant discontinuation-emergent effects, fluoxetine-treated patients do not, a disparity likely due to differences in the half-life of these medications (Judge et al. 2002; Michelson et al. 2000).

To mitigate the emergence of withdrawal symptoms, practitioners are advised to gradually taper the dose of paroxetine when discontinuing this medication in their patients. Despite the potential for withdrawal reactions after abrupt discontinuation, there is no clinical evidence for dose escalation, craving, or drug-seeking behavior associated with dependence or addiction (Inman et al. 1993; Johnson et al. 1998; Sharma et al. 2000).

Overdoses with paroxetine are rarely associated with morbidity or mortality, which is in sharp contrast to the situation with the TCAs or venlafaxine (Buckley et al. 2003; Cheeta et al. 2004). In the clinical trials program prior to FDA registration of paroxetine, 16 patients had ingested an overdose (doses of up to 850 mg of paroxetine); all patients recovered uneventfully (Jenner 1992). An extensive review of the literature (including adverse events databases) revealed a total of 28 fatalities involving paroxetine overdoses; however, in nearly all cases, either coingestants were involved or causality could not be ascertained (Barbey and Roose 1998).

Pregnancy and Lactation

A more complete discussion of the use of psychotropic medications during pregnancy appears elsewhere in this volume (see Chapter 41, "Psychopharmacology During Pregnancy and Lactation"); however, because paroxetine is the only SSRI to be allocated to FDA Pregnancy Category D ("There is positive evidence of human fetal risk based on adverse reaction data from investigational or marketing experience or studies in humans, but potential benefits may warrant use of the drug in pregnant women despite potential risks"), it warrants specific discussion here.

Spontaneous abortion has been linked both to depression and to antidepressants; the risk may be even greater for women who are treated with paroxetine or venlafaxine (Nakhai-Pour et al. 2010).

Compared with other SSRIs, paroxetine has lower transmission across the placenta, and cord blood concentrations do not correlate with maternal dosing (Hendrick et al. 2003b). Maternal CYP2D6 polymorphisms appear to affect the pharmacokinetics of paroxetine. Women characterized as extensive metabolizers show decreases in paroxetine plasma levels over the course of pregnancy, whereas women characterized as intermediate or poor metabolizers show increased paroxetine levels (Ververs et al. 2009). It is possible that this effect may translate to a greater risk of teratogenicity in women who are poor or intermediate metabolizers (Ververs et al. 2009).

Teratogenicity is a major concern when prescribing medications to women of childbearing age. The results of an unpublished study by GlaxoSmithKline (Paxil) led the FDA to warn that paroxetine may increase the risk of major congenital malformations (GlaxoSmithKline 2005). Several organ systems, including the gastrointestinal, genitourinary, and central nervous systems, were affected; the most common cardiovascular anomalies were ventricular septal defects. A recent meta-analysis, also completed by GlaxoSmithKline, found a prevalence odds ratio of 1.46 for combined cardiac defects with exposure to paroxetine in the first trimester. Considering a background prevalence of cardiac defects in the unexposed population of 1%, this would represent a 50% increase for the paroxetine-exposed population (Wurst et al. 2010).

A cohort study comparing rates of major congenital malformations in pregnant women treated with paroxetine, fluvoxamine, or sertraline found no significant differences among the medication groups compared with control groups (Kulin et al. 1998). In another study comparing paroxetine, fluoxetine, and sertraline, rates of neonatal complications and congenital malformations in antidepressant-treated women were lower (1.4%) than rates in the general population, with no significant differences among medications (Hendrick et al. 2003a). Whereas one prospective controlled observational study found no increased risk of cardiac defects from paroxetine exposure (Diav-Citrin et al. 2008), a case-control study of data from a population-based birth defects registry in the Netherlands did find an increased risk of atrial septal defects with first-trimester paroxetine exposure (adjusted odds ratio = 5.7, 95% confidence interval = 1.4–23.7) (Bakker et al. 2010). Frequently, studies of teratogenicity are complicated by the effects of depression itself or of polypharmacy (e.g., concurrent use of benzodiazepines) (Yonkers et al. 2009).

Clinical studies of paroxetine in the setting of pregnancy suggest that gestational exposure might have transient negative effects on the newborn infant, particularly if the mother is treated during the third trimester. Third-trimester paroxetine exposure is associated with significant increases in neonatal distress compared with infants not exposed to paroxetine in the third trimester (Costei et al. 2002). Neonatal symptoms described following in utero exposure to SSRIs include tremor, hypertonicity, irritability, weak or absent cry, seizures, and poor feeding; these symptoms typically resolve within 2 weeks (Knoppert et al. 2006; Yonkers et al. 2009). There remains debate among neonatologists as to whether the newborn distress is a manifestation of serotonin excess or serotonin withdrawal (Laine et al. 2004; Stiskal 2005, 2006).

Although not specific to paroxetine, another issue that has received much media attention is the development of persistent pulmonary hypertension of the newborn (PPHN) in neonates exposed to SSRIs late (>20 weeks) in gestation. A rare condition associated with significant morbidity, PPHN has an estimated base rate in the United States of 1–2 per 1,000 births (Andrade et al. 2009). One large case-control epidemiological study found an odds ratio of developing PPHN of 6.1 for infants exposed to SSRIs after gestational week 20 (Chambers et al. 2006). However, a more recent retrospective review did not find a significant difference in risk of developing PPHN with exposure to SSRIs; in fact, the authors found a higher prevalence in the nonexposed group (Andrade et al. 2009).

If a woman opts to continue antidepressant treatment during pregnancy, the clinician is advised to monitor for relapse, given that higher dosages are often needed, especially in the early third trimester, to achieve or maintain disease remission (Hostetter et al. 2000).

Paroxetine is secreted into breast milk, with greater concentrations found in hindmilk than foremilk (Ohman et al. 1999; Stowe et al. 2000). However, in a study in which the sera of nursing infants were analyzed for the presence of paroxetine after 10 days of maternal treatment with paroxetine at a stable daily dose of 10–50 mg, the drug was undetectable in all infants (Stowe et al. 2000).

Drug-Drug Interactions

As noted previously, paroxetine is primarily dependent on the CYP2D6 enzyme for conversion into its inactive metabolites (Hiemke and Härtter 2000). Paroxetine is not only a substrate of this system but also an inhibitor; therefore, other drugs that are metabolized by this hepatic enzyme are potentially subject to decreased clearance and subsequent increased plasma concentrations (Sindrup et al. 1992b). Concern is greatest for potential drug-drug interactions when the medication in question has a low therapeutic index. (See Table 4–1 for the important drug-drug interactions with paroxetine.)

Medications that are CYP2D6 dependent include many antipsychotics, TCAs, type IC antiarrhythmics, β-adrenergic agents, trazodone, and dextromethorphan (Nemeroff et al. 1996). Most reports of interactions between these medications and paroxetine are published as case reports (Lane 1996).

Paroxetine does not appear to potentiate the sedative effects of haloperidol (Cooper et al. 1989); however, dystonia has been reported with the combination (Budman et al. 1995). In one prospective study, clozapine serum levels increased by an average of 40% when clozapine was coadministered with SSRIs, including paroxetine at a mean dosage of 31.2 mg/day (Centorrino et al. 1996). In another study that used a lower dosage of paroxetine (20 mg/day), no significant increase in clozapine concentrations was noted (Wetzel et al. 1998). Case reports have described possible exaggerated extrapyramidal side effects when paroxetine was coadministered with perphenazine (Ozdemir et al. 1997), molindone (Malek-Ahmadi and Allen 1995), or pimozide (Horrigan and Barnhill 1994).

Paroxetine is highly protein bound and has the potential to increase free drug levels of other medications that are bound to

TABLE 4–1. Potential drug-drug interactions involving paroxetine

Monoamine oxidase inhibitors	Clinically significant
Tricyclic antidepressants	Clinically significant
Type IC antiarrhythmics	Probably significant
β-Adrenergic antagonists	Probably significant
Antiepileptic agents	Probably significant
Cimetidine	Probably significant
Typical antipsychotics	Possibly significant
Warfarin	Possibly significant
Clozapine	Inconclusive
Lithium	Not clinically significant
Digoxin	Not clinically significant

plasma proteins, such as warfarin, lithium, and digoxin, although this effect is rarely clinically meaningful (Bannister et al. 1989; Haenen et al. 1995; Preskorn 1993).

In prospective studies involving valproate, carbamazepine, and phenytoin, coadministration with paroxetine did not cause any significant changes in plasma levels of these drugs (Andersen et al. 1991; Kaye et al. 1989). By contrast, both phenytoin and carbamazepine have been shown to decrease plasma paroxetine concentrations (Hiemke and Härtter 2000; Kaye et al. 1989). Valproate may increase plasma paroxetine concentrations (Andersen et al. 1991). Cimetidine, which is a potent inhibitor of the CYP 2D6 isoenzyme, has been shown to result in a 50% elevation of paroxetine concentrations (Bannister et al. 1989). The clinical significance of these variations in paroxetine concentrations is minor because of the wide interindividual pharmacokinetic variability, high therapeutic index, and lack of a concentration-efficacy relationship with paroxetine (Gunasekara et al. 1998).

Paroxetine does not potentiate the psychomotor effects of amobarbital, oxazepam, diazepam, or alcohol (Bannister et al. 1989; Cooper et al. 1989).

Combinations of medications that enhance serotonergic activity may result in serotonin toxicity, manifesting as agitation, myoclonus, hyperreflexia, diarrhea, diaphoresis, delirium, fever, and possibly death (Weiner et al. 1997). Concomitant use of MAOIs with any of the SSRIs is absolutely contraindicated, and a washout period of 14 days is recommended when switching from one agent to another (Gunasekara et al. 1998; Weiner et al. 1997). Evidence of serotonin toxicity has been documented in case reports describing coadministration of paroxetine with moclobemide (Hawley et al. 1996), nefazodone (John et al. 1997), dextromethorphan (Skop et al. 1994), imipramine (Weiner et al. 1997), trazodone (Reeves and Bullen 1995), or other agents. The combination of SSRIs and sumatriptan, a serotonin$_{1D}$ (5-HT$_{1D}$) receptor agonist used in the treatment of migraine, was previously discouraged because of the theoretical risk of precipitation of serotonin toxicity; however, a series of six cases, one involving paroxetine, of concurrent sumatriptan and SSRI administration demonstrated no such adverse events (Leung and Ong 1995).

References

Aberg-Wistedt A, Agren H, Ekselius L, et al: Sertraline versus paroxetine in major depression: clinical outcome after six months of continuous therapy. J Clin Psychopharmacol 20:645–652, 2000

Ahrold TK, Meston CM: Effects of SNS activation on SSRI-induced sexual side effects differ by SSRI. J Sex Marital Ther 35:311–319, 2009

Andersen BB, Mikkelsen M, Vesterager A, et al: No influence of the antidepressant paroxetine on carbamazepine, valproate and phenytoin. Epilepsy Res 10:201–204, 1991

Andrade SE, McPhillips H, Loren D, et al: Antidepressant medication use and risk of persistent pulmonary hypertension of the newborn. Pharmacoepidemiol Drug Saf 18:246–252, 2009

Artigas F, Perez V, Alvarez E: Pindolol induces a rapid improvement of depressed patients treated with serotonin reuptake inhibitors. Arch Gen Psychiatry 51:248–251, 1994

Bakker A, van Dyck R, Spinhoven P, et al: Paroxetine, clomipramine, and cognitive therapy in the treatment of panic disorder. J Clin Psychiatry 60:831–838, 1999

Bakker MK, Kerstjens-Frederikse WS, Buys CH, et al: First-trimester use of paroxetine and congenital heart defects: a population-based case-control study. Birth Defects Res A Clin Mol Teratol 88:94–100, 2010

Baldwin DS, Hawley CJ, Abed RT, et al: A multicenter double-blind comparison of nefazodone and paroxetine in the treatment of outpatients with moderate-to-severe depression. J Clin Psychiatry 57 (suppl 2):46–52, 1996

Baldwin DS, Bobes J, Stein DJ, et al: Paroxetine in social phobia/social anxiety disorder. Br J Psychiatry 175:120–126, 1999

Baldwin DS, Cooper JA, Huusom AK, et al: A double-blind, randomized, parallel-group, flexible-dose study to evaluate the tolerability, efficacy and effects of treatment discontinuation with escitalopram and paroxetine in patients with major depressive disorder. Int Clin Psychopharmacol 21:159–169, 2006

Ballenger JC, Wheadon DE, Steiner M, et al: Double-blind, fixed dose, placebo-controlled study of paroxetine in the treatment of panic disorder. Am J Psychiatry 155:36–42, 1998

Bannister SJ, Houser VP, Hulse JD, et al: Evaluation of the potential for interaction of paroxetine with diazepam, cimetidine, warfarin, and digoxin. Acta Psychiatr Scand Suppl 350:102–106, 1989

Barbey JT, Roose SP: SSRI safety in overdose. J Clin Psychiatry 59 (suppl 15):42–48, 1998

Barbui C, Furukawa TA, Cipriani A: Effectiveness of paroxetine in the treatment of acute major depression in adults: a systematic re-examination of published and unpublished data from randomized trials. CMAJ 178:296–305, 2008

Bauer M, Zaninelli R, Müller-Oerhlinghausen B, et al: Paroxetine and amitriptyline augmentation of lithium in the treatment of major depression: a double-blind study. J Clin Psychopharmacol 19:164–171, 1999

Bayer AJ, Roberts NA, Allen EA, et al: The pharmacokinetics of paroxetine in the elderly. Acta Psychiatr Scand Suppl 350:152–155, 1989

Benkert O, Szegedi A, Kohnen R: Mirtazapine compared with paroxetine in major depression. J Clin Psychiatry 61:656–663, 2000

Bielski RJ, Bose A, Chang CC: A double-blind comparison of escitalopram and paroxetine in the long-term treatment of generalized anxiety. Ann Clin Psychiatry 17:65–69, 2005

Bird H, Broggini M: Paroxetine versus amitriptyline for the treatment of depression associated with rheumatoid arthritis: a randomized, double blind, parallel group study. J Rheumatol 27:2791–2797, 2000

Blier P, Bergeron R: Effectiveness of pindolol with selected antidepressant drugs in the treatment of major depression. J Clin Psychopharmacol 15:217–222, 1995

Blier P, de Montigny C, Chaput Y: A role for the serotonin system in the mechanism of action of antidepressant treatments: preclinical evidence. J Clin Psychiatry 51 (suppl 4):14–20, 1990

Bordet R, Thomas P, Dupuis B: Effect of pindolol on onset of action of paroxetine in the treatment of major depression: intermediate analysis of a double-blind, placebo-controlled trial. Reseau de Recherche et d'Experimentation Psychopharmacologique. Am J Psychiatry 155:1346–1351, 1998

Borgherini G: The Bioequivalence and Therapeutic Efficacy of Generic Versus Brand-Name Psychoactive Drugs. Clin Therapeutics 25:1578–1593, 2003

Boulenger JP, Huusom AK, Florea I, et al: A comparative study of the efficacy of long-term treatment with escitalopram and paroxetine in severely depressed patients. Curr Med Res Opin 22:1331–1341, 2006

Boyer WF, Blumhardt CL: The safety profile of paroxetine. J Clin Psychiatry 53 (suppl 2):61–66, 1992

Bremner JD, Vermetten E, Charney DS, et al: Long-term treatment with paroxetine increases verbal declarative memory and hippocampal volume in post traumatic stress disorder. Biol Psychiatry 54:693–702, 2003

Brent DA: Paroxetine and the FDA [comment]. J Am Acad Child Adolesc Psychiatry 43:127–128, 2004

Buckley NA, Whyte IM, Dawson AH: Relative toxicity of venlafaxine and selective serotonin reuptake inhibitors in overdose compared to tricyclic antidepressants. Q J Med 96:369–374, 2003

Budman CL, Sherling M, Bruun RD: Combined pharmacotherapy risk. J Am Acad Child Adolesc Psychiatry 34:263–264, 1995

Bump GM, Mulsant BH, Pollock BG, et al: Paroxetine versus nortriptyline in the continuation and maintenance treatment of depression in the elderly. Depress Anxiety 13:38–44, 2001

Carney RM, Blumenthal JA, Freedland KE, et al: Low heart rate variability partially explains the effect on post-MI mortality. Arch Intern Med 165:1486–1491, 2005

Cassano GB, Puca F, Scapicchio PL, et al: Paroxetine and fluoxetine effects on mood and cognitive functions in depressed nondemented elderly patients. J Clin Psychiatry 63:396–402, 2002

Centers for Disease Control and Prevention: Suicide trends among youths and young adults aged 10–24—United States, 1990–2004. MMWR Morb Mortal Wkly Rep 56:905–908, 2007

Centorrino F, Baldessarini RJ, Frankenburg FR, et al: Serum levels of clozapine and norclozapine in patients treated with selective serotonin reuptake inhibitors. Am J Psychiatry 153:820–822, 1996

Chambers CD, Hernandez-Diaz S, Van Marter LJ, et al: Selective serotonin-reuptake inhibitors and risk of persistent pulmonary hypertension of the newborn. N Engl J Med 354:579–587, 2006

Chaput Y, de Montigny C, Blier P, et al: Presynaptic and postsynaptic modifications of the serotonin system by long-term administration of antidepressant treatments. Neuropsychopharmacology 5:219–229, 1991

Charlier C, Broly F, Plomteux G, et al: Polymorphisms in the CYP 2D6 gene: association with plasma concentrations of fluoxetine and paroxetine. Ther Drug Monit 25:738–742, 2003

Cheeta S, Schifano F, Oyefeso A, et al: Antidepressant-related deaths and antidepressant prescriptions in England and Wales, 1998–2000. Br J Psychiatry 184:41–47, 2004

Chouinard G, Saxena B, Belanger MC, et al: A Canadian multicenter, double-blind study of paroxetine and fluoxetine in major depressive disorder. J Affect Disord 54:39–48, 1999

Clayton AH, Pradko JF, Croft HA, et al: Prevalence of sexual dysfunction among newer antidepressants. J Clin Psychiatry 63:357–366, 2002

Cohen LS, Soares CN, Steiner M, et al: Paroxetine controlled release for premenstrual dysphoric disorder: a double-blind, placebo-controlled trial. Psychosom Med 66:707–713, 2004

Cooper SM, Jackson D, Loudon JM, et al: The psychomotor effects of paroxetine alone and in combination with haloperidol, amylobarbitone, oxazepam or alcohol. Acta Psychiatr Scand Suppl 350:53–55, 1989

Costei AM, Kozer E, Koren G, et al: Perinatal outcome following third trimester exposure to paroxetine. Arch Pediatric Adolesc Med 156:1129–1132, 2002

Crewe HK, Lennard MS, Tucker GT, et al: The effect of selective serotonin re-uptake inhibitors on cytochrome P450 2D6 (CYP2D6) activity in human liver microsomes. Br J Clin Pharmacol 34:262–265, 1992

Cubeddu A, Giannini A, Bucci F, et al: Paroxetine increases brain-derived neurotrophic factor in postmenopausal women. Menopause 17:338–343, 2010

Cutler NR, Kramer MS, Reines SA, et al: Single site results from a multicenter study of efficacy and safety of MK-869, an NK-1 antagonist, in patients with major depressive disorder (abstract S.05.4). Int J Neuropsychopharmacol 3 (suppl 1):S7, 2000

Dalhoff K, Almadi TP, Bjerrum K, et al: Pharmacokinetics of paroxetine in patients with cirrhosis. Eur J Clin Pharmacol 41:351–354, 1991

DeVane CL: Pharmacokinetics, drug interactions, and tolerability of paroxetine and paroxetine CR. Psychopharmacol Bull 37 (suppl 1):29–41, 2003

De Wilde J, Spiers R, Mertens C, et al: A double-blind, comparative, multicentre study comparing paroxetine with fluoxetine in depressed patients. Acta Psychiatr Scand 87:141–145, 1993

Diav-Citrin O, Shechtman S, Weinbaum D, et al: Paroxetine and fluoxetine in pregnancy: a prospective, multicentre, controlled, observational study. Br J Clin Pharmacol 66:695–705, 2008

Dimmock PW, Wyatt KM, Jones PW, et al: Efficacy of selective serotonin-reuptake inhibitors in premenstrual syndrome: a systematic review. Lancet 356:1131–1136, 2000

Doyle GD, Laher M, Kelly JG, et al: The pharmacokinetics of paroxetine in renal impairment. Acta Psychiatr Scand Suppl 350:89–90, 1989

Duboff EA: Long-term treatment of major depressive disorder with paroxetine. J Clin Psychopharmacol 13 (suppl 2):28–33, 1993

Dunner DL, Dunbar GC: Optimal dose regimen for paroxetine. J Clin Psychiatry 53 (suppl 2):21–26, 1992

Emslie GJ, Wagner KD, Wilkinson C, et al: Paroxetine treatment in children and adolescents with major depressive disorder: a randomized, multicenter, double-blind, placebo-controlled trial. J Am Acad Child Adolesc Psychiatry 45:709–719, 2006

Eriksson E, Hedberg HA, Andersch B, et al: The serotonin reuptake inhibitor paroxetine is superior to the noradrenaline reuptake inhibitor maprotiline in the treatment of premenstrual syndrome. Neuropsychopharmacology 12:167–176, 1995

Fabian TJ, Amico JA, Pollock BG, et al: Paroxetine-induced hyponatremia in older adults: a 12-week prospective study. Arch Intern Med 164:327–332, 2004

Fang Y, Yuan C, Xu Y, et al: Comparisons of the efficacy and tolerability of extended-release venlafaxine, mirtazapine, and paroxetine in treatment-resistant depression: a double-blind, randomized pilot study in a Chinese population. OPERATION Study Team. J Clin Psychopharmacol 30:357–364, 2010

Fava M, Amsterdam JD, Deltito JA, et al: A double-blind study of paroxetine, fluoxetine, and placebo in outpatients with major depression. Ann Clin Psychiatry 10:145–150, 1998

Fava M, Rosenbaum JF, Hoog SL, et al: Fluoxetine versus sertraline and paroxetine in major depression: tolerability and efficacy in anxious depression. J Affect Disord 59:119–126, 2000

Findling RL, Reed MD, Myers C, et al: Paroxetine pharmacokinetics in depressed children and adolescents. J Am Acad Child Adolesc Psychiatry 38:952–959, 1999

Finley PR: Selective serotonin reuptake inhibitors: pharmacologic profiles and potential therapeutic distinctions. Ann Pharmacother 28:1359–1369, 1994

Frazer A: Serotonergic and noradrenergic reuptake inhibitors: prediction of clinical effects from in vitro potencies. J Clin Psychiatry 62 (suppl 12): 16–23, 2001

Geller DA, Wagner KD, Gardiner C, et al: Paroxetine treatment in children and adolescents with obsessive-compulsive disorder: a randomized, multicenter, double-blind, placebo-controlled trial. J Am Acad Child Adolesc Psychiatry 43:1387–1396, 2004

Geretsegger C, Böhmer F, Ludwig M: Paroxetine in the elderly depressed patient: randomized comparison with fluoxetine of efficacy, cognitive and behavioural effects. Int Clin Psychopharmacol 9:25–29, 1994

Geretsegger C, Stuppaeck CH, Mair M, et al: Multicenter double blind study of paroxetine and amitriptyline in elderly depressed inpatients. Psychopharmacology 199:277–281, 1995

Geretsegger C, Bitterlich W, Stelzig R, et al: Paroxetine with pindolol augmentation: a double-blind, randomized, placebo-controlled study in depressed patients. Eur Neuropsychopharmacol 18:141–146, 2008

Gilmor ML, Owens MJ, Nemeroff CB: Inhibition of norepinephrine uptake in patients with major depression treated with paroxetine. Am J Psychiatry 159:1702–1710, 2002

GlaxoSmithKline: Important Prescribing Information. December 2005. Available at: http://www.gsk.com/media/paroxetine/paxil_letter_e3.pdf. Accessed October 2012.

GlaxoSmithKline: Paroxetine Adult Suicidality Analysis: Major Depressive Disorder and Non-Major Depressive Disorder. Briefing Document. Updated April 5, 2006. Available at: http://www.gsk.com/media/paroxetine/briefing_doc.pdf. Accessed October 2012.

Golden RN, Nemeroff CB, McSorley P, et al: Efficacy and tolerability of controlled-release and immediate-release paroxetine in the treatment of depression. J Clin Psychiatry 63:577–584, 2002

Goldstein DJ, Lu Y, Demitrack MA, et al: Duloxetine in the treatment of depression: a double-blind placebo-controlled comparison with paroxetine. J Clin Psychopharmacol 24:389–399, 2004

Gorman JM, Sloan RP: Heart rate variability in depression and anxiety disorders. Am Heart J 140:77–83, 2000

Greist JH, Jefferson JW, Kobak KA, et al: Efficacy and tolerability of serotonin transport inhibitors in obsessive-compulsive disorder. Arch Gen Psychiatry 52:53–60, 1995

Guillibert E, Pelicier Y, Archambault JC, et al: A double-blind, multicentre study of paroxetine versus clomipramine in depressed elderly patients. Acta Psychiatr Scand Suppl 350:132–134, 1989

Gunasekara NS, Noble S, Benfield P: Paroxetine: an update of its pharmacology and therapeutic use in depression and a review of its use in other disorders. Drugs 55:85–120, 1998

Haenen J, DeBleeker E, Mertens C, et al: An interaction study of paroxetine on lithium levels in depressed patients on lithium therapy. Eur J Clin Res 7:161–167, 1995

Hawley CJ, Quick SJ, Ratnam S, et al: Safety and tolerability of combined treatment with moclobemide and SSRIs: a systemic study of 50 patients. Int Clin Psychopharmacol 11:187–191, 1996

Heim C, Nemeroff CB: The impact of early adverse experiences on brain systems involved in the pathophysiology of anxiety and affective disorders. Biol Psychiatry 46:1509–1522, 1999

Hendrick V, Smith LM, Altshuler L, et al: Birth outcomes after prenatal exposure to antidepressant medication. Am J Obstet Gynecol 188:812–815, 2003a

Hendrick V, Stowe ZN, Haynes D, et al: Placental passage of antidepressant medications. Am J Psychiatry 160:993–996, 2003b

Hiemke C, Härtter S: Pharmacokinetics of selective serotonin reuptake inhibitors. Pharmacol Ther 85:11–28, 2000

Hirschfeld RMA: Panic disorder: diagnosis, epidemiology, and clinical course. J Clin Psychiatry 57 (suppl 10):3–8, 1996

Horrigan JP, Barnhill LJ: Paroxetine-pimozide drug interaction. J Am Acad Child Adolesc Psychiatry 33:1060–1061, 1994

Hostetter A, Stowe ZN, Strader JR, et al: Dose of selective serotonin uptake inhibitors across pregnancy: clinical implications. Depress Anxiety 11:51–57, 2000

Hutchinson DR, Tong S, Moon CA, et al: Paroxetine in the treatment of elderly depressed patients in general practice: a double-blind comparison with amitriptyline. Int Clin Psychopharmacol 6 (suppl 4):43–51, 1992

Hyttel J: Pharmacological characterization of selective serotonin reuptake inhibitors (SSRIs). Int Clin Psychopharmacol 9 (suppl 1):19–26, 1994

Inman W, Kubota K, Pearce G, et al: PEM report number 6: paroxetine. Pharmacoepidemiol Drug Saf 2:393–422, 1993

Jenner PN: Paroxetine: an overview of dosage, tolerability, and safety. Int Clin Psychiatry 6 (suppl 4): 69–80, 1992

John L, Perreault M, Tao T: Serotonin syndrome associated with nefazodone and paroxetine. Ann Emerg Med 29:287–289, 1997

Johnson H, Bouman WP, Lawton J: Withdrawal reaction associated with venlafaxine. BMJ 317:787, 1998

Judge R, Parry MG, Quail D, Jacobson JG: Discontinuation symptoms: comparison of brief interruption in fluoxetine and paroxetine treatment. Int Clin Psychopharmacol 17:217–225, 2002

Kasper S, Baldwin DS, Larsson Lonn S, et al: Superiority of escitalopram to paroxetine in the treatment of depression. Eur Neuropsychopharmacol 19:229–237, 2009

Kaye CM, Haddock RE, Langley PF, et al: A review of the metabolism and pharmacokinetics of paroxetine in man. Acta Psychiatr Scand Suppl 350:60–75, 1989

Keller MB, Ryan ND, Strober M, et al: Efficacy of paroxetine in the treatment of adolescent major depression: a randomized, controlled trial. J Am Acad Child Adolesc Psychiatry 40:762–772, 2001

Kelly CM, Juurlink DN, Gomes T, et al: Selective serotonin reuptake inhibitors and breast cancer mortality in women receiving tamoxifen: a population based cohort study. BMJ 340:c693, 2010

Kent JM, Coplan JD, Lombardo I, et al: Occupancy of brain serotonin transporters during treatment with paroxetine in patients with social phobia: a positron emission tomography study with [11C] McN 5652. Psychopharmacology (Berl) 164:341–348, 2002

Kim Y, Asukai N, Konishi T, et al: Clinical evaluation of paroxetine in post-traumatic stress disorder (PTSD): 52-week, non-comparative open-label study for clinical use experience. Psychiatry Clin Neurosci 62:646–652, 2008

Knoppert DC, Nimkar R, Principi T, et al: Paroxetine toxicity in a newborn after in utero exposure: clinical symptoms correlate with serum levels. Ther Drug Monit 28:5–7, 2006

Kraus JE, Horrigan JP, Carpenter DJ, et al: Clinical features of patients with treatment-emergent suicidal behavior following initiation of paroxetine therapy. J Affect Disord 120:40–47, 2010

Kulin NA, Pastuszak A, Sage SR, et al: Pregnancy outcome following maternal use of the new selective serotonin reuptake inhibitors. JAMA 279:609–610, 1998

Laine K, Kytola J, Bertilsson L: Severe adverse effects in a newborn with two defective CYP2D6 alleles after exposure to paroxetine during late pregnancy. Ther Drug Monit 26:685–687, 2004

Landen M, Nissbrandt H, Allgulander C, et al: Placebo-controlled trial comparing intermittent and continuous paroxetine in premenstrual dysphoric disorder. Neuropsychopharmacology 32:153–161, 2007

Landen M, Erlandsson H, Bengtsson F, et al: Short onset of action of a serotonin reuptake inhibitor when used to reduce premenstrual irritability. Neuropsychopharmacology 34:585–592, 2009

Lane RM: Pharmacokinetic drug interaction potential of selective serotonin reuptake inhibitors. Int Clin Psychopharmacol 11 (suppl 5):31–61, 1996

Lecrubier Y, Judge R: Long-term evaluation of paroxetine, clomipramine and placebo in panic disorder. Collaborative Paroxetine Panic Study Investigators. Acta Psychiatr Scand 95:153–160, 1997

Lecrubier Y, Bakker A, Dunbar G, et al: A comparison of paroxetine, clomipramine and placebo in the treatment of panic disorder. Acta Psychiatr Scand 95:145–152, 1997

Leung M, Ong M: Lack of an interaction between sumatriptan and selective serotonin reuptake inhibitors. Headache 35:488–489, 1995

Liebowitz MR, Gelenberg AJ, Munjack D: Venlafaxine extended release vs placebo and paroxetine in social anxiety disorder. Arch Gen Psychiatry 62:190–198, 2005

Liston HL, DeVane CL, Goldman J, et al: Differential time course of cytochrome P450 2D6 enzyme inhibition by fluoxetine, sertraline, and paroxetine in healthy volunteers. J Clin Psychopharmacol 22:169–173, 2002

Lotrich FE, Pollock BG, Kirshner M, et al: Serotonin transporter genotype interacts with paroxetine plasma levels to influence depression treatment response in geriatric patients. J Psychiatry Neurosci 33:123–130, 2008

Lydiard RB, Bobes J: Therapeutic advances: paroxetine for the treatment of social anxiety disorder. Depress Anxiety 11:99–104, 2000

Magnussen I, Tønder K, Engbaek F: Paroxetine, a potent selective long-acting inhibitor of synaptosomal 5-HT uptake in mice. J Neural Transm 55:217–226, 1982

Malek-Ahmadi P, Allen SA: Paroxetine-molindone interaction. J Clin Psychiatry 56:82–83, 1995

Mancini C, van Amerigen M: Paroxetine in social phobia. J Clin Psychiatry 57:519–522, 1996

Marshall RD, Schneier FR, Fallow BA, et al: An open trial of paroxetine in patients with noncombat-related, chronic posttraumatic stress disorder. J Clin Psychiatry 18:10–18, 1998

Marshall RD, Beebe KL, Oldham M, et al: Efficacy and safety of paroxetine treatment for chronic PTSD: a fixed dose, placebo-controlled study. Am J Psychiatry 158:1982–1988, 2001

Martinez D, Broft A, Laruelle M: Pindolol augmentation of antidepressant treatment: recent contributions from brain imaging studies. Biol Psychiatry 48:844–853, 2000

Masand PS, Gupta S, Schwartz T, et al: Paroxetine in patients with irritable bowel syndrome (IBS): a pilot open-label study. Paper presented at the New Clinical Drug Evaluation Unit (NCDEU), Phoenix, AZ, May 2001

Meston CM: A randomized, placebo-controlled, crossover study of ephedrine for SSRI-induced female sexual dysfunction. J Sex Marital Ther 30:57–68, 2004

Meyer JH, Wilson AA, Ginovart N, et al: Occupancy of serotonin transporters by paroxetine and citalopram during treatment of depression: a [11C]DASB PET imaging study. Am J Psychiatry 158:1843–1849, 2001

Michelson D, Fava M, Amsterdam J, et al: Interruption of selective serotonin reuptake inhibitor treatment. Br J Psychiatry 176:363–368, 2000

Montejo-Gonzalez AL, Llorca G, Izquierdo JA, et al: SSRI-induced sexual dysfunction: fluoxetine, paroxetine, sertraline, and fluvoxamine in a prospective, multicenter, and descriptive clinical study of 344 patients. J Sex Marital Ther 23:176–194, 1997

Montgomery SA: A meta-analysis of the efficacy and tolerability of paroxetine versus tricyclic antidepressants in the treatment of major depression. Int Clin Psychopharmacol 16:169–178, 2001

Montgomery SA, Dunbar G: Paroxetine is better than placebo in relapse prevention and the prophylaxis of recurrent depression. Int Clin Psychopharmacol 8:189–195, 1993

Montgomery SA, Kennedy SH, Burrows GD, et al: Absence of discontinuation symptoms with agomelatine and occurrence of discontinuation symptoms with paroxetine: a randomized, double-blind, placebo-controlled discontinuation study. Int Clin Psychopharmacol 19:271–280, 2004

Murphy GM Jr, Kremer C, Rodrigues HE, et al: Pharmacogenetics of antidepressant medication intolerance. Am J Psychiatry 160:1830–1835, 2003

Murphy GM Jr, Hollander SB, Schatzberg AF, et al: Effects of the serotonin transporter gene promoter polymorphism on mirtazapine and paroxetine efficacy and adverse events in geriatric major depression. Arch Gen Psychiatry 61:1163–1169, 2004

Musselman DL, Lawson DH, Gumnick JF, et al: Paroxetine for the prevention of depression induced by high-dose interferon alpha. N Engl J Med 344:961–966, 2001

Nakhai-Pour HR, Broy P, Berard A: Use of antidepressants during pregnancy and the risk of spontaneous abortion. CMAJ 182:1031–1037, 2010

Nardi AE, Freire RC, Mochcovitch MD, et al: A randomized, naturalistic, parallel-group study for the long-term treatment of panic disorder with clonazepam or paroxetine. J Clin Psychopharmacol 32:120–126, 2012

Nebes RD, Pollock BG, Mulsant BH, et al: Cognitive effects of paroxetine in older depressed patients. J Clin Psychiatry 60 (suppl 20):26–29, 1999

Nemeroff CB: Paroxetine: an overview of the efficacy and safety of a new selective serotonin reuptake inhibitor in the treatment of depression. J Clin Psychopharmacol 13 (suppl 2):10–17, 1993

Nemeroff CB: The corticotropin-releasing factor (CRF) hypothesis of depression. Mol Psychiatry 1:336–342, 1996

Nemeroff CB, DeVane CL, Pollock BG: Newer antidepressants and the cytochrome P450 system. Am J Psychiatry 153:311–320, 1996

Nemeroff CB, Evans DL, Laszlo G, et al: Double-blind, placebo-controlled comparison of imipramine and paroxetine in the treatment of bipolar depression. Am J Psychiatry 158:906–912, 2001

Nemeroff CB, Etsuah AR, Willard LB, et al: Venlafaxine and SSRIs: pooled remission analysis (New Research Abstract NR263). Program and abstracts of the American Psychiatric Association 156th Annual Meeting, San Francisco, CA, May 17–22, 2003

Nemeroff CB, Kalali A, Schatzberg A, et al: Impact of publicity concerning pediatric suicidality data on physician practice patterns in the United States. Arch Gen Psychiatry 64:466–472, 2007

Newport J, Stowe ZN, Nemeroff CB: Parental depression: animal models of an adverse life event. Am J Psychiatry 158:1265–1283, 2002

Oehrberg S, Christiansen PE, Behnke K, et al: Paroxetine in the treatment of panic disorder. Br J Psychiatry 167:374–379, 1995

Ohman R, Hägg S, Carleborg L, et al: Excretion of paroxetine into breast milk. J Clin Psychiatry 60:519–523, 1999

Owens MJ, Morgan WN, Plott SJ, et al: Neurotransmitter receptor and transporter binding profiles of antidepressants and their metabolites. J Pharmacol Exp Ther 283:1305–1322, 1997

Owens MJ, Krulewicz S, Simon JS, et al: Estimates of serotonin and norepinephrine transporter inhibition in depressed patients treated with paroxetine or venlafaxine. Neuropsychopharmacology 33:3201–3212, 2008

Ozdemir V, Naranjo CA, Herrmann N, et al: Paroxetine potentiates central nervous system side effects of perphenazine: contribution of cytochrome P4502D6 inhibition in vivo. Clin Pharmacol Ther 62:334–347, 1997

Paxil (package insert). Research Triangle Park, NC, GlaxoSmithKline, 2001

Paxil CR (package insert). Research Triangle Park, NC, GlaxoSmithKline, 2002

Perez V, Soler J, Puigdemont D, et al: A double-blind, randomized, placebo-controlled trial of pindolol augmentation in depressive patients resistant to serotonin reuptake inhibitors. Grup de Recerca en Trastorns Afectius. Arch Gen Psychiatry 56:375–379, 1999

Piccinelli M, Pini S, Bellantuono C, et al: Efficacy of drug treatment in OCD: a meta-analysis review. Br J Psychiatry 166:424–443, 1995

Poirier MF, Boyer P: Venlafaxine and paroxetine in treatment-resistant depression. Br J Psychiatry 175:12–16, 1999

Pollack MH, Rocco Z, Goddard A, et al: Paroxetine in the treatment of generalized anxiety disorder: results of a placebo-controlled, flexible-dosage trial. J Clin Psychiatry 62:350–357, 2001

Preskorn SH: Pharmacokinetics of antidepressants: why and how they are relevant to treatment. J Clin Psychiatry 54 (suppl 9):14–34, 1993

Price JS, Waller PC, Wood SM, et al: A comparison of the post-marketing safety of four selective serotonin re-uptake inhibitors including the investigation of symptoms occurring on withdrawal. Br J Clin Psychopharmacol 42:757–763, 1996

Rapaport MH, Lydiard RB, Pitts CD, et al: Low doses of controlled-release paroxetine in the treatment of late-life depression: a randomized, placebo-controlled trial. J Clin Psychiatry 70:46–57, 2009

Rasmussen SA, Eisen JL, Pato MT: Current issues in the pharmacologic management of obsessive compulsive disorder. J Clin Psychiatry 54 (suppl 6):4–9, 1993

Rechlin T: The effect of amitriptyline, doxepin, fluvoxamine and paroxetine treatment on heart rate variability. J Clin Psychopharmacol 14:392–395, 1994

Reeves R, Bullen J: Serotonin syndrome produced by paroxetine and low-dose trazodone. Psychosomatics 36:159–160, 1995

Reynolds CF III, Dew MA, Kupfer DJ, et al: Maintenance treatment of major depression in old age. N Engl J Med 354:1130–1138, 2006

Richard IH, McDermott MP, Kurlan R, et al: A randomized, double-blind, placebo-controlled trial of antidepressants in Parkinson disease. SAD-PD Study Group. Neurology 78:1229–1236, 2012

Rickels K, Zaninelli R, Sheehan D, et al: Paroxetine treatment of generalized anxiety disorder: a double-blind, placebo-controlled study. Am J Psychiatry 160:749–756, 2003

Riddle MA: Paroxetine and the FDA [comment]. J Am Acad Child Adolesc Psychiatry 43:128–130, 2004

Rocca P, Fonzo V, Scotta M, et al: Paroxetine efficacy in the treatment of generalized anxiety disorder. Acta Psychiatr Scand 95:444–450, 1997

Roose SP, Laghrissi-Thode F, Kennedy JS, et al: Comparison of paroxetine and nortriptyline in depressed patients with ischemic heart disease. JAMA 279:287–291, 1998

Rosen RC, Lane RM, Menza M: Effects of SSRIs on sexual function: a critical review. J Clin Psychiatry 19:67–85, 1999

Rosenbaum JF, Fava M, Hoog SL, et al: Selective serotonin reuptake inhibitor discontinuation syndrome: a randomized clinical trial. Biol Psychiatry 44:77–87, 1998

Ruhe HG, Booij J, v Weert H, et al: Evidence why paroxetine dose escalation is not effective in major depressive disorder: a randomized controlled trial with assessment of serotonin transporter occupancy. Neuropsychopharmacology 34:999–1010, 2009a

Ruhe HG, Ooteman W, Booij J, et al: Serotonin transporter gene promoter polymorphisms modify the association between paroxetine serotonin transporter occupancy and clinical response in major depressive disorder. Pharmacogenet Genomics 19:67–76, 2009b

Sachs GS, Nierenberg MD, Thase ME, et al: Effectiveness of adjunctive antidepressant treatment for bipolar depression. N Engl J Med 356:1711–1722, 2007

Safarinejad MR: Comparison of dapoxetine versus paroxetine in patients with premature ejaculation: a double-blind, placebo-controlled, fixed-dose, randomized study. Clin Neuropharmacol 29:243–252, 2006

Schneeweiss S, Patrick AR, Solomon DH, et al: Comparative safety of antidepressant agents for children and adolescents regarding suicidal acts. Pediatrics 125:876–888, 2010a

Schneeweiss S, Patrick AR, Solomon DH, et al: Variation in the risk of suicide attempts and completed suicides by antidepressant agent in adults: a propensity score-adjusted analysis of 9 years' data. Arch Gen Psychiatry 67:497–506, 2010b

Schneier FR, Neria Y, Pavlicova M, et al: Combined prolonged exposure therapy and paroxetine for PTSD related to the World Trade Center attack: a randomized controlled trial. Am J Psychiatry 169:80-88, 2012

Schöne W, Ludwig M: A double-blind study of paroxetine compared with fluoxetine in geriatric patients with major depression. J Clin Psychopharmacol 13 (6, suppl 2):34S–39S, 1993

Sharma A, Goldberg MJ, Cerimele BJ: Pharmacokinetics and safety of duloxetine, a dual serotonin and norepinephrine reuptake inhibitor. J Clin Pharmacol 40:161–167, 2000

Shelton C, Entsuah R, Padmanabhan SK, et al: Venlafaxine XR demonstrates higher rates of sustained remission compared to fluoxetine, paroxetine or placebo. Int Clin Psychopharmacol 20:233–238, 2005

Sindrup SH, Brøsen K, Gram LF: Pharmacokinetics of the selective serotonin reuptake inhibitor paroxetine: nonlinearity and relation to the sparteine oxidation polymorphism. Clin Pharmacol Ther 51:288–295, 1992a

Sindrup SH, Brøsen K, Gram LF, et al: The relationship between paroxetine and sparteine oxidation polymorphism. Clin Pharmacol Ther 51:278–287, 1992b

Skop BP, Finkelstein JA, Mareth TR: The serotonin syndrome associated with paroxetine, an over-the-counter cold remedy, and vascular disease. Am J Emerg Med 12:642–644, 1994

Soares CN, Joffe H, Cohen LS, et al: Paroxetine versus placebo for women in midlife after hormone therapy discontinuation. Am J Med 121:159–162, 2008

Stearns V, Isaacs C, Rowland J, et al: A pilot trial assessing the efficacy of paroxetine hydrochloride (Paxil) in controlling hot flashes in breast cancer survivors. Ann Oncol 11:17–22, 2000

Stearns V, Beebe KL, Iyengar M, et al: Paroxetine controlled release in the treatment of menopausal hot flashes: a randomized controlled trial. JAMA 289:2827–2834, 2003

Stearns V, Slack R, Isaacs C, et al: Paroxetine is an effective treatment for hot flashes: results from a prospective randomized clinical trial. J Clin Oncol 23:6919–6930, 2005

Stein DJ, Versiani M, Hair T, et al: Efficacy of paroxetine for relapse prevention in social anxiety disorder: a 24-week study. Arch Gen Psychiatry 59:1111–1118, 2002

Stein MB, Chartier MJ, Hazen AL, et al: Paroxetine in the treatment of generalized social phobia: open-label treatment and double-blind, placebo-controlled discontinuation. J Clin Psychopharmacol 16:218–222, 1996

Stein MB, Liebowitz MR, Lydiard RB, et al: Paroxetine treatment of generalized social phobia (social anxiety disorder): a randomized controlled trial. JAMA 280:708–713, 1998

Steiner M, Hirschberg AL, Van Erp E, et al: Luteal phase dosing with paroxetine controlled release (CR) in the treatment of premenstrual dysphoric disorder. Am J Obstet Gynecol 193:352–360, 2005

Steiner M, Ravindran AV, LeMelledo JM, et al: Luteal phase administration of paroxetine for the treatment of premenstrual dysphoric disorder: a randomized, double-blind, placebo-controlled trial in Canadian women. J Clin Psychiatry 69:991–998, 2008

Stiskal JA: Defective alleles may not have contributed to adverse effects. Ther Drug Monit 27:683, 2005

Stiskal JA: Defective alleles may not have contributed to adverse effects [comment]. Ther Drug Monit 28:142, 2006

Stocchi F, Nordera G, Jokinen RH, et al: Efficacy and tolerability of paroxetine for the long-term treatment of generalized anxiety disorder. Paroxetine Generalized Anxiety Disorder Study Team. J Clin Psychiatry 64:250–258, 2003

Stowe ZN, Cohen L, Hostetter A, et al: Paroxetine in human breast milk and nursing infants. Am J Psychiatry 157:185–189, 2000

Strachan J, Shepherd J: Hyponatremia associated with the use of selective serotonin re-uptake inhibitors. Aust N Z J Psychiatry 32:295–298, 1998

Sunblad C, Wikander I, Andersch B, et al: A naturalistic study of paroxetine in premenstrual syndrome: efficacy and side-effects during ten cycles of treatment. Eur Neuropsychopharmacol 7:201–206, 1997

Tanrikut C, Feldman AS, ALtemus M, et al: Adverse effect of paroxetine on sperm. Fertil Steril 94: 1021–1026, 2010

Tasker TCG, Kaye CM, Zussman BD, et al: Paroxetine plasma levels: lack of correlation with efficacy or adverse events. Acta Psychiatr Scand Suppl 350:152–155, 1989

Thomas DR, Nelson DR, Johnson AM: Biochemical effects of the antidepressant paroxetine, a specific 5-hydroxytryptamine uptake inhibitor. Psychopharmacology (Berl) 93:193–200, 1987.

Tignol J: A double-blind, randomized, fluoxetine-controlled, multicenter study of paroxetine in the treatment of depression. J Clin Psychopharmacol 13 (suppl 2):18–22, 1993

Tome MB, Isaac MT, Harte R, et al: Paroxetine and pindolol: a randomized trial of serotonergic receptor blockade in the reduction of antidepressant latency. Int Clin Psychopharmacol 12:81–89, 1997.

Tucker P, Zaninelli R, Yehuda R, et al: Paroxetine in the treatment of chronic posttraumatic stress disorder: results of a placebo-controlled, flexible dosage trial. J Clin Psychiatry 62:860–868, 2001

Tucker P, Beebe KL, Nawar O, et al: Paroxetine treatment of depression with posttraumatic stress disorder: effects on autonomic reactivity and cortisol secretion. J Clin Psychopharmacol 24:131–140, 2004

Tulloch IF, Johnson AM: The pharmacologic profile of paroxetine, a new selective serotonin reuptake inhibitor. J Clin Psychiatry 53 (suppl):7–12, 1992

U.S. Food and Drug Administration: FDA Statement Regarding the Antidepressant Paxil for Pediatric Population. June 19, 2003. Available at: http://www.fda.gov/bbs/topics/ANSWERS/2003/ANS01230.html. Accessed September 2008.

U.S. Food and Drug Administration: New Warnings Proposed for Antidepressants. May 3, 2007. (FDA Consumer Health Information, Consumer Updates archive) Available at: http://www.fda.gov/consumer/updates/antidepressants050307.html. Accessed September 2008.

Ververs FF, Voorbij HA, Zwarts P, et al: Effect of cytochrome P450 2D6 genotype on maternal paroxetine plasma concentrations during pregnancy. Clin Pharmacokinet 48:677–683, 2009

Wagner KD, Berard R, Machin A, et al: A multicenter, randomized, double-blind, placebo-controlled trial of paroxetine in children and adolescents with social anxiety disorder. Arch Gen Psychiatry 61:1153–1162, 2004

Wagstaff AJ, Cheer SM, Matheson AJ, et al: Paroxetine: an update of its use in psychiatric disorders in adults. Drugs 62:655–703, 2002

Waldinger MD, Hengeveld MW, Zwinderman AH, et al: Effect of SSRI antidepressants on ejaculation: a double-blind, randomized, placebo-controlled study with fluoxetine, fluvoxamine, paroxetine, and sertraline. J Clin Psychopharmacol 18:274–281, 1998

Waldinger MD, Zwinderman AH, Olivier B: Antidepressants and ejaculation: a double-blind, randomized, fixed-dose study with mirtazapine and paroxetine. J Clin Psychopharmacol 23:467–470, 2003

Weihs KL, Settle EC, Batey SR, et al: Bupropion sustained-release versus paroxetine for the treatment of depression in the elderly. J Clin Psychiatry 61:196–202, 2000

Weiner AL, Tilden FF, McKay CA: Serotonin syndrome: case report and review of the literature. Conn Med 61:717–721, 1997

Weitzner MA, Moncello J, Jacobsen PB, et al: A pilot trial of paroxetine in the treatment of hot flashes and associated symptoms associated with breast cancer. J Pain Symptom Manage 23:337–345, 2002

West CHK, Ritchie JC, Weiss JM: Paroxetine-induced increase in activity of locus coeruleus neurons in adolescent rats: implication of a countertherapeutic effect of an antidepressant. Neuropsychopharmacology 35:1653–1663, 2010

Wetzel H, Anghelescu I, Szegedi A, et al: Pharmacokinetic interactions of clozapine with selective serotonin reuptake inhibitors: differential effects of fluvoxamine and paroxetine in a prospective study. J Clin Psychopharmacol 18:2–9, 1998

Wu KY, Liu CY, Hsiao MC: Six month paroxetine treatment of premenstrual dysphoric disorder: continuous versus intermittent treatment protocols. Psychiatry Clin Neurosci 62:109–114, 2008

Wurst KE, Poole C, Ephross SA, et al: First trimester paroxetine use and the prevalence of congenital, specifically cardiac, defects: a meta-analysis of epidemiological studies. Birth Defects Res A Clin Mol Teratol 88:159–170, 2010

Yonkers KA, Gullion C, Williams BA, et al: Paroxetine as a treatment for premenstrual dysphoric disorder. J Clin Psychopharmacol 16:3–8, 1996

Yonkers KA, Wisner KL, Stewart DE, et al: The management of depression during pregnancy: a report from the American Psychiatric Association and the American College of Obstetricians and Gynecologists. Gen Hosp Psychiatry 31:403–413, 2009

Zanardi R, Franchini L, Gasperini M, et al: Double-blind controlled trial of sertraline versus paroxetine in the treatment of delusional depression. Am J Psychiatry 153:1631–1633, 1996

Zanardi R, Artigas F, Franchini L, et al: How long should pindolol be associated with paroxetine to improve the antidepressant response? J Clin Psychopharmacol 17:446–450, 1997

Zanardi R, Benedetti F, Smeraldi E, et al: Efficacy of paroxetine in depression is influenced by a functional polymorphism within the promoter of the serotonin transporter gene. J Clin Psychopharmacol 20:105–107, 2000

Zis AP, Grof P, Webster M, et al: Prediction of relapse in recurrent affective disorder. Psychopharmacol Bull 16:47–49, 1980

Zohar J, Judge R: Paroxetine versus clomipramine in the treatment of obsessive-compulsive disorder. Br J Psychiatry 169:468–474, 1996

CHAPTER 5

Fluvoxamine

Elias Aboujaoude, M.D.

Lorrin M. Koran, M.D.

Structure-Activity Relations

Fluvoxamine was the first selective serotonin reuptake inhibitor (SSRI) to reach the market (Buchberger and Wagner 2002). It belongs to the 2-aminoethyl oxime ethers of the aralkyl ketones and is chemically identified as 5-methoxy-4′-(trifluoromethyl) valerophenone-(E)-O-(2-aminoethyl) oxime maleate (1:1). Fluvoxamine's empirical formula is C15H21O2N2F3.C4H4O4, and it does not have a chiral center or exist in stereoisomers. Because of local irritant properties, fluvoxamine cannot be administered parenterally (Physicians' Desk Reference 2002).

Mechanism of Action

Like other SSRIs, fluvoxamine binds to the presynaptic serotonin transporter (SERT) and prevents it from absorbing serotonin back into the presynaptic terminals. This increases the amount of serotonin in the synaptic cleft. How this increase translates into efficacy remains unclear, but it has been hypothesized to involve downstream effects, including serotonin$_{1A}$ (5-HT$_{1A}$) autoreceptor desensitization (Stahl 1998); increased sensitivity of dopamine$_2$ (D$_2$)-like receptors in the nucleus accumbens (Gershon et al. 2007), enhanced neurogenesis (Dranovsky and Hen 2006), and individual pharmacogenomic factors involving SERT gene variants (Mancama and Kerwin 2003). Furthermore, sigma-1 receptors appear to modulate several neurotransmitter pathways, and evidence suggests that fluvoxamine's affinity for the sigma-1 receptor exceeds that of all other SSRIs (Ishikawa et al. 2007).

Pharmacological Profile

Fluvoxamine is a more potent inhibitor of serotonin reuptake than the tricyclic antidepressants, including clomipramine, but is less potent than the other SSRIs. It is highly selective for the serotonin transporter (K_i = 2.3 nmol/L) and has minimal affinity for the norepinephrine and dopamine transporters, or the muscarinic, α_1-adrenergic, histaminic, and 5-HT$_{2C}$ receptors. It possesses no monoamine oxidase–inhibiting properties (Lapierre et al. 1983; Owens et al. 2001; Palmer and Benfield 1994; Ware 1997).

Pharmacokinetics and Disposition

Fluvoxamine is almost entirely absorbed from the gastrointestinal tract, regardless of the presence of food (Van Harten 1995). Still, first-pass metabolism limits oral bioavailability to 53% (DeVane 2003; DeVane and Gill 1997). Peak plasma concentrations occur within 2–8 hours, and steady-state concentration is achieved within 10 days (Van Harten 1995). Plasma concentration shows no consistent correlation with efficacy or side effects, thus limiting the value of monitoring concentration.

The mean half-life of fluvoxamine is 15 hours, making twice-daily dosing preferable. Despite fluvoxamine's relatively short half-life, a discontinuation syndrome is rare (Buchberger and Wagner 2002), possibly because of the drug's slower elimination from the brain (Strauss et al. 1998).

Because fluvoxamine is widely distributed and reaches higher concentrations in the brain and other organs than in plasma (Benfield and Ward 1986), patients receiving hemodialysis do not require replacement doses; re-equilibration should occur (DeVane and Gill 1997).

Compared with other SSRIs, fluvoxamine's rate of protein binding is relatively low (77%) (DeVane and Gill 1997), which implies less risk of interactions from drug displacement.

At least 11 products of fluvoxamine metabolism are known, but none seems pharmacologically active (DeVane and Gill 1997; Palmer and Benfield 1994). Metabolism is thought to occur primarily through oxidative demethylation. Only minimal amounts of fluvoxamine (3%) are excreted unchanged by the kidneys, suggesting that renal impairment should not significantly alter fluvoxamine's pharmacokinetics (Van Harten 1995).

Because hepatic clearance is decreased in patients with liver disease and in elderly patients, dosage adjustments are sometimes necessary (DeVane and Gill 1997; Van Harten et al. 1993). No gender-based differences in concentration seem to exist in adults (DeVane and Gill 1997). Pharmacokinetics studies in children report a higher area under the curve (AUC) than in adolescents, with the difference being more pronounced in females, suggesting lower dosages may be sufficient in children. No appreciable pharmacokinetic differences were observed between adolescents and adults (Physicians' Desk Reference 2002).

In the United States, fluvoxamine is available in both immediate-release and controlled-release formulations.

Indications and Efficacy

Depression

The first trial of fluvoxamine treatment of depression dates to 1976. Since then, several randomized, single- or double-blind studies conducted have tested fluvoxamine's antidepressant efficacy against placebo, SSRIs, serotonin–norepinephrine reuptake inhibitors, tricyclic antidepressants, tetracyclic antidepressants, and a reversible inhibitor of monoamine oxidase. The trials vary in design but, taken together, support the efficacy and safety of fluvoxamine in treating depression—including psychotic depression—across all age groups (Fukuchi and Kanemoto 2002; Haffmans et al. 1996; Kiev and Feiger 1997; Otsubo et al. 2005; Rapaport et al. 1996; Rossini et al. 2005; Ware 1997; Zanardi et al. 2000; Zohar et al. 2003). Study durations ranged from 4 to 7 weeks, and dosages ranged from 50 to 300 mg/day. Further, benefits from fluvoxamine seem to be sustained over at least 1 year (Terra and Montgomery 1998).

In a well-designed recent analysis of 54 randomized controlled trials (N = 5,122), no strong evidence was found to indicate that fluvoxamine was either superior or inferior to other antidepressants regarding response and remission (Omori et al. 2010). However, differing side-effect profiles were evident, especially with regard to worse nausea and vomiting when compared to some other antidepressants.

Finally, because of fluvoxamine's potent sigma-1 agonist action and the putative antipsychotic property such action might confer, some authors have suggested that fluvoxamine monotherapy might be a useful alternative to combined treatment with an antidepressant and an antipsychotic in cases of psychotic depression (Furuse and Hashimoto 2009).

Obsessive-Compulsive Disorder in Adults

The first formal test of fluvoxamine in the treatment of obsessive-compulsive disorder (OCD) took place in 1987 (Price et al. 1987). Since then, multiple randomized studies have established fluvoxamine's efficacy and safety in treating OCD. These trials have compared fluvoxamine with placebo, clomipramine, and other SSRIs.

In randomized, double-blind comparisons with placebo, subjects were given fluvoxamine 100–300 mg/day for 6–10 weeks. Significant improvements in Yale-Brown Obsessive Compulsive Scale (Y-BOCS) scores were observed, and response rates ranged from 38% to 52% (vs. 0% to 18% for placebo) (Figgitt and McClellan 2000).

We identified five published double-blind comparisons of fluvoxamine and clomipramine, both dosed at ≤300 mg/day, involving a total of 531 subjects and lasting 9–10 weeks (Figgitt and McClellan 2000; Freeman et al. 1994; Koran et al. 1996; Milanfranchi et al. 1997; Mundo et al. 2000, 2001). All studies demonstrated equal efficacy for the two agents (range of response rates: 56%–85% for fluvoxamine and 53%–83% for clomipramine). One small published study compared fluvoxamine with other SSRIs. This 10-week single-blind study of 30 subjects randomly assigned to fluvoxamine, paroxetine, or citalopram suggested similar efficacy (Mundo et al. 1997).

Long-term maintenance treatment with fluvoxamine seems to protect against relapse. A 2-year open-label follow-up study enrolling 130 subjects who had responded to fluvoxamine 300 mg/day, clomipramine 150 mg/day, or fluoxetine 40 mg/day showed that maintenance treatment at full or half dosages was significantly superior to treatment discontinuation in preventing relapse (Ravizza et al. 1996).

Obsessive-Compulsive Disorder in Children and Adolescents

Fluvoxamine 50–200 mg/day was tested in a 10-week double-blind, placebo-controlled study involving 120 subjects ages 8–17 years with OCD. Response was defined as a reduction of at least 25% in the Children's Yale-Brown Obsessive Compulsive Scale (CY-BOCS) score. Mean scores were significantly lower in the fluvoxamine group as early as week 1 ($P<0.05$). End-of-study response rates were 42% for the fluvoxamine group versus 26% for the placebo group ($P=0.065$). The most common side effects were insomnia and asthenia (Riddle et al. 2001).

Panic Disorder

The largest randomized, double-blind, placebo-controlled study to test fluvoxamine in the treatment of panic disorder involved 188 subjects who were assigned to 8 weeks of fluvoxamine 100–300 mg/day or placebo. At study end, significantly more subjects in the fluvoxamine group were free from panic attacks (69% vs. 46%, $P=0.002$) (Figgitt and McClellan 2000).

Limited data suggest similar efficacy between fluvoxamine and the tricyclic antidepressant imipramine, as well as a possible potentiating effect of fluvoxamine when combined with cognitive or exposure therapy (Figgitt and McClellan 2000).

Social Anxiety Disorder

The largest double-blind, placebo-controlled study to assess the effectiveness of fluvoxamine (50–300 mg/day) in social anxiety disorder recruited 92 subjects with social phobia (Stein et al. 1999). Significantly more subjects assigned to fluvoxamine responded (43% vs. 23%, $P=0.04$), as determined by a rating of much or very much improved on the global improvement item of the Clinical Global Impressions Scale. More recently, a controlled-release (CR) formulation of fluvoxamine showed similarly good results in two randomized, double-blind studies (Davidson et al. 2004; Westenberg et al. 2004). This formulation was approved in the United States in 2008 for the treatment of social anxiety disorder and OCD.

Posttraumatic Stress Disorder

Small open-label studies suggest a role for fluvoxamine in treating posttraumatic stress disorder (PTSD) (Davidson et al. 1998; Figgitt and McClellan 2000; Marmar et al. 1996; Tucker et al. 2000). Twenty-four Dutch veterans of World War II with chronic PTSD showed significant improvement on a PTSD self-rating scale after a 12-week course of fluvoxamine at ≤300 mg/day ($P=0.04$) (De Boer et al. 1992). More recently, a 14-week open-label trial of fluvoxamine (100–300 mg/day) in 15 U.S. veterans with combat-related PTSD reported a statistically significant decrease in the Clinician-Administered PTSD Scale (CAPS) total score ($P<0.001$) (Escalona et al. 2002).

Obsessive-Compulsive Spectrum Disorders

Three open-label trials of fluvoxamine, involving a total of 75 subjects with body dysmorphic disorder, reported response rates of 63%–67% (Perugi et al. 1996; Phillips et al. 1998, 2001).

Like other SSRIs, fluvoxamine has produced inconsistent results when tested in impulse-control disorders considered part of the obsessive-compulsive spectrum. Despite encouraging open-label data in compulsive buying disorder (Black et al. 1997), two double-blind, placebo-controlled studies failed to show benefit over placebo (Black et al. 2000; Ninan et al. 2000).

Similarly, two small studies in pathological gambling suggested that fluvoxamine might be beneficial (Hollander et al. 1998, 2000). However, a larger 6-month double-blind, placebo-controlled study failed to show separation from placebo (Blanco et al. 2002).

Furthermore, a 12-week open-label study of fluvoxamine in 21 subjects with trichotillomania produced only minor improvement (Stanley et al. 1997).

Eating Disorders

In another study, 72 subjects with bulimia nervosa who had been treated successfully with psychotherapy were randomly assigned to receive fluvoxamine (100–300 mg/day) or placebo and were followed for 12 weeks. Fluvoxamine was significantly superior in preventing relapse ($P<0.05$) (Fichter et al. 1996). A small 12-week double-blind, placebo-controlled study in 12 subjects with acute bulimia nervosa suggested that fluvoxamine 200 mg/day was superior to placebo (Milano et al. 2005).

A 9-week double-blind, placebo-controlled study in 85 subjects with binge-eating disorder found that fluvoxamine (50–300 mg/day) was significantly more effective than placebo in reducing binge frequency (Hudson et al. 1998).

Delirium

Delirium, especially in hospitalized older patients, is associated with increased morbidity and mortality, prolonged hospital stays, and cognitive deterioration. Antipsychotic drugs have been widely used for treating delirium but are associated with sedation, extrapyramidal side effects, and cardiac arrhythmias.

Furthermore, there is an elevated risk of mortality in older patients treated with atypical antipsychotics. The endoplasmic reticulum protein sigma-1 receptors are thought to play a key role in calcium signaling and cell survival and may regulate a number of neurotransmitter systems implicated in the pathophysiology of delirium. Several recent case reports have suggested that fluvoxamine, because of its potent sigma-1 receptor agonism, may be effective in the treatment of delirium (Furuse and Hashimoto 2010a, 2010b, 2010c).

Side Effects and Toxicology

Data from 34,587 patients enrolled in postmarketing fluvoxamine studies were combined in a database to assess safety. Dosages ranged from 50 to 300 mg/day taken over 4–52 weeks (Wagner et al. 1994). Overall, 14% of participants discontinued treatment because of side effects, most frequently nausea and vomiting (4.6% and 1.7%, respectively). The adverse events reported at greater than 5% incidence were nausea, somnolence, and asthenia (15.7%, 6.4%, and 5.1%, respectively). The rate of weight gain was only 1%. Sexual side effects were not mentioned in the analysis (only side effects with >1% incidence were listed), although a separate open-label study designed to assess SSRI-induced sexual dysfunction in men and women showed statistically similar rates for fluvoxamine, fluoxetine, sertraline, and paroxetine (range: 54.4%–64.7%) (Montejo-Gonzalez et al. 1997).

Another postmarketing surveillance review covering 17 years (Buchberger and Wagner 2002) analyzed 6,658 individual reports, including 16,110 adverse drug reactions. The frequency of death was calculated at 0.9 per 100,000 patients. Suicide, mostly by overdose, was the cause of death in nearly half, but only 1.2% of overdoses involved fluvoxamine alone. The rate of suicidality (ideation, attempts, and completed suicides) was estimated at 2.81 events per 100,000 patients. Drug interactions were reported at a rate of 0.85 case per 100,000 patients, most commonly with clozapine. Cases of switch to mania and discontinuation syndrome were also rare, occurring at rates of 0.47 and 0.38 events per 100,000 patients, respectively. Serotonin syndrome was even less frequent.

Two studies found no consistent treatment-related changes in laboratory values or vital signs in fluvoxamine-exposed subjects (Wagner et al. 1994).

Drug-Drug Interactions

Fluvoxamine is a potent inhibitor of cytochrome P450 (CYP) 1A2. Drugs partially metabolized by CYP1A2 whose levels may rise as a result of fluvoxamine's inhibition of this isozyme include tizanidine, tertiary-amine tricyclic antidepressants (imipramine, amitriptyline, clomipramine), clozapine, tacrine, theophylline, propranolol, and caffeine. Doses of theophylline and clozapine should be reduced if coadministered with fluvoxamine (DeVane and Gill 1997).

Fluvoxamine also inhibits CYP2C19 and CYP3A4. CYP2C19 metabolizes warfarin, and elevations in warfarin concentration have been reported in patients taking fluvoxamine. As a result, closer monitoring of anticoagulation status is indicated in these patients. Alprazolam and diazepam are metabolized in part through CYP3A4, and fluvoxamine has been shown to prolong their elimination (DeVane and Gill 1997). Carbamazepine is partially metabolized through CYP3A4, and elevated carbamazepine levels have been documented in patients concomitantly taking fluvoxamine (Palmer and Benfield 1994). Other drugs whose metabolism through CYP3A4 may be affected by fluvoxamine include pimozide, methadone, and thioridazine. Also, because of the serious QT interval prolongation that can occur when terfenadine or astemizole is combined with the potent CYP3A4 inhibitor ketoconazole, it is recommended that fluvoxamine be avoided in patients who require these antihistamines (DeVane and Gill 1997). Fluvoxamine is contraindicated for use with thioridazine, tizanidine, pimozide, alosetron, ramelteon, and monoamine oxidase inhibitors (MAOIs) (Jazz Pharmaceuticals 2011).

Pregnancy and Lactation

Only limited fluvoxamine-specific data in pregnancy exist to help guide clinicians and patients. One study tried to assess teratogenic or perinatal effects relating to fluvoxamine exposure in utero in 92 pregnant women, 37 of whom were taking concomitant medications. No significant difference in adverse events was seen compared with the control group (Gentile 2005). The U.S. Food and Drug Administration (FDA) lists fluvoxamine under Category C.

Very limited information is available on infants exposed to fluvoxamine through lactation (Gentile 2005). In the eight cases published, no adverse events have been reported.

References

Benfield P, Ward A: Fluvoxamine: a review of its pharmacodynamic and pharmacokinetic properties, and therapeutic efficacy in depressive illness. Drugs 32:313–334, 1986

Black DW, Monahan P, Gabel J: Fluvoxamine in the treatment of compulsive buying. J Clin Psychiatry 58:159–163, 1997

Black DW, Gabel J, Hansen J, et al: A double-blind comparison of fluvoxamine versus placebo in the treatment of compulsive buying disorder. Ann Clin Psychiatry 12:205–211, 2000

Blanco C, Petkova E, Ibanez A, et al: A pilot placebo-controlled study of fluvoxamine for pathological gambling. Ann Clin Psychiatry 14:9–15, 2002

Buchberger R, Wagner W: Fluvoxamine: safety profile in extensive post-marketing surveillance. Pharmacopsychiatry 35:101–108, 2002

Davidson JR, Weisler RH, Malik M, et al: Fluvoxamine in civilians with posttraumatic stress disorder. J Clin Psychopharmacol 18:93–95, 1998

Davidson J, Yaryura-Tobias J, DuPont R, et al: Fluvoxamine controlled-release formulation for the treatment of generalized social anxiety disorder. J Clin Psychopharmacol 24:118–125, 2004

De Boer M, Op den Velde W, Falger PJ, et al: Fluvoxamine treatment for chronic PTSD: a pilot study. Psychother Psychosom 57:158–163, 1992

DeVane CL: Pharmacokinetics, drug interactions and tolerability of paroxetine and paroxetine CR. Psychopharmacol Bull 37 (suppl 1):29–41, 2003

DeVane CL, Gill HS: Clinical pharmacokinetics of fluvoxamine: applications to dosage regimen design. J Clin Psychiatry 58 (suppl 5):7–14, 1997

Dranovsky A, Hen R: Hippocampal neurogenesis: regulation by stress and antidepressants. Biol Psychiatry 59:1136–1143, 2006

Escalona R, Canive JM, Calais LA, et al: Fluvoxamine treatment in veterans with combat-related post-traumatic stress disorder. Depress Anxiety 15:29–33, 2002

Fichter MM, Kruger R, Rief W, et al: Fluvoxamine in prevention of relapse in bulimia nervosa: effects on eating-specific psychopathology. J Clin Psychopharmacol 16:9–18, 1996

Figgitt DP, McClellan KJ: Fluvoxamine: an updated review of its use in the management of adults with anxiety disorders. Drugs 60:925–954, 2000

Freeman CP, Trimble MR, Deakin JF, et al: Fluvoxamine versus clomipramine in the treatment of obsessive compulsive disorder: a multicenter, randomized, double-blind, parallel group comparison. J Clin Psychiatry 55:301–305, 1994

Fukuchi T, Kanemoto K: Differential effects of milnacipran and fluvoxamine, especially in patients with severe depression and agitated depression: a case-control study. Int Clin Psychopharmacol 17:53–58, 2002

Furuse T, Hashimoto K: Fluvoxamine monotherapy for psychotic depression: the potential role for sigma-1 receptors. Ann Gen Psychiatry 8:26, 2009

Furuse T, Hashimoto K: Sigma-1 agonist fluvoxamine for delirium in intensive care units: report of five cases. Ann Gen Psychiatry 9:18, 2010a

Furuse T, Hashimoto K: Sigma-1 receptor agonist fluvoxamine for delirium in patients with Alzheimer's disease. Ann Gen Psychiatry 9:6, 2010b

Furuse T, Hashimoto K: Sigma-1 receptor agonist fluvoxamine for postoperative delirium in older patients: report of three cases. Ann Gen Psychiatry 9:28, 2010c

Gentile S: The safety of newer antidepressants in pregnancy and breastfeeding. Drug Saf 28:137–152, 2005

Gershon AA, Vishne T, Grunhaus L: Dopamine D2-like receptors and the antidepressant response. Biol Psychiatry 61:145–153, 2007

Haffmans PM, Timmerman L, Hoogduin CA: Efficacy and tolerability of citalopram in comparison with fluvoxamine in depressed outpatients: a double-blind, multicentre study. The LUCIFER Group. Int Clin Psychopharmacol 11:157–164, 1996

Hollander E, DeCaria CM, Mari E, et al: Short-term single-blind fluvoxamine treatment of pathological gambling. Am J Psychiatry 155:1781–1783, 1998

Hollander E, DeCaria CM, Finkell JN, et al: A randomized double-blind fluvoxamine/placebo crossover trial in pathologic gambling. Biol Psychiatry 47:813–817, 2000

Hudson JI, McElroy SL, Raymond NC, et al: Fluvoxamine in the treatment of binge-eating disorder: a multicenter placebo-controlled, double-blind trial. Am J Psychiatry 155:1756–1762, 1998

Ishikawa M, Ishiwata K, Ishii K, et al: High occupancy of sigma-1 receptors in the human brain after single oral administration of fluvoxamine: a positron emission tomography study using [(11)C]SA4503. Biol Psychiatry 62:878–883, 2007

Jazz Pharmaceuticals: Luvox CR (fluvoxamine maleate) extended-release capsules for oral administration (package insert). Palo Alto, CA, Jazz Pharmaceuticals Inc., May 2011. Available at: http://www.luvoxcr.com/LUVOX-CR-PI.pdf. Accessed July 2012.

Kiev A, Feiger A: A double-blind comparison of fluvoxamine and paroxetine in the treatment of depressed outpatients. J Clin Psychiatry 58:146–152, 1997

Koran LM, McElroy SL, Davidson JR, et al: Fluvoxamine versus clomipramine for obsessive-compulsive disorder: a double-blind comparison. J Clin Psychopharmacol 16:121–129, 1996

Lapierre YD, Rastoqi RB, Singhal RL: Fluvoxamine influences serotonergic system in the brain: neurochemical evidence. Neuropsychobiology 10:213–216, 1983

Mancama D, Kerwin RW: Role of pharmacogenomics in individualizing treatment with SSRIs. CNS Drugs 17:143–151, 2003

Marmar CR, Schoenfeld F, Weiss DS, et al: Open trial of fluvoxamine treatment for combat-related posttraumatic stress disorder. J Clin Psychiatry 57 (suppl 8):66–70, 1996

Milanfranchi A, Ravagli S, Lensi P, et al: A double-blind study of fluvoxamine and clomipramine in the treatment of obsessive-compulsive disorder. Int Clin Psychopharmacol 12:131–136, 1997

Milano W, Siano C, Putrella C, et al: Treatment of bulimia nervosa with fluvoxamine: a randomized controlled trial. Adv Ther 22:278–283, 2005

Montejo-Gonzalez AL, Llorca G, Izquierdo JA, et al: SSRI-induced sexual dysfunction: fluoxetine, paroxetine, sertraline, and fluvoxamine in a prospective, multicenter, and descriptive clinical study of 344 patients. J Sex Marital Ther 23:176–194, 1997

Mundo E, Bianchi L, Bellodi L: Efficacy of fluvoxamine, paroxetine, and citalopram in the treatment of obsessive-compulsive disorder: a single-blind study. J Clin Psychopharmacol 17:267–271, 1997

Mundo E, Maina G, Uslenghi C: Multicenter, double-blind comparison of fluvoxamine and clomipramine in the treatment of obsessive-compulsive disorder. Int Clin Psychopharmacol 15:69–76, 2000

Mundo E, Rouillon F, Figuera ML, et al: Fluvoxamine in obsessive-compulsive disorder: similar efficacy but superior tolerability in comparison with clomipramine. Hum Psychopharmacol 16:461–468, 2001

Ninan PT, McElroy SL, Kane CP, et al: Placebo-controlled study of fluvoxamine in the treatment of patients with compulsive buying. J Clin Psychopharmacol 20:362–366, 2000

Omori IM, Watanabe N, Nakagawa A, et al: Fluvoxamine versus other anti-depressive agents for depression. Cochrane Database Syst Rev (3):CD006114, 2010

Otsubo T, Akimoto Y, Yamada H, et al: A comparative study of the efficacy and safety profiles between fluvoxamine and nortriptyline in Japanese patients with major depression. Pharmacopsychiatry 38:30–35, 2005

Owens JM, Knight DL, Nemeroff CB: Second generation SSRIs: human monoamine transporter binding profile of escitalopram and R-fluoxetine. Biol Psychiatry 50:345–350, 2001

Palmer KJ, Benfield P: Fluvoxamine: an overview of its pharmacological properties and review of its therapeutic potential in nondepressive disorders. CNS Drugs 1:57–87, 1994

Perugi G, Giannotti D, Di Vaio S, et al: Fluvoxamine in the treatment of body dysmorphic disorder (dysmorphophobia). Int Clin Psychopharmacol 11:247–254, 1996

Phillips KA, Dwight MM, McElroy SL: Efficacy and safety of fluvoxamine in body dysmorphic disorder. J Clin Psychiatry 59:165–171, 1998

Phillips KA, McElroy SL, Dwight MM, et al: Delusionality and response to open-label fluvoxamine in body dysmorphic disorder. J Clin Psychiatry 62:87–91, 2001

Physicians' Desk Reference, 56th Edition. Montvale, NJ, Medical Economics Company, 2002

Price LH, Goodman WK, Charney DS, et al: Treatment of severe obsessive-compulsive disorder with fluvoxamine. Am J Psychiatry 144:1059–1061, 1987

Rapaport M, Coccaro E, Sheline Y, et al: A comparison of fluvoxamine and fluoxetine in the treatment of major depression. J Clin Psychopharmacol 16:373–378, 1996

Ravizza L, Barzega G, Bellino S, et al: Drug treatment of obsessive-compulsive disorder (OCD): long-term trial with clomipramine and selective serotonin reuptake inhibitors (SSRIs). Psychopharmacol Bull 32:167–173, 1996

Riddle MA, Reeve EA, Yaryura-Tobias JA, et al: Fluvoxamine for children and adolescents with obsessive compulsive disorder: a randomized, controlled, multicenter trial. J Am Acad Child Adolesc Psychiatry 40:222–229, 2001

Rossini D, Serretti A, Franchini L, et al: Sertraline versus fluvoxamine in the treatment of elderly patients with major depression: a double-blind, randomized trial. J Clin Psychopharmacol 25: 471–475, 2005

Stahl SM: Mechanism of action of selective serotonin reuptake inhibitors: serotonin receptors and pathways mediate therapeutic effects and side effects. J Affect Disord 51:215–235, 1998

Stanley MA, Breckenridge JK, Swann AC, et al: Fluvoxamine treatment of trichotillomania. J Clin Psychopharmacol 17:278–283, 1997

Stein MB, Fyer AJ, Davidson JR, et al: Fluvoxamine treatment of social phobia (social anxiety disorder): a double-blind, placebo-controlled study. Am J Psychiatry 156:756–760, 1999

Strauss WL, Layton ME, Dager SR: Brain elimination half-life of fluvoxamine measured by 19F magnetic resonance spectroscopy. Am J Psychiatry 155:380–384, 1998

Terra JL, Montgomery SA: Fluvoxamine prevents recurrence of depression: results of a long-term, double-blind, placebo-controlled study. Int Clin Psychopharmacol 13:55–62, 1998

Tucker P, Smith KL, Marx B, et al: Fluvoxamine reduces physiologic reactivity to trauma scripts in posttraumatic stress disorder. J Clin Psychopharmacol 20:367–372, 2000

Van Harten J: Overview of the pharmacokinetics of fluvoxamine. Clin Pharmacokinet 29 (suppl 1): 1–9, 1995

Van Harten J, Duchier J, Devissaguet JP, et al: Pharmacokinetics of fluvoxamine maleate in patients with liver cirrhosis after single-dose oral administration. Clin Pharmacokinet 24:177–182, 1993

Wagner W, Zaborny BA, Gray TE: Fluvoxamine: a review of its safety in world-wide studies. Int Clin Psychopharmacol 9:223–227, 1994

Ware MR: Fluvoxamine: a review of the controlled trials in depression. J Clin Psychiatry 58 (suppl 5):15–23, 1997

Westenberg HG, Stein DJ, Yang H, et al: A double-blind placebo-controlled study of controlled release fluvoxamine for the treatment of generalized social anxiety disorder. J Clin Psychopharmacol 24:49–55, 2004

Zanardi R, Franchini L, Serretti A, et al: Venlafaxine versus fluvoxamine in the treatment of delusional depression: a pilot double-blind controlled study. J Clin Psychiatry 61:26–29, 2000

Zohar J, Keegstra H, Barrelet L: Fluvoxamine as effective as clomipramine against symptoms of severe depression: results from a multicentre, double-blind study. Hum Psychopharmacol 18:113–119, 2003

CHAPTER 6

Citalopram and S-Citalopram

Patrick H. Roseboom, Ph.D.

Ned H. Kalin, M.D.

Citalopram (Celexa) and its pharmacologically active enantiomer, *S*-citalopram (Lexapro), are among the most selective serotonin reuptake inhibitors available. Both drugs are widely prescribed and have been shown in large-scale, controlled trials to be effective in the treatment of depression; *S*-citalopram has also been shown to be effective in the treatment of anxiety disorders. In addition, both drugs are well tolerated in patients and show a low potential for pharmacokinetic drug-drug interactions. Citalopram and *S*-citalopram have similar efficacy in the treatment of depression, with some studies suggesting a modest superiority of *S*-citalopram over citalopram in some measures of efficacy, including a possibly faster onset of therapeutic effect for *S*-citalopram. Antagonism of the effects of *S*-citalopram by *R*-citalopram has been invoked to explain the purported therapeutic differences between the two drugs. In addition, the affinity of citalopram for histamine receptors appears to reside in the *R*-enantiomer, suggesting that *S*-citalopram has a decreased potential for antihistaminergic side effects. Whether the postulated superiority of *S*-citalopram over citalopram is clinically meaningful in psychiatric practice requires further study.

History and Discovery

The pharmacology of citalopram was first described in 1977 (Christensen et al. 1977; Hyttel 1977). Citalopram was shown to be a very potent inhibitor of serotonin (5-HT) reuptake in both in vitro and in vivo models (Hyttel 1977, 1978). It was subsequently discovered that all of the inhibitory activity of citalopram on 5-HT reuptake resides in the *S*-(+)-enantiomer (*S*-citalopram) (Hyttel et al. 1992). Originally introduced in Denmark in 1989, citalopram was approved by the U.S. Food and Drug Administration (FDA) for the treatment of depression in July 1998. *S*-Citalopram received FDA approval for the treatment of major depressive disorder in August 2002 and for the treatment of generalized anxiety disorder (GAD) in December 2003. S-Citalopram also received FDA approval in March 2009 for the treatment of major depressive disorder in adolescents ages 12–17 years.

Structure-Activity Relations

Citalopram has a single chiral center (Figure 6–1). A chiral center is an atom surrounded by an asymmetrical arrangement of atoms such that the three-dimensional configuration is not superimposable on its mirror image. At this chiral center, there are two possible stereoisomers. Often, drugs are produced as a mixture of both stereoisomers, referred to as the *racemate*. However, because desired pharmacological activity or unwanted toxicity may reside in only one of the stereoisomers, a stereoisomer-selective formulation may be superior (Agranat et al. 2002). Citalopram was originally characterized and marketed as the racemate, but subsequently the single stereoisomer of citalopram, S-citalopram, has been developed for the treatment of depression and other psychiatric disorders. Preclinical studies indicate that inhibition of 5-HT transporter activity resides in the S-enantiomer (Hyttel et al. 1992), with S-citalopram being 30-fold more potent than R-citalopram at inhibiting 5-HT transport (Owens et al. 2001).

A possible explanation for the postulated modest superiority of S-citalopram over citalopram in some measures of antidepressant efficacy is provided by the evidence that the R-enantiomer of citalopram may interfere with the activity of the S-enantiomer, as evidenced in several behavioral and physiological assays (for a review, see Sanchez 2006). This antagonism has been hypothesized to result from a kinetic interaction at the level of the 5-HT transporter (Storustovu et al. 2004).

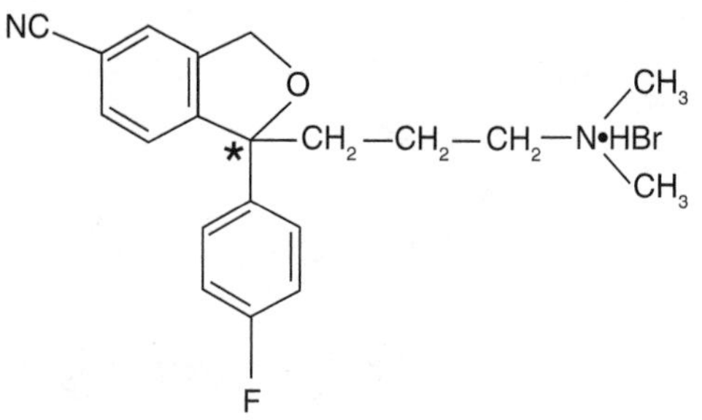

FIGURE 6–1. Chemical structure of citalopram.

Asterisk (*) indicates chiral center.

Pharmacological Profile

Citalopram

Of the selective serotonin reuptake inhibitors (SSRIs) approved to date, citalopram is one of the most selective, with a 524-fold lower potency for inhibiting the human norepinephrine (NE) transporter and a >10,000-fold lower potency for inhibiting the human dopamine (DA) transporter (Owens et al. 2001). In addition, citalopram has low affinity for a wide variety of neurotransmitter receptors (for a review, see Hyttel et al. 1995). Citalopram has been reported to have submicromolar affinity for the histamine$_1$ (H_1) receptor (Hyttel 1994; Richelson and Nelson 1984), but this appears to be true only for the R-enantiomer (Owens et al. 2001). Citalopram does not show significant inhibition of monoamine oxidase (MAO) (Hyttel 1977). Behavioral studies in rats and mice have shown citalopram to be a potent and selective inhibitor of 5-HT reuptake (Christensen et al. 1977; Hyttel 1994). In contrast, citalopram is ineffective in models that reflect in vivo inhibition of DA and NE reuptake (Hyttel 1994). Citalopram is active in various behavioral models related to antidepressant activity (Martin et al. 1990; Sanchez and Meier 1997) and anxiolytic activity (Inoue 1993; Sanchez 1995).

S-Citalopram

S-Citalopram is also a highly potent inhibitor of 5-HT reuptake, with a K_i for binding to the human 5-HT transporter of 1.1 nM compared with a K_i of 1.9 nM for citalopram and 36 nM for *R*-citalopram (Owens et al. 2001). *S*-Citalopram is the most selective SSRI approved for clinical use, with a 2,600-fold lower potency for inhibiting the human NE transporter and a >45,000-fold lower potency for inhibiting the human DA transporter. *S*-Citalopram also has no appreciable binding affinity for a large number of other neurotransmitter receptors (Owens et al. 2001; Sanchez et al. 2003). *S*-Citalopram also has potent activity in various in vivo paradigms, including a model of 5-HT reuptake inhibition and behavioral models of antidepressant, antiaggressive, and anxiolytic activity (for a review, see Sanchez et al. 2003). In these in vivo paradigms, the potency of *S*-citalopram ranges from similar to citalopram to approximately twofold greater than citalopram. In contrast, in the majority of these paradigms, *R*-citalopram is severalfold less potent than either *S*-citalopram or citalopram.

Pharmacokinetics and Disposition

Citalopram

Citalopram is well absorbed after oral administration, with an absolute bioavailability of 80% for citalopram tablets (Joffe et al. 1998). The peak plasma concentration is normally observed 2–4 hours following an oral dose (Kragh-Sorensen et al. 1981). The bioavailability of citalopram is not affected by food (Baumann and Larsen 1995), and it is subject to very little first-pass metabolism (Kragh-Sorensen et al. 1981). The apparent volume of distribution is 12–16 L/kg (Kragh-Sorensen et al. 1981; Overo 1982), which indicates that the drug distributes widely. There is a linear relationship between steady-state plasma concentration and dose (Bjerkenstedt et al. 1985), and plasma protein binding is approximately 80% (Baumann and Larsen 1995). Systemic clearance of citalopram is 0.3–0.4 L/minute (Baumann and Larsen 1995), and renal clearance of citalopram is approximately 0.05–0.08 L/minute (Sindrup et al. 1993).

Racemic citalopram undergoes *N*-demethylation by the hepatic cytochrome P450 (CYP) system to the major metabolite, monodesmethylcitalopram (DCT). CYP enzymes 2C19, 3A4, and 2D6 all contribute approximately equally to the formation of DCT (Kobayashi et al. 1997; Rochat et al. 1997; von Moltke et al. 1999). DCT also undergoes *N*-demethylation to the minor metabolite didesmethylcitalopram (DDCT) by the actions of CYP2D6 (Sindrup et al. 1993; von Moltke et al. 2001). Clinical studies indicate that the half-lives for citalopram, DCT, and DDCT are approximately 36 hours, 50 hours, and 100 hours, respectively (Dalgaard and Larsen 1999; Kragh-Sorensen et al. 1981; Overo 1982). Citalopram is metabolized by human cytochromes that display genetic polymorphisms, and metabolism of citalopram and DCT is impaired in subjects who show poor metabolism via the CYP2C19 and the CYP2D6 pathways (Baumann et al. 1996; Sindrup et al. 1993; Yu et al. 2003).

S-Citalopram

The clinical pharmacokinetic characteristics of *S*-citalopram have been reviewed and are similar to those described for citalopram (Rao 2007). The pharmacokinetic characteristics of *S*-citalopram are essentially the same regardless of whether patients are given a single oral dose of 20 mg of *S*-citalopram or 40 mg of racemic citalopram (which contains 20 mg of *S*-citalopram). This indicates that there is no pharmacokinetic interaction or interconversion between *R*-citalopram and *S*-citalopram (Rao 2007).

Mechanism of Action

The majority of studies on mechanism of action have focused on citalopram, with a relatively limited number of studies using S-citalopram. Because the antidepressant activity of citalopram results from S-citalopram, the majority of the conclusions from these studies pertain to both citalopram and S-citalopram.

Citalopram is a potent and selective inhibitor of 5-HT reuptake and acts by binding directly to the 5-HT transporter. Citalopram selectively inhibits radioligand binding to the 5-HT transporter (K_i=0.75 nM) versus the NE transporter (K_i=3,042 nM) in rat cortical membranes. A similar selectivity was found for inhibiting the binding of the same radioligands to the cloned human 5-HT and NE transporters expressed in transfected cells and for inhibiting [^{3}H]5-HT (K_i=8.9 nM) and [^{3}H]NE (K_i=30,285 nM) reuptake into these transfected cells (Owens et al. 1997).

Several studies have described how repeated dosing alters the effects of citalopram on serotonergic neuronal function. Much as with other SSRIs, the ability of citalopram to inhibit the firing of 5-HT neurons in the dorsal raphe nucleus is greatly reduced after 14 days of repeated administration (Chaput et al. 1986). This is associated with an increase in the ability of citalopram to elevate the extracellular levels of 5-HT in the cortex (Invernizzi et al. 1994). These two effects appear to result from a desensitization of 5-HT_{1A} autoreceptors (Chaput et al. 1986; Cremers et al. 2000; Invernizzi et al. 1994). This adaptive change of 5-HT_{1A} receptors following repeated administration of citalopram, as well as other SSRIs, has been postulated to underlie the slow onset of antidepressant efficacy that is observed clinically (Blier and de Montigny 1994).

Evidence suggests that a variety of antidepressants, including those that block monoamine reuptake or metabolism, produce their therapeutic response in part by overcoming depression-associated decreases in neurogenesis and synaptogenesis, possibly through effects on brain-derived neurotrophic factor (BDNF) expression. Citalopram, like several other antidepressants, has been shown to increase the levels of BDNF mRNA in various subregions of the rat ventral hippocampus (Russo-Neustadt et al. 2004) and to induce signaling through the BDNF receptor TrkB (Rantamaki et al. 2007). Interestingly, this effect of antidepressants on TrkB appears to be independent of BDNF release and 5-HT transporter blockade and does not involve a direct binding of the antidepressant to TrkB (Rantamaki et al. 2011). A recent clinical study demonstrated that S-citalopram treatment can affect circulating BDNF levels. In this study, depressed subjects (n=18) showed elevated plasma levels of BDNF and decreased platelet levels of BDNF compared with healthy control subjects (n=14), and these differences were normalized with 24 weeks of S-citalopram (10–40 mg/day) treatment (Serra-Millas et al. 2011). Finally, there are preliminary clinical data suggesting that a polymorphism within the coding region for BDNF (Val66Met) is associated with therapeutic response to citalopram (Choi et al. 2006).

A number of studies have implicated the 5-HT_{2A} receptor in a variety of neuropsychiatric disorders (Norton and Owen 2005), and there is evidence implicating the 5-HT_{2A} receptor in the mechanism of action of antidepressants, including citalopram (Chen and Lawrence 2003; Peremans et al. 2005). Also, a large-scale clinical study involving 1,953 patients who participated in the Sequenced Treatment Alternatives to Relieve Depression (STAR*D) trial identified a significant association between a polymorphism contained in the second intron of the gene for the 5-HT_{2A} receptor (rs7997012) and treatment response to citalopram (McMahon et al. 2006). While perhaps relevant to clinical work, the functional significance of this intronic polymorphism on the 5-HT_{2A} receptor has yet to be determined.

Finally, several cellular and in vivo animal model studies have shown that antidepressants can increase glucocorticoid receptor (GR) translocation, induce GR downregulation, and decrease GR agonist–mediated effects (Anacker et al. 2011; Carvalho and Pariante 2008). A recent study suggests that similar effects occur in vivo in humans. Four days of citalopram treatment (20 mg/day) was associated with a diminished ability of cortisol to increase electroencephalogram alpha power and to impair working memory (Pariante et al. 2012). These results suggest that GR activation by antidepressants does occur in the human brain.

Indications and Efficacy

Depression

Citalopram

The efficacy of citalopram (dosage range 20–80 mg/day) in the treatment of depression has been shown in at least 11 placebo-controlled clinical trials (for a review, see Keller 2000). In addition, meta-analyses of multiple placebo-controlled studies reported similar findings (Bech and Cialdella 1992; Montgomery et al. 1994). In the United States, three large, multicenter clinical trials have demonstrated citalopram's efficacy in the treatment of major depression (Feighner and Overo 1999; Mendels et al. 1999; Stahl 2000). Most recently, citalopram (20 mg/day; $n=274$) was shown to be equally effective compared with the NE reuptake inhibitor reboxetine (4 mg twice daily; $n=272$) in the treatment of severe depression (≥15 on Beck Depression Inventory) in primary care patients in the United Kingdom (Wiles et al. 2012).

STAR*D trial. The effectiveness of citalopram has also been demonstrated in a study designed to simulate real-world conditions for the treatment of depression. The STAR*D trial was a large-scale multicenter study that enrolled 4,041 patients with nonpsychotic major depression in a test of various antidepressant therapies (Rush et al. 2004). The mean daily dose of citalopram at study exit was 41.8 mg, the remission rates were 28% (when remission was defined as a score of ≤7 on the 17-item Hamilton Rating Scale for Depression [Ham-D_{17}]) and 33% (using definition of a score of ≤5 on the 16-item Quick Inventory of Depressive Symptomatology, Self-Report [QIDS-SR]), and the response rate was 47% (using definition of a ≥50% reduction in QIDS-SR score) (Trivedi et al. 2006). These response and remission rates are comparable to those found in 8-week controlled clinical trials examining the efficacy of acute antidepressant treatment.

Long-term treatment with citalopram. Two placebo-controlled studies indicate that citalopram may be effective in continuation therapy to prevent depression relapse. Both studies showed that for patients with an acute therapeutic response to citalopram, continuation of citalopram therapy at the same dosage (20, 40, or 60 mg/day) for an additional 24 weeks significantly decreased the relapse rate compared with placebo (Montgomery et al. 1993; Robert and Montgomery 1995). Two additional studies suggest that citalopram may be beneficial in patients with a history of recurrent depression. Long-term (at least 48 weeks) administration of citalopram at the same fixed dosage at which patients initially showed therapeutic response (20–60 mg/day) can significantly increase the time before depression recurs in adult patients (18–65 years) and in the elderly (≥65 years) (Hochstrasser et al. 2001; Klysner et al. 2002).

S-Citalopram

A number of placebo-controlled clinical trials and retrospective analyses have demonstrated the efficacy of S-citalopram (dosage range 10–20 mg/day) in the treatment of major depression (Burke et al. 2002; Lepola et al. 2003; Montgomery et al. 2001b; Wade et al. 2002). There are also a large number of retrospective pooled analyses that have compared S-citalopram with other SSRIs (Einarson 2004; Kennedy et al. 2006; Llorca et al. 2005). In general, S-citalopram was at least as effective as other widely used antidepressants, and in some clinical trials it has been suggested to be superior to other antidepressants based on modestly greater changes in various depression rating scales, especially in severely depressed patients. In addition, also based on depression rating scales, S-citalopram has been suggested in a few clinical trials to possibly have a faster onset of therapeutic effect, occurring as early as 1 week. It remains to be demonstrated whether the modest differences between S-citalopram and other antidepressants in controlled clinical trials translate into a therapeutically meaningful difference in the treatment of depression in psychiatric practice.

Major depression with severe asthma. Major depression is often seen in asthmatic individuals, and depression may be a risk factor for asthma-related morbidity. In a recent proof-of-concept, placebo-controlled, randomized, double-blind trial (Brown et al. 2012), S-citalopram was evaluated for the treatment of depression in patients (10–20 mg/day; $n=25$) with asthma. Improvement in depression symptoms was seen in both placebo and S-citalopram groups from week 1 to study exit at week 12, with a trend favoring S-citalopram for depression remission based on changes in the Ham-D score (Brown et al. 2012).

Long-term treatment with S-citalopram. S-Citalopram (10–20 mg/day; $n=181$) was shown to be effective in preventing relapse following resolution of a depressive episode in a 36-week placebo-controlled ($n=93$) clinical trial (Rapaport et al. 2004). Additionally, the effectiveness of long-term S-citalopram therapy in the prevention of recurrence of depression was also demonstrated in a group of patients who had been diagnosed with recurrent major depressive disorder (Kornstein et al. 2006). Treatment with S-citalopram (10 or 20 mg/day; $n=73$) in this 52-week study significantly prolonged the time to recurrence compared with placebo ($n=66$).

Depression in Children and Adolescents

Fluoxetine is currently the only FDA-approved medication for the treatment of depression in both children and adolescents (ages 8 years and older). S-Citalopram was recently approved for the treatment of depression in adolescents (ages 12–17 years) but not in younger children (as detailed below). In addition, the FDA has mandated the placement of black box warnings on product labels to indicate that there is a potential for increased suicidality associated with the use of SSRIs in patients younger than 25 years. Nevertheless, a meta-analysis of pediatric trials conducted between 1988 and 2006 indicated that the benefits of antidepressant treatment of the young outweigh the risks (Bridge et al. 2007).

Citalopram

Only a limited number of clinical studies have examined the effectiveness of citalopram in the treatment of depression in the young. In one double-blind trial involving children and adolescents (ages 7–17 years; $n=174$), citalopram (20 mg/day) showed a modest superiority over placebo in the treatment of depression (Wagner et al. 2004). Conversely, citalopram (10–40 mg/day) was not superior to placebo in a clinical trial involving adolescents (ages 13–18 years; $n=244$) receiving treatment for 12 weeks (von Knorring et al. 2006). Clearly, additional clinical trials are required to establish the efficacy and safety of citalopram in the treatment of childhood depression.

S-Citalopram

In addition to the treatment of depression in adults, in 2009 the FDA approved S-citalopram for the treatment of depression in adolescents. This decision was based on two clinical trials. In the first study, S-citalopram was shown to be effective in the treatment of depression in adolescents (ages 12–17 years) in a randomized, double-blind, placebo-controlled multicenter clinical trial (Emslie et al. 2009). In this study, S-citalopram (10–20 mg/day; $n = 155$) was superior to placebo ($n = 157$) based on a change from baseline to week 8 in the Children's Depression Rating Scale–Revised. In the second study, the effectiveness of S-citalopram was inferred from a successful clinical trial using citalopram (20–40 mg/day) to treat depression, as is described in the preceding paragraph (Wagner et al. 2004). This study included both children (ages 7–11 years) and adolescents (ages 12–17 years), but the FDA noted that the positive outcome of the study was carried primarily by the adolescents.

Obsessive-Compulsive Disorder

Citalopram

To date, a limited number of clinical studies have evaluated the effectiveness of citalopram in the treatment of obsessive-compulsive disorder (OCD). In the only published large-scale ($n = 401$) double-blind, placebo-controlled study of citalopram in the treatment of OCD, all three dosages of citalopram (20, 40, and 60 mg/day) given for 12 weeks were significantly more effective than placebo in relieving the symptoms of OCD (Montgomery et al. 2001a). Citalopram appears to be effective in treating both obsessions and compulsions.

S-Citalopram

The effectiveness of S-citalopram in the treatment of OCD has been demonstrated in a 24-week double-blind, placebo-controlled multicenter clinical trial (Stein et al. 2007). In this study, S-citalopram at 20 mg/day ($n = 116$) and paroxetine at 40 mg/day ($n = 119$) produced a significant improvement compared with placebo, and by week 24, all treatments, including S-citalopram at 10 mg/day ($n = 116$), were superior to placebo ($n = 115$). Long-term treatment with S-citalopram was shown in one large-scale study to prevent relapse of OCD in patients who had responded to initial treatment (Fineberg et al. 2007). Patients treated with S-citalopram (10 or 20 mg/day; $n = 163$) showed a significantly greater time to relapse compared with those receiving placebo ($n = 157$).

Generalized Anxiety Disorder

Citalopram

There are no published large-scale, randomized, double-blind clinical trials examining the effectiveness of citalopram in the treatment of GAD. As described in the next section, all large-scale trials have focused on the development of S-citalopram for the treatment of GAD.

S-Citalopram

The efficacy of S-citalopram in the treatment of GAD has been established is several randomized controlled clinical trials (Baldwin and Nair 2005). S-Citalopram's effectiveness in acute treatment (up to 12 weeks) of GAD was shown in three double-blind, placebo-controlled clinical trials that were also subjected to pooled analysis. These studies demonstrated that S-citalopram (10–20 mg/day administered for 8–12 weeks) was superior to placebo (Davidson et al. 2004; Goodman et al. 2005; Stein et al. 2005). The efficacy of S-citalopram (10–20 mg/day) in the long-term treatment of GAD was demonstrated in two 24-week controlled clinical trials, one open label (Davidson et al. 2005) and the other double-blind (Bielski et al. 2005). S-Citalopram also showed efficacy in the prevention of GAD relapse for an additional 24–76 weeks (Allgulander et al. 2006).

Panic Disorder

Citalopram

Few well-controlled studies have evaluated the effectiveness of citalopram in the treatment of panic disorder. In a 1-year placebo-controlled, double-blind study, patients (*n*=279) assigned to citalopram (20–30 mg/day or 40–60 mg/day) or clomipramine (60–90 mg/day) showed significantly greater improvement compared with placebo on a variety of anxiety rating scales including the Clinical Anxiety Scale (CAS) panic attack item. The authors concluded that citalopram in the dosage range of 20–60 mg/day was an effective long-term therapy for the management of panic disorder (Lepola et al. 1998).

S-Citalopram

S-Citalopram (5–10 mg/day) was shown to be effective in the treatment of panic disorder in a 10-week randomized, double-blind, placebo-controlled, flexible-dosage study in patients with a diagnosis of panic disorder with or without agoraphobia (Stahl et al. 2003). The relative panic attack frequency was significantly lower in the S-citalopram group (*n*=125) compared with the placebo group (*n*=114), and at the end of the study, there was a greater proportion of patients with zero panic attacks in the S-citalopram group (50%) compared with the placebo group (38%) that was marginally significant (P=0.051).

Social Anxiety Disorder

Citalopram

A large-scale, double-blind, placebo-controlled study demonstrated that paroxetine is effective in the treatment of social anxiety disorder, suggesting that other SSRIs may be effective in the treatment of this disorder (Stein et al. 1998). While there are no such published large-scale placebo-controlled studies with citalopram, case reports indicate that citalopram may have efficacy in the treatment of social anxiety disorder (Bouwer and Stein 1998; Lepola et al. 1994, 1996; Simon et al. 2001). In addition, one 12-week small-scale (*n*=21) flexible-dose, open-label study demonstrated the effectiveness of citalopram (20–60 mg/day) in relieving the symptoms of social anxiety disorder in patients who suffered from comorbid depression (Schneier et al. 2003).

S-Citalopram

Two large-scale, multinational, multicenter clinical trials have demonstrated the effectiveness of S-citalopram in the treatment of social anxiety disorder. In a 24-week fixed-dosage trial in patients with a diagnosis of social anxiety disorder, S-citalopram (5 mg/day [*n*=167], 10 mg/day [*n*=167], or 20 mg/day [*n*=170]) and paroxetine (20 mg/day [*n*=169]) each showed a statistically superior therapeutic effect compared with placebo (*n*=166) by week 12 (Lader et al. 2004). Further improvement was seen by week 24 for all dosages of S-citalopram and for paroxetine, and 20 mg/day S-citalopram was superior to 20 mg/day paroxetine. In a second study of 12 weeks, S-citalopram (10–20 mg/day; *n*=181) produced a superior therapeutic response compared with placebo (*n*=177) based on mean change from baseline in the Liebowitz Social Anxiety Scale score (Kasper et al. 2005). In a long-term study, S-citalopram treatment (10 or 20 mg/day) for up to 24 weeks was shown to be effective in preventing relapse of social anxiety disorder following successful short-term therapy, with relapse being 2.8 times more likely with placebo treatment (*n*=181) than with S-citalopram treatment (*n*=190) (Montgomery et al. 2005).

Anxiety Associated With Major Depression

Citalopram

A retrospective study of 2,000 depressed patients enrolled in eight double-blind, placebo-controlled clinical trials revealed that citalopram was effective in relieving the symptoms of anxiety in depressed patients based on a greater decrease in the anxiety factor of the Ham-D compared with placebo (Flicker et al. 1998). Another double-blind, placebo-controlled study in 323 patients with a diagnosis of major depression revealed a significant antianxiety effect of citalopram (20–60 mg/day) compared with placebo based on decreases in the Hamilton Anxiety Scale (Ham-A) score (Stahl 2000).

S-Citalopram

The effectiveness of S-citalopram in the treatment of anxiety symptoms associated with major depressive disorder has been evaluated in a pooled analysis of five clinical trials (Bandelow et al. 2007). These placebo-controlled trials were originally designed to examine the effectiveness of S-citalopram in treating major depression. In the pooled analysis, S-citalopram (10–20 mg/day; $n=$ 850) was consistently superior to placebo ($n=737$) in relieving the anxious symptoms associated with depression as revealed in several different assessments of anxiousness. The analyses presented in this pooled study indicate that S-citalopram is effective in relieving anxiety symptoms in depressed patients.

Side Effects and Toxicology

Citalopram

In a meta-analysis of 746 depressed patients involved in several short-term clinical trials, the most common adverse events associated with citalopram were nausea and vomiting (20%), increased sweating (18%), and dry mouth and headache (17%) (Baldwin and Johnson 1995). Analysis of an integrated safety database, which includes data from 3,107 patients enrolled in 24 clinical trials, indicated that in placebo-controlled trials, nausea, dry mouth, somnolence, increased sweating, tremor, diarrhea, and ejaculatory failure of mild to moderate severity occurred with significantly greater frequency with citalopram compared with placebo (Muldoon 1996). The incidences of these adverse events were less than 10% above those seen with placebo and were comparable to those seen with other SSRIs. Citalopram had a tolerability that was superior to that of the tricyclic antidepressants (TCAs), with the exception that nausea and ejaculatory failure occurred with a 5% greater frequency with citalopram (Keller 2000).

S-Citalopram

In general, the side effects associated with S-citalopram are similar to those observed with citalopram. In the three placebo-controlled clinical trials that have been performed with S-citalopram, a dosage of 10 mg/day produced rates of discontinuation due to adverse events that did not differ from those in the placebo group (Burke et al. 2002; Montgomery et al. 2001b; Wade et al. 2002). In the one trial that included an S-citalopram dosage of 20 mg/day, the rate of discontinuation was 10.4%, which was greater than the placebo rate of 2.5% (Burke et al. 2002). In addition, the rate of adverse events overall in the 20 mg/day S-citalopram group (85.6%) was significantly greater than that in the placebo group (70.5%). Regardless of dose, the adverse events that have been reported to occur more frequently with S-citalopram compared with placebo are nausea, diarrhea, insomnia, dry mouth, and ejaculatory disorder, with nausea being reported most frequently, at a rate of 15% (McRae 2002). No published studies have reported clinically significant findings in laboratory test values, vital signs, weight gain or loss, or electrocardiogram values.

Specific Effects and Syndromes

Hyponatremia

Citalopram and S-citalopram have been shown to produce hyponatremia in case reports involving the elderly, and this information has been reviewed (Jacob and Spinler 2006). In addition to advanced age, other factors that may increase the likelihood of hyponatremia include female gender, concurrent diuretic use, low body weight, and recent pneumonia. Treatment of SSRI-induced hyponatremia usually involves fluid restriction and/or administration of a loop diuretic such as furosemide and may include discontinuation of the SSRI.

Discontinuation Syndrome

The abrupt cessation of antidepressant therapy can result in a discontinuation syndrome characterized by dizziness, nausea and vomiting, lethargy, and flu-like symptoms. This syndrome is more common with short-half-life SSRIs such as paroxetine and less common with long-half-life SSRIs such as fluoxetine. The data obtained from clinical trials suggest that the adverse events associated with discontinuation of citalopram or S-citalopram tend to be mild and transient (Baldwin et al. 2007; Markowitz et al. 2000; Montgomery et al. 1993). Dose tapering is recommended for patients discontinuing treatment.

Treatment-Emergent Suicidal Ideation and Suicide

Considerable attention has been focused in recent years on the possibility that antidepressant drugs, especially SSRIs, may lead to an increase in suicidal ideation in some patients, particularly at the onset of therapy (Jick et al. 2004). This issue is of great concern in young patients and was described earlier in the chapter (see section "Depression in Children and Adolescents"). In the case of citalopram, analyses of data obtained from 17 controlled clinical trials involving 5,000 patients indicate that the group of patients receiving citalopram had the lowest rate of suicide compared with the groups receiving placebo, TCAs, or other SSRIs (Nemeroff 2003). The risk of suicide associated with S-citalopram was evaluated based on data contained in the Summary Basis of Approval reports obtained from the FDA (Khan and Schwartz 2007). This study did not detect a significantly greater rate of suicide in the S-citalopram group compared with either the citalopram or the placebo group. There was also no indication that S-citalopram increased suicidal behavior in major depressive disorder and anxiety disorders in a meta-analysis of the S-citalopram clinical trials database consisting of 2,277 S-citalopram-treated patients and 1,814 placebo-treated patients (Pedersen 2005).

Drug-Drug Interactions

Even though the majority of a dose of citalopram is metabolized in the liver (75%), because multiple P450 enzymes (CYP2C19, CYP3A4, and CYP2D6) contribute equally to the metabolism of citalopram and S-citalopram, inhibition of any one of these enzymes by another drug is unlikely to significantly impact the overall metabolism of citalopram or S-citalopram. Consistent with this, there are relatively few reports in the literature of drug-drug interactions involving citalopram or S-citalopram. Because of the possibility of a potentially fatal pharmacodynamic interaction resulting in the serotonin syndrome, neither citalopram nor S-citalopram should be administered with an MAO inhibitor or within 14 days of discontinuing an MAO inhibitor.

Conclusion

Citalopram and S-citalopram are highly selective 5-HT reuptake inhibitors that are well tolerated and effective in the treatment of depression, with S-citalopram also having proven efficacy in large-scale clinical trials in the treatment of GAD. While the use of citalopram and S-citalopram in the treatment of other psychiatric conditions has not been as thoroughly studied, the few well-controlled trials that have been completed suggest that both drugs may have a significant role in treating a wide range of psychiatric illnesses, including panic disorder, GAD, social anxiety disorder, anxiety associated with depression, and OCD. An advantage of citalopram and S-citalopram compared with some other common SSRIs is a relatively weak inhibition of liver cytochrome P450 enzymes, which reduces the potential for adverse pharmacokinetic drug-drug interactions. In addition, because S-citalopram does not share with citalopram a modest affinity for the histamine H_1 receptor, it may have a lower potential for antihistaminergic side effects compared with citalopram, a difference that has yet to be demonstrated in a clinical trial. There are a number of clinical trials comparing S-citalopram with a variety of other antidepressants, including citalopram and venlafaxine, that suggest that S-citalopram may have a faster onset of antidepressant efficacy and modest superiority in the treatment of the severely depressed. More extensive experience with S-citalopram is necessary to conclusively determine whether its statistically significant superiority to citalopram and other SSRIs in clinical studies translates into the "real world" of psychiatric practice.

References

Agranat I, Caner H, Caldwell J: Putting chirality to work: the strategy of chiral switches. Nat Rev Drug Discov 1:753–768, 2002

Allgulander C, Florea I, Huusom AK: Prevention of relapse in generalized anxiety disorder by escitalopram treatment. Int J Neuropsychopharmacol 9:495–505, 2006

Anacker C, Zunszain PA, Cattaneo A: Antidepressants increase human hippocampal neurogenesis by activating the glucocorticoid receptor. Mol Psychiatry 16:738–750, 2011

Baldwin D, Johnson FN: Tolerability and safety of citalopram. Rev Contemp Pharmacother 6:315–325, 1995

Baldwin DS, Nair RV: Escitalopram in the treatment of generalized anxiety disorder. Expert Rev Neurother 5:443–449, 2005

Baldwin DS, Montgomery SA, Nil R, et al: Discontinuation symptoms in depression and anxiety disorders. Int J Neuropsychopharmacol 10:73–84, 2007

Bandelow B, Andersen HF, Dolberg OT: Escitalopram in the treatment of anxiety symptoms associated with depression. Depress Anxiety 24:53–61, 2007

Baumann P, Larsen F: The pharmacokinetics of citalopram. Rev Contemp Pharmacother 6:287–295, 1995

Baumann P, Nil R, Souche A, et al: A double-blind, placebo-controlled study of citalopram with and without lithium in the treatment of therapy-resistant depressive patients: a clinical, pharmacokinetic, and pharmacogenetic investigation. J Clin Psychopharmacol 16:307–314, 1996

Bech P, Cialdella P: Citalopram in depression—meta-analysis of intended and unintended effects. Int Clin Psychopharmacol 6 (suppl 5): 45–54, 1992

Bielski RJ, Bose A, Chang CC: A double-blind comparison of escitalopram and paroxetine in the long-term treatment of generalized anxiety disorder. Ann Clin Psychiatry 17:65–69, 2005

Bjerkenstedt L, Flyckt L, Overo KF, et al: Relationship between clinical effects, serum drug concentration and serotonin uptake inhibition in depressed patients treated with citalopram. A double-blind comparison of three dose levels. Eur J Clin Pharmacol 28:553–557, 1985

Blier P, de Montigny C: Current advances and trends in the treatment of depression. Trends Pharmacol Sci 15:220–226, 1994

Bouwer C, Stein DJ: Use of the selective serotonin reuptake inhibitor citalopram in the treatment of generalized social phobia. J Affect Disord 49:79–82, 1998

Bridge JA, Iyengar S, Salary CB, et al: Clinical response and risk for reported suicidal ideation and suicide attempts in pediatric antidepressant treatment: a meta-analysis of randomized controlled trials. JAMA 297:1683–1696, 2007

Brown ES, Howard C, Khan DA, et al: Escitalopram for severe asthma and major depressive disorder: a randomised, double-blind, placebo-controlled proof-of-concept study. Psychosomatics 53:75–80, 2012

Burke WJ, Gergel I, Bose A: Fixed-dose trial of the single isomer SSRI escitalopram in depressed outpatients. J Clin Psychiatry 63:331–336, 2002

Carvalho LA, Pariante CM: In vitro modulation of the glucocorticoid receptor by antidepressants. Stress 11:411–424, 2008

Chaput Y, de Montigny C, Blier P: Effects of a selective 5-HT reuptake blocker, citalopram, on the sensitivity of 5-HT autoreceptors: electrophysiological studies in the rat brain. Naunyn Schmiedebergs Arch Pharmacol 333:342–348, 1986

Chen F, Lawrence AJ: The effects of antidepressant treatment on serotonergic and dopaminergic systems in Fawn-Hooded rats: a quantitative autoradiography study. Brain Res 976:22–29, 2003

Choi MJ, Kang RH, Lim SW, et al: Brain-derived neurotrophic factor gene polymorphism (Val66 Met) and citalopram response in major depressive disorder. Brain Res 1118:176–182, 2006

Christensen AV, Fjalland B, Pedersen V, et al: Pharmacology of a new phthalane (Lu 10-171), with specific 5-HT uptake inhibiting properties. Eur J Pharmacol 41:153–162, 1977

Cremers TI, Spoelstra EN, de Boer P, et al: Desensitisation of 5-HT autoreceptors upon pharmacokinetically monitored chronic treatment with citalopram. Eur J Pharmacol 397:351–357, 2000

Dalgaard L, Larsen C: Metabolism and excretion of citalopram in man: identification of O-acyl- and N-glucuronides. Xenobiotica 29:1033–1041, 1999

Davidson JR, Bose A, Korotzer A, et al: Escitalopram in the treatment of generalized anxiety disorder: double-blind, placebo controlled, flexible-dose study. Depress Anxiety 19:234–240, 2004

Davidson JR, Bose A, Wang Q: Safety and efficacy of escitalopram in the long-term treatment of generalized anxiety disorder. J Clin Psychiatry 66:1441–1446, 2005

Einarson TR: Evidence based review of escitalopram in treating major depressive disorder in primary care. Int Clin Psychopharmacol 19:305–310, 2004

Emslie GJ, Ventura D, Korotzer A, et al: Escitalopram in the treatment of adolescent depression: a randomized placebo-controlled multisite trial. J Am Acad Child Adolesc Psychiatry 48:721–729, 2009

Feighner JP, Overo K: Multicenter, placebo-controlled, fixed-dose study of citalopram in moderate-to-severe depression. J Clin Psychiatry 60:824–830, 1999

Fineberg NA, Tonnoir B, Lemming O, et al: Escitalopram prevents relapse of obsessive-compulsive disorder. Eur Neuropsychopharmacol 17:430–439, 2007

Flicker C, Hakkarainen H, Tanghoj P: Citalopram in anxious depression: anxiolytic effects and lack of activation. Biol Psychiatry 43 (8, suppl 1): 106S, 1998

Goodman WK, Bose A, Wang Q: Treatment of generalized anxiety disorder with escitalopram: pooled results from double-blind, placebo-controlled trials. J Affect Disord 87:161–167, 2005

Hochstrasser B, Isaksen PM, Koponen H, et al: Prophylactic effect of citalopram in unipolar, recurrent depression: placebo-controlled study of maintenance therapy. Br J Psychiatry 178:304–310, 2001

Hyttel J: Neurochemical characterization of a new potent and selective serotonin uptake inhibitor: Lu 10-171. Psychopharmacology (Berl) 51:225–233, 1977

Hyttel J: Effect of a specific 5-HT uptake inhibitor, citalopram (Lu 10-171), on 3H-5-HT uptake in rat brain synaptosomes in vitro. Psychopharmacology (Berl) 60:13–18, 1978

Hyttel J: Pharmacological characterization of selective serotonin reuptake inhibitors (SSRIs). Int Clin Psychopharmacol 9 (suppl 1):19–26, 1994

Hyttel J, Bogeso KP, Perregaard J, et al: The pharmacological effect of citalopram resides in the (S)-(+)-enantiomer. J Neural Transm Gen Sect 88:157–160, 1992

Hyttel J, Arnt J, Sanchez C: The pharmacology of citalopram. Rev Contemp Pharmacother 6:271–285, 1995

Inoue T: Effects of conditioned fear stress on monoaminergic systems in the rat brain. Hokkaido Igaku Zasshi 68:377–390, 1993

Invernizzi R, Bramante M, Samanin R: Chronic treatment with citalopram facilitates the effect of a challenge dose on cortical serotonin output: role of presynaptic 5-HT1A receptors. Eur J Pharmacol 260:243–246, 1994

Jacob S, Spinler SA: Hyponatremia associated with selective serotonin-reuptake inhibitors in older adults. Ann Pharmacother 40:1618–1622, 2006

Jick H, Kaye JA, Jick SS: Antidepressants and the risk of suicidal behaviors. JAMA 292:338–343, 2004

Joffe P, Larsen FS, Pedersen V, et al: Single-dose pharmacokinetics of citalopram in patients with moderate renal insufficiency or hepatic cirrhosis compared with healthy subjects. Eur J Clin Pharmacol 54:237–242, 1998

Kasper S, Stein DJ, Loft H, et al: Escitalopram in the treatment of social anxiety disorder: randomised, placebo-controlled, flexible-dosage study. Br J Psychiatry 186:222–226, 2005

Keller MB: Citalopram therapy for depression: a review of 10 years of European experience and data from US clinical trials. J Clin Psychiatry 61:896–908, 2000

Kennedy SH, Andersen HF, Lam RW: Efficacy of escitalopram in the treatment of major depressive disorder compared with conventional selective serotonin reuptake inhibitors and venlafaxine XR: a meta-analysis. J Psychiatry Neurosci 31:122–131, 2006

Khan A, Schwartz K: Suicide risk and symptom reduction in patients assigned to placebo in duloxetine and escitalopram clinical trials: analysis of the FDA Summary Basis of Approval reports. Ann Clin Psychiatry 19:31–36, 2007

Klysner R, Bent-Hansen J, Hansen HL, et al: Efficacy of citalopram in the prevention of recurrent depression in elderly patients: placebo-controlled study of maintenance therapy. Br J Psychiatry 181:29–35, 2002

Kobayashi K, Chiba K, Yagi T, et al: Identification of cytochrome P450 isoforms involved in citalopram N-demethylation by human liver microsomes. J Pharmacol Exp Ther 280:927–933, 1997

Kornstein SG, Bose A, Li D, et al: Escitalopram maintenance treatment for prevention of recurrent depression: a randomized, placebo-controlled trial. J Clin Psychiatry 67:1767–1775, 2006

Kragh-Sorensen P, Overo KF, Petersen OL, et al: The kinetics of citalopram: single and multiple dose studies in man. Acta Pharmacol Toxicol (Copenh) 48:53–60, 1981

Lader M, Stender K, Burger V, et al: Efficacy and tolerability of escitalopram in 12- and 24-week treatment of social anxiety disorder: randomised, double-blind, placebo-controlled, fixed-dose study. Depress Anxiety 19:241–248, 2004

Lepola U, Koponen H, Leinonen E: Citalopram in the treatment of social phobia: a report of three cases. Pharmacopsychiatry 27:186–188, 1994

Lepola U, Leinonen E, Koponen H: Citalopram in the treatment of early onset panic disorder and school phobia. Pharmacopsychiatry 29:30–32, 1996

Lepola UM, Wade AG, Leinonen EV, et al: A controlled, prospective, 1-year trial of citalopram in the treatment of panic disorder. J Clin Psychiatry 59:528–534, 1998

Lepola UM, Loft H, Reines EH: Escitalopram (10–20 mg/day) is effective and well tolerated in a placebo-controlled study in depression in primary care. Int Clin Psychopharmacol 18:211–217, 2003

Llorca PM, Azorin JM, Despiegel N, et al: Efficacy of escitalopram in patients with severe depression: a pooled analysis. Int J Clin Pract 59:268–275, 2005

Markowitz JS, DeVane CL, Liston HL, et al: An assessment of selective serotonin reuptake inhibitor discontinuation symptoms with citalopram. Int Clin Psychopharmacol 15:329–333, 2000

Martin P, Soubrie P, Puech AJ: Reversal of helpless behavior by serotonin uptake blockers in rats. Psychopharmacology (Berl) 101:403–407, 1990

McMahon FJ, Buervenich S, Charney D, et al: Variation in the gene encoding the serotonin 2A receptor is associated with outcome of antidepressant treatment. Am J Hum Genet 78:804–814, 2006

McRae AL: Escitalopram. Curr Opin Investig Drugs 3:1225–1229, 2002

Mendels J, Kiev A, Fabre LF: Double-blind comparison of citalopram and placebo in depressed outpatients with melancholia. Depress Anxiety 9:54–60, 1999

Montgomery SA, Rasmussen JG, Tanghoj P: A 24-week study of 20 mg citalopram, 40 mg citalopram, and placebo in the prevention of relapse of major depression. Int Clin Psychopharmacol 8:181–188, 1993

Montgomery SA, Pedersen V, Tanghoj P, et al: The optimal dosing regimen for citalopram—a meta-analysis of nine placebo-controlled studies. Int Clin Psychopharmacol 9 (suppl 1):35–40, 1994

Montgomery SA, Kasper S, Stein DJ, et al: Citalopram 20 mg, 40 mg and 60 mg are all effective and well tolerated compared with placebo in obsessive-compulsive disorder. Int Clin Psychopharmacol 16:75–86, 2001a

Montgomery SA, Loft H, Sanchez C, et al: Escitalopram (S-enantiomer of citalopram): clinical efficacy and onset of action predicted from a rat model. Pharmacol Toxicol 88:282–286, 2001b

Montgomery SA, Nil R, Durr-Pal N, et al: A 24-week randomized, double-blind, placebo-controlled study of escitalopram for the prevention of generalized social anxiety disorder. J Clin Psychiatry 66:1270–1278, 2005

Muldoon C: The safety and tolerability of citalopram. Int Clin Psychopharmacol 11 (suppl 1): 35–40, 1996

Nemeroff CB: Overview of the safety of citalopram. Psychopharmacol Bull 37:96–121, 2003

Norton N, Owen MJ: HTR2A: association and expression studies in neuropsychiatric genetics. Ann Med 37:121–129, 2005

Overo KF: Kinetics of citalopram in man: plasma levels in patients. Prog Neuropsychopharmacol Biol Psychiatry 6:311–318, 1982

Owens MJ, Morgan WN, Plott SJ, et al: Neurotransmitter receptor and transporter binding profile of antidepressants and their metabolites. J Pharmacol Exp Ther 283:1305–1322, 1997

Owens MJ, Knight DL, Nemeroff CB: Second-generation SSRIs: human monoamine transporter binding profile of escitalopram and R-fluoxetine. Biol Psychiatry 50:345–350, 2001

Pariante CM, Alhaj HA, Arulnathan VE, et al: Central glucocorticoid receptor-mediated effects of the antidepressant, citalopram, in humans: a study using EEG and cognitive testing. Psychoneuroendocrinology 37:618–628, 2012

Pedersen AG: Escitalopram and suicidality in adult depression and anxiety. Int Clin Psychopharmacol 20:139–143, 2005

Peremans K, Audenaert K, Hoybergs Y, et al: The effect of citalopram hydrobromide on 5-HT2A receptors in the impulsive-aggressive dog, as measured with 123I-5-I-R91150 SPECT. Eur J Nucl Med Mol Imaging 32:708–716, 2005

Rantamaki T, Hendolin P, Kankaanpaa A, et al: Pharmacologically diverse antidepressants rapidly activate brain-derived neurotrophic factor receptor TrkB and induce phospholipase-C gamma signaling pathways in mouse brain. Neuropsychopharmacology 32:2152–2162, 2007

Rantamaki T, Vesa L, Antila H, et al: Antidepressant drugs transactivate TrkB neurotrophin receptors in adult rodent brain independently of BDNF and monoamine transporter blockade. PloS One 6:e20567, 2011

Rao N: The clinical pharmacokinetics of escitalopram. Clin Pharmacokinet 46:281–290, 2007

Rapaport MH, Bose A, Zheng H: Escitalopram continuation treatment prevents relapse of depressive episodes. J Clin Psychiatry 65:44–49, 2004

Richelson E, Nelson A: Antagonism by antidepressants of neurotransmitter receptors of normal human brain in vitro. J Pharmacol Exp Ther 230:94–102, 1984

Robert P, Montgomery SA: Citalopram in doses of 20–60 mg is effective in depression relapse prevention: a placebo-controlled 6 month study. Int Clin Psychopharmacol 10 (suppl 1):29–35, 1995

Rochat B, Amey M, Gillet M, et al: Identification of three cytochrome P450 isozymes involved in N-demethylation of citalopram enantiomers in human liver microsomes. Pharmacogenetics 7:1–10, 1997

Rush AJ, Fava M, Wisniewski SR, et al: Sequenced treatment alternatives to relieve depression (STAR*D): rationale and design. Control Clin Trials 25:119–142, 2004

Russo-Neustadt AA, Alejandre H, Garcia C, et al: Hippocampal brain-derived neurotrophic factor expression following treatment with reboxetine, citalopram, and physical exercise. Neuropsychopharmacology 29:2189–2199, 2004

Sanchez C: Serotonergic mechanisms involved in the exploratory behaviour of mice in a fully automated two-compartment black and white text box. Pharmacol Toxicol 77:71–78, 1995

Sanchez C: The pharmacology of citalopram enantiomers: the antagonism by R-citalopram on the effect of S-citalopram. Basic Clin Pharmacol Toxicol 99:91–95, 2006

Sanchez C, Meier E: Behavioral profiles of SSRIs in animal models of depression, anxiety and aggression: are they all alike? Psychopharmacology (Berl) 129:197–205, 1997

Sanchez C, Bergqvist PB, Brennum LT, et al: Escitalopram, the S-(+)-enantiomer of citalopram, is a selective serotonin reuptake inhibitor with potent effects in animal models predictive of antidepressant and anxiolytic activities. Psychopharmacology (Berl) 167:353–362, 2003

Schneier FR, Blanco C, Campeas R, et al: Citalopram treatment of social anxiety disorder with comorbid major depression. Depress Anxiety 17:191–196, 2003

Serra-Millas M, Lopez-Vilchez I, Navarro V, et al: Changes in plasma and platelet BDNF levels induced by S-citalopram in major depression. Psychopharmacology 216:1–8, 2011

Simon NM, Sharma SG, Worthington JJ, et al: Citalopram for social phobia: a clinical case series. Prog Neuropsychopharmacol Biol Psychiatry 25:1469–1474, 2001

Sindrup SH, Brosen K, Hansen MG, et al: Pharmacokinetics of citalopram in relation to the sparteine and the mephenytoin oxidation polymorphisms. Ther Drug Monit 15:11–17, 1993

Stahl SM: Placebo-controlled comparison of the selective serotonin reuptake inhibitors citalopram and sertraline. Biol Psychiatry 48:894–901, 2000

Stahl SM, Gergel I, Li D: Escitalopram in the treatment of panic disorder: a randomized, double-blind, placebo-controlled trial. J Clin Psychiatry 64:1322–1327, 2003

Stein DJ, Andersen HF, Goodman WK: Escitalopram for the treatment of GAD: efficacy across different subgroups and outcomes. Ann Clin Psychiatry 17:71–75, 2005

Stein DJ, Andersen EW, Tonnoir B, et al: Escitalopram in obsessive-compulsive disorder: a randomized, placebo-controlled, paroxetine-referenced, fixed-dose, 24-week study. Curr Med Res Opin 23:701–711, 2007

Stein MB, Liebowitz MR, Lydiard RB, et al: Paroxetine treatment of generalized social phobia (social anxiety disorder): a randomized controlled trial. JAMA 280:708–713, 1998

Storustovu S, Sanchez C, Porzgen P, et al: R-citalopram functionally antagonises escitalopram in vivo and in vitro: evidence for kinetic interaction at the serotonin transporter. Br J Pharmacol 142:172–180, 2004

Trivedi MH, Rush AJ, Wisniewski SR, et al: Evaluation of outcomes with citalopram for depression using measurement-based care in STAR*D: implications for clinical practice. Am J Psychiatry 163:28–40, 2006

von Knorring AL, Olsson GI, Thomsen PH, et al: A randomized, double-blind, placebo-controlled study of citalopram in adolescents with major depressive disorder. J Clin Psychopharmacol 26:311–315, 2006

von Moltke LL, Greenblatt DJ, Grassi JM, et al: Citalopram and desmethylcitalopram in vitro: human cytochromes mediating transformation, and cytochrome inhibitory effects. Biol Psychiatry 46:839–849, 1999

von Moltke LL, Greenblatt DJ, Giancarlo GM, et al: Escitalopram (S-citalopram) and its metabolites in vitro: cytochromes mediating biotransformation, inhibitory effects, and comparison to R-citalopram. Drug Metab Dispos 29:1102–1109, 2001

Wade A, Michael Lemming O, Bang Hedegaard K: Escitalopram 10 mg/day is effective and well tolerated in a placebo-controlled study in depression in primary care. Int Clin Psychopharmacol 17:95–102, 2002

Wagner KD, Robb AS, Findling RL, et al: A randomized, placebo-controlled trial of citalopram for the treatment of major depression in children and adolescents. Am J Psychiatry 161:1079–1083, 2004

Wiles NJ, Mulligan J, Peters TJ, et al: Severity of depression and response to antidepressants: GENPOD randomised controlled trial. Br J Psychiatry 200:130–136, 2012

Yu BN, Chen GL, He N, et al: Pharmacokinetics of citalopram in relation to genetic polymorphism of CYP2C19. Drug Metab Dispos 31:1255–1259, 2003

CHAPTER 7

Monoamine Oxidase Inhibitors

K. Ranga Rama Krishnan, M.D.

History and Discovery

Monoamine oxidase inhibitors (MAOIs) were first identified as effective antidepressants in the late 1950s. An early report suggested that iproniazid, an antitubercular agent, had mood-elevating properties in patients who had been treated for tuberculosis (Bloch et al. 1954). Following these observations, two studies confirmed that iproniazid did indeed have antidepressant properties (Crane 1957; Kline 1958). Zeller (1963) reported that iproniazid caused potent inhibition of monoamine oxidase (MAO) enzymes both in vivo and in vitro in the brain. He also reported that the medication reversed some of the actions of reserpine. Because reserpine produced significant depression as a side effect, it was suggested that iproniazid might have mood-elevating properties.

The use of iproniazid soon fell into disfavor because of its significant hepatotoxicity. Other MAOIs, both hydrazine derivatives (e.g., isocarboxazid and phenylhydrazine) and nonhydrazine derivatives (e.g., tranylcypromine), were introduced. These MAOIs were not specific for any subtype of MAO enzyme, and they were irreversible inhibitors of MAO (see next section, "Monoamine Oxidase"). Their use has been rather limited because hypertensive crisis by the MAOIs may occur in some patients from potentiation of the pressor effects of amines (such as tyramine) in food (Blackwell et al. 1967).

In the past few years, there has been a resurgence of interest in the development of new MAOIs—that is, in development of MAOIs that are more selective for specific subtypes of MAO enzyme and that are reversible in nature. Newer MAOIs, such as L-deprenyl (selegiline hydrochloride), a monoamine oxidase B (MAO-B) inhibitor, have been introduced (Table 7–1). Reversible monoamine oxidase A (MAO-A) inhibitors, such as moclobemide, have been introduced in Europe but are not yet available in the United States.

TABLE 7–1. Classification of monoamine oxidase inhibitor (MAOI) drugs by structure, selectivity, and reversibility

DRUG	HYDRAZINE	SELECTIVE	REVERSIBLE
Phenelzine	Yes	No	No
Isocarboxazid	Yes	No	No
Tranylcypromine	No	No	No
Selegiline	No	Yes[a,b]	No
Moclobemide	No	Yes[c]	Yes
Brofaromine	No	Yes[c]	Yes

[a]Selective for MAO-B at lower doses.
[b]Becomes nonselective at higher doses.
[c]Selective for MAO-A.

Monoamine Oxidase

A and B Isoenzymes

MAO is widely distributed in mammals. Two isoenzymes, MAO-A and MAO-B, are of special interest (Cesura and Pletscher 1992). Both are present in the central nervous system (CNS) and in some peripheral organs. For example, MAO-A is present in the liver, heart, and pancreas, and MAO-B is present in the liver, posterior pituitary, renal tubules, and endocrine pancreas (Saura et al. 1992). Both MAO-A and MAO-B are present in discrete cell populations within the CNS. MAO-A is present in both dopamine (DA) and norepinephrine (NE) neurons, whereas MAO-B is present to a greater extent in serotonin (5-HT)–containing neurons. They are also present in nonaminergic neurons in various subcortical regions of the brain. Glial cells also express MAO-A and MAO-B (Cesura and Pletscher 1992).

The physiological functions of these two isoenzymes have not been fully elucidated. The main substrates for MAO-A are epinephrine, NE, and 5-HT. The main substrates for MAO-B are phenylethylamine, phenylethanolamine, tyramine, and benzylamine. DA and tryptamine are metabolized by both isoenzymes. The localization of the MAO subtypes does not fully correspond to the neurons containing the substrates. The reason for this discrepancy is unknown. The occurrence of the MAO-B form in 5-HT neurons may actually protect these neurons from amines (other than 5-HT) that could be toxic to them (Cesura and Pletscher 1992).

The primary structures of MAO-A and MAO-B have been fully described. MAO-A has 527 amino acids, and MAO-B has 520 amino acids. About 70% of the amino acid sequence of the two forms is homologous. The genes for both isoenzymes are located on the short arm of the human X chromosome. MAO-A and MAO-B are linked and have been located in the XP11.23–P11 and XP22.1 regions, respectively. The genes are about 70 kilobases and consist of about 15 exons and 14 introns. MAO-A has two messenger RNA (mRNA) transcripts of 2.1 and 5.0 kilobytes in length. MAO-B has a 3-kb mRNA single transcript (Cesura and Pletscher 1992). A rare inherited disorder, Norrie's disease, is characterized by deletion of both genes; patients with this disorder have very severe mental retardation and blindness.

The subunit composition of MAO is unknown. The enzyme is primarily found in the outer mitochondrial membrane; flavin adenine dinucleotide (FAD) is a cofactor for both MAO-A and MAO-B.

Because the cofactor domain is the same for both of the MAO isoenzymes, the structural differences responsible for substrate specificity are believed to lie in regions of the protein that bind to the hydrophobic moiety of the substrate. Although DA is considered to be a mixed substrate for both MAO-A and MAO-B, the breakdown of DA in the striatal regions of the brain is preferentially by MAO-B. In other regions, MAO-A may be more important. There may be regional differences as to which isoenzyme is responsible for the metabolism of other biogenic amines that are substrates for both forms of MAO (Cesura and Pletscher 1992).

Enzyme Kinetics

The enzyme kinetics of MAO-A have not been well studied. The enzyme kinetics for MAO-B, for which more information is available, depend on the nature of the substrate. Some substrates (e.g., tyramine) go through ping-pong mechanisms characterized by first oxidation of the amine to the imine form that is subsequently released from the reduced enzyme before reoxidation of the latter occurs. Other substrates (e.g., benzylamine) involve formation of a tertiary complex with the enzyme and oxygen (Husain et al. 1982; Pearce and Roth 1985; Ramsay and Singer 1991).

Positron Emission Tomographic Studies of MAO-A in Psychiatric Disorders

[^{11}C]Harmine is a selective reversible positron emission tomography (PET) radiotracer with high brain uptake that binds with high affinity to MAO-A. A study using this tracer reported highly significant elevations in brain MAO-A binding during episodes of major depression that persisted even after selective serotonin reuptake inhibitor (SSRI) treatment (Meyer et al. 2009). Interestingly, subjects with higher MAO-A levels had a higher rate of major depressive episode recurrence (Meyer et al. 2009).

Mechanism of Action

The target function of MAOIs is regulation of the monoamine content within the nervous system. Because MAO is bound to the outer surface of the plasma membrane of the mitochondria, in neurons MAO is unable to deaminate amines that are present inside stored vesicles and can metabolize only amines that are present in the cytoplasm. As a result, MAO maintains a low cytoplasmic concentration of amines within the cells. Inhibition of neuronal MAO produces an increase in the amine content in the cytoplasm. Initially, it was believed that the therapeutic action of MAOIs was a result of this amine accumulation (Finberg and Youdim 1984; Murphy et al. 1984, 1987). More recently, it has been suggested that secondary adaptive mechanisms may be important for the antidepressant action of these agents.

After several weeks of treatment, MAOIs produce effects such as a reduction in the number of β-adrenoreceptors, α_1- and α_2-adrenoreceptors, and serotonin$_1$ (5-HT$_1$) and serotonin$_2$ (5-HT$_2$) receptors. These changes are similar to those produced by the chronic use of tricyclic antidepressants (TCAs) and other antidepressant treatment (DaPrada et al. 1984, 1989).

MAOIs can be subdivided on the basis of not only the particular type of enzyme inhibition but also the type of inhibition they produce (reversible or irreversible). The reversible MAOIs are basically chemically inert substrate analogs. MAOIs are recognized as substrates by the enzyme and are converted into intermediates by the normal mechanism. These converted compounds react to the inactive site of the enzyme and form a stable bound enzyme. This effect occurs gradually, and there is usually a correlation between the plasma concentration of the reversible inhibitors and pharmacological action.

Pharmacological Profile

The classic MAOIs inhibit both forms of the enzyme and are divided into two main subtypes: hydrazine and nonhydrazine derivatives. The hydrazine derivatives, two of which (phenelzine and isocarboxazid) are currently available, are related to iproniazid. The nonhydrazine irreversible MAOI is tranylcypromine. Clorgyline is an example of an irreversible inhibitor of MAO-A, whereas selegiline is an irreversible inhibitor of MAO-B. The only commercially available reversible inhibitor of MAO-A is moclobemide.

Three classic MAOIs (i.e., tranylcypromine, phenelzine, and isocarboxazid) are of clinical interest. Clinicians must recognize that these drugs not only inhibit MAO but also exert other actions that may be clinically relevant. Thus, these compounds can block MAO uptake—tranylcypromine more than isocarboxazid or phenelzine. In addition, because tranylcypromine is structurally similar to amphetamine, it is believed to exert stimulant-like actions in the brain. Many issues are common to all three of these MAOIs. The reversible MAOI moclobemide is not available in the United States.

Indications and Efficacy

Major and Atypical Depression

Many studies have examined the efficacy of MAOIs in the treatment of different types of depression. MAOIs have been effective in the treatment of major depression or atypical depression (Davidson et al. 1987a; Himmelhoch et al. 1982, 1991; Johnstone 1975; Johnstone and Marsh 1973; McGrath et al. 1986; Paykel et al. 1982; Quitkin et al. 1979, 1990, 1991; Rowan et al. 1981; Thase et al. 1992; Vallejo et al. 1987; White et al. 1984; Zisook et al. 1985). Although early studies of relatively low-dose regimens suggested that the efficacy of MAOIs was lower than that of TCAs, more recent studies have documented that their efficacy is comparable (Table 7–2).

Quitkin et al. (1979, 1991) reviewed both phenelzine and tranylcypromine studies in patients with either atypical neurotic depression or melancholic depression. The authors reported that phenelzine appeared to be effective for the treatment of atypical depression.

Relatively few studies of endogenous depression in patients have been done. From the limited number of initial patient studies, it is difficult to conclude that phenelzine is effective in the treatment of these patients. In addition, very few well-controlled studies of tranylcypromine, compared with placebo, have been done. Three of the four studies that compared tranylcypromine with placebo showed that tranylcypromine was more effective. In one study, a nonsignificant trend was found favoring tranylcypromine. More recently, studies have documented the efficacy of tranylcypromine in treating anergic depression and, at high doses, treatment-resistant depression (Himmelhoch et al. 1982, 1991; Thase et al. 1992; White et al. 1984). In the Sequenced Treatment Alternatives to Relieve Depression (STAR*D) study, patients who had failed to respond to at least three treatment options were randomly assigned to tranylcypromine or a combination of venlafaxine and mirtazapine. Remission rates were modest for both the tranylcypromine group and the extended-release venlafaxine plus mirtazapine group, and the rates were not statistically different between groups (McGrath et al. 2006).

The heterogeneity of acetylation rate may account for some of the variance in response to phenelzine (Johnstone 1975; Johnstone and Marsh 1973; Paykel et al. 1982; Rowan et al. 1981). One-half of the patients in a given population are often slow acetylators. An initial study by Johnstone and Marsh (1973) suggested that slow acetylators improve more with phenelzine than do fast acetylators.

TABLE 7–2. Indications for use of monoamine oxidase inhibitors (MAOIs)

Definitely effective	**Other possible uses**
Atypical depression	OCD
Major depression	Narcolepsy
Dysthymia	Headache
Melancholia	Chronic pain syndrome
Panic disorder	GAD
Bulimia	
Atypical facial pain	
Anergic depression	
Treatment-resistant depression	
Parkinson's disease[a]	

Note. GAD=generalized anxiety disorder; OCD=obsessive-compulsive disorder.
[a]Selegiline is the only MAOI that is useful in the treatment of Parkinson's disease.

Other groups have been unable to confirm the relation between acetylation, acetylator type, and response to MAOIs.

MAOIs are used in a wide range of psychiatric disorders. Early studies suggested that MAOIs are particularly effective in patients who have atypical depression, originally defined as depression with anxiety or chronic pain, reversed vegetative symptoms, and rejection sensitivity (Quitkin et al. 1990).

The concept of atypical depression remains controversial and has not been completely validated. In general, patients with atypical depression have an earlier age at onset than do patients with melancholic depression, and the prevalence of dysthymia, alcohol abuse, sociopathy, and atypical depression is increased in the relatives of patients with atypical depression. The best differentiating criterion appears to be that phenelzine and other irreversible MAOIs are more effective than TCAs in treating these patients (Cesura and Pletscher 1992; Quitkin et al. 1990; Zisook et al. 1985). A metareview noted evidence that MAOIs are superior to TCAs, but not SSRIs, in treating atypical depression (Cipriani et al. 2007).

Some studies have also suggested that MAOIs are effective in treating typical major depression and melancholic depression (Davidson et al. 1987a; McGrath et al. 1986; Vallejo et al. 1987). In a Cochrane review, Lima and Moncrieff (2000) noted that MAOIs were comparable in efficacy to other classes of antidepressants in treating dysthymia.

Panic Disorder

Both single- and double-blind studies have found that phenelzine and iproniazid are effective in treating panic disorder (Lydiard et al. 1989; Quitkin et al. 1990; Tyrer et al. 1973). About 50%–60% of patients with panic disorder respond to MAOIs. In the early stages of treatment, patients may have a worsening of symptoms. This is reduced in clinical practice by combining the MAOI with a benzodiazepine for the initial phase of the study. It has been suggested that in addition to its antipanic effect, phenelzine has an antiphobic action (Kelly et al. 1971). The time course of effect and the dose used are similar to those for major depression.

Social Phobia

Liebowitz et al. (1992) reported that phenelzine is effective in treating social phobia.

In an open-label study, Versiani et al. (1988) suggested that tranylcypromine is effective. Versiani et al. (1992) also demonstrated the efficacy of moclobemide in a double-blind study. In clinical experience, about 50% of patients respond to MAOIs, and the onset of response is gradual (usually about 2–3 weeks). A Cochrane review of pharmacotherapy for social phobia noted that whereas traditional MAOIs were comparable in efficacy to SSRIs, reversible inhibitors were less efficacious (Stein et al. 2004).

Obsessive-Compulsive Disorder

Although initial case reports suggested that MAOIs may be effective in obsessive-compulsive disorder (Jenike 1981), no double-blind studies have indicated efficacy.

Posttraumatic Stress Disorder

The classic MAOI phenelzine has been proven effective for the treatment of posttraumatic stress disorder (PTSD) in single-blind trials (Davidson et al. 1987b) and a double-blind crossover trial (Kosten et al. 1991).

Generalized Anxiety Disorder

MAOIs are not usually used to treat generalized anxiety disorder (GAD) because the risk–benefit ratio favors the use of selective serotonin reuptake inhibitors (SSRIs), azaspirones, or benzodiazepines. When they are used, MAOIs are used primarily for treating treatment-resistant GAD.

Bulimia Nervosa

Both phenelzine and isocarboxazid have been shown to be effective in treating some symptoms of bulimia nervosa (Kennedy et al. 1988; McElroy et al. 1989; Walsh et al. 1985, 1987).

Premenstrual Dysphoria

Preliminary studies and clinical experience suggest that MAOIs may be effective in the treatment of premenstrual dysphoria (Glick et al. 1991).

Chronic Pain

MAOIs are believed to be effective in the treatment of atypical facial pain and other chronic pain syndromes. However, only limited data on these conditions are available.

Neurological Diseases

The classic MAOIs have not been found to be effective for treating neurological disorders such as Parkinson's disease and Alzheimer's dementia. However, the MAO-B inhibitor selegiline has been shown to be effective in slowing the progression of Parkinson's disease (Cesura and Pletscher 1992), but the mechanism underlying this effect is unknown.

Side Effects and Toxicology

The side effects of MAOIs are generally not more severe or frequent than those of other antidepressants (Zisook 1984). The most frequent side effects include dizziness, headache, dry mouth, insomnia, constipation, blurred vision, nausea, peripheral edema, forgetfulness, fainting spells, trauma, urinary hesitancy, weakness, and myoclonic jerks. Loss of weight and appetite may occur with isocarboxazid use (Davidson and Turnbull 1982). Hepatotoxicity is rare with the currently available MAOIs, compared with iproniazid. However, liver enzymes, such as aspartate transaminase (AST) and alanine transaminase (ALT), are elevated in 3%–5% of patients. Liver function tests must be done when patients have symptoms like malaise, jaundice, and excessive fatigue.

Some side effects first emerge during maintenance treatment (Evans et al. 1982). These side effects include weight gain (which occurs in almost one-half of patients), edema, muscle cramps, carbohydrate craving, sexual dysfunction (usually anorgasmia), pyridoxine deficiency (see Goodheart et al. 1991), hypoglycemia, hypomania, urinary retention, and disorientation. Peripheral neuropathy (Goodheart et al. 1991) and speech blockage (Goldstein and Goldberg 1986) are rare side effects of MAOIs. Weight gain is more of a problem with hydrazine compounds, such as phenelzine, than with tranylcypromine. Therefore, weight gain that is caused by hydrazine derivatives is an indication to switch to tranylcypromine. Edema is also more common with phenelzine than with tranylcypromine.

The management of some of these side effects can be difficult. Orthostatic hypotension is common with MAOIs. Addition of salt and salt-retaining steroids such as fludrocortisone (9-α-fluorohydrocortisone) is sometimes effective in treating orthostatic hypotension. Elastic support stockings are also helpful. Small amounts of coffee or tea taken during the day also keep the blood pressure elevated. The dose of fluorohydrocortisol should be adjusted carefully because in elderly patients it could provoke cardiac failure resulting from fluid retention.

Sexual dysfunction that occurs with these compounds is also difficult to treat. Common problems include anorgasmia, decreased libido, impotence, and delayed ejaculation (Harrison et al. 1985; Jacobson 1987). Cyproheptadine is sometimes effective in treating sexual dysfunction like anorgasmia. Bethanechol may also be effective in some patients.

Insomnia occasionally occurs as an intermediate or late side effect of these compounds. Changing the time of administration does not seem to help much, although dosage reduction may be helpful. Adding trazodone at bedtime is effective, but this should be done with caution. Myoclonic jerks, peripheral neuropathy, and paresthesia, when present, are also difficult to treat. When a patient has paresthesia, the clinician should evaluate for peripheral neuropathy and pyridoxine deficiency. In general, patients taking MAOIs should also receive concomitant pyridoxine therapy. When myoclonic jerks occur, patients can be treated with cyproheptadine.

MAOIs also have the potential to suppress anginal pain; therefore, coronary artery disease could be overlooked or underestimated.

Patients with hyperthyroidism are more sensitive to MAOIs because of their overall sensitivity to pressor amines. MAOIs can also worsen hypoglycemia in patients taking hypoglycemic agents like insulin.

Dietary Interactions

After the introduction of MAOIs, several reports of severe headaches in patients who were taking these compounds were published ("Cheese and Tranylcypromine" 1970; Cronin 1965; Hedberg et al. 1966; Simpson and Gratz 1992). These headaches were caused by a drug-food interaction. The risk of such an interaction is highest for tranylcypromine and lower for phenelzine, provided that the dose of the latter remains low. However, it must be kept in mind that this interaction can occur even at low doses with any of the traditional MAOIs. The interaction of MAOIs with food has been attributed to increased tyramine levels. Tyramine, which has a pressor action, is present in a number of foodstuffs. It is normally broken down by the MAO enzymes and has both direct and indirect sympathomimetic actions. The classic explanation of this side effect may not be entirely accurate; in fact, it has been suggested that the potentiation of tyramine by an MAOI may be secondary to increased release of NE rather than to the MAOI. Adrenaline would increase the indirect sympathetic activity of tyramine. The spontaneous occurrence of hypertensive crises in a few patients lends support to this hypothesis (O'Brien et al. 1992; Zajecka and Fawcett 1991).

The tyramine effect of food is potentiated by MAOIs 10- to 20-fold. A mild tyramine interaction occurs with about 6 mg of tyramine; 10 mg can produce a moderate episode, and 25 mg can produce a severe episode that is characterized by hypertension, occipital headache, palpitations, nausea, vomiting, apprehension, occasional chills, sweating, and restlessness. On examination, neck stiffness, pallor, mild pyrexia, dilated pupils, and motor agitation may be seen. The reaction usually develops within 20–60 minutes after ingestion of food. Occasionally, the reaction can be very severe and may lead to alteration of consciousness, hyperpyrexia, cerebral hemorrhage, and death. Death is exceedingly rare and has been calculated to be about 0.01%–0.02% for all patients taking tranylcypromine.

The classic treatment of the hypertensive reaction is phentolamine (5 mg) administered intravenously (Youdim et al. 1987; Zisook 1984). More recently, nifedipine, a calcium channel blocker, has been shown to be effective. Nifedipine has an onset of action of about 5 minutes, and it lasts approximately 3–5 hours; in fact, some clinicians have suggested that patients should carry nifedipine with them for immediate use in the event of a hypertensive crisis.

Because of the drug interaction of the classic MAOIs with food, clinicians usually make several dietary recommendations (Table 7–3). These recommendations are quite varied.

All of the MAOI diets recommend restriction of cheese (with the exception of cream cheese and cottage cheese), red wine, sherry, liqueurs, pickled fish, overripe (aged) fruit, brewer's yeast, fava beans, beef and chicken liver, and fermented products. Other diets also recommend restriction of all alcoholic beverages, coffee, chocolate, colas, tea, yogurt, soy sauce, avocados, and bananas. Furthermore, many of the restricted foods—for example, avocados and bananas—rarely cause hypertensive crisis. For example, an interaction may occur only if overripe fruit is eaten or, in the case of bananas, if the skin is eaten (which is an uncommon practice in the United States). Similarly, unless a person ingests large amounts of caffeine, the interaction is usually not clinically significant. Although there is greater risk of noncompliance with highly restrictive diets, it is nevertheless advisable to emphasize the need to adhere to dietary restrictions and the potential risks that arise by breaking the diet when discussing restrictions and cautions with the patient.

In evaluating patients who may have had a drug-food reaction, it is important to evaluate the hypertensive reaction and differentiate it from histamine headache, which can occur with an MAOI. Histamine headaches are usually accompanied by hypotension, colic, loose stools, salivation, and lacrimation (Cooper 1967). The clinician should provide oral instructions, as well as printed cards outlining these instructions, to patients who are taking classic MAOIs.

In addition to the food interaction, drug interactions are extremely important (see next section, "Drug-Drug Interactions"). Each patient should be given a card indicating that he or she is taking an MAOI and instructions that the card should be carried at all times. A medical bracelet indicating that the wearer takes an MAOI is also a good idea.

Drug-Drug Interactions

The extensive inhibition of MAO enzymes by MAOIs raises the potential for a number of drug interactions (Table 7–4). Of particular importance, many over-the-counter medications can interact with MAOIs. These medications include cough syrups containing sympathomimetic agents, which in the presence of an MAOI can precipitate a hypertensive crisis.

Another area of caution is the use of MAOIs in patients who need surgery. In this situation, interactions include those with narcotic drugs, especially meperidine (Pethidine). Meperidine administered with MAOIs can produce a syndrome characterized by coma, hyperpyrexia, and hypertension. This syndrome has been reported primarily with phenelzine; however, it has also been reported

TABLE 7–3. Food restrictions for monoamine oxidase inhibitors (MAOIs)

To be avoided	To be used in moderation
Cheese (except for cream cheese and cottage cheese)	Coffee
Overripe (aged) fruit (e.g., banana peel)	Chocolate
Fava beans	Colas
Sausage, salami	Tea
Sherry, liqueurs	Soy sauce
Sauerkraut	Beer, other wines
Monosodium glutamate	
Pickled fish	
Brewer's yeast	
Beef and chicken livers	
Fermented products	
Red wine	

with tranylcypromine (Mendelson 1979; Stack et al. 1988). Stack et al. (1988) noted that this syndrome is most likely to occur with meperidine and that it may be related to that drug's serotonergic properties. Similar reactions have not been reported to any significant extent with other narcotic analgesics such as morphine and codeine. In fact, many patients probably receive these medications without problems. Only a small fraction of patients may have this interaction, and it could reflect an idiosyncratic effect. In general, current opinion favors the use of morphine or fentanyl when intra- or postoperative narcotics are needed in patients taking MAOIs.

The issue of whether directly acting sympathomimetic amines interact with MAOIs is more controversial. Intravenous administration of sympathomimetic amines to patients receiving MAOIs does not provoke hypertension. When a bolus infusion of catecholamines is given to healthy volunteer subjects who have been taking phenelzine or tranylcypromine for 1 week, a potentiation of the pressor effect of phenylephrine occurs, but no clinically significant potentiation of cardiovascular effects of NE, epinephrine, or isoproterenol occurs (Wells 1989).

In general, direct sympathomimetic amine-MAOI interactions do not appear to produce significant cardiovascular problems. However, there is a low incidence of hypertensive episodes in the presence of indirect sympathomimetics. Ideally, these compounds should not be used in those patients who are receiving MAOIs. A direct-acting compound is preferable to an indirect-acting compound.

Caution should be exercised when using MAOIs in patients with pheochromocytoma or with cardiovascular, cerebrovascular, or hepatic disease. Because phenelzine tablets contain gluten, they should not be given to patients with celiac disease.

Specific Monoamine Oxidase Inhibitors

Phenelzine

Phenelzine, a hydrazine derivative, is a potent MAOI and the best studied among the MAOIs.

TABLE 7–4. Drug interactions with monoamine oxidase inhibitors (MAOIs)

DRUG	INTERACTION	COMMENT
Other MAOIs (e.g., furazolidone, pargyline, procarbazine)	Potentiation of side effects; convulsions possible	Allow at least 1 week before changing to another MAOI
Tricyclic antidepressants (TCAs) (e.g., maprotiline, bupropion)	Severe side effects, such as hypertension and convulsions, possible	Allow at least 2 weeks before changing to an MAOI; combinations have been used occasionally for refractory depression
Carbamazepine	Low possibility of interaction; similar to TCAs	Same as for TCAs
Cyclobenzaprine	Low possibility of interaction; similar to TCAs	Same as for TCAs
Selective serotonin reuptake inhibitors (SSRIs)	Serotonin syndrome	Avoid combinations; allow at least 2 weeks before changing to an MAOI and 5 weeks if switching from fluoxetine to an MAOI
Stimulants (e.g., methylphenidate, dextroamphetamine)	Potential for increased blood pressure (hypertension)	Avoid combination
Buspirone	Potential for increased blood pressure (hypertension)	Avoid use; if used, monitor blood pressure
Meperidine	Severe, potentially fatal interaction possible (see text)	Avoid combination
Dextromethorphan	Reports of brief psychosis	Avoid high doses
Direct sympathomimetics (e.g., L-dopa)	Increased blood pressure	Avoid use if possible; if they need to be used, use with caution
Indirect sympathomimetics	Hypertensive crisis possible	Avoid use
Oral hypoglycemics (e.g., insulin)	Worsening of hypoglycemia possible	Monitor blood sugar levels and adjust medications
Fenfluramine	Serotonin syndrome possible	Avoid use
L-Tryptophan	Serotonin syndrome possible	Avoid use

Pharmacokinetics

Phenelzine is a substrate as well as an inhibitor of MAO, and major identified metabolites of phenelzine include phenylacetic acid and *p*-hydroxyphenylacetic acid. Phenelzine undergoes acetylation, and therefore drug levels are lower in fast acetylators than in slow acetylators. However, because phenelzine is an irreversible inhibitor, plasma concentrations are not relevant. The antidepressant effect, the degree of inhibition of MAO, and the amount of free phenelzine excreted in the urine are all significantly greater in slow acetylators than in fast acetylators (Baker et al. 1999).

Efficacy

Phenelzine is useful in the treatment of major depression, atypical depression, panic disorder, social phobia, and atypical facial pain (see section "Indications and Efficacy" presented earlier in this chapter).

Side Effects

The primary side effects of phenelzine are similar to those of other MAOIs. Hepatitis secondary to phenelzine may occur. This effect is quite rare (<1 in 30,000). The most difficult side effect, often leading to discontinuation, is postural hypotension.

Contraindications

The contraindications to phenelzine include known sensitivity to the drug, pheochromocytoma, congestive heart failure, and history of liver disease. (In addition, see sections "Dietary Interactions" and "Drug-Drug Interactions" presented earlier in this chapter.)

Isocarboxazid

Isocarboxazid is a hydrazine type of MAOI.

Pharmacokinetics

Isocarboxazid is rapidly absorbed from the gastrointestinal tract and is metabolized in the liver. It is primarily excreted as hippuric acid. Its half-life is of little interest because it is an irreversible MAOI. Chemically, isocarboxazid is 5-methyl-3-isoxazolecarboxylic acid 2-benzylhydrazide. Isocarboxazid is a colorless crystalline substance with very little taste.

Efficacy

Isocarboxazid is the least studied of the MAOIs. Its indications are similar to those of the other MAOIs.

Side Effects

The side effects of isocarboxazid are similar to those of phenelzine. Postural hypotension is the most common problem.

Contraindications

The contraindications to isocarboxazid are similar to those of phenelzine.

Tranylcypromine

Tranylcypromine, a nonhydrazine reversible MAOI, increases the concentration of NE, epinephrine, and 5-HT in the CNS. When tranylcypromine is discontinued, about 5 days are needed for recovery of MAO function. Tranylcypromine has a mild stimulant effect.

Pharmacokinetics

Limited data exist on pharmacokinetics. Tranylcypromine is excreted within 24 hours. The dynamic effect lasts for up to 5 days after withdrawal. There is considerable debate about whether tranylcypromine is metabolized to amphetamine; most studies in the literature indicate that this does not occur.

Efficacy

Tranylcypromine's indications are similar to those of other MAOIs (see section "Indications and Efficacy" presented earlier in this chapter).

Side Effects

The side effects of tranylcypromine are similar to those of other MAOIs. In addition, problems with physical dependence on tranylcypromine have been reported. Thus, withdrawal symptoms, such as anxiety, restlessness, depression, and headache, may occur. Syndrome of inappropriate antidiuretic hormone (SIADH) has been reported with tranylcypromine. Rare cases of toxic hepatitis have been reported. Tranylcypromine can lead to increased agitation, insomnia, and restlessness, compared with phenelzine.

Contraindications

The contraindications to tranylcypromine are the same as those for phenelzine. In addition, in view of the greater potential for hypertensive episodes, tranylcypromine should be used with particular caution in patients with cerebrovascular or cardiovascular disease.

Moclobemide

Moclobemide, a reversible inhibitor of MAO-A enzyme (Amrein et al. 1989), has a higher potency in vivo than in vitro. Therefore, it has been suggested that moclobemide is a prodrug and that it is metabolized to a form with higher affinity for MAO-A than the parent compound. After single- or repeated-dose administration of moclobemide, the recovery of MAO-A activity is much quicker than that seen with other MAOIs, including clorgyline, an irreversible inhibitor of MAO-A. One of the metabolites of moclobemide does inhibit MAO-B; however, this action is minimally significant in humans. When administered to rats, moclobemide increases the concentration of 5-HT, NE, epinephrine, and DA in rat brain (see Haefely et al. 1992). These effects are short-lasting, and they parallel the time course of MAO-A inhibition. In addition, unlike irreversible inhibitors, repeated administration does not increase the inhibition.

In animals, moclobemide only partially potentiates the blood pressor effect of oral tyramine. This is because it is a reversible inhibitor with a low affinity for the MAO isoenzymes and is easily displaced by the pressor amines ingested in food. On the basis of these studies, moclobemide is thought to be safer than irreversible MAOIs.

Pharmacokinetics

After oral administration of moclobemide, peak plasma concentrations are reached within 1 hour. The drug is about 50% bound to plasma proteins and is extensively metabolized; only 1% of the compound is excreted (unchanged) in the urine. The half-life of the compound is approximately 12 hours. Moclobemide is extensively metabolized; 95% of the administered dose is excreted in the urine. The metabolites are pharmacologically inactive. The presence of food reduces the rate (but not the extent) of moclobemide absorption.

Efficacy

Moclobemide has been studied in all types of depressive disorders (Gabelic and Kuhn 1990; Larsen et al. 1991; Rossel and Moll 1990). Controlled trials have found that it is superior to placebo. In addition, moclobemide has been found to be as effective as imipramine, desipramine, clomipramine, and amitriptyline in the treatment of depression. The dosage required is 300–600 mg/day.

Unlike the classic MAOIs, moclobemide has been found to be effective in treating both endogenous and nonendogenous depression. In addition, in combination with antipsychotics, the drug seems to be effective in treating psychotic depression (Amrein et al. 1989). Moclobemide has also been effective in treating bipolar endogenous depression.

Versiani et al. (1992) compared phenelzine, moclobemide, and placebo and reported that both phenelzine and moclobemide were superior to placebo in treating patients with social phobia. Given the efficacy of classic MAOIs in the treatment of other psychiatric disorders, such as bulimia, panic disorder, and PTSD, it is likely that patients with such disorders would respond to the reversible MAOIs. Additional trials of moclobemide are required to confirm its utility in other psychiatric disorders.

Side Effects

Nausea was the only side effect noted to be greater in patients taking moclobemide than in patients taking placebo. Thus, the profile of moclobemide seems to be ideal in that it causes few or no major side effects. Case reports have shown no toxicity after overdoses of up to 20 g (Amrein et al. 1989).

Dietary Interactions

Intravenous tyramine pressor tests indicate that a single dose of moclobemide increases tyramine sensitivity (Cusson et al. 1991). However, this increase is marginal, compared with the increase associated with other MAOIs. Under most conditions, there appears to be limited drug-food interaction. However, to minimize even mild tyramine pressor effects, it would be preferable to administer moclobemide after a meal rather than before it. In a study in which tyramine was administered in doses of up to 100 mg, inpatients pretreated with moclobemide had no significant changes in blood pressure. The drug also has minimal effect on cognitive performance and no effect on body weight or hematological parameters (Wesnes et al. 1989; Youdim et al. 1987).

Drug-Drug Interactions

Several studies have examined potential drug-drug interactions with moclobemide (Amrein et al. 1992). No drug interaction with lithium or in combination with TCAs has been reported. Moclobemide has also been combined with fluoxetine and other SSRIs with no significant interaction. No interactions with benzodiazepines or neuroleptics have been reported (Amrein et al. 1992). Parallel data suggest that moclobemide can potentiate the effects of meperidine; therefore, the narcotic-MAOI interaction may occur. Until proven otherwise, it would be prudent to avoid the combination of moclobemide with opiates like meperidine. A pharmacokinetic interaction has been observed with cimetidine that requires the reduction of the moclobemide dose because cimetidine reduces the clearance of moclobemide.

Selegiline Hydrochloride

Selegiline hydrochloride is an irreversible MAO-B inhibitor (Cesura and Pletscher 1992). Its primary use is in the treatment of Parkinson's disease, as an adjunct to L-dopa and carbidopa. The average dosage for Parkinson's disease is 5–10 mg/day. The exact mechanism of action of MAO-B in Parkinson's disease is unknown (Gerlach et al. 1996; Hagan et al. 1997; Lyytinen et al. 1997).

Pharmacokinetics

Selegiline is metabolized to levoamphetamine, methamphetamine, and *N*-desmethylselegiline. Selegiline hydrochloride undergoes significant first-pass metabolism following oral administration. Transdermal delivery avoids the first-pass effect and provides greater levels of unchanged drug and reduced levels of metabolites compared with the oral regimen. The time to reach the peak is less than 1 hour. The elimination half-life of selegiline is about 1.5 hours. There is at least a threefold increase in the area under the curve (AUC) of selegiline with food (Mahmood 1997).

Efficacy

The efficacy of selegiline in treating depression has not been well studied. The few studies that have examined its utility have been equivocal. The dose required for treating depression may be much higher than that required to treat Parkinson's disease. Clinical experience suggests that dosages of 20–40 mg/day are needed. At these dosages, dietary interactions could occur. Early studies have reported that selegiline is of modest benefit in patients with Alzheimer's disease (Lawlor et al. 1997). Quitkin et al. (1984) showed that L-deprenyl was superior to 6 weeks of placebo administered to patients with depression in a separate double-blind study. Dosages of more than 10–20 mg/day were needed.

Side Effects

Selegiline has been found to have no adverse effects when combined with other antidepressants during treatment of depression in patients with Parkinson's disease. The few side effects that have been noted with selegiline include nausea, dizziness, and lightheadedness. When the drug is abruptly discontinued, nausea, hallucinations, and confusion have been reported.

Dietary Interactions

Because MAO-B is not involved in the intestinal tyramine interaction, dietary interaction with selegiline (at low dosages, i.e., 5–10 mg/day) would probably be minimal; therefore, no drug interactions have been reported. An interaction between selegiline and narcotics has been reported and should be kept in mind.

Selegiline Transdermal System

The selegiline transdermal system (STS) was developed to overcome limitations of orally administered MAOIs, particularly dietary tyramine restrictions. The system does not overcome drug-drug interactions. It bypasses the gut, thereby reducing drug-food interactions. The pharmacokinetic and pharmacodynamic properties promote the inhibition of MAO-A and MAO-B in the CNS while avoiding significant inhibition of intestinal and liver MAO-A enzymes. Three different strengths of Emsam patch are currently marketed: 20 mg/20 cm^2, 30 mg/30 cm^2, and 40 mg/40 cm^2. The three patch sizes deliver 24-hour doses of selegiline averaging 6 mg, 9 mg, and 12 mg, respectively. Use of the lowest-dosage Emsam 6-mg/24-hour patch does not call for dietary modification. A restricted "MAOI diet" is advised for the higher-dosage Emsam 9-mg/24-hour patch and the 12-mg/24-hour patch to avoid any risk of hypertensive crisis. Patients are strongly advised to follow these restrictions.

Pharmacokinetics

Following dermal application of the selegiline patch, 25%–30% of the selegiline content on average is delivered systemically over 24 hours. Consequently, the degree of drug absorption is one-third higher than the average amounts of 6–12 mg/24 hours. In comparison with oral dosing, transdermal dosing results in substantially higher exposure to selegiline and lower exposure to metabolites.

Efficacy

The efficacy of STS as a treatment for major depressive disorder was established in two placebo-controlled studies of 6 and 8 weeks' duration in adult outpatients with major depressive disorder. In both studies, patients were randomly assigned to double-blind treatment with drug patch or placebo. The 6-week trial showed that 6 mg/24 hours was significantly more effective than placebo, as assessed by scores on the 17-item Hamilton Rating Scale for Depression (Ham-D) (Amsterdam 2003). In an 8-week dosage titration trial, depressed patients receiving the drug patch (starting dosage was 6 mg/24 hours, with possible increases to 9 mg/24 hours or 12 mg/24 hours based on clinical response) showed significant improvement compared with those receiving placebo on the primary outcome measure, the 28-item Ham-D total score (Feiger et al. 2006). In another trial, 322 patients meeting DSM-IV-TR (American Psychiatric Association 2000) criteria for major depressive disorder who had responded during an initial 10-week open-label treatment phase were randomly assigned either to continuation at the same dose or to placebo under double-blind conditions for observation of relapse. In this double-blind phase, patients receiving continued transdermal selegiline experienced a significantly longer time to relapse (Amsterdam and Bodkin 2006).

Drug-Drug Interactions

Potential drug interactions for STS are the same as for other MAOIs.

Conclusion

Various MAOIs have been shown to be effective in treating a wide variety of psychiatric disorders, including depression, panic disorder, social phobia, and PTSD. The classic MAOIs are currently used only rarely as first-line medication because of potential dietary interactions and other long-term side effects. The reversible inhibitors of MAO-A enzyme, such as moclobemide, which have fewer side effects and no dietary restrictions compared with classic MAOIs, are unlikely to be introduced in the United States. In fact, the risk-benefit ratio for these compounds is highly favorable, compared with other antidepressants. The MAO-B inhibitor selegiline is used to reduce the progression of Parkinson's disease. Its utility in treating other degenerative disorders is currently being assessed. The selegiline transdermal system reduces dietary interactions when used at low doses and is now approved for the treatment of major depression. New applications and a wider use of these compounds may be found in the near future.

References

American Psychiatric Association: Diagnostic and Statistical Manual of Mental Disorders, 4th Edition, Text Revision. Washington, DC, American Psychiatric Association, 2000

Amrein R, Allen SR, Guentert TW, et al: Pharmacology of reversible MAOIs. Br J Psychiatry 144:66–71, 1989

Amrein R, Guntert TW, Dingemanse J, et al: Interactions of moclobemide with concomitantly administered medication: evidence from pharmacological and clinical studies. Psychopharmacology (Berl) 106 (suppl):S24–S31, 1992

Amsterdam JD: A double-blind, placebo-controlled trial of the safety and efficacy of selegiline transdermal system without dietary restrictions in patients with major depressive disorder. J Clin Psychiatry 64:208–214, 2003

Amsterdam JD, Bodkin JA: Selegiline transdermal system in the prevention of relapse of major depressive disorder: a 52-week, double-blind, placebo-substitution, parallel-group clinical trial. J Clin Psychopharmacol 26:579–586, 2006

Baker GB, Urichuk LJ, McKenna KF, et al: Metabolism of monoamine oxidase inhibitors. Cell Mol Neurobiol 19:411–426, 1999

Blackwell B, Marley E, Price J, et al: Hypertensive interactions between monoamine oxidase inhibitors and food stuffs. Br J Psychiatry 113:349–365, 1967

Bloch RG, Doonief AS, Buchberg AS, et al: The clinical effect of isoniazid and iproniazid in the treatment of pulmonary tuberculosis. Ann Intern Med 40:881–900, 1954

Cesura AM, Pletscher A: The new generation of monoamine oxidase inhibitors. Prog Drug Res 38:171–297, 1992

Cheese and tranylcypromine (letter). BMJ 3(5718): 354, 1970

Cipriani A, Geddes JR, Furukawa TA, et al: Metareview on short-term effectiveness and safety of antidepressants for depression: an evidence-based approach to inform clinical practice. Can J Psychiatry 52:553–562, 2007

Cooper AJ: MAO inhibitors and headache (letter). BMJ 2:420, 1967

Crane GE: Iproniazid (Marsilid) phosphate, a therapeutic agent for mental disorders and debilitating disease. Psychiatr Res Rep 8:142–152, 1957

Cronin D: Monoamine-oxidase inhibitors and cheese (letter). BMJ 5469:1065, 1965

Cusson JR, Goldenberg E, Larochelle P: Effect of a novel monoamine oxidase inhibitor, moclobemide, on the sensitivity to intravenous tyramine and norepinephrine in humans. J Clin Pharmacol 31:462–467, 1991

DaPrada M, Kettler R, Burkard W, et al: Moclobemide, an antidepressant with short-lasting MAO-A inhibition: brain catecholamines/tyramine pressor effects in rats, in Monoamine Oxidase and Disease. Edited by Tipton K, Dostert P, Strolin Benedetti M. New York, Academic Press, 1984, pp 137–154

DaPrada M, Kettler R, Keller HH, et al: Neurochemical profile of moclobemide, a short-acting and reversible inhibitor of monoamine oxidase type A. J Pharmacol Exp Ther 248:400–414, 1989

Davidson J, Turnbull C: Loss of appetite and weight associated with the monoamine oxidase inhibitor isocarboxazid. J Clin Psychopharmacol 2:263–266, 1982

Davidson J, Raft D, Pelton S: An outpatient evaluation of phenelzine and imipramine. J Clin Psychiatry 48:143–146, 1987a

Davidson J, Walker JI, Kilts C: A pilot study of phenelzine in the treatment of post-traumatic stress disorder. Br J Psychiatry 150:252–255, 1987b

Evans DL, Davidson J, Raft D: Early and late side effects of phenelzine. J Clin Psychopharmacol 2:208–210, 1982

Feiger AD, Rickels K, Rynn MA, et al: Selegiline transdermal system for the treatment of major depressive disorder: an 8-week, double-blind, placebo-controlled, flexible-dose titration trial. J Clin Psychiatry 67:1354–1361, 2006

Finberg JPM, Youdim MBH: Reversible monoamine oxidase inhibitors and the cheese effect, in Monoamine Oxidase and Disease: Prospects for Therapy With Reversible Inhibitors. Edited by Tipton KF, Dostert P, Strolin Benedetti M. New York, Academic Press, 1984, pp 479–485

Gabelic I, Kuhn B: Moclobemide (Ro 11–1163) versus tranylcypromine in the treatment of endogenous depression (abstract). Acta Psychiatr Scand Suppl 360:63, 1990

Gerlach M, Youdim MB, Riederer P: Pharmacology of selegiline. Neurology 47 (6, suppl 3):S137–S145, 1996

Glick R, Harrison W, Endicott J, et al: Treatment of premenstrual dysphoric symptoms in depressed women. J Am Med Womens Assoc 46:182–185, 1991

Goldstein DM, Goldberg RL: Monoamine oxidase inhibitor-induced speech blockage (case report). J Clin Psychiatry 47:604, 1986

Goodheart RS, Dunne JW, Edis RH: Phenelzine associated peripheral neuropathy: clinical and electrophysiologic findings. Aust N Z J Med 21:339–340, 1991

Haefely W, Burkard WP, Cesura AM, et al: Biochemistry and pharmacology of moclobemide: a prototype RIMA. Psychopharmacology (Berl) 106 (suppl):S6–S15, 1992

Hagan JJ, Middlemiss DN, Sharpe PC, et al: Parkinson's disease: prospects for improved drug therapy. Trends Pharmacol Sci 18:156–163, 1997

Harrison WM, Stewart J, Ehrhardt AA, et al: A controlled study of the effects of antidepressants on sexual function. Psychopharmacol Bull 21:85–88, 1985

Hedberg DL, Gordon MW, Glueck BC Jr: Six cases of hypertensive crisis in patients on tranylcypromine after eating chicken livers. Am J Psychiatry 122:933–937, 1966

Himmelhoch JM, Fuchs CZ, Symons BJ: A double-blind study of tranylcypromine treatment of major anergic depression. J Nerv Ment Dis 170:628–634, 1982

Himmelhoch JM, Thase ME, Mallinger AG, et al: Tranylcypromine versus imipramine in anergic bipolar depression. Am J Psychiatry 148:910–916, 1991

Husain M, Edmondson DE, Singer TP: Kinetic studies on the catalytic mechanism of liver monoamine oxidase. Biochemistry 21:595–600, 1982

Jacobson JN: Anorgasmia caused by an MAOI (letter). Am J Psychiatry 144:527, 1987

Jenike MA: Rapid response of severe obsessive-compulsive disorder to tranylcypromine. Am J Psychiatry 138:1249–1250, 1981

Johnstone EC: Relationship between acetylator status and response to phenelzine. Mod Probl Pharmacopsychiatry 10:30–37, 1975

Johnstone EC, Marsh W: The relationship between response to phenelzine and acetylator status in depressed patients. Proc R Soc Lond B Biol Sci 66:947–949, 1973

Kelly D, Mitchell-Heggs N, Sherman D: Anxiety and the effects of sodium lactate assessed clinically and physiologically. Br J Psychiatry 119:129–141, 1971

Kennedy SH, Warsh JJ, Mainprize E, et al: A trial of isocarboxazid in the treatment of bulimia. J Clin Psychopharmacol 8:391–396, 1988

Kline NS: Clinical experience with iproniazid (Marsilid). J Clin Exp Psychopathol 19 (suppl 1):72–78, 1958

Kosten TR, Frank JB, Dan E, et al: Pharmacotherapy for posttraumatic stress disorder using phenelzine or imipramine. J Nerv Ment Dis 179:366–370, 1991

Larsen JK, Gjerris A, Holm P, et al: Moclobemide in depression: a randomized, multicentre trial against isocarboxazide and clomipramine emphasizing atypical depression. Acta Psychiatr Scand 84:564–570, 1991

Lawlor BA, Aisen PS, Green C, et al: Selegiline in the treatment of behavioural disturbance in Alzheimer's disease. Int J Geriatr Psychiatry 12:319–322, 1997

Liebowitz MR, Schneier F, Campeas R, et al: Phenelzine vs atenolol in social phobia: a placebo-controlled comparison. Arch Gen Psychiatry 49:290–300, 1992

Lima MS, Moncrieff J: Drugs versus placebo for dysthymia. Cochrane Database Syst Rev (4): CD001130, 2000

Lydiard RB, Laraia MT, Howell EF, et al: Phenelzine treatment of panic disorder: lack of effect on pyridoxal phosphate levels. J Clin Psychopharmacol 9:428–431, 1989

Lyytinen J, Kaakkola S, Ahtila S, et al: Simultaneous MAO-B and COMT inhibition in L-dopa-treated patients with Parkinson's disease. Mov Disord 12:497–505, 1997

Mahmood I: Clinical pharmacokinetics and pharmacodynamics of selegiline: an update. Clin Pharmacokinet 33:91–102, 1997

McElroy SL, Keck PE Jr, Pope HG Jr, et al: Pharmacological treatment of kleptomania and bulimia nervosa. J Clin Psychopharmacol 9:358–360, 1989

McGrath PJ, Stewart JW, Harrison W, et al: Phenelzine treatment of melancholia. J Clin Psychiatry 47:420–422, 1986

McGrath PJ, Stewart JW, Fava M, et al: Tranylcypromine versus venlafaxine plus mirtazapine following three failed antidepressant medication trials for depression: a STAR*D report. Am J Psychiatry 163:1531–1541, 2006

Mendelson G: Narcotics and monoamine oxidase inhibitors (letter). Med J Aust 1:400, 1979

Meyer JH, Wilson AA, Sagrati S, et al: Brain monoamine oxidase A binding in major depressive disorder: relationship to selective serotonin reuptake inhibitor treatment, recovery, and recurrence. Arch Gen Psychiatry 66:1304–1312, 2009

Murphy DL, Garrick NA, Aulakh CS, et al: New contribution from basic science of understanding the effects of monoamine oxidase inhibiting antidepressants. J Clin Psychiatry 45:37–43, 1984

Murphy DL, Sunderland T, Garrick NA, et al: Selective amine oxidase inhibitors: basic to clinical studies and back, in Clinical Pharmacology in Psychiatry. Edited by Dahl SG, Gram A, Potter W. Berlin, Springer-Verlag, 1987, pp 135–146

O'Brien S, McKeon P, O'Regan M, et al: Blood pressure effects of tranylcypromine when prescribed singly and in combination with amitriptyline. J Clin Psychopharmacol 12:104–109, 1992

Paykel ES, West PS, Rowan PR, et al: Influence of acetylator phenotype on antidepressant effects of phenelzine. Br J Psychiatry 141:243–248, 1982

Pearce LB, Roth JA: Human brain monoamine oxidase type B: mechanism of deamination as probed by steady-state methods. Biochemistry 24:1821–1826, 1985

Quitkin F, Rifkin A, Klein DF: Monoamine oxidase inhibitors: a review of antidepressant effectiveness. Arch Gen Psychiatry 36:749–760, 1979

Quitkin FM, Liebowitz MR, Stewart JW, et al: L-Deprenyl in atypical depressives. Arch Gen Psychiatry 41:777–781, 1984

Quitkin FM, McGrath PJ, Stewart JW, et al: Atypical depression, panic attacks, and response to imipramine and phenelzine: a replication. Arch Gen Psychiatry 47:935–941, 1990

Quitkin FM, Harrison W, Stewart JW, et al: Response to phenelzine and imipramine in placebo nonresponders with atypical depression: a new application of the crossover design. Arch Gen Psychiatry 48:319–323, 1991

Ramsay RR, Singer TP: The kinetic mechanisms of monoamine oxidases A and B. Biochem Soc Trans 19:219–223, 1991

Rossel L, Moll E: Moclobemide versus tranylcypromine in the treatment of depression. Acta Psychiatr Scand Suppl 360:61–62, 1990

Rowan PR, Paykel ES, West PS, et al: Effects of phenelzine and acetylator phenotype. Neuropharmacology 20(12B):1353–1354, 1981

Saura J, Kettler R, Da Prada M, et al: Quantitative enzyme radioautography with 3H-Ro 41-1049 and 3H-Ro 19-6327 in vitro: localization and abundance of MAO-A and MAO-B in rat CNS, peripheral organs, and human brain. J Neurosci 12:1977–1999, 1992

Simpson GM, Gratz SS: Comparison of the pressor effect of tyramine after treatment with phenelzine and moclobemide in healthy male volunteers. Clin Pharmacol Ther 52:286–291, 1992

Stack CG, Rogers P, Linter SPK: Monoamine oxidase inhibitors and anaesthesia: a review. Br J Anaesth 60:222–227, 1988

Stein DJ, Ipser JC, Balkom AJ: Pharmacotherapy for social phobia. Cochrane Database Syst Rev (4):CD001206, 2004

Thase ME, Mallinger AG, McKnight D, et al: Treatment of imipramine-resistant recurrent depression, IV: a double-blind crossover study of tranylcypromine for anergic bipolar depression. Am J Psychiatry 149:195–198, 1992

Tyrer PJ, Candy J, Kelly D: A study of the clinical effects of phenelzine and placebo in the treatment of phobic anxiety. Psychopharmacologia 32:237–254, 1973

Vallejo J, Gasto C, Catalan R, et al: Double-blind study of imipramine versus phenelzine in melancholias and dysthymic disorders. Br J Psychiatry 151:639–642, 1987

Versiani M, Mundim FD, Nardi AE, et al: Tranylcypromine in social phobia. J Clin Psychopharmacol 8:279–283, 1988

Versiani M, Nardi AE, Mundim FD, et al: Pharmacotherapy of social phobia: a controlled study with moclobemide and phenelzine. Br J Psychiatry 161:353–360, 1992

Walsh BT, Stewart JW, Roose SP, et al: A double-blind trial of phenelzine in bulimia. J Psychiatr Res 19:485–489, 1985

Walsh BT, Gladis M, Roose SP, et al: A controlled trial of phenelzine in bulimia. Psychopharmacol Bull 23:49–51, 1987

Wells DG: MAOI revisited. Can J Anaesth 36:64–74, 1989

Wesnes KA, Simpson PM, Christmas L, et al: Acute cognitive effects of moclobemide and trazodone, alone and in combination with alcohol, in the elderly. Br J Clin Pharmacol 27:647P–648P, 1989

White K, Razani J, Cadow B, et al: Tranylcypromine vs nortriptyline vs placebo in depressed outpatients: a controlled trial. Psychopharmacology (Berl) 82:258–262, 1984

Youdim MBH, DaPrada M, Amrein R (eds): The cheese effect and new reversible MAO-A inhibitors. Proceedings of the Round Table of the International Conference on New Directions in Affective Disorders, Jerusalem, Israel, April 5–9, 1987

Zajecka J, Fawcett J: Susceptibility to spontaneous MAOI hypertensive episodes (letter). J Clin Psychiatry 52:513–514, 1991

Zeller EA: Diamine oxidase, in The Enzymes, 2nd Edition, Vol 8. Edited by Boyer PD, Lardy H, Myrback K. London, Academic Press, 1963, pp 313–335

Zisook S: Side effects of isocarboxazid. J Clin Psychiatry 45 (7, part 2):53–58, 1984

Zisook S, Braff DL, Click MA: Monoamine oxidase inhibitors in the treatment of atypical depression. J Clin Psychopharmacol 5:131–137, 1985

CHAPTER 8

Trazodone and Nefazodone

Robert N. Golden, M.D.

Karon Dawkins, M.D.

Linda Nicholas, M.D.

Trazodone was among the earliest "second generation" antidepressants to become available for clinical use in the United States in the early 1980s. Its side-effect profile and potential toxicity were considerably different from—and in many instances preferable to—those of the original antidepressants (i.e., the monoamine oxidase inhibitors [MAOIs] and tricyclic antidepressants [TCAs]). Several years later, trazodone's pharmacological "cousin," nefazodone, also became available.

Trazodone

History and Discovery

Trazodone was first synthesized in Italy about four decades ago, and clinical studies began in the United States in 1978. In sharp contrast to most other antidepressants available at the time, trazodone showed minimal effects on muscarinic cholinergic receptors.

In 1982, trazodone was introduced for clinical use in the United States under the brand name Desyrel. The medication is now available in generic formulation and also in an extended-release preparation (Oleptro).

Pharmacological Profile

Trazodone is a relatively weak SSRI; however, it is relatively *specific* for serotonin (5-HT) uptake inhibition, with minimal effects on norepinephrine (NE) or dopamine reuptake (Hyttel 1982). Trazodone appears to increase extracellular 5-HT concentrations through a combination of mechanisms involving the 5-HT transporter (5-HTT) and the serotonin$_{2A/2C}$ (5-HT$_{2A/2C}$) receptors (Pazzagli et al. 1999). In addition, trazodone has some 5-HT receptor antagonist activity (Haria et al. 1994). Its active metabolite, *m*-chlorophenylpiperazine (m-CPP), is a potent direct 5-HT agonist. Thus, trazodone can be viewed as a mixed serotonergic agonist–antagonist, with the relative amount of m-CPP accumulation affecting the relative degree of the predominant agonist activity. Sustained administration is associated with enhanced serotonergic neurotransmission in vivo in the rat brain (Ghanbari et al. 2010).

In vivo, trazodone is virtually devoid of anticholinergic activity, and in clinical studies, the incidence of anticholinergic side effects is similar to that seen with placebo. Trazodone is a relatively potent antagonist of postsynaptic α_1-adrenergic receptors, and it has a propensity to cause orthostatic hypotension. Trazodone has moderate antihistaminergic (histamine$_1$ [H_1] receptor) activity.

Pharmacokinetics and Disposition

Trazodone is well absorbed after oral administration, with peak blood levels occurring about 1–2 hours after dosing. Trazodone is 89%–95% bound to plasma protein. Elimination appears to be biphasic; the initial alpha and subsequent beta phases have half-lives of 3–6 and 5–9 hours, respectively. Bioavailability is not influenced by age or food intake.

Trazodone undergoes extensive hepatic metabolism. The active metabolite m-CPP is cleared more slowly than the parent compound (4- to 14-hour half-life) and reaches higher concentrations in the brain than in plasma (Caccia et al. 1981). The cytochrome P450 (CYP) 2D6 and 3A microsomal enzyme systems also appear to play a role in trazodone metabolism. The relation between steady-state blood levels and clinical response to trazodone is not well defined.

Mechanism of Action

The ultimate mechanism of action of trazodone remains unclear. Although the drug is described as a 5-HT reuptake inhibitor, its effects on this neurotransmitter system are complex. Trazodone has relative selectivity for 5-HT reuptake sites (Hyttel 1982); however, in vivo, it blocks the head twitch response induced by classic 5-HT agonists in animals. The potent 5-HT agonist properties of trazodone's major metabolite, m-CPP, may play a role in the mechanism of action of the parent compound. Trazodone, unlike the vast majority of antidepressants, does not produce downregulation of β-adrenergic receptors in rat cortex (Sulser 1983).

Indications and Efficacy

The primary indication for trazodone is the treatment of major depression. In an early review of double-blind studies, Schatzberg (1987) found the therapeutic efficacy of trazodone to be similar to that of TCAs in patients with either endogenous or nonendogenous depression. A review of European open and double-blind trials (Lader 1987) found that trazodone's antidepressant efficacy was similar to that of amitriptyline, doxepin, or mianserin.

Questions have been raised about the effectiveness of trazodone in treating severely ill patients, especially those with prominent psychomotor retardation. Shopsin et al. (1981) pointed out that in several unpublished double-blind, controlled studies, the rates of clinical response to trazodone were low (i.e., 10%–20%).

The performance of trazodone, in direct comparisons with other second-generation antidepressants, has been mixed. In a double-blind, placebo-controlled comparison with venlafaxine, the final response rates were 55% for placebo, 60% for trazodone, and 72% for venlafaxine. Trazodone was more effective than venlafaxine in ameliorating sleep disturbances and was associated with the most dizziness and somnolence (Cunningham et al. 1994). In a double-blind comparison, response rates for trazodone and bupropion were 46% and 58%, respectively (Weisler et al. 1994). In a double-blind study of 200 hospitalized patients with moderate to severe major depressive episode, mirtazapine yielded greater reductions in depression ratings than did trazodone (van Moffaert et al. 1995).

Three double-blind studies reported that trazodone has antidepressant efficacy similar to that of other antidepressants in geriatric patients (Gerner 1987). However, trazodone's association with orthostatic hypotension may increase the risk of falls, with devastating consequences in elderly patients. Still, trazodone is often helpful for geriatric patients with depression who have severe agitation and insomnia. A survey of British geropsychiatrists identified trazodone as one of their most popular adjuncts or alternatives to atypical antipsychotics in the management of behavioral symptoms in the elderly (Condren and Cooney 2001). A Cochrane Database review found insufficient evidence to support trazodone as a treatment for the behavioral and psychological symptoms of dementia, although the review could not conclude that trazodone was ineffective, given the limited number of eligible studies (Martinon-Torres et al. 2004).

In a randomized, double-blind, placebo-controlled trial, the anxiolytic efficacy of trazodone was comparable to that of diazepam in weeks 3–8 of treatment for generalized anxiety disorder, although patients treated with diazepam had greater improvement during the first 2 weeks of treatment (Rickels et al. 1993).

Many clinicians use low-dose trazodone as an alternative to benzodiazepines for the treatment of insomnia. Trazodone is the second most prescribed agent for primary insomnia, even though there is minimal evidence to support its use for this indication (Mendelson 2005; Rosenberg 2006). Controlled trials have confirmed trazodone's efficacy (at doses of 50–100 mg) in treating antidepressant-associated insomnia (Nierenberg et al. 1994). A retrospective analysis at a Department of Veterans Affairs (VA) medical center found that approximately 24% of patients receiving trazodone were taking other primary antidepressants (Clark and Alexander 2000). Another VA study of patients with posttraumatic stress disorder (PTSD) found that of those patients who were able to tolerate trazodone (60 of 72 patients), 92% reported that it improved sleep onset and 78% reported that it improved sleep maintenance (Warner et al. 2001).

Trazodone is more effective than placebo when added to antipsychotic medication in the treatment of the negative symptoms of schizophrenia (Singh et al. 2010; Watanabe 2011). A recent double-blind, placebo-controlled trial found trazodone to be effective in treating neuroleptic-induced akathisia (Stryjer et al. 2010).

Trazodone should be initiated at a low dose and increased gradually, based on clinical response and tolerance to side effects. For the treatment of a major depressive episode, the suggested initial dosage is 150 mg/day, with increases of 50-mg increments every 3–4 days. Doses may be divided, although many patients prefer bedtime dosing because of the sedating effects. The maximum dosage recommended for outpatients is 400 mg/day, although for inpatients with more severe depression, dosages up to 600 mg/day have been used. When trazodone is prescribed as a hypnotic agent, the usual dose is 50 mg at bedtime, although some patients may require as little as 25 mg or as much as 200–300 mg.

Side Effects and Toxicology

Because of its lack of anticholinergic side effects, trazodone is especially useful for patients with prostatic hypertrophy, closed-angle glaucoma, or severe constipation. Trazodone's propensity to cause sedation is a dual-edged sword. For many patients, the relief from agitation, anxiety, and insomnia can be rapid; for others, including those with psychomotor retardation and low energy, trazodone may not be tolerable.

Trazodone was found to be among the top three medications associated with orthostatic hypotension in patients attending a VA geriatric clinic (Poon and Braun 2005). More than 200 cases of trazodone-associated priapism have been reported (Thompson et al. 1990), and the manufacturer estimates that the incidence of any abnormal erectile function is approximately 1 in 6,000 male patients. The risk appears to be greatest during the first month of treatment at low dosages (<150 mg/day). Early recognition of any abnormal erectile function is important and should prompt immediate discontinuation of trazodone treatment.

In overdose situations, trazodone appears to be *relatively* safer than TCAs, MAOIs, and a few of the other second-generation antidepressants, especially when it is the only agent taken. Fatalities are rare, and uneventful recoveries have been reported after ingestion of doses as high as 6,000–9,200 mg (Ayd 1984). When trazodone overdoses occur, clinicians should carefully monitor for hypotension.

Drug-Drug Interactions

Trazodone can potentiate the effects of other central nervous system (CNS) depressants. Patients should be warned about increased drowsiness and sedation when trazodone is combined with other CNS depressants, including alcohol.

The combination of trazodone with an MAOI, as with other antidepressants, should be handled with great caution, although there are case reports of the successful combination of trazodone with an MAOI. Development of the serotonin syndrome has been associated with the combination of trazodone with other proserotonergic agents. Trazodone inhibits the antihypertensive effects of clonidine. Trazodone can cause hypotension, especially orthostatic hypotension, and concomitant administration of trazodone with antihypertensive therapy may require a reduction in the dose of the antihypertensive agent.

Clinically significant cases of suspected trazodone-warfarin interactions have been described.

Nefazodone

History and Discovery

Trazodone's sedative properties and association with orthostatic hypotension inspired an effort to discover a modified molecule that would possess a more desirable pharmacological profile. This led to the development of nefazodone, which became available in the United States in 1994. Nefazodone and trazodone share a common active metabolite.

In 2004, the manufacturer of Serzone (nefazodone) announced that it was discontinuing the drug's sale in the United States, citing declining sales. The drug had been banned in many countries because of its association with liver toxicity, and lawsuits against that manufacturer and the FDA had been initiated in this country. Nefazodone continues to be available in the United States as a generic medication.

Pharmacological Profile

Nefazodone is a 5-HT_2 receptor antagonist and a weak inhibitor of 5-HT and NE reuptake. It has little affinity for α_2-adrenergic, β-adrenergic, or 5-HT_{1A} receptors, and its affinity for the α_1-adrenergic receptor is less than that of trazodone. Nefazodone is inactive at most other receptor-binding sites (Taylor et al. 1986).

Nefazodone demonstrates several of the classic preclinical characteristics of antidepressants. In humans, nefazodone does not suppress rapid eye movement (REM) sleep, in contrast to most other antidepressants (Sharpley et al. 1996).

Pharmacokinetics and Disposition

Nefazodone is rapidly and completely absorbed and is then extensively metabolized, resulting in a low (about 20%) and variable absolute bioavailability. The plasma half-life is only 2–4 hours. Nefazodone has three active metabolites: triazole dione, hydroxynefazodone, and m-CPP. Triazole dione is a specific 5-HT_2 antagonist with weaker affinity for that receptor than the parent compound and no appreciable effects on 5-HT reuptake. With a plasma half-life of 18 hours, triazole dione predominates in the plasma, occurring at concentrations approaching four times that of the parent compound. Hydroxynefazodone has similar affinities for the 5-HT_2 receptor and 5-HT reuptake site as the parent compound. Its plasma half-life is between 1.5 and 4 hours, and at steady state, plasma concentrations are approximately 40% of those of the parent compound. m-CPP is a direct agonist at the 5-HT_1, 5-HT_2, and serotonin$_3$ (5-HT_3) receptors, with one order of magnitude higher affinity for 5-HT_{2C} receptors. m-CPP has a plasma half-life of 4–8 hours, and its plasma concentrations are only 7% of those seen with the parent compound (DeVane et al. 2002). However, the ratios of m-CPP to nefazodone concentrations in the brain are 47:1 and 10:1 in the mouse and rat, respectively. Brain concentrations of hydroxynefazodone in the rat are less than 10% of those in plasma, suggesting very poor blood-brain barrier penetration. Thus, despite its relatively lower plasma concentrations, m-CPP has substantial presence in the brain, whereas the in vivo activity of hydroxynefazodone may be mostly the result of its biotransformation to m-CPP (Nacca et al. 1998).

Nefazodone has nonlinear kinetics, which result in greater than proportional mean plasma concentrations with higher doses. Nefazodone is extensively (99%) but loosely protein bound (Bristol-Myers Squibb 2003). In patients with hepatic cirrhosis, single-dose nefazodone and hydroxynefazodone levels are about twice as high as in healthy volunteers, but the difference decreases to approximately 25% at steady state. Exposure to m-CPP is about two- to threefold greater in patients with cirrhosis, and exposure to triazole dione is similar after a single dose and at steady state (Barbhaiya et al. 1995).

Mechanism of Action

The mechanism of action of nefazodone is poorly understood. The manufacturer has indicated that nefazodone antagonizes 5-HT_2 receptors and also inhibits neuronal uptake of both 5-HT and NE (Bristol-Myers Squibb 2003). Several reviews refer to nefazodone as a "dual acting" antidepressant, suggesting that it enhances both serotonergic and noradrenergic neurotransmission via uptake blockade. Although nefazodone has similar effects on the 5-HT and NE transporters, this observation is potentially misleading. Nefazodone's inhibition of NE reuptake is weaker than that of the SSRI fluoxetine and is approximately three orders of magnitude weaker than what is seen with conventional NE reuptake inhibitors. Furthermore, nefazodone's inhibition of 5-HT reuptake is nearly identical to that of desipramine and more than 100-fold less than that of fluoxetine (Bolden-Watson and Richelson 1993). Thus, the "dual action" of nefazodone refers to minimal, albeit equal, effects on 5-HT and NE reuptake inhibition.

In humans, therapeutic doses of nefazodone do not cause sustained 5-HT uptake inhibition at the platelet 5-HTT (Narayan et al. 1998). The active metabolite m-CCP, which appears to predominate in the brain because of greater penetration of the blood-brain barrier (Nacca et al. 1998), may play an important role in the mechanism of action.

Indications and Efficacy

In three of four Phase III imipramine- and placebo-controlled studies, nefazodone was found to be an effective antidepressant with similar efficacy to imipramine; in one of these studies, neither active drug had significantly greater efficacy than did placebo. The incidence of premature treatment discontinuation and side effects was higher for the imipramine group than for the nefazodone treatment group (Rickels et al. 1995). In double-blind studies without placebo control groups, there were no significant differences in the clinical responses to nefazodone and sertraline or paroxetine in outpatients with depression (Feiger et al. 1996). Hospitalized patients with severe major depression achieved higher response rates to nefazodone, compared with placebo (Feighner et al. 1998). In patients with moderate to severe major depression, the efficacy of amitriptyline was clearly superior to that of nefazodone (Ansseau et al. 1994). Keller et al. (2000) compared nefazodone, cognitive-behavioral therapy (CBT), and a combination of these two treatments in a double-blind study of patients with chronic major depressive disorder. Each monotherapy yielded a response rate of 48%, whereas the combined treatment had a greater efficacy (73%). When patients who failed to respond to 12 weeks of treatment with either nefazodone or cognitive-behavioral analysis system psychotherapy are then switched to the other treatment, significant symptom improvement is achieved (Schatzberg et al. 2005). Nefazodone has also been shown to be effective in the continuation phase of treatment in double-blind studies (Baldwin et al. 2001; Feiger et al. 1999).

In a double-blind, placebo-controlled study, nefazodone was found to be safe and effective in the treatment of depression in patients with alcohol dependence, although it did not add any advantage over psychoeducational group intervention in terms of drinking outcomes (Roy-Byrne et al. 2000). A double-blind, controlled study found that nefazodone was not efficacious for the treatment of alcohol dependence (Kranzler et al. 2000). A randomized, placebo-controlled, double-blind multicenter study compared nefazodone versus placebo and CBT versus nondirective group counseling (GC) for relapse prevention in alcohol dependence. Two hundred forty-two male patients received either nefazodone plus GC or CBT or placebo plus GC or CBT. There were no differences among the four groups in cumulative days of abstinence or amount of alcohol consumed during specified time periods during the initial 12-week study phase. After 1 year, the only significant difference among the groups was higher alcohol consumption in the nefazodone plus GC group, raising concerns that nefazodone may potentially increase the risk of relapse (Wetzel et al. 2004).

The usual starting dosage of nefazodone is 200 mg/day in two divided doses. The suggested dosage range is 300–600 mg/day. Increases should be in increments of 100–200 mg/day at weekly intervals. The starting dosage in elderly or debilitated patients should be lowered to 100 mg/day, taken in two divided doses, and the rate of titration should be adjusted accordingly (Bristol-Myers Squibb 2003). Zajecka et al. (2002) reported that in studies comparing low-dosage (50–250 mg/day) and high-dosage (100–500 mg/day) nefazodone, better clinical response was obtained in the latter group, and the mean effective dosage ranged from 375 mg/day to 460 mg/day. A lower starting dose should be considered when switching to nefazodone from an SSRI if a full washout has not been completed. Once-daily bedtime dosing appears to be well tolerated and effective.

Side Effects and Toxicology

In initial clinical trials that included approximately 2,250 patients, side effects more frequently associated with nefazodone than with placebo included dizziness, asthenia, dry mouth, nausea, and constipation (Fontaine 1993).

Preskorn (1995) found that the total cumulative incidence of treatment-emergent adverse effects for nefazodone was lower than that of imipramine or fluoxetine. The most common placebo-adjusted adverse effects associated with nefazodone were dry mouth, somnolence, dizziness, nausea, constipation, blurred vision, and postural hypotension. Nefazodone appears to have advantages over SSRIs in terms of treatment-associated sexual dysfunction (Clayton et al. 2002; Ferguson et al. 2001).

There are now well-publicized concerns regarding the association of nefazodone with liver toxicity and liver failure, including fatalities (Choi 2003). In 2001 the manufacturer added a black box warning to the package insert, describing a reported rate of life-threatening liver failure in this country of 1 case per 250,000–300,000 patient-years of nefazodone treatment. In 2004 Serzone was withdrawn from the U.S. market, following its withdrawal from several international markets. The generic drug remains available in the United States. In a review of 1,338 humans with exposure to nefazodone overdoses, there were no reported deaths. The most common serious clinical effect was hypotension, reported in 1.6% of cases (Benson et al. 2000).

Drug-Drug Interactions

The manufacturer of triazolam warns that its concurrent use with nefazodone is contraindicated. Increases in the plasma concentration of digoxin occur with concurrent nefazodone administration. Nefazodone increases the plasma concentrations of terfenadine and loratadine (with associated QTc prolongation), carbamazepine, and cyclosporine.

Conclusion

Trazodone was one of the earliest second-generation antidepressants. Its lack of anticholinergic effects provided an advantage over the TCAs for many patients; its sedative properties are helpful for some patients but problematic for others; and orthostatic hypotension is a concern for elderly patients. Nefazodone is related to trazodone, and the two drugs share an active metabolite, m-CPP, that may play an important role in their mechanism of action. The risk of serious liver damage led to Serzone's removal from the market in several countries, although generic nefazodone is currently available in the United States.

References

Ansseau M, Darimont P, Lecoq A, et al: Controlled comparison of nefazodone and amitriptyline in major depressive inpatients. Psychopharmacology (Berl) 115:254–260, 1994

Ayd FJ Jr: Pharmacology update: which antidepressant to choose, II: the overdose factor. Psychiatric Annals 14:212–214, 1984

Baldwin DS, Hawley CJ, Mellors K, et al: A randomized, double-blind controlled comparison of nefazodone and paroxetine in the treatment of depression: safety, tolerability and efficacy in continuation phase treatment. J Psychopharmacol 15:161–165, 2001

Barbhaiya RJ, Sukla UA, Matarakam CS, et al: Single- and multiple-dose pharmacokinetics of nefazodone in patients with hepatic cirrhosis. Clin Pharmacol Ther 58:390–398, 1995

Benson BE, Mathiason M, Dahl B, et al: Toxicities and outcomes associated with nefazodone poisoning: an analysis of 1,338 exposures. Am J Emerg Med 18:587–592, 2000

Bolden-Watson C, Richelson E: Blockade by newly developed antidepressants of biogenic amine uptake into rat brain synaptosomes. Life Sci 52:1023–1029, 1993

Bristol-Myers Squibb: Serzone (nefazodone hydrochloride) tablets [packet insert]. Revised September 2003. Available at: http://www.fda.gov/ohrms/dockets/ac/04/briefing/4006B1_11_Serzone-Label.pdf. Accessed July 2012.

Caccia S, Ballabio M, Fanelli R, et al: Determination of plasma and brain concentrations of trazodone and its metabolite, 1-m-chlorophenylpiperazine, by gas-liquid chromatography. J Chromatogr 210:311–318, 1981

Choi S: Nefazodone (serzone) withdrawn because of hepatotoxicity. CMAJ 169:1187, 2003

Clark NA, Alexander B: Increased rate of trazodone prescribing with bupropion and selective serotonin reuptake inhibitors versus tricyclic antidepressants. Ann Pharmacother 34:1007–1012, 2000

Clayton AH, Pradko JF, Croft HA, et al: Prevalence of sexual dysfunction among newer antidepressants. J Clin Psychiatry 63:357–366, 2002

Condren CM, Cooney C: Use of drugs by old age psychiatrists in the treatment of psychotic and behavioural symptoms in patients with dementia. Aging Ment Health 5:235–241, 2001

Cunningham LA, Borison RL, Carman JS, et al: A comparison of venlafaxine, trazodone, and placebo in major depression. J Clin Psychopharmacol 14:99–106, 1994

DeVane CL, Grothe DR, Smith SL: Pharmacology of antidepressants: focus on nefazodone. J Clin Psychiatry 63 (suppl 1):10–17, 2002

Feiger A, Kiev A, Shriastava RK, et al: Nefazodone versus sertraline in outpatients with major depression: focus on efficacy, tolerability, and effects on sexual function and satisfaction. J Clin Psychiatry 57 (suppl 2):53–62, 1996

Feiger AD, Bielski RJ, Bremner J, et al: Double-blind, placebo substitution study of nefazodone in the prevention of relapse during continuation treatment of outpatients with major depression. Int Clin Psychopharmacol 14:19–28, 1999

Feighner J, Targum SD, Bennett ME, et al: A double-blind, placebo-controlled trial of nefazodone in the treatment of patients hospitalized for major depression. J Clin Psychiatry 59:246–253, 1998

Ferguson JM, Shrivastava RK, Stahl SM, et al: Reemergence of sexual dysfunction in patients with major depressive disorder: double-blind comparison of nefazodone and sertraline. J Clin Psychiatry 62:24–29, 2001

Fontaine R: Novel serotonergic mechanisms and clinical experience with nefazodone. Clin Neuropharmacol 16 (suppl 3): S45–S50, 1993

Gerner RH: Geriatric depression and treatment with trazodone. Psychopathology 20:82–91, 1987

Ghanbari R, El Mansari M, Blier P: Sustained administration of trazodone enhances serotonergic neurotransmission: in vivo electrophysiological study in rat brain. J Pharmacol Exp Ther 335: 197–206, 2010

Haria M, Fitton A, McTavish D: Trazodone: a review of its pharmacology, therapeutic use in depression and therapeutic potential in other disorders. Drugs Aging 4:331–335, 1994

Hyttel J: Citalopram—pharmacologic profile of a specific serotonin uptake inhibitor with antidepressant activity. Prog Neuropsychopharmacol Biol Psychiatry 6:277–295, 1982

Keller MB, McCullough JP, Klein DN, et al: A comparison of nefazodone, the cognitive behavioral-analysis system of psychotherapy, and their combination for the treatment of chronic depression. N Engl J Med 342:1462–1470, 2000

Kranzler HR, Modesto-Lowe V, Van Kirk J: Naltrexone vs nefazodone for treatment of alcohol dependence: a placebo controlled trial. Neuropsychopharmacology 22:493–503, 2000

Lader M: Recent experience with trazodone. Psychopathology 20 (suppl 1):39–47, 1987

Martinon-Torres G, Fioravanti M, Grimley EJ: Trazodone for agitation in dementia. Cochrane Database Syst Rev (4):CD004990, 2004

Mendelson WB: A review of the evidence for the efficacy and safety of trazodone in insomnia. J Clin Psychiatry 66:469–476, 2005

Nacca A, Guiso G, Fracasso C, et al: Brain-to-blood partition and in vivo inhibition of 5-hydroxytryptamine reuptake and quipazine-mediated behaviour of nefazodone and its main active metabolites in rodents. Br J Pharmacol 125:1617–1623, 1998

Narayan M, Anderson G, Cellar J, et al: Serotonin transporter-blocking properties of nefazodone assessed by measurement of platelet serotonin. J Clin Psychopharmacol 18:67–71, 1998

Nierenberg A, Adler LA, Peselow E, et al: Trazodone for antidepressant-associated insomnia. Am J Psychiatry 151:1069–1072, 1994

Pazzagli M, Giovannini MG, Pepeu G: Trazodone increases extracellular serotonin levels in the frontal cortex of rats. Eur J Pharmacol 383:249–257, 1999

Poon IO, Braun U: High prevalence of orthostatic hypotension and its correlation with potentially causative medications among elderly veterans. J Clin Ther 30:173–178, 2005

Preskorn SH: Comparison of the tolerability of bupropion, fluoxetine, imipramine, nefazodone, paroxetine, sertraline, and venlafaxine. J Clin Psychiatry 56 (suppl):12–21, 1995

Rickels K, Downing R, Schweizer E, et al: Antidepressants for the treatment of generalized anxiety disorder: a placebo-controlled comparison of imipramine, trazodone, and diazepam. Arch Gen Psychiatry 50:884–895, 1993

Rickels K, Robinson DS, Schweizer E, et al: Nefazodone: aspects of efficacy. J Clin Psychiatry 56 (suppl 6):43–46, 1995

Rosenberg RP: Sleep maintenance insomnia: strengths and weaknesses of current pharmacologic therapies. Ann Clin Psychiatry 18:49–56, 2006

Roy-Byrne PP, Pages KP, Russo JE, et al: Nefazodone treatment of major depression in alcohol-dependent patients: a double-blind, placebo-controlled trial. J Clin Psychopharmacol 20:129–136, 2000

Schatzberg AF: Trazodone: a 5-year review of antidepressant efficacy. Psychopathology 20 (suppl 1): 48–56, 1987

Schatzberg AF, Rush AJ, Arnow BA, et al: Chronic depression: medication (nefazodone) or psychotherapy (CBASP) is effective when the other is not. Arch Gen Psychiatry 62:513–520, 2005

Sharpley AL, Williamson DJ, Attenburrow ME, et al: The effects of paroxetine and nefazodone on sleep: a placebo controlled trial. Psychopharmacology (Berl) 126:50–54, 1996

Shopsin B, Cassano GB, Conti L: An overview of new "second generation" antidepressant compounds: research and treatment implications, in Antidepressants: Neurochemical, Behavioral and Clinical Perspectives. Edited by Enna SJ, Molick J, Richelson E. New York, Raven, 1981, pp 219–251

Singh SP, Singh V, Kar N, et al: Efficacy of antidepressants in treating the negative symptoms of chronic schizophrenia: meta-analysis. Br J Psychiatry 197:174–179, 2010

Stryjer R, Rosenzcwaig S, Bar F, et al: Trazodone for the treatment of neuroleptic-induced acute akathisia: a placebo-controlled, double-blind, crossover study. Clin Neuropharmacol 33:219–222, 2010

Sulser F: Mode of action of antidepressant drugs. J Clin Psychiatry 44 (5 pt 2):14–20, 1983

Taylor DP, Smith DW, Hyslop DK, et al: Receptor binding and atypical antidepressant drug discovery, in Receptor Binding in Drug Research. Edited by O'Brien RA. New York, Marcel Dekker, 1986, pp 151–165

Thompson JW Jr, Ware MR, Blashfield RK: Psychotropic medication and priapism: a comprehensive review. J Clin Psychiatry 51:430–433, 1990

van Moffaert M, de Wilde J, Vereecken A, et al: Mirtazapine is more effective than trazodone: a double-blind controlled study in hospitalized patients with major depression. Int Clin Psychopharmacol 10:3–9, 1995

Warner MD, Dorn MR, Peabody CA: Survey on the usefulness of trazodone in patients with PTSD with insomnia or nightmares. Pharmacopsychiatry 34:128–131, 2001

Watanabe N: Fluoxetine, trazodone and ritanserin are more effective than placebo when used as add-on therapies for negative symptoms of schizophrenia. Evid Based Ment Health 14:21, 2011

Weisler RH, Johnston JA, Lineberry CG, et al: Comparison of bupropion and trazodone for the treatment of major depression. J Clin Psychopharmacol 14:170–179, 1994

Wetzel H, Szegedi A, Scheurich A, et al: Combination treatment with nefazodone and cognitive-behavioral therapy for relapse prevention in alcohol-dependent men: a randomized controlled study. J Clin Psychiatry 65:1406–1413, 2004

Zajecka J, McEnany GW, Lusk KM: Antidepressant dosing and switching guidelines: focus on nefazodone. J Clin Psychiatry 63:42–47, 2002

CHAPTER 9

Bupropion

Anita H. Clayton, M.D.

Elizabeth H. Gillespie, D.O.

Justin B. Smith, M.D.

History and Discovery

Bupropion was discovered more than 40 years ago when investigators were searching for an antidepressant with a novel mechanism of action and safer side-effect profile. It first received U.S. Food and Drug Administration (FDA) approval in 1985 and was on the brink of release when a study by Horne et al. (1988) reported that 4 of 55 subjects with bulimia experienced seizures during treatment with the medication. Further research revealed that the risk of seizures increased from 0.3% to 0.4% at dosages of 450 mg/day to almost 2% at dosages of 600 mg/day. Bupropion was reintroduced in 1989 with a maximum recommended dosage of 450 mg/day (Davidson 1989). The original immediate-release (IR) formulation of bupropion was dosed three times daily. In an effort to improve tolerability and safety, a sustained-release (SR) formulation of bupropion, dosed twice daily, was subsequently introduced, and a once-daily extended-release (XL) formulation became available in 2003.

Structure-Activity Relations

Bupropion, 2-(tert-butylamino)-1-(3′-chlorophenyl)propan-1-one, is a monocyclic antidepressant and member of the aminoketone group. It works as an organic base with a high degree of both water and lipid solubility, resulting in good systemic absorption. Bupropion's benign side-effect profile in comparison with that of tricyclic and tetracyclic antidepressants is due to the absence of heterocyclic rings as well as other common functional groups (Mehta 1983).

Pharmacological Profile

Bupropion inhibits the reuptake of dopamine (DA) and norepinephrine (NE) by acting as a nonselective inhibitor of the dopamine transporter (DAT) and the norepinephrine transporter (NET). Studies show that bupropion also acts as an antagonist to nicotinic acetylcholine (nACh) receptors. Alternatively, bupropion does not act as an inhibitor of monoamine oxidase A or B, nor are the effects of bupropion mediated by serotonin (Ascher et al. 1995).

Although it resembles amphetamine in certain structural aspects, bupropion does not increase the spontaneous release of catecholamines in rat striatum and hypothalamus. A study by Griffith et al. (1983) examining the effect of bupropion and amphetamine in previous amphetamine abusers concluded that bupropion had little abuse potential in humans.

Pharmacokinetics and Disposition

Bupropion is rapidly absorbed in the gastrointestinal tract after oral administration. Peak plasma levels occur within 2 hours for the IR preparation. As expected, absorption is prolonged for the SR and XL formulations, for which peak plasma concentrations occur at 3 and 5 hours, respectively. Food does not impair absorption, and protein binding ranges from 82% to 88%. The elimination half-life for bupropion is 21(±9) hours, and the half-life for hydroxybupropion, the major metabolite of bupropion, is close to 20 (±5) hours. Finally, excretion in the urine occurs with 0.5% of the drug unchanged (Jefferson et al. 2005).

Bupropion is extensively metabolized by the liver. The major metabolite, hydroxybupropion, is formed by cytochrome P450 (CYP) 2B6. Although CYP2B6 is the primary isoenzyme involved in bupropion's metabolism, other isoforms, including 1A2, 2A6, 2CP, 2D6, 2E1, and 3A4, play a small role (Hesse et al. 2000; Kirchheiner et al. 2003).

In examining the pharmacokinetics of bupropion in regard to gender, age, and smoking status, no significant effect has been found, and definitive results have been inconclusive (Jefferson et al. 2005). Nevertheless, it is prudent to monitor elderly patients more closely as they often have greater clinical issues with tolerability. For patients with impaired renal and/or hepatic function, dosing should be initiated at lower levels, given the finding that levels of bupropion and its metabolites are increased in these populations relative to controls (DeVane et al. 1990; Jefferson et al. 2005; Worrall et al. 2004).

Mechanism of Action

Bupropion is the only newer antidepressant without substantial serotonergic activity (Ascher et al. 1995; Richelson 1996; Stahl et al. 2004). Most researchers believe, and there is strong evidence to support, that the neurochemical mechanisms mediating the antidepressant effects of bupropion are from DA and NE reuptake inhibition, as the efficacy of bupropion and hydroxybupropion has been shown to decrease in animal models when NE- or DA-blocking drugs are administered (Cooper et al. 1980; Dwoskin et al. 2006).

Indications and Efficacy

Primary Indications

Depression

The efficacy of all three forms of bupropion for the treatment of major depressive disorder (MDD) is supported by numerous clinical trials (Fabre et al. 1983; Lineberry et al. 1990). Comparison trials have demonstrated that bupropion is as effective as other classes of antidepressants, including tricyclic antidepressants (TCAs) and selective serotonin reuptake inhibitors (SSRIs) (Branconnier et al. 1983; Clayton et al. 2006; Coleman et al. 1999, 2001; Croft et al. 1999; Feighner et al. 1986; Kavoussi et al. 1997; Mendels et al. 1983; Thase et al. 2005; Weihs et al. 2000). A 2006 study comparing the efficacy of bupropion versus the serotonin-norepinephrine reuptake inhibitor (SNRI) venlafaxine found that higher dosages of bupropion XL (300–450 mg/day) resulted in significantly higher remission rates for bupropion XL relative to low-dose venlafaxine XR (Thase et al. 2006). In contrast, two more recent studies by Hewett et al. (2009, 2010) found venlafaxine XR (75–150 mg/day) superior to low-dose bupropion XL (150–300 mg/day). Of note in these studies, bupropion XL was not superior to placebo.

It is also important to note that for patients who are unable to tolerate or fail to respond to SSRIs, bupropion may be added. Studies have shown bupropion to be efficacious for treatment of MDD not only as monotherapy but also as an augmenting agent with SSRIs or SNRIs (Bodkin et al. 1997; DeBattista et al. 2003; Fava et al. 2003; Ferguson et al. 1994; Lam et al. 2004; Rush et al. 2006; Spier 1998; Stern et al. 1983; Trivedi et al. 2006). In addition, bupropion has been found to be an effective and well-tolerated antidepressant in elderly patients (Birrer and Vemuri 2004; Branconnier et al. 1983; Weihs et al. 2000).

Bupropion XL has been studied specifically in patients with a retarded-anergic profile. Jefferson et al. (2006) showed that bupropion XL was more effective than placebo in treatment of patients with decreased energy, pleasure, and interest. The unique norepinephrine-dopamine reuptake inhibitor (NDRI) mechanism of action of bupropion may play a role in its effectiveness in treating these symptoms (Jefferson et al. 2006). A study examining gender- and age-related differences in treatment of depressive symptoms, anxious and somatic symptoms, and insomnia found SSRIs and bupropion to be equally effective (Papakostas et al. 2007).

Bupropion and SSRIs appear to be equally effective in reducing symptoms of anxiety associated with MDD in the general population and in the elderly (Feighner et al. 1991; Weihs et al. 2000). A meta-analysis comparing efficacy of bupropion and SSRIs for treatment of anxious symptoms in major depressive disorder came to the conclusion that both classes of medication led to a similar degree of improvement in anxiety symptoms, with no significant difference in the severity of residual anxiety symptoms (Papakostas et al. 2008).

A small number of early studies demonstrated the advantages of bupropion in the treatment of depression in bipolar disorder (Haykal and Akiskal 1990; Shopsin 1983; Wright et al. 1985). Although these investigations yielded positive results, they were limited by small numbers of subjects and were uncontrolled. Several more recent trials have examined the risk of treatment-emergent mania with adjunctive bupropion use in bipolar disorder. There appears to be a lower risk of mania with bupropion and SSRIs than with the SNRI venlafaxine, although findings regarding bupropion's efficacy for depressive symptoms in bipolar disorder are mixed (Leverich et al. 2006; Post et al. 2006; Sachs et al. 2007).

Bupropion XL also has a labeled indication for the preventive treatment of seasonal affective disorder (SAD). In 2005, Modell et al. published results of three prospective randomized, placebo-controlled prevention trials involving 1,042 outpatients with a diagnosis of SAD. Patients received 150–300 mg/day of bupropion XL or placebo in autumn while they were still well. Bupropion XL reduced the frequency of emergence of SAD by 44% and protected against the recurrence of seasonal major depressive episodes. Furthermore, there was no noticeable increase in major depressive episodes following discontinuation of bupropion in the springtime (Modell et al. 2005).

Smoking Cessation

A meta-analysis (Eisenberg et al. 2008) and a randomized controlled trial (Piper et al. 2009) have confirmed the efficacy of bupropion in smoking cessation, an indication for which it first received FDA approval in 1997. Recommended dosages are 150 mg/day for 3 days, with an increase to 150 mg two times a day for 7–12 weeks. The patient should set a quit date of 1–2 weeks after treatment has been initiated.

Other Uses

Attention-Deficit/Hyperactivity Disorder

Although bupropion does not have an FDA indication for attention-deficit/hyperactivity disorder (ADHD), studies have demonstrated that it may be helpful in treating symptoms of ADHD in both children and adults (Barrickman et al. 1995; Conners et al. 1996; Peterson et al. 2008; Simeon et al. 1986; Wilens et al. 2001). Currently, bupropion is thought of as a useful second-line agent in the treatment of ADHD. Outcomes may be more favorable with comorbid conduct disorder or substance abuse. More studies are needed to further establish the efficacy of bupropion for use in this condition.

Sexual Dysfunction

Several clinical trials have demonstrated bupropion's efficacy in treating hypoactive sexual desire disorder (HSDD) in women (Segraves et al. 2001, 2004). Bupropion has also been studied as an antidote to SSRI-induced sexual dysfunction. A placebo-controlled comparative trial of bupropion SR treatment in 42 patients with SSRI-induced sexual dysfunction concluded that bupropion SR improved both desire to engage in sexual activity and frequency of engaging in sexual activity relative to placebo (Clayton et al. 2004). A meta-analysis of bupropion for SSRI-induced sexual dysfunction published in 2008 found limited evidence that bupropion can reverse SSRI-induced dysfunction, although the dosages used in several of the relevant studies may have been inadequate (Demyttenaere and Jaspers 2008).

Side Effects and Toxicology

Thousands of clinical trials and millions of patient exposures reveal bupropion to be a safe and generally well-tolerated medication across populations. Because of its unique mechanism of action and structure, its reported side effects are somewhat different than those of other antidepressants.

In a series of large randomized, placebo-controlled multicenter trials evaluating the safety of bupropion SR in the treatment of depressed outpatients, Settle et al. (1999) found that the most commonly reported adverse events (occurring in >5% of subjects) were headache, dry mouth, nausea, insomnia, constipation, and dizziness. Only three of these—dry mouth, nausea, and insomnia—occurred at higher rates in patients taking bupropion SR than in those receiving placebo. The rate of discontinuation due to adverse events was low: 7% for bupropion SR, compared with 4% for placebo. Rash, nausea, agitation, and migraine were the most common adverse effects leading to discontinuation (Settle et al. 1999). Similarly favorable safety and tolerability findings were reported for continuation-phase bupropion SR treatment in a longer-term (up to 44 weeks) relapse prevention trial (Weihs et al. 2002).

A review by Fava et al. (2005) concluded that bupropion causes much less somnolence than SSRIs. Moreover, insomnia, a known adverse effect of bupropion, occurs at rates similar to those seen with SSRIs (Fava et al. 2005).

Other important adverse events that have been reported with bupropion may include seizures, allergic reactions, or vital sign changes. These are less common but could possibly be more harmful. Allergic reactions, including rash, arthralgias, fever, and serum sickness–like reactions, have all been reported (Kanani et al. 2000; McCollom et al. 2000). In light of these data, it is important to fully evaluate any reports of hypersensitivity when administering bupropion.

Because high dosages of bupropion were found to be associated with seizures in hospitalized bulimia patients (Horne et al. 1988), screening for a history of seizure disorder or other organic brain disease should be performed before commencing a trial of bupropion. Seizure has been reported at a rate of 0.1% at dosages up to 300 mg/day with bupropion SR, with a dose-related effect (Dunner et al. 1998). This rate is similar to that of other newer antidepressants, such as SSRIs and mirtazapine, but lower than the rate associated with therapeutic doses of TCAs (Montgomery 2005).

Although cases of spontaneous hypertension with bupropion therapy have been reported, clinical trials across the approved dosage range have shown minimal changes in heart rate and blood pressure, even among patients with hypertension (Jorenby et al. 1999; Settle et al. 1999; Thase et al. 2008). However, clinicians should be aware that elevated blood pressure is a possibility with bupropion therapy and should monitor patients accordingly.

In regard to sexual functioning, bupropion has a favorable side-effect profile comparable to that of placebo and superior to that of the SSRIs and the SNRIs (Clayton et al. 2002, 2006; Croft et al. 2002; Jefferson et al. 2006; Modell et al. 2005; Thase et al. 2006).

Many agents used to treat depression have been associated with weight gain. Studies have shown bupropion XL to be associated with a loss of 0.1–1.1 kg in the short term, compared with placebo, which was linked with a small gain of 0.1–0.8 kg (Jefferson et al. 2006; Modell et al. 2005; Thase et al. 2006). In a longer-term depression relapse prevention study, Croft et al. (2002) observed that patients with a higher body mass index at baseline experienced greater weight loss with bupropion XL.

Although safe in general, bupropion can be fatal with high blood levels. Serious medical consequences such as hypertension, acidosis, sinus tachycardia, seizures, cardiotoxicity with QRS widening, and even death have all been reported with overdoses of bupropion (Bhattacharjee et al. 2001; Curry et al. 2005; Shrier et al. 2000).

On initiation of bupropion therapy, it is usually not necessary to obtain routine laboratory evaluations, although cases of elevated serum transaminase (Oslin and Duffy 1993) and rare cases of hepatitis (Hu et al. 2000) have been reported. Other unexpected changes in laboratory values have also occurred with bupropion therapy and include false-positive urine amphetamine screening results (Weintraub and Linder 2000).

Unfortunately, there is little available evidence about the safety of bupropion in pregnancy. In a study by Cole et al. (2007), bupropion exposure in the first trimester was not associated with teratogenic effects.

Drug-Drug Interactions

The main enzyme responsible for the metabolism of bupropion is CYP2B6. Competitive inhibition of metabolism could occur with other drugs processed by this enzyme (Hesse et al. 2000; Jefferson et al. 2005).

Bupropion and its major metabolite hydroxybupropion are also inhibitors of CYP2D6, an enzyme that plays a role in the metabolism of several classes of medications, including antidepressants, β-blockers, and antiarrhythmic agents (Wilkinson 2005). Studies of the effects of bupropion on CYP2D6 activity are limited, but those that have been done suggest that bupropion may increase blood levels of drugs metabolized by CYP2D6, including desipramine and venlafaxine (Jefferson et al. 2005; Kennedy et al. 2002). Other agents known to induce various metabolic pathways have also been shown to affect the metabolism of bupropion. Carbamazepine, which induces CYP2B6, 3A4, and 1A2 activity, has been shown to decrease bupropion concentrations but increase hydroxybupropion concentrations (Ketter et al. 1995).

Bupropion should also be used with caution if coadministered with other agents that can lower the seizure threshold, such as tramadol, other antidepressants, or antipsychotics (Delanty et al. 1998; Gardner et al. 2000). It should also be used with caution in patients who abuse alcohol, as this population may have increased risk for seizures (Dunner et al. 1998). In addition, because bupropion increases DA reuptake, additive effects with other dopaminergic agents (e.g., levodopa) have been observed (Goetz et al. 1984).

Conclusion

Bupropion is unique in that it works as a DA and NE reuptake inhibitor and acts as an antagonist of nACh receptors. Unlike other newer agents, it has very little serotonergic activity and therefore produces a different side-effect profile. Bupropion may be the antidepressant of choice for patients who cannot tolerate or do not respond to SSRIs. While currently indicated for MDD, for tobacco dependence, and for prevention of SAD, bupropion has also proven useful in many other circumstances, such as child and adult ADHD, obesity, and sexual disorders. For more specific treatment of depression associated with decreased energy and interest, for depression with concomitant anxiety, and for bipolar depression, bupropion may be beneficial. Bupropion may also be used to augment other antidepressants in the treatment of MDD and to reverse SSRI-induced side effects. Greater tolerability, including low risk of weight gain, less sedation, and fewer sexual side effects, adds to its value as an effective antidepressant.

References

Ascher JA, Cole JO, Colin JN, et al: Bupropion: a review of its mechanism of antidepressant activity. J Clin Psychiatry 56:395–401, 1995

Barrickman LL, Perry PJ, Allen AJ, et al: Bupropion versus methylphenidate in the treatment of attention-deficit hyperactivity disorder. J Am Acad Child Adolesc Psychiatry 34:649–657, 1995

Bhattacharjee C, Smith M, Todd F, et al: Bupropion overdose: a potential problem with the new "miracle" anti-smoking drug. Int J Clin Pract 55:221–222, 2001

Birrer RB, Vemuri SP: Depression in later life: a diagnostic and therapeutic challenge. Am Fam Physician 69:2375–2382, 2004

Bodkin JA, Lasser RA, Wines JD Jr, et al: Combining serotonin reuptake inhibitors and bupropion in partial responders to antidepressant monotherapy. J Clin Psychiatry 58:137–145, 1997

Branconnier RJ, Cole JO, Ghazvinian S, et al: Clinical pharmacology of bupropion and imipramine in elderly depressives. J Clin Psychiatry 44:130–133, 1983

Clayton AH, Pradko JF, Croft HA, et al: Prevalence of sexual dysfunction among newer antidepressants. J Clin Psychiatry 63:357–366, 2002

Clayton AH, Warnock JK, Kornstein SG, et al: A placebo-controlled trial of bupropion SR as an antidote for selective serotonin reuptake inhibitor–induced sexual dysfunction. J Clin Psychiatry 65:62–67, 2004

Clayton AH, Croft HA, Horrigan JP, et al: Bupropion extended release compared with escitalopram: effects on sexual functioning and antidepressant efficacy in 2 randomized, double-blind, placebo-controlled studies. J Clin Psychiatry 67:736–746, 2006

Cole JA, Modell JG, Haight BR, et al: Bupropion in pregnancy and the prevalence of congenital malformations. Pharmacoepidemiol Drug Saf 16:474–484, 2007

Coleman CC, Cunningham LA, Foster VJ, et al: Sexual dysfunction associated with the treatment of depression: a placebo-controlled comparison of bupropion sustained release and sertraline treatment. Ann Clin Psychiatry 11:205–215, 1999

Coleman CC, King BR, Bolden-Watson C, et al: A placebo-controlled comparison of the effects on sexual functioning of bupropion sustained release and fluoxetine. Clin Ther 23:1040–1058, 2001

Conners CK, Casat CD, Gualtieri CT, et al: Bupropion hydrochloride in attention deficit disorder with hyperactivity. J Am Acad Child Adolesc Psychiatry 35:1314–1321, 1996

Cooper BR, Hester TJ, Maxwell RA: Behavioral and biochemical effects of the antidepressant bupropion (Wellbutrin): evidence for selective blockade of dopamine uptake in vivo. J Pharmacol Exp Ther 215:127–134, 1980

Croft H, Settle E Jr, Houser T, et al: A placebo-controlled comparison of the antidepressant efficacy and effects on sexual functioning of sustained-release bupropion and sertraline. Clin Ther 21:643–658, 1999

Croft H, Houser TL, Jamerson BD, et al: Effect on body weight of bupropion sustained-release in patients with major depression treated for 52 weeks. Clin Ther 24:662–672, 2002

Curry SC, Kashani JS, LoVecchio F, et al: Intraventricular conduction delay after bupropion overdose. J Emerg Med 29:299–305, 2005

Davidson J: Seizures and bupropion: a review. J Clin Psychiatry 50:256–261, 1989

DeBattista C, Solvason HB, Poirier J, et al: A prospective trial of bupropion SR augmentation of partial and non-responders to serotonergic antidepressants. J Clin Psychopharmacol 23:27–30, 2003

Delanty N, Vaughan CJ, French JA: Medical causes of seizures. Lancet 352:383–390, 1998

Demyttenaere K, Jaspers L: Review: bupropion and SSRI-induced side effects. J Psychopharmacol 22:792–804, 2008

DeVane CL, Laizure SC, Stewart JT, et al: Disposition of bupropion in healthy volunteers and subjects with alcoholic liver disease. J Clin Psychopharmacol 10:328–332, 1990

Dunner DL, Zisook S, Billow AA, et al: A prospective safety surveillance study for bupropion sustained-release in the treatment of depression. J Clin Psychiatry 59:366–373, 1998

Dwoskin LP, Rauhut AS, King-Pospisil KA, et al: Review of the pharmacology and clinical profile of bupropion, an antidepressant and tobacco use cessation agent. CNS Drug Rev 12:178–207, 2006

Eisenberg MJ, Filion KB, Yavin D, et al: Pharmacotherapies for smoking cessation: a meta-analysis of randomized controlled trials. CMAJ 179: 135–144, 2008; erratum in CMAJ 179:802, 2008

Fabre LF, Brodie HK, Garver D, et al: A multicenter evaluation of bupropion versus placebo in hospitalized depressed patients. J Clin Psychiatry 44:88–94, 1983

Fava M, Papakostas GI, Petersen T, et al: Switching to bupropion in fluoxetine-resistant major depressive disorder. Ann Clin Psychiatry 15:17–22, 2003

Fava M, Rush AJ, Thase ME, et al: 15 years of clinical experience with bupropion HCl: from bupropion to bupropion SR to bupropion XL. Prim Care Companion J Clin Psychiatry 7:106–113, 2005

Feighner J, Hendrickson G, Miller L, et al: Double-blind comparison of doxepin versus bupropion in outpatients with a major depressive disorder. J Clin Psychopharmacol 6:27–32, 1986

Feighner JP, Gardner EA, Johnston JA, et al: Double-blind comparison of bupropion and fluoxetine in depressed outpatients. J Clin Psychiatry 52:329–335, 1991

Ferguson J, Cunningham L, Merideth C, et al: Bupropion in tricyclic antidepressant nonresponders with unipolar major depressive disorder. Ann Clin Psychiatry 6:153–160, 1994

Gardner JS, Blough D, Drinkard CR, et al: Tramadol and seizures: a surveillance study in a managed care population. Pharmacotherapy 20:1423–1431, 2000

Goetz CG, Tanner CM, Klawans HL: Bupropion in Parkinson's disease. Neurology 34:1092–1094, 1984

Griffith JD, Carranza J, Griffith C, et al: Bupropion: clinical assay for amphetamine-like abuse potential. J Clin Psychiatry 44:206–208, 1983

Haykal RF, Akiskal HS: Bupropion as a promising approach to rapid cycling bipolar II patients. J Clin Psychiatry 51:450–455, 1990

Hesse LM, Venkatakrishnan K, Court MH, et al: CYP2B6 mediates the in vitro hydroxylation of bupropion: potential drug interactions with other antidepressants. Drug Metab Dispos 28:1176–1184, 2000

Hewett K, Chrzanowski W, Schmitz M, et al: Eight-week, placebo-controlled, double-blind comparison of the antidepressant efficacy and tolerability of bupropion XR and venlafaxine XR. J Psychopharmacol 23:531–538, 2009

Hewett K, Gee MD, Krishen A, et al: Double-blind, placebo-controlled comparison of the antidepressant efficacy and tolerability of bupropion XR and venlafaxine XR. J Psychopharmacol 24:1209–1216, 2010

Horne RL, Ferguson JM, Pope HG Jr, et al: Treatment of bulimia with bupropion: a multicenter controlled trial. J Clin Psychiatry 49:262–266, 1988

Hu KQ, Tiyyagura L, Kanel G, et al: Acute hepatitis induced by bupropion. Dig Dis Sci 45:1872–1873, 2000

Jefferson JW, Pradko JF, Muir KT: Bupropion for major depressive disorder: pharmacokinetic and formulation considerations. Clin Ther 27:1685–1695, 2005

Jefferson JW, Rush AJ, Nelson JC, et al: Extended-release bupropion for patients with major depressive disorder presenting with symptoms of reduced energy, pleasure, and interest: findings from a randomized, double-blind, placebo-controlled study. J Clin Psychiatry 67:865–873, 2006

Jorenby DE, Leischow SJ, Nides MA, et al: A controlled trial of sustained-release bupropion, a nicotine patch, or both for smoking cessation. N Engl J Med 340:685–691, 1999

Kanani AS, Kalicinsky C, Warrington RJ, et al: Serum sickness–like reaction with bupropion sustained release. Can J Allergy Clin Immunol 5:27–29, 2000

Kavoussi RJ, Segraves RT, Hughes AR, et al: Double-blind comparison of bupropion sustained release and sertraline in depressed outpatients. J Clin Psychiatry 58:532–537, 1997

Kennedy SH, McCann SM, Masellis M, et al: Combining bupropion SR with venlafaxine, paroxetine, or fluoxetine: a preliminary report on pharmacokinetic, therapeutic, and sexual dysfunction effects. J Clin Psychiatry 63:181–186, 2002

Ketter TA, Jenkins JB, Schroeder DH, et al: Carbamazepine but not valproate induces bupropion metabolism. J Clin Psychopharmacol 15:327–333, 1995

Kirchheiner J, Klein C, Meineke I, et al: Bupropion and 4-OH-bupropion pharmacokinetics in relation to genetic polymorphisms in CYP2B6. Pharmacogenetics 13:619–626, 2003

Lam RW, Hossie H, Solomons K, et al: Citalopram and bupropion-SR: combining versus switching in patients with treatment-resistant depression. J Clin Psychiatry 65:337–340, 2004

Leverich GS, Altshuler LL, Frye MA, et al: Risk of switch in mood polarity to hypomania or mania in patients with bipolar depression during acute and continuation trials of venlafaxine, sertraline, and bupropion as adjuncts to mood stabilizers. Am J Psychiatry 163:232–239, 2006

Lineberry CG, Johnston JA, Raymond RN, et al: A fixed-dose (300 mg) efficacy study of bupropion and placebo in depressed outpatients. J Clin Psychiatry 51:194–199, 1990

McCollom RA, Elbe DH, Ritchie AH: Bupropion-induced serum sickness–like reaction. Ann Pharmacother 34:471–473, 2000

Mehta NB: The chemistry of bupropion. J Clin Psychiatry 44:56–59, 1983

Mendels J, Amin MM, Chouinard G, et al: A comparative study of bupropion and amitriptyline in depressed outpatients. J Clin Psychiatry 44:118–120, 1983

Modell JG, Rosenthal NE, Harriett AE, et al: Seasonal affective disorder and its prevention by anticipatory treatment with bupropion XL. Biol Psychiatry 58:658–667, 2005

Montgomery SA: Antidepressants and seizures: emphasis on newer agents and clinical implications. Int J Clin Pract 59:1435–1440, 2005

Oslin DW, Duffy K: The rise of serum aminotransferases in a patient treated with bupropion. J Clin Psychopharmacol 13:364–365, 1993

Papakostas GI, Kornstein SG, Clayton AH, et al: Relative antidepressant efficacy of bupropion and the selective serotonin reuptake inhibitors in major depressive disorder: gender-age interactions. Int Clin Psychopharmacol 22:226–229, 2007

Papakostas GI, Trivedi MH, Alpert JE, et al: Efficacy of bupropion and the selective serotonin reuptake inhibitors in the treatment of anxiety symptoms in major depressive disorder: a meta-analysis of individual patient data from 10 double-blind, randomized clinical trials. J Psychiatr Res 42:134–140, 2008

Peterson K, McDonagh MS, Fu R: Comparative benefits and harms of competing medications for adults with attention-deficit hyperactivity disorder: a systematic review and indirect comparison meta-analysis. Psychopharmacology 197:1–11, 2008

Piper ME, Smith SS, Schlam TR, et al: A randomized placebo-controlled clinical trial of 5 smoking cessation pharmacotherapies. Arch Gen Psychiatry 66:1253–1262, 2009; erratum in Arch Gen Psychiatry 67:77, 2010

Post RM, Altshuler LL, Leverich GS, et al: Mood switch in bipolar depression: comparison of adjunctive venlafaxine, bupropion and sertraline. Br J Psychiatry 189:124–131, 2006

Richelson E: Synaptic effects of antidepressants. J Clin Psychopharmacol 16:1S–7S; discussion 7S–9S, 1996

Rush AJ, Trivedi MH, Wisniewski SR, et al: Bupropion-SR, sertraline, or venlafaxine-XR after failure of SSRIs for depression. N Engl J Med 354:1231–1242, 2006

Sachs GS, Nierenberg AA, Calabrese JR, et al: Effectiveness of adjunctive antidepressant treatment for bipolar depression. N Engl J Med 356:1711–1722, 2007

Segraves RT, Croft H, Kavoussi R, et al: Bupropion sustained release (SR) for the treatment of hypoactive sexual desire disorder (HSDD) in nondepressed women. J Sex Marital Ther 27:303–316, 2001

Segraves RT, Clayton AH, Croft H, et al: Bupropion sustained release for the treatment of hypoactive sexual desire disorder in premenopausal women. J Clin Psychopharmacol 24:339–342, 2004

Settle EC, Stahl SM, Batey SR, et al: Safety profile of sustained-release bupropion in depression: results of three clinical trials. Clin Ther 21:454–463, 1999

Shopsin B: Bupropion's prophylactic efficacy in bipolar affective illness. J Clin Psychiatry 44:163–169, 1983

Shrier M, Diaz JE, Tsarouhas N: Cardiotoxicity associated with bupropion overdose. Ann Emerg Med 35:100, 2000

Simeon JG, Ferguson HB, Van Wyck Fleet J: Bupropion effects in attention deficit and conduct disorders. Can J Psychiatry 31:581–585, 1986

Spier SA: Use of bupropion with SRIs and venlafaxine. Depress Anxiety 7:73–75, 1998

Stahl SM, Pradko JF, Haight BR, et al: A review of the neuropharmacology of bupropion, a dual norepinephrine and dopamine reuptake inhibitor. Prim Care Companion J Clin Psychiatry 6:159–166, 2004

Stern WC, Harto-Truax N, Bauer N: Efficacy of bupropion in tricyclic-resistant or intolerant patients. J Clin Psychiatry 44:148–152, 1983

Thase ME, Haight BR, Richard N, et al: Remission rates following antidepressant therapy with bupropion or selective serotonin reuptake inhibitors: a meta-analysis of original data from 7 randomized controlled trials. J Clin Psychiatry 66: 974–981, 2005

Thase ME, Clayton AH, Haight BR, et al: A double-blind comparison between bupropion XL and venlafaxine XR: sexual functioning, antidepressant efficacy, and tolerability. J Clin Psychopharmacol 26:482–488, 2006

Thase ME, Haight BR, Johnson MC, et al: A randomized, double-blind, placebo-controlled study of the effect of sustained-release bupropion on blood pressure in individuals with mild untreated hypertension. J Clin Psychopharmacol 28:302–307, 2008

Trivedi MH, Fava M, Wisniewski SR, et al: Medication augmentation after the failure of SSRIs for depression. N Engl J Med 354:1243–1252, 2006

Weihs KL, Settle EC Jr, Batey SR, et al: Bupropion sustained release versus paroxetine for the treatment of depression in the elderly. J Clin Psychiatry 61:196–202, 2000

Weihs KL, Houser TL, Batey SR, et al: Continuation phase treatment with bupropion SR effectively decreases the risk for relapse of depression. Biol Psychiatry 51:753–761, 2002

Weintraub D, Linder MW: Amphetamine positive toxicology screen secondary to bupropion. Depress Anxiety 12:53–54, 2000

Wilens TE, Spencer TJ, Biederman J, et al: A controlled clinical trial of bupropion for attention deficit hyperactivity disorder in adults. Am J Psychiatry 158:282–288, 2001

Wilkinson GR: Drug metabolism and variability among patients in drug response. N Engl J Med 352:2211–2221, 2005

Worrall SP, Almond MK, Dhillon S: Pharmacokinetics of bupropion and its metabolites in hemodialysis patients who smoke: a single dose study. Nephron Clin Pract 97:c83–c89, 2004

Wright G, Galloway L, Kim J, et al: Bupropion in the long-term treatment of cyclic mood disorders: mood stabilizing effects. J Clin Psychiatry 46:22–25, 1985

CHAPTER 10

Mirtazapine

Alan F. Schatzberg, M.D.

History and Discovery

Mirtazapine, originally known as ORG 3770, was first synthesized in the Netherlands by the Department of Medicinal Chemistry of NV Organon (Kaspersen et al. 1989). First approved for use in major depression in the Netherlands in 1994, mirtazapine was introduced in the United States in 1996.

Structure-Activity Relations

Mirtazapine is a member of the piperazino-azepines, a class of chemical compounds that is unrelated to any other class used in the treatment of psychiatric conditions (Maris et al. 1999). Mirtazapine is also known by its chemical name, 1,2,3,4,10,14b-hexahydro-2-methylpyrazino[2,1-a]pyridol[2,3-c]benzazepine (Dahl et al. 1997; Dodd et al. 2000).

Pharmacological Profile

Mirtazapine is described as a noradrenergic and specific serotonergic antidepressant (NaSSA) (Holm and Markham 1999; Kent 2000; Nutt 1998). It is a potent serotonin$_2$ (5-HT$_2$), serotonin$_3$ (5-HT$_3$), and central α_2-adrenergic receptor antagonist (De Boer 1996; De Boer et al. 1995; Kooyman et al. 1994). Antagonism of 5-HT$_2$ and 5-HT$_3$ receptors results in an increase in serotonin$_{1A}$ (5-HT$_{1A}$) receptor–mediated transmission and, thus, a more specific effect on serotonergic transmission, relative to the selective serotonin reuptake inhibitor (SSRI) class of antidepressants (Bengtsson et al. 2000; Berendsen and Broekkamp 1997; Kent 2000). In addition, because α_2-adrenergic receptors normally act to inhibit transmission at serotonergic and noradrenergic axon terminals, mirtazapine acts to increase the release of both serotonin (5-HT) and norepinephrine via blockade of central α_2 receptors (Numazawa et al. 1995).

Mirtazapine has no significant affinity for dopamine receptors, low affinity for muscarinic cholinergic receptors (De Boer 1996), and high affinity for histamine$_1$ (H$_1$) receptors (De Boer 1996). Mirtazapine appears to have no effect on 5-HT and dopamine reuptake and only a minimal effect on norepinephrine reuptake (De Boer 1996; Kent 2000). The drug appears to significantly reduce cortisol levels (Laakmann et al. 2004; Schmid et al. 2006).

Pharmacokinetics and Disposition

Absorption

Mirtazapine is well absorbed from the gastrointestinal tract, and bioavailability does not appear to be affected by the presence of food in the stomach (Fawcett and Barkin 1998b). An oral rapidly disintegrating tablet has been available since 2001 (Benkert et al. 2006).

Distribution

Mirtazapine appears to be 85% bound to plasma proteins (Fawcett and Barkin 1998b).

Metabolism

Mirtazapine is primarily metabolized by the liver via demethylation and hydroxylation, followed by glucuronidation (Fawcett and Barkin 1998b; Remeron package insert 2002). Its major metabolite, desmethylmirtazapine, is weakly active but is present in lower serum concentrations than the parent compound (Fawcett and Barkin 1998b; Kent 2000). Mirtazapine lacks both autoinduction and autoinhibition of hepatic cytochrome P450 (CYP) enzymes (Fawcett and Barkin 1998b). Although in vitro studies do not demonstrate an inhibitory effect, mirtazapine is a substrate for CYP1A2, 2D6, and 3A4 (Fawcett and Barkin 1998b; Remeron package insert 2002). Mirtazapine is a mild competitive inhibitor of CYP2D6 (Barkin et al. 2000; Fawcett and Barkin 1998b). A pharmacogenetic study of CYP2D6 in geriatric depressed patients failed to reveal that slow and intermediate metabolizers demonstrate increased dropout rates due to side effects of the drug (Murphy et al. 2003b). These findings suggest that mirtazapine is well tolerated in individuals who are slow metabolizers of CYP2D6.

Elimination

Mirtazapine and its metabolites are eliminated primarily in the urine (up to 75%) and feces (up to 15%) (Fawcett and Barkin 1998b). The elimination half-life of mirtazapine is 20–40 hours (Fawcett and Barkin 1998b; Remeron package insert 2002; Stimmel et al. 1997). Of note, the clearance of mirtazapine may be affected by hepatic or renal impairment (Fawcett and Barkin 1998b). The elimination half-life may increase by 30%–40% in patients with hepatic impairment (Fawcett and Barkin 1998b; Kent 2000). In patients with moderate to severe renal impairment, the clearance of mirtazapine may be decreased by 30%–50% (Fawcett and Barkin 1998b; Kent 2000; Remeron package insert 2002).

Indications and Efficacy

Major Depression

Pooled data from the 6-week U.S. clinical trials that were part of the new drug application showed that approximately 50% of mirtazapine-treated patients and 20% of placebo-controlled patients achieved at least a 50% improvement in scores on the Hamilton Rating Scale for Depression (Ham-D) (Fawcett and Barkin 1998b).

In a randomized, double-blind, placebo-controlled study of 90 outpatients with a major depressive episode, mirtazapine treatment resulted in clinically significant reductions in Ham-D scores by study endpoint at 6 weeks, although improvement was noted as early as the first week (Claghorn and Lesem 1995).

A meta-analysis of four randomized, double-blind 6-week studies demonstrated mirtazapine to be as effective as amitriptyline in the treatment of major depression, but with significantly fewer anticholinergic, serotonergic, and cardiovascular adverse effects (Stahl et al. 1997).

In a randomized, double-blind multicenter study comparing mirtazapine and fluoxetine, both medications were found to be well tolerated in the treatment of major depression, although the former was noted to demonstrate a significantly greater improvement in Ham-D scores, beginning in the third week of treatment (Wheatley et al. 1998).

When mirtazapine was compared with paroxetine in a randomized, double-blind study of 275 patients with major depression, the two drugs were found to be, overall, equally well tolerated and efficacious, but mirtazapine was noted to result in significantly lower Ham-D and Hamilton Anxiety Scale (Ham-A) scores at week 1 (Benkert et al. 2000).

Similarly, when compared with citalopram in an 8-week randomized, double-blind multicenter study of 270 patients with major depression, mirtazapine was equally well tolerated and efficacious at study endpoint but was significantly more effective (as assessed by Ham-A, Montgomery-Åsberg Depression Rating Scale [MADRS], and Clinical Global Impression [CGI] Scale scores) at week 2 (Leinonen et al. 1999).

Of interest, in an 8-week randomized, double-blind multicenter study comparing two antidepressants with both serotonergic and noradrenergic activity, mirtazapine was found to be equal in efficacy to venlafaxine in the treatment of major depression with melancholic features, although it demonstrated a trend (not statistically significant) toward a higher percentage of responders and remitters (Guelfi et al. 2001).

In a meta-analysis of 15 studies comparing mirtazapine with an SSRI, Thase et al. (2010) concluded that mirtazapine was significantly more likely than the SSRI to induce remission at weeks 1, 2, 4, and 6. At week 2, the remission rates with mirtazapine were more than 70% higher than those with the SSRI, suggesting more rapid effects.

A recent report noted that mirtazapine coadministered with fluoxetine was significantly more effective than fluoxetine alone. Similarly high rates of remission were also observed for mirtazapine combined with bupropion and mirtazapine combined with venlafaxine (Blier et al. 2010).

The sleep effects of mirtazapine in major depression were reported by Steiger's group (Schmid et al. 2006). Mirtazapine improved sleep continuity by day 2 of therapy, and the effect was sustained for at least 4 weeks. At day 28, significant increases in slow-wave and low-delta sleep were also observed.

Treatment Failure With a Selective Serotonin Reuptake Inhibitor

In an 8-week open-label study of 103 outpatients with DSM-IV (American Psychiatric Association 1994) major depressive disorder complicated by failure to respond to (or intolerance of) treatment with fluoxetine, paroxetine, or sertraline, approximately one-half of the outpatients demonstrated a 50% reduction in the 17-item Ham-D (Ham-D-17) score when switched to treatment with mirtazapine (Fava et al. 2001).

In a 4-week study of patients with persistent major depression despite adequate antidepressant monotherapy, augmentation with mirtazapine resulted in a 45% remission rate, compared with a 13% remission rate among patients receiving placebo (Carpenter et al. 2002). Of note, in this study there were no significant differences in side effects between drug and placebo (Carpenter et al. 2002).

In level 3 of the Sequenced Treatment Alternatives to Relieve Depression (STAR*D) trial, mirtazapine was compared with nortriptyline in patients who had failed to respond to two previous consecutive antidepressant trials (Fava et al. 2006). Level 1 of STAR*D employed citalopram; level 2 employed a switch to another drug or augmentation. Nortriptyline produced higher remission rates than did mirtazapine (19.8% vs. 12.3%); however, the difference was not statistically significant.

Patients With Depression and Sexual Dysfunction

In an open-label study of 103 patients with depression treated with mirtazapine, 54% of patients who had reported poor or very poor sexual functioning during prior treatment with an SSRI described an improvement in sexual functioning by study endpoint (Fava et al. 2001).

Similarly, Gelenberg et al. (2000) reported that 58% of patients with prior SSRI-induced sexual dysfunction had a return of normal sexual functioning when they switched to treatment with mirtazapine.

In contrast, augmentation with mirtazapine was no more effective than placebo augmentation in reversing SSRI-associated sexual side effects in patients with fluoxetine-associated sexual dysfunction (Michelson et al. 2002).

Depression in Elderly Patients

In a 6-week study of 150 outpatients (ages between 55 and 80 years) with moderate to severe depression, mirtazapine was found to be effective and well tolerated (Halikas 1995). Half of the mirtazapine-treated patients and 35% of the placebo-treated patients demonstrated at least a 50% reduction in Ham-D score (Halikas 1995). In another blinded study, mirtazapine was significantly more effective than paroxetine at weeks 1, 2, 3, and 6, but not at week 8, in subjects older than 65 years (Schatzberg et al. 2002). Differences were observed primarily on measures of anxiety and sleep. Apolipoprotein epsilon 4 (*ApoE-ε4*) carrier status predicted a positive response to mirtazapine (Murphy et al. 2003a).

An oral disintegrating tablet has been studied in the elderly and appears to be well tolerated (Nelson et al. 2007; Varia et al. 2007).

Patients With Comorbid and Primary Symptoms of Anxiety

Meta-analyses of placebo-controlled studies of patients with depression and associated symptoms of anxiety have demonstrated that mirtazapine-treated patients exhibit significantly greater improvement in symptoms of anxiety (Fawcett and Barkin 1998a; Nutt 1998), beginning as early as the first week of treatment (Fawcett and Barkin 1998a).

In an 8-week open-label study of 10 patients with major depressive disorder and comorbid generalized anxiety disorder, mirtazapine treatment resulted in significant decreases in Ham-D and Ham-A scores, with improvement beginning as early as the first week of treatment (Goodnick et al. 1999).

Dysthymia

In a 10-week open-label trial of the use of mirtazapine in 15 patients with dysthymic disorder, 8 patients demonstrated at least a 40% reduction in Ham-D scores, and 4 of these 8 patients showed symptom remission by study endpoint (Dunner et al. 1999).

Posttraumatic Stress Disorder

In an 8-week open-label study of 6 patients with severe chronic posttraumatic stress disorder (PTSD), mirtazapine treatment resulted in one-half of the patients demonstrating at least a 50% reduction in CGI score and significant reductions on scales of PTSD severity (Connor et al. 1999).

In a 6-week double-blind comparison study, mirtazapine was compared with sertraline in Korean veterans with PTSD (Chung et al. 2004). At study endpoint, mirtazapine was statistically significantly superior to sertraline on several measures. Efficacy was apparently maintained to 24 weeks (Kim et al. 2005).

Social Phobia

Mirtazapine was compared with placebo in a 10-week double-blind comparison study in 66 women with social phobia. Mirtazapine appeared to separate from placebo on several primary measures of social phobia symptoms (Muehlbacher et al. 2005).

Generalized Anxiety Disorder

In an open-label trial of mirtazapine treatment in 44 adult patients with generalized anxiety disorder, response criteria were achieved in 80% of patients (Gambi et al. 2005). Controlled trial data are not available.

Obsessive-Compulsive Disorder

Koran et al. (2005) reported on a two-phase study (a 12-week open-label phase followed by an 8-week double-blind discontinuation phase) of mirtazapine (maximum dosage of 60 mg/day) in 30 patients with obsessive-compulsive disorder (OCD). In the 8-week discontinuation phase, mirtazapine was significantly more effective than placebo in preventing symptom recurrence.

Mirtazapine augmentation of citalopram was assessed in 49 nondepressed OCD patients (Pallanti et al. 2004). Subjects were treated with citalopram plus placebo or citalopram plus mirtazapine under single-blind conditions. Mirtazapine appeared to speed the response to citalopram but not to improve overall response.

Sleep Disorders

Because of its sedating properties in depression, mirtazapine has been studied in patients with primary sleep disorders. In a double-blind crossover study in 7 patients with obstructive sleep apnea, mirtazapine dosages of 4.5 and 15 mg/day produced significantly greater reductions (on the order of 46%–52%) in apnea-hypopnea index (AHI) scores in comparison with placebo (Carley et al. 2007). However, because of concerns regarding weight gain and sedation, the authors concluded that mirtazapine could not at present be recommended as a primary therapy in this disorder.

Chronic or Recurrent Pain

A number of case reports indicate that mirtazapine could be beneficial in chronic or recurrent pain (Brannon and Stone 1999; Brannon et al. 2000; Kuiken et al. 2005; Nutt 1999).

A large series of 600 patients with comorbid pain and depression treated with mirtazapine has been reported in Germany (Freynhagen et al. 2006). The drug appeared to reduce pain effectively in this sample, with a relatively low-order risk of side effects (7%) at a mean dosage of 35 mg/day.

Mirtazapine at 15–30 mg/day was also reported to be effective in a double-blind crossover study in 24 nondepressed patients with chronic tension headaches (Bendtsen and Jensen 2004). Area under the curve (intensity times duration) for headache was significantly lower for mirtazapine than for placebo.

Chemotherapy- or Anesthesia-Related Nausea

A case series of 20 breast and gynecological cancer patients treated with mirtazapine demonstrated a significant reduction in symptoms of depression, anxiety, nausea, anorexia, and insomnia in 19 of the patients, as well as a lack of adverse drug interactions when combined with oncology treatment regimens, including chemotherapy (Thompson 2000).

A 7-week open-label crossover trial of mirtazapine in 20 patients with cancer revealed significant improvements in mood, anxiety, insomnia, appetite, weight, and pain symptoms by study endpoint (Theobold et al. 2002).

It has been suggested that mirtazapine could prove to be a safe and effective adjunct to cancer chemotherapy because of its ability to treat nausea via a 5-HT_3 receptor antagonism effect; insomnia, anorexia, and weight loss via H_1 receptor antagonism; symptoms of depression via enhanced 5-HT and noradrenergic transmission by way of α_2, 5-HT_2, and 5-HT_3 receptor blockade; and symptoms of anxiety via 5-HT_2 and 5-HT_3 receptor antagonism (Kast 2001). A recent study reported that the incidence of nausea and vomiting after spinal anesthesia with intrathecal morphine was significantly lower in orthopedic surgery patients who received preoperative mirtazapine (30 mg) than in those who received placebo (Chang et al. 2010).

Obstetrics/Gynecology

A review of 7 cases of pregnant patients with treatment-refractory hyperemesis gravidarum and symptoms of depression and anxiety determined that treatment with mirtazapine produced resolution of symptoms without adverse impact on the newborns (Saks 2001).

Waldinger et al. (2000) described 4 cases in which women (ages between 39 and 60 years) experienced a near-complete resolution of symptoms of hot flushes and perspiration within the first week of treatment with mirtazapine.

An 8-week open-label trial of mirtazapine in 22 menopausal patients receiving estrogen replacement therapy who had major depression demonstrated an almost 90% remission rate among the study completers (Joffe et al. 2001).

Pediatric Depression and Anxiety

Mirtazapine has been assessed in several trials involving children or adolescents with major depression or anxiety disorders. In one trial of 24 adolescents with major depression, patients responded well to the drug, with no dropouts due to side effects (Haapasalo-Pesu et al. 2004). In another small open-label trial in 18 patients with social phobia, mirtazapine also demonstrated efficacy (Mrakotsky et al. 2008). Although there was a very high dropout rate, most of the discontinuations were not due to side effects.

Pervasive Developmental Disorders

In an open-label study on the use of mirtazapine in 26 patients with pervasive developmental disorders, 35% of subjects demonstrated significant improvement on CGI scores with respect to symptoms of aggression, self-injury, irritability, hyperactivity, anxiety, depression, and insomnia (Posey et al. 2001).

Depression in Alzheimer's Disease

Raji and Brady (2001) described 3 cases of patients with comorbid Alzheimer's dementia (Mini-Mental State Exam [MMSE] scores of 21/30, 11/30, and 18/30) and depressive symptomatology who were treated safely with mirtazapine. The patients demonstrated significant improvement in appetite, weight loss, sleep disturbances, anxiety, mood, anhedonia, and energy level. However, in a recent large-scale trial comparing sertraline (up to 150 mg/day), mirtazapine (up to 45 mg/day), and placebo in Alzheimer's disease patients with depression, there were no differences between the three groups in reduction of depression symptoms (Banerjee et al. 2011). Given these negative findings of benefit and the heightened risk of side effects from these drugs, the authors recommended that the current practice of prescribing antidepressants in this group of patients be reconsidered.

Add-On Therapy in Schizophrenia

The utility of mirtazapine in the treatment of the negative symptoms of schizophrenia has been examined in several studies. In a 6-week double-blind, randomized, placebo-controlled trial, addition of mirtazapine to haloperidol in the treatment of schizophrenia demonstrated a statistically significant reduction in Positive and Negative Syndrome Scale (PANSS) scores, as well as in CGI–Severity and CGI–Improvement scores (Berk et al. 2001). In addition, PANSS negative symptom scores in this study were found to be reduced by 42% in the group of patients who received adjunctive mirtazapine, compared with the group who received placebo (Berk et al. 2001). Furthermore, the latter finding was not correlated with Ham-D scores at study endpoint, suggesting that the effect of mirtazapine on diminution of negative symptoms in schizophrenia was not a result of improvement in mood symptoms (Berk et al. 2001).

In a subsequent study, Berk et al. (2009) compared mirtazapine 30 mg with placebo add-on in schizophrenia patients treated with atypical antipsychotics. Mirtazapine's effects on negative symptoms or cognition failed to separate from those of placebo.

Several positive studies have followed the mixed findings of Berk and colleagues. Abbasi et al. (2010) reported that mirtazapine add-on at 30 mg/day was significantly more effective than placebo in reducing negative symptoms and total PANSS scores in schizophrenia patients being treated with risperidone. Similarly, Cho et al. (2011) noted that mirtazapine augmentation separated from placebo in improving negative symptoms and cognition in patients undergoing treatment with risperidone. Neuropsychological testing results likewise showed significantly greater improvement with mirtazapine. Stenberg et al. (2010) reported that patients who were not sufficiently improved on first-generation antipsychotics showed significantly greater improvement in cognition with mirtazapine than with placebo.

Akathisia

Poyurovsky et al. (2003, 2006) conducted two double-blind, placebo-controlled studies of mirtazapine treatment of antipsychotic-induced akathisia in patients with schizophrenia. In the first study (Poyurovsky et al. 2003), mirtazapine 15 mg/day was compared with placebo in 26 patients. The drug was significantly superior to placebo. In the second study (Poyurovsky et al. 2006), mirtazapine at the same dose was compared with propranolol 80 mg/day or placebo in 90 patients. Both drugs separated from placebo, but propranolol was associated with significantly greater bradycardia and hypotension.

Side Effects and Toxicology

In a double-blind, placebo-controlled study of outpatients with depression, the most commonly reported side effects associated with mirtazapine treatment were somnolence, increased appetite, and weight gain (Claghorn and Lesem 1995).

In a review of data from the clinical development program for mirtazapine, the only adverse effects that occurred at a higher incidence with mirtazapine versus placebo were excessive sedation, increased appetite, weight gain, and dry mouth (Montgomery 1995). Also reported in this review was the observation that these side effects were typically mild and transient in nature and that they decreased with time and often diminished with increased dose (Montgomery 1995).

Side effects typical of SSRIs, such as nausea, diarrhea, and sexual dysfunction, appear to occur less frequently in patients treated with mirtazapine (Boyarsky et al. 1999; Farah 1998; Montgomery 1995; Stimmel et al. 1997).

Mirtazapine also appears to be well tolerated in elderly patients. The most common side effects reported, including somnolence, increased appetite, weight gain, and dry mouth, are of the same type as those reported in younger adults (Fawcett and Barkin 1998b; Halikas 1995).

Mirtazapine appears to have a very low incidence of causing clinically relevant laboratory abnormalities, such as transient rise in liver enzymes (2%) and severe neutropenia (0.1%) (Claghorn and Lesem 1995; Fawcett and Barkin 1998b; Kent 2000; Montgomery 1995).

Mirtazapine appears to have no clinically significant effects on seizure threshold or on the cardiovascular system (Claghorn and Lesem 1995; Fawcett and Barkin 1998b; Kent 2000; Montgomery 1995).

Of note, the noradrenergic effects of mirtazapine appear to be dose dependent and increase significantly at dosages >15 mg/day. As such, sedation associated with the affinity for H_1 receptors and typically experienced at dosages of ≤15 mg/day may be counteracted by an increasing noradrenergic neurotransmission at dosages ≥30 mg/day (Claghorn and Lesem 1995; Kent 2000). Likewise, it is also hypothesized that the risk of weight gain with mirtazapine is diminished at dosages ≥30 mg/day (Barkin et al. 2000; Fawcett and Barkin 1998b).

Use During Pregnancy and Lactation

A study conducted across six countries (Djulus et al. 2006) assessed the risk associated with exposure to mirtazapine during pregnancy. Birth outcomes were examined for three groups: pregnant women taking mirtazapine, disease-matched pregnant women taking other antidepressants, and pregnant women exposed to nonteratogens. There were approximately 100 patients per group. The rate of spontaneous abortions in the mirtazapine group (19%) was similar to that in the other antidepressant group (17%) and in the nonteratogen control group (11%). The rate of prematurity was significantly higher in the mirtazapine group (10%) versus the nonteratogen group (2%). The prematurity rate in the group taking other antidepressants was 7%. The rate of major malformations was not elevated in the mirtazapine group.

In a study of 8 women taking mirtazapine while breast-feeding, concentrations of mirtazapine or desmethylmirtazapine were measured in milk and plasma (Kristensen 2007). Low infant doses were observed, leading the authors to conclude that the drug is safe for lactating women who breast-feed.

Overdose

Mirtazapine appears to be safe in overdose. In one report (Holzbach et al. 1998), the cases of 2 patients who had overdosed with 30–50 times the average daily dose of mirtazapine were presented. In each case, the patient recovered fully and without any complications.

Symptoms reported in cases of mirtazapine overdose include disorientation, drowsiness, impaired memory, and tachycardia (Fawcett and Barkin 1998b; Kent 2000; Montgomery 1995; Stimmel et al. 1997).

A review of 117 mirtazapine overdoses (average ingestion: 450 mg) in Scotland revealed the adverse consequences to be relatively mild (Waring et al. 2007). Decreased consciousness was seen in 27% of subjects; 30% demonstrated tachycardia.

A more recent study of overdoses seen at six general hospitals in the United Kingdom between 2000 and 2006 indicated that mirtazapine was of intermediate toxicity between tricyclic antidepressants and venlafaxine, on the one hand, and SSRIs, on the other (Hawton et al. 2010).

Drug-Drug Interactions

In vitro data suggest that mirtazapine is unlikely to have clinically significant effects on the metabolism of drugs by CYP enzymes (Barkin et al. 2000; Fawcett and Barkin 1998b; Kent 2000). Analyses of data from the clinical development program for mirtazapine and postmarketing surveillance reveal no clinically relevant drug-drug interactions occurring with the concomitant use of medications such as opiates, anticonvulsants, analgesics, antihypertensives, diuretics, or nonsteroidal anti-inflammatory drugs (NSAIDs) (Barkin et al. 2000; Fawcett and Barkin 1998b). However, few formal drug interaction studies involving mirtazapine have been conducted (Barkin et al. 2000; Fawcett and Barkin 1998b; Holm and Markham 1999). Of note, a study of elderly patients with depression allowed for patients to be on drugs that are CYP2D6 substrates (Schatzberg et al. 2002). In this study, no increase in side effects was observed in these patients, compared with patients who were not taking CYP2D6 substrate agents (Schatzberg et al. 2002).

Conclusion

Mirtazapine is derived from the piperazino-azepine class of compounds and, as such, is structurally unrelated to any other psychotropic medications. Mirtazapine is also unique as an antidepressant because of its 5-HT_2, 5-HT_3, and α_2 receptor antagonist pharmacodynamic profile, which results in enhancement of noradrenergic and serotonergic transmission. It is an antidepressant that has been shown to be efficacious and well tolerated in the treatment of depression, and there are suggestions that it may be effective in a number of other medical and psychiatric conditions. Mirtazapine has also been suggested as a treatment intervention that may offer a more rapid amelioration of symptoms of depression and anxiety, compared with other antidepressants. The most common side effects reported with mirtazapine are somnolence, increased appetite, weight gain, and dry mouth. It otherwise appears to be free of many of the adverse effects typical of the SSRIs, especially sexual dysfunction.

Furthermore, mirtazapine appears to be well tolerated and effective in the treatment of geriatric depression and to have positive effects as an add-on agent in schizophrenia. In addition, mirtazapine is considered to be relatively safe in overdose, with case reports documenting complete and uncomplicated recovery following ingestion of up to 50 times the average daily dose. Finally, mirtazapine appears devoid of clinically significant drug-drug interactions, although larger formal clinical trials are still needed to verify this.

References

Abbasi SH, Behpournia H, Ghoreshi A, et al: The effect of mirtazapine add on therapy to risperidone in the treatment of schizophrenia: a double-blind randomized placebo-controlled trial. Schizophr Res 116:101–106, 2010

American Psychiatric Association: Diagnostic and Statistical Manual of Mental Disorders, 4th Edition. Washington, DC, American Psychiatric Association, 1994

Banerjee S, Hellier J, Dewey M, et al: Sertraline or mirtazapine for depression in dementia (HTA-SADD): a randomised, multicentre, double-blind, placebo-controlled trial. Lancet 378:403–411, 2011

Barkin RL, Schwer W, Barkin SJ: Recognition and management of depression in primary care: a focus on the elderly: a pharmacotherapeutic overview of the selection process among the traditional and new antidepressants. Am J Ther 7:205–226, 2000

Bendtsen L, Jensen R: Mirtazapine is effective in the prophylactic treatment of chronic tension-type headache. Neurology 62:1706–1711, 2004

Bengtsson HJ, Kele J, Johansson J, et al: Interaction of the antidepressant mirtazapine with α2-adrenoceptors modulating the release of 5-HT in different rat brain regions in vivo. Naunyn Schmiedebergs Arch Pharmacol 362:406–412, 2000

Benkert O, Szegedi A, Kohnen R: Mirtazapine compared with paroxetine in major depression. J Clin Psychiatry 61:656–663, 2000

Benkert O, Szegedi A, Philipp M, et al: Mirtazapine orally disintegrating tables versus venlafaxine extended release: a double-blind, randomized multicenter trial comparing the onset of antidepressant response in patients with major depressive disorder. J Clin Psychopharmacol 26:75–78, 2006

Berendsen HH, Broekkamp CL: Indirect in vivo 5-HT1A-agonistic effects of the new antidepressant mirtazapine. Psychopharmacology (Berl) 133:275–282, 1997

Berk M, Ichim C, Brook S: Efficacy of mirtazapine add on therapy to haloperidol in the treatment of the negative symptoms of schizophrenia: a double-blind randomized placebo-controlled study. Int Clin Psychopharmacol 16:87–92, 2001

Berk M, Gama CS, Sundram S, et al: Mirtazapine add-on therapy in the treatment of schizophrenia with atypical antipsychotics: a double-blind, randomised, placebo-controlled clinical trial. Hum Psychopharmacol 24:233–238, 2009

Blier P, Ward HE, Tremblay P, et al: Combination of antidepressant medications from treatment initiation for major depressive disorder: a double-blind randomized study. Am J Psychiatry 167:281–288, 2010

Boyarsky BK, Haque W, Rouleau MR, et al: Sexual functioning in depressed outpatients taking mirtazapine. Depress Anxiety 9:175–179, 1999

Brannon GE, Stone KD: The use of mirtazapine in a patient with chronic pain. J Pain Symptom Manage 18:382–385, 1999

Brannon GE, Rolland PD, Gary JM: Use of mirtazapine as prophylactic treatment for migraine headache. Psychosomatics 41:153–154, 2000

Carley DW, Olopade C, Ruigt GS, et al: Efficacy of mirtazapine in obstructive sleep apnea syndrome. Sleep 30:35–41, 2007

Carpenter LL, Yasmin S, Price L: A double-blind, placebo-controlled study of antidepressant augmentation with mirtazapine. Biol Psychiatry 51:183–188, 2002

Chang FL, Ho ST, Sheen MJ: Efficacy of mirtazapine in preventing intrathecal morphine-induced nausea and vomiting after orthopedic surgery. Anaesthesia 65:1206–1211, 2010

Cho SJ, Yook K, Kim B, et al: Mirtazapine augmentation enhances cognitive and reduces negative symptoms in schizophrenia patients treated with risperidone: a randomized controlled trial. Prog Neuropsychopharmacol Biol Psychiatry 35:208–211, 2011

Chung MY, Min KH, Jun YJ, et al: Efficacy and tolerability of mirtazapine and sertraline in Korean veterans with posttraumatic stress disorder: a randomized open label trial. Hum Psychopharmacol 19:489–494, 2004

Claghorn JL, Lesem MD: A double-blind placebo-controlled study of Org 3770 in depressed outpatients. J Affect Disord 34:165–171, 1995

Connor KM, Davidson JRT, Weisler RH, et al: A pilot study of mirtazapine in post-traumatic stress disorder. Int Clin Psychopharmacol 14:29–31, 1999

Dahl ML, Voortman G, Alm C, et al: In vitro and in vivo studies on the disposition of mirtazapine in humans. Clin Drug Invest 13:37–46, 1997

De Boer T: The pharmacologic profile of mirtazapine. J Clin Psychiatry 57 (suppl 4):19–25, 1996

De Boer T, Ruigt GC, Berendsen HH: The α2 adrenoceptor antagonist Org 3770 (mirtazapine, Remeron®) enhances noradrenergic and serotonergic transmission. Hum Psychopharmacol Clin Exp 10 (suppl):S107–S118, 1995

Djulus J, Koren G, Einarson TR, et al: Exposure to mirtazapine during pregnancy: a prospective, comparative study of birth outcomes. J Clin Psychiatry 67:1280–1284, 2006

Dodd S, Burrows GD, Norman TR: Chiral determination of mirtazapine in human blood plasma by high-performance liquid chromatography. J Chromatogr B Biomed Sci Appl 748:439–443, 2000

Dunner DL, Hendrickson HE, Bea C, et al: Dysthymic disorder: treatment with mirtazapine. Depress Anxiety 10:68–72, 1999

Farah A: Lack of sexual adverse effects with mirtazapine. Am Health Syst Pharm 55:2195–2196, 1998

Fava M, Dunner DL, Greist JH, et al: Efficacy and safety of mirtazapine in major depressive disorder patients after SSRI treatment failure: an open-label trial. J Clin Psychiatry 62:413–420, 2001

Fava M, Rush AJ, Wisniewski SR, et al: A comparison of mirtazapine and nortriptyline following two consecutive failed medication treatments for depressed outpatients: a STAR*D report. Am J Psychiatry 163:1161–1172, 2006

Fawcett J, Barkin RL: A meta-analysis of eight randomized, double-blind controlled clinical trials of mirtazapine for the treatment of patients with major depression and symptoms of anxiety. J Clin Psychiatry 59:123–127, 1998a

Fawcett J, Barkin RL: Review of the results from clinical studies on the efficacy, safety and tolerability of mirtazapine for the treatment of patients with major depression. J Affect Disord 51:267–285, 1998b

Freynhagen R, Muth-Selbach U, Lipfert P, et al: The effect of mirtazapine in patients with chronic pain and concomitant depression. Curr Med Res Opin 22:257–264, 2006

Gambi F, De Berardis D, Campanello D, et al: Mirtazapine treatment of generalized anxiety disorder: a fixed dose, open label study. J Psychopharmacol 19:483–487, 2005

Gelenberg AJ, Laukes C, McGauhey C, et al: Mirtazapine substitution in SSRI-induced sexual dysfunction. J Clin Psychiatry 61:356–360, 2000

Goodnick PJ, Puig A, DeVane CL, et al: Mirtazapine in major depression with comorbid generalized anxiety disorder. J Clin Psychiatry 60:446–448, 1999

Guelfi JD, Ansseau M, Timmerman L, et al: Mirtazapine versus venlafaxine in hospitalized severely depressed patients with melancholic features. J Clin Psychopharmacol 21:425–431, 2001

Haapasalo-Pesu KM, Vuola T, Lahelma L, et al: Mirtazapine in the treatment of adolescents with major depression: an open-label, multicenter pilot study. J Child Adolesc Psychopharmacol 14:175–184, 2004

Halikas JA: Org 3770 (mirtazapine) versus trazodone: a placebo controlled trial in depressed elderly patients. Hum Psychopharmacol 10:125–133, 1995

Hawton K, Bergen H, Simkin S, et al: Toxicity of antidepressants: rates of suicide relative to prescribing and non-fatal overdose. Br J Psychiatry 196:354–358, 2010

Holm KJ, Markham A: Mirtazapine: a review of its use in major depression. Drugs 57:607–631, 1999

Holzbach R, Jahn H, Pajonk FG, et al: Suicide attempts with mirtazapine overdose without complications. Biol Psychiatry 44:925–926, 1998

Joffe H, Groninger H, Soares C, et al: An open trial of mirtazapine in menopausal women with depression unresponsive to estrogen replacement therapy. J Womens Health Gend Based Med 10:999–1004, 2001

Kaspersen FM, van Rooij FA, Sperling EM: The synthesis of Org 3770 labeled with 3-H, 13-C and 14-C. J Labelled Comp Radiopharma 27:1055–1068, 1989

Kast RE: Mirtazapine may be useful in treating nausea and insomnia of cancer chemotherapy. Support Care Cancer 9:469–470, 2001

Kent JM: SNaRIs, NaSSAs, and NaRIs: new agents for the treatment of depression. Lancet 355:911–918, 2000

Kim W, Pae CU, Chae JH, et al: The effectiveness of mirtazapine in the treatment of post-traumatic stress disorder: a 24-week continuation therapy. Psychiatry Clin Neurosci 59:743–747, 2005

Kooyman AR, Zwart R, Vanderheijden PM, et al: Interaction between enantiomers of mianserin and Org 3770 at 5-HT3 receptors in cultured mouse neuroblastoma cells. Neuropsychopharmacology 33:501–510, 1994

Koran LM, Gamel NN, Choung HW, et al: Mirtazapine for obsessive-compulsive disorder: an open trial followed by double-blind discontinuation. J Clin Psychiatry 66:515–520, 2005

Kristensen JH, Ilett KF, Rampono J, et al: Transfer of the antidepressant mirtazapine into breast milk. Br J Clin Pharmacol 63:322–327, 2007

Kuiken TA, Schechtman L, Harden RN: Phantom limb pain treatment with mirtazapine: a case series. Pain Pract 5:356–360, 2005

Laakmann G, Hennig J, Baghai T, et al: Mirtazapine acutely inhibits salivary cortisol concentrations in depressed patients. Ann N Y Acad Sci 1032:279–282, 2004

Leinonen E, Skarstein J, Behnke K, et al: Efficacy and tolerability of mirtazapine versus citalopram: a double-blind, randomized study in patients with major depressive disorder. Int Clin Psychopharmacol 14:329–337, 1999

Maris FA, Dingler E, Niehues S: High-performance liquid chromatographic assay with fluorescence detection for the routine monitoring of the antidepressant mirtazapine and its desmethyl metabolite in human plasma. J Chromatogr B Biomed Sci Appl 721:309–316, 1999

Michelson D, Kociban K, Tamura R, et al: Mirtazapine, yohimbine or olanzapine augmentation therapy for serotonin reuptake-associated female sexual dysfunction: a randomized, placebo controlled trial. J Psychiatr Res 36:147–152, 2002

Montgomery SA: Safety of mirtazapine: a review. Int Clin Psychopharmacol 10 (suppl 4):37–45, 1995

Mrakotsky C, Masek B, Biederman J, et al: Prospective open-label pilot trial of mirtazapine in children and adolescents with social phobia. J Anxiety Disord 22:88–97, 2008

Muehlbacher M, Nickel MK, Nickel C, et al: Mirtazapine treatment of social phobia in women: a randomized, double-blind, placebo-controlled study. J Clin Psychopharmacol 25:580–582, 2005

Murphy GM, Kremer C, Rodrigues H, et al: The apolipoprotein E epsilon4 allele and antidepressant efficacy in cognitively intact elderly depressed patients. Biol Psychiatry 54:665–673, 2003a

Murphy GM Jr, Kremer C, Rodrigues HE, et al: Pharmacogenetics of antidepressant medication intolerance. Am J Psychiatry 160:1830–1835, 2003b

Nelson JC, Holden K, Roose S, et al: Are there predictors of outcome in depressed elderly nursing home residents during treatment with mirtazapine orally disintegrating tablets? Int J Geriatr Psychiatry 22:999–1003, 2007

Numazawa R, Yoshioka M, Matsumoto M, et al: Pharmacological characterization of $\alpha 2$ adrenoceptor regulated serotonin release in the rat hippocampus. Neurosci Lett 192:161–164, 1995

Nutt DJ: Efficacy of mirtazapine in clinically relevant subgroups of depressed patients. Depress Anxiety 7 (suppl 1):7–10, 1998

Nutt D: Treatment of cluster headache with mirtazapine. Headache 39:586–587, 1999

Pallanti S, Quercioli L, Bruscoli M: Response acceleration with mirtazapine augmentation of citalopram in obsessive-compulsive disorder patients without comorbid depression: a pilot study. J Clin Psychiatry 65:1394–1399, 2004

Posey DJ, Guenin KD, Kohn AE, et al: A naturalistic open-label study of mirtazapine in autistic and other pervasive developmental disorders. J Child Adolesc Psychopharmacol 11:267–277, 2001

Poyurovsky M, Epshtein S, Fuchs C, et al: Efficacy of low-dose mirtazapine in neuroleptic-induced akathisia: a double-blind randomized placebo-controlled pilot study. J Clin Psychopharmacol 23:305–308, 2003

Poyurovsky M, Pashinian A, Weizman R, et al: Low-dose mirtazapine: a new option in the treatment of antipsychotic-induced akathisia: a randomized, double-blind, placebo- and propranolol-controlled trial. Biol Psychiatry 59:1071–1077, 2006

Raji MA, Brady SR: Mirtazapine for treatment of depression and comorbidities in Alzheimer's disease. Ann Pharmacother 35:1024–1027, 2001

Remeron (package insert). Physicians' Desk Reference, 56th Edition. Montvale, NJ, Medical Economics Company, 2002

Saks BR: Mirtazapine: treatment of depression, anxiety, and hyperemesis gravidarum in the pregnant patient: a report of 7 cases. Arch Women Ment Health 3:165–170, 2001

Schatzberg AF, Kremer C, Rodrigues HE, et al: Double-blind randomized comparison of mirtazapine and paroxetine in elderly depressed patients. Am J Geriatr Psychiatry 10:541–550, 2002

Schmid DA, Wichniak A, Uhr M, et al: Changes of sleep architecture, spectral composition of sleep EEG, the nocturnal secretion of cortisol, ACTH, GH, prolactin, melatonin, ghrelin, and leptin, and the DEX-CRH test in depressed patients during treatment with mirtazapine. Neuropsychopharmacology 31:832–844, 2006

Stahl S, Zivkov M, Reimitz PE, et al: Meta-analysis of randomized, double-blind, placebo-controlled, efficacy and safety studies of mirtazapine versus amitriptyline in major depression. Acta Psychiatr Scand Suppl 391:22–30, 1997

Stenberg JH, Terevnikov V, Joffe M, et al: Effects of add-on mirtazapine on neurocognition in schizophrenia: a double-blind, randomized, placebo-controlled study. Int J Neuropsychopharmacol 13:433–441, 2010

Stimmel GL, Dopheide JA, Stahl SM: Mirtazapine: an antidepressant with noradrenergic and specific serotonergic effects. Pharmacotherapy 17:10–21, 1997

Thase ME, Nierenberg AA, Vrijland P, et al: Remission with mirtazapine and selective serotonin reuptake inhibitors: a meta-analysis of individual patient data from 15 controlled trials of acute phase treatment of major depression. Int Clin Psychopharmacol 25:189–198, 2010

Theobold DE, Kirsh KE, Holtszclaw E, et al: An open-label, crossover trial of mirtazapine (15 and 30 mg) in cancer patients with pain and other distressing symptoms. J Pain Symptom Manage 23:442–447, 2002

Thompson DS: Mirtazapine for the treatment of depression and nausea in breast and gynecological oncology. Psychosomatics 41:356–359, 2000

Varia I, Venkataraman S, Hellegers C, et al: Effect of mirtazapine orally disintegrating tablets on health-related quality of life in elderly depressed patients with comorbid medical disorders: a pilot study. Psychopharmacol Bull 40:47–56, 2007

Waldinger MD, Berendsen HH, Schweitzer DH: Treatment of hot flushes with mirtazapine: four case reports. Maturitas 36:165–168, 2000

Waring WS, Good AM, Bateman DN: Lack of significant toxicity after mirtazapine overdose: a five-year review of cases admitted to a regional toxicology unit. Clin Toxicol (Phila) 45:45–50, 2007

Wheatley DP, Van Moffaert M, Timmerman L, et al: Mirtazapine: efficacy and tolerability in comparison with fluoxetine in patients with moderate to severe major depressive disorder. J Clin Psychiatry 59:306–312, 1998

CHAPTER 11

Venlafaxine and Desvenlafaxine

Michael E. Thase, M.D.

History and Discovery

Venlafaxine was first identified as a relatively selective serotonin-norepinephrine reuptake inhibitor (SNRI) in the 1980s and early 1990s (Bolden-Watson and Richelson 1993; Muth et al. 1986). Several early randomized controlled trials (RCTs) confirmed that venlafaxine had antidepressant effects comparable to those of tricyclic antidepressants (TCAs), with fewer side effects attributable to anticholinergic and antihistaminergic activity (see, for example, Einarson et al. 1999). An immediate-release (IR) form of venlafaxine was approved by the U.S. Food and Drug Administration (FDA) for treatment of depression in 1994. The more widely used extended-release (XR) formulation was introduced in 1997. Generic formulations of both products are now available.

O-Desmethylvenlafaxine (ODV), the primary active metabolite of venlafaxine, was developed in an extended-release formulation as desvenlafaxine succinate (DVS) and was approved by the FDA for treatment of depression in 2008. Like venlafaxine, DVS is classified as an SNRI and was developed in the hope of improving on the strengths of the parent drug. In comparison with venlafaxine, DVS has somewhat greater potency for blockade of norepinephrine transporters, and the formulation results in greater bioavailability (Deecher et al. 2006).

Structure-Activity Relations and Pharmacological Profile

Venlafaxine and desvenlafaxine are bicyclic phenylethylamine compounds and are structurally and chemically unrelated to all other available antidepressants and anxiolytics. Venlafaxine and desvenlafaxine inhibit the neuronal reuptake of serotonin (5-HT) and norepinephrine (NE) in in vitro and ex vivo experimental paradigms (Bolden-Watson and Richelson 1993; Muth et al. 1986; Owens et al. 1997); do not inhibit monoamine oxidase; and have little or no in vitro affinity for muscarinic, cholinergic, histaminergic H_1, and α-adrenergic receptors (Bolden-Watson and Richelson 1993; Muth et al. 1986).

Pharmacokinetics and Disposition

Venlafaxine and desvenlafaxine are well absorbed from the gastrointestinal tract after oral ingestion and undergo extensive first-pass hepatic metabolism. ODV is the only major metabolite of venlafaxine with relevant activity; desvenlafaxine has no active metabolites. Peak plasma concentrations are achieved within 2 hours for venlafaxine and within 3 hours for ODV following ingestion of the IR formulation (Troy et al. 1995). Venlafaxine XR is absorbed more slowly than the IR formulation (peak plasma concentrations are achieved within 5.5 hours for venlafaxine and within 9 hours for ODV), resulting in lower peak and higher trough plasma concentrations. Steady-state plasma concentrations of both venlafaxine and ODV are reached within 3–4 days of therapy. For normal and extensive metabolizers, ODV accounts for about 70% of the total drug concentration at steady state (Klamerus et al. 1992). Venlafaxine exhibits linear kinetics over a dosage range of 75–450 mg/day (Klamerus et al. 1992). The same is true for DVS across a range of 50–400 mg/day. Renal elimination is the primary route of excretion for both drugs (Howell et al. 1993). Clearance of ODV (half-life = 10 hours) is slower than that of venlafaxine (half-life = 4 hours). Both venlafaxine and ODV are minimally bound to plasma albumin.

The recommended starting dosage of venlafaxine is 75 mg/day (either divided doses [IR] or once daily [XR]), which is the minimum effective dose. A lower starting dosage (i.e., 37.5 mg/day) may be used when treating patients who are elderly or who have a history of tolerability problems. The maximum approved dosage of the IR formulation is 375 mg/day, whereas 225 mg/day is the highest approved dosage for the XR formulation. The recommended starting dose of desvenlafaxine is 50 mg/day, which is also the minimum effective dosage; 100 mg/day is the maximum approved daily dosage. Lower dosages of both drugs are recommended for patients with renal insufficiency; lower dosages of venlafaxine are also recommended for patients with liver disease.

Unlike most newer antidepressants, venlafaxine shows a dose-response relationship for efficacy in major depressive disorder (MDD) (Kelsey 1996; Khan et al. 1998; Rudolph et al. 1998; Thase et al. 2006). Whereas the original form of venlafaxine was approved for treatment at dosages of up to 375 mg/day (divided bid or tid), the recommended maximum daily dose of XR was "capped" at 225 mg because of a lack of data on safety and tolerability at higher doses. By contrast, DVS does not exhibit a positive dose-response curve in MDD: drug versus placebo differences on 50 mg/day are as large as those observed on higher dosages (Thase et al. 2009). It has not been determined whether patients who do not respond to 50 mg/day will benefit from upward titration.

Mechanism of Action

Venlafaxine and DVS are potent inhibitors of 5-HT reuptake at minimum therapeutic doses; inhibition of NE reuptake is lower at these doses (Bolden-Watson and Richelson 1993; Deecher et al. 2006; Vaishnavi et al. 2004). It has long been suggested that this relationship underpins the ascending dose-response relationship of venlafaxine (Kelsey 1996). Although experimental (Harvey et al. 2000) and clinical (Davidson et al. 2005; Entsuah and Gao 2002; Rudolph et al. 1998; Thase 1998; Thase et al. 2006) data are consistent with this hypothesis, significant effects on autonomic measures of noradrenergic function are evident at 37.5- and 75-mg/day dosages (Bitsios et al. 1999; Siepmann et al. 2007). As of yet, studies that image NE transporter occupancy in vivo during treatment with venlafaxine or DVS have not been undertaken.

Indications and Efficacy

Venlafaxine is approved by the FDA for the treatment of MDD, generalized anxiety disorder (GAD), social anxiety disorder, and panic disorder. Desvenlafaxine is approved only for the treatment of MDD.

Major Depressive Disorder

The efficacy of venlafaxine at dosages ranging from 75 mg/day to 375 mg/day has been established in a large number of RCTs (see Thase and Sloan 2006). Meta-analyses of studies using active comparators have determined that venlafaxine therapy is, at the least, one of the more effective newer-generation antidepressants (Cipriani et al. 2009; Nemeroff et al. 2008; Schueler et al. 2011; Smith et al. 2002; Thase et al. 2001), although evidence of its superiority over the selective serotonin reuptake inhibitors (SSRIs) as a class is largely dependent on the sizable subgroup of studies using fluoxetine (Cipriani et al. 2009; Nemeroff et al. 2008), and there is no evidence of its superiority over escitalopram (Kennedy et al. 2009).

The antidepressant efficacy of DVS has been established against placebo at dosages ranging from 50 mg/day to 400 mg/day (Thase et al. 2009). To date, DVS (100–200 mg/day) has been compared with an SSRI in only one study, which found it to be comparable in efficacy to escitalopram (10–20 mg/day) (Soares et al. 2010). In the two studies that directly compared DVS (200–400 mg/day) with venlafaxine XR (75–150 or 150–225 mg/day), the drugs were comparably effective, although tolerability indices tended to favor the older drug (Lieberman et al. 2008).

With respect to other newer antidepressants, venlafaxine has been compared with mirtazapine (Benkert et al. 2006; Guelfi et al. 2001), bupropion (Hewett et al. 2010; Thase et al. 2006), duloxetine (Perahia et al. 2008), and agomelatine (Kennedy et al. 2008). Overall, the results of these studies suggest that whereas the various non-SSRI antidepressants are generally comparable in efficacy, their tolerability profiles differ markedly. For example, mirtazapine and agomelatine are associated with less residual insomnia than venlafaxine, and agomelatine and bupropion are associated with less treatment-emergent sexual dysfunction.

Neither venlafaxine nor DVS has established efficacy in bipolar depression. In two comparative studies that enrolled patients with bipolar I depression who were being treated with mood stabilizers, adjunctive venlafaxine therapy was associated with somewhat higher rates of treatment-emergent affective switches than was paroxetine (Vieta et al. 2002) or sertraline and bupropion (Post et al. 2006). Interestingly, a randomized open-label study comparing venlafaxine and lithium as monotherapy in outpatients with bipolar II depression (Amsterdam and Shults 2008) found significant advantages for the SNRI, even among the subset of patients with a history of rapid cycling.

In an era in which most patients with depression are first treated with an SSRI, venlafaxine has for more than a decade been one of the preferred second-line choices for patients who do not respond to SSRI treatment (Thase et al. 2000). A meta-analysis of randomized trials of patients with SSRI-resistant depression comparing venlafaxine with other second-line antidepressants confirmed a modest advantage for switching to the SNRI (Papakostas et al. 2008).

Both venlafaxine and DVS have demonstrated sustained efficacy in studies of longer-term therapy. Results of a pooled analysis of the extension phases of four double-blind RCTs in outpatients with major depression demonstrated that the rate of relapse at 6 months and 1 year was significantly lower in the venlafaxine-treated group than in the placebo-treated group (Entsuah et al. 1996). Double-blind, placebo-controlled studies subsequently confirmed the efficacy of venlafaxine treatment for prevention of relapse during 6 months of continuation treatment (Simon et al. 2004) and for prevention of recurrence during 12 months (Kocsis et al. 2007) and 24 months (Keller et al. 2007) of maintenance-phase therapy. In the latter study, which included an active comparison group treated with fluoxetine, an interesting trend emerging during the second year of maintenance therapy suggested greater efficacy for venlafaxine versus the SSRI (Thase et al. 2011). To date, the efficacy of DVS continuation therapy has been studied only for dosages higher than those currently recommended (Rickels et al. 2010a).

Generalized Anxiety Disorder

Venlafaxine XR was approved by the FDA for treatment of GAD on the basis of a series of placebo-controlled RCTs (see Thase and Sloan 2006). Across studies, efficacy was established for dosages ranging from 75 mg/day to 225 mg/day, with little evidence of a dose-response relationship. Sustained efficacy across 12 months was subsequently demonstrated in one study using a classic placebo-controlled discontinuation design (Rickels et al. 2010b). With respect to comparative efficacy, superiority to buspirone was found on some—although not all—measures in one study (Davidson et al. 1999), and neither venlafaxine nor diazepam was found to be effective in the only study to use a benzodiazepine comparison group (Hackett et al. 2003). Venlafaxine XR was found to be comparably effective to duloxetine (Allgulander et al. 2008) and escitalopram (Bose et al. 2008) in the only studies of GAD to use antidepressant comparators.

Social Anxiety Disorder

Venlafaxine XR was approved for treatment of social anxiety disorder on the basis of a series of RCTs that confirmed its efficacy and safety relative to placebo across up to 6 months of double-blind therapy (see Thase and Sloan 2006). As was the case in GAD, effective dosages ranged from 75 mg/day to 225 mg/day, with little evidence of an ascending dose-response relationship. In the two studies that included paroxetine as an active comparator, the SSRI and the SNRI were comparably effective and similarly well tolerated (Allgulander et al. 2004; Liebowitz et al. 2005).

Panic Disorder

The efficacy of venlafaxine XR in panic disorder was demonstrated in three placebo-controlled studies of acute-phase therapy (Bradwejn et al. 2005; Pollack et al. 2007a, 2007b). These studies, which used a 37.5-mg starting dose to minimize early side effects, established an effective dosage range of 75–225 mg/day. In the studies that included paroxetine (40 mg/day) as an active comparator (Pollack et al. 2007a, 2007b), the two fixed dosages of venlafaxine XR (75 mg/day and 150 mg/day) were comparable to paroxetine in both efficacy and tolerability. In the single RCT that included a fixed-dose 225-mg/day arm, the higher dose of venlafaxine therapy was significantly more effective than paroxetine on several secondary outcome measures, including the proportion of patients who experienced complete relief from full-symptom panic attacks (70% vs. 58%) (Pollack et al. 2007b). A fourth study demonstrated sustained efficacy across 6 months of therapy using a classic relapse prevention design (Ferguson et al. 2007).

Other Anxiety Disorders

The efficacy of venlafaxine therapy in posttraumatic stress disorder (PTSD) was established in two large placebo-controlled studies (Davidson et al. 2006a, 2006b). Although no pivotal studies of venlafaxine therapy were conducted in obsessive-compulsive disorder, the results of a 12-week single-blind study indicated that venlafaxine might be at least as effective as clomipramine and significantly better tolerated (Albert et al. 2002).

Premenstrual Dysphoric Disorder

A double-blind RCT evaluated the efficacy of venlafaxine IR for the treatment of premenstrual dysphoric disorder in 157 women treated across four menstrual cycles (Freeman et al. 2001). Dosages ranged from 50 mg/day to 200 mg/day, with adjustments for adverse events or lack of efficacy early in each cycle. Analysis of daily symptom rating scores revealed significantly greater improvement in the venlafaxine group compared with the placebo group at endpoint in the primary factors of emotion, function, physical symptoms, and pain.

Treatment of Children and Adolescents

Neither venlafaxine XR nor desvenlafaxine is approved for treatment of individuals younger than 18 years. Nevertheless, five studies of venlafaxine XR have been completed in pediatric populations; these include a pair of studies in MDD (Emslie et al. 2007), two RCTs in GAD (Rynn et al. 2007), and one study in social anxiety disorder (March et al. 2007). Results in the depression studies (pooled $N=334$) were mixed: venlafaxine XR was significantly more effective than placebo among participants ages 12–17 years but not among those ages 7–11 years (Emslie et al. 2007). In the pooled data set, venlafaxine XR therapy was associated with an increased risk of treatment-emergent suicidal and aggressive behaviors compared with placebo. In the pair of GAD studies (pooled $N=330$), venlafaxine XR was significantly more effective than placebo in the pooled data set; one study was unequivocally positive, but the second study failed to separate between drug and placebo on the primary outcome measure (Rynn et al. 2007). In the social anxiety disorder study ($N=293$), venlafaxine XR was significantly more effective than placebo on both primary and secondary outcome measures (March et al. 2007).

Side Effects and Toxicology

The tolerability profiles of venlafaxine and desvenlafaxine include all of the characteristic side effects associated with 5-HT uptake inhibition (i.e., nausea, insomnia, tremor, and sexual dysfunction) as well as side effects attributable to NE reuptake inhibition (i.e., sweating and dry mouth); therefore, therapy with these SNRIs is associated with a somewhat higher side-effect burden than is usual with the SSRIs (Schueler et al. 2011; Thase and Sloan 2006). In the meta-analysis of Nemeroff et al. (2008), for example, 11% of the venlafaxine-treated patients withdrew from therapy because of adverse events, compared with 9% of patients treated with SSRIs. The results of several studies suggest that venlafaxine and the SSRIs are associated with similar risks of sexual side effects (Clayton et al. 2002; Kennedy et al. 2000; Montejo et al. 2001; Serretti and Chiesa 2009).

Venlafaxine and desvenlafaxine do not adversely affect cardiac conduction or lower seizure threshold at therapeutic doses. Both drugs are associated with small average increases in pulse rate and dose-dependent increases in the risk of elevated blood pressure (Clayton et al. 2009; Thase 1998). It is recommended that patients receiving these medications have regular monitoring of blood pressure.

Venlafaxine and desvenlafaxine are classified as pregnancy Category C, indicating that there are no adequate and well-controlled studies in pregnant women and that the drugs should be used during pregnancy only if they are clearly clinically indicated. Venlafaxine and desvenlafaxine are excreted in human breast milk and therefore should not be taken by women who are breast-feeding.

It is well known that abrupt withdrawal of venlafaxine can result in "discontinuation-emergent" symptoms such as dizziness, dry mouth, insomnia, nausea, nervousness, sweating, anorexia, diarrhea, somnolence, and sensory disturbances (Haddad 2001). Available evidence suggests that desvenlafaxine may have somewhat less problematic discontinuation-emergent symptoms (Montgomery et al. 2009). To minimize discontinuation symptoms, therapy should be tapered over several weeks when possible.

Clinicians should counsel patients about the possibility of adverse effects following abrupt discontinuation of treatment.

A number of fatal overdoses of venlafaxine have been reported; there is less clinical experience with overdoses of desvenlafaxine. In nonfatal overdoses of venlafaxine, electrocardiogram changes (e.g., prolongation of QT interval, bundle branch block, QRS prolongation), sinus and ventricular tachycardia, bradycardia, hypotension, altered level of consciousness (ranging from somnolence to coma), serotonin syndrome, and seizures have been reported (Howell et al. 2007; Whyte et al. 2003). Some pharmacoepidemiological data collected in the United Kingdom suggest that venlafaxine may have greater toxicity in overdose than SSRIs (Buckley and McManus 2002; Hawton et al. 2010). However, these data are subject to bias, as the patients who were selected for venlafaxine therapy in this era tended to have more severe and treatment-resistant psychiatric illness, and thus were at greater inherent suicide risk, than the patients treated with SSRIs (Mines et al. 2005; Rubino et al. 2007).

Drug-Drug Interactions

Venlafaxine undergoes extensive metabolism in the liver by the cytochrome P450 (CYP) enzyme system, particularly by the CYP2D6 isoenzyme, which is the pathway for conversion of venlafaxine into O-desmethylvenlafaxine. People who are poor metabolizers of CYP2D6 thus have unusually low plasma levels of the ODV metabolite (Preskorn et al. 2009) and may be somewhat less likely to benefit from treatment with the parent drug than patients who are normal or extensive metabolizers (Lobello et al. 2010; Shams et al. 2006). Such patients thus could potentially be better candidates for therapy with desvenlafaxine than the parent drug.

Venlafaxine and ODV are weak inhibitors of CYP2D6 (Alfaro et al. 2000; Amchin et al. 2001; Ball et al. 1997; Oganesian et al. 2009). In vitro and in vivo studies have shown that venlafaxine and ODV cause little or no inhibition of other CYP isoenzymes, including 1A2, 2C9, 2C19, and 3A4 (Ball et al. 1997; Oganesian et al. 2009; Owen and Nemeroff 1998).

Both venlafaxine and desvenlafaxine are contraindicated in patients taking monoamine oxidase inhibitors (MAOIs), because of the risk of serotonin syndrome. This is as true for the newer transdermally delivered formulation of selegiline as it is with the older agents. As with cyclic antidepressants and SSRIs, venlafaxine or desvenlafaxine treatment should not be initiated until 2 weeks after discontinuation of an MAOI, and MAOI therapy should not be initiated until at least 7 days after discontinuation of venlafaxine or desvenlafaxine.

Conclusion

Venlafaxine, the first widely used member of the SNRI class, is among the most effective of the newer-generation antidepressants, with an overall safety profile that is intermediate between the SSRIs and the TCAs. There is evidence of a modest efficacy advantage compared with fluoxetine and perhaps to the SSRIs as a class, although a significant efficacy advantage has not been demonstrated against all members of the class, most particularly escitalopram. Venlafaxine also has established efficacy for treatment of GAD, social anxiety disorder, and panic disorder. Generic formulations of venlafaxine IR and XR are available. Desvenlafaxine succinate, which is available only in a branded formulation and is approved only for the treatment of MDD, has several advantages relative to venlafaxine XR, including a lower starting dose, a narrower dosing range, and a metabolism not dependent on CYP 2D6. For the time being, it seems likely that therapy with a generic formulation of venlafaxine XR is the more cost-effective option for all patients except those who are poor 2D6 metabolizers.

References

Albert U, Aguglia E, Maina G, et al: Venlafaxine versus clomipramine in the treatment of obsessive-compulsive disorder: a preliminary single-blind, 12-week, controlled study. J Clin Psychiatry 63:1004–1009, 2002

Alfaro CL, Lam YW, Simpson J, et al: CYP2D6 inhibition by fluoxetine, paroxetine, sertraline, and venlafaxine in a crossover study: intraindividual variability and plasma concentration correlations. J Clin Pharmacol 40:58–66, 2000

Allgulander C, Mangano R, Zhang J, et al: Efficacy of venlafaxine ER in patients with social anxiety disorder: a double-blind, placebo-controlled, parallel-group comparison with paroxetine. SAD 388 Study Group. Hum Psychopharmacol 19:387–396, 2004

Allgulander C, Nutt D, Detke M, et al: A non-inferiority comparison of duloxetine and venlafaxine in the treatment of adult patients with generalized anxiety disorder. J Psychopharmacol 22:417–425, 2008

Amchin J, Ereshefsky L, Zarycranski W, et al: Effect of venlafaxine versus fluoxetine on metabolism of dextromethorphan, a CYP2D6 probe. J Clin Pharmacol 41:443–451, 2001

Amsterdam JD, Shults J: Comparison of short-term venlafaxine versus lithium monotherapy for bipolar II major depressive episode: a randomized open-label study. J Clin Psychopharmacol 28:171–181, 2008

Ball SE, Ahern D, Scatina J, et al: Venlafaxine: in vitro inhibition of CYP2D6 dependent imipramine and desipramine metabolism: comparative studies with selected SSRIs, and effects on human hepatic CYP3A4, CYP2C9 and CYP1A2. Br J Clin Pharmacol 43:619–626, 1997

Benkert O, Szegedi A, Philipp M, et al: Mirtazapine orally disintegrating tablets versus venlafaxine extended release: a double-blind, randomized multicenter trial comparing the onset of antidepressant response in patients with major depressive disorder. J Clin Psychopharmacol 26:75–78, 2006

Bitsios P, Szabadi E, Bradshaw CM: Comparison of the effects of venlafaxine, paroxetine and desipramine on the pupillary light reflex in man. Psychopharmacology (Berl) 143:286–292, 1999

Bolden-Watson C, Richelson E: Blockade by newly developed antidepressants of biogenic amine uptake into rat brain synaptosomes. Life Sci 52:1023–1029, 1993

Bose A, Korotzer A, Gommoll C, et al: Randomized placebo-controlled trial of escitalopram and venlafaxine XR in the treatment of generalized anxiety disorder. Depress Anxiety 25:854–861, 2008

Bradwejn J, Ahokas A, Stein DJ, et al: Venlafaxine extended-release capsules in panic disorder: flexible-dose, double-blind, placebo-controlled study. Br J Psychiatry 187:352–359, 2005

Buckley NA, McManus PR: Fatal toxicity of serotoninergic and other antidepressant drugs: analysis of United Kingdom mortality data. BMJ 325:1332–1333, 2002

Cipriani A, Furukawa TA, Salanti G, et al: Comparative efficacy and acceptability of 12 new-generation antidepressants: a multiple-treatments meta-analysis. Lancet 373:746–758, 2009

Clayton AH, Pradko JF, Croft HA, et al. Prevalence of sexual dysfunction among newer antidepressants. J Clin Psychiatry 63:357–366, 2002

Clayton AH, Kornstein SG, Rosas G, et al: An integrated analysis of the safety and tolerability of desvenlafaxine compared with placebo in the treatment of major depressive disorder. CNS Spectr 14:183–195, 2009

Davidson JR, DuPont RL, Hedges D, et al: Efficacy, safety, and tolerability of venlafaxine extended release and buspirone in outpatients with generalized anxiety disorder. J Clin Psychiatry 60:528–535, 1999

Davidson J, Watkins L, Owens M, et al: Effects of paroxetine and venlafaxine XR on heart rate variability in depression. J Clin Psychopharmacol 25:480–484, 2005

Davidson J, Baldwin D, Stein DJ, et al: Treatment of posttraumatic stress disorder with venlafaxine extended release: a 6-month randomized controlled trial. Arch Gen Psychiatry 63:1158–1165, 2006a

Davidson J, Rothbaum BO, Tucker P, et al: Venlafaxine extended release in posttraumatic stress disorder: a sertraline- and placebo-controlled study. J Clin Psychopharmacol 26:259–267, 2006b

Deecher DC, Beyer CE, Johnston G, et al: Desvenlafaxine succinate: a new serotonin and norepinephrine reuptake inhibitor. J Pharmacol Exp Ther 318:657–665, 2006

Einarson TR, Arikian SR, Casciano J, et al: Comparison of extended-release venlafaxine, selective serotonin reuptake inhibitors, and tricyclic antidepressants in the treatment of depression: a meta-analysis of randomized controlled trials. Clin Ther 21:296–308, 1999

Emslie GJ, Findling RL, Yeung PP, et al: Venlafaxine ER for the treatment of pediatric subjects with depression: results of two placebo-controlled trials. J Am Acad Child Adolesc Psychiatry 46:479–488, 2007

Entsuah AR, Rudolph RL, Hackett D, et al: Efficacy of venlafaxine and placebo during long-term treatment of depression: a pooled analysis of relapse rates. Int Clin Psychopharmacol 11:137–145, 1996

Entsuah R, Gao B: Global benefit-risk evaluation of antidepressant action: comparison of pooled data for venlafaxine, SSRIs, and placebo. CNS Spectr 7:882–888, 2002

Ferguson JM, Khan A, Mangano R, et al: Relapse prevention of panic disorder in adult outpatient responders to treatment with venlafaxine extended release. J Clin Psychiatry 68:58–68, 2007

Freeman EW, Rickels K, Yonkers KA, et al: Venlafaxine in the treatment of premenstrual dysphoric disorder. Obstet Gynecol 98:737–744, 2001

Guelfi JD, Ansseau M, Timmerman L, et al: Mirtazapine versus venlafaxine in hospitalized severely depressed patients with melancholic features. J Clin Psychopharmacol 21:425–431, 2001

Hackett D, Haudiquet V, Salinas E: A method for controlling for a high placebo response rate in a comparison of venlafaxine XR and diazepam in the short-term treatment of patients with generalised anxiety disorder. Eur Psychiatry 18:182–187, 2003

Haddad PM: Antidepressant discontinuation syndromes. Drug Saf 24:183–197, 2001

Harvey AT, Rudolph RL, Preskorn SH: Evidence of the dual mechanisms of action of venlafaxine. Arch Gen Psychiatry 57:503–509, 2000

Hawton K, Bergen H, Simkin S, et al: Toxicity of antidepressants: rates of suicide relative to prescribing and non-fatal overdose. Br J Psychiatry 196:354–358, 2010

Hewett K, Gee MD, Krishen A, et al: Double-blind, placebo-controlled comparison of the antidepressant efficacy and tolerability of bupropion XR and venlafaxine XR. J Psychopharmacol 24:1209–1216, 2010

Howell C, Wilson AD, Waring WS: Cardiovascular toxicity due to venlafaxine poisoning in adults: a review of 235 consecutive cases. Br J Clin Pharmacol 64:192–197, 2007

Howell SR, Husbands GE, Scatina JA, et al: Metabolic disposition of 14C-venlafaxine in mouse, rat, dog, rhesus monkey and man. Xenobiotica 23:349–359, 1993

Keller MB, Trivedi MH, Thase ME, et al: The Prevention of Recurrent Episodes of Depression with Venlafaxine for Two Years (PREVENT) Study: outcomes from the 2-year and combined maintenance phases. J Clin Psychiatry 68:1246–1256, 2007

Kelsey JE: Dose-response relationship with venlafaxine. J Clin Psychopharmacol 16:21S–26S, 1996

Kennedy SH, Eisfeld BS, Dickens SE, et al: Antidepressant-induced sexual dysfunction during treatment with moclobemide, paroxetine, sertraline, and venlafaxine. J Clin Psychiatry 61: 276–281, 2000

Kennedy SH, Rizvi S, Fulton K, et al: A double-blind comparison of sexual functioning, antidepressant efficacy, and tolerability between agomelatine and venlafaxine XR. J Clin Psychopharmacol 28:329–333, 2008

Kennedy SH, Andersen HF, Thase ME: Escitalopram in the treatment of major depressive disorder: a meta-analysis. Curr Med Res Opin 25:161–175, 2009

Khan A, Upton GV, Rudolph RL, et al: The use of venlafaxine in the treatment of major depression and major depression associated with anxiety: a dose-response study. J Clin Psychopharmacol 18:19–25, 1998

Klamerus KJ, Maloney K, Rudolph RL, et al: Introduction of a composite parameter to the pharmacokinetics of venlafaxine and its active O-desmethyl metabolite. J Clin Pharmacol 32:716–724, 1992

Kocsis JH, Thase ME, Trivedi MH, et al: Prevention of recurrent episodes of depression with venlafaxine ER in a 1-year maintenance phase from the PREVENT Study. J Clin Psychiatry 68:1014–1023, 2007

Lieberman DZ, Montgomery SA, Tourian KA, et al: A pooled analysis of two placebo-controlled trials of desvenlafaxine in major depressive disorder. Int Clin Psychopharmacol 23:188–197, 2008

Liebowitz MR, Gelenberg AJ, Munjack D: Venlafaxine extended release vs placebo and paroxetine in social anxiety disorder. Arch Gen Psychiatry 62:190–198, 2005

Lobello KW, Preskorn SH, Guico-Pabia CJ, et al: Cytochrome P450 2D6 phenotype predicts antidepressant efficacy of venlafaxine: a secondary analysis of 4 studies in major depressive disorder. J Clin Psychiatry 71:1482–1487, 2010

March JS, Entusah AR, Rynn M, et al: A randomized controlled trial of venlafaxine ER versus placebo in pediatric social anxiety disorder. Biol Psychiatry 62:1149–1154, 2007

Mines D, Hill D, Yu H, et al: Prevalence of risk factors for suicide in patients prescribed venlafaxine, fluoxetine, and citalopram. Pharmacoepidemiol Drug Saf 14:367–372, 2005

Montejo AL, Llorca G, Izquierdo JA, et al: Incidence of sexual dysfunction associated with antidepressant agents: a prospective multicenter study of 1022 outpatients. J Clin Psychiatry 62:10–21, 2001

Montgomery SA, Fava M, Padmanabhan SK, et al: Discontinuation symptoms and taper/poststudy-emergent adverse events with desvenlafaxine treatment for major depressive disorder. Int Clin Psychopharmacol 24:296–305, 2009

Muth EA, Haskins JT, Moyer JA, et al: Antidepressant biochemical profile of the novel bicyclic compound Wy-45,030, an ethyl cyclohexanol derivative. Biochem Pharmacol 35:4493–4497, 1986

Nemeroff CB, Entsuah R, Benattia I, et al: Comprehensive Analysis of Remission (COMPARE) with venlafaxine versus SSRIs. Biol Psychiatry 63:424–434, 2008

Oganesian A, Shilling AD, Young-Sciame R, et al: Desvenlafaxine and venlafaxine exert minimal in vitro inhibition of human cytochrome P450 and P-glycoprotein activities. Psychopharmacol Bull 42:47–63, 2009

Owen JR, Nemeroff CB: New antidepressants and the cytochrome P450 system: focus on venlafaxine, nefazodone, and mirtazapine. Depress Anxiety 7 (suppl 1):24–32, 1998

Owens MJ, Morgan WN, Plott SJ, et al: Neurotransmitter receptor and transporter binding profile of antidepressants and their metabolites. J Pharmacol Exp Ther 283:1305–1322, 1997

Papakostas GI, Fava M, Thase ME: Treatment of SSRI-resistant depression: a meta-analysis comparing within- versus across-class switches. Biol Psychiatry 63:699–704, 2008

Perahia DG, Pritchett YL, Kajdasz DK, et al: A randomized, double-blind comparison of duloxetine and venlafaxine in the treatment of patients with major depressive disorder. J Psychiatr Res 42:22–34, 2008

Pollack MH, Lepola U, Koponen H, et al: A double-blind study of the efficacy of venlafaxine extended-release, paroxetine, and placebo in the treatment of panic disorder. Depress Anxiety 24:1–14, 2007a

Pollack M, Mangano R, Entsuah R, et al: A randomized controlled trial of venlafaxine ER and paroxetine in the treatment of outpatients with panic disorder. Psychopharmacology (Berl) 194:233–342, 2007b

Post RM, Altshuler LL, Leverich GS, et al: Mood switch in bipolar depression: comparison of adjunctive venlafaxine, bupropion and sertraline. Br J Psychiatry 189:124–131, 2006

Preskorn S, Patroneva A, Silman H, et al: Comparison of the pharmacokinetics of venlafaxine extended release and desvenlafaxine in extensive and poor cytochrome P450 2D6 metabolizers. J Clin Psychopharmacol 29:39–43, 2009

Rickels K, Etemad B, Khalid-Khan S, et al: Time to relapse after 6 and 12 months' treatment of generalized anxiety disorder with venlafaxine extended release. Arch Gen Psychiatry 67:1274–1281, 2010a

Rickels K, Montgomery SA, Tourian KA, et al: Desvenlafaxine for the prevention of relapse in major depressive disorder: results of a randomized trial. J Clin Psychopharmacol 30:18–24, 2010b

Rubino A, Roskell N, Tennis P, et al: Risk of suicide during treatment with venlafaxine, citalopram, fluoxetine, and dothiepin: retrospective cohort study. BMJ 334:242, 2007

Rudolph RL, Fabre LF, Feighner JP, et al: A randomized, placebo-controlled, dose-response trial of venlafaxine hydrochloride in the treatment of major depression. J Clin Psychiatry 59:116–122, 1998

Rynn MA, Riddle MA, Yeung PP, et al: Efficacy and safety of extended-release venlafaxine in the treatment of generalized anxiety disorder in children and adolescents: two placebo-controlled trials. Am J Psychiatry 164:290–300, 2007

Schueler YB, Koesters M, Wieseler B, et al: A systematic review of duloxetine and venlafaxine in major depression, including unpublished data. Acta Psychiatr Scand 123:247–265, 2011

Serretti A, Chiesa A: Treatment-emergent sexual dysfunction related to antidepressants: a meta-analysis. J Clin Psychopharmacol 29:259–266, 2009

Shams ME, Arneth B, Hiemke C, et al: CYP2D6 polymorphism and clinical effect of the antidepressant venlafaxine. J Clin Pharmacol Ther 31:493–502, 2006

Siepmann T, Ziemssen T, Mueck-Weymann M, et al: The effects of venlafaxine on autonomic functions in healthy volunteers. J Clin Psychopharmacol 27:687–691, 2007

Simon JS, Aguiar LM, Kunz NR, et al: Extended-release venlafaxine in relapse prevention for patients with major depressive disorder. J Psychiatr Res 38:249–257, 2004

Smith D, Dempster C, Glanville J, et al: Efficacy and tolerability of venlafaxine compared with selective serotonin reuptake inhibitors and other antidepressants: a meta-analysis. Br J Psychiatry 180:396–404, 2002

Soares CN, Thase ME, Clayton A, et al: Desvenlafaxine and escitalopram for the treatment of postmenopausal women with major depressive disorder. Menopause 17:700–711, 2010

Thase ME: Effects of venlafaxine on blood pressure: a meta-analysis of original data from 3744 depressed patients. J Clin Psychiatry 59:502–508, 1998

Thase ME, Sloan DME: Venlafaxine, in Essentials of Clinical Psychopharmacology, 2nd Edition. Edited by Schatzberg AF, Nemeroff CB. Washington, DC, American Psychiatric Publishing. 2006, pp 159–170

Thase ME, Friedman ES, Howland RH: Venlafaxine and treatment-resistant depression. Depress Anxiety 12:55–62, 2000

Thase ME, Entsuah AR, Rudolph RL: Remission rates during treatment with venlafaxine or selective serotonin reuptake inhibitors. Br J Psychiatry 178:234–241, 2001

Thase ME, Shelton RC, Khan A: Treatment with venlafaxine extended release after SSRI nonresponse or intolerance: a randomized comparison of standard- and higher-dosing strategies. J Clin Psychopharmacol 26:250–258, 2006

Thase ME, Kornstein SG, Germain JM, et al: An integrated analysis of the efficacy of desvenlafaxine compared with placebo in patients with major depressive disorder. CNS Spectr 14:144–154, 2009

Thase ME, Gelenberg A, Kornstein SG, et al: Comparing venlafaxine extended release and fluoxetine for preventing the recurrence of major depression: results from the PREVENT study. J Psychiatr Res 45:412–420, 2011

Troy SM, Parker VD, Fruncillo RJ, et al: The pharmacokinetics of venlafaxine when given in a twice-daily regimen. J Clin Pharmacol 35:404–409, 1995

Vaishnavi SN, Nemeroff CB, Plott SJ, et al: Milnacipran: a comparative analysis of human monoamine uptake and transporter binding affinity. Biol Psychiatry 55:320–322, 2004

Vieta E, Martinez-Aran A, Goikolea JM, et al: A randomized trial comparing paroxetine and venlafaxine in the treatment of bipolar depressed patients taking mood stabilizers. J Clin Psychiatry 63:508–512, 2002

Whyte IM, Dawson AH, Buckley NA: Relative toxicity of venlafaxine and selective serotonin reuptake inhibitors in overdose compared to tricyclic antidepressants. QJM 96:369–374, 2003

Chapter 12

Duloxetine and Milnacipran

Daniel Zigman, M.D.
Sandhaya Norris, M.D.
Pierre Blier, M.D., Ph.D.

Duloxetine was approved by the U.S. Food and Drug Administration (FDA) for the treatment of major depressive disorder and diabetic neuropathy in 2004. Duloxetine has subsequently received approval in most countries worldwide. Milnacipran was approved in France for the treatment of depression in 1996. It has been available in several countries worldwide but was only recently approved in North America for the treatment of fibromyalgia.

Structure-Activity Relations

Duloxetine at 60 mg/day is a potent reuptake inhibitor of serotonin (5-hydroxytryptamine; 5-HT) (Takano et al. 2006). The exact degree of norepinephrine (NE) reuptake inhibition occurring in humans from duloxetine 60 mg/day remains controversial, but duloxetine clearly achieves physiologically relevant NE reuptake inhibition at 120 mg/day (Chalon et al. 2003; Turcotte et al. 2001; Vincent et al. 2004).

Milnacipran appears to preferentially block NE reuptake, whereas robust 5-HT reuptake inhibition (>80% transporter blockade) in humans appears to be achieved only with supratherapeutic doses (i.e., 300–400 mg; Palmier et al. 1989).

Mechanism of Action

Serotonin-norepinephrine reuptake inhibitors (SNRIs) produce rapid inhibition of reuptake transporters in the brain, but antidepressant effects are generally not seen for at least 2 weeks (see Blier 2006 for a review). This delay may occur because, as a result of 5-HT transporter (5-HTT) inhibition, 5-HT reuptake inhibitors initially suppress the firing of 5-HT neurons through the activation of 5-HT_{1A} autoreceptors on 5-HT neuron cell bodies. After 2–3 weeks of sustained reuptake inhibition, 5-HT_{1A} autoreceptors desensitize, and 5-HT neuronal firing rate returns to normal. At this point, there is a net enhancement of 5-HT transmission in the forebrain (Bel and Artigas 1993; Blier and de Montigny 1983; Rueter et al. 1998a, 1998b). Similarly, blockade of the NE transporter (NET) leads to activation of the α_2-adrenergic autoreceptors on their cell bodies and the firing rate of NE neurons is promptly diminished. After 2–3 weeks of sustained administration, α_2-adrenergic autoreceptors on NE terminals generally desensitize, and this leads to a net enhancement of NE transmission in the forebrain in presence of sustained NE reuptake inhibition (Invernizzi and Garattini 2004; Rueter et al. 1998a, 1998b; Szabo and Blier 2001).

SNRIs produce pain relief in depression and in a variety of pain syndromes, including fibromyalgia (Stahl et al. 2005). SNRIs likely relieve pain by increasing 5-HT and NE, leading to increased activity of central descending inhibitory pain pathways (Mainguy 2009).

Pharmacokinetics

Duloxetine is rapidly absorbed after oral administration, and its absorption is not altered by food. Its plasma level is proportional to dose, up to a maximum of 60 mg twice daily. Duloxetine is about 90% protein bound. Its plasma elimination half-life is approximately 12 hours (Sharma et al. 2000). With repeated administration, duloxetine takes approximately 3 days to reach steady-state levels.

Milnacipran has low plasma protein binding. It is rapidly absorbed after oral administration and has high bioavailability, and its absorption is not affected by food intake. Milnacipran possesses no active metabolite and has an elimination half-life of 8 hours. Steady-state levels are achieved within 3 days, and the drug is cleared from the body within 3 days of treatment cessation. Milnacipran is eliminated by the kidneys essentially as the parent compound and the inactive glucuronic acid conjugate (Puozzo and Leonard 1996).

Metabolic Pathways

Duloxetine is metabolized mainly by cytochrome P450 (CYP) 1A2 and 2D6 (Skinner et al. 2003). Its metabolites are not believed to contribute to its therapeutic activity.

Milnacipran is metabolized mainly via Phase II conjugation and not through the CYP system (Briley 1998). Approximately 50%–60% of the drug is recovered in the urine as the parent compound and 20% as its glucuronide conjugate (Puozzo et al. 2002).

Indications and Efficacy

Duloxetine has been FDA approved for major depressive disorder, generalized anxiety disorder, fibromyalgia, diabetic peripheral neuropathic pain, and chronic musculoskeletal pain. In Europe, it is also approved for stress urinary incontinence.

Milnacipran has been FDA approved for fibromyalgia. In other countries, it is indicated for major depressive disorder. It has also been used off-label for neuropathic pain and chronic pain.

Major Depressive Disorder

Duloxetine was evaluated for the treatment of major depressive disorder in 12 randomized controlled trials (RCTs) using dosages of 40–120 mg/day (Table 12–1). These trials indicated that duloxetine is an effective antidepressant with efficacy equal to the selective serotonin reuptake inhibitors (SSRIs) fluoxetine and paroxetine at 20 mg/day. For patients with moderate to severe symptoms, remission rates with duloxetine were statistically significantly higher than remission rates with SSRIs (Thase et al. 2007).

Milnacipran was more effective than placebo for treatment of depression in three RCTs at dosages of 50 and 100 mg twice daily (Lecrubier et al. 1996; Macher et al. 1989) (Table 12–2). Milnacipran has equal efficacy but superior tolerability to imipramine (Puech et al. 1997). In short-term studies, milnacipran also has efficacy similar to that of SSRIs (Papakostas and Fava 2007).

Generalized Anxiety Disorder

Duloxetine at dosages of 60–120 mg/day is more effective than placebo and of similar efficacy to venlafaxine in reducing symptoms of generalized anxiety disorder (Carter and McCormack 2009). Medication-placebo differences emerge as early as week 1 or 2. In RCTs, patients taking duloxetine also reported improvements in anxiety-related disability and quality of life (Carter and McCormack 2009).

Neuropathic Pain and Chronic Pain Syndromes

In an 8-week RCT, duloxetine at a fixed dosage of 60 mg/day significantly reduced pain measures compared with placebo (Brecht et al. 2007). Similarly, elderly patients with depression treated with duloxetine for 8 weeks reported improvement in back pain scores and amount of time in pain, as compared with placebo (Raskin et al. 2007). In one RCT, duloxetine 60 mg/day provided greater efficacy than placebo in reducing overall, shoulder, and back pain, as well as time spent with pain (Detke et al. 2002b). Overall pain severity and back pain improved the most.

Preliminary open trials and case series suggest that milnacipran may also improve chronic pain syndromes, but RCTs are lacking (Ito et al. 2010).

Fibromyalgia

RCTs of duloxetine at dosages of 60 and 120 mg/day in patients with fibromyalgia with or without depression found significant improvement in pain, sleep, and quality of life compared with placebo regardless of the extent of accompanying depression. There was also a trend toward improved fatigue (Hauser et al. 2011).

Similarly, multiple RCTs have shown milnacipran at dosages of 100 and 200 mg/day to be both safe and effective for treatment of fibromyalgia, with improvement beginning as early as week 1. Milnacipran improved pain, fatigue, and overall functioning, but not sleep (Hauser et al. 2011).

Stress Urinary Incontinence

Duloxetine at 40 mg twice daily reduced the frequency of stress urinary incontinence episodes and improved quality of life but rarely led to remission of symptoms (Mariappan et al. 2007). Serotonin and NE increase excitatory glutamate transmission in the Onuf nucleus in the sacral spinal cord, which facilitates urethral sphincter contraction (Thor 2003). This is presumably the mechanism for the beneficial effect of duloxetine on incontinence.

Safety and Tolerability

Drug-Drug Interactions

Inhibitors of CYP1A2 increase plasma levels of duloxetine. When duloxetine is coadministered with a CYP2D6 inhibitor of moderate potency, duloxetine levels may increase. Generally, however, such alterations of duloxetine levels are not clinically significant.

Duloxetine moderately inhibits the activity of the 2D6 cytochrome. If duloxetine is prescribed with agents metabolized by CYP2D6, clinicians should use doses that are approximately half those usually recommended for the concomitant medication.

Milnacipran is not metabolized by CYP pathways, and it does not produce pharmacokinetic drug-drug interactions.

Both duloxetine and milnacipran have the potential to interact lethally with monoamine oxidase inhibitors (MAOIs) due to the risk of serotonin syndrome. To avoid this risk, MAOIs must not be started until 5 days after stopping duloxetine or milnacipran. A longer elimination period than that expected from

TABLE 12–1. Duloxetine versus placebo and/or active SSRI or SNRI comparator in acute studies (≤12 weeks) of depression

Study	Duration (weeks)	Sample size	Duloxetine dosage (mg/day)	Comparator used	Comparator dosage (mg/day)	Placebo?	Results
Goldstein et al. 2002	8	173	120	Fluoxetine	20	Yes	Duloxetine>placebo No difference with fluoxetine
Nemeroff et al. 2002[a]	8	194	120	Fluoxetine	20	Yes	No difference in remission rates at endpoint
Nemeroff et al. 2002[a]	8	354	40, 80	Paroxetine	20	Yes	No difference in remission rates at endpoint
Detke et al. 2002a	9	245	60	None	—	Yes	Duloxetine>placebo
Detke et al. 2002b	9	267	60	None	—	Yes	Duloxetine>placebo
Goldstein et al. 2004	8	353	40, 80	Paroxetine	20	Yes	Duloxetine 80 (but not 40)>placebo No difference between duloxetine 80 and paroxetine
Detke et al. 2004	8	354	80, 120	Paroxetine	20	Yes	Duloxetine (80 and 120)>placebo Paroxetine=placebo
Perahia et al. 2006	8	392	80, 120	Paroxetine	20	Yes	Duloxetine (80 and 120)>placebo Paroxetine=placebo
Raskin et al. 2007	8	311	60	None	—	Yes	Duloxetine>placebo
Nierenberg et al. 2007	8	684	60	Escitalopram	10	Yes	No difference between any groups at endpoint
Khan et al. 2007	8	278	60	Escitalopram	10–20	No	Escitalopram>duloxetine
Brecht et al. 2007	8	327	60	None	—	Yes	Duloxetine>placebo
Lee et al. 2007	8	478	60	Paroxetine	20	No	Duloxetine=paroxetine
Perahia et al. 2008	12	667	120	Venlafaxine	225	No	Duloxetine=venlafaxine

Note. SNRI=serotonin-norepinephrine reuptake inhibitor; SSRI=selective serotonin reuptake inhibitor. ">" denotes significantly greater effect; "=" denotes no difference.
[a]These failed studies were reported in this review but were not conducted by Dr. Nemeroff.

TABLE 12–2. Milnacipran versus placebo and/or active SSRI comparator in acute studies (≤12 weeks) of depression

Study	Duration (weeks)	Sample size	Milnacipran dosage (mg/day)	Comparator used	Comparator dosage (mg/day)	Placebo?	Results
Macher et al. 1989	4	58	100	None	—	Yes	Milnacipran > placebo
Ansseau et al. 1991	4	127	150–300	Fluvoxamine	200	No	Milnacipran = fluvoxamine
Ansseau et al. 1994	6	190	100[a]	Fluoxetine	20	No	Fluoxetine > milnacipran
Lecrubier et al. 1996[b]	6–8	644	50–200	None	—	Yes	Milnacipran 100 and 200 (but not 50) > placebo
Guelfi et al. 1998	12	289	100–200	Fluoxetine	20	No	Milnacipran = fluoxetine
Clerc 2001	6	113	100	Fluvoxamine	200	No	Milnacipran > fluvoxamine
Sechter et al. 2004	6	302	100	Paroxetine	20	No	Milnacipran = paroxetine
Lee et al. 2005	6	70	100	Fluoxetine	20	No	Milnacipran = fluoxetine

Note. SSRI = selective serotonin reuptake inhibitor. "=" denotes no difference.

[a]Milnacipran was given once daily in contrast to the other studies in which it was administered on a twice-daily basis.

[b]This is a composite of two positive controlled studies.

plasma half-life is recommended, as brain elimination generally lags behind plasma elimination. At least a 14-day washout of MAOIs must be respected before starting any SNRI.

Side Effects and Toxicology

Duloxetine

The safety and tolerability of duloxetine at a dosage range of 40–120 mg/day have been assessed in clinical trials. In an 8-month study, the most common treatment-emergent adverse events were nausea, dry mouth, vomiting, yawning, and night sweats (Pigott et al. 2007). Most of these emerged early, within the first 8 weeks. Other studies have reported insomnia, somnolence, headaches, ejaculation disorders, diarrhea, constipation, and dizziness as common adverse events with duloxetine (Detke et al. 2002a, 2002b; Khan et al. 2007; Nierenberg et al. 2007).

Rates of nausea with duloxetine are comparable to those reported with other SSRIs and with SNRIs. Nausea is usually transient. A starting dosage of 60 mg/day appears to provide the best combination of clinical response and tolerability (Bech et al. 2006; Pritchett et al. 2007). Clinicians may, however, consider starting at a lower dosage, 30 mg/day, for patients for whom tolerance is a concern. One study indicated that duloxetine's tolerability at an initial dosage of 60 mg/day can be improved if it is taken with food, to the point of being comparable to the tolerability of an initial dosage of 30 mg/day (Whitmyer et al. 2007).

Duloxetine rarely causes weight gain and may even produce slight weight loss compared with placebo (Nierenberg et al. 2007). Changes in blood pressure and heart rate are rarely clinically significant (Schatzberg 2003). In RCTs, rates of sexual dysfunction, including anorgasmia, erectile dysfunction, delayed ejaculation, and decreased libido, appeared to be low (Pigott et al. 2007), but this side effect may still be problematic in clinical practice.

Rates of discontinuation due to adverse events for duloxetine have been similar to those for placebo or active comparators in acute or longer-term studies. However, patients who discontinued duloxetine because of adverse effects often did so early in treatment (Nierenberg et al. 2007; Perahia et al. 2008; Pigott et al. 2007), which may suggest poorer initial tolerability for duloxetine.

Milnacipran

The side-effect profile of milnacipran is similar to that of SSRIs, except that the SSRIs have a higher frequency of nausea and anxiety, whereas milnacipran has a higher incidence of dysuria (Puech et al. 1997). Weight gain is uncommon, but sedation may be reported. Rates of sexual dysfunction with milnacipran have not been reported but are estimated to be lower than rates with venlafaxine and much lower than rates with SSRIs (Stahl et al. 2005).

Blood pressure increases are minimal with milnacipran dosages of 100 and 200 mg/day (Guelfi et al. 1998). Tachycardia, a heart rate greater than 100 beats per minute, occurs in 3% of patients on milnacipran 100 mg/day and 6% of patients on milnacipran 200 mg/day. There has been no cardiotoxicity reported from overdoses of up to 2.8 g/day, which is 28 times the recommended daily dosage (Montgomery et al. 1996).

Most adverse effects from milnacipran appear within the first 3 months of treatment, with the incidence decreasing steadily thereafter. No emergent adverse events developed during a long-term treatment study (Puech et al. 1997).

Conclusion

At their minimal effective dosages, duloxetine (60 mg/day) and milnacipran (100 mg/day) potently block the reuptake of 5-HT and NE, respectively. Duloxetine at its maximum recommended dosage (120 mg/day) and milnacipran at the upper end of its therapeutic range (200 mg/day) are dual reuptake inhibitors. Duloxetine has demonstrated efficacy for the treatment of depression, chronic musculoskeletal pain, fibromyalgia, generalized anxiety disorder, and stress urinary incontinence. Milnacipran has demonstrated efficacy for depression and fibromyalgia.

Duloxetine and milnacipran are generally well tolerated, with most adverse events occurring early in treatment, being of mild to moderate severity, and having a tendency to decrease or disappear with continued treatment.

Because they are not toxic in overdose, either of these two medications may be used as a first-line treatment for depression, and they can be administered at therapeutic dosages from treatment initiation onward with minimal side effects. Furthermore, data suggest that treatment with a dual reuptake inhibitor is superior to treatment with an antidepressant with only one mechanism of action, such as an SSRI (Nemeroff et al. 2008; Poirier and Boyer 1999; Thase et al. 2007). Consequently, duloxetine and milnacipran may be useful in patients with SSRI-resistant conditions, provided that they are prescribed at dosages at the upper end of the therapeutic range.

References

Ansseau M, von Frenckell R, Gérard MA, et al: Interest of a loading dose of milnacipran in endogenous depressive inpatients: comparison with the standard regimen and with fluvoxamine. Eur Neuropsychopharmacol 1:113–121, 1991

Ansseau M, Pampart P, Troisfontaines B, et al: Controlled comparison of milnacipran and fluoxetine in major depression. Psychopharmacology (Berl) 114:131–137, 1994

Bech P, Kajdasz DK, Porsdal V: Dose-response relationship of duloxetine in placebo-controlled clinical trials in patients with major depressive disorder. Psychopharmacology (Berl) 188:273–280, 2006

Bel N, Artigas F: Chronic treatment with fluvoxamine increases extracellular serotonin in frontal cortex but not in raphe nuclei. Synapse 15:243–245, 1993

Blier P: Dual serotonin and norepinephrine reuptake inhibitors: focus on their differences. International Journal of Psychiatry in Clinical Practice 10 (suppl 2):22–32, 2006

Blier P, de Montigny C: Electrophysiological investigations on the effect of repeated zimelidine administration on serotonergic neurotransmission in the rat. J Neurosci 3:1270–1278, 1983

Brecht S, Courtecuisse C, Debieuvre C, et al: Efficacy and safety of duloxetine 60 mg once daily in the treatment of pain in patients with major depressive disorder and at least moderate pain of unknown etiology: a randomized controlled trial. J Clin Psychiatry 68:1707–1716, 2007

Briley M: Milnacipran, a well tolerated specific serotonin and norepinephrine reuptake inhibiting antidepressant. CNS Drug Rev 4:137–148, 1998

Carter NJ, McCormack PL: Duloxetine: a review of its use in the treatment of generalized anxiety disorder. CNS Drugs 23:523–541, 2009

Chalon SA, Granier LA, Vandenhende FR, et al: Duloxetine increases serotonin and norepinephrine availability in healthy subjects: a double-blind, controlled study. Neuropsychopharmacology 28:1685–1693, 2003

Clerc G; Milnacipran/Fluvoxamine Study Group: Antidepressant efficacy and tolerability of milnacipran: a dual serotonin and noradrenaline reuptake inhibitor: a comparison with fluvoxamine. Int Clin Psychopharmacol 16:145–151, 2001

Detke MJ, Lu Y, Goldstein DJ, et al: Duloxetine, 60 mg once daily, for major depressive disorder: a randomized double-blind placebo-controlled trial. J Clin Psychiatry 63:308–315, 2002a

Detke MJ, Lu Y, Goldstein DJ, et al: Duloxetine 60 mg once daily dosing versus placebo in the acute treatment of major depression. J Psychiatr Res 36:383–390, 2002b

Detke MJ, Wiltse CG, Mallinckrodt CH, et al: Duloxetine in the acute and long-term treatment of major depressive disorder: a placebo- and paroxetine-controlled trial. Eur Neuropsychopharmacol 14:457–470, 2004

Goldstein DJ, Mallinckrodt CH, Lu Y, et al: Duloxetine in the treatment of major depressive disorder: a double-blind clinical trial. J Clin Psychiatry 63:225–231, 2002

Goldstein DJ, Lu Y, Detke MJ, et al: Duloxetine in the treatment of depression: a double-blind placebo-controlled comparison with paroxetine. J Clin Psychopharmacol 24:389–399, 2004

Guelfi JD, Ansseau M, Corruble E, et al: A double-blind comparison of the efficacy and safety of milnacipran and fluoxetine in depressed inpatients. Int Clin Psychopharmacol 13:121–128, 1998

Hauser W, Petzke F, Üçeyler N, et al: Comparative efficacy and acceptability of amitriptyline, duloxetine and milnacipran in fibromyalgia syndrome: a systematic review with meta-analysis. Rheumatology (Oxford) 50:532–543, 2011

Invernizzi RW, Garattini S: Role of presynaptic alpha2-adrenoceptors in antidepressant action: recent findings from microdialysis studies. Prog Neuropsychopharmacol Biol Psychiatry 28:819–827, 2004

Ito M, Kimura H, Yoshida K, et al: Effectiveness of milnacipran for the treatment of chronic pain in the orofacial region. Clin Neuropharmacol 33:79–83, 2010

Khan A, Bose A, Alexopoulos GS, et al: Double-blind comparison of escitalopram and duloxetine in the acute treatment of major depressive disorder. Clin Drug Investig 27:481–492, 2007

Lecrubier Y, Pletan Y, Solles A, et al: Clinical efficacy of milnacipran: placebo-controlled trials. Int Clin Psychopharmacol 11 (suppl 4):29–33, 1996

Lee MS, Ham BJ, Kee BS, et al: Comparison of efficacy and safety of milnacipran and fluoxetine in Korean patients with major depression. Curr Med Res Opin 21:1369–1375, 2005

Lee P, Shu L, Xu X, et al: Once-daily duloxetine 60 mg in the treatment of major depressive disorder: multicenter, double-blind, randomized, paroxetine-controlled, non-inferiority trial in China, Korea, Taiwan and Brazil. Psychiatry Clin Neurosci 61:295–307, 2007

Macher JP, Sichel JP, Serre C, et al: Double-blind placebo-controlled study of milnacipran in hospitalized patients with major depressive disorders. Neuropsychobiology 22:77–82, 1989

Mainguy Y: Functional magnetic resonance imagery (fMRI) in fibromyalgia and the response to milnacipran. Hum Psychopharmacol 24 (suppl 1): S19–S23, 2009

Mariappan P, Alhasso A, Ballantyne Z, et al: Duloxetine, a serotonin and noradrenaline reuptake inhibitor (SNRI) for the treatment of stress urinary incontinence: a systematic review. Eur Urol 51:67–74, 2007

Montgomery SA, Prost JF, Solles A, et al: Efficacy and tolerability of milnacipran: an overview. Int Clin Psychopharmacol 11 (suppl 4):47–51, 1996

Nemeroff CB, Schatzberg AF, Goldstein DJ, et al: Duloxetine for the treatment of major depressive disorder. Psychopharmacol Bull 36:106–132, 2002

Nemeroff CB, Entsuah R, Benattia I, et al: Comprehensive analysis of remission (COMPARE) with venlafaxine versus SSRIs. Biol Psychiatry 63:424–434, 2008

Nierenberg AA, Greist JH, Mallinckrodt CH, et al: Duloxetine versus escitalopram and placebo in the treatment of patients with major depressive disorder: onset of antidepressant action, a non-inferiority study. Curr Med Res Opin 23:401–416, 2007

Palmier C, Puozzo C, Lenehan T, et al: Monoamine uptake inhibition by plasma from healthy volunteers after single oral doses of the antidepressant milnacipran. Eur J Clin Pharmacol 37:235–238, 1989

Papakostas GI, Fava M: A meta-analysis of clinical trials comparing milnacipran, a serotonin-norepinephrine reuptake inhibitor, with a selective serotonin reuptake inhibitor for the treatment of major depressive disorder. Eur Neuropsychopharmacol 17:32–36, 2007

Perahia DG, Wang F, Mallinckrodt CH, et al: Duloxetine in the treatment of major depressive disorder: a placebo- and paroxetine-controlled trial. Eur Psychiatry 21:367–378, 2006

Perahia DG, Pritchett YL, Kajdasz DK, et al: A randomized, double-blind comparison of duloxetine and venlafaxine in the treatment of patients with major depressive disorder. J Psychiatr Res 42:22–34, 2008

Pigott TA, Prakash A, Arnold LM, et al: Duloxetine versus escitalopram and placebo: an 8 month, double-blind trial in patients with major depressive disorder. Curr Med Res Opin 23:1303–1318, 2007

Poirier MF, Boyer P: Venlafaxine and paroxetine in treatment-resistant depression: double-blind, randomised comparison. Br J Psychiatry 175:12–16, 1999

Pritchett YL, Marciniak MD, Corey-Lisle PK, et al: Use of effect size to determine optimal dose of duloxetine in major depressive disorder. J Psychiatr Res 41:311–318, 2007

Puech A, Montgomery SA, Prost JF, et al: Milnacipran, a new serotonin and noradrenaline reuptake inhibitor: an overview of its antidepressant activity and clinical tolerability. Int Clin Psychopharmacol 12:99–108, 1997

Puozzo C, Leonard BE: Pharmacokinetics of milnacipran in comparison with other antidepressants. Int Clin Psychopharmacol 2 (suppl 4): 15–27, 1996

Puozzo C, Panconi E, Deprez D: Pharmacology and pharmacokinetics of milnacipran. Int Clin Psychopharmacol 17 (suppl 1): S25–S35, 2002

Raskin J, Wiltse CG, Siegal A, et al: Efficacy of duloxetine on cognition, depression, and pain in elderly patients with major depressive disorder: an 8-week, double-blind, placebo-controlled trial. Am J Psychiatry 164:900–909, 2007

Rueter LE, de Montigny C, Blier P: Electrophysiological characterization of the effect of long-term duloxetine administration on the rat serotonergic and noradrenergic systems. J Pharmacol Exp Ther 285:404–412, 1998a

Rueter LE, Kasamo K, de Montigny C, et al: Effect of long-term administration of duloxetine on the function of serotonin and noradrenaline terminals in the rat brain. Naunyn Schmiedebergs Arch Pharmacol 357:600–610, 1998b

Schatzberg AF: Efficacy and tolerability of duloxetine, a novel dual reuptake inhibitor, in the treatment of major depressive disorder. J Clin Psychiatry 64 (suppl 13):30–37, 2003

Sechter D, Vandel P, Weiller E, et al: A comparative study of milnacipran and paroxetine in outpatients with major depression. J Affect Disord 83:233–236, 2004

Sharma A, Goldberg MJ, Cerimele BJ: Pharmacokinetics and safety of duloxetine, a dual-serotonin and norepinephrine reuptake inhibitor. J Clin Pharmacol 40:161–167, 2000

Skinner MH, Kuan HY, Pan A, et al: Duloxetine is both an inhibitor and a substrate of cytochrome P450 2D6 in healthy volunteers. Clin Pharmacol Ther 73:170–177, 2003

Stahl S, Grady M, Moret C, et al: SNRIs: their pharmacology, clinical efficacy, and tolerability in comparison with other classes of antidepressants. CNS Spectr 10:732–747, 2005

Szabo ST, Blier P: Effect of the selective noradrenergic reuptake inhibitor reboxetine on the firing activity of noradrenaline and serotonin neurons. Eur J Neurosci 13:2077–2087, 2001

Takano A, Suzuki K, Kosaka J, et al: A dose-finding study of duloxetine based on serotonin transporter occupancy. Psychopharmacology (Berl) 185:395–399, 2006

Thase ME, Pritchett YL, Ossanna MJ, et al: Efficacy of duloxetine and selective serotonin reuptake inhibitors: comparisons as assessed by remission rates in patients with major depressive disorder. J Clin Psychopharmacol 27:672–676, 2007

Thor KB: Serotonin and norepinephrine involvement in efferent pathways to the urethral rhabdosphincter: implications for treating stress urinary incontinence. Urology 62 (suppl 1):3–9, 2003

Turcotte JE, Debonnel G, de Montigny C, et al: Assessment of the serotonin and norepinephrine reuptake blocking properties of duloxetine in healthy subjects. Neuropsychopharmacology 24:511–521, 2001

Vincent S, Bieck PR, Garland EM, et al: Clinical assessment of norepinephrine transporter blockade through biochemical and pharmacological profiles. Circulation 109:3202–3207, 2004

Whitmyer VG, Dunner DL, Kornstein SG, et al: A comparison of initial duloxetine dosing strategies in patients with major depressive disorder. J Clin Psychiatry 68:1921–1930, 2007

CHAPTER 13

Benzodiazepines

David V. Sheehan, M.D., M.B.A.

B. Ashok Raj, M.D.

History and Discovery

In spite of adverse publicity and a problematic public image, the most widely prescribed psychiatric medication in the United States over the past decade is not an antidepressant, an atypical antipsychotic, or a mood stabilizer but the benzodiazepine alprazolam, with 31 million prescriptions issued in 2001 (see Stahl 2002).

The first benzodiazepine, chlordiazepoxide (Librium), was patented in 1959. Diazepam was introduced in 1963, and numerous derivatives of this drug have since been introduced into the market. The triazolobenzodiazepine alprazolam was introduced in 1981 and revolutionized the treatment of anxiety disorders when it was shown to be effective in the treatment of panic disorder (Chouinard et al. 1982; Sheehan et al. 1982). It was the first benzodiazepine to be approved by the U.S. Food and Drug Administration (FDA) for the treatment of panic disorder. Since then, clonazepam, another high-potency benzodiazepine, has also received approval from the FDA for the treatment of panic disorder.

Benzodiazepines were widely prescribed in the 1960s, 1970s, and 1980s for pathological anxiety by psychiatrists, family practitioners, and internists who knew the drugs were effective and relatively safe when compared with prior anxiolytic medications such as the barbiturates and meprobamate. However, since the 1990s, benzodiazepines have increasingly been displaced by the selective serotonin reuptake inhibitors (SSRIs) as the clinician's first choice for the treatment of anxiety disorders (Kramer 1993). The SSRIs are safer and better tolerated than the tricyclic antidepressants and have been shown to be efficacious in a number of different anxiety disorders. In addition, they do not have the dependence, withdrawal, alcohol interaction, and abuse liability of the benzodiazepines.

Despite these drawbacks, benzodiazepines are often used as an adjunctive treatment with an SSRI or as the primary treatment for the patient with no response or only a partial response to the SSRI. The net result is only a small decline in the recommendation for a benzodiazepine (Uhlenhuth et al. 1999). One user in four uses the benzodiazepine for a year or longer. Among those using it as a hypnotic, 14% reported long-term use (Balter 1991). Rates of use increase with age. Persons older than 65 years account for 27% of all benzodiazepine prescriptions and 38% of all benzodiazepine hypnotics (IMS America 1991). In recent years, there has been a shift to the use of short-half-life benzodiazepines.

Structure-Activity Relations

Currently marketed benzodiazepines are similar in that they have the 1,4-benzodiazepine ring system. Modification of this ring system results in benzodiazepines with somewhat different properties.

Pharmacokinetics and Disposition

Knowledge of benzodiazepine pharmacokinetics helps the clinician choose the most appropriate benzodiazepine for the patient and also guides in its correct use. Benzodiazepines differ in their pharmacokinetic properties, such as absorption, distribution, and elimination (Table 13–1). On the other hand, all benzodiazepines are similar in that to some degree they all exhibit anxiolytic, muscle-relaxant, sedative-hypnotic, and anticonvulsant properties. The belief that one benzodiazepine is primarily anxiolytic while another is primarily hypnotic is not based on scientific evidence (Greenblatt et al. 1983a, 1983b). The preferential selection of a benzodiazepine for one market over another is usually dictated by its pharmacokinetic properties.

Rate of Absorption

Benzodiazepines that are rapidly absorbed from the gastrointestinal tract enter and peak in the circulation quickly and have a quicker onset of action than those that are absorbed more slowly. Diazepam and clorazepate are rapidly absorbed and act quickly, chlordiazepoxide and lorazepam have intermediate rates of absorption and onset of action, and prazepam is slowly absorbed and has a slower onset of action.

Gastrointestinal absorption of benzodiazepines is dictated by intrinsic physiochemical properties of the drug and characteristics of the formulation such as particle size (Greenblatt et al. 1983a, 1983b). Benzodiazepine absorption when given intramuscularly is dictated by other factors. For example, chlordiazepoxide and lorazepam when given orally are absorbed at similar rates in the gastrointestinal tract. When given intramuscularly, lorazepam is more reliably, rapidly, and completely absorbed than chlordiazepoxide (Greenblatt et al. 1979, 1982b, 1983a, 1983b).

Lipophilicity

The lipid solubility (lipophilicity) of a benzodiazepine at physiological pH influences the rate at which it crosses the blood-brain barrier by passive diffusion from the circulation, and this, in turn, determines the rapidity of onset of action and intensity of effect (Greenblatt et al. 1983a, 1983b). Highly lipophilic drugs cross the blood-brain barrier rapidly, and although all benzodiazepines are highly lipophilic, they differ in their degree of lipophilicity. Because diazepam is more lipophilic than lorazepam or chlordiazepoxide, it provides more rapid anxiety reduction and onset of side effects.

Duration of Action

With benzodiazepines, the duration of therapeutic action is determined mainly by the rate and extent of drug distribution rather than by the rate of elimination. Benzodiazepine distribution is largely determined by its lipophilicity. Diazepam, which has a longer half-life than lorazepam, has a shorter duration of clinical action after a single dose. The

TABLE 13–1. Pharmacokinetics of benzodiazepines

GROUP	MEDICATION	METABOLISM	CYP ENZYME(S)	$T_{1/2}$, HOURS	K_I
Desmethyldiazepam	Diazepam	Oxidation	2C19, 3A4	26–50	9.6
	Bromazepam	Oxidation	3A4	1–5	NA
	Prazepam	Oxidation		>21	NA
	Chlordiazepoxide	Oxidation	3A4	>21	NA
Desalkylflurazepam	Flurazepam	Oxidation		40–120	NA
	Clonazepam	Oxidation		24–56	0.5
Triazolobenzodiazepine	Triazolam	Oxidation	3A4	2–4	0.4
	Alprazolam	Oxidation	3A4	10–15	4.8
Imidazobenzodiazepine	Midazolam	Oxidation	3A4	1–3	0.4
Thienodiazepine	Brotizolam	Oxidation	3A4	4–8	0.9
	Nitrazepam	Reduction	3A4, 2D6	20–50	11.5
	Flunitrazepam	Reduction		10–25	3.8
Oxazolobenzodiazepine	Oxazepam	Glucuronidation		5–15	17.2
	Lorazepam	Glucuronidation		10–20	3.8
	Temazepam	Glucuronidation		6–16	23.0

Note. CYP = cytochrome P450; K_i = kinetic inhibition constant value (nM); NA = not available.

reason for this is that diazepam, because of its greater lipid solubility, is more extensively distributed to peripheral sites, particularly to fat tissue. Consequently, it is more rapidly moved out of the blood and brain into inactive storage sites, and its central nervous system (CNS) effects end more rapidly. Conversely, less lipophilic benzodiazepines maintain their effective brain concentrations longer because they are less extensively distributed to the periphery (Greenblatt et al. 1983a, 1983b).

Rate of Elimination

The rate of elimination (elimination half-life) influences the speed and extent of accumulation and the time to reach a steady state. It also influences the time for drug washout after termination of multiple doses. Accumulation is slow and extensive when the half-life is long. When the rate of metabolic removal equals the rate of ingestion, the drug is said to have reached steady state. A useful rule of thumb is that when treatment has been in progress for at least four to five times as long as the elimination half-life, then the accumulation process is more than 90% complete (Greenblatt et al. 1983a, 1983b). When drugs with long elimination half-lives are stopped, they are washed out slowly, and the symptoms recur gradually over a period of days, with less intense or sudden rebound phenomena (Greenblatt et al. 1981, 1982a; Kales et al. 1982). Side effects from long-term treatment with long-half-life benzodiazepines last longer than with short-half-life benzodiazepines. Because of greater drug accumulation with long-half-life benzodiazepines, frequent drowsiness and sedation are a theoretical concern (Greenblatt et al. 1981). Tolerance to sedation occurs with long-term use, even though the plasma drug level remains the same. However, as a matter of caution, it is prudent to choose a benzodiazepine with a shorter or intermediate half-life for the elderly (Greenblatt et al. 1982c), individuals operating equipment, and those engaging in high-level intellectual tasks.

Biotransformation Pathway

Benzodiazepines are metabolized in the liver by microsomal oxidation or by glucuronide conjugation. The oxidation pathway is influenced by hepatic disease, age, several medical illnesses, and a number of drugs that impair oxidizing capacity, such as cimetidine, estrogens, and the hydrazine monoamine oxidase inhibitors (MAOIs). These factors usually magnify the side effects of the benzodiazepine. Consequently, in the elderly and in individuals with liver disease, benzodiazepines that are conjugated (e.g., temazepam, oxazepam, and lorazepam) are safer than benzodiazepines that are metabolized by oxidation (e.g., diazepam and alprazolam).

Dosing: Sustained-Release Formulations

Dosing schedules of benzodiazepines should be dictated by knowledge about the rate of distribution rather than by information about elimination half-life. Sustained-release formulations of several benzodiazepines have been introduced to provide 24 hours of anxiolysis. In our experience, the sustained-release forms of alprazolam, clorazepate, diazepam, and adinazolam have a duration of therapeutic action of approximately 12 hours, not 24 hours. Standard alprazolam has a duration of action of 4–6 hours, clonazepam has a duration of action of 7 hours, and other standard-formulation benzodiazepines are within this 4- to 7-hour range.

Mechanism of Action

Benzodiazepines produce anxiolysis by their effect on the γ-aminobutyric acid (GABA)–benzodiazepine receptor complex. GABA is synthesized from glutamic acid, which is also the most abundant free amino acid in the CNS. Like serotonin, norepinephrine, and dopamine neurons, the presynaptic GABA neuron has a reuptake pump that transports GABA from the synapse for storage or destruction by GABA transaminase. GABA has two target receptors, $GABA_A$ and $GABA_B$. The chloride ion channel is controlled by $GABA_A$.

Four distinct pharmacological properties have been described for the benzodiazepine receptor: anxiolytic, hypnotic, anticonvulsant, and muscle relaxation effects. Anxiolytic and sedative-hypnotic actions are mediated mainly by the ω_1 receptor and muscle relaxation through the benzodiazepine$_2$ (ω_2) receptor. Most benzodiazepines interact with both these receptor subtypes. Typically, when GABA occupies the $GABA_A$ receptor site, the chloride channel is opened up a little, and this effect is inhibitory. If at the same time a benzodiazepine binds to the nearby benzodiazepine receptor, the $GABA_A$ receptor is allosterically modulated, and GABA exerts a greater effect on the chloride channel and conductance. Although GABA works alone at the GABA receptor, it works better in the presence of a benzodiazepine. The benzodiazepine, on the other hand, in the absence of GABA cannot influence the chloride channel by itself.

Therapeutic Uses

Because of their multiple pharmacological actions, benzodiazepines have been found useful in many areas of medical practice, such as induction of anesthesia, use as a muscle relaxant, and control of seizures. It is beyond the scope of this chapter to elaborate on these uses.

In psychiatry, benzodiazepines are used to control anxiety, to treat insomnia, and to acutely manage agitation and withdrawal syndromes. In the treatment of anxiety disorders, benzodiazepines have a greater impact in some disorders than others. In panic disorder, they have a significant impact on all dimensions of the illness, with the exception of depression. Alprazolam, for example, has been shown to be effective in panic disorder at a mean dosage of 5.7 mg/day (range = 1–10 mg/day) (Ballenger et al. 1988; Chouinard et al. 1982; Cross National Collaborative Panic Study 1992; Sheehan et al. 1982, 1984, 1993). Rapid improvement was seen within the first week in the form of decreased panic attacks, phobic fears and avoidance, anticipatory anxiety, and disability. These benefits were shown to persist during a follow-up period of 8 months (Schweizer et al. 1993). Efficacy has also been demonstrated for lorazepam (Rickels and Schweizer 1986) and clonazepam (Pollack et al. 1993; Tesar et al. 1991). In the latter studies, clonazepam 2.5 mg/day was as effective and well tolerated as alprazolam 5.3 mg/day.

Despite the well-documented efficacy of benzodiazepines in panic disorder, they have been displaced in clinical practice by the SSRIs. However, it is common practice to initiate treatment with both classes of drug simultaneously and then withdraw the benzodiazepine after 6 weeks. The benefits and practicality of this approach to treating panic disorder have been reinforced by the findings from two studies (Goddard et al. 2001, 2008). The American Psychiatric Association (1998) guidelines for the treatment of panic disorder recommending SSRI monotherapy as the treatment of first choice have failed to achieve traction, since more than two-thirds of the SSRI prescriptions were accompanied by a concomitant benzodiazepine. The above studies by Goddard et al. (2008) lend justification to the rationale for using the combination treatment more frequently and blessing it as a reasonable alternative first-line treatment for many patients with panic disorder.

Three double-blind studies have shown efficacy for benzodiazepines in the treatment of social phobia (Davidson et al. 1993; Gelernter et al. 1991; Versiani et al. 1997).

In a double-blind, placebo-controlled study, Rickels et al. (1993) found that the tricyclic antidepressant imipramine was better than diazepam in the treatment of nondepressed generalized anxiety disorder (GAD) patients over 8 weeks. Imipramine showed a trend to be significantly better on the primary outcome measure scale (the Hamilton

Anxiety Scale [Ham-A]) and was statistically superior to diazepam on the Psychic Anxiety factor of the Ham-A. Psychic anxiety includes the items of worry, anxious mood, tension, fears, and concentration problems. Diazepam and imipramine had identical endpoint Ham-A Somatic Anxiety factor scores, suggesting that they are equally effective against the somatic anxiety symptoms in GAD. This suggests that imipramine is a better "anti-worry" medication than the benzodiazepine. Patients being treated with diazepam had an earlier response than those taking imipramine.

Generally, benzodiazepines are thought to be ineffective in the treatment of obsessive-compulsive disorder (OCD).

The strongest evidence for effective pharmacotherapy in posttraumatic stress disorder (PTSD) is with SSRIs. A meta-analysis of medications in treating PTSD found effect sizes of 0.49 and 1.38 for benzodiazepines and SSRIs, respectively (Van Etten and Taylor 1998).

Intramuscular clonazepam has been compared with intramuscular haloperidol in the management of acute psychotic agitation. Clonazepam use reduced agitation, but haloperidol use had a more rapid onset (Chouinard et al. 1993). Individuals with schizophrenia have high levels of anxiety and frequently experience panic attacks. Overall, it appears that benzodiazepines have a role in the acute management of agitation, and their use can reduce the need for or the dose of antipsychotics used.

Side Effects and Toxicology

Benzodiazepines are among the safest of drugs, but unwanted effects do occur. The first 1,4-benzodiazepines, such as diazepam and flurazepam, had slow rates of elimination and low receptor-binding affinities. Their main side effect was excessive daytime sleepiness. The late 1970s saw the introduction of the 1,4-benzodiazepines flunitrazepam and lorazepam, which had shorter half-lives and were more potent. These drugs were associated with enhanced efficacy but also with more rapid development of tolerance and significant withdrawal problems. The triazolobenzodiazepines were introduced in the 1980s and were even more potent and had even shorter half-lives. They have also been found to be associated with amnesia, daytime anxiety, early-morning insomnia, and withdrawal problems such as rebound insomnia, anxiety, and seizures (Noyes et al. 1986).

Sedation and drowsiness are common, occurring in 4%–9% of patients taking benzodiazepines. Ataxia occurs in up to 2%. The drowsiness tends to disappear with time or a reduction in dose (Greenblatt et al. 1982b; Miller 1973; Svenson and Hamilton 1966). Benzodiazepines may impair psychomotor performance. Most benzodiazepines, shortly after administration at their peak concentration, cause anterograde amnesia (Lister et al. 1988). These effects are dependent on potency and route of administration (Bixler et al. 1979). Overall, this memory impairment does appear to be independent of the degree of sedation produced by the drug (Scharf et al. 1988). Benzodiazepine-treated subjects are often unaware or underestimate the extent of their memory impairment (Roach and Griffiths 1985, 1987).

Hyperexcitability phenomena such as early-morning awakening and rebound anxiety and nervousness are more likely with the short-half-life, high-potency benzodiazepines such as triazolam, alprazolam, lorazepam, and brotizolam (Kales et al. 1983, 1986, 1987; Vela-Bueno et al. 1983). Treatment-emergent hostility (Rosenbaum et al. 1984) may be seen in up to 10% of patients being treated with benzodiazepines. This is most likely to happen early in treatment, is unrelated to pretreatment impulsivity, and has been reported with all benzodiazepines with the exception of oxazepam. Treatment-emergent mania has been reported with alprazolam (Goodman and Charney 1987; Pecknold and Fleury 1986; Strahan et al. 1985).

Since the 1960s, benzodiazepines have been known to produce anterograde amnesia, even with oral dosing (Lister 1985). The deficit is one of disrupted consolidation and not impairment of memory retrieval. The degree of amnesia can range from minimal inability to retain isolated pieces of information to total inability to recall any activities that occurred during a specific period. Whether some benzodiazepines are more likely than others to produce amnesia remains an unresolved question.

Another area of concern is that the long-term use of benzodiazepines may lead to cognitive and other impairments that persist long after the drugs have been discontinued. Abnormal computed tomography (CT) scans were reported in long-term users of benzodiazepines in one study (Lader et al. 1984) but not in others (Poser et al. 1983; Rickels 1985). Busto et al. (2000) found no difference in the CT brain scans of patients taking benzodiazepines compared with control subjects. Long-term benzodiazepine users have been compared with control subjects and found to have cognitive impairments that reversed on reexamination after taper (Golombok et al. 1988; Lucki et al. 1986; Rickels et al. 1999; Sakol and Power 1988). Another study found that after long-term use, if the benzodiazepine is stopped, there was only partial recovery even after 6 months (Tata et al. 1994).

Drug-Drug Interactions

Antacids slow benzodiazepine absorption, as aluminum delays gastric emptying (Greenblatt et al. 1983a, 1983b). An acid medium is needed for conversion of clorazepate to desmethyldiazepam, the active metabolite, which is then absorbed (Shader et al. 1978).

In the liver, benzodiazepines are metabolized by oxidation, reduction, or conjugation. Alprazolam, diazepam, clorazepate, prazepam, chlordiazepoxide, bromazepam, and halazepam are metabolized by oxidation; nitrazepam by reduction; and lorazepam, oxazepam, and temazepam by conjugation. Inhibitors of the oxidase system prolong the half-life of benzodiazepines that are metabolized by this system. This accentuates the side effects, notably the sedation, ataxia, slurred speech, and imbalance. A decrease in dosage may solve this problem, or a switch to a benzodiazepine that is metabolized by conjugation may be needed. MAOIs, cimetidine (Greenblatt et al. 1984), and oral contraceptives inhibit the oxidative system. There is a decline in this system with age or liver disease. In the elderly, there is a 50% decrease in clearance, with a four- to ninefold increase in half-life and a two- to fourfold increase in the volume of distribution (Peppers 1996). Heparinized patients (Routledge et al. 1980) should have partial thromboplastin time (PTT) monitored more closely, as PTT is prolonged by benzodiazepines. Because antidepressants like fluoxetine, paroxetine, and nefazodone and protease inhibitors like indinavir sulfate inhibit the cytochrome P450 enzyme 3A4, they inhibit the metabolism of triazolobenzodiazepines such as midazolam, alprazolam, and triazolam.

Clinical Issues

Despite decades of research, the optimal extent and duration of appropriate benzodiazepine use in the treatment of anxiety and related disorders remain unresolved. This is primarily because of concerns expressed by prescribers, regulators, and the public about issues such as tolerance, dependence, and abuse liability of this class of medications.

Tolerance

In a study of persistent users of alprazolam and lorazepam, Romach et al. (1995) found that most were not abusing these benzodiazepines, nor were they addicted to them; rather, they were using them appropriately for a chronic disorder and at a constant or a decreasing dose. Soumerai et al. (2003) found a lack of relationship between long-term use of benzodiazepines and escalation to high doses in 2,440 long-term (at least 2 years) users of benzodiazepines and that escalation to a high dose was very rare.

The cross-tolerance between the benzodiazepines, although good, is not perfect, and it is preferable to switch patients gradually from one benzodiazepine to another and to use comparable doses of each during the switch. One milligram of alprazolam is approximately equivalent to 0.7 milligram of clonazepam, 10 milligrams of diazepam, or 1 milligram of lorazepam.

Withdrawal

A withdrawal syndrome is defined as a predictable constellation of signs and symptoms involving altered CNS activity (e.g., tremor, convulsions, or delirium) after the abrupt discontinuation of, or rapid decrease in, dosing of the drug (Rinaldi et al. 1988). Typically, a withdrawal syndrome from short-half-life benzodiazepines will intensify by the second day, will usually have peaked by day 5, and will begin to decrease and taper off by day 10. After 2 weeks, withdrawal symptoms have usually become minimal or are absent. Drug factors associated with withdrawal symptoms include length of use, dose, potency, and rate of discontinuation. The most common are anxiety, restlessness, irritability, insomnia, agitation, muscle tension, weakness, aches and pains, blurred vision, and racing heart, in that order (O'Brien 2005). Nausea, sweating, runny nose, hypersensitivity to stimuli, and tremor are less frequent. Severe withdrawal symptoms, such as psychosis, seizures, hallucinations, paranoid delusions, and persistent tinnitus, are relatively rare and are more likely to occur in abrupt withdrawal from high doses of high-potency benzodiazepines and in the elderly (American Psychiatric Association 1990; Lader 1990; Petturson and Lader 1991).

The minimum duration of use after which clinically significant withdrawal symptoms can be expected has not been definitively determined. At the end of any course of treatment with therapeutic doses and of duration greater than 3–6 weeks, withdrawal of the benzodiazepine should be done as a slow taper. This reduces the risk of unpleasant withdrawal symptoms and the danger of withdrawal seizures and minimizes rebound reactivation of the underlying anxiety disorder (Fontaine et al. 1984; Pecknold et al. 1988; Power et al. 1985).

In a 3-year follow-up of patients who tapered successfully in a benzodiazepine taper program, 73% remained benzodiazepine free. Among those who were able to reduce intake by 50%, only 39% were benzodiazepine free at the end of 3 years. In the group that could not tolerate taper at all, only 14% were benzodiazepine free (Rickels et al. 1991).

Addiction Potential

In our zeal to heal an anxiety disorder, are we creating a population of addicts? There is much misinformation and concern generated because terms like *addiction* are used without precise definition and pejoratively. Terms such as *addiction*, *physical dependency*, and *withdrawal syndrome* are often used interchangeably. There is a presumption that a medicine being associated with a withdrawal syndrome is evidence that the medicine is addicting. Some clinicians believe that benzodiazepines that require frequent dosing during the day are more addicting than those that require less frequent dosing. In fact, frequency of dosing is a function of the duration of therapeutic action of the drug rather than of any innate addiction potential of the drug.

DSM-IV-TR (American Psychiatric Association 2000) defines *substance (drug) dependence* as a maladaptive pattern of substance use leading to clinically significant impairment or distress, as manifested by the presence of three (or more) of seven criteria at any time in the same 12-month period. *Addiction*, in contrast, is defined as a chronic disorder associated with compulsive use of a drug, resulting in physical, psychological, or social harm to the user and continued use despite that harm (Rinaldi et al. 1988). Addiction involves both intense drug-seeking behavior and difficulty in stopping the drug use. If these criteria are used, benzodiazepines are not addictive drugs. *Physical dependence* is different from addiction and is defined as a physiological state of adaptation to a drug, with the development of tolerance to the drug's effects and the emergence of a withdrawal syndrome during prolonged abstinence. During withdrawal after chronic use, biochemical, physiological, or behavioral problems may be triggered. When used on a regular schedule, benzodiazepines are associated with physical dependence, as opposed to drug dependence or DSM-IV-TR "substance dependence," and have a withdrawal syndrome.

Abuse

Studies of abuse use four criteria for benzodiazepine abuse. A benzodiazepine is being abused if it is used 1) to get high, 2) to promote psychological regression, 3) at doses higher than prescribed, and 4) after the medical indication has passed (Dietch 1983). On the basis of this definition, the data suggest that the incidence of benzodiazepine abuse in clinical practice is low.

The incidence of benzodiazepine dependence in the therapeutic setting (among those for whom the drug is medically correctly prescribed) was estimated to be 1 case in 50 million patient-months (Marks 1978). Of these cases, 92% were associated with alcohol or other drugs of abuse. This estimate is probably on the low side since it is based on the number of published cases of dependence from 1961 to 1977.

In Basel, Switzerland, with a catchment area of 300,000 people, physicians were surveyed on the prevalence of benzodiazepine abuse in their patients. Only 31 patients were identified—a prevalence of 0.01%, or 1 in 10,000. An additional 88 polysubstance abusers were identified (Ladewig and Grossenbacher 1988). In a random sample of all psychiatric hospitalizations over 15 years (1967–1983) in Sweden (n=32,679), Allgulander (1989) found only 38 admissions for substance dependence on sedative-hypnotics. Twenty-one of the 38 had polysubstance abuse, and 17 had sedative-hypnotic abuse.

In another study of all medical and psychiatric hospitalizations (n=1.6 million) in Stockholm County, Allgulander (1996) found that 0.04% of "prescribed medication" users (including benzodiazepines) were ever admitted for medical problems relating to their drug use. In a study of 5,426 physicians randomly selected from the U.S. physicians American Medical Association database, Hughes et al. (1992) found that although 11.9% had used benzodiazepines in the past year, only 0.6% met DSM-III-R (American Psychiatric Association 1987) criteria for benzodiazepine abuse and 0.5% met criteria for benzodiazepine dependence. In 1990, the American Psychiatric Association task force concluded that benzodiazepines were not normally drugs of abuse but noted that people who abused alcohol, cocaine, and opiates were at increased risk for benzodiazepine abuse (Salzman 1991).

A number of studies have noted no increase in dosage with chronic therapy of duration from 1 to 2.5 years, even though many of the patients had residual symptoms that would have benefited from a dose increase or more intensive or additional treatment strategies (Pollack et al. 1986; Sheehan 1987). Nonanxious subjects and those with low anxiety levels find benzodiazepines dysphoric (Reed et al. 1965), prefer placebo to diazepam (Johanson and Uhlenhuth 1978, 1980), or rate their mood as less happy and pleasant after they were given 10 mg of diazepam (Svensson et al. 1980).

Although the data suggest that the prevalence of benzodiazepine abuse or dependence is generally low, this is not true among those who abuse alcohol and other drugs. In a study of chronic alcoholic individuals who were high consumers of benzodiazepines, 17% got their benzodiazepines from nonmedical sources (Busto et al. 1983). In a study of 1,000 admissions to an alcohol treatment unit, 35% of patients used benzodiazepines, but only 10% of the total sample were considered abusers or misusers (Ashley et al. 1978). A study of 427 patients seeking treatment in Toronto who met DSM-III (American Psychiatric Association 1980) criteria for alcohol abuse or dependence found that 40% were recent users and 20% had a lifetime history of benzodiazepine abuse or dependence. On the other hand, only 5% of 108 alcoholic patients treated for a year with benzodiazepines for anxiety and tension showed evidence of abuse, and 94% felt it helped them function and remain out of the hospital (Rothstein et al. 1976).

Benzodiazepines were the primary drug of abuse in one-third of polydrug abusers (Busto et al. 1986), in 29% of 113 drug abusers admitting to the street purchase of diazepam in the previous month (Woody et al. 1975b), and in 40% of patients at a methadone maintenance clinic (Woody et al. 1975a). The principal reasons for benzodiazepine use among drug addicts are self-treatment of withdrawal symptoms, relief from rebound dysphoria, or potentiation of alcohol or street drug effects (Petera et al. 1987). In one study at an addictions treatment center, 100% of urine samples tested were positive for benzodiazepines and 44% were positive for multiple nonprescribed benzodiazepines (Igochi et al. 1993). A survey of patients at three different methadone maintenance clinics found that 78%–94% admitted to a lifetime use of benzodiazepines and 44%–66% admitted to use in the prior 6 months. Snorting of benzodiazepines by cocaine addicts has been reported (Sheehan et al. 1991), primarily as a means of blunting the anxiogenic effect of cocaine and allowing for a more pleasant and "less edgy" high from that drug. Overall, the existing evidence suggests that the prevalence of benzodiazepine abuse is uncommon, except among those individuals who abuse alcohol and or other drugs.

Despite extensive data and discussion on this topic, the issue remains and will continue to be controversial, with strong opinions held by opposing camps. Klerman characterized these camps as "pharmacological Calvinism" and "psychotropic hedonism," respectively (Klerman 1972; Rosenbaum 2005). The middle ground suggests that we should not hesitate to prescribe benzodiazepines when it is reasonable but that we should exercise restraint in using them when we see any evidence of abuse (Pomeranz 2007).

Medicolegal Issues

In addition to issues of dependence and withdrawal described in the previous section, there are a number of potential medicolegal pitfalls in using benzodiazepines. These include issues of teratogenicity, injury, and interaction with substances.

Benzodiazepines and Pregnancy

Since anxiety disorders have their highest incidence in women during their childbearing years, the clinician may have to advise patients who are planning a pregnancy or who become pregnant while taking a benzodiazepine.

First and Second Trimesters

An important concern in the first and second trimesters is the possibility of teratogenic effects. Diazepam and desmethyldiazepam cross the placental barrier easily, and concentrations are higher in fetal blood than in maternal blood (Idanpaan-Heikkila et al. 1971). Early concern over benzodiazepine exposure in pregnancy arose because benzodiazepines act on GABA receptors and GABA is involved in palate shelf reorientation (Wee and Zimmerman 1983; Zimmerman and Wee 1984). The teratogenic effects of benzodiazepines, however, are a matter of controversy. Exposure to benzodiazepines has been associated with teratogenic effects, including facial clefts and skeletal anomalies in the newborn in some animal studies (Miller and Becker 1975; Walker and Patterson 1974; Wee and

Zimmerman 1983; Zimmerman 1984; Zimmerman and Wee 1984) but not in others (Beall 1972; Chesley et al. 1991). Early studies in humans, including retrospective and case-control studies, reported an increased risk of oral clefts associated with diazepam (Aarskog 1975; Livezey et al. 1986; Safra and Oakley 1975; Saxen 1975; Saxen and Lahti 1974). These results, however, have been criticized on methodological grounds and are contradicted by more recent prospective studies, case-control studies, and meta-analyses that show no increased risk of oral clefts related to benzodiazepine use in pregnancy (Altshuler et al. 1996; Bracken 1986; Czeizel 1988; Dolovich et al. 1998; Ornoy et al. 1998; Pastuszak et al. 1996; Rosenberg et al. 1983; Shiono and Mills 1984).

Pooled data from seven cohort studies, however, do not support an association between fetal exposure to benzodiazepines and major malformations (Dolovich et al. 1998).

Third Trimester and Labor

Two concerns associated with benzodiazepine use in the last trimester and through delivery are the possibilities of CNS depression and a withdrawal syndrome. Signs of CNS depression may include hypotonia, lethargy, sucking difficulties, decreased fetal movements, loss of cardiac beat-to-beat variability, respiratory depression, and thermogenesis. These symptoms in the neonate are more likely with higher doses and longer duration of benzodiazepine use by the mother. There have been numerous reports of "floppy infant syndrome" in babies born to women taking diazepam long term during pregnancy (Gillberg 1977; Haram 1977; Rowlatt 1978; Spreight 1977). Neonatal withdrawal symptoms may include hyperactivity and irritability. The occurrence of neonatal withdrawal symptoms is well documented (Barry and St. Clair 1987; Briggs et al. 1998; Cree et al. 1973; Fisher et al. 1985; Gillberg 1977; Haram 1977). Symptoms may be present at birth or appear weeks later and may continue for a period of time (Schardein 1993).

Diazepam in isolated doses is safe during labor (Briggs et al. 1998). There are conflicting reports on the effect of benzodiazepines on Apgar scores. Lowered Apgar scores have been reported with benzodiazepine use in some studies (Berdowitz et al. 1981; McElhatton 1994). One study found that diazepam reduced Apgar scores only when doses greater than 30 mg were administered during labor (Cree et al. 1973).

Breast-Feeding

Neonates have only limited capacity to metabolize diazepam (Morselli et al. 1973). Benzodiazepines are excreted in breast milk (Llewellyn and Stowe 1998). Because of the neonate's limited capacity to metabolize these drugs, they can potentially accumulate and cause sedation, lethargy, and loss of weight in the nursing infant. Although the extent to which benzodiazepines actually accumulate in the serum of breast-feeding infants is a matter of debate (Birnbaum et al. 1999), and three decades of studies support a low incidence of toxicity and adverse effects (Birnbaum et al. 1999; Llewellyn and Stowe 1998), caution taking benzodiazepines while breast-feeding is advised.

Psychomotor Impairment

Another area of risk of benzodiazepine use relates to issues of psychomotor impairment resulting in injury. An examination of the medical records of a group of benzodiazepine users and nonusers revealed that the benzodiazepine users were more likely to experience at least one episode of accident-related health care and a greater number of accident-related inpatient days and also utilized significantly more non-accident-related health care services than did nonusers. Accident-related utilization of health care was more likely in the first month after the drug was prescribed (Oster et al. 1987). In the elderly, the issue of benzodiazepine use increasing the risk for falls and fractures is of great concern because hip fractures are associated with increased morbidity and mortality. A number of studies (Boston Collaborative Drug Surveillance Program 1973; Cummings et al. 1995; Greenblatt et al. 1977; Hemmelgarn et al. 1997; Ray et al. 1992; Roth et al. 1980) have found a greater risk for falls with the use of long-half-life benzodiazepines, and others (Cumming and Klineberg 1993; Herings et al. 1995; Leipzig et al. 1999) have found the risk to be greater with short-half-life drugs. A more recent study (Wang et al. 2001) found the risk for hip fracture in the elderly to be the same with the use of short- or long-half-life benzodiazepines. The researchers did find that the risk increased when benzodiazepine dosages were >3 mg/day in diazepam equivalents. They also found the greatest risk to be shortly after initiation of therapy and after 1 month of continuous use. A 5-year prospective cohort study followed a large group of elderly people newly exposed to benzodiazepines (Tamblyn et al. 2005). The elderly using benzodiazepines are at greater risk of a motor vehicle accident (Hemmelgarn et al. 1997). On the other hand, a study of the effect of New York State requiring triplicate forms for prescribing benzodiazepines showed that despite a 50% drop in the number of prescriptions written, there was no significant change in age-adjusted risk for hip fractures (Wagner et al. 2007).

Patients receiving benzodiazepines are nearly five times more likely than nonusers to experience a serious motor vehicle accident (Skegg et al. 1979). In the first 2 weeks after persons start using benzodiazepines, there is a several-fold excess risk for hospitalization related to accidental injury compared with persons using antidepressants or antipsychotics (Neutel 1995).

The best protection is a discussion of these issues with the patient prior to prescribing a benzodiazepine. This discussion, including cautionary statements about driving or using dangerous appliances, should be documented in the chart at the start of therapy. The patient should be educated about potentiation by alcohol or other sedating drugs. He or she should be strongly advised never to abruptly discontinue the medicine because of a risk of seizures (Noyes et al. 1986), and this should be documented. Prescribing benzodiazepines for patients with a current or lifetime history of substance abuse or dependence should be done infrequently and only after documenting a risk-benefit discussion in the chart. It is good practice to routinely screen for substance abuse before prescribing a benzodiazepine and to document that this was done.

Conclusion

Benzodiazepines, if given in adequate doses, are effective in the treatment of anxiety. They have a lower mortality and morbidity per million prescriptions than some of the alternatives (Girdwood 1974). Benzodiazepines are quicker in onset of action, easier for the clinician to use, associated with better compliance, and less subjectively disruptive for the patient than any of the other medication alternatives. Until benzodiazepines are replaced by another class of medicine that is safer, better tolerated, and as rapidly effective, it is likely that they will continue to be prescribed to a significant proportion of patients.

References

Aarskog D: Associations between maternal intake of diazepam and oral clefts (letter). Lancet 2(7941): 921, 1975

Allgulander C: Psychoactive drug use in a general population sample, Sweden: correlates with perceived health, psychiatric diagnoses, and mortality in an automated record-linkage study. Am J Public Health 79:1006–1010, 1989

Allgulander C: Addiction in sedative-hypnotics. Hum Psychopharmacol 119:S49–S54, 1996

Altshuler LL, Cohen L, Szuba MP, et al: Pharmacologic management of psychiatric illness during pregnancy: dilemmas and guidelines. Am J Psychiatry 153:592–606, 1996

American Psychiatric Association: Diagnostic and Statistical Manual of Mental Disorders, 3rd Edition. Washington, DC, American Psychiatric Association, 1980

American Psychiatric Association: Diagnostic and Statistical Manual of Mental Disorders, 3rd Edition, Revised. Washington, DC, American Psychiatric Association, 1987

American Psychiatric Association: Benzodiazepine Dependence, Toxicity, and Abuse: A Task Force Report of the American Psychiatric Association. Washington, DC, American Psychiatric Association, 1990

American Psychiatric Association: Practice guideline for the treatment of patients with panic disorder. Am J Psychiatry 155 (suppl 5):1–34, 1998

American Psychiatric Association: Diagnostic and Statistical Manual of Mental Disorders, 4th Edition, Text Revision. Washington, DC, American Psychiatric Association, 2000

Ashley MJ, LeRiche WH, Olin GS, et al: "Mixed" (drug abusing) and "pure" alcoholics: a sociomedical comparison. Br J Addict 73:19–34, 1978

Ballenger JC, Burrows G, Dupont RL, et al: Alprazolam in panic disorder and agoraphobia: results from a multicenter study. Arch Gen Psychiatry 45:413–422, 1988

Balter MB: Prevalence of medical use of prescription drugs. Presentation at Evaluation of the Impact of Prescription Drug Diversion Control Systems on Medical Practice and Patient Care: Possible Implications for Future Research (NIDA Technical Review), Bethesda, MD, 1991

Barry WS, St. Clair SM: Exposure to benzodiazepines in utero. Lancet 1(8547):1436–1437, 1987

Beall JR: Study of the teratogenic potential of oral diazepam and SCH 12041. Can Med Assoc J 106:1061, 1972

Berdowitz RL, Coustan DR, Mochizuke T (eds): Handbook for Prescribing Medications During Pregnancy. Boston, MA, Little, Brown, 1981

Birnbaum CS, Cohen LS, Bailey JW, et al: Serum concentrations of antidepressants and benzodiazepines in nursing infants: a case series. Pediatrics 104(1):e11, 1999

Bixler EO, Scharf MB, Soldatos CR, et al: Effects of hypnotic drugs on memory. Life Sci 25:1379–1388, 1979

Boston Collaborative Drug Surveillance Program: Clinical depression of the central nervous system due to diazepam and chlordiazepoxide in relation to cigarette smoking and age. N Engl J Med 288:277–280, 1973

Bracken MB: Drug use in pregnancy and congenital heart disease in offspring (letter). N Engl J Med 314:1120, 1986

Briggs GG, Yaffe SJ, Freeman RK: Drugs in Pregnancy and Lactation: A Reference Guide to Fetal and Neonatal Risk, 5th Edition. Baltimore, MD, Williams & Wilkins, 1998

Busto U, Simpkins J, Sellers EM, et al: Objective determination of benzodiazepine use and abuse in alcoholics. Br J Addict 78:429–435, 1983

Busto U, Sellers EM, Naranjo CA, et al: Patterns of benzodiazepine abuse and dependence. Br J Addict 81:87–94, 1986

Busto UE, Bremner KE, Knight K, et al: Long-term benzodiazepine therapy does not result in brain abnormalities. J Clin Psychopharmacol 20:2–6, 2000

Chesley S, Lumpkin M, Schatzki A, et al: Prenatal exposure to benzodiazepine, I: prenatal exposure to lorazepam in mice alters open-field activity and GABA receptor function. Neuropharmacology 30:53–58, 1991

Chouinard G, Annable L, Fontaine R, et al: Alprazolam and the treatment of generalized anxiety and panic disorders: a double-blind placebo controlled study. Psychopharmacology (Berl) 77:229–233, 1982

Chouinard G, Annable L, Turnier L, et al: Double blind randomized clinical trial of rapid tranquilization with IM clonazepam and IM haloperidol in agitated psychotic patients with manic symptoms. Can J Psychiatry 38 (suppl 4):S114–S120, 1993

Cree JE, Meyer J, Hailey DM: Diazepam in labor: its metabolism and effect on the clinical condition of thermogenesis of the newborn. BMJ 4:251–255, 1973

Cross National Collaborative Panic Study, Second Phase Investigators: Drug treatment of panic disorder: comparative efficacy of alprazolam, imipramine, and placebo. Br J Psychiatry 160:191–201, 1992

Cumming RG, Klineberg RJ: Psychotropics, thiazide diuretics and hip fracture in the elderly. Med J Aust 158:414–417, 1993

Cummings SR, Nevitt MC, Browner WS, et al: Risk factors for hip fracture in white women. N Engl J Med 332:767–773, 1995

Czeizel A: Lack of evidence of teratogenicity of benzodiazepine drugs in Hungary. Reprod Toxicol 1(3):183–188, 1988

Davidson JRT, Potts NLS, Richichi E, et al: Treatment of social phobia with clonazepam and placebo. J Clin Psychopharmacol 13:423–428, 1993

Dietch J: The nature and extent of benzodiazepine abuse: an overview of recent literature. Hosp Community Psychiatry 34:1139–1145, 1983

Dolovich LR, Addis A, Vaillancourt JM, et al: Benzodiazepine use in pregnancy and major malformations or oral cleft: meta-analysis of cohort and case-control studies. BMJ 317:839–843, 1998

Fisher JB, Edgren BE, Mammel MC, et al: Neonatal apnea associated with maternal clonazepam therapy: a case report. Obstet Gynecol 66 (suppl):34–35, 1985

Fontaine RG, Chouinard G, Annable L: Rebound anxiety in anxious patients after abrupt withdrawal of benzodiazepine treatment. Am J Psychiatry 141:848–852, 1984

Gelernter CS, Uhde TW, Cimbolic P, et al. Cognitive-behavioral and pharmacologic treatment of social phobia: a controlled study. Arch Gen Psychiatry 48:938–945, 1991

Gillberg C: "Floppy infant syndrome" and maternal diazepam (letter). Lancet 2(8031):244, 1977

Girdwood RH: Death after taking medicaments. BMJ 1(5906):501–504, 1974

Goddard AW, Brouette T, Almai A, et al: Early coadministration of clonazepam with sertraline for panic disorder. Arch Gen Psychiatry 58:681–686, 2001

Goddard AW, Sheehan DV, Rickels K: A Double blind placebo controlled study comparing sertraline plus placebo and sertraline plus alprazolam XR in the treatment of panic disorder. Presented at Anxiety Disorders Association of America annual meeting, Savannah, GA, March 2008

Golombok S, Moodley P, Lader M: Cognitive impairment in long-term benzodiazepine users. Psychol Med 18:365–374, 1988

Goodman WK, Charney DS: A case of alprazolam but not lorazepam inducing manic symptoms. J Clin Psychiatry 48:117–118, 1987

Greenblatt DJ, Allen MD, Shader RI: Toxicity of high dose flurazepam in the elderly. Clin Pharmacol Ther 21:355–361, 1977

Greenblatt DJ, Shader RI, Franke K, et al: Pharmacokinetics and bioavailability of intravenous, intramuscular, and oral lorazepam in humans. J Pharm Sci 68:57–63, 1979

Greenblatt DJ, Divoll M, Harmatz JS, et al: Kinetics and clinical effects of flurazepam in young and elderly noninsomniacs. Clin Pharmacol Ther 30:475–486, 1981

Greenblatt DJ, Divoll M, Abernethy DR, et al: Benzodiazepine hypnotics: kinetic and therapeutic options. Sleep 5 (suppl 1):S18–S27, 1982a

Greenblatt DJ, Divoll M, Harmatz JS, et al: Pharmacokinetic comparison of sublingual lorazepam with intravenous, intramuscular, and oral lorazepam. J Pharm Sci 71:248–252, 1982b

Greenblatt DJ, Sellers EM, Shader RI: Drug therapy: drug distribution in old age. N Engl J Med 306:1081–1088, 1982c

Greenblatt DJ, Shader RI, Abernethy DR: Drug therapy: current status of benzodiazepines, part 1. N Engl J Med 309:354–358, 1983a

Greenblatt DJ, Shader RI, Abernethy DR: Drug therapy: current status of benzodiazepines, part 2. N Engl J Med 309:410–416, 1983b

Greenblatt DJ, Abernethy DR, Morse DS, et al: Clinical importance of the interaction of diazepam and cimetidine. N Engl J Med 310:1639–1643, 1984

Haram K: Floppy infant syndrome and maternal diazepam. Lancet 2(8038):612–613, 1977

Hemmelgarn B, Suissa S, Huang A, et al: Benzodiazepine use and the risk of motor vehicle crash in the elderly. JAMA 278:27–31, 1997

Herings RM, Stricker BH, de Boer A, et al: Benzodiazepines and the risk of falling leading to femur fractures: dosage more important than elimination half-life. Arch Intern Med 155:1801–1807, 1995

Hughes PH, Brandenburg N, Baldwin DC, et al: Prevalence of substance use among US physicians. JAMA 267:2333–2339, 1992

Idanpaan-Heikkila JE, Jouppila PI, Puolakka JO, et al: Placental transfer in fetal metabolism of diazepam in early human pregnancy. Am J Obstet Gynecol 109:1011–1016, 1971

Igochi MY, Handelsman L, Bickel WK, et al: Benzodiazepine and sedative use/abuse by methadone maintenance clients. Drug Alcohol Depend 32:257–266, 1993

IMS America: National Disease and Therapeutic Index (NDTI). Plymouth Meeting, PA, IMS America, 1991

Johanson CE, Uhlenhuth EH: Drug self-administration in humans. NIDA Res Monogr (20):68–85, 1978

Johanson CE, Uhlenhuth EH: Drug preference and mood in humans: diazepam. Psychopharmacology (Berl) 71:269–273, 1980

Kales A, Bixler EO, Soldatos CR, et al: Quazepam and flurazepam: long-term use and extended withdrawal. Clin Pharmacol Ther 32:781–788, 1982

Kales A, Soldatos CR, Bixler EO, et al: Early morning insomnia with rapidly eliminated benzodiazepines. Science 220:95–97, 1983

Kales A, Bixler EO, Soldatos CR, et al: Lorazepam: effects on sleep and withdrawal phenomena. Pharmacology 32:121–130, 1986

Kales A, Bixler EO, Vela-Bueno A, et al: Alprazolam: effects on sleep and withdrawal phenomena. J Clin Pharmacol 27:508–515, 1987

Klerman GL: Psychotropic hedonism vs. pharmacological Calvinism. Hastings Cent Rep 2:1–3, 1972

Kramer PD: Listening to Prozac. New York, Penguin Books, 1993

Lader M: Benzodiazepine withdrawal, in Handbook of Anxiety, Vol 4. Edited by Noyer R, Roth M, Burrows GD. Amsterdam, Elsevier, 1990, pp 57–71

Lader MH, Ron M, Petursson H: Computed axial brain tomography in long term benzodiazepine users. Psychol Med 14:203–206, 1984

Ladewig D, Grossenbacher H: Benzodiazepine abuse in patients of doctors in domiciliary practice in the Basle area. Pharmacopsychiatry 21:104–108, 1988

Leipzig RM, Cumming RG, Tinetti ME: Drugs and falls in older people: a systematic review and meta-analysis, I: psychotropic drugs. J Am Geriatr Soc 47:30–39, 1999

Lister RG: The amnestic action of benzodiazepines in man. Neurosci Biobehav Rev 9:87–94, 1985

Lister RG, Weingartner H, Eckhardt MJ, et al: Clinical relevance of effects of benzodiazepines on learning and memory. Psychopharmacol Ser 6: 117–127, 1988

Livezey GT, Marczynski TJ, McGrew EA, et al: Prenatal exposure to diazepam: late postnasal teratogenic effect. Neurobehav Toxicol Teratol 8:433–440, 1986

Llewellyn A, Stowe ZN: Psychotropic medications in lactation. J Clin Psychiatry 59 (suppl 2):41–52, 1998

Lucki I, Rickels K, Geller AM: Chronic use of benzodiazepines and psychomotor and cognitive test performance. Psychopharmacology (Berl) 88:426–433, 1986

Marks J: The Benzodiazepines. Lancaster, UK, MTP Press, 1978

McElhatton PR: The effects of benzodiazepine use during pregnancy and lactation. Reprod Toxicol 8:461–475, 1994

Miller RP, Becker BA: Teratogenicity of oral diazepam and diphenylhydantoin in mice. Toxicol Appl Pharmacol 32:53–61, 1975

Miller RR: Drug surveillance utilizing epidemiologic methods: a report from the Boston Collaborative Drug Surveillance Program. Am J Hosp Pharm 30:584–592, 1973

Morselli PL, Principi N, Tognoni G, et al: Diazepam elimination and premature and full-term infants and children. J Perinat Med 1(2):133–141, 1973

Neutel CI: Risk of traffic accident injury after a prescription for a benzodiazepine. Ann Epidemiol 5:239–244, 1995

Noyes R Jr, Perry PJ, Crowe RR, et al: Seizures following the withdrawal of alprazolam. J Nerv Ment Dis 174:50–52, 1986

O'Brien CP: Benzodiazepine use, abuse, and dependence. J Clin Psychiatry 66 (suppl 2):28–33, 2005

Ornoy A, Arnon J, Shechtman S, et al: Is benzodiazepine use during pregnancy really teratogenic? Reprod Toxicol 12:511–515, 1998

Oster G, Russell MW, Huse DM, et al: Accident- and injury-related health-care utilization among benzodiazepine users and nonusers. J Clin Psychiatry 48 (12, suppl):17–21, 1987

Pastuszak A, Milich V, Chan S, et al: Prospective assessment of pregnancy outcome following first trimester exposure to benzodiazepines. Can J Clin Pharmacol 3:167–171, 1996

Pecknold JC, Fleury D: Alprazolam-induced manic episode in two patients with panic disorder. Am J Psychiatry 143:652–653, 1986

Pecknold JC, Swinson RP, Kuch K, et al: Alprazolam in panic disorder and agoraphobia: results from a multicenter trial, III: discontinuation effects. Arch Gen Psychiatry 45:429–436, 1988

Peppers MP: Benzodiazepines for alcohol withdrawal in the elderly and in patients with liver disease. Pharmacotherapy 16:49–58, 1996

Petera KM, Tulley M, Jenner FA: The use of benzodiazepines among street drug addicts. Br J Addict 82:511–515, 1987

Petturson H, Lader MH: Withdrawal from long term benzodiazepine treatment. BMJ 283:643–645, 1991

Pollack MH, Tesar GE, Rosenbaum JF, et al: Clonazepam in the treatment of panic disorder and agoraphobia: a one-year follow-up. J Clin Psychopharmacol 6:302–304, 1986

Pollack MH, Otto MW, Tesar GE, et al: Long-term outcome after acute treatment with alprazolam or clonazepam for panic disorder. J Clin Psychopharmacol 13:257–263, 1993

Pomeranz JM: Risk versus benefit of benzodiazepines. Psychiatric Times 22–26, August 2007

Poser W, Poser S, Roscher D, et al: Do benzodiazepines cause cerebral atrophy (letter)? Lancet 1(8326 Pt 1):715, 1983

Power KG, Jerrom DWA, Simpson RJ, et al: Controlled study of withdrawal symptoms and rebound anxiety after a six week course of diazepam for generalized anxiety disorder. BMJ 290:1246–1248, 1985

Ray WA, Fought RL, Decker MD: Psychoactive drugs and the risk of injurious motor vehicle crashes in elderly drivers. Am J Epidemiol 136:873–883, 1992

Reed CF, Witt PN, Peakall DB: Freehand copying of a geometric pattern as a test for sensory-motor disturbance. Percept Mot Skills 20:941–951, 1965

Rickels K: Clinical management of benzodiazepine dependence (letter). BMJ 291:1649, 1985

Rickels K, Schweizer EE: Benzodiazepines for treatment of panic attacks: a new look. Psychopharmacol Bull 23:93–99, 1986

Rickels K, Case WG, Schweizer E, et al: Long-term benzodiazepine users 3 years after participation in a discontinuation program. Am J Psychiatry 148:757–761, 1991

Rickels K, Downing R, Schweizer E, et al: Antidepressants for the treatment of generalized anxiety disorder: a placebo-controlled comparison of imipramine, trazodone, and diazepam. Arch Gen Psychiatry 50:884–895, 1993

Rickels K, Lucki I, Schweizer E, et al: Psychomotor performance of long term benzodiazepine users, before, during and after benzodiazepine discontinuation. J Clin Psychopharmacol 19:107–113, 1999

Rinaldi RD, Steindler EM, Wilford BB, et al: Clarification and standardization of substance abuse terminology. JAMA 259:555–557, 1988

Roach JD, Griffiths RR: Comparison of triazolam and pentobarbital: performance impairment, subjective effects and abuse liability. J Pharmacol Exp Ther 234:120–133, 1985

Roach JD, Griffiths RR: Lorazepam and meprobamate dose effects in humans: behavioral effects and abuse liability. J Pharmacol Exp Ther 243:978–988, 1987

Romach M, Busto U, Somer MA, et al: Clinical aspects of the chronic use of alprazolam and lorazepam. Am J Psychiatry 152:1161–1167, 1995

Rosenbaum JF: Attitudes towards benzodiazepines over the years. J Clin Psychiatry 66 (suppl 2):4–8, 2005

Rosenbaum JF, Woods SW, Groves JE, et al: Emergence of hostility during alprazolam treatment. Am J Psychiatry 141:792–793, 1984

Rosenberg L, Mitchell AA, Parsells JL, et al: Lack of relation of oral clefts to diazepam use during pregnancy. N Engl J Med 309:1282–1285, 1983

Roth T, Hartse KM, Saab PG, et al: The effects of flurazepam, lorazepam and triazolam on sleep and memory. Psychopharmacology (Berl) 70:231–237, 1980

Rothstein E, Cobble JC, Sampson N: Chlordiazepoxide: long-term use in alcoholism. Ann N Y Acad Sci 273:381–384, 1976

Routledge PA, Kitchell BB, Bjornson TD, et al: Diazepam and N-desmethyldiazepam redistribution after heparin. Clin Pharmacol Ther 27:528–532, 1980

Rowlatt RJ: Effective maternal diazepam on the newborn (letter). BMJ 1(6118):985, 1978

Safra MJ, Oakley GP: Association between cleft lip with or without cleft palate and prenatal exposure to diazepam. Lancet 2(7933):478–480, 1975

Sakol MS, Power KG: The effects of long term benzodiazepine treatment and graded withdrawal on psychomotor performance. Psychopharmacology (Berl) 95:135–138, 1988

Salzman C: APA Task Force report on benzodiazepine dependence, toxicity, and abuse. Am J Psychiatry 148:151–152, 1991

Saxen I: Associations between oral clefts and drugs taken during pregnancy. Int J Epidemiol 4:37–44, 1975

Saxen I, Lahti A: Cleft lip and palate in Finland: incidence, secular, seasonal, and geographical variations. Teratology 9:217–224, 1974

Schardein JL (ed): Chemically Induced Birth Defects, 2nd Edition. New York, Marcel Dekker, 1993

Scharf MB, Fletcher K, Graham JP: Comparative amnesic effects of benzodiazepine hypnotic agents. J Clin Psychiatry 49:134–137, 1988

Schweizer E, Rickels K, Weiss S, et al: Maintenance drug treatment of panic disorder, I: results of a prospective, placebo controlled comparison of alprazolam and imipramine. Arch Gen Psychiatry 50:51–60, 1993

Shader RI, Georgotas A, Greenblatt DJ, et al: Impaired absorption of desmethyldiazepam from clorazepate by magnesium aluminum hydroxide. Clin Pharmacol Ther 24:308–315, 1978

Sheehan DV: Benzodiazepines in panic disorder and agoraphobia. J Affect Disord 13:169–181, 1987

Sheehan DV, Uzogara E, Coleman JH, et al: The treatment of panic attacks with agoraphobia with alprazolam and ibuprofen: a controlled study. Presentation at the annual meeting of the American Psychiatric Association, Toronto, Canada, May 1982

Sheehan DV, Coleman JH, Greenblatt DJ, et al: Some biochemical correlates of panic attacks with agoraphobia and their response to a new treatment. J Clin Psychopharmacol 4:66–75, 1984

Sheehan DV, Raj BA, Harnett-Sheehan K, et al: The relative efficacy of high dose buspirone and alprazolam in the treatment of panic disorder: a double blind placebo controlled study. Acta Psychiatr Scand 88:1–11, 1993

Sheehan MF, Sheehan DV, Torres A, et al: Snorting benzodiazepines. Am J Drug Alcohol Abuse 17:457–468, 1991

Shiono PH, Mills JL: Oral clefts and diazepam use during pregnancy. N Engl J Med 311:919–920, 1984

Skegg DCG, Richards SM, Doll R: Minor tranquilizers and road accidents. BMJ 1(6168):917–919, 1979

Soumerai AB, Simoni-Wastila L, Singer C, et al: Lack of relationship between long-term use of benzodiazepines and escalation to high dosages. Psychiatr Serv 54:1006–1011, 2003

Spreight AN: Floppy-infant syndrome and maternal diazepam and/or nitrazepam (letter). Lancet 2(8043):878, 1977

Stahl SM: Don't ask, don't tell, but benzodiazepines are still the leading treatments for anxiety disorder. J Clin Psychiatry 63:756–757, 2002

Strahan A, Rosenthal J, Kaswan M, et al: Three case reports of acute paroxysmal excitement associated with alprazolam treatment. Am J Psychiatry 142:859–861, 1985

Svenson SE, Hamilton RG: A critique of overemphasis on side effects with the psychotropic drugs: an analysis of 18,000 chlordiazepoxide-treated cases. Curr Ther Res 8:455–464, 1966

Svensson E, Persson LO, Sjöberg L: Mood effects of diazepam and caffeine. Psychopharmacology (Berl) 67:73–80, 1980

Tamblyn R, Abrahamowicz M, du Berger R, et al: A 5-year prospective assessment of the risk associated with individual benzodiazepines and doses in new elderly users. J Am Geriatr Soc 53:233–241, 2005

Tata PR, Rollings J, Collins M, et al: Lack of cognitive recovery following withdrawal from benzodiazepine use. Psychol Med 24:203–213, 1994

Tesar GE, Rosenbaum JF, Pollack MH, et al: Double-blind, placebo-controlled comparison of clonazepam and alprazolam for panic disorder. J Clin Psychiatry 52:69–76, 1991

Uhlenhuth EH, Balter MB, Ban TA, et al: International study of expert judgment on therapeutic use of benzodiazepines and other psychotherapeutic medications, VI: trends in recommendations for the pharmacotherapy of anxiety disorders, 1992–1997. Depress Anxiety 9:107–116, 1999

Van Etten ML, Taylor S: Comparative efficacy of treatments for posttraumatic stress disorder: a meta-analysis. Clin Psychol Psychother 5:126–144, 1998

Vela-Bueno A, Oliveros JC, Dobladez-Blanco B, et al: Brotizolam: a sleep laboratory evaluation. Eur J Clin Pharmacol 25:53–56, 1983

Versiani M, Nardi AE, Figueira I, et al: Double blind placebo controlled trial with bromazepam in social phobia. Serie Psicofarmacologia J Bras Psiquiatr 46:167–171, 1997

Wagner AK, Ross-Degnan D, Gurwitz JH, et al: Effect of New York State regulatory action on benzodiazepine prescribing and hip fracture rates. Ann Intern Med 146:96–103, 2007

Walker BE, Patterson A: Induction of cleft palate in mice by tranquillizers and barbiturates. Teratology 10:159–163, 1974

Wang PS, Bohn RL, Glynn RJ, et al: Hazardous benzodiazepine regimens in the elderly: effects of half-life, dosage, and duration on risk of hip fracture. Am J Psychiatry 158:892–898, 2001

Wee EL, Zimmermann EF: Involvement of GABA in palate morphogenesis and its relation to diazepam teratogenesis in two mouse strains. Teratology 28:15–22, 1983

Woody GE, Mintz G, O'Hare K, et al: Diazepam use by patients in a methadone program: how serious a problem? J Psychedelic Drugs 7:373–379, 1975a

Woody GE, O'Brien CP, Greenstein R: Misuse and abuse of diazepam: an increasingly common medical problem. Int J Addict 10:843–848, 1975b

Zimmermann EF: Neuropharmacologic teratogenesis and neurotransmitter regulation of palate development. Am J Ment Defic 88:548–558, 1984

Zimmermann EF, Wee EL: Role of neurotransmitters in palate development. Curr Top Dev Biol 19:37–63, 1984

CHAPTER 14

Buspirone

Donald S. Robinson, M.D.

Karl Rickels, M.D.

Evidence of altered central serotonergic function exists for several psychiatric disorders, especially mood and anxiety disorders. Discovery of the serotonin$_{1A}$ (5-HT$_{1A}$) receptor linked modulation of serotonin neurotransmission to anxiety symptoms.

The notion that serotonin (5-HT) plays a role in the treatment of anxiety arose from the discovery that both acute and chronic administration of benzodiazepines reduced brain turnover of 5-HT and that administration of para-chlorophenylalanine (pCPA), an inhibitor of serotonin synthesis, mimics the effects of benzodiazepines in behavioral models of anxiety. Characterization of subtypes of 5-HT receptors and discovery of the 5-HT$_{1A}$ receptor partial agonist buspirone indicated that serotonin plays a key role in anxiolysis (Eison and Eison 1994). Because both the benzodiazepines and buspirone reduce 5-HT impulse flow, albeit by different mechanisms, it was hypothesized that altered serotonergic tone might be an underlying factor in the etiology of anxiety disorders.

The 5-HT$_{1A}$ Receptor

The development of specific pharmacological ligands led to the identification of multiple 5-HT receptor subtypes (Hoyer et al. 2002). The 5-HT$_{1A}$ receptor is the most extensively studied 5-HT receptor for several reasons: 1) identification of the selective agonists, including 8-OH-DPAT (Hamon et al. 1984) and the azapirones, and specific receptor antagonists (Fletcher et al. 1996) has allowed for strict pharmacological classification; 2) it was the first 5-HT receptor to be cloned and sequenced (Fargin et al. 1988; Kobilka et al. 1987); 3) polyclonal antibodies have been generated for subcellular distribution studies in brain (Azmetia et al. 1996; El

Mestikawy et al. 1990); and 4) human, rat, and mouse receptors have been cloned and sequenced (Albert et al. 1998; Charest et al. 1993; Fargin et al. 1988).

Studies utilizing the full agonist [^{3}H]8-OH-DPAT (8-hydroxy-2-[*N*-dipropylamino]-tetralin) and the putative 5-HT_{1A} receptor antagonist ligand [^{3}H]WAY-100635 reveal high levels of specific binding in hippocampus, raphe nuclei, amygdala, hypothalamus, and cortex (Burnet et al. 1997; Palacios et al. 1990). At the subcellular level, the receptor is localized on cell bodies and dendrites of 5-HT-containing neurons projecting to limbic brain regions. In limbic regions receiving input from 5-HT-containing neurons, particularly hippocampus and cortex, 5-HT_{1A} receptors are located predominantly postsynaptically (Palacios et al. 1990; Riad et al. 2000). The high regional density of 5-HT_{1A} receptors in midbrain, hippocampus, and limbic areas of the brain is consistent with the notion that 5-HT neurotransmission modulates mood and anxiety. These brain regions of high density of 5-HT_{1A} receptors control thermoregulation, endocrine function, appetite, aggressive and sexual behavior, and mood. Mice lacking the 5-HT_{1A} receptor gene exhibit various manifestations of anxious behavior (Parks et al. 1998; Pattij et al. 2002). 5-HT_{1A} receptors on 5-HT neurons in midbrain raphe regions modulate release of 5-HT at synapses in forebrain. These somatodendritic autoreceptors control impulse flow (Yocca 1990), synthesis (Yocca 1990), and release (Sharp et al. 1989) of neurotransmitter from ascending 5-HT-containing neurons.

Given the large body of work implicating 5-HT in affective disorders and the role of the 5-HT_{1A} receptor in 5-HT neurotransmission, it is not surprising that drugs targeting this receptor hold interest for the treatment of mood disorders. There is a region-dependent difference in responses to 5-HT_{1A} agonists at pre- and postsynaptic 5-HT_{1A} receptors. This may be attributable to differences in regional receptor reserve (Meller et al. 1990; Yocca et al. 1992). Therefore, the proper degree of agonism at both pre- and postsynaptic 5-HT_{1A} receptors may be critical to achieving anxiolytic efficacy.

History and Development

Buspirone hydrochloride, an azaspirodecanedione derivative, was synthesized in 1968 in the laboratories of Mead Johnson by Wu et al. (1969). Based on positive findings in conditioned-avoidance testing in rats, buspirone was originally studied as a putative antipsychotic agent, but clinical trials failed to demonstrate efficacy in schizophrenia (Sathananthan et al. 1975). Single doses of buspirone had a marked taming effect in aggressive monkeys (Tompkins et al. 1980), and buspirone showed activity in various behavioral models of anxiety (Riblet et al. 1982). Buspirone displaced [^{3}H]spiperone from dopamine D_2 receptors in rat striatal membranes and demonstrated a right shift in binding activity in the presence of guanosine triphosphate (GTP), characteristics of a D_2 agonist (Riblet et al. 1982). Until the subsequent finding of buspirone's high-affinity binding to the newly discovered 5-HT_{1A} receptor some 4 years later, the anxiolytic activity of buspirone was presumed to be dopaminergic.

A Phase II proof-of-concept study in patients with DSM-II (American Psychiatric Association 1968) anxiety disorder demonstrated significant anxiolytic treatment effects of buspirone compared with placebo (Goldberg and Finnerty 1979) and led to its clinical development as an antianxiety agent (Robinson 1991).

Pharmacological Profile

Buspirone is relatively inactive in receptor binding studies in vitro at noradrenergic, cholinergic, and histaminergic sites and does not displace [^{3}H]diazepam or [^{3}H]nitrazepam from the benzodiazepine receptor complex (Riblet et al. 1982). Although buspirone does displace [^{3}H]spiperone from rat striatal membranes at high concentrations (Mennini et al. 1986, 1987), dopamine receptor binding is believed to play no role in either the therapeutic or side effects of buspirone (Eison et al. 1991).

The discovery that nanomolar quantities of buspirone displaced [^{3}H]5-HT from hippocampal membranes (Glaser and Traber 1983) led to elucidation of interactions of buspirone with specific central 5-HT receptors. Buspirone was found to inhibit [^{3}H]5-HT binding to cortical and hippocampal membranes (Skolnick et al. 1985) and to selectively displace [^{3}H]8-OH-DPAT from 5-HT_{1A} receptor binding sites in rat hippocampal membranes with high affinity (24 nM) (Yocca 1990).

The antianxiety properties of buspirone appear to be exerted through its actions at both pre- and postsynaptic 5-HT_{1A} receptors (Eison and Eison 1994; Yocca 1990). At presynaptic 5-HT_{1A} receptors located in the dorsal raphe, buspirone acts as a full agonist, inhibiting neuronal 5-HT synthesis and firing, whereas at postsynaptic receptors in hippocampus and cortex, it functions as a partial agonist. Buspirone differs from benzodiazepines in that it does not affect motor coordination or spontaneous motor activity but does induce the serotonin syndrome in rats (Barrett and Witkin 1991; Eison et al. 1991). Buspirone lacks abuse potential and does not impair psychomotor performance either alone or in combination with ethanol, unlike the benzodiazepines (Smiley 1987; Sussman and Chow 1988).

Of interest, 5-HT_{1A} agonists show antidepressant-like activity in the forced-swim test used as an animal model of depression (Wieland and Lucki 1990). The finding of activity in a preclinical model of depression comports with results from clinical studies of buspirone that indicate antidepressant effects (Rickels et al. 1991; Robinson et al. 1989).

Pharmacokinetics and Mechanism of Action

With oral administration, buspirone undergoes extensive first-pass metabolism by cytochrome P450 3A4 enzymes, with an elimination half-life of 3 to 4 hours (mean) (Gammans and Johnston 1991). Ingestion of food prolongs the elimination half-life of buspirone, as does hepatic and renal impairment. The pharmacokinetics of buspirone in elderly patients do not differ from those in young adults (Gammans et al. 1989).

Buspirone has three metabolites with varying pharmacological activity: 5-hydroxybuspirone (5-OH-Bu), 8-hydroxybuspirone (8-OH-Bu), and 1-(2-pyrimidinyl) piperazine (1-PP). It is postulated that unwanted noradrenergic effects of 1-PP may be deleterious in patients experiencing benzodiazepine withdrawal or panic attacks.

Conversion of buspirone to the metabolite 6-hydroxybuspirone (6-OH-Bu) has now been identified as the predominant metabolic pathway in the hepatic clearance of buspirone (Zhu et al. 2005). Plasma levels of 6-OH-Bu are 40-fold greater than those of buspirone in humans (Dockens et al. 2006). In vitro, 6-OH-Bu has high affinity (25 nM) and partial agonist activity for the 5-HT_{1A} receptor; in vivo, it exhibits anxiolytic activity (Robinson et al. 2009). The pharmacokinetics of 6-OH-Bu are similar to those of buspirone, except that bioavailability is greater (19% for 6-OH-Bu vs. 1.4% for buspirone; Wong et al. 2007). 6-OH-Bu demonstrates in vivo occupancy of 5-HT_{1A} receptors (Wong et al. 2007). These findings suggest that 6-OH-Bu contributes significantly to the therapeutic effect of buspirone.

It appears that the anxiolytic effects of buspirone are mediated by its actions on 5-HT receptors in the limbic system (Eison and Eison 1994; Yocca 1990). Buspirone has unrelated neuroendocrine effects. 5-HT_{1A} receptors regulate neuroendocrine hormones, such as growth hormone, adrenocorticotropic hormone (ACTH) release, and corticosterone (Gilbert et al. 1988; Pan and Gilbert 1992; Van de Kar et al. 1985). Buspirone, ipsapirone, and gepirone all increase plasma cortisol, prolactin, and growth hormone and decrease body temperature (Cowen et al. 1990; Meltzer et al. 1991). Buspirone stimulation of prolactin and corticosterone secretion in the rat is enhanced by pretreatment with pCPA, whereas spiperone inhibits buspirone-induced increases in corticosterone secretion (Meltzer et al. 1991). Pindolol, a 5-HT_{1A} antagonist, does not block the buspirone-induced increase in prolactin (Meltzer et al. 1991). These findings suggest that the neuroendocrine effects of buspirone are complex, exhibiting pharmacological properties indicative of both a dopamine antagonist and a 5-HT_{1A} agonist.

Switching From Benzodiazepine Therapy to Buspirone

Therapeutic response to buspirone differs significantly in anxious patients naive to benzodiazepine treatment compared with patients previously treated with a benzodiazepine (DeMartinis et al. 2000; Schweizer and Rickels 1986). Meta-analysis of placebo-controlled efficacy trials of buspirone revealed that generalized anxiety disorder (GAD) patients with either no prior benzodiazepine treatment or temporally remote benzodiazepine treatment (>6 months previously) improved more with buspirone therapy than did patients recently treated with a benzodiazepine. This difference in response may reflect an unrecognized benzodiazepine withdrawal syndrome (possibly exacerbated by 1-PP). Patients previously treated with benzodiazepines may be preconditioned by the benzodiazepines' euphoriant and sedating properties and benefit when benzodiazepine treatment is reinstituted due to amelioration of an unrecognized (subclinical) withdrawal syndrome.

Indications and Efficacy

Generalized Anxiety Disorder

The clinical development program of buspirone as an anxiolytic agent was undertaken after positive findings in a placebo-controlled proof-of-concept study in anxious patients (Goldberg and Finnerty 1979). In a series of Phase III placebo-controlled clinical trials comparing buspirone and diazepam, the efficacy of these two anxiolytics was comparable in patients fulfilling diagnostic criteria for DSM-II anxiety neurosis (Boehm et al. 1990a; Goldberg and Finnerty 1982; Rickels et al. 1982).

By the time the U.S. Food and Drug Administration (FDA) granted marketing approval of buspirone in 1986, the newer DSM classification system, DSM-III (American Psychiatric Association 1980), had replaced anxiety neurosis with the diagnostic category of GAD. Analyses of Hamilton Anxiety Scale (Ham-A; Hamilton 1959) and other symptom ratings were consistent with a diagnosis of DSM-III GAD, so buspirone received FDA-approved labeling for this clinical indication.

Buspirone was noted to have a slightly slower onset of therapeutic effect than the benzodiazepines (Enkelmann 1991; Pecknold et al. 1989; Rickels 1990). This slower onset of effect was attributable to differences between buspirone and benzodiazepines in early relief of somatic anxiety but not psychic anxiety. It was postulated that lack of sedation with buspirone contributed to a perception of more gradual onset of anxiolysis, because relief of somatic anxiety, particularly insomnia, was only manifest with buspirone treatment after psychic anxiety symptoms had abated, whereas the immediate sedating properties of benzodiazepines accounted for a perception of faster onset of therapeutic benefit. A similar slower onset of effectiveness in anxiety disorders occurs with imipramine (Rickels et al. 1993) and selective serotonin reuptake inhibitor (SSRI) treatment (Rickels et al. 2003).

A longer-term (6-month) double-blind comparative trial of buspirone and benzodiazepines found a similar slower onset of anxiolytic effect with buspirone compared with clorazepate during the first 4 weeks of treatment (Rickels et al. 1988). However, with ongoing treatment, the therapeutic response to the two drugs was similar. On double-blind termination of treatment after 6 months, patients who stopped clorazepate abruptly relapsed during a 4-week observation period, whereas the buspirone group experienced no symptom changes. These findings confirmed the observation of others (Fontaine et al. 1984; Noyes et al. 1988) that rapid return of symptoms on discontinuation of clorazepate is attributable to a benzodiazepine withdrawal syndrome and not to recrudescence of symptoms of the underlying anxiety disorder, because this did not occur with abrupt discontinuation of buspirone.

Acute treatment of chronically anxious patients is often best managed initially with a benzodiazepine; however, longer-term use of a benzodiazepine can lead to physical dependence and symptom chronicity. For this reason, some patient populations are inappropriate for benzodiazepine therapy due to history of substance abuse or risk of cognitive impairment. When initiating therapy with buspirone, one should inform the patient that it is less sedating, with a gradual onset of action. Patients can be reassured that buspirone will not lead to physical dependence or withdrawal symptoms on discontinuation and will not impair cognition or ability to acquire new coping skills (Rickels and Schweizer 1990).

Long-term follow-up at 40 months of patients who completed a prior 6-month controlled trial comparing buspirone and clorazepate revealed that none of the buspirone-treated patients required anxiolytic medication, whereas more than 50% of patients originally treated with clorazepate still required benzodiazepine therapy (Rickels and Schweizer 1990). The therapeutic advantages of buspirone treatment in elderly anxious patients include the fact the drug both is nonsedating and spares cognitive and memory functions. Buspirone has been studied in elderly patients with anxiety symptoms in a double-blind, placebo-controlled trial and shown to be safe and effective (Boehm et al. 1990b). Meta-analyses of several multicenter trials of buspirone in elderly patients also indicated that the drug is very safe and well tolerated by older patients (Ritchie and Cox 1993; Robinson et al. 1988).

Mixed Anxiety-Depression and Major Depressive Disorder

It was observed in early trials of patients with anxiety disorder and subsyndromal depression that depressive symptoms improved significantly during buspirone treatment (Feighner et al. 1982; Goldberg and Finnerty 1979). This finding generated interest in the potential antidepressant properties of buspirone because of the high comorbidity of GAD and major depressive disorder (MDD) (Brown and Barlow 1992). It has been suggested that GAD and MDD may represent differing clinical manifestations of a single underlying diathesis. Roy-Byrne (2008) reviewed the relationship of MDD and GAD and their therapy.

Several placebo-controlled trials of buspirone have been conducted in patients with MDD and significant associated anxiety symptoms (Rickels et al. 1991; Robinson et al. 1990). Patients with MDD were eligible for inclusion in these studies if their Hamilton Rating Scale for Depression (Ham-D; Hamilton 1960) and Ham-A scores were 18 or greater and 15 or greater, respectively. The daily dosage in these dosage titration studies ranged up to a maximum of buspirone 90 mg/day (mean of ~50 mg/day). Buspirone treatment was found to be superior to placebo treatment, with a global response rate based on a Clinical Global Impressions–Improvement (CGI-I) scale score of 70% for buspirone and 35% for placebo (Rickels et al. 1991). In a subsequent placebo-controlled study involving 177 geriatric depressed outpatients, Schweizer et al. (1998) compared buspirone and imipramine treatment for 8 weeks. There was a statistically significant treatment effect for both buspirone (mean daily dose of ~50 mg) and imipramine (mean daily dose of ~90 mg) compared with placebo treatment.

Open-label augmentation of SSRI treatment of partially responding depressed patients leads to further improvement (Dimitriou and Dimitriou 1998; Gonul et al. 1999; Jacobsen 1991; Landren et al. 1998). These findings were confirmed in a report of the Sequenced Treatment Alternatives to Relieve Depression (STAR*D) program. Patients who initially failed an adequate therapeutic trial with an SSRI responded when their medication was augmented with either buspirone or bupropion (Trivedi et al. 2006).

Nonapproved Clinical Indications

Potential clinical indications for buspirone treatment unapproved by the FDA were reviewed by Rickels et al. (2003); only a few studies are mentioned here. Two small double-blind clinical trials indicated modest efficacy of buspirone over placebo in the symptomatic treatment of postmenopausal syndrome (Brown et al. 1990; Rickels et al. 1989). Several placebo-controlled trials showed that smoking cessation is facilitated by buspirone therapy (Hilleman et al. 1992; West et al. 1991); its main effect, however, is in smokers who are also highly anxious (Cinciripini et al. 1995). Buspirone has been assessed in a few double-blind, placebo-controlled trials involving anxious outpatients with coexisting alcohol use disorders and found to be efficacious (Rickels et al. 2003). Because buspirone lacks abuse potential and has negligible additive effects on psychomotor and cognitive functions when coadministered with alcohol (Mattila et al. 1982), it has therapeutic benefit in the management of alcohol abuse and dependence.

Dosage and Administration

The recommended dosage of buspirone for the treatment of GAD is 15–20 mg/day initially, prescribed in divided doses, with increases to 30 mg/day if indicated and a maximum dosage of 60 mg/day. It should be mentioned that in the double-blind MDD trials (described earlier), the maximal dosage was 90 mg/day. Thus, higher dosages than those prescribed for anxiety disorders may be required in the treatment of MDD, either as monotherapy or as augmentation of an SSRI.

Side Effects and Toxicology

Newton et al. (1986), summarizing data from 17 clinical trials, reported the incidence of frequently reported adverse events during buspirone treatment: dizziness (12%), drowsiness (10%), nausea (8%), headache (6%), nervousness (5%), fatigue (4%), insomnia (3%), light-headedness (3%), dry mouth (3%), and excitement (2%).

Buspirone lacks abuse potential, unlike alcohol and benzodiazepines (Balster 1991). Psychomotor function studies, including evaluation of complex motor driving skills and memory tasks, document an absence of impairment with buspirone administration, unlike the case with alcohol and the benzodiazepines (Boulenger et al. 1989; Greenblatt et al. 1994; Lucki et al. 1987; Smiley and Moskowitz 1986). Since buspirone's use in clinical practice, no deaths attributable to buspirone overdose alone have occurred to our knowledge. Buspirone remains an unusually safe and well-tolerated medication with no abuse liability.

Buspirone does not inhibit P450 enzymes, although it causes modest elevations of haloperidol and cyclosporin A levels. It has few pharmacodynamic interactions with other psychotropic drugs, except for a potential risk of serotonin syndrome with monoamine oxidase inhibitors.

Conclusion

Discovery of the 5-HT_{1A} receptor was instrumental in linking modulation of 5-HT neurotransmission to anxiety symptoms. Buspirone, a partial agonist of the 5-HT_{1A} receptor, is the first of a new class of antianxiety agents approved for treatment of GAD and anxiety with associated depressive symptoms.

References

Albert PR, Morris SJ, Ghahremani MH, et al: A putative α-helical Gβγ-coupling domain in the second intracellular loop of the 5-HT1A receptor. Ann N Y Acad Sci 861:146–161, 1998

American Psychiatric Association: Diagnostic and Statistical Manual of Mental Disorders, 2nd Edition. Washington, DC, American Psychiatric Association, 1968

American Psychiatric Association: Diagnostic and Statistical Manual of Mental Disorders, 3rd Edition. Washington, DC, American Psychiatric Association, 1980

Azmetia EC, Gannon PJ, Kheck NM, et al: Cellular localization of the 5-HT1A receptor in primate brain neurons and glial cells. Neuropsychopharmacology 14:35–46, 1996

Balster RL: Preclinical studies of the abuse potential of buspirone, in Buspirone: Mechanisms and Clinical Aspects. Edited by Tunnicliff G, Eison AS, Taylor DP. New York, Academic Press, 1991, pp 97–107

Barrett JE, Witkin JM: Buspirone in animal models of anxiety, in Buspirone: Mechanisms and Clinical Aspects. Edited by Tunnicliff G, Eison AS, Taylor DP. New York, Academic Press, 1991, pp 37–79

Boehm C, Placchi M, Stallone R, et al: A double-blind comparison of buspirone, clobazam, and placebo in patients with anxiety treated in a general practice setting. J Clin Psychopharmacol 10:385–425, 1990a

Boehm C, Robinson DS, Gammans RE, et al: Buspirone therapy in anxious elderly patients: a controlled clinical trial. J Clin Psychopharmacology 10 (suppl):47–51, 1990b

Boulenger JP, Gram LF, Jolicouer FB, et al: Repeated administration of buspirone: absence of pharmacodynamic or pharmacokinetic interaction with triazolam. Hum Psychopharmacol 8:117–124, 1989

Brown CS, Ling FW, Farmer RG, et al: Buspirone in the treatment of premenstrual syndrome. Drug Ther Bull 8 (suppl):112–116, 1990

Brown TA, Barlow D: Comorbidity among anxiety disorders: implications for treatment and DSM-IV. J Consult Clin Psychol 60:835–844, 1992

Burnet PW, Eastwood SL, Harrison PJ: [3H]WAY-100635 for 5-HT1A receptor autoradiography in human brain: a comparison with [3H]8-OH-DPAT and demonstration of increased binding in the frontal cortex in schizophrenia. Neurochem Int 30:565–574, 1997

Charest A, Wainer BH, Albert PR: Cloning and differentiation-induced expression of a murine serotonin1A receptor in a septal cell line. J Neurosci 13:5164–5171, 1993

Cinciripini PM, Lapitsky L, Seay S, et al: A placebo-controlled evaluation of the effects of buspirone on smoking cessation: differences between high- and low-anxiety smokers. J Clin Psychopharmacol 15:182–191, 1995

Cowen PJ, Anderson IM, Grahame-Smith DG: Neuroendocrine effects of azapirones. J Clin Psychopharmacol 10 (suppl):21S–25S, 1990

DeMartinis N, Rynn M, Rickels K, et al: Prior benzodiazepine use and buspirone response in the treatment of generalized anxiety disorder. J Clin Psychiatry 61:91–94, 2000

Dimitriou EC, Dimitriou CE: Buspirone augmentation of antidepressant therapy. J Clin Psychopharmacol 18:465–469, 1998

Dockens RC, Salazar DE, Fulmor E, et al: Pharmacokinetics of a newly identified active metabolite of buspirone after administration of buspirone over its therapeutic range. J Clin Pharmacol 46:1308–1312, 2006

Eison AS, Eison MS: Serotonergic mechanisms in anxiety. Prog Neuropsychopharmacol Biol Psychiatry 18:47–62, 1994

Eison AS, Yocca FD, Taylor DP: Mechanism of action of buspirone: current perspectives, in Buspirone: Mechanisms and Clinical Aspects. Edited by Tunnicliff G, Eison AS, Taylor DP. New York, Academic Press, 1991, pp 3–17

El Mestikawy S, Riad M, Laport AM: Production of specific anti-rat 5-HT1A receptor antibodies in rabbits injected with a synthetic peptide. Neurosci Lett 118:189–192, 1990

Enkelmann R: Alprazolam vs buspirone in the treatment of outpatients with generalized anxiety disorder. Psychopharmacology 105:428–432, 1991

Fargin A, Raymond JR, Lohse MJ, et al: The genomic clone G-21 which resembles a β-adrenergic receptor sequence encodes the 5-HT1A receptor. Nature 335:358–360, 1988

Feighner JP, Merideth CH, Hendrickson GA: A double-blind comparison of buspirone and diazepam in outpatients with generalized anxiety disorder. J Clin Psychiatry 43:103–107, 1982

Fletcher A, Forster EA, Bill DJ, et al: Electrophysiology, biochemical, neurohormonal and behavioral studies with WAY-100635, a potent, selective and silent 5-HT1A receptor antagonist. Behav Brain Res 73:337–353, 1996

Fontaine R, Chouinard G, Annable L: Rebound anxiety in anxious patients after abrupt withdrawal of benzodiazepine treatment. Am J Psychiatry 141:848–852, 1984

Gammans RE, Johnston RE: Metabolism, pharmacokinetics, and toxicology of buspirone, in Buspirone: Mechanisms and Clinical Aspects. Edited by Tunnicliff G, Eison AS, Taylor DP. New York, Academic Press, 1991, pp 233–260

Gammans RE, Westrick ML, Shea JP, et al: Pharmacokinetics of buspirone in elderly subjects. J Clin Pharmacol 29:72–78, 1989

Gilbert F, Dourish CT, Brazell C: Relationship of increased food intake and plasma ACTH levels to 5-HT1A receptor activation in rats. Psychoneuroendocrinology 13:471–478, 1988

Glaser HL, Traber J: Buspirone: action on serotonergic receptors in calf hippocampus. Eur J Pharmacol 88:137–138, 1983

Goldberg HL, Finnerty R: The comparative efficacy of buspirone and diazepam in the treatment of anxiety. Am J Psychiatry 136:1184–1187, 1979

Goldberg HL, Finnerty R: Comparison of buspirone in two separate studies. J Clin Psychiatry 43:87–91, 1982

Gonul AS, Oguz A, Yabanoglu I, et al: Buspirone and pindolol in augmentation therapy of treatment-resistant depression. Eur J Neuropsychopharmacology 9 (suppl):S215, 1999

Greenblatt DJ, Harmatz JS, Gouthro TA, et al: Distinguishing a benzodiazepine agonist (triazolam) from a nonagonist anxiolytic (buspirone) by electroencephalography: kinetic studies. Clin Pharmacol Ther 56:100–111, 1994

Hamilton M: The assessment of anxiety states by rating. J Med Psychol 32:50–55, 1959

Hamilton M: A rating scale for depression. J Neurol Neurosurg Psychiatry 23:56–62, 1960

Hamon M, Bourgoin S, Gozlan H, et al: Biochemical evidence for the 5-HT agonist properties of PAT (8-hydroxy-2-(di-n-propylamino)tetralin) in the rat brain. Eur J Pharmacol 100:263–276, 1984

Hilleman DE, Mohiuddin SM, Del Core MG, et al: Effect of buspirone on withdrawal symptoms associated with smoking cessation. Arch Gen Psychiatry 152:73–77, 1992

Hoyer D, Hannon JP, Martin GR: Molecular, pharmacological and functional diversity of 5-HT receptors. Pharmacol Biochem Behav 71:533–554, 2002

Jacobsen FM: Possible augmentation of antidepressant response by buspirone. J Clin Psychiatry 52:217–220, 1991

Kobilka BK, Frielle T, Collins S, et al: An intronless gene encoding a potential member of the family of receptors coupled to guanine nucleotide regulatory proteins. Nature 329:75–79, 1987

Landren M, Bjorling G, Agren H, et al: A randomized, double-blind, placebo-controlled trial of buspirone in combination with an SSRI in patients with treatment-refractory depression. J Clin Psychiatry 59:664–668, 1998

Lucki I, Rickels K, Giesecke A, et al: Differential effects of the anxiolytic drugs, diazepam and buspirone on memory function. Br J Clin Pharmacol 23:207–211, 1987

Mattila MJ, Aranko K, Seppala T: Acute effects of buspirone and alcohol on psychomotor skills. J Clin Psychiatry 43:56–60, 1982

Meller E, Goldstein M, Bohmaker K: Receptor reserve for 5-hydroxtryptamine1A-mediated inhibition of serotonin synthesis: possible relationship to the anxiolytic properties of 5-hydroxytryptamine1A agonists. Mol Pharmacol 37:231–237, 1990

Meltzer HY, Gudelsky GA, Lowy MT, et al: Neuroendocrine effects of buspirone: mediation by dopaminergic and serotonergic mechanisms, in Buspirone: Mechanisms and Clinical Aspects. Edited by Tunnicliff G, Eison AS, Taylor DP. New York, Academic Press, 1991, pp 177–192

Mennini T, Gobbi M, Ponzio F, et al: Neurochemical effects of buspirone in rat hippocampus: evidence for selective activation of 5HT neurons. Arch Int Pharmacodyn Ther 279:40–49, 1986

Mennini T, Caccia C, Garattini S: Mechanism of action of anxiolytic drugs. Prog Drug Res 31:315–347, 1987

Newton RE, Maruncyz JD, Alderdice MT, et al: Review of the side effect profile of buspirone. Am J Med 80 (suppl):17–21, 1986

Noyes R, Garvey MJ, Cooke BL, et al: Benzodiazepine withdrawal: a review of the evidence. J Clin Psychiatry 49:383–389, 1988

Palacios JM, Waeber C, Hoyer D, et al: Distribution of serotonin receptors. Ann N Y Acad Sci 600:36–52, 1990

Pan LH, Gilbert F: Activation of 5-HT1A receptor subtype in the paraventricular nuclei of the hypothalamus induces CRH and ACTH release in the rat. Neuroendocrinology 56:797–802, 1992

Parks CL, Robinson PS, Sibille E, et al: Increased anxiety of mice lacking the serotonin1A receptor. Proc Natl Acad Sci U S A 95:10734–10739, 1998

Pattij T, Groenick L, Hijzen TH, et al: Autonomic changes associated with enhanced anxiety in 5-HT1A receptor knockout mice. Neuropsychopharmacology 27:380–390, 2002

Pecknold JC, Matas M, Howarth BG, et al: Evaluation of buspirone as an antianxiety agent: buspirone and diazepam versus placebo. Am J Psychiatry 34:766–771, 1989

Riad M, Garcia S, Watkins KC, et al: Somatodendritic localization of 5-HT1A and pre-terminal axonal localization of 5-HT1B serotonin receptors in adult rat brain. J Comp Neurol 417:181–194, 2000

Riblet LA, Taylor DP, Eison MS, et al: Pharmacology and neurochemistry of buspirone. J Clin Psychiatry 43:81–86, 1982

Rickels K: Buspirone in clinical practice. J Clin Psychiatry 51 (suppl):51–54, 1990

Rickels K, Schweizer E: The clinical course and long-term management of generalized anxiety disorder. J Clin Psychopharmacol 19:101S–105S, 1990

Rickels K, Weisman K, Norstad M, et al: Buspirone and diazepam in anxiety: a controlled study. J Clin Psychiatry 43:81–86, 1982

Rickels K, Schweizer E, Csanalosi I, et al: Long-term treatment of anxiety and risk of withdrawal. Arch Gen Psychiatry 45:444–450, 1988

Rickels K, Freeman E, Sondheimer S: Buspirone in treatment of premenstrual syndrome. Lancet 1(8641):777, 1989

Rickels K, Amsterdam JD, Clary C, et al: Buspirone in major depression: a controlled study. J Clin Psychiatry 52:34–38, 1991

Rickels K, Downing R, Schweizer E, et al: Antidepressants for the treatment of generalized anxiety disorder: a placebo-controlled comparison of imipramine, trazodone, and diazepam. Arch Gen Psychiatry 50:884–895, 1993

Rickels K, Khalid-Kahn S, Rynn M: Buspirone in the treatment of anxiety disorders, in Anxiety Disorders. Edited by Nutt DJ, Ballenger JC. Oxford, UK, Blackwell Publishing, 2003, pp 381–397

Ritchie LD, Cox J: A multicenter study of buspirone in the treatment of anxiety disorders in the elderly. Br J Clin Res 4:131–139, 1993

Robinson DS: Buspirone in the treatment of anxiety, in Buspirone: Mechanisms and Clinical Aspects. Edited by Tunnicliff G, Eison AS, Taylor DP. New York, Academic Press, 1991, pp 3–17

Robinson DS, Napoliello MJ, Schenk J: The safety and usefulness of buspirone as an anxiolytic drug in elderly versus young patients. Clin Ther 10:740–746, 1988

Robinson DS, Alms DR, Shrotriya RC, et al: Serotonergic anxiolytics and treatment of depression. Psychopathology 22 (suppl):27–36, 1989

Robinson DS, Rickels K, Feighner J, et al: Clinical effects of the 5-HT1A partial agonists in depression: a composite analysis of buspirone in the treatment of depression. J Clin Psychopharmacol 10:67S–76S, 1990

Robinson DS, Rickels K, Yocca FD: Buspirone and gepirone, in The American Psychiatric Publishing Textbook of Psychopharmacology, 4th Edition. Edited by Schatzberg AF, Nemeroff CB. Arlington, VA, American Psychiatric Publishing, 2009, pp 487–501

Roy-Byrne PP: Comorbid MDD and GAD: revisiting the concept of "anxious depression." Psychiatric Times Supplement 1 (Perspectives in Psychiatry: A Clinical Update; August):25–30, 2008

Sathananthan GL, Sanghvi I, Phillips N, et al: Correlation between neuroleptic potential and stereotypy. Curr Ther Res 18:701–705, 1975

Schweizer E, Rickels K: Failure of buspirone to manage benzodiazepine withdrawal. Am J Psychiatry 143:12, 1986

Schweizer E, Rickels K, Hassman, et al: Buspirone and imipramine for the treatment of major depression in the elderly. J Clin Psychiatry 59:175–183, 1998

Sharp T, Bramwell SR, Grahame-Smith DG: 5-HT1A agonists reduce 5-hydroxytryptamine release in rat hippocampus in vivo as determined by brain microdialysis. Br J Pharmacol 96:283–290, 1989

Skolnick P, Weissman BA, Youdim MBH: Monoaminergic involvement in the pharmacologic actions of buspirone. Br J Pharmacol 86:637–644, 1985

Smiley A: Effects of minor tranquilizers and antidepressants on psychomotor performance. J Clin Psychiatry 49 (suppl):22–28, 1987

Smiley A, Moskowitz H: The effect of chronically administered buspirone and diazepam on driver steering control. Am J Med 80:22–29, 1986

Sussman N, Chow JC: Current issues in benzodiazepine use of anxiety disorders. Psychiatr Ann 18:139–145, 1988

Tompkins EC, Clemento AJ, Taylor DP, et al: Inhibition of aggressive behavior in rhesus monkeys by buspirone. Res Commun Psychol Psychiatr Res 5:337–352, 1980

Trivedi M, Fava M, Wiesnewski SR, et al: Medication augmentation after failure of SSRIs for depression. N Engl J Med 354:1243–1252, 2006

Van de Kar LD, Karteszi M, Bethea CL, et al: Serotonergic stimulation of prolactin and corticosterone secretion is mediated by different pathways from the mediobasal hypothalamus. Neuroendocrinology 41:380–384, 1985

West R, Hajek P, McNeill A: Effect of buspirone on cigarette withdrawal symptoms and short-term abstinence rates in a smokers' clinic. Psychopharmacology 104:91–96, 1991

Wieland S, Lucki I: Antidepressant-like activity of 5-HT1A agonists measured with the forced swim test. Psychopharmacology 101:497–504, 1990

Wong H, Dockens RA, Pajor L, et al: 6-Hydroxybuspirone is a major active metabolite of buspirone: assessment of pharmacokinetics and 5-hydroxytryptamine1A receptor occupancy in rats. Drug Metab Dispos 35:1387–1392, 2007

Wu YH, Smith KR, Rayburn JW, et al: Psychosedative agents: N-(4-phenyl-1-piperazinylalkyl)-substituted cyclic imides. J Med Chem 12:876–881, 1969

Yocca FD: Neurochemistry and neurophysiology of buspirone and gepirone: interactions at presynaptic and postsynaptic 5-HT1A receptors. J Clin Psychiatry 10:6S–12S, 1990

Yocca FD, Iben L, Meller E: Lack of apparent receptor reserve at postsynaptic 5-HT1A receptors negatively coupled to adenylyl cyclase activity in rat hippocampal membranes. Mol Pharmacol 41:1066–1072, 1992

Zhu M, Zhao W, Jimenez H, et al: Cytochrome P450 3A-mediated metabolism of buspirone in human liver microsomes. Drug Metab Dispos 33:500–507, 2005

Antipsychotics

CHAPTER 15

Classic Antipsychotic Medications

Henry A. Nasrallah, M.D.

Rajiv Tandon, M.D.

History and Discovery

Prior to the introduction of classic antipsychotic medications in the 1950s, treatment for psychotic disorders primarily consisted of institutional confinement and supportive care with minimal control of psychotic symptoms. The discovery of chlorpromazine, the first of the "classic" antipsychotics, was serendipitous and owes much to the observations of a French surgeon, Henri Laborit, who noted that chlorpromazine, when used as an adjunct to anesthesia, calmed patients significantly following surgery. Laborit recommended its use to two French psychiatrists, Jean Delay and Pierre Deniker, who used it successfully in psychotic patients. Heinz Lehmann was the first to use chlorpromazine in North America (in Montreal, Canada). In the early 1960s, the first large-scale placebo-controlled trials were conducted within the U.S. Veterans Administration system.

After the successes of chlorpromazine, numerous other phenothiazines were synthesized by modifying the side chains on the phenothiazine rings. Subsequently, several nonphenothiazine antipsychotics, such as haloperidol, were introduced. The last of these drugs approved by the U.S. Food and Drug Administration (FDA) was molindone, introduced in 1975. Of 51 classic antipsychotic drugs (representing 8 different chemical classes) available in the world, 10 are currently available in the United States.

The ability of chlorpromazine and other conventional antipsychotics to suppress psychotic symptoms (delusions, hallucinations, and bizarre behavior) had a profound impact on chronically hospitalized psychiatric populations worldwide. Massive numbers of psychiatric patients were discharged from state hospitals to the community. This period of deinstitutionalization led to a decrease in the number of patients in state and county mental hospitals in the United States from 559,000 in 1955 to 338,000 in 1970 to 107,000 in 1988, an 80% decrease over 30 years. Initially, this led to enthusiasm about the possibility that patients with schizophrenia and other psychoses would be able to function well in the community. However, it soon became apparent that improvement with antipsychotic treatment was incomplete. In addition, poor treatment adherence—with subsequent relapses—led to frequent rehospitalization (i.e., the "revolving door" phenomenon).

As psychiatrists began using chlorpromazine, they observed that treated patients frequently manifested signs and symptoms of parkinsonism. Along with other side effects such as dystonia and akathisia, these symptoms are collectively referred to as *extrapyramidal side effects* (EPS). Because of the high prevalence of these movement disorders in patients receiving antipsychotic treatment, many psychiatrists believed EPS to be an unavoidable accompaniment of antipsychotic action; in fact, the onset of some EPS was considered to indicate the minimal effective antipsychotic dose (i.e., the "neuroleptic threshold"). The first report of persistent orobuccal movements (later labeled *tardive dyskinesia*) came from France in 1959. The pervasiveness of debilitating short-term and long-term motor side effects associated with classic antipsychotic drugs led to a search for agents that would be at least as efficacious but without the risk of EPS.

Clozapine, a dibenzodiazepine synthesized in 1959, was the first antipsychotic drug without EPS (i.e., atypical). It was initially marketed in Europe in 1972 but was withdrawn in some countries in 1975 after several reports of fatalities secondary to agranulocytosis. Clozapine was not introduced in the United States until 1989, after convincing studies demonstrated its efficacy in neuroleptic-refractory schizophrenia. Other atypical agents (also referred to as second-generation antipsychotics [SGAs]) have been launched in the past 15 years and are reported to be associated with lower levels of EPS and a broader spectrum of efficacy; of the 14 SGAs currently being marketed, 10 are available in the United States (see Chapters 16–24 in this volume). Since the introduction of these newer agents, use of the classic antipsychotics (also referred to as traditional, conventional, or first-generation antipsychotics [FGAs]) has declined, especially in the United States—FGAs currently aggregate less than 10% of all antipsychotic prescriptions in the country. Results of several government-sponsored effectiveness studies—for example, the Clinical Antipsychotic Trials of Intervention Effectiveness (CATIE)—in the past decade have challenged the prevailing worldview of the greater effectiveness of SGAs over FGAs and have reinvigorated interest in the utility and clinical applicability of classic antipsychotics.

Structure-Activity Relations

Phenothiazines

Members of the phenothiazine class of classic antipsychotics share the same basic phenothiazine ring but differ in substitutions at both their R1 and R2 positions (Figure 15–1). Based on the side chain attached to the nitrogen atom in the middle ring (R1), the phenothiazines are further subdivided into three subtypes: aliphatic, piperidine, and piperazine phenothiazines.

Aliphatic Phenothiazines

The aliphatic phenothiazines share a dimethylamide substitution at their tenth carbon. Chlorpromazine (Thorazine or Largactil) is the prototypical member of this class and remains the aliphatic phenothiazine most widely used throughout the world. With a chlorine atom attached to its second carbon, chlorpromazine is heavily sedating because of its high level of anticholinergic, anti-α-adrenergic, and antihistaminergic actions.

Piperidine Phenothiazines

Piperidine phenothiazines—for example, thioridazine (Mellaril) and its metabolite, mesoridazine (Serentil)—are named for the presence of a piperidine ring at their tenth carbon. Although members of this group have similar efficacy and side effects compared with aliphatic phenothiazines, they are notable for having a less potent effect on nigrostriatal dopamine$_2$ (D_2) receptors and a higher level of anticholinergic activity; consequently they are associated with a lower frequency of EPS. The use of these agents has been virtually extinguished by a black box warning about significant QTc prolongation that was added to their product label in 2000.

Piperazine Phenothiazines

With a substitution of a piperazine group at the tenth carbon of a phenothiazine, the piperazines have greatly increased D_2 blockade and a lower affinity to muscarinic, α-adrenergic, and histaminergic receptors. Some of the most potent conventional antipsychotics available in the United States, including fluphenazine (Prolixin), perphenazine (Trilafon), and trifluoperazine (Stelazine), belong to this class. The well-known antiemetic prochlorperazine (Compazine) is also part of this class; although approved for the treatment of psychosis, it is rarely utilized as an antipsychotic.

Thioxanthenes

Structurally and pharmacologically similar to the phenothiazines, the thioxanthenes also differ widely in their pharmacological profiles based on similar side-chain substitutions (see Figure 15–1). For instance, chlorprothixene shares the same dimethylamide and chloride substitution as chlorpromazine, with which it also shares its pharmacological profile. Thiothixene (Navane) has both a piperazine side chain and a strongly electrophilic substitution [$SO_2N(CH_3)CH_3$], thus sharing the pharmacological profile of the piperazines.

Butyrophenones

The butyrophenone class has a piperidine ring with a three-carbon chain ending in a carbonyl-substituted p-fluorobenzene ring. Haloperidol, arguably the best-known classic antipsychotic, is the most widely used member of this class. Haloperidol and other members of this class are strong dopamine receptor antagonists and show little antimuscarinic, antihistaminergic, and antiadrenergic activity.

Dibenzoxazepines

Loxapine, the only FDA-approved agent within the dibenzoxazepine class, is composed of a tricyclic ring structure with a seven-member central ring. It has a piperazine side chain and chlorine at position R2 (see Figure 15–1). It exhibits an intermediate level of D_2 blockade, as well as some serotonin$_2$ (5-HT_2) antagonism. Its side-effect profile is characterized by intermediate sedation and autonomic effects. Loxapine has the distinction of being the most "atypical" of the classic antipsychotics because it is structurally similar to the dibenzodiazepine clozapine. Another notable feature of loxapine is that one of its metabolites, amoxapine, is marketed as an antidepressant.

Dihydroindoles

Molindone is the only member of the dihydroindoles available in the United States. Sharing a similar structure with the indoleamines (see Figure 15–1), such as serotonin, molindone has the distinction of being the only classic antipsychotic not associated with any weight gain or a lowering of the seizure threshold.

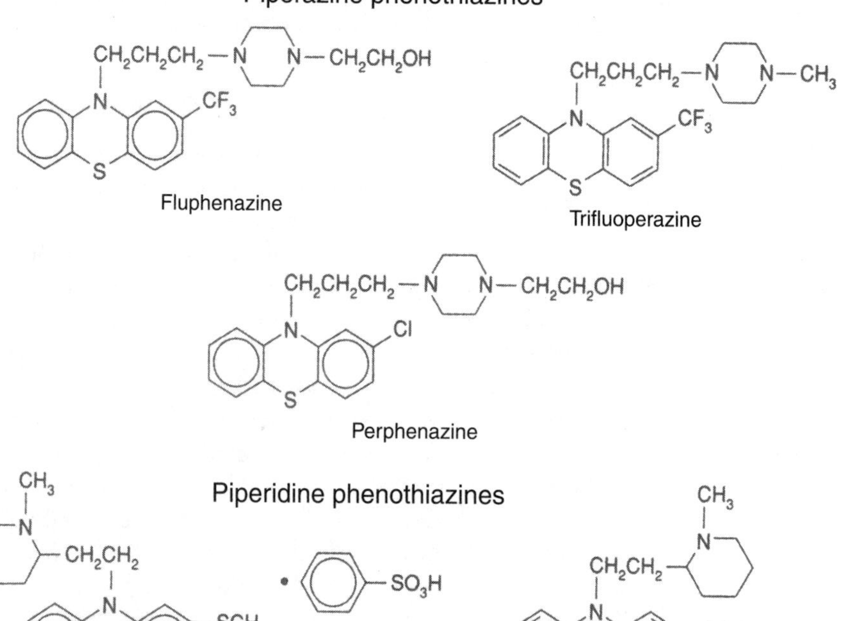

FIGURE 15–1. Chemical structures of various classic antipsychotics.

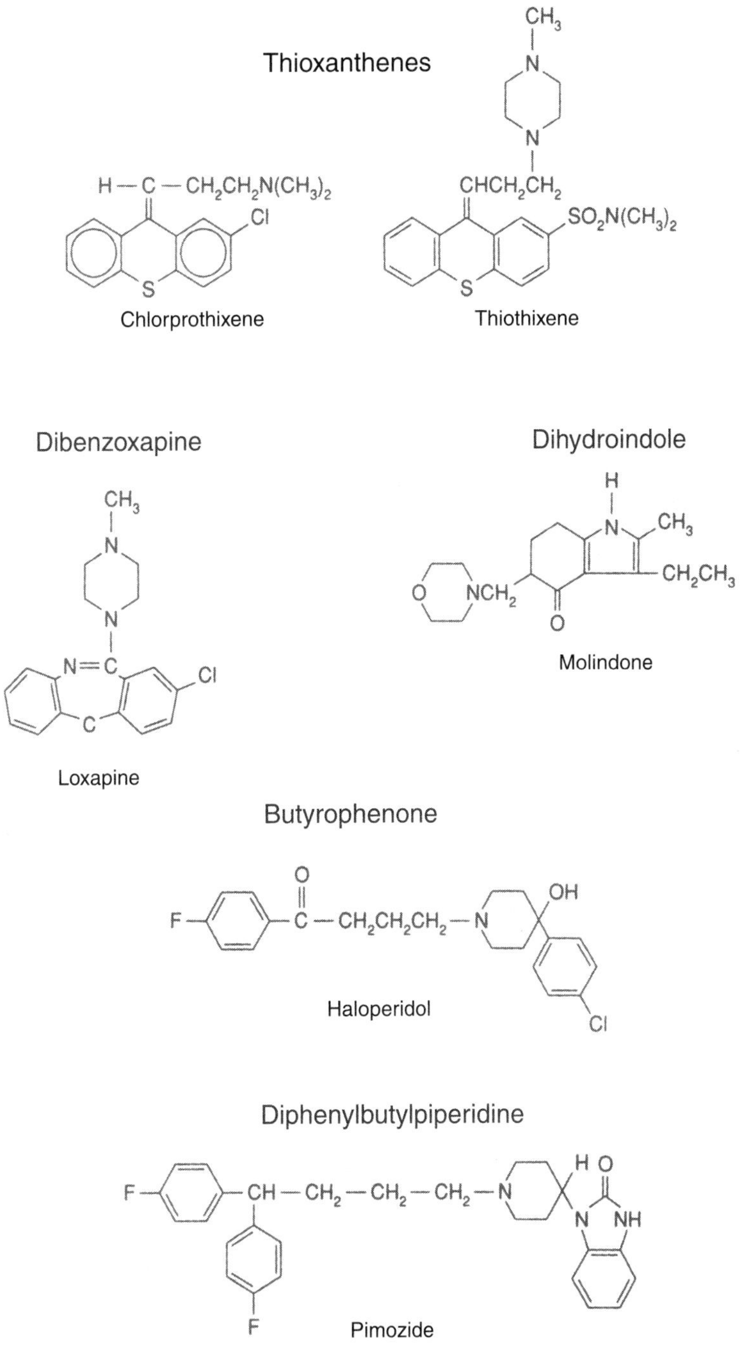

FIGURE 15–1. Chemical structures of various classic antipsychotics (*continued*).

Diphenylbutylpiperidines

Pimozide, the only agent within the diphenylbutylpiperidine class available in the United States, is approved only for the treatment of Tourette's syndrome and has the distinction of possessing the highest selectivity and potency for dopamine D_2 receptors among the conventional antipsychotics. It significantly prolongs the QTc interval, and this has limited its utilization. Derived from benperidol, pimozide shares many characteristics of the butyrophenones (see Figure 15–1).

Benzamides and Iminodibenzyl Agents

Sulpiride, the prototypical substituted benzamide, is a relatively selective dopamine D_2 antagonist and lacks significant activity on cholinergic, histaminergic, or noradrenergic receptors. Because of this relative selectivity and a lower propensity to cause EPS, sulpiride is one of the more common classic antipsychotics utilized in Europe. No classic antipsychotic agent from either the benzamide or the iminodibenzyl classes is available in the United States.

Pharmacological Profile

The classic conventional antipsychotic drugs have a multitude of effects on various physiological variables through their actions on different neurotransmitter systems. The antipsychotic effects of these agents are believed to occur primarily through antagonism of D_2-type dopaminergic receptors. Therapeutic and adverse effects of D_2 antagonism have been conceptualized in the context of the major dopaminergic tracts present in the brain, which include the mesocortical, mesolimbic (A10), tuberoinfundibular (A12), and nigrostriatal (A8 and A9) tracts.

The effect of D_2 blockade on the mesolimbic dopaminergic systems is believed to represent the putative mechanism of action of conventional antipsychotics, but D_2 blockade in other tracts is believed to result in a number of adverse cognitive and behavioral side effects. Such side effects are frequently observed in both animals and human subjects. D_2 receptor antagonism in the mesocortical dopaminergic pathway leads to a blunting of cognition (bradyphrenia) and avolition-apathy (sometimes referred to as the *neuroleptic-induced deficit syndrome*), which can be difficult to differentiate from the primary negative symptoms of schizophrenic illness itself.

Blockade of the tuberoinfundibular tract projecting to the hypothalamus and pituitary gland results in multiple neuroendocrine side effects processed through the pituitary gland. Although dopamine is involved in enhancing the release of most pituitary hormones, it is actually responsible for the tonic inhibition of prolactin release. With significant dopaminergic blockade of the tuberoinfundibular tract, prolactin release is no longer prevented, and the release of other pituitary hormones is no longer enhanced. High levels of prolactin combined with decreased levels of follicle-stimulating hormone and luteinizing hormone often result in amenorrhea, galactorrhea, gynecomastia, decreased bone density, impaired libido, and erectile dysfunction.

High levels (exceeding 78%) of D_2 dopaminergic blockade within the nigrostriatal system, which projects to the basal ganglia and caudate, produce some of the most undesirable side effects of conventional antipsychotics. Movement disorders or EPS such as akathisia, rigidity, and hypokinesia were once believed to be necessary "evidence" of a therapeutic antipsychotic dosage. However, the advent of the new-generation antipsychotics that are associated with minimal EPS conclusively dispensed with this misconception. At higher levels of D_2 blockade, one may also observe dystonia, catalepsy, and a rigid, immobile catatonic state.

Classic antipsychotic agents have varying degrees of activity at serotonergic, cholinergic, noradrenergic, histaminergic, and other nondopaminergic receptors. Although it is unclear whether any of these activities contribute to or interfere with their efficacy in the treatment of psychotic symptoms, they clearly result in a variety of adverse effects. Because of differences in the pharmacological activity of different classic antipsychotic agents at these receptors, there are predictable differences in their side-effect profiles.

Pharmacokinetics

Generally, the pharmacokinetic profiles of the conventional antipsychotics remain poorly understood. Even for some of the more extensively studied agents, many hundreds of potential metabolites remain undiscovered, and the physiological activity of several metabolites has yet to be adequately defined. Nonetheless, certain general statements can be made concerning the classic antipsychotics as a group.

Administration and Absorption

Many of the conventional antipsychotics are available in both oral and intramuscular formulations. Although relatively common in the past, intravenous usage of parenteral formulations of antipsychotics is not FDA approved. Peak plasma levels with oral preparations are generally reached in 1–4 hours, with these levels being reached slightly more rapidly with liquid concentrates. Oral preparations are extensively metabolized in the liver during their first pass through portal circulation by undergoing a range of transformations, including glucuronidation, oxidation, reduction, and methylation. Steady-state levels are reached in a period of four to five times the half-life of the drug in question.

Intramuscular administration results in faster, more predictable absorption, with peak plasma levels in 30–60 minutes and clinical efficacy as rapidly as 15 minutes. With intramuscular or intravenous administration, plasma levels may be as much as four times the levels of the oral route because of circumvention of the hepatic first-pass metabolism.

Although 10 classic antipsychotics are available in a long-acting (depot) formulation around the world, haloperidol and fluphenazine are the only classic antipsychotics currently available in such a formulation in the United States. The currently available decanoate forms of both haloperidol and fluphenazine are administered through injection into a major muscle, and the drug is slowly released to the bloodstream over time. As the esterified version of the drug diffuses into other tissues, the ester chain is hydrolyzed, resulting in the smooth release of the drug in question. Fluphenazine decanoate can be given every 2–3 weeks on the basis of its half-life of 7–10 days, whereas haloperidol decanoate may be given every 4 weeks because of its longer half-life. The bioavailability of intramuscular relative to oral administration is twofold greater.

Distribution

Most of the conventional antipsychotics are highly protein bound (85%–90%). This feature is of importance when other highly protein-bound medications are used concomitantly because of the risk of increasing levels of free or unbound drugs into the toxic range. The antipsychotic drugs are highly lipophilic, which allows unbound portions of the drug to readily cross the blood-brain barrier with concentrations twofold higher in the brain than in the peripheral circulation. The drugs also readily cross the placenta to the fetus in pregnancy.

Metabolism

The conventional antipsychotics are metabolized in the liver by hydroxylation and demethylation to forms that are more soluble and readily excreted by the kidneys and in the feces. Many of these compounds undergo further glucuronidation and remain active as dopamine receptor antagonists. Because of the many active metabolites of the antipsychotic agents, it has not been possible to obtain meaningful correlations between plasma levels and clinical response. Variables such as age, genetic variability among individuals, and coadministration of other drugs cause plasma levels to vary 10- to 20-fold across individuals. The majority of conventional antipsychotics are metabolized by the cytochrome P450 (CYP) enzyme subfamilies. Since CYP2D6 is important for the metabolism of many of these antipsychotics, genetic variation in the rate of 2D6 metabolism should be considered. CYP1A2 and 3A4 subfamily enzymes are also involved in the metabolism of some classic antipsychotics, and this may be relevant to understanding drug-drug interactions of those agents.

Excretion

The major routes of excretion of the classic antipsychotics are through urine and feces by way of bile. These drugs are also excreted in sweat, saliva, tears, and breast milk. Elimination half-life varies from 18 to 40 hours for these drugs. Lower doses of antipsychotics are generally needed in elderly patients because of decreased renal clearance. Because of the long elimination half-lives of the classic antipsychotics, once-a-day dosing is possible for each of these agents following stabilization.

Mechanism of Action

Dopamine has been at the center of neurobiological theories of psychosis for the past half-century, and even today, all agents approved as antipsychotics share the single common attribute of dopamine D_2 receptor antagonism. Amphetamine intoxication served as a drug-induced model of the positive symptoms of schizophrenia. Drugs that blocked dopaminergic receptors, specifically the D_2 receptor, were noted to have greater efficacy and potency as antipsychotics. Since dopaminergic agonists exacerbate psychosis and dopaminergic blockade treats it, dopamine has held central importance in our conceptualization of the neuropharmacology of schizophrenia.

Indications and Efficacy

Schizophrenia and Schizoaffective Disorder

Classic antipsychotics are best known for the acute and maintenance treatment of the psychotic (also known as positive) symptoms of schizophrenia and schizoaffective disorder. The major putative mechanism of action is through D_2 blockade of the mesolimbic and mesocortical tracts. In many individuals, this blockade results in a measurable decrease in the positive symptoms of schizophrenia, including hallucinations, delusions, and behavioral disorganization. However, negative and cognitive symptoms of schizophrenia respond less robustly. In fact, they may be worsened by blockade of mesocortical tracts that play roles in cognition and hedonic reinforcement.

The failure to improve the negative symptoms of schizophrenia is one of the major drawbacks of the classic antipsychotics. In fact, the EPS induced by the FGAs can worsen negative and cognitive symptoms by inducing bradykinesia and bradyphrenia. Another major limitation is the lack of improvement of positive symptoms (i.e., refractoriness) in about 25% of schizophrenia patients and partial response (i.e., treatment resistance) in another 25%.

Substance-Induced Psychosis

As noted previously, conventional agents can reverse the psychosis associated with acute and chronic amphetamine intoxication as well as that associated with cocaine use. However, the risk of acute dystonia must be considered in these populations, as dopamine receptor downregulation is common, resulting in greater sensitivity to rapid D_2 blockade. Results in treatment of psychosis secondary to drugs acting in nondopaminergic mechanisms (such as hallucinogens) are less satisfactory, although there may be some role for the classic antipsychotics in treating phencyclidine (PCP) psychosis.

Personality Disorders

Although any personality disorder can be associated with transient psychotic features emerging under stressful conditions, Cluster B disorders are most often associated with this phenomenon. Treatment for the transient psychotic episodes has included short-term use of a high-potency antipsychotic. Although some symptoms of personality disorders may be amenable to such pharmacological treatment, long-term conventional antipsychotic treatment is not recommended.

Affective Disorders

The utility of antipsychotic agents in the treatment of affective disorders with psychotic features is well known. However, their utility in the treatment of nonpsychotic depression and bipolar disorder is described as well. Several conventional antipsychotics (such as thioridazine) are FDA approved for the treatment of depression and anxiety without overt psychosis. However, they are not used for this purpose anymore because of the availability of other, more effective, and better-tolerated agents. The utility of conventional agents as adjuncts to mood stabilizers in the treatment of patients with bipolar spectrum disorders has been well described, both in the acute management of mania and in the maintenance of severe and psychotic bipolar disorder. However, the newer atypical antipsychotics have largely replaced conventional antipsychotics in the management of bipolar disorder.

Tourette Syndrome

The tics present within Tourette syndrome are believed to be due to a hyperdopaminergic state that is amenable to treatment by dopamine receptor antagonists. Pimozide is the only conventional antipsychotic with this indication, which is its only FDA-approved indication.

Huntington's Disease

Although there is no cure for Huntington's disease, the psychosis and choreiform movements associated with this disease may be ameliorated by dopamine receptor antagonism. Several conventional antipsychotics carry FDA indications for treatment of this disease.

Nausea, Emesis, and Hiccups

The lower-potency antipsychotics exert a potent antiemetic effect through histamine$_1$ (H_1) receptor antagonism. This effect is closely related to their original role in reducing perioperative stress and emesis. Many well-known antiemetics, such as promethazine (Phenergan), are phenothiazines with a short-chain substitution. In addition, chlorpromazine is approved for oral or intramuscular therapy of intractable hiccups.

Side Effects and Toxicology

As noted earlier, side-effect profile—rather than efficacy in treating psychosis—is used to differentiate the conventional antipsychotics. These agents serve as antagonists at four major neurotransmitter receptor systems in the central nervous system (CNS): the dopamine type 2 receptor family (D_2, D_3, and D_4), muscarinic cholinergic receptors (M_1), α-adrenergic receptors (α_1 and α_2), and histamine receptors (H_1) (Table 15–1).

The therapeutic action of classic antipsychotics in ameliorating the positive symptoms of schizophrenia is believed to be due to D_2 blockade in the mesolimbic dopamine tract. Blockade of D_2 receptors in the mesocortical, nigrostriatal, and tuberoinfundibular systems leads to the tract-related side effects described earlier in this chapter (see section "Pharmacological Profile"). Lower-

TABLE 15–1. Relative affinities of classic antipsychotics to various neurotransmitter receptors

	Chlorpromazine	Thioridazine	Perphenazine	Trifluoperazine	Fluphenazine	Thiothixene	Haloperidol	Loxapine	Molindone
D_1	High	—	High	High	High	Moderate	High	High	Low
D_2	High	Very high	Very high	Very high	Very high	Very high	Very high	Very high	Very high
D_3	High	Very high	Unknown	Unknown	Very high	Unknown	Very high	Unknown	Unknown
D_4	High	Very high	Unknown	High	Very high	Unknown	Very high	Very high	Low
H_1	High	High	Moderate	Moderate	High	Moderate	Low	High	Very low
M_1	High	High	Low	Low	Low	Low	Low	Moderate	None
α_1	Very high	Very high	High	High	High	Moderate	Low	High	Low
α_2	Moderate	Very high	Moderate	Low	Low	Moderate	Low	Low	Moderate
5-HT_1	Low	Low	Low	Low	Low	Low	Low	Low	Low
5-HT_2	High	High	Moderate	Moderate	Moderate	Moderate	Moderate	Very high	Low

potency agents have greater antihistaminergic, anticholinergic, and antiadrenergic actions. However, they have fewer D_2-related side effects because of their lower affinity to D_2 receptors and relatively high anticholinergic activity. Higher-potency agents, such as haloperidol, produce more D_2-related movement disorders and prolactin elevation but otherwise have a cleaner side-effect profile, having fewer anticholinergic, antiadrenergic, and antihistaminergic side effects. Anticholinergic action often leads to dry mouth (xerostomia), blurred vision (mydriasis), constipation, urinary retention, sinus tachycardia, confusion, impaired cognition, paralytic ileus, exacerbation of open-angle glaucoma, and drowsiness. Antagonism of α_1-adrenergic receptors is associated with orthostatic hypotension, QTc prolongation, reflex tachycardia, dizziness, incontinence, and sedation. Antagonism of α_2 receptors can be associated with retrograde ejaculation and priapism. Antagonism of H_1 receptors leads to sedation, drowsiness, and weight gain.

The frequencies of adverse reactions of classic antipsychotic agents are summarized in Table 15–2.

Cognitive Side Effects

CNS side effects of classic antipsychotics can be subclassified into cognitive and neuromuscular side effects. Cognitive effects include sedation, confusion, disturbed concentration, memory impairment, and delirium. Antihistaminergic and anticholinergic actions lead to sedation and slowed mentation. These effects, which are most pronounced with lower-potency agents (e.g., chlorpromazine), are most severe earlier in treatment, with some tolerance developing over time. Anticholinergic delirium is the most common cause of medication-induced delirium. Because delirium results in high rates of morbidity and mortality (over 20% mortality), this potential side effect is important, especially in populations of individuals who are more sensitive to anticholinergic medications, such as the elderly. In addition, every antipsychotic—especially the low-potency agents—can potentially lower the seizure threshold.

Extrapyramidal Side Effects

Neuromuscular CNS side effects are due to antagonism of D_2 receptors in the nigrostriatal dopaminergic pathway. Generally, antipsychotics manifest EPS when dopaminergic blockade exceeds 75%–80% of D_2 receptors. EPS effects are most frequent with the high-potency agents such as haloperidol.

Acute-Onset EPS

Acute-onset EPS include medication-induced parkinsonism, acute dystonia, and akathisia. *Antipsychotic-induced parkinsonism* occurs in 15% of patients after several weeks of treatment. It is more common in patients older than 40 years, although it can occur at any age. Symptoms are identical to those of Parkinson's disease and include muscle stiffness ("lead-pipe" rigidity), cogwheel rigidity, shuffling gait, stooped posture, drooling, bradykinesia, resting tremor, masked facies, and akinesia. Slowed, restricted movements of the body and face (*akinesia*) may be mistakenly diagnosed as being due to depression or the negative symptoms of schizophrenia.

It is estimated that up to 10% of patients may experience an acute dystonic episode, which usually occurs within the first few hours or days of treatment. It is more common in youth, in recent cocaine users, and with intramuscular doses of high-potency antipsychotics. *Dystonia* is an acute, sustained, painful muscular contraction. Potential areas of involvement include the tongue (protrusions, twisting), jaw, neck (spasmodic retrocollis or torticollis), and back (opisthotonos). If the dystonia involves the eyes, it results in a symmetrical or unilateral upward lateral movement called an *oculogyric crisis*. Laryngeal dystonia can result in sudden death secondary to a patient's inability to breathe. Dystonia can be extremely uncomfortable and frightening for patients and can lead to

TABLE 15–2. Incidence of adverse reactions to classic antipsychotics at therapeutic doses

	Phenothiazines						Butyrophenone	Dibenzoxazepine	Dihydroindole	Diphenylbutylpiperidine	Thioxanthene
	Chlorpromazine	**Mesoridazine**	**Thioridazine**	**Fluphenazine**	**Perphenazine**	**Trifluoperazine**	**Haloperidol**	**Loxapine**	**Molindone**	**Pimozide**	**Thiothixene**
Cognitive effects											
Drowsiness, sedation	High	High	High	Low	Moderate	Low	Low	High	High	Moderate	Moderate
Insomnia, agitation	Low	Low	Low	Low	Low	Low	Moderate	Low	Low	Low	Moderate
Extrapyramidal effects											
Parkinsonism	Low to Moderate	Low to Moderate	Low	High	Moderate	Moderate to High	High	Moderate	Moderate to High	Moderate	High
Akathisia	Low	Moderate	Low	High	Moderate	High	High	Moderate	High	Moderate	High
Dystonic reactions	Low	Low	Low	High	Moderate	Moderate	High	Moderate	Moderate	Low	Low
Cardiovascular effects											
Orthostatic hypotension	High	High	High	Low	Low	Low to Moderate	Low	Low	Low	Low	Low
Tachycardia	Moderate	Moderate	High	Low	Low	Low	Low	Moderate	Low	Low	Low
ECG abnormalities	Moderate	Low	Moderate	Low	Low	Low	Low	Low	Low	Low	Low
Cardiac arrhythmias	Low	Moderate	Moderate	Low	Low	Low	Moderate	Low	Low	Low	Low
Anticholinergic effects											
	High	High	High	Low	Low	Low	Low	Moderate	Moderate	Low	Low

TABLE 15–2. Incidence of adverse reactions to classic antipsychotics at therapeutic doses *(continued)*

	Phenothiazines						Butyrophenone	Dibenzoxazepine	Dihydroindole	Diphenylbutylpiperidine	Thioxanthene
	Chlorpromazine	Mesoridazine	Thioridazine	Fluphenazine	Perphenazine	Trifluoperazine	Haloperidol	Loxapine	Molindone	Pimozide	Thiothixene
Endocrine effects											
Sexual dysfunction	Moderate	Moderate	High	Moderate	Moderate	Moderate	Moderate	Low	Low	Low	Low
Galactorrhea	Moderate	Moderate	Moderate	High	Moderate	Moderate	High	Moderate	Moderate	Low	Low
Weight gain	High	High	High	Moderate	Moderate	Moderate	Low	Moderate	Low	Low	Moderate
Skin reactions											
Photosensitivity	Moderate	Low	Moderate	Low	Low	Low	Low	Low	Low	—	Low
Rashes	Moderate	Low	Moderate	Low	Low	Low	Low	Low	Low	Low	Low
Pigmentation	High	Low	Low	Low	Low	Low	Low	Low	Low	—	Low
Ocular effects											
Lenticular pigmentation	Low	Low	Low	Low	Low	Low	Low	Low	Low	Low	Low
Pigmentary retinopathy	Low	Low	Moderate	Low	Low	Low	Low	Low	Low	—	Low
Other effects											
Blood dyscrasias	Low to Moderate	Low	Low	Low	Low	Low	Low	Low	Low	Low	Low
Hepatic disorder	Low	Low	Low	Low	Low	Low	Low	Low	Low	Low	Low
Seizures	Moderate	Moderate	Moderate	Low	Low	Low	Low	Low	Low	Low	Low

noncompliance with medication for fear of recurrence. Treatment of dystonia requires rapid diagnosis and intravenous administration of antihistaminergic or anticholinergic agents. Anticholinergic agents are often initiated with high-potency antipsychotics in an effort to avoid this side effect.

Akathisia is a subjective feeling of motor restlessness in which patients feel an irresistible urge to move continuously. It is described as an unpleasant sensation and may result in dysphoria. Akathisia can occur at any time during treatment and is the most prevalent of the EPS. It frequently leads to noncompliance with medications and is believed to increase suicide risk in some patients.

Late-Onset EPS

Tardive dyskinesia is characterized by a persistent syndrome of involuntary choreoathetoid movements of the head, limbs, and trunk. It generally takes at least 3–6 months of exposure to antipsychotics before the disorder develops. Perioral movements involving buccolingual masticatory musculature are the most common early manifestation of tardive dyskinesia. Tardive dyskinesia has an estimated yearly incidence of 5% among adults and as high as 25% in the elderly who receive continuous conventional antipsychotic therapy and has been a major source of litigation in past psychiatric practice. The risk of developing tardive dyskinesia is reported to increase with age and to be higher in certain ethnic groups; female gender, presence of mood disorders, and early onset of EPS have also been associated with increased risk of tardive dyskinesia.

Tardive dyskinesia may be masked by continuing dopamine blockade and has a variable course following development. Over time, spontaneous resolution or improvement has been described in some individuals. There is no single effective treatment, although treatment with clozapine has been reported to improve symptoms. Cases of tardive dyskinesia have been described with every antipsychotic. Other tardive syndromes include tardive dystonia, tardive akathisia, and tardive pain.

Neuroleptic Malignant Syndrome

Neuroleptic malignant syndrome (NMS) is a poorly understood syndrome that usually appears within hours or days of initiation of antipsychotic treatment. This syndrome is characterized by muscular rigidity, hyperpyrexia, autonomic instability (hypo- or hypertension, tachycardia, diaphoresis, pallor), and altered consciousness. NMS has an estimated incidence of 0.02%–2% and carries a mortality rate of 20%–30%. Death most often occurs secondary to dysrhythmias, renal failure secondary to rhabdomyolysis, aspiration pneumonia, or respiratory failure. Laboratory findings include elevated creatine phosphokinase, elevated white blood cell count, elevated liver enzymes, myoglobinemia, and myoglobinuria. The syndrome can last up to 10–14 days.

Treatment requires immediate discontinuation of the offending antipsychotic and supportive care with aggressive intravenous hydration. In the past, mild cases of NMS were treated with intravenous bromocriptine, while more severe cases were treated with intravenous dantrolene. However, evidence-based studies of NMS treatment have never been performed because of its infrequent occurrence.

Cardiac Effects

α-Adrenergic antagonism is associated with orthostatic hypotension with reflex tachycardia, with tolerance possibly developing later in the treatment course. Orthostasis is important because of an increase in falls and related injuries.

Recent studies involving several antipsychotics have drawn attention to the risk of cardiac dysrhythmias, which is especially prominent with use of lower-potency conventional antipsychotics. High dosage, rapid titration, intramuscular administration, and especially intravenous administration may be associated with a lengthening of the QTc interval, with resulting risk of serious dysrhythmias such as torsades de pointes and ventricular fibrillation. Studies with thioridazine have raised concerns about piperidine antipsychotics, leading to a decrease in the use of this class. In reality, torsades de pointes is rarely encountered during treatment with conventional antipsychotics, although some have speculated that a syndrome of unexplained sudden death described with all conventional antipsychotics may be related to sudden dysrhythmias.

Gastrointestinal Side Effects

The anticholinergic actions of conventional agents include dry mouth, nausea, vomiting, and constipation that can progress to paralytic ileus. Antihistaminergic action is associated with medication-related weight gain, which greatly increases the patient's risk of developing diabetes.

Cholestatic jaundice is a hypersensitivity reaction described with the aliphatic phenothiazines, especially chlorpromazine (incidence of 0.1%). This reaction typically manifests during the first 1–2 months of treatment and presents with nausea, malaise, fever, pruritus, abdominal pain, and jaundice, with resulting elevations in levels of bilirubin and alkaline phosphatase. This condition rarely lasts more than 2–4 weeks after discontinuation.

Weight Gain, Diabetes Mellitus, and Dyslipidemia

With the introduction of atypical antipsychotics, several of which cause significant weight gain, there is renewed awareness of the metabolic side effects associated with antipsychotic therapy such as obesity, elevated cholesterol and triglyceride levels, and an increased risk of diabetes mellitus. These metabolic changes increase the risk of ischemic heart disease and contribute to the increased mortality observed in schizophrenia. Antihistaminergic action is associated with medication-related weight gain, which greatly increases the patient's risk of developing diabetes. Diabetes is currently described as a worldwide epidemic. Serotonin 5-HT_{2C} receptor blockade also significantly contributes to weight gain; anticholinergic and 5-HT_{2A} antagonism may likewise contribute. There are significant differences among classic antipsychotics with reference to their propensity to cause these metabolic adverse effects. Molindone is the least likely to cause weight gain, whereas thioridazine and chlorpromazine are among the most likely to do so. In general, high-potency agents cause less weight gain than do low-potency agents.

Genitourinary Side Effects

Renal effects secondary to blockade of M_1 receptors include urinary hesitancy or retention, which can lead to a comparable increase in urinary tract infections in both genders. As mentioned previously, antagonism of tuberoinfundibular dopaminergic tracts increases prolactin secretion. Hyperprolactinemia causes both endocrine and sexual side effects, including gynecomastia, galactorrhea, diminished libido, erectile dysfunction, amenorrhea, decreased bone density, menstrual irregularities, infertility, delayed ovulation, anorgasmia, and possibly increased risk of breast cancer. Sexual difficulties, including erectile dysfunction, retrograde ejaculation (due to blockade of α_2-adrenergic receptors), anorgasmia, and occasionally priapism, can also occur.

Hematological Side Effects

Hematological effects of conventional antipsychotics include transient leukopenia (white blood cell [WBC] count $<3,500/\text{mm}^3$), which is common but not usually problematic, and agranulocytosis (WBC count $<500/\text{mm}^3$), a life-threatening problem. Agranulocytosis occurs most often during the first 3 months of treatment, with an incidence of 1 in 500,000. Aliphatic and piperidine phenothiazines are the most common causal agents among the conventional antipsychotics. Rarely, thrombocytopenic or nonthrombocytopenic purpura, hemolytic anemia, and pancytopenia may occur.

Ocular Side Effects

In addition to direct anticholinergic ocular effects such as blurred vision (mydriasis and cycloplegia) and exacerbation of open-angle glaucoma, direct optic toxicity has been described. The conventional antipsychotics are associated with several kinds of optical pathology involving the lens, cornea, and retina. Lenticular opacities have been reported with some phenothiazines, including perphenazine, chlorpromazine, and thioridazine. An irreversible increase in retinal pigmentation has been described with thioridazine when high dosages (>800 mg/day) are used. This retinal pigmentation, which can progress even after drug discontinuation, can lead to reduced visual acuity and even blindness. Early symptoms include poor night vision and secondary nocturnal confusion.

Dermatological Side Effects

Cutaneous side effects of conventional antipsychotics involve hypersensitivity rashes—most commonly maculopapular erythematous rashes of the trunk, face, neck, and extremities—and photosensitivity reactions that can lead to severe sunburn. Care must be taken with injectable versions of many antipsychotics because of direct dermatological toxicity if the skin or subcutaneous layers are exposed. Prolonged use of chlorpromazine can lead to blue-gray discoloration in body areas exposed to sunlight.

Drug-Drug Interactions

Careful consideration of a patient's existing drug regimen should be given prior to the initiation of antipsychotic therapy.

Protein Binding

Because conventional antipsychotics are tightly protein bound, care must be taken when these medications are administered with other highly protein-bound medications. Mutual displacement of medications such as phenytoin, digoxin, warfarin, and valproate could lead to a short-term increase in serum levels of these drugs and of the conventional antipsychotic.

Cytochrome P450 Inhibition

As mentioned previously, conventional antipsychotics are primarily hepatically metabolized through the CYP2D6 and 3A4 enzymes. In addition, each inhibits the 2D6 enzyme to some degree. Care must be taken when conventional agents are coadministered with potent CYP2D6 inhibitors such as fluoxetine, paroxetine, cimetidine, erythromycin, and certain class IC antiarrhythmics (e.g., quinidine). Similarly, potent CYP3A4 inhibitors such as nefazodone, fluvoxamine, and ketoconazole should be used with care. Inhibitors of CYP2D6 and 3A4, as well as competitive substrates, should be used carefully with conventional antipsychotics because of their potential to increase plasma levels. CYP1A2, induced by nicotine and inhibited by estrogen, plays a role in metabolizing some antipsychotics.

Neurotoxicity

More than two dozen studies published between 1988 and 2012 have reported neurotoxicity—including induction of apoptosis, increased levels of reactive species, and reduced levels of neurotrophins such as brain-derived neurotrophic factor (BDNF)—with the classic antipsychotics (Abekawa et al. 2011; Pillai et al. 2008; Ukai et al. 2004). No similar findings have been reported with the atypical class. Given such neurotoxic effects, some have questioned whether the conventional agents should be used in the treatment of psychosis.

Conclusion

The classic antipsychotics revolutionized the practice of psychiatry and the treatment of the severely mentally ill throughout the world. Second-generation "atypical" antipsychotics have commercially eclipsed these first-generation agents to a large extent, in that more than 90% of patients with schizophrenia and related psychoses in the United States are currently receiving one of the atypical oral agents. In regard to long-acting (depot) agents, use of classic antipsychotic injectables such as haloperidol decanoate and fluphenazine decanoate is still higher than use of second-generation injectable agents, but this may change in the near future as several new atypical long-acting formulations become available. The landmark National Institute of Mental Health–funded CATIE study, which compared four SGA oral agents (olanzapine, quetiapine, risperidone, and ziprasidone) against one FGA oral agent (perphenazine), showed that there was no difference between the two generations in clinical effectiveness (defined as all-cause discontinuation). However, the CATIE study excluded subjects with tardive dyskinesia from random assignment to perphenazine and instead assigned them to one of the atypical agents. This methodological stipulation may have confounded the findings, because the 231 subjects with tardive dyskinesia were later found to have a higher severity of psychopathology and a much greater likelihood of substance use, both of which could have influenced the primary outcome. Nonetheless, both classic antipsychotics and atypical antipsychotics can cause serious side effects, with neurological adverse events being much more likely with the FGAs and metabolic complications being more common with the SGAs.

Conventional antipsychotics will always be remembered for their critical role as the foundation of antipsychotic pharmacotherapy and as the main impetus for the remarkable neuropharmacological progress in psychiatric neuroscience over the second half of the twentieth century. They retain an important, if limited, role in the antipsychotic armamentarium of the twenty-first century.

References

Abekawa T, Ito K, Nakagawa S, et al: Effects of aripiprazole and haloperidol on progression to schizophrenia-like behavioural abnormalities and apoptosis in rodents. Schizophr Res 125:77–87, 2011

Pillai A, Dhandapani KM, Pillai BA, et al: Erythropoietin prevents haloperidol treatment-induced neuronal apoptosis through regulation of BDNF. Neuropsychopharmacology 33:1942–1951, 2008

Ukai W, Ozawa H, Tateno M, et al: Neurotoxic potential of haloperidol in comparison with risperidone: implication of Akt-mediated signal changes by haloperidol. J Neural Transm 111: 667–681, 2004

Suggested Reading

Correll CU, Leucht S, Kane JM: Lower risk of tardive dyskinesia associated with second-generation antipsychotics: a systematic review. Am J Psychiatry 161:414–425, 2004

Glazer WM: Review of incidence studies of tardive dyskinesia associated with typical antipsychotics. J Clin Psychiatry 61 (suppl):15–20, 2000

Janicak PA, Davis JM, Preskorn SH, et al: Principles and Practice of Psychopharmacotherapy, 4th Edition. Philadelphia, PA, Lippincott Williams & Wilkins, 2006

Jeste DV, Lacro JP, Palmer B, et al: Incidence of tardive dyskinesia in early stages of low-dose treatment with typical neuroleptics in older patients. Am J Psychiatry 156:309–311, 1999

Kapur S, Seeman P: Does fast dissociation from the dopamine D2 receptor explain the action of atypical antipsychotics? A new hypothesis. Am J Psychiatry 158:360–369, 2001

Lee JW: Catatonic variants, hyperthermic extrapyramidal reactions, and subtypes of neuroleptic malignant syndrome. Ann Clin Psychiatry 19:9–16, 2007

Lieberman JA, Stroup ST, McEvoy JP, et al: Effectiveness of antipsychotic drugs in patients with chronic schizophrenia. N Engl J Med 353:1209–1233, 2005

Meyer JM, Nasrallah HA (eds): Medical Illness and Schizophrenia, 2nd Edition. Washington, DC, American Psychiatric Publishing, 2010

Nasrallah HA: CATIE's surprises: in antipsychotics' standoff, were there winners or losers? Curr Psychiatry 5:11–19, 2006

Nasrallah HA, Smeltzer D: Contemporary Diagnosis and Management of Schizophrenia, 2nd Edition. Newtown, PA, Handbooks in Health Care, 2011

Sachdev PS: Neuroleptic-induced movement disorders: an overview. Psychiatr Clin North Am 28:255–274, 2005

Sadock BJ, Sadock V (eds): Comprehensive Textbook of Psychopharmacology. Philadelphia, PA, Lippincott Williams & Wilkins, 2000

Smith D, Pantelis S, McGrath J, et al: Ocular abnormalities in chronic schizophrenia: clinical implications. Aust N Z J Psychiatry 31:252–256, 1997

Tandon R, Moller H-J, Belmaker RH, et al: World Psychiatric Association Pharmacopsychiatry Section Statement on Comparative Effectiveness of Antipsychotics in the Treatment of Schizophrenia. Schizophr Res 100:20–38, 2008

Tandon R, Nasrallah HA, Keshavan MS: Schizophrenia, "Just the facts" 4: Clinical features and conceptualization. Schizophr Res 110:1–23, 2009

Tandon R, Nasrallah HA, Keshavan MS: Schizophrenia, "Just the facts" 5: Treatment and prevention: past, present, and future. Schizophr Res 122:1–23, 2010

CHAPTER 16

Clozapine

Stephen R. Marder, M.D.
Donna Ames, M.D.

History and Discovery

Clozapine has played a critical role in the history of therapeutics for psychosis. When clozapine was initially developed in the 1960s (following its synthesis in 1958 in Switzerland), there was skepticism as to whether an agent that barely caused catalepsy in rodents could be an effective antipsychotic. According to Hippius (1999), there was limited enthusiasm for this drug because its profile was inconsistent with the "neuroleptic dogma" that extrapyramidal side effects (EPS) were an essential feature of an antipsychotic agent. Nevertheless, Hippius and others challenged this dogma and supported clozapine's development in Germany. As a result, clozapine was eventually marketed in a number of countries in Europe.

Enthusiasm about clozapine's unique profile turned to despair when it was reported that 13 patients in Finland developed agranulocytosis during treatment with clozapine and that 8 of these patients died (Griffith and Saameli 1975). This news led to a near-halt in research on clozapine and attempts to switch patients to other antipsychotic agents. However, some individuals demonstrated substantial deterioration when they were switched (Hippius 1999). These patients were changed back to clozapine and carefully monitored with regular white blood cell (WBC) counts. It was subsequently confirmed that clozapine-induced agranulocytosis was reversible. If clozapine was discontinued before patients developed infections, the drug could be readministered safely (Honigfeld et al. 1998). Moreover, studies revealed that clozapine was particularly effective for patients who were severely ill and for patients who had failed to respond to treatment with conventional antipsychotics.

The discovery that clozapine was an effective antipsychotic with minimal EPS led to a reassessment of models for developing antipsychotic agents. This reassessment, in turn, led to the later development of a new generation of antipsychotics. Moreover, attempts to understand clozapine's mechanism of action have had important effects on current views of the pharmacology of schizophrenia.

Structure-Activity Relations

Clozapine belongs to the group of tricyclic antipsychotics known as the dibenzepines. This group is characterized by a seven-member central ring. The antipsychotic dibenzepines include a loxapine-like group of compounds (the dibenzoxazepines) and a clozapine-like group (the dibenzodiazepines). Substitutions in the clozapine group resulted in the development of both quetiapine and olanzapine.

Pharmacological Profile

Animal behavioral models have been of limited use in schizophrenia. The primary problem is that there is not a well-accepted animal model for psychopathology in schizophrenia. A number of models—including latent inhibition of the conditioned response, prepulse inhibition, and P_{50} gating—are being studied, and these models suggest unique properties of clozapine that may be clinically relevant. The models used in the development of antipsychotics over the years were empirical models based on dopamine blockade. Criteria for antipsychotic action included the ability of the agent to cause catalepsy at higher doses as well as its antagonism of stereotypies in animals resulting from the administration of amphetamine. Although clozapine meets neither of these criteria, it does block the conditioned avoidance response, suggesting that it has antipsychotic activity.

Pharmacokinetics and Disposition

Peak plasma levels of clozapine are reached approximately 2 hours after oral administration. The elimination half-life is about 12 hours. Patients will usually reach steady-state plasma concentrations within 1 week. The coadministration of highly protein-bound drugs may lead to increased free clozapine levels, although the total (free plus bound) levels may be unchanged. Clozapine's volume of distribution is lower than that of other antipsychotic drugs but is nonetheless large, with a mean of 2.0–5.1 L/kg (range: 1.0–10.2 L/kg).

Clozapine undergoes extensive first-pass metabolism in the liver and gut. Although clozapine is predominately metabolized by cytochrome P450 (CYP) 1A2, CYP2D6 and CYP3A3 also contribute (Buur-Rasmussen and Brosen 1999).

Plasma concentrations of clozapine average about 10–80 ng/mL per mg of drug given per kg of weight. Thus, a typical daily dose of 300–400 mg (about 5 mg/kg) is associated with plasma levels ranging between 200 and 400 ng/mL. However, there is considerable variability among individuals treated with clozapine. A number of studies have focused on the clinical implications of this variation in plasma concentrations. These studies, when taken together, indicate that patients are more likely to do well when their plasma levels are greater than 350 ng/mL (Bell et al. 1998; Kronig et al. 1995; Miller 1996; Miller et al. 1994; Potkin et al. 1994). If patients have not responded after 6 weeks with a plasma level of 250 ng/mL, the clinician should increase the level to approximately 350 ng/mL. High levels, such as 600 ng/mL, are not associated with a greater likelihood of improvement than are moderate levels, and they may be associated with a higher incidence of side effects. Therefore, patients with high levels and side effects may benefit from having the dosage reduced. In interpreting plasma concentrations of clozapine, it is important for clinicians to consider whether the laboratory is reporting just the parent drug or clozapine plus norclozapine. If it is the combination, levels will be higher.

Mechanism of Action

The explanation for clozapine's unique effectiveness remains controversial. As mentioned earlier, clozapine was the first agent to challenge the dogma that antipsychotic efficacy required high levels of EPS. There are a number of characteristics of clozapine that could explain how it can reduce psychosis without causing EPS.

Clozapine's low incidence of EPS could be explained by its low occupancy of dopamine$_2$ (D_2) receptors at therapeutic doses. Studies using positron emission tomography (PET) with selective D_2 receptor ligands, such as raclopride, make it possible to determine the proportion of D_2 receptors that are occupied by an antipsychotic in a particular individual at a particular time. These studies found that conventional antipsychotics are effective when approximately 80% of receptors are occupied (Farde et al. 1992). Higher levels of occupancy may increase EPS, but they do not result in greater efficacy. In contrast, clozapine is effective when it occupies 20%–67% of D_2 receptors. This observation may help explain two important properties of clozapine: its tendency to cause very few EPS and the suggestion that its effectiveness is associated with something more than just D_2 receptor occupancy.

It has also been suggested that clozapine's properties are associated with its combination of relatively low affinity for D_2 receptors and high affinity for other receptors, including 5-HT_{2A}, 5-HT_{1C}, adrenergic, and cholinergic receptors. Most of the attention has focused on clozapine's high ratio of 5-HT_{2A} to D_2 receptors, because this property is shared by nearly all of the second-generation antipsychotics (SGAs). Moreover, serotonin can modulate dopamine neurons in the substantia nigra, which in turn may decrease EPS. Clozapine also has a very high affinity for the dopamine$_4$ (D_4) receptor. The D_4 receptor is widely distributed in the cortex and less so in striatal areas. However, other agents with high D_4 receptor activity have failed to demonstrate antipsychotic activity.

Another theory—supported by both Seeman (2002) and Kapur and Seeman (2001)—hypothesizes that the lack of EPS with clozapine and other SGAs is related to their fast dissociation from the D_2 receptor. Conventional antipsychotics tend to bind more tightly to dopamine receptors than to dopamine itself. Nearly all of the SGAs, including clozapine, bind more loosely and tend to come off the receptor more readily in the presence of dopamine. As a result, these newer agents may block these receptors more transiently, coming off the receptor to permit more normal dopamine transmission.

Indications and Efficacy

Acute Schizophrenia and Schizoaffective Disorder

Because of its side-effect profile, clozapine should not be administered as a first-line agent for schizophrenia or schizoaffective disorder. However, this does not mean that clozapine is ineffective in these disorders. Early trials comparing clozapine with haloperidol and chlorpromazine indicated that clozapine was at least as effective as the other agents for acutely psychotic patients.

Treatment-Refractory Schizophrenia

Early studies suggested that clozapine was particularly effective in patients with more severe treatment-refractory forms of schizophrenia. This was important when it was discovered that clozapine was associated with a risk of agranulocytosis. Given that clozapine was viewed as an agent that might be helpful for patients who had failed to respond to other antipsychotics, a study was designed to test whether there was a role for clozapine in this population. The result was the design of a multicenter study comparing clozapine with chlorpromazine in severely ill patients with treatment-refractory schizophrenia (Kane et al. 1988). Treatment-refractory illness was characterized on the basis of a history of drug nonresponsiveness and a failure to improve during a 6-week trial of up to 60 mg of haloperidol. Clozapine resulted in greater improvement in nearly every dimension of psychopathology. Thirty percent of the clozapine-treated patients met stringent improvement criteria, compared with only 4% of those treated with chlorpromazine.

Other studies suggest that the proportion of patients improving with clozapine treatment will be higher if clozapine is continued for a longer time. For example, a 16-week trial by Pickar et al. (1992) found a 38% improvement rate. A more recent report (Kane et al. 2001) found that 60% of patients with treatment-refractory illness improved after a 29-week trial on clozapine.

Two large trials compared clozapine with SGAs in patients with treatment-resistant illness. In the United States, the National Institute of Mental Health (NIMH) Clinical Antipsychotic Trials of Intervention Effectiveness (CATIE) compared clozapine with risperidone, olanzapine, or quetiapine in patients with schizophrenia who had failed to show response in an earlier phase of the study because of a lack of efficacy (Stroup et al. 2006). Clozapine was administered open label, whereas the other antipsychotics were administered double-blind. Patients assigned to clozapine had the lowest discontinuation rates, with 56% of patients on clozapine discontinuing treatment, compared with 71% of those on olanzapine, 86% of those on risperidone, and 93% of those on quetiapine. Clozapine-treated patients also showed greater symptom improvements than those receiving the other agents. Another trial in the United Kingdom, the Cost Utility of the Latest Antipsychotic Drugs in Schizophrenia Study—band 2 (CUtLASS-2) (Lewis et al. 2006), randomly assigned 136 patients who had responded poorly to two prior antipsychotics to either clozapine or an SGA selected prior to the randomization. Patients who received clozapine demonstrated greater improvement than those on the comparison drugs.

A large body of evidence indicates that clozapine has an important role in the treatment of patients who have failed to respond to either first-generation antipsychotics (FGAs) or other SGAs. Clozapine's advantages are clearest in patients who have failed to respond to FGAs but are still apparent in those who have had an inadequate response to other SGAs. Because clozapine is associated with a risk of agranulocytosis and other side effects (summarized later in this chapter under section "Side Effects and Toxicology"), patients should probably receive a trial of one or two other SGAs before receiving a trial of clozapine. Clinical guidelines (Lehman et al. 2004a, 2004b; Marder et al. 2002; Miller et al. 2004) differ to a minor degree on the number of trials that should precede a trial with clozapine, but most recommend at least two agents, one of which is an SGA. There is a consensus that patients should not be considered to have treatment-refractory illness until they have received an adequate treatment trial with clozapine.

Hostile and Aggressive Behavior in Schizophrenia

Clozapine may have other advantages for patients with schizophrenia. A number of studies suggest that clozapine may decrease hostility and aggression, compared with other agents. In a study of 157 inpatients (Citrome et al. 2001), clozapine resulted in greater reductions in the hostility item from the Positive and Negative Syndrome Scale (PANSS) than did the FGAs and other SGAs. A study by Chengappa et al. (2003) found significant reductions in the rates of seclusion and restraint among schizophrenia patients who received clozapine during the first 3 years after its introduction. Other randomized studies have consistently found that patients treated with clozapine exhibit less hostility and less aggressive behavior than patients on comparators (Essock et al. 2000; Kane et al. 1988). These findings suggest that clozapine may be of particular benefit to patients with treatment-refractory illness who demonstrate hostile and aggressive behavior.

Schizophrenia Patients at High Risk for Suicide

Clozapine may also be a preferred agent for patients with schizophrenia who are at a higher risk for suicide. Large epidemiological studies have found that mortality from suicide is reduced among individuals taking clozapine (Reid et al. 1998; Walker et al. 1997). Meltzer and Okayli (1995) followed patients who were changed to clozapine and found a reduction in the number of serious suicide attempts as well as in expressed depression and hopelessness. The most convincing study was a comparison of clozapine and olanzapine in 980 patients with schizophrenia who were considered at risk for suicide. In that study, clozapine was more effective in reducing the risk of suicide (Meltzer 2002).

Clozapine may also offer advantages for patients with polydipsia-hyponatremia syndrome (Canuso and Goldman 1999). Patients with this syndrome tend to intoxicate themselves through excessive water drinking. Hyponatremia may result in seizures.

Schizophrenia With Comorbid Substance Abuse

Although the effectiveness of clozapine in patients with comorbid substance abuse has not been demonstrated in randomized controlled trials, there is some supporting evidence from naturalistic studies. One retrospective study (Green et al. 2003) found that patients treated with clozapine were more likely than those treated with risperidone to abstain from alcohol and cannabis use. A prospective study (Green et al. 2007) found that patients treated with clozapine were often able to reduce their substance abuse. This finding was supported by other prospective studies (Brunette et al. 2006; Drake et al. 2000), indicating that clozapine is effective for reducing substance abuse.

Supplemental Antipsychotic Treatment in Partial Responders to Clozapine

A number of studies have evaluated augmentation strategies for individuals who are partial responders to clozapine. A recent meta-analysis (Sommer et al. 2012) reviewed 29 double-blind randomized trials of agents used to augment the effects of clozapine. The most-studied antipsychotics added to clozapine were risperidone and aripiprazole, and the most-studied mood stabilizer was lamotrigine. Although some of the studies reported positive findings, none of the strategies was viewed as having adequate empirical support.

Maintenance Therapy in Schizophrenia

Clozapine use has largely been confined to patients with treatment-refractory schizophrenia. As a result, clozapine has not been studied in traditional relapse prevention designs in which patients who are stable are randomly assigned to either clozapine or a comparator. Nevertheless, there are substantial data supporting clozapine's long-term effectiveness. Breier et al. (2000) evaluated the outcomes of 30 patients with schizophrenia who received clozapine for 1 year. Patients taking clozapine experienced fewer relapses and rehospitalizations than they did in the year prior to being changed to clozapine. A study in the state hospitals in Connecticut compared patients who were assigned to clozapine with patients who were maintained on their usual antipsychotics (Essock et al. 2000). Although clozapine did not result in a greater likelihood of hospital discharge, patients who were treated with clozapine had a higher likelihood of remaining in the community following discharge. This finding supports the observation that clozapine is associated with a reduced risk of relapse compared with conventional antipsychotics.

A study from the U.S. Department of Veterans Affairs (VA) Cooperative Studies Program compared haloperidol and clozapine in patients with treatment-refractory schizophrenia (Rosenheck et al. 1997). This study was not designed as a relapse prevention trial but rather as a comparison of the two agents in individuals who were poor responders to conventional therapy. However, the 1-year study is somewhat informative about the usefulness of the two drugs in patients living in the community. Fifty-seven percent of the patients taking clozapine completed the study, compared with only 28% of the patients taking haloperidol (P<0.001). Using 20% improvement on the PANSS as the criterion for response, the investigators found that 42% of patients treated with clozapine and 31% of patients treated with haloperidol were responders (P=0.09). In addition, clozapine-treated patients had fewer mean days of hospitalization (143.8 days) compared with haloperidol-treated patients (168.1 days; P=0.03).

Mania in Bipolar Disorder

Given that all available antipsychotics are effective in reducing manic symptoms, it is not surprising that clozapine is effective in bipolar mania. However, accumulating evidence suggests that clozapine is particularly effective for manic symptoms that are not responsive to other agents. McElroy et al. (1991) were among the first to observe clozapine's unique effects in patients with bipolar disorder. Subsequent studies have confirmed clozapine's effectiveness as monotherapy and as a supplementation medication for mania in bipolar disorder. In an open-label randomized trial in acutely manic patients (Barbini et al. 1997), clozapine was as effective as chlorpromazine and had a more rapid onset of action. Suppes et al. (1999) randomly assigned patients with schizoaffective or bipolar illness to either supplemental clozapine or treatment as usual during a 1-year open-label trial. Among both groups of patients, those treated with clozapine demonstrated greater improvements.

Depression With Psychotic Features

Limited evidence suggests that clozapine is effective as monotherapy and as an adjunctive treatment for patients with major depression with psychotic features. This evidence is currently confined to case reports with relatively small numbers of cases (Ranjan and Meltzer 1996; Rothschild 1996).

Psychosis in Parkinson's Disease

Psychosis with delusions and hallucinations occurs in approximately 25% of patients with Parkinson's disease (Wolters and Berendse 2001). These symptoms frequently appear in patients who are receiving dopaminomimetic drugs but may also occur as a result of a cholinergic deficit. Three double-blind studies (French Clozapine Parkinson Study Group 1999; Jones and Stoukides 1992; Parkinson Study Group 1999; Pollak et al. 2004) found that clozapine at doses as low as 25–50 mg was effective in reducing psychotic symptoms. Moreover, these doses were not associated with an increase in tremor and rigidity. A report from the American Academy of Neurology (Miyasaki et al. 2006) recommended clozapine as a preferred agent for psychosis in Parkinson's disease.

Schizophrenia in Children and Adolescents

Two randomized controlled trials from NIMH have evaluated the effectiveness of clozapine in childhood-onset schizophrenia. The first (Kumra et al. 1996) compared clozapine and haloperidol in individuals with a mean age of about 14 years who had done poorly on FGAs. Clozapine was superior for both positive and negative symptoms. A more recent double-blind study (Shaw et al. 2006) compared clozapine and olanzapine in subjects with a mean age of about 12 years. The results from this study were less clear. Although there were substantial differences favoring clozapine, the differences were statistically significant only for negative symptoms. The small sample ($n = 12$ for clozapine and $n = 13$ for olanzapine) was a limiting factor for obtaining statistical significance. Both studies found that this younger population appeared to be particularly vulnerable to clozapine's side effects. Nevertheless, these studies suggest an important role for clozapine in younger patients with schizophrenia with refractory symptoms.

Side Effects and Toxicology

Hematological Effects

The side effects of clozapine make it one of the most challenging medications for psychiatrists to prescribe. The main factor that limits its use is the potential serious side effect of agranulocytosis. Agranulocytosis is defined as a drop in absolute neutrophil count (ANC) to levels below $500/mm^3$. In 1975, there were 17 cases of agranulocytosis in Finland, and widespread use of the medication for the treatment of schizophrenia was temporarily halted (Amsler et al. 1977; de la Chapelle et al. 1977). Agranulocytosis is a potentially lethal side effect that occurs in less than 1% of patients treated in the United States (Alvir et al. 1993). In the United States, all patients who are taking clozapine are entered into a national registry. Through the national registry, patients are prescribed the medication only if their WBC count shows no signs of clinically meaningful suppression (Honigfeld 1996). In a review of the morbidity and mortality of clozapine-treated patients (Honigfeld et al. 1998) over a 5-year period, 99,502 patients were registered through the Clozaril National Registry. Of these, 2,931 (2.95%) patients developed leukopenia (WBC count = $3{,}500/mm^3$), and 382 (0.38%) patients developed agranulocytosis (ANC $<500/mm^3$). Twelve of the cases of agranulocytosis (0.012%) were fatal.

When clozapine treatment is discontinued upon identification of marked leukopenia, patients usually recover within 14–24 days and without any long-term consequences. However, rechallenging patients who have experienced agranulocytosis almost always leads to reoccurrence of the problem. The onset of the second episode is more aggressive than that of the first. In nine patients who were known to be rechallenged, the average time to onset of the second episode was 10 weeks shorter (14 weeks) than for the first episode (24 weeks) (Safferman et al. 1992). Agranulocytosis has been successfully treated by discontinuing the medication, providing supportive measures, and administering granulocyte colony–stimulating factor, a medication that is commonly prescribed to patients with medical illnesses that precipitate WBC count suppression (Raison et al. 1994; Weide et al. 1992; Wickramanayake et al. 1995).

In January 2006, Novartis and the U.S. Food and Drug Administration (FDA) issued a notification to clinicians regarding modifications to the recommended monitoring schedule for patients receiving clozapine (available at www.pharma.us.novartis.com/product/pi/pdf/Clozaril.pdf). Under the new monitoring guidelines, a patient beginning clozapine treatment must have a baseline WBC count of no less than $3{,}500/mm^3$ and an ANC of no less than $2{,}000/mm^3$. Weekly WBC and ANC levels must be obtained for 6 months, at which time the frequency can be reduced to every 2 weeks, provided that treatment and monitoring have not been interrupted and WBC counts and ANCs have remained within acceptable ranges. After 1 year, monitoring can be reduced to monthly blood tests. There are specific recommendations for intensified monitoring following discontinuation of clozapine therapy, particularly if therapy is interrupted because of blood dyscrasias. Studies focused on identifying genetic groups associated with an increased risk of agranulocytosis are currently under way and may provide guidance to clinicians in the near future (Athanasiou et al. 2011).

Cardiac Effects

Well-known side effects of clozapine on the cardiovascular system include tachycardia and orthostatic hypotension. Tachycardia is thought to be attributable to the anticholinergic activity of the medication, whereas hypotension is due to α-adrenergic blockade. Reports of clozapine-associated myocarditis and cardiomyopathy have raised concern that clozapine may be associated with other forms of cardiovascular toxicity. In January 2002, Novartis reported that there had been 213 cases of myocarditis, 85% of which occurred at recommended dosages of clozapine within the first 2 months of therapy. The presence of eosinophilia in many of the reported cases indicates that an immunoglobulin E (IgE)–mediated hypersensitivity reaction may be involved (Killian et al. 1999). Novartis (2002) also reported 178 cases of clozapine-associated cardiomyopathy, 80% of which were in patients younger than 50 years. Almost 20% of the incidents resulted in death, an alarming figure that may reflect delay in diagnosis and treatment. The detection of cardiac toxicity is particularly challenging, because its manifestations (tachycardia, fatigue, and orthostatic hypotension) are frequently observed in clozapine-treated patients, particularly when alterations in dosage are made (Lieberman and Safferman 1992). The poor specificity of signs for cardiac toxicity demands that patients with any personal or family history of heart disease be identified, and the threshold for medical evaluation of patients developing respiratory and cardiovascular symptoms must be low (Wooltorton 2002). The etiology of the myocarditis and cardiomyopathy remains unclear at this time.

For hypotension caused by clozapine, we also recommend a slow upward titration of the medication and monitoring of orthostatic vital signs during the first weeks of therapy. Patients should be educated about the risk of orthostatic hypotension and should be taught to rise slowly from supine positions. Concomitant treatment with β-blocking agents may be necessary for persistent tachycardia. However, the use of β-blockers may exacerbate the hypotensive effects of clozapine and should be used cautiously.

Metabolic Effects

Weight Gain

Weight gain has been observed in both premarketing and postmarketing trials of clozapine (Henderson 2001; Simpson and Varga 1974; Wirshing et al. 1998, 1999). Allison et al. (1999) performed a meta-analysis of the weight-gain data in short-term trials of medications. The average weight gain observed with clozapine was 4.45 kg, which exceeded the weight gain observed with all of the other medications in the study, including the conventional agent thioridazine (3.19 kg), a medication known for its weight-gain liability. The weight gain observed with clozapine seems to occur for a prolonged period of time—up to 40 weeks. In one naturalistic study, Henderson (2001) observed patients in a clozapine clinic for 5 years and noted weight gain occurring for up to 46 months in some patients.

Phase II of CATIE provided an opportunity to compare weight gain among patients assigned to clozapine, olanzapine, risperidone, and quetiapine (McEvoy et al. 2006). The numbers of patients assessed in the analyses were small, with only 45 patients in the clozapine group, 17 in the olanzapine group, 14 in the quetiapine group, and 14 in the risperidone group. Although the differences in weight gain among these agents were not statistically significant, they were interesting, with patients on clozapine gaining a mean of 0.5 lb per month, compared with 1.0 lbs on olanzapine, –0.4 lb on quetiapine, and 0.5 lb on risperidone.

Diabetes

The weight gain observed with clozapine can place patients at risk for significant health problems. Diabetes is naturally the most concerning potential sequela of this weight gain. Numerous case reports have linked clozapine with new-onset diabetes (Wirshing et al. 1998). In Henderson's (2001) naturalistic study of 81 patients observed over a 5-year period, 36.6% of the patients developed diabetes.

Patients treated with clozapine should be routinely screened for diabetes and other metabolic abnormalities, including raised lipid levels. Patients with risk factors for diabetes should be monitored more closely. Reports and clinical experience suggest that in a case of antipsychotic-associated diabetes or diabetic ketoacidosis, discontinuation of the antipsychotic agent may result in reversal of the hyperglycemia and diabetes. During clozapine therapy, we recommend monitoring fasting glucose, cholesterol, and lipids at baseline and every 6 months thereafter.

Prevention of weight gain with clozapine, through nutrition and diet counseling, is recommended. Caloric restriction and exercise for 30 minutes per day should be recommended. Screening questions by physicians that we find useful include the following: "Have you noticed if your belt or pants size has changed?" "Have you noticed an increase in thirst or urinary frequency?" We strongly recommend weighing patients at each visit and monitoring blood pressure.

Dyslipidemias

Clozapine treatment is associated with dyslipidemias, including elevations in triglycerides and cholesterol, particularly low-density lipoprotein (LDL) cholesterol (McEvoy et al. 2006; Wirshing et al. 2002a).

In 2004, in response to growing concern that the majority of antipsychotic medications may be associated with weight gain and other metabolic changes, the American Diabetes Association and other groups published a set of guidelines for monitoring weight, glucose, and lipids (American Diabetes Association et al. 2004). Also in 2004, a very comprehensive literature review was conducted by Marder et al.) to provide guidance to clinicians regarding monitoring of weight, glucose, lipids, and other parameters of physical health in patients with schizophrenia. Labeling changes were made for all antipsychotic medications, including clozapine, regarding these metabolic risk factors.

Seizures

A well-known side effect of clozapine treatment is the risk for seizures, which are thought to occur in 5%–10% of patients treated with this medication (Welch et al. 1994). The cause of seizures is unclear, but it is generally thought that rapid escalations in dosage and possibly high plasma levels of clozapine may account for the development of seizures (Klimke and Klieser 1995). Clozapine-associated seizures occur most often at dosages greater than 600 mg/day. The relationship between clozapine plasma levels and seizures is somewhat inconsistent in the literature (Simpson and Cooper 1978; Vailleau et al. 1996).

The anticonvulsant agents sodium valproate, gabapentin, and topiramate have been used successfully to treat clozapine-induced seizures (Navarro et al. 2001; Toth and Frankenburg 1994; Usiskin et al. 2000). Topiramate has an advantage over sodium valproate in that it is associated with very little weight gain. In cases in our clinic where patients have developed seizures while taking clozapine, we institute rapid loading with anticonvulsant medication and temporarily discontinue the clozapine treatment. We then slowly reintroduce and retitrate the clozapine once the patient is taking an adequate dose of anticonvulsant medication.

Constipation

A truly problematic consequence of clozapine's anticholinergic activity is its propensity to cause significant constipation. This can be a difficult side effect to manage in severely mentally ill individuals, who may not complain about the problem until a medical emergency, such as acute bowel obstruction, occurs. In institutional settings and in prisons, where patients may have little access to exercise and where monitoring of patients' fluid intake is not performed, constipation from clozapine can be serious or even fatal (Drew and Herdson 1997; Hayes and Gibler 1995;

Levin et al. 2002). Typically, constipation can be avoided by proactive modifications in patients' diets and education about adequate fluid intake and exercise. The medical treatment that we favor is prophylactic therapy with sorbitol. We are less inclined to recommend treatments involving bulking agents, particularly in the setting of poor fluid intake. High-fiber diets can also be beneficial.

Other Side Effects

Sedation is one of the most difficult and common side effects of clozapine to manage. Patients often do not want their doses increased in the setting of increased sedation and will complain of sedation as one of the most annoying consequences of clozapine treatment (Angermeyer et al. 2001). In our experience, sedation is usually the limiting factor controlling both the rate at which the dosage of clozapine can be increased and the maximum dosage the patient can tolerate. However, no rigorous studies have been published.

There have been several reports of respiratory arrest or depression during the early stages of treatment with clozapine (Novartis 2002). Two of the patients who experienced respiratory arrest were concomitantly taking benzodiazepines.

Sialorrhea is a commonly reported side effect of clozapine (occurring in over 50% of patients) that can be problematic for patients. The etiology of sialorrhea is unclear, but the condition does not seem to be caused by the dopamine blockade. It may be mediated through α-adrenergic receptor blockade. Case series and small pilot studies indicate that treating sialorrhea with antiadrenergic agents, such as the clonidine patch, or anticholinergic agents, such as benztropine and intranasal ipratropium bromide, may be successful (Calderon et al. 2000). We generally recommend that patients sleep with a towel on their pillow, as this side effect seems to be most bothersome during the night. Unfortunately, the use of concomitant antiadrenergic or anticholinergic agents adds to the potential side-effect burdens of hypotension and constipation, respectively.

Neuroleptic malignant syndrome (NMS), a syndrome of unknown etiology that includes hyperthermia, autonomic instability, and severe rigidity, has been reported in several patients treated with clozapine (Anderson and Powers 1991). The etiology of NMS that occurs in the context of clozapine use, as well as that occurring with use of conventional antipsychotics, remains unclear.

Hepatotoxicity has been reported with clozapine, especially in the setting of polypharmacy (Macfarlane et al. 1997; Wirshing et al. 1997). Asymptomatic elevation of transaminase levels was observed most commonly, affecting between 30% and 50% of patients treated with clozapine. Icteric hepatitis was uncommonly seen in Macfarlane et al.'s (1997) review of clozapine-related hepatotoxicity and was noted in 84 of 136,000 patients (0.06%). Fatal acute fulminant hepatitis has been documented in 2 patients (0.001%). Although serious toxicity is rare, prescribers of clozapine should be aware of its hepatotoxic potential.

Sexual side effects, including priapism and impotence, have been reported with clozapine. Urinary retention and bladder dysfunction can also result from clozapine. In a study surveying patients' sexual side effects, we found that clozapine-treated patients actually had fewer sexual complaints than patients on other antipsychotic medications (fluphenazine and risperidone) (Wirshing et al. 2002b).

Although this daunting array of side effects—along with the management of the risk of agranulocytosis—makes the treatment of patients with clozapine complex, it is common for patients to report a sense of relief from the dysphoric moods they experienced while taking conventional drugs. Additionally, the freedom from EPS may account for the enhanced sense of well-being in patients treated with clozapine.

Drug-Drug Interactions

As previously mentioned, clozapine is predominately metabolized by CYP1A2, although CYP2D6 and CYP3A3 also contribute to its metabolism (Buur-Rasmussen and Brosen 1999). Smoking, which induces CYP 1A2, lowers clozapine plasma levels. Fluvoxamine, a potent inhibitor of CYP1A2, dramatically increases plasma levels of clozapine (Heeringa et al. 1999), and on occasion, adverse effects are seen (Koponen et al. 1996). This phenomenon can lead to clozapine intoxication in patients receiving high doses of fluvoxamine. Other reports suggest that inhibitors of CYP2D6, including paroxetine and fluoxetine, can elevate clozapine levels (Joos et al. 1997; Spina et al. 1998).

Conclusion

Clozapine maintains an important place in the treatment of severe psychosis. Side effects, including agranulocytosis, seizures, sedation, and weight gain, make it the most difficult antipsychotic to prescribe. For this reason, clozapine should be reserved for patients who have failed to respond to other antipsychotics. The difficulty in administering clozapine has led many patients and their clinicians to resist its use. As a result, this effective treatment is underutilized in most communities. This is unfortunate, because patients should never be deemed "treatment refractory" or "partial responders" until they have received an adequate trial of clozapine.

References

Allison DB, Mentore JL, Heo M, et al: Antipsychotic-induced weight gain: a comprehensive research synthesis. Am J Psychiatry 156:1686–1696, 1999

Alvir JM, Lieberman JA, Safferman AZ, et al: Clozapine-induced agranulocytosis: incidence and risk factors in the United States. N Engl J Med 329:162–167, 1993

American Diabetes Association; American Psychiatric Association; American Association of Clinical Endocrinologists; North American Association for the Study of Obesity: Consensus development conference on antipsychotic drugs and obesity and diabetes. Diabetes Care 27: 596–601, 2004

Amsler HA, Teerenhovi L, Barth E, et al: Agranulocytosis in patients treated with clozapine: a study of the Finnish epidemic. Acta Psychiatr Scand 56:241–248, 1977

Anderson ES, Powers PS: Neuroleptic malignant syndrome associated with clozapine use. J Clin Psychiatry 52:102–104, 1991

Angermeyer MC, Loffler W, Muller P, et al: Patients' and relatives' assessment of clozapine treatment. Psychol Med 31:509–517, 2001

Athanasiou MC, Dettling M, Cascorbi I, et al: Candidate gene analysis identifies a polymorphism in HLA-DQB1 associated with clozapine-induced agranulocytosis. J Clin Psychiatry 72: 458–463, 2011

Barbini B, Scherillo P, Benedetti F, et al: Response to clozapine in acute mania is more rapid than that of chlorpromazine. Int Clin Psychopharmacol 12:109–112, 1997

Bell R, McLaren A, Galanos J, et al: The clinical use of plasma clozapine levels. Aust N Z J Psychiatry 32:567–574, 1998

Breier A, Buchanan R, Irish D, et al: Clozapine treatment of outpatients with schizophrenia: outcome and long-term response patterns, 1993. Psychiatr Serv 51:1249–1253, 2000

Brunette MF, Drake RE, Xie H, et al: Clozapine use and relapses of substance use disorder among patients with co-occurring schizophrenia and substance use disorders. Schizophr Bull 32:637–643, 2006

Buur-Rasmussen B, Brosen K: Cytochrome P450 and therapeutic drug monitoring with respect to clozapine. Eur Neuropsychopharmacol 9:453–459, 1999

Calderon J, Rubin E, Sobota WL: Potential use of ipratropium bromide for the treatment of clozapine-induced hypersalivation: a preliminary report. Int Clin Psychopharmacol 15:49–52, 2000

Canuso CM, Goldman MB: Clozapine restores water balance in schizophrenic patients with polydipsia-hyponatremia syndrome. J Neuropsychiatry Clin Neurosci 11:86–90, 1999

Chengappa KN, Goldstein JM, Greenwood M, et al: A post hoc analysis of the impact on hostility and agitation of quetiapine and haloperidol among patients with schizophrenia. Clin Ther 25:530–541, 2003

Citrome L, Volavka J, Czobor P, et al: Effects of clozapine, olanzapine, risperidone, and haloperidol on hostility among patients with schizophrenia. Psychiatr Serv 52:1510–1514, 2001

de la Chapelle A, Kari C, Nurminem M, et al: Clozapine-induced agranulocytosis: a genetic and epidemiologic study. Hum Genet 37:183–194, 1977

Drake RE, Xie H, McHugo GJ, et al: The effects of clozapine on alcohol and drug use disorders among patients with schizophrenia. Schizophr Bull 26:441–449, 2000

Drew L, Herdson P: Clozapine and constipation: a serious issue. Aust N Z J Psychiatry 31:149–150, 1997

Essock SM, Frisman LK, Covell NH, et al: Cost-effectiveness of clozapine compared with conventional antipsychotic medication for patients in state hospitals. Arch Gen Psychiatry 57:987–994, 2000

Farde L, Nordstrom AL, Wiesel FA, et al: Positron emission tomographic analysis of central D and D1 and D2 dopamine receptor occupancy in patients treated with classical neuroleptics and clozapine: relation to extrapyramidal side effects. Arch Gen Psychiatry 49:538–544, 1992

French Clozapine Parkinson Study Group: Clozapine in drug-induced psychosis in Parkinson's disease. Lancet 353:2041–2042, 1999

Green AI, Burgess ES, Dawson R, et al: Alcohol and cannabis use in schizophrenia: effects of clozapine vs risperidone. Schizophr Res 60:81–85, 2003

Green AI, Drake RE, Brunette MF, et al: Schizophrenia and co-occurring substance use disorder. Am J Psychiatry 164:402–408, 2007

Griffith RW, Saamerli K: Clozapine and agranulocytosis. Lancet 2(7936):657, 1975

Hayes G, Gibler B: Clozapine-induced constipation. Am J Psychiatry 152:298, 1995

Heeringa M, Beurskens R, Schouten W, et al: Elevated plasma levels of clozapine after concomitant use of fluvoxamine. Pharm World Sci 21:243–244, 1999

Henderson D: Clozapine: diabetes mellitus, weight gain, and lipid abnormalities. J Clin Psychiatry 62 (suppl 23):39–44, 2001

Hippius H: A historical perspective of clozapine. J Clin Psychiatry 60 (suppl 12):22–23, 1999

Honigfeld G: Effects of the clozapine national registry system on incidence of deaths related to agranulocytosis. Psychiatr Serv 47:52–56, 1996

Honigfeld G, Arellano F, Sethi J, et al: Reducing clozapine-related morbidity and mortality: 5 years of experience with the Clozaril National Registry. J Clin Psychiatry 59 (suppl 3):3–7, 1998

Jones KM, Stoukides CA: Clozapine in treatment of Parkinson's disease. Ann Pharmacother 26: 1386–1377, 1992

Joos AA, Konig F, Frank UG, et al: Dose-dependent pharmacokinetic interaction of clozapine and paroxetine in an extensive metabolizer. Pharmacopsychiatry 30:266–270, 1997

Kane J, Honigfeld G, Singer J, et al: Clozapine for the treatment-resistant schizophrenic: a double-blind comparison with chlorpromazine. Arch Gen Psychiatry 45:789–796, 1988

Kane JM, Marder SR, Schooler NR, et al: Clozapine and haloperidol in moderately refractory schizophrenia: a 6-month randomized and double-blind comparison. Arch Gen Psychiatry 58: 965–972, 2001

Kapur S, Seeman P: Does fast dissociation from the dopamine D2 receptor explain the action of atypical antipsychotics? A new hypothesis. Am J Psychiatry 158:360–369, 2001

Killian JG, Kerr K, Lawrence C, et al: Myocarditis and cardiomyopathy associated with clozapine. Lancet 354:1841–1845, 1999

Klimke A, Klieser E: [The atypical neuroleptic clozapine (Leponex)—current knowledge and recent clinical aspects.] Fortschr Neurol Psychiatr 63:173–193, 1995

Koponen HJ, Leinonen E, Lepola U: Fluvoxamine increases the clozapine serum levels significantly. Eur Neuropsychopharmacol 6:69–71, 1996

Kronig MH, Munne RA, Szymanski S, et al: Plasma clozapine levels and clinical response for treatment-refractory schizophrenic patients. Am J Psychiatry 152:179–182, 1995

Kumra S, Frazier JA, Jacobsen LK, et al: Childhood-onset schizophrenia: a double-blind clozapine-haloperidol comparison. Arch Gen Psychiatry 53:1090–1097, 1996

Lehman AF, Kreyenbuhl J, Buchanan RW, et al: The Schizophrenia Patient Outcomes Research Team (PORT): updated treatment recommendations 2003. Schizophr Bull 30:193–217, 2004a

Lehman AF, Lieberman JA, Dixon LB, et al: Practice guideline for the treatment of patients with schizophrenia, second edition. Am J Psychiatry 161 (2 suppl):1–56, 2004b

Levin TT, Barrett J, Mendelowitz A: Death from clozapine-induced constipation: case report and literature review. Psychosomatics 43:71–73, 2002

Lewis SW, Barnes TR, Davies L, et al: Randomized controlled trial of effect of prescription of clozapine versus other second-generation antipsychotic drugs in resistant schizophrenia. Schizophr Bull 32:715–723, 2006

Lieberman JA, Safferman AZ: Clinical profile of clozapine: adverse reactions and agranulocytosis. Psychiatr Q 63:51–70, 1992

Macfarlane B, Davies S, Mannan K, et al: Fatal acute fulminant liver failure due to clozapine: a case report and review of clozapine-induced hepatotoxicity. Gastroenterology 112:1707–1709, 1997

Marder SR, Essock SM, Miller AL, et al: The Mount Sinai conference on the pharmacotherapy of schizophrenia. Schizophr Bull 28:5–16, 2002

Marder SR, Essock SM, Miller AL, et al: Physical health monitoring of patients with schizophrenia. Am J Psychiatry 161:1334–1349, 2004

McElroy SL, Dessain EC, Pope HG Jr, et al: Clozapine in the treatment of psychotic mood disorders, schizoaffective disorder, and schizophrenia. J Clin Psychiatry 52:411–414, 1991

McEvoy JP, Lieberman JA, Stroup TS, et al: Effectiveness of clozapine versus olanzapine, quetiapine, and risperidone in patients with chronic schizophrenia who did not respond to prior atypical antipsychotic treatment. Am J Psychiatry 163:600–610, 2006

Meltzer HY: Suicidality in schizophrenia: a review of the evidence for risk factors and treatment options. Curr Psychiatry Rep 4:279–283, 2002

Meltzer HY, Okayli G: Reduction of suicidality during clozapine treatment of neuroleptic-resistant schizophrenia: impact on risk-benefit assessment. Am J Psychiatry 152:183–190, 1995

Miller AL, Hall CS, Buchanan RW, et al: The Texas Medication Algorithm Project antipsychotic algorithm for schizophrenia: 2003 update. J Clin Psychiatry 65:500–508, 2004

Miller DD: The clinical use of clozapine plasma concentrations in the management of treatment-refractory schizophrenia. Ann Clin Psychiatry 8:99–109, 1996

Miller DD, Fleming F, Holman TL, et al: Plasma clozapine concentrations as a predictor of clinical response: a follow-up study. J Clin Psychiatry 55 (suppl B):117–121, 1994

Miyasaki JM, Shannon K, Voon V, et al: Practice parameter: evaluation and treatment of depression, psychosis, and dementia in Parkinson disease (an evidence-based review): report of the Quality Standards Subcommittee of the American Academy of Neurology. Neurology 66:996–1002, 2006

Navarro V, Pons A, Romero A, et al: Topiramate for clozapine-induced seizures. Am J Psychiatry 158:968–969, 2001

Novartis: Clozaril (clozapine) tablets: prescribing information. Hanover, NJ, Novartis Pharmaceuticals, July 2002

Parkinson Study Group: Low-dose clozapine for the treatment of drug-induced psychosis in Parkinson's disease. N Engl J Med 340:757–763, 1999

Pickar D, Owen RR, Litman RE, et al: Clinical and biologic response to clozapine in patients with schizophrenia: crossover comparison with fluphenazine. Arch Gen Psychiatry 49:345–353, 1992

Pollak P, Tison F, Rascol O, et al: Clozapine in drug induced psychosis in Parkinson's disease: a randomised, placebo controlled study with open follow up. J Neurol Neurosurg Psychiatry 75: 689–695, 2004

Potkin SG, Bera R, Gulasekaram B, et al: Plasma clozapine concentrations predict clinical response in treatment resistant schizophrenia. J Clin Psychiatry 55 (9, suppl B):117–121, 1994

Raison CL, Guze BH, Kissell RL, et al: Successful treatment of clozapine-induced agranulocytosis with granulocyte colony-stimulating factor. J Clin Psychopharmacol 14:285–286, 1994

Ranjan R, Meltzer HY: Acute and long-term effectiveness of clozapine in treatment-resistant psychotic depression. Biol Psychiatry 40:253–258, 1996

Reid WH, Mason M, Hogan T: Suicide prevention effects associated with clozapine therapy in schizophrenia and schizoaffective disorder. Psychiatr Serv 49:1029–1033, 1998

Rosenheck R, Cramer J, Xu W, et al: A comparison of clozapine and haloperidol in hospitalized patients with refractory schizophrenia. Department of Veterans Affairs Cooperative Study Group on Clozapine in Refractory Schizophrenia. N Engl J Med 337:809–815, 1997

Rothschild AJ: Management of psychotic, treatment-resistant depression. Psychiatr Clin North Am 19:237–252, 1996

Safferman AZ, Lieberman JA, Alvir JM, et al: Rechallenge in clozapine-induced agranulocytosis (letter). Lancet 339:1296–1297, 1992

Seeman P: Atypical antipsychotics: mechanism of action. Can J Psychiatry 47:27–38, 2002

Shaw P, Sporn A, Gogtay N, et al: Childhood-onset schizophrenia: a double-blind, randomized clozapine-olanzapine comparison. Arch Gen Psychiatry 63:721–730, 2006

Simpson GM, Cooper TA: Clozapine plasma levels and convulsions. Am J Psychiatry 135:99–100, 1978

Simpson GM, Varga E: Clozapine—a new antipsychotic agent. Curr Ther Res Clin Exp 16:679–686, 1974

Sommer IE, Begemann MJ, Temmerman A, et al: Pharmacological augmentation strategies for schizophrenia patients with insufficient response to clozapine: a quantitative literature review. Schizophr Bull 38:1003–1011, 2012

Spina E, Avenoso A, Facciola G, et al: Effect of fluoxetine on the plasma concentrations of clozapine and its major metabolites in patients with schizophrenia. Int Clin Psychopharmacol 13: 141–145, 1998

Stroup TS, Lieberman JA, McEvoy JP, et al: Effectiveness of olanzapine, quetiapine, risperidone, and ziprasidone in patients with chronic schizophrenia following discontinuation of a previous atypical antipsychotic. Am J Psychiatry 163:611–622, 2006

Suppes T, Webb A, Paul B, et al: Clinical outcome in a randomized 1-year trial of clozapine versus treatment as usual for patients with treatment-resistant illness and a history of mania. Am J Psychiatry 156:1164–1169, 1999

Toth P, Frankenburg FR: Clozapine and seizures: a review. Can J Psychiatry 39:236–238, 1994

Usiskin SI, Nicolson R, Lenane M, et al: Gabapentin prophylaxis of clozapine-induced seizures. Am J Psychiatry 157:482–483, 2000

Vailleau JL, Jeanny B, Chomard P, et al: [Importance of determining clozapine plasma level in follow-up of schizophrenic patients.] Encephale 22:103–109, 1996

Walker AM, Lanzall LL, Arellano F, et al: Mortality in current and former users of clozapine. Epidemiology 8:671–677, 1997

Weide R, Koppler H, Heymanns J, et al: Successful treatment of clozapine induced agranulocytosis with granulocyte–colony-stimulating factor (G-CSF). Br J Haematol 80:557–559, 1992

Welch J, Manschreck T, Redmond D: Clozapine-induced seizures and EEG changes. J Neuropsychiatry Clin Neurosci 6:250–256, 1994

Wickramanayake PD, Scheid C, Josting A, et al: Use of granulocyte colony-stimulating factor (filgrastim) in the treatment of non-cytotoxic drug-induced agranulocytosis. Eur J Med Res 1:153–156, 1995

Wirshing DA, Spellberg BJ, Erhart SM, et al: Novel antipsychotics and new onset diabetes. Biol Psychiatry 44:778–783, 1998

Wirshing DA, Wirshing WC, Kysar L, et al: Novel antipsychotics: comparison of weight gain liabilities. J Clin Psychiatry 60:358–363, 1999

Wirshing DA, Boyd J, Meng LR: The effects of novel antipsychotics on glucose and lipid levels. J Clin Psychiatry 63:856–865, 2002a

Wirshing DA, Pierre JM, Marder SR, et al: Sexual side effects of novel antipsychotic medications. Schizophr Res 56:25–30, 2002b

Wirshing W, Ames D, Bisheff S, et al: Hepatic encephalopathy associated with combined clozapine and divalproex sodium treatment. J Clin Psychopharmacol 17:120–121, 1997

Wolters EC, Berendse HW: Management of psychosis in Parkinson's disease. Curr Opin Neurol 14:499–504, 2001

Wooltorton E: Antipsychotic clozapine (Clozaril): myocarditis and cardiovascular toxicity. CMAJ 166:1185–1186, 2002

CHAPTER 17

Olanzapine

Jacob S. Ballon, M.D.

Donna Ames, M.D.

S. Charles Schulz, M.D.

History and Discovery

The story of specific antipsychotic medications for patients with schizophrenia and other severe psychiatric illnesses began in the early 1950s, when chlorpromazine was first given to psychotic patients in France (Delay and Bernitzer 1952). The antipsychotic qualities of this compound, as well as its "tranquilizing" effect, were dramatic and substantial. Studies performed around the world during the 1950s showed the usefulness of this new compound and the others that followed. As is well known, multicenter trials of antipsychotic medications found that the approved medications were substantially and significantly better than placebo (Cole et al. 1964). Furthermore, despite the range of chemical structures, the clinical effects were similar. In addition, the need to investigate the new medications for psychiatric illness led to improved clinical trial methodology for the field. During the 1960s, randomized and placebo-controlled trials became the standard for assessing the new medications for schizophrenia. These trials led to the neuroleptic medications becoming the standard somatic treatment for schizophrenia.

However, over time, the adverse effects of the neuroleptic medications began to be recognized as more troublesome (Table 17–1). For example, many patients complained of iatrogenic parkinsonism, dystonias, slowed thinking, blunted affect, akathisia, and tardive dyskinesia. These side effects were uncomfortable for patients taking the neuroleptic medications and, in many cases, led to poor adherence with treatment.

Looking for ways to achieve treatment benefit but with decreased side effects, investigators at Eli Lilly were screening numerous compounds for psychotropic properties. In 1990, the company applied for and received a patent for the compound olanzapine. It is interesting to note that the new compound

TABLE 17–1. Shortcomings of traditional antipsychotic medications

Significant response in only 60%–70% of patients
Movement disorder side effects
Dystonia
Parkinsonism
Tardive dyskinesia
Akathisia
Slowed thinking ("cognitive parkinsonism")
Secondary negative symptoms

had many structural similarities to clozapine, which in 1989 had been approved for use in treating refractory schizophrenia. Hailed as a novel second-generation antipsychotic drug, clozapine was thought to have potential for schizophrenia, mania, and anxiety. Clozapine was noted for its efficacy as well as its freedom from neurological side effects.

Olanzapine was first given to patients with schizophrenia in 1995 (Baldwin and Montgomery 1995). The patients in the study experienced a substantial decrease in their symptoms while receiving 5–30 mg/day of the compound. The study researchers noted a low degree of extrapyramidal side effects (EPS), although concern was raised regarding elevation of liver enzymes, as one patient had to discontinue the study for that reason.

The initial testing of olanzapine had useful results and led to a program of four pivotal trials of olanzapine. These first four controlled studies examined the differences between olanzapine (10 mg/day fixed dosage) and placebo (Beasley et al. 1996a), olanzapine and haloperidol or placebo (Beasley et al. 1996b), olanzapine (low, medium, or high dose) and olanzapine 1.0 mg/day or haloperidol 15 mg/day (Beasley et al. 1997), and olanzapine and haloperidol in a large international study (Tollefson et al. 1997). The positive results for olanzapine led to U.S. Food and Drug Administration (FDA) approval in 1997 and then widespread use in the United States and around the world.

Structure-Activity Relations

Olanzapine is a thiobenzodiazepine derivative that bears a close structural resemblance to clozapine. The formal chemical name of olanzapine is 2-methyl-4-(4-methyl-1-piperazinyl)-10*H*-thieno[2,3-*b*] [1,5]benzodiazepine. Structurally, olanzapine differs from clozapine by two additional methyl groups and the lack of a chloride moiety. The in vitro receptor binding profiles of olanzapine and clozapine are relatively similar. According to the package insert, olanzapine is known to have a high affinity for selective dopaminergic (D), serotonergic (5-HT), histaminergic (H), and α-adrenergic receptors, with weaker affinity for muscarinic (M) receptors and weak activity at benzodiazepine, γ-aminobutyric acid type A ($GABA_A$), and β-adrenergic receptors (Eli Lilly 2006).

Pharmacological Profile

In vitro and preclinical behavioral studies of olanzapine predicted significant antipsychotic activity with a low propensity to induce EPS. Because clozapine is the prototype for second-generation antipsychotic action, similarity to its effects relative to those of classic antipsychotics is evidence for the "atypicality" of comparator compounds such as olanzapine.

One possible mechanism for lowering risk for EPS is nonselective dopamine receptor binding. Classic antipsychotics selectively block D_2-like (D_2, D_3, and D_4) receptors over D_1-like (D_1 and D_5) receptors—for example, haloperidol has a D_2-to-D_1 binding ratio of 25:1. Clozapine nonselectively binds all five dopamine receptor subtypes, with a D_2-to-D_1 ratio of 0.7:1, whereas olanzapine is only partially selective for the D_2-like group, with a D_2-to-D_1 ratio of approximately 3:1, intermediate between those of haloperidol and clozapine.

In animal models predictive of antipsychotic efficacy, olanzapine produces effects indicating dopamine antagonism, with a low propensity to produce EPS. For example, in rats, olanzapine reduces climbing behavior induced by apomorphine and antagonizes stimulant-induced hyperactivity, both characteristic of antipsychotic effects. The ratio of the dose needed to produce catalepsy to the dose needed to inhibit conditioned avoidance, another model for atypical efficacy, is higher for olanzapine than for conventional agents (Moore 1999).

Another potential mechanism whereby dopamine antagonists may exert antipsychotic effects with minimal EPS is through selective activity in the A10 dopaminergic tracts from the ventral tegmentum to mesolimbic areas compared with effects antagonizing the A9 nigrostriatal projections that mediate EPS. Olanzapine in chronic administration, like clozapine, selectively inhibits firing of A10 neurons without significant inhibition of A9 tracts (Stockton and Rasmussen 1996a). Olanzapine shows increased c-fos activity in the nucleus accumbens relative to the dorsolateral striatum, thus demonstrating selective blockade of the mesolimbic dopamine tract compared with the nigrostriatal tract (Robertson and Fibiger 1996).

The current leading theory regarding atypicality relates to the fleeting effects of atypical antipsychotics at the D_2 receptor, coupled with regional selectivity of these compounds (Seeman 2002). Olanzapine has been shown to have a D_2 receptor occupancy saturation that is between that of clozapine and haloperidol and may be responsible for a decreased risk of EPS (Tauscher et al. 1999). However, as the current second-generation antipsychotic medications have substantially differing effects at many of the targets thought to play a role in atypicality, consensus is not there regarding the true rationale for "atypicality" compared with the first-generation antipsychotics (Farah 2005).

Amphetamine administration in rats is often used as a model for psychosis. The sympathomimetic activity and dopamine release provide a target for testing antipsychotic medications. Olanzapine disrupts the activity of amphetamines in rats (Gosselin et al. 1996). Olanzapine was shown in a rat model to decrease dopamine release in the A10 dopaminergic neurons of the ventral tegmentum greater than the A9 dopaminergic neurons of the striatum after chronic administration and after an amphetamine challenge (Stockton and Rasmussen 1996a, 1996b). Olanzapine does not induce catalepsy in rats at doses needed for antipsychotic efficacy.

Another model of psychosis in rats is produced by administration of the glutamatergic *N*-methyl-D-aspartate (NMDA) receptor antagonist phencyclidine (PCP). Chronic PCP use in humans is associated with symptoms similar to those in schizophrenia, including negative symptoms, thus making it a putative model for schizophrenia (Krystal et al. 1994). Olanzapine has been shown to decrease the hyperactivity of NMDA receptors under chronic PCP administration, which may have a bearing on the effect on negative symptoms (Ninan et al. 2003). With chronic administration, glutamatergic activity continues to be affected by olanzapine (Jardemark et al. 2000). Despite these findings, olanzapine has no direct affinity for the NMDA receptor (Stephenson and Pilowsky 1999).

Effects on other systems show that olanzapine has a broad range of neurotransmitter effects. Although olanzapine has potent muscarinic M_{1-5} receptor affinity in vitro (another contributor to putative anti-EPS effects), in practice few patients have anticholinergic side effects that are clinically significant. α_1-Adrenergic and H_1 histaminergic antagonism contribute to olanzapine's adverse-effect profile of orthostatic hypotension (α_1), sedation (H_1), and possibly weight gain (H_1). Olanzapine has little or no effect on α_2- and β-adrenergic, H_2, nicotinic, GABA, opioid, sigma, or benzodiazepine receptors.

Pharmacokinetics and Disposition

Olanzapine is well absorbed after oral administration, with peak concentrations in most people occurring 4–6 hours after ingestion (Kassahun et al. 1997). Approximately 40% of a given dose undergoes first-pass metabolism and therefore does not reach the systemic circulation, and food has little effect on olanzapine's bioavailability (Callaghan et al. 1999; Eli Lilly 2006; Kassahun et al. 1997).

Two bioequivalent oral formulations of olanzapine are currently available: a standard oral tablet and an oral disintegrating tablet. The oral disintegrating tablets are intended for swallowing and absorption through the gut; however, sublingual administration has also been favored by some. Markowitz et al. (2006) discovered that while the oral disintegrating preparation of olanzapine is more quickly absorbed than a standard oral tablet, it is absorbed at an equal rate if taken sublingually or if swallowed conventionally. In either case, the onset of action with the oral dissolving tablet is faster than with the standard oral tablet. After a 12.5-mg oral dose of ^{14}C-labeled olanzapine, approximately 57% of the radiocarbon was recovered in urine and 30% in feces. In vitro studies suggest that olanzapine is approximately 93% protein bound, binding primarily to albumin and α_1-acid glycoprotein (Kassahun et al. 1997).

Olanzapine is available as an intramuscular preparation, intended for treatment of the acute agitation typically seen in schizophrenia or acute manic episodes of bipolar disorder. The peak plasma concentration is typically reached between 15 and 45 minutes after administration. The potency of intramuscular olanzapine is nearly five times greater than that of the orally administered drug, based on plasma levels. Clinical antipsychotic onset with intramuscular olanzapine is evident within 2 hours of administration, with benefits lasting for at least 24 hours (Kapur et al. 2005).

Olanzapine is also available in a long-acting injectable (LAI) preparation composed of a dihydrate form of olanzapine pamoate. As a dihydrate molecule, it is less soluble in water than a monohydrate and thus has the longer half-life required for a depot formulation. This formulation is designed to be dosed once every 4 weeks (Mamo et al. 2008).

Finally, olanzapine is available in a combined preparation with fluoxetine. The olanzapine-fluoxetine combination (OFC) tablet provides fixed doses of olanzapine and fluoxetine. Overall, few pharmacokinetic differences result from adding fluoxetine to olanzapine, and those present are generally related to cytochrome P450 (CYP) 2D6 inhibition. There is no change in the overall half-life of olanzapine. While there are minor yet statistically significant differences in the concentration of olanzapine when taken in combination with fluoxetine, these changes are not clinically significant and do not change the side-effect profile of olanzapine (Gossen et al. 2002).

Olanzapine is extensively metabolized to multiple metabolites but primarily to 10-*N*-glucuronide and 4′-*N*-desmethylolanzapine (Macias et al. 1998). In vitro studies assessing the oxidative metabolism of olanzapine suggest that CYP1A2 is the enzyme primarily responsible for the formation of 4′-*N*-desmethylolanzapine, flavin-containing monooxygenase-3 (FMO3) is responsible for the formation of 4′-*N*-oxide olanzapine, and CYP2D6 is the primary enzyme responsible for the formation of 2-hydroxymethyl olanzapine (Ring et al. 1996b). Although CYP1A2 appears to be a major route of metabolism, olanzapine clearance in one study was not significantly correlated with salivary paraxanthine-to-caffeine ratio (thought to be a measure of CYP1A2 activity) (Hagg et al. 2001). Another analysis, however, found that the 4′-*N*-desmethylolanzapine–to–olanzapine plasma metabolic ratio significantly correlated with olanzapine clearance (Callaghan et al. 1999). Olanzapine pharmacokinetic parameters do not differ significantly between extensive and poor metabolizers of CYP2D6 (see Hagg et al. 2001).

Olanzapine shows linear pharmacokinetics within the recommended dosage range (Aravagiri et al. 1997; Bergstrom et al. 1995; Callaghan et al. 1999). Mean half-life was 36 hours, mean clearance was 29.4 L/hour, mean volume of distribution was 19.2 L/kg, and area under the concentration-time curve over 24 hours (AUC_{0-24}) was 333 ng*hour/mL. The half-lives of the two major metabolites (4′-*N*-desmethylolanzapine and 10-*N*-glucuronide) were 92.6 and 39.6 hours, respectively (Macias et al. 1998). Other analyses also have found the mean half-life of olanzapine to be approximately 30 hours and the mean apparent clearance to be approximately 25 L/hour (Callaghan et al. 1999; Eli Lilly 2006; Kassahun et al. 1997). Once-daily administration of olanzapine produces steady-state concentrations in about a week that are approximately twofold higher than concentrations after single doses (Callaghan et al. 1999).

Clearance of olanzapine is approximately 25%–30% lower in women than in men, based on results of population pharmacokinetic analyses (Callaghan et al. 1999; Patel et al. 1995, 1996). A study of 20 male and 7 female patients with schizophrenia receiving olanzapine also found that women had higher trough concentrations after receiving 1 week of olanzapine 12.5 mg/day (Kelly et al. 1999). Despite the differences in clearance and plasma levels, there is no difference between sexes in incidence of EPS or other movement disorders (Aichhorn et al. 2006).

Olanzapine's pharmacokinetics in the elderly and in children differ from those in adults. In the elderly, olanzapine clearance is approximately 30% lower than in younger individuals, and the half-life is approximately 50% longer (Callaghan et al. 1999; Patel et al. 1995). A study of eight children and adolescents (ages 10–18 years) found pharmacokinetic parameters similar to those reported in nonsmoking adults, with an average T_{max} (time required to reach the maximal plasma concentration) of 4.7 hours, an average apparent oral clearance of 9.6 L/hour, and an average half-life of 37.2 hours (Grothe et al. 2000). The highest concentrations were seen when smaller-sized patients received dosages greater than 10 mg/day; therefore, dosing should take into consideration the size of the child.

Impairment in either hepatic or renal function has not been associated with altered olanzapine disposition. In a study of four healthy individuals and eight patients with hepatic cirrhosis, no significant differences in olanzapine pharmacokinetics were found, although urinary concentrations of olanzapine 10-*N*-glucuronide were increased in patients with cirrhosis (Callaghan et al. 1999). A study comparing olanzapine pharmacokinetics in six subjects with normal renal function, six subjects with renal failure who received an olanzapine dose 1 hour before hemodialysis, and six subjects with renal failure who received an olanzapine dose during their 48-hour interdialytic interval did not find any significant differences. These data suggest that olanzapine dosage does not need to be adjusted in patients with renal or hepatic disease (Callaghan et al. 1999).

Mechanism of Action

In discussing the mechanism of action for olanzapine in the treatment of schizophrenia, it should be noted that there is no established molecular mechanism to unify the symptoms of schizophrenia. No precise animal or in vitro model for the illness exists, nor is there a consensus on the precise etiology or pathophysiology. Numerous neurochemical hypotheses exist and include abnormalities in dopaminergic, glutamatergic, serotonergic, and other systems such as neurotensin (Boules et al. 2007) and neuregulin (Benzel et al. 2007). Furthermore, other theories about the etiology and pathophysiology of schizophrenia include the possibility of abnormal development of the brain resulting in postulated changes in the relation of one part of the brain to the other (e.g., the prefrontal cortex to limbic areas) (Weinberger 1987). Further complicating these theories of pathophysiology of schizophrenia has been the understanding of the multiple different types of receptors for the same neurotransmitters that exist in the brain. Therefore, it is no longer possible to simply discuss hypotheses such as increased dopamine as a comprehensive theory for the etiology of schizophrenia.

Despite the caveats noted above regarding the rudimentary knowledge of the nature of schizophrenia, it is important to note that all approved antipsychotic medications have an important effect on the dopaminergic system, largely through the blockade of D_2 receptors (Kapur and Remington 2001). Even though there are substantial differences in affinities to the D_2 receptor among the traditional antipsychotic medications and the atypical antipsychotics, they all are full antagonists or are partial agonists at the D_2 receptor. Of interest is the evolving research indicating the importance for blockade of other receptors by the atypical antipsychotic medication class. As these systems have been investigated in the neuropsychopharmacology of schizophrenia, evidence is emerging that the action of second-generation antipsychotics, and olanzapine specifically, may improve different parts of the schizophrenia syndrome through effects on 5-HT receptors, by multiple-receptor binding, by region-specific and more fleeting binding to dopamine receptors, by effects on glutamate neurotransmission, and perhaps by influence on neuroprotein neurotransmitters. Each of these specific ideas for the mechanism of action of olanzapine is discussed in order.

In clinical investigations with positron emission tomography (PET) imaging, Kapur et al. (1998) showed that olanzapine at a wide range of doses blocks a high percentage (95% or greater) of 5-HT_{2A} receptors and blocks dopamine receptors in a dose-dependent fashion—crossing the putative antipsychotic blockade line at doses commonly used to diminish psychotic symptoms of schizophrenia. This study indicated that olanzapine's primary mechanism was related to the blockade of dopamine receptors and additionally noted that olanzapine showed stronger affinity for 5-HT_{2A} receptors than for dopamine receptors at all dosage ranges.

A more compelling hypothesis regarding the atypicality of olanzapine has emerged from the in vivo PET scanning work being performed in a series of experiments at the University of Toronto and in Sweden. Results of the initial PET scanning studies of patients receiving clozapine indicated that there was atypical dopamine receptor binding (Farde and Nordstrom 1992; Farde et al. 1992; Kapur et al. 2000). The group subsequently found similar results for quetiapine and, to some degree, olanzapine (Kapur et al. 1998). The authors indicated that the successful reduction of psychotic symptoms in schizophrenic patients without movement disorder side effects may be the result of a "fast off" property of some of the atypical antipsychotic medications. They argued that for medicines that block the dopamine receptor but leave that receptor quickly, there may be an effect at the receptor to decrease psychosis but that a "physiological" dopamine activity at the receptor remains. Thus, for olanzapine, this may contribute to the treatment of schizophrenia while causing fewer EPS at standard doses. From a clinical view, it is important to note that at higher dosages of olanzapine (30 mg/day), higher dopamine receptor blockade is seen, and movement disorder side effects, such as akathisia, are more likely to occur.

In recent years, there has been substantial interest in the role of glutamate, an excitatory neurotransmitter, in the pathophysiology of schizophrenia (see, e.g., Javitt and Zukin 1991; Krystal et al. 1994; Lahti et al. 1995). This theory is supported by the psychotomimetic properties of glutamate antagonists such as PCP and ketamine. These NMDA receptor antagonists lead to a group of behaviors that often have closer parallels to schizophrenia than do those of the dopamine sympathomimetic agents, in both mice and humans. Clinical trial evidence points to the usefulness of glutamatergic agonists (e.g., D-cycloserine) in treating schizophrenia (Goff et al. 1995). One way of examining the possible effect of olanzapine on glutamatergic measures was addressed in a study of rats with isolation-induced disruption of prepulse inhibition. Prepulse inhibition, a measure of sensory motor gating, is believed to be abnormal in patients with schizophrenia. In a study by Bakshi et al. (1998), both quetiapine and olanzapine reversed the isolation-induced prepulse inhibition deficit.

In summary, olanzapine works at least at the dopamine, acetylcholine, histamine, 5-HT, and glutamate receptors. At this time, dopamine receptor–blocking capabilities appear to be a necessary but not sufficient characteristic of an antipsychotic medication. The other studied mechanisms, when taken in total, may be the factors leading to olanzapine's broad efficacy and side-effect profile.

Indications and Efficacy

Olanzapine received FDA approval initially for the treatment of psychosis. Currently, it has multiple indications, including treatment of schizophrenia; acute treatment of manic or mixed states in bipolar disorder; and maintenance treatment of bipolar disorder, both as monotherapy and as an adjunct to mood stabilizer therapy. The OFC preparation has an FDA indication for bipolar depression. Intramuscular olanzapine carries an indication for acute agitation in schizophrenia and bipolar mania. Olanzapine is approved for adults and for children ages 13–18 years. Olanzapine has been studied, and at times used with limited evidence, in several other illnesses. In this section, we present the evidence base that supports the use of olanzapine for its FDA-indicated usages as well as for other off-label usages.

Schizophrenia

As noted earlier, olanzapine was originally developed as a medication with potential for treating schizophrenia, mania, and anxiety. To gain FDA approval for the treatment of schizophrenia, olanzapine was tested in four pivotal studies to assess the compound for efficacy, safety, and dose ranging. The earliest testing of olanzapine was an assessment of olanzapine in doses of 5–30 mg following an initial starting dose of 10 mg. Brief Psychiatric Rating Scale (BPRS) scores were reduced substantially for the participants in the study, and EPS were low (Baldwin and Montgomery 1995). These encouraging results led to further studies and pointed to a dose range to be tested.

Efficacy Studies

The first pivotal study examined a dose of 10 mg of olanzapine. The study showed that 10 mg of olanzapine was statistically significantly superior to placebo on objective rating scales (Beasley et al. 1996a). The next step was a dose-ranging study of olanzapine compared with haloperidol and placebo. The dosage ranges were 1) low (5 ± 2.5 mg/day), 2) medium (10 ± 2.5 mg/day), and 3) high (15 ± 2.5 mg/day). Haloperidol was dosed to 15 ± 2.5 mg/day. The medium and high doses of olanzapine and haloperidol led to significant improvements compared with placebo (Beasley et al. 1996b). Tollefson and Sanger (1997), after analysis of these early data, pointed out that the effect on negative symptoms by olanzapine was independent of movement disorders.

Another large international multicenter trial used a flexible dosing strategy to show a statistical superiority of olanzapine over haloperidol. In this study, patients were started on olanzapine or haloperidol at dosages ranging from 5 to 20 mg/day. Ultimately, patients received olanzapine 13 mg/day compared with haloperidol 11.8 mg/day (Tollefson et al. 1997).

The third pivotal study included an interesting arm—olanzapine 1 mg/day—in comparison to low-, medium-, and high-dose olanzapine and haloperidol (15±5 mg/day). This study established the statistical efficacy of low- and high-dose olanzapine compared with 1 mg/day of olanzapine (Beasley et al. 1997).

The group of studies described above led to the approval of olanzapine for psychosis (later changed to schizophrenia). Several other studies have reinforced olanzapine's efficacy for the treatment of schizophrenia. Coupled with its efficacy and substantially fewer movement disorder side effects, olanzapine has become an important addition to the armamentarium of the psychiatrist treating schizophrenia. Leucht et al. (1999) reported that olanzapine was statistically more effective than placebo (moderate effect) and also more effective than haloperidol (small effect) on global schizophrenia symptomatology.

A large National Institute of Mental Health (NIMH)–funded trial was completed that sought to compare the atypical antipsychotics olanzapine, risperidone, quetiapine, and ziprasidone with perphenazine in order to understand the efficacy and side-effect profiles of the newer versus older antipsychotic medications (Lieberman et al. 2005). The study, Clinical Antipsychotic Trials of Intervention Effectiveness (CATIE), was designed to provide a double-blind yet reasonably naturalistic way for clinicians to treat patients, using the time to discontinuation as a primary outcome variable. Olanzapine demonstrated the longest time to discontinuation in the trial, based on all-cause discontinuation. Olanzapine had the highest rate of discontinuation due to metabolic complications such as weight gain, while perphenazine had the highest rate of discontinuation for EPS. Overall, however, the discontinuation rate was high for all medications, with nearly 75% of patients changing medications within the 18-month study duration. Much has been written since the initial findings were published, including analyses of cost-effectiveness (Rosenheck et al. 2006), psychosocial functioning (Swartz et al. 2007), and switching of medications (Essock et al. 2006), as well as numerous editorials about the treatment implications from the study.

Schizophrenia is often not fully responsive to first-generation antipsychotic treatment. Assessment of olanzapine in patients with treatment-refractory illness did not indicate usefulness in a stringent nonresponder protocol (Conley et al. 1998). However, in an Eli Lilly–sponsored double-blind noninferiority multicenter trial, olanzapine's effect in lowering Positive and Negative Syndrome Scale (PANSS) scores was comparable to that of clozapine (Tollefson et al. 2001). A second phase of CATIE examined the use of clozapine in patients with treatment-refractory illness and found, based on the time to discontinuation, that clozapine was a superior treatment for patients who had failed to respond to other atypical medications (McEvoy et al. 2006).

Olanzapine has often been linked to improvements in the negative symptoms and cognitive symptoms of schizophrenia, albeit with less potency than for positive symptoms. The efficacy of olanzapine for negative symptoms was first reported by Tollefson et al. (1997), following completion of a large double-blind trial of olanzapine and haloperidol. When all symptom improvements were taken into consideration, olanzapine-treated subjects had greater improvement in negative symptoms on both the Scale for the Assessment of Negative Symptoms (SANS) and the BPRS negative symptom subscore. In a flexible-dose comparison between risperidone and olanzapine in patients followed for 1 year, olanzapine-treated patients showed significantly greater improvement on SANS scores than did risperidone-treated patients (Alvarez et al. 2006). Interestingly, in a study by researchers from Eli Lilly that followed patients taking either quetiapine or olanzapine for 6 months, the two groups showed similar improvements on the SANS at study completion (Kinon et al. 2006).

Cognitive functioning may be an important prognostic indicator for schizophrenia (Green 2006). In a 1-year comparison of olanzapine with risperidone, both groups showed modest benefits on a cognitive function battery (Gurpegui et al. 2007). In a study conducted over a 1-year period by Eli Lilly researchers in Spain, olanzapine showed greater benefit on social functioning than did risperidone, as assessed by scores on the Social Functioning Scale (SFS). The greatest difference was in occupation/employment, but improvements were also seen on measures of independence, social engagement, and recreation (Ciudad et al. 2006). The LAI formulation of olanzapine was assessed in an 8-week double-blind, placebo-controlled study, and a statistically significant difference in PANSS ratings was noted by 7 days (Lauriello et al. 2008). Another study that assessed a longer period of olanzapine LAI treatment—24 weeks—found that a high percentage of subjects remained exacerbation free (Kane et al. 2010). The published report of this study also discussed the relationship between oral and LAI olanzapine dosing and noted that the potential for accidental intravascular injection—which can cause sedation and/or delirium—requires that patients be observed for 3 hours after injection.

Olanzapine has been studied for some time as a treatment for serious psychiatric illness in adolescents. In a recent systematic review of the literature in children, second-generation antipsychotics were shown to be beneficial overall for targeting psychotic symptoms, although there is still a need for research on the long-term safety profile of these agents (Jensen et al. 2007). A double-blind, flexible-dose study conducted in North Carolina demonstrated similar efficacy for risperidone, olanzapine, and haloperidol in psychotic young people (Sikich et al. 2004). In subsequent research comparing first- and second-generation antipsychotic medications, the olanzapine arm was discontinued because of weight gain (Sikich et al. 2008). A further study of olanzapine in adolescents demonstrated a statistically significant difference in symptom improvement ratings for olanzapine over placebo. As in previous studies, there was significantly more weight gain in the adolescents on olanzapine (Kryzhanovskaya et al. 2009). In late 2009, olanzapine received FDA approval for the treatment of schizophrenia in teenagers, but with the recommendation that clinicians first consider the use of other agents.

The use of olanzapine in a population considered to be at risk for schizophrenia but not yet meeting full symptom criteria was evaluated in a double-blind multicenter study. The olanzapine group demonstrated a decreased rate of conversion to psychosis compared with the placebo group, although the difference did not quite reach statistical significance. However, a number of factors, including high dropout rates in both groups, the lack of a systematic method for diagnosing Axis I disorders, and the method of patient selection, limited the generalizability and reliability of the findings (McGlashan et al. 2006). The number needed to treat, a measure of effect size, was 4.5 in this study; thus, early medication treatment may benefit some patients. Nonetheless, given the long-term side-effect consequences of antipsychotics, much further refinement, including greater precision in identifying appropriate candidates for treatment, is required before presyndromal medication therapy can be considered to be evidence based.

At the other end of the age spectrum, olanzapine has been tested in the treatment of several syndromes in the elderly. Olanzapine, like all antipsychotic medications, carries a black box warning regarding use in the elderly and increased risk for stroke. Further discussion of the use of olanzapine in dementia is provided in a separate subsection (see "Dementia-Related Agitation and Psychosis," later in chapter). A study of a group of older patients with chronic schizophrenia showed a statistical advantage for olanzapine (Barak et al. 2002). For a broad group of psychotic patients, Hwang et al. (2003) reported reduction in BPRS symptoms in 94 acutely ill patients, some with organic psychosis, thus illustrating the usefulness of olanzapine in this older patient group. As in any treatment with the elderly, special care must be taken for cardiovascular complications. With olanzapine, orthostatic hypotension, oversedation, and thus the risk of falls must be factored into the dosing decision (Gareri et al. 2006).

Treatment Approaches

Early studies of olanzapine assessed dosages ranging from 5 to 30 mg/day. When olanzapine was initially released, it was recommended that it be started at a dosage of 10 mg/day—frequently as a bedtime dose. Subsequently, clinicians have used average dosages higher than 10 mg/day (e.g., approximately 13 mg/day). In CATIE, the average daily dose in the flexible-dose segment (available doses were 7.5, 15.0, 22.5, and 30.0 mg) was 20.1 mg (Lieberman et al. 2005). For inpatient use, clinicians often will give patients 5 mg of olanzapine in the morning and 10 mg at bedtime (Schulz 1999). Some patients appear to have an inadequate response to olanzapine at the recommended doses, so clinicians have assessed the usefulness of olanzapine at dosages above the recommended 20 mg/day. Many inpatient clinicians employ a loading strategy with olanzapine, particularly in patients presenting with agitation, using up to 40 mg/day for the first 2 days and gradually decreasing the dose to a goal of 20–30 mg/day (Baker et al. 2003; Brooks et al. 2008). While sedation and hypotension must be watched for in any individual patient, increased rates of those side effects were not seen in a study comparing the loading-dose strategy with conventional 10-mg/day dosing (Baker et al. 2003).

Typically, agitated patients are best treated with the rapid-dissolving preparation of olanzapine. Given their faster onset of action compared with the conventional pill form and their decreased risk for "cheeking" of the medication, rapid-dissolving tablets are preferable in the acute setting, particularly when some sedation is also needed. When patients are severely agitated, use of injectable olanzapine is often necessary. The intramuscular preparation also has a rapid onset of action, similar to that of dissolvable tablets, and a certainty of delivery that is imperative in an emergency. The injectable preparation has been shown to be superior to placebo at doses of 10 mg and as effective as haloperidol, with significantly fewer side effects (Breier et al. 2002). Case reports, however, caution against use of olanzapine in conjunction with intramuscular lorazepam because of hypotension (Zacher and Roche-Desilets 2005).

For chronic patients, olanzapine LAI can be useful for a once-monthly administration schedule. Because of concerns regarding the delirium and even coma seen in initial studies, patients receiving olanzapine LAI must be observed for 3 hours after the injection.

Bipolar Disorder and Major Depressive Disorder

In the past, before the introduction of atypical antipsychotic medications, it was well known that traditional antipsychotic medications were useful in the treatment of mania. An assessment of the effect of olanzapine on symptoms of schizoaffective disorder provided a rationale for studying olanzapine in bipolar patients. When the results for the schizoaffective disorder patients were analyzed, those patients who received olanzapine had a superior outcome, compared with patients who received haloperidol, on many, but not all, measures (Tran et al. 1999).

The first controlled study of olanzapine in bipolar disorder was a 21-day comparison of olanzapine with placebo (Tohen et al. 1999). An analysis of the Young Mania Rating Scale (YMRS) showed a significant score reduction for patients taking olanzapine compared with those taking placebo. No difference was seen in the outcomes for depression. In this study, EPS were not more frequent in the olanzapine-treated patients than in the patients taking placebo (Tohen et al. 1999). These findings were confirmed by a second pivotal study showing an advantage of olanzapine over placebo (Tohen et al. 2000). An open-label follow-up (49 weeks) added valuable information, especially noting that decreases in YMRS scores continued. For the longer term, depression scores also improved. Importantly, for the patients who were exposed to olanzapine at a mean dosage of approximately 14 mg/day, no cases of tardive dyskinesia occurred (Sanger et al. 2001).

An important question of practical interest is how olanzapine compares with conventional mood stabilizers. In a double-blind trial conducted by Eli Lilly, olanzapine was compared with lithium in the maintenance treatment of bipolar disorder (Tohen et al. 2005). In the study, patients were stabilized on a combination of lithium and olanzapine and then randomly assigned to receive one or the other for 52 weeks. In the noninferiority analysis, olanzapine was shown to prevent depression relapse as well as lithium, and in fact it had a lower rate of mixed or manic relapse over the 52-week follow-up. Weight gain was higher in the olanzapine group (Tohen et al. 2005).

Further studies confirmed the equivalent efficacy of olanzapine and the most widely used anticonvulsant mood stabilizer, divalproex (Tohen et al. 2002). The group of studies focusing on olanzapine's use in treating mania that showed reduction of manic as well as psychotic symptoms led to the approval of olanzapine by the FDA for the treatment of manic symptoms. A review of the mood-stabilizing properties of olanzapine has recently reported on its efficacy (Schulz and Cornelius 2010). Mean dosages of olanzapine used in monotherapy are similar to those used in schizophrenia: 13 mg/day. For acute mania, a study has shown the usefulness of intramuscular olanzapine in treating agitated bipolar patients (Meehan et al. 2001).

The treatment of bipolar depression is often complicated. Monotherapy with antidepressants is associated with an increased risk of switching into mania. Olanzapine packaged with fluoxetine—OFC—has been studied in the treatment of depression in bipolar disorder. In an 8-week double-blind trial conducted by Eli Lilly, OFC was compared against olanzapine monotherapy and placebo in patients with bipolar I disorder in a depressed phase. While both treatments were more effective than placebo, OFC was significantly more effective than either olanzapine or placebo in treating depressive symptoms. OFC-treated patients showed greater improvement in mood compared with olanzapine-treated patients by the fourth week of the study (Tohen et al. 2003). Benefits were also seen in the subjects' health-related quality of life (Shi et al. 2004). OFC was also compared with lamotrigine in a 7-week study (Brown et al. 2006). Although OFC demonstrated a statistical separation from lamotrigine by the first week, it is difficult to make a full comparison in such a short study. As lamotrigine requires slow titration to decrease the risk of serious rash, it was received at the target dosage (200 mg/day) only for the last 2 weeks of the study, whereas the OFC dosage could be titrated to therapeutic levels much more quickly. Although the rapid titration of OFC is helpful when a more urgent approach is required, further study is needed to determine whether OFC's greater benefits persist once lamotrigine has had an opportunity to remain at a therapeutic dose for a longer period of time (Brown et al. 2006). Rates of treatment-emergent mania with OFC were low and did not significantly differ from rates with placebo or olanzapine monotherapy (Amsterdam and Shults 2005; Tohen et al. 2003).

OFC has been studied in treatment-refractory major depressive disorder. Thase et al. (2007) conducted a study comparing OFC against olanzapine or fluoxetine monotherapy in patients who had failed to respond to at least two prior trials with antidepressants. In the pooled analysis (Thase et al. 2007), OFC showed improvement over olanzapine or fluoxetine monotherapy on the Montgomery-Åsberg Depression Rating Scale (MADRS). In a double-blinded trial sponsored by Eli Lilly that compared olanzapine, fluoxetine, OFC, and venlafaxine, all treatments showed similar rates of efficacy (Corya et al. 2006).

The second-generation antipsychotic medications have found a role in treating not only mania but also depression. Olanzapine has demonstrated efficacy in both acute and maintenance phases of bipolar disorder, and when combined with fluoxetine in the OFC formulation, it has shown benefit in treating depression in bipolar I disorder. Particularly in cases where psychosis is prominent with mania, olanzapine is a reasonable first-line agent, although consideration must be given to the potential metabolic consequences. In depression, olanzapine has been studied primarily in treatment-refractory cases, and given its metabolic side-effect profile, it is appropriate for use only in such cases.

In bipolar I adolescents, Tohen et al. (2007) reported significantly greater improvement in mania ratings with olanzapine than with placebo. Of note is that olanzapine is approved by the FDA for treatment of bipolar I disorder in adolescents.

Dementia-Related Agitation and Psychosis

Olanzapine does not have an FDA-approved indication for the treatment of dementia. Because elderly people are generally more sensitive to the EPS and tardive dyskinesia associated with first-generation antipsychotic medications, the second-generation medications are often preferred when antipsychotics are needed.

A large placebo-controlled trial of olanzapine in Alzheimer's patients showed that the lower dosages of olanzapine (5–10 mg/day) were significantly better than placebo in treating target symptoms of agitation, hallucinations, and delusions (Street et al. 2000, 2001). The FDA placed a black box warning on the prescribing information of antipsychotic medications calling attention to the increased risk of death, primarily from cardiovascular and infectious complications. According to the warning, second-generation antipsychotic use over a 10-week period carries a 1.6- to 1.7-fold increased risk of mortality based on data from 17 placebo-controlled trials of atypical antipsychotics in dementia-related psychosis. Ultimately, clinical judgment and thorough documentation are important, as in certain situations the hazards of untreated psychotic agitation may outweigh the potential risks of treatment.

Several studies have examined olanzapine in the treatment of dementia without agitation (Brooks and Hoblyn 2007). A placebo-controlled multicenter trial conducted by researchers at Eli Lilly evaluated olanzapine at low fixed dosages (1.0, 2.5, 5.0, and 7.5 mg/day) in the treatment of dementia-related psychosis (De Deyn et al. 2004). Although olanzapine did not separate from placebo on the primary outcome measure, Hallucinations and Delusions items of the Neuropsychiatric Inventory—Nursing Home edition (NPI/NH), improvements were seen in each of the dosage groups studied. All patients who received dosages of 2.5 mg/day or greater were initially started on 2.5 mg/day, with the dosage titrated upward by 2.5 mg/week (as indicated based on their assigned study group), and there was an overall difference from placebo in the acute phase of the study, suggesting that a 2.5-mg dose was an effective starting dose in the more acute setting. On some secondary outcome measures, the greatest improvement was seen with the highest olanzapine dosage (7.5 mg/day), suggesting that for some patients, an increase to 7.5 mg/day is beneficial. Because no higher dosages were used in the study, it is unclear whether continuing to increase the dosage would lead to greater efficacy (De Deyn et al. 2004).

In treatment of cognitive decline, acetylcholine has been the focus of treatments aimed at protecting people with dementia from undergoing as rapid a deterioration as they would naturally. Cholinesterase inhibitors have been used on that basis. Olanzapine may have beneficial effects on prefrontal cortex cholinergic and serotonergic neurons that may facilitate acetylcholine release to that region. However, in a double-blind study conducted by researchers at Eli Lilly, olanzapine was shown to worsen cognitive functioning, as assessed on the Alzheimer's Disease Assessment Scale for Cognition (ADAS-Cog), and there was no statistical difference between the olanzapine and placebo groups in scores on the Clinician's Interview-Based Impression of Change (CIBIC) scale (Kennedy et al. 2005). Patients in the olanzapine group also showed worsening on the Mini-Mental State Examination (MMSE). Previous studies have found little to no benefit on cognition from olanzapine treatment in nonagitated patients with dementia (De Deyn et al. 2004; Street et al. 2000).

The CATIE studies described earlier also had an Alzheimer's disease component in which olanzapine, risperidone, and quetiapine were compared with placebo for the treatment of psychosis and agitation in outpatients (Schneider et al. 2006b). Patients were included if they had psychotic symptoms and lived either in an assisted living facility or at home, but they were excluded for skilled nursing needs or primary psychotic disorders. Patients who were to receive cholinesterase inhibitors or antidepressants were also excluded from the study. Like the schizophrenia portion of CATIE, the primary outcome variable was time to discontinuation. No difference was found among the groups in time to discontinuation, and no benefit was seen on the Alzheimer's Disease Cooperative Study–Clinical Global Impression of Change (ADCS-CGIC). The average time to discontinuation ranged between 5 and 8 weeks among the treatments. Discontinuation because of lack of efficacy occurred sooner for placebo or quetiapine than for risperidone or olanzapine. Side effects such as parkinsonism, sedation, and higher body mass index were all increased with the study medications over placebo (Schneider et al. 2006b).

Overall, there are limited data to support the effectiveness of second-generation antipsychotics in the treatment of dementia. Risks for worsened cognitive function and metabolic concerns must be considered when use of antipsychotic medications is contemplated. Nonetheless, there are times when behavioral consequences and patient safety require more aggressive treatment, and antipsychotic medication may be warranted. Ultimately, a painstaking evaluation of the risk-benefit ratio of antipsychotic medications must precede any decision to prescribe these agents, in both the acute and the long-term time frames. Further study is needed, however, regarding the use of second-generation antipsychotic medications in this population (Schneider et al. 2006a).

Borderline Personality Disorder

Borderline personality disorder is a severe psychiatric illness that afflicts nearly 1% of the population (Torgersen et al. 2001). Based on earlier studies indicating that low doses of traditional antipsychotic medications may be useful for borderline personality disorder (Goldberg et al. 1986; Soloff et al. 1986), Schulz et al. (1999) reported on an open-label study that found that olanzapine led to a substantial decrease in Symptom Checklist–90 symptoms, as well as objective measures of impulsivity and aggression. Of the 11 patients entered in the trial, 9 (82%) completed the study. The design of the trial allowed for early flexible dosing, and the subjects ended the 8-week trial taking olanzapine at an average dosage of approximately 7.5 mg/day, usually at bedtime. Zanarini and Frankenburg (2001) extended this open-label trial and showed superiority of olanzapine over placebo in a longer-term (26-week) study. This interesting study of only women indicated that lower dosages (5 mg/day) of olanzapine can be useful and are associated with only minimal weight gain.

In a study comparing olanzapine, fluoxetine, and OFC in women with borderline personality disorder, olanzapine monotherapy was found to be more effective in treating the depressive symptoms of borderline personality disorder than either fluoxetine or OFC, as assessed on the MADRS. Additionally, olanzapine was superior to fluoxetine in treating symptoms of impulsivity and aggression, as measured by the Overt Aggression Scale (OAS). Weight gain was seen in a greater percentage of olanzapine-treated patients than fluoxetine-treated patients (Zanarini et al. 2004). More recently, two large placebo-controlled studies have evaluated olanzapine for borderline personality disorder with mixed results. Schulz et al. (2008) reported no significant advantage for olanzapine compared with placebo in a flexible dosing design, whereas Zanarini et al. (2011) noted a statistical advantage for olanzapine in a fixed-dose trial comparing low-dose olanzapine, higher-dose olanzapine, and placebo. These latest studies have led to controversy in the field about the use of antipsychotic medications in borderline personality disorder.

Dialectical behavioral therapy (DBT) is a mainstay of current treatment for borderline personality disorder. In a double-blind, placebo-controlled trial, olanzapine was studied as an adjunctive agent in patients receiving DBT. Impulsive and aggressive behaviors were found to be lower in the group who received olanzapine than in the placebo group. The average olanzapine dosage in the trial was 8.8 mg/day. Statistically significant levels of weight gain and dyslipidemia were observed in the olanzapine group compared with the placebo group (Soler et al. 2005). Therefore, with consideration for side effects, olanzapine may be helpful for a broader range of illnesses, particularly when used in conjunction with psychotherapy.

Anorexia Nervosa

Anorexia nervosa is a common and severe psychiatric illness that may well have the highest mortality of all mental disorders. Among the symptoms of this illness is severe restriction of food intake, leading to low weight; however, patients also have psychotic-like levels of self-perception of body size and appearance and unusual ideas about food and metabolism. Some investigators have begun to explore the possibility that olanzapine may help with this patient group. Initially, reports were largely from pilot studies, including case series, but data are now emerging from small controlled trials.

In an open-label trial, 17 patients hospitalized for anorexia nervosa were given olanzapine in conjunction with concurrent cognitive-behavioral therapy (CBT) and DBT group treatment (Barbarich et al. 2004). Olanzapine was initiated at a dosage of 1.25–5.00 mg/day, with upward titration as needed, balancing sedation and side effects with efficacy. Although patients showed improvement in weight as well as in Beck Depression Inventory (BDI) and Spielberger State-Trait Anxiety Inventory (STAI) scores, the lack of a control group limits the validity of these results (Barbarich et al. 2004). In a more recent double-blind, placebo-controlled trial in women with anorexia nervosa (Bissada et al. 2008), olanzapine-treated patients showed significant increases in weight and reductions in obsessive symptoms. A case series evaluating low-dose olanzapine treatment in adolescent girls with anorexia nervosa (Leggero et al. 2010) found improvement in weight and a decrease in hyperactivity.

Because olanzapine has weight gain as a significant side effect, the utility of that effect and the mechanism behind it have become a target for research. Ghrelin and leptin are hormones associated with satiety. In a double-blind, placebo-controlled trial, olanzapine was given concurrently with CBT in patients with anorexia, and ghrelin and leptin levels were assessed over 3 months. While both the olanzapine patients and the placebo patients gained weight, there was no statistical difference between groups in amount of weight gained or in leptin or ghrelin levels, which remained unchanged over the course of the study (Brambilla et al. 2007).

Side Effects and Toxicology

The adverse effects of olanzapine in clinical use are consistent with the preclinical studies predicting few neurological effects. In Phase II and III clinical trials, olanzapine-treated groups generally showed an improvement in EPS from baseline, reflecting the fact that most of the subjects had previously taken typical antipsychotics. In a large multinational comparison study (Tollefson et al. 1997), olanzapine produced fewer treatment-emergent neurological adverse effects than haloperidol for parkinsonism (14% vs. 38%) and akathisia (12% vs. 40%). In another study (Volavka et al. 2002), antiparkinsonian agents were prescribed to 13% of both clozapine- and olanzapine-treated subjects, compared with 32% of risperidone-treated patients.

The reduction of EPS is predictive of decreased risk of tardive dyskinesia, the most problematic of the common adverse effects of classic antipsychotics. The accumulated experience with atypical antipsychotics indicates that tardive dyskinesia is 10- to 15-fold less common, at an annual rate of 0.52% of olanzapine-treated patients compared with 7.45% of haloperidol-treated patients, based on pooled data from long-term comparison trials (Beasley et al. 1999).

A major adverse effect found during treatment with olanzapine is weight gain. This is a serious concern because persons with schizophrenia are more likely than the general population to be obese, and weight gain may contribute to nonadherence to antipsychotic treatment, leading to increased risk for relapse. With the decrease in neurological side effects with second-generation antipsychotic agents, metabolic effects have emerged as a major risk for patients and a focus of consideration for clinicians. The relative degree of weight gain associated with first- and second-generation antipsychotics was studied in a comprehensive meta-analysis by Allison et al. (1999). Estimates of weight change associated with standardized doses over 10 weeks were calculated from published data from 81 studies. Clozapine produced the greatest weight gain (4.45 kg), followed by olanzapine (4.15 kg). By comparison, risperidone was associated with a gain of 2.1 kg, haloperidol was associated with a gain of 1.08 kg, and patients lost 0.74 kg while taking placebo. In long-term treatment, 30%–50% of patients may gain more than 7% of body weight, with low pretreatment weight and good clinical response associated with more weight gain.

Small studies using metformin, an agent known to decrease hepatic glucose output, have tested the possibility that it may help patients either lose weight or remain at the same weight while receiving olanzapine or other second-generation antipsychotics. In a double-blind, placebo-controlled trial (Baptista et al. 2006), patients were given 10 mg of olanzapine and randomly assigned to receive either metformin or placebo for 14 weeks. No differences between groups were seen in body mass index or waist circumference. There was a modest improvement in overall glucose levels and in measures of glucose homeostasis (homeostasis model assessment for insulin resistance [HOMA-IR]), but no change was seen in lipid levels. A follow-up study conducted by the same group (Baptista et al. 2007) demonstrated similar results, although in the second study, small differences in weight gain between the groups were found, with the metformin group losing an average of 1.5 kg and showing decreased leptin levels while the placebo group maintained a consistent weight. In a double-blind, placebo-controlled trial in adolescents who had gained weight after 1 year of treatment with a second-generation antipsychotic (olanzapine, risperidone, or quetiapine), the addition of metformin resulted in statistical differences in waist circumference, body mass index, and overall weight gain (Klein et al. 2006). HOMA-IR scores were significantly decreased, and the number of subjects requiring referral for a glucose tolerance test was reduced, among the subjects who received metformin. These equivocal results suggest that further research is needed on adjunctive agents to help with the metabolic complications often seen with olanzapine.

Weight gain is an even greater concern in the treatment of children and adolescents, who may be exposed to medication for a longer time and are concerned with body image. After 12 weeks of treatment with olanzapine, hospitalized adolescent patients gained 7.2±6.3 kg, approximately twice the weight gain experienced by those taking risperidone; 19 of 21 patients (90%) gained more than 7% of their body weight (Ratzoni et al. 2002).

In addition to weight gain, other metabolic effects have been noted. Reports of glucose intolerance, hyperglycemia, hyperlipidemia, diabetes, and diabetic ketoacidosis (DKA) have surfaced, mostly associated with clozapine and olanzapine therapy (Wirshing et al. 2002). Cases reported to the FDA Drug Surveillance System and published cases of olanzapine-associated diabetes and hyperglycemia were reviewed by Koller and Doriswamy (2002). Two hundred eighty-nine cases were identified, of which 225 (78%) were new-onset diabetes, 100 (35%) involved ketosis or acidosis, and 23 (8%) patients died. Most cases developed within 6 months of initiation of olanzapine therapy. Many cases occurred in the first month of therapy, indicating that weight gain alone did not mediate the occurrence of diabetes-related problems. On the basis of the temporal relation between metabolic changes and the introduction and withdrawal of olanzapine, the young age of patients affected, and the number of reports, the authors concluded that the data suggested that olanzapine was causally related to the development or worsening of diabetes. A similar conclusion about clozapine and diabetes was reported earlier (Koller et al. 2001). Because case studies and reports by clinicians to regulatory agencies may reflect reporting bias, controlled studies comparing the development of metabolic disorders are needed to clarify whether these are related to the underlying psychosis, causally related to drug treatment in general, or specifically related to individual agents.

Studies that used large health system databases have been published linking use of antipsychotics with subsequent diagnoses of diabetes or use of hypoglycemic agents. These studies show increased risk of development of type 2 diabetes following the use of olanzapine and clozapine relative to the use of risperidone or typical antipsychotics or compared with matched untreated persons (Gianfrancesco et al. 2002; Koro et al. 2002a; Sernyak et al. 2002).

While olanzapine has been associated with weight gain and type 2 diabetes, there have also been reports of DKA, a condition more often associated with type 1 diabetes mellitus. These reports first appeared in the literature in 1999 (Gatta et al. 1999; Goldstein et al. 1999; Lindenmayer and Patel 1999). In a review of California Medicaid data on cases of risperidone- and olanzapine-associated DKA, Ramaswamy et al. (2007) found a higher incidence of DKA for olanzapine than for risperidone and noted that the risk increased with duration of treatment with olanzapine.

Another metabolic adverse effect seen with olanzapine is the development of dyslipidemia, often in association with weight gain. In a large British patient database, olanzapine conferred a fivefold increase in the rates of dyslipidemia over an untreated control condition and a threefold increase over conventional antipsychotics, whereas risperidone did not increase the risk (Koro et al. 2002b).

Among other side effects, sedation is frequent at the start of therapy with olanzapine but diminishes as patients develop tolerance for this side effect. In long-term treatment, the incidence of sedation is about 15%, similar to that of haloperidol. Prolactin elevations observed during olanzapine treatment occur early in the course of treatment, and levels are much lower than those seen with risperidone or classic antipsychotic treatment. Leukopenia is rare and occurs at a rate similar to that seen with other typical and atypical antipsychotics, but olanzapine does not cause agranulocytosis, even in patients who developed this effect while taking clozapine. In animal toxicology studies and in clinical trials, no QTc prolongation was observed, and other cardiovascular effects are rarely of clinical importance.

Drug-Drug Interactions

Olanzapine is metabolized primarily via glucuronidation and via oxidation by CYP1A2 (see section "Pharmacokinetics and Disposition" earlier in this chapter). Other drugs that affect the activity of these metabolic pathways would therefore be expected to affect olanzapine pharmacokinetics. Indeed, drugs that inhibit CYP1A2 activity have been shown to decrease olanzapine clearance, thereby increasing olanzapine plasma concentrations.

Fluvoxamine, a known inhibitor of CYP1A2, has been shown to inhibit olanzapine metabolism in several studies. A study of 10 healthy male smokers receiving 11 days of fluvoxamine administration (50–100 mg) resulted in an 84% increase in maximal olanzapine concentrations (C_{max}) and a 119% increase in AUC_{0-24} compared with olanzapine administered with placebo. No change in half-life was observed in either olanzapine or 4′-*N*-desmethylolanzapine, suggesting that fluvoxamine inhibited olanzapine's first-pass metabolism (Maenpaa et al. 1997).

Fluoxetine and imipramine, although not known to be significant inhibitors of CYP1A2, when coadministered with olanzapine have been associated with statistically significant but small changes in olanzapine pharmacokinetics. Coadministration of fluoxetine resulted in a 15% decrease in olanzapine clearance and an 18% increase in C_{max}, with no significant difference in the half-life of olanzapine (Callaghan et al. 1999). Coadministration of imipramine resulted in an approximately 14% increase in olanzapine C_{max} and a non–statistically significant increase in AUC of 19% (Callaghan et al. 1997).

Inducers of the CYP1A2 enzyme increase olanzapine clearance, thereby decreasing olanzapine systemic exposure. Carbamazepine, an inducer of several CYP enzymes (including 1A2), affects olanzapine disposition. A study in healthy volunteers showed that 18 days of carbamazepine therapy resulted in significantly higher clearance and apparent volume of distribution but significantly lower C_{max}, AUC, and half-life after a single 10-mg dose of olanzapine (Lucas et al. 1998).

Smoking, also known to induce CYP1A2, can affect olanzapine disposition. A study comparing 19 male smokers with 30 male nonsmokers found that olanzapine clearance in smokers was 23% higher than that in nonsmokers (Callaghan et al. 1999). A population pharmacokinetic analysis of 910 patients receiving olanzapine found that clearance among nonsmokers was 37% lower in men and 48% lower in women than it was in the corresponding group of smokers (Patel et al. 1996). A smaller analysis of healthy volunteers also found higher drug clearances among smokers (Patel et al. 1995). The polycyclic aromatic hydrocarbons in cigarette smoke are responsible for inducing the aryl hydrocarbon hydroxylases and thus lead to enzymatic induction (Desai et al. 2001). Thus, dosage adjustments might be needed when a patient who smokes is placed in a smoke-free inpatient unit, even if adequate nicotine replacement is provided.

In vitro studies suggest that olanzapine does not significantly inhibit the activity of the CYP enzymes 1A2, 3A, 2D6, 2C9, or 2C19 (Ring et al. 1996a). In vivo studies suggest that olanzapine does not affect the disposition of aminophylline (Macias et al. 1998), diazepam, alcohol, imipramine (Callaghan et al. 1997), warfarin, biperiden, or lithium (Callaghan et al. 1999; Demolle et al. 1995).

Conclusion

After review of the research focused on olanzapine, it is clear that this compound, which has been approved for use in the United States since 1997, has wide utility and is a step forward from the traditional antipsychotic medications. In addition to the positive effect on a broad group of symptoms of schizophrenia, olanzapine has now been approved for treatment of mania, both acute and long term, in bipolar disorder. Recent research has shown that there may be benefit to disorders beyond psychosis (e.g., borderline personality disorder, anorexia, PTSD, OCD, Tourette's syndrome) with olanzapine. The extension of uses of olanzapine is in many ways allowed by the low rates of movement disorders. The lack of dystonia, parkinsonism, and tardive dyskinesia leads to greater acceptability in chronic schizophrenia and has encouraged clinicians and investigators to find patients earlier in the course of the illness, thus reducing the duration of untreated psychosis and perhaps decreasing the number of patients who develop psychosis (McGlashan et al. 2003). The low rate of movement disorders has been a major factor in moving forward with treatment of mood disorders and nonpsychotic illnesses.

As noted in the section titled "Side Effects and Toxicology," olanzapine is not free of adverse effects, even though they are outside the movement disorder arena. Weight gain and metabolic disturbances are of significant concern and are the objects of intense research—in areas of both pathophysiology and prevention/treatment.

In addition to providing better treatment for schizophrenia and other disorders, olanzapine promotes actions in the brain that have provided new avenues of research in the exploration of pathophysiology of psychiatric disease. As noted earlier in this chapter, olanzapine's effects on glutamate measures and neurotensin may open new avenues of treatment.

References

Aichhorn W, Whitworth AB, Weiss EM, et al: Second-generation antipsychotics: is there evidence for sex differences in pharmacokinetic and adverse effect profiles? Drug Saf 29:587–598, 2006

Allison D, Mentore JL, Heo M, et al: Antipsychotic-induced weight gain: a comprehensive research synthesis. Am J Psychiatry 156:1686–1696, 1999

Alvarez E, Ciudad A, Olivares JM, et al: A randomized, 1-year follow-up study of olanzapine and risperidone in the treatment of negative symptoms in outpatients with schizophrenia. J Clin Psychopharmacol 26:238–249, 2006

Amsterdam JD, Shults J: Comparison of fluoxetine, olanzapine, and combined fluoxetine plus olanzapine initial therapy of bipolar type I and type II major depression—lack of manic induction. J Affect Disord 87:121–130, 2005

Aravagiri M, Ames D, Wirshing WC, et al: Plasma level monitoring of olanzapine in patients with schizophrenia: determination by high-performance liquid chromatography with electrochemical detection. Ther Drug Monit 19:307–313, 1997

Baker RW, Kinon BJ, Maguire GA, et al: Effectiveness of rapid initial dose escalation of up to forty milligrams per day of oral olanzapine in acute agitation. J Clin Psychopharmacol 23:342–348, 2003

Bakshi VP, Swerdlow NR, Braff DL, et al: Reversal of isolation rearing-induced deficits in prepulse inhibition by Seroquel and olanzapine. Biol Psychiatry 43:436–445, 1998

Baldwin DS, Montgomery SA: First clinical experience with olanzapine (LY 170053): results of an open-label safety and dose-ranging study in patients with schizophrenia. Int Clin Psychopharmacol 10:239–244, 1995

Baptista T, Martinez J, Lacruz A, et al: Metformin for prevention of weight gain and insulin resistance with olanzapine: a double-blind placebo-controlled trial. Can J Psychiatry 51:192–196, 2006

Baptista T, Rangel N, Fernandez V, et al: Metformin as an adjunctive treatment to control body weight and metabolic dysfunction during olanzapine administration: a multicentric, double-blind, placebo-controlled trial. Schizophr Res 93:99–108, 2007

Barak Y, Shamir E, Zemishlani H, et al: Olanzapine vs. haloperidol in the treatment of elderly chronic schizophrenic patients. Prog Neuropsychopharmacol Biol Psychiatry 26:1199–1202, 2002

Barbarich NC, McConaha CW, Gaskill J, et al: An open trial of olanzapine in anorexia nervosa. J Clin Psychiatry 65:1480–1482, 2004

Beasley CM Jr, Sanger T, Satterlee W, et al: Olanzapine versus placebo: results of a double-blind, fixed-dose olanzapine trial. Psychopharmacology (Berl) 124:159–167, 1996a

Beasley CM Jr, Tollefson G, Tran P, et al: Olanzapine versus placebo and haloperidol: acute phase results of the North American double-blind olanzapine trial. Neuropsychopharmacology 14:111–123, 1996b

Beasley CM Jr, Hamilton SH, Crawford AM, et al: Olanzapine versus haloperidol: acute phase results of the international double-blind olanzapine trial. Eur Neuropsychopharmacol 7:125–137, 1997

Beasley CM, Dellva MA, Tamura RN, et al: Randomised double-blind comparison of the incidence of tardive dyskinesia in patients with schizophrenia during long-term treatment with olanzapine or haloperidol. Br J Psychiatry 174:23–30, 1999

Benzel I, Bansal A, Browning BL, et al: Interactions among genes in the ErbB-Neuregulin signalling network are associated with increased susceptibility to schizophrenia. Behav Brain Funct 3:31, 2007

Bergstrom RF, Callaghan JT, Cerimele BJ, et al: Pharmacokinetics of olanzapine in elderly and young (abstract). Pharm Res 12 (9, suppl):S358, 1995

Bissada H, Tasca GA, Barber AM, et al: Olanzapine in the treatment of low body weight and obsessive thinking in women with anorexia nervosa: a randomized, double-blind, placebo-controlled trial. Am J Psychiatry 165:1281–1288, 2008

Boules M, Shaw A, Fredrickson P, et al: Neurotensin agonists: potential in the treatment of schizophrenia. CNS Drugs 21:13–23, 2007

Brambilla F, Monteleone P, Maj M: Olanzapine-induced weight gain in anorexia nervosa: involvement of leptin and ghrelin secretion? Psychoneuroendocrinology 32:402–406, 2007

Breier A, Meehan K, Kirkett M, et al: A double-blind, placebo-controlled dose-response comparison of intramuscular olanzapine and haloperidol in the treatment of acute agitation in schizophrenia. Arch Gen Psychiatry 59:441–448, 2002

Brooks JO, Hoblyn JC: Neurocognitive costs and benefits of psychiatric medication in older adults: invited review. J Geriatr Psychiatr Neurol 20:199–214, 2007

Brooks JO, Karnik N, Hoblyn JC: High initial dosing of olanzapine for stabilization of acute agitation: a retrospective case series. J Pharm Technol 24:7–11, 2008

Brown EB, McElroy SL, Keck PE Jr, et al: A 7-week, randomized, double-blind trial of olanzapine/fluoxetine combination versus lamotrigine in the treatment of bipolar I depression. J Clin Psychiatry 67:1025–1033, 2006

Callaghan JT, Cerimele BJ, Kassahun KJ, et al: Olanzapine: interaction study with imipramine. J Clin Pharmacol 37:971–978, 1997

Callaghan JT, Bergstrom RF, Ptak LR, et al: Olanzapine: pharmacokinetic and pharmacodynamic profile. Clin Pharmacokinet 37:177–193, 1999

Ciudad A, Olivares JM, Bousono M, et al: Improvement in social functioning in outpatients with schizophrenia with prominent negative symptoms treated with olanzapine or risperidone in a 1 year randomized, open-label trial. Prog Neuropsychopharmacol Biol Psychiatry 30:1515–1522, 2006

Cole JO, Goldberg SC, Klerman GL: Phenothiazine in treatment of acute schizophrenia. Arch Gen Psychiatry 10:246–261, 1964

Conley RR, Tamminga CA, Bartko JJ, et al: Olanzapine compared with chlorpromazine in treatment-resistant schizophrenia. Am J Psychiatry 155:914–920, 1998

Corya SA, Williamson D, Sanger TM, et al: A randomized, double-blind comparison of olanzapine/fluoxetine combination, olanzapine, fluoxetine, and venlafaxine in treatment-resistant depression. Depress Anxiety 23:364–372, 2006

De Deyn PP, Carrasco MM, Deberdt W, et al: Olanzapine versus placebo in the treatment of psychosis with or without associated behavioral disturbances in patients with Alzheimer's disease. Int J Geriatr Psychiatry 19:115–126, 2004

Delay J, Bernitzer P: Le traitment des psychoses par une methode neuroleptique derivee de l'hibernotherapie, in Congres de Medecins Alienistes et Neurologistes de France. Edited by Ossa PC. Paris, Masson, 1952, pp 497–502

Demolle D, Onkelinx C, Miller-Oerlinghausen B: Interaction between olanzapine and lithium in healthy male volunteers (abstract 486). Therapie 50 (suppl), 1995

Desai HD, Seabolt J, Jann MW: Smoking in patients receiving psychotropic medications: a pharmacokinetic perspective. CNS Drugs 15:469–494, 2001

Eli Lilly: Zyprexa (olanzapine) tablets: prescribing information. Indianapolis, IN, Eli Lilly, 2006

Essock SM, Covell NH, Davis SM, et al: Effectiveness of switching antipsychotic medications. Am J Psychiatry 163:2090–2095, 2006

Farah A: Atypicality of atypical antipsychotics. Prim Care Companion J Clin Psychiatry 7:268–274, 2005

Farde L, Nordstrom AL: PET analysis indicates atypical central dopamine receptor occupancy in clozapine-treated patients. Br J Psychiatry 17 (suppl):30–33, 1992

Farde L, Nordstrom AL, Wiesel FA, et al: Positron emission tomographic analysis of central D1 and D2 dopamine receptor occupancy in patients treated with classical neuroleptics and clozapine: relation to extrapyramidal side effects. Arch Gen Psychiatry 49:538–544, 1992

Gareri P, De Fazio P, De Fazio S, et al: Adverse effects of atypical antipsychotics in the elderly: a review. Drugs Aging 23:937–956, 2006

Gatta B, Rigalleau V, Gin H: Diabetic ketoacidosis with olanzapine treatment. Diabetes Care 22:1002–1003, 1999

Gianfrancesco FD, Grogg AL, Mahmoud RA, et al: Differential effects of risperidone, olanzapine, clozapine, and conventional antipsychotics on type 2 diabetes: findings from a large health plan database. J Clin Psychiatry 63:920–930, 2002

Goff DC, Tsai G, Manoach DS, et al: Dose-finding trial of D-cycloserine added to neuroleptics for negative symptoms in schizophrenia. Am J Psychiatry 152:1213–1215, 1995

Goldberg SC, Schulz SC, Schulz PM, et al: Borderline and schizotypal personality disorders treated with low-dose thiothixene vs placebo. Arch Gen Psychiatry 43:680–686, 1986

Goldstein LE, Sporn J, Brown S, et al: New-onset diabetes mellitus and diabetic ketoacidosis associated with olanzapine treatment. Psychosomatics 40:438–443, 1999

Gosselin G, Oberling P, Di Scala G: Antagonism of amphetamine-induced disruption of latent inhibition by the atypical antipsychotic olanzapine in rats. Behav Pharmacol 7:820–826, 1996

Gossen D, de Suray JM, Vandenhende F, et al: Influence of fluoxetine on olanzapine pharmacokinetics. AAPS PharmSci 4(2):E11, 2002

Green MF: Cognitive impairment and functional outcome in schizophrenia and bipolar disorder. J Clin Psychiatry 67(10):e12, 2006

Grothe DR, Calis KA, Jacobsen L, et al: Olanzapine pharmacokinetics in pediatric and adolescent inpatients with childhood-onset schizophrenia. J Clin Psychopharmacol 20:220–225, 2000

Gurpegui M, Alvarez E, Bousono M, et al: Effect of olanzapine or risperidone treatment on some cognitive functions in a one-year follow-up of schizophrenia outpatients with prominent negative symptoms. Eur Neuropsychopharmacol 17:725–734, 2007

Hagg S, Spigset O, Lakso HA, et al: Olanzapine disposition in humans is unrelated to CYP1A2 and CYP2D6 phenotypes. Eur J Clin Pharmacol 57:493–497, 2001

Hwang J, Yang CH, Lee TW, et al: The efficacy and safety of olanzapine for the treatment of geriatric psychosis. J Clin Psychopharmacol 23:113–118, 2003

Jardemark KE, Liang X, Arvanov V, et al: Subchronic treatment with either clozapine, olanzapine or haloperidol produces a hyposensitive response of the rat cortical cells to N-methyl-D-aspartate. Neuroscience 100:1–9, 2000

Javitt DC, Zukin SR: Recent advances in the phencyclidine model of schizophrenia. Am J Psychiatry 148:1301–1308, 1991

Jensen PS, Buitelaar J, Pandina GJ, et al: Management of psychiatric disorders in children and adolescents with atypical antipsychotics: a systematic review of published clinical trials. Eur Child Adolesc Psychiatry 16:104–120, 2007

Kane JM, Detke HC, Naber D, et al: Olanzapine long-acting injection: a 24-week, randomized, double-blind trial of maintenance treatment in patients with schizophrenia. Am J Psychiatry 167:181–189, 2010

Kapur S, Remington G: Dopamine D(2) receptors and their role in atypical antipsychotic action: still necessary and may even be sufficient. Biol Psychiatry 50:873–883, 2001

Kapur S, Zipursky RB, Remington G, et al: 5-HT2 and D2 receptor occupancy of olanzapine in schizophrenia: a PET investigation. Am J Psychiatry 155:921–928, 1998

Kapur S, Zipursky R, Jones C, et al: A positron emission tomography study of quetiapine in schizophrenia: a preliminary finding of an antipsychotic effect with only transiently high dopamine D2 receptor occupancy. Arch Gen Psychiatry 57:553–559, 2000

Kapur S, Arenovich T, Agid O, et al: Evidence for onset of antipsychotic effects within the first 24 hours of treatment. Am J Psychiatry 162:939–946, 2005

Kassahun K, Mattiuz E, Nyhart E Jr, et al: Disposition and biotransformation of the antipsychotic agent olanzapine in humans. Drug Metab Dispos 25:81–93, 1997

Kelly DL, Conley RR, Tamminga CA: Differential olanzapine plasma concentrations by sex in a fixed-dose study. Schizophr Res 40:101–104, 1999

Kennedy J, Deberdt W, Siegal A, et al: Olanzapine does not enhance cognition in non-agitated and non-psychotic patients with mild to moderate Alzheimer's dementia. Int J Geriatr Psychiatry 20:1020–1027, 2005

Kinon BJ, Noordsy DL, Liu-Seifert H, et al: Randomized, double-blind 6-month comparison of olanzapine and quetiapine in patients with schizophrenia or schizoaffective disorder with prominent negative symptoms and poor functioning. J Clin Psychopharmacol 26:453–461, 2006

Klein DJ, Cottingham EM, Sorter M, et al: A randomized, double-blind, placebo-controlled trial of metformin treatment of weight gain associated with initiation of atypical antipsychotic therapy in children and adolescents. Am J Psychiatry 163:2072–2079, 2006

Koller E, Doriswamy PM: Olanzapine-associated diabetes mellitus. Pharmacotherapy 22:841–845, 2002

Koller E, Schneider B, Bennett K, et al: Clozapine-associated diabetes. Am J Med 111:716–723, 2001

Koro C, Fedder DO, L'Italien GL, et al: Assessment of independent effect of olanzapine and risperidone on risk of diabetes among patients with schizophrenia: population based nested case-control study. BMJ 325:243, 2002a

Koro C, Fedder DO, L'Italien GL, et al: An assessment of the independent effects of olanzapine and risperidone exposure on the risk of hyperlipidemia in schizophrenic patients. Arch Gen Psychiatry 59:1021–1026, 2002b

Krystal JH, Karper LP, Seibyl JP, et al: Subanesthetic effects of the noncompetitive NMDA antagonist, ketamine, in humans: psychotomimetic, perceptual, cognitive, and neuroendocrine responses. Arch Gen Psychiatry 51:199–214, 1994

Kryzhanovskaya L, Schulz SC, McDougle C, et al: Olanzapine versus placebo in adolescents with schizophrenia: a 6-week randomized, double-blind, placebo-controlled trial. J Am Acad Child Adolesc Psychiatry 48:60–70, 2009

Lahti AC, Koffel B, LaPorte D, et al: Subanesthetic doses of ketamine stimulate psychosis in schizophrenia. Neuropsychopharmacology 13:9–19, 1995

Lauriello J, Lambert T, Andersen S, et al: An 8-week, double-blind, randomized, placebo-controlled study of olanzapine long-acting injection in acutely ill patients with schizophrenia. J Clin Psychiatry 69:790–799, 2008

Leggero C, Masi G, Brunori E, et al: Low-dose olanzapine monotherapy in girls with anorexia nervosa, restricting subtype: focus on hyperactivity. J Child Adolesc Psychopharmacol 20:127–133, 2010

Leucht S, Pitschel-Walz G, Abraham D, et al: Efficacy and extrapyramidal side-effects of the new antipsychotics olanzapine, quetiapine, risperidone, and sertindole compared to conventional antipsychotics and placebo: a meta-analysis of randomized controlled trials. Schizophr Res 35:51–68, 1999

Lieberman JA, Stroup TS, McEvoy JP, et al: Effectiveness of antipsychotic drugs in patients with chronic schizophrenia. N Engl J Med 353:1209–1223, 2005

Lindenmayer JP, Patel R: Olanzapine-induced ketoacidosis with diabetes mellitus. Am J Psychiatry 156:1471, 1999

Lucas RA, Gilfillan DJ, Bergstrom RF: A pharmacokinetic interaction between carbamazepine and olanzapine. Eur J Clin Pharmacol 54:639–643, 1998

Macias WL, Bergstrom RF, Cerimele BJ, et al: Lack of effect of olanzapine on the pharmacokinetics of a single aminophylline dose in healthy men. Pharmacotherapy 18:1237–1248, 1998

Maenpaa J, Wrighton S, Bergstrom R, et al: Pharmacokinetic (PK) and pharmacodynamic (PD) interactions between fluvoxamine and olanzapine (abstract). Clin Pharmacol Ther 61:225, 1997

Mamo D, Kapur S, Keshavan M, et al: D(2) Receptor occupancy of olanzapine pamoate depot using positron emission tomography: an open-label study in patients with schizophrenia. Neuropsychopharmacology 33:298–304, 2008

Markowitz JS, DeVane CL, Malcolm RJ, et al: Pharmacokinetics of olanzapine after single-dose oral administration of standard tablet versus normal and sublingual administration of an orally disintegrating tablet in normal volunteers. J Clin Pharmacol 46:164–171, 2006

McEvoy JP, Lieberman JA, Stroup TS, et al: Effectiveness of clozapine versus olanzapine, quetiapine, and risperidone in patients with chronic schizophrenia who did not respond to prior atypical antipsychotic treatment. Am J Psychiatry 163:600–610, 2006

McGlashan T, Zipursky RB, Perkins DO, et al: Olanzapine versus placebo treatment of the schizophrenia prodrome: one year results (abstract). Schizophr Res 60 (suppl):295, 2003

McGlashan TH, Zipursky RB, Perkins D, et al: Randomized, double-blind trial of olanzapine versus placebo in patients prodromally symptomatic for psychosis. Am J Psychiatry 163:790–799, 2006

Meehan K, Zhang F, David S, et al: A double-blind, randomized comparison of the efficacy and safety of intramuscular injections of olanzapine, lorazepam, or placebo in treating acutely agitated patients diagnosed with bipolar mania. J Clin Psychopharmacol 21:389–397, 2001

Moore NA: Behavioural pharmacology of the new generation of antipsychotic agents. Br J Psychiatry 174 (suppl 138):5–11, 1999

Ninan I, Jardemark KE, Wang RY: Olanzapine and clozapine but not haloperidol reverse subchronic phencyclidine-induced functional hyperactivity of N-methyl-D-aspartate receptors in pyramidal cells of the rat medial prefrontal cortex. Neuropharmacology 44:462–472, 2003

Patel BR, Nyhart EH, Callaghan JT, et al: Combined population pharmacokinetic analysis of olanzapine in healthy volunteers (abstract). Pharm Res 12:S360, 1995

Patel BR, Kurtz DL, Callaghan JT, et al: Effects of smoking and gender on population pharmacokinetics of olanzapine (OL) in a phase III clinical trial (abstract). Pharm Res 13 (9, suppl): S408, 1996

Ramaswamy K, Kozma CM, Nasrallah H: Risk of diabetic ketoacidosis after exposure to risperidone or olanzapine. Drug Saf 30:589–599, 2007

Ratzoni G, Gothelf D, Brand-Gothelf A, et al: Weight gain associated with olanzapine and risperidone in adolescent patients: a comparative prospective study. J Am Acad Child Adolesc Psychiatry 41:337–343, 2002

Ring BJ, Binkley SN, Vandenbranden M, et al: In vitro interaction of the antipsychotic agent olanzapine with human cytochromes P450 CYP2C9, CYP2C19, CYP2D6 and CYP3A. Br J Clin Pharmacol 41:181–186, 1996a

Ring BJ, Catlow J, Lindsay TJ, et al: Identification of the human cytochromes P450 responsible for the in vitro formation of the major oxidative metabolites of the antipsychotic agent olanzapine. J Pharmacol Exp Ther 276:658–666, 1996b

Robertson GS, Fibiger HC: Effects of olanzapine on regional c-fos expression in rat forebrain. Neuropsychopharmacology 14:105–110, 1996

Rosenheck RA, Leslie DL, Sindelar J, et al: Cost-effectiveness of second-generation antipsychotics and perphenazine in a randomized trial of treatment for chronic schizophrenia. Am J Psychiatry 163:2080–2089, 2006

Sanger T, Grundy S, Gibson PJ, et al: Long-term olanzapine therapy in the treatment of bipolar I disorder: an open-label continuation phase study. J Clin Psychiatry 62:273–281, 2001

Schneider LS, Dagerman K, Insel PS: Efficacy and adverse effects of atypical antipsychotics for dementia: meta-analysis of randomized, placebo-controlled trials. Am J Geriatr Psychiatry 14:191–210, 2006a

Schneider LS, Tariot PN, Dagerman KS, et al: Effectiveness of atypical antipsychotic drugs in patients with Alzheimer's disease. N Engl J Med 355:1525–1538, 2006b

Schulz SC: Pharmacologic treatment of schizophrenia. Psychiatr Clin North Am 6:51–71, 1999

Schulz SC, Cornelius K: Second-generation antipsychotics are effective mood stabilizers. Curr Psychiatry 9 (suppl):S37–S43, 2010

Schulz SC, Camlin KL, Berry SA, et al: Olanzapine safety and efficacy in patients with borderline personality disorder and comorbid dysthymia. Biol Psychiatry 46:1429–1435, 1999

Schulz SC, Zanarini MC, Bateman A, et al: Olanzapine for the treatment of borderline personality disorder: variable dose 12-week randomised double-blind placebo-controlled study. Br J Psychiatry 193:485–492, 2008

Seeman P: Atypical antipsychotics: mechanism of action. Can J Psychiatry 47:27–38, 2002

Sernyak M, Leslie DL, Alarcon RD, et al: Association of diabetes mellitus with use of atypical neuroleptics in the treatment of schizophrenia. Am J Psychiatry 159:561–566, 2002

Shi L, Namjoshi MA, Swindle R, et al: Effects of olanzapine alone and olanzapine/fluoxetine combination on health-related quality of life in patients with bipolar depression: secondary analyses of a double-blind, placebo-controlled, randomized clinical trial. Clin Ther 26:125–134, 2004

Sikich L, Hamer RM, Bashford RA, et al: A pilot study of risperidone, olanzapine, and haloperidol in psychotic youth: a double-blind, randomized, 8-week trial. Neuropsychopharmacology 29:133–145, 2004

Sikich L, Frazier JA, McClellan J, et al: Double-blind comparison of first- and second-generation antipsychotics in early-onset schizophrenia and schizoaffective disorder: findings from the treatment of early-onset schizophrenia spectrum disorders (TEOSS) study. Am J Psychiatry 165:1420–1431, 2008

Soler J, Pascual JC, Campins J, et al: Double-blind, placebo-controlled study of dialectical behavior therapy plus olanzapine for borderline personality disorder. Am J Psychiatry 162:1221–1224, 2005

Soloff P, George A, Nathan RS, et al: Progress in pharmacotherapy of borderline disorders. Arch Gen Psychiatry 43:691–697, 1986

Stephenson C, Pilowsky LS: Psychopharmacology of olanzapine: a review. Br J Psychiatry 174 (suppl 38):52–58, 1999

Stockton ME, Rasmussen K: Electrophysiological effects of olanzapine, a novel atypical antipsychotic, on A9 and A10 dopamine neurons. Neuropsychopharmacology 14:97–105, 1996a

Stockton ME, Rasmussen K: Olanzapine, a novel atypical antipsychotic, reverses d-amphetamine-induced inhibition of midbrain dopamine cells. Psychopharmacology 124:50–56, 1996b

Street JS, Clark WS, Gannon KS, et al: Olanzapine treatment of psychotic and behavioral symptoms in patients with Alzheimer disease in nursing care facilities: a double-blind, randomized, placebo-controlled trial. The HGEU Study Group. Arch Gen Psychiatry 57:968–976, 2000

Street JS, Clark WS, Kadam DL, et al: Long-term efficacy of olanzapine in the control of psychotic and behavioral symptoms in nursing home patients with Alzheimer's dementia. Int J Geriatr Psychiatry 16 (suppl 1):S62–S70, 2001

Swartz MS, Perkins DO, Stroup TS, et al: Effects of antipsychotic medications on psychosocial functioning in patients with chronic schizophrenia: findings from the NIMH CATIE study. Am J Psychiatry 164:428–436, 2007

Tauscher J, Kufferle B, Asenbaum S, et al: In vivo 123I IBZM SPECT imaging of striatal dopamine-2 receptor occupancy in schizophrenic patients treated with olanzapine in comparison to clozapine and haloperidol. Psychopharmacology (Berl) 141:175–181, 1999

Thase ME, Corya SA, Osuntokun O, et al: A randomized, double-blind comparison of olanzapine/fluoxetine combination, olanzapine, and fluoxetine in treatment-resistant major depressive disorder. J Clin Psychiatry 68:224–236, 2007

Tohen M, Sanger TM, McElroy SL, et al: Olanzapine versus placebo in the treatment of acute mania. Olanzapine HGEH Study Group. Am J Psychiatry 156:702–709, 1999

Tohen M, Jacobs TG, Grundy SL, et al: Efficacy of olanzapine in acute bipolar mania: a double-blind, placebo-controlled study. The Olanzapine HGGW Study Group. Arch Gen Psychiatry 57:841–849, 2000

Tohen M, Baker RW, Altshuler LL, et al: Olanzapine versus divalproex in the treatment of acute mania. Am J Psychiatry 159:1011–1017, 2002

Tohen M, Vieta E, Calabrese J, et al: Efficacy of olanzapine and olanzapine-fluoxetine combination in the treatment of bipolar I depression. Arch Gen Psychiatry 60:1079–1088, 2003

Tohen M, Greil W, Calabrese JR, et al: Olanzapine versus lithium in the maintenance treatment of bipolar disorder: a 12-month, randomized, double-blind, controlled clinical trial. Am J Psychiatry 162:1281–1290, 2005

Tohen M, Kryzhanovskaya L, Carlson G, et al: Olanzapine versus placebo in the treatment of adolescents with bipolar mania. Am J Psychiatry 164:1547–1556, 2007

Tollefson GD, Sanger TM: Negative symptoms: a path analytic approach to a double-blind, placebo- and haloperidol-controlled clinical trial with olanzapine. Am J Psychiatry 154:466–474, 1997

Tollefson GD, Beasley CM Jr, Tran PV, et al: Olanzapine versus haloperidol in the treatment of schizophrenia and schizoaffective and schizophreniform disorders: results of an international collaborative trial. Am J Psychiatry 154:457–465, 1997

Tollefson GD, Birkett MA, Kiesler GM, et al: Double-blind comparison of olanzapine versus clozapine in schizophrenic patients clinically eligible for treatment with clozapine. Biol Psychiatry 49:52–63, 2001

Torgersen S, Kringlen E, Cramer V: The prevalence of personality disorders in a community sample. Arch Gen Psychiatry 58:590–596, 2001

Tran PV, Tollefson GD, Sanger TM, et al: Olanzapine versus haloperidol in the treatment of schizoaffective disorder: acute and long-term therapy. Br J Psychiatry 174:15–22, 1999

Volavka J, Czobor P, Sheitman B, et al: Clozapine, olanzapine, risperidone, and haloperidol in the treatment of patients with chronic schizophrenia and schizoaffective disorder. Am J Psychiatry 159:255–262, 2002

Weinberger DR: Implications of normal brain development for the pathogenesis of schizophrenia. Arch Gen Psychiatry 44:660–669, 1987

Wirshing DA, Boyd JA, Meng LR, et al: The effects of novel antipsychotics on glucose and lipid levels. J Clin Psychiatry 63:856–865, 2002

Zacher JL, Roche-Desilets J: Hypotension secondary to the combination of intramuscular olanzapine and intramuscular lorazepam. J Clin Psychiatry 66:1614–1615, 2005

Zanarini MC, Frankenburg FR: Olanzapine treatment of female borderline personality disorder patients: a double-blind, placebo-controlled pilot study. J Clin Psychiatry 62:849–854, 2001

Zanarini MC, Frankenburg FR, Parachini EA: A preliminary, randomized trial of fluoxetine, olanzapine, and the olanzapine-fluoxetine combination in women with borderline personality disorder. J Clin Psychiatry 65:903–907, 2004

Zanarini MC, Schulz SC, Detke HC, et al: A dose comparison of olanzapine for the treatment of borderline personality disorder: a 12-week randomized, double-blind, placebo-controlled study. J Clin Psychiatry 72:1353–1362, 2011

CHAPTER 18

Quetiapine

Peter F. Buckley, M.D.

Adriana E. Foster, M.D.

Matthew Byerly, M.D.

History and Discovery

Quetiapine is a second-generation antipsychotic (SGA) developed and subsequently marketed by AstraZeneca. In preclinical trials, quetiapine showed the features associated with antipsychotic efficacy, as well as a low rate of motor effects (Goldstein 1999; Nemeroff et al. 2002). Quetiapine was approved in 1997 by the U.S. Food and Drug Administration (FDA) for the treatment of schizophrenia; it was subsequently approved in Europe and in other countries worldwide. Additional approvals and indications for quetiapine's use in bipolar disorder, as well as approval of an extended-release formulation of quetiapine, have followed (Möller et al. 2007; Peuskens et al. 2007). The extended-release formulation has an additional indication as adjunctive treatment for major depression in patients who show inadequate response to antidepressants alone.

Structure-Activity Relations

Quetiapine is an SGA of the dibenzothiazepine class. Its complex neuropharmacology includes a relatively low binding profile for dopamine type 2 (D_2) receptors (Kapur et al. 2000). Indeed, considering the idea that an antipsychotic needs to occupy 60% or more of D_2 receptors in order to be clinically efficacious (Kapur et al. 2000), quetiapine's low D_2 binding—typically approximately 30%—is noteworthy.

In attempting to reconcile this apparently subtherapeutic D_2 receptor antagonism with the well-recorded efficacy of quetiapine as an antipsychotic, Kapur et al. (2000) proposed an elegant *kiss and run hypothesis* to explain quetiapine's mechanisms of action. In a series of studies, they found that when D_2 receptor occupancy with quetiapine was measured with positron emission tomography (PET) at shorter intervals (4 hours and 6 hours) than the conventional 12 hours after the last dose was taken, quetiapine did indeed show high D_2 occupancy. In contrast to other antipsychotics, quetiapine demonstrated a more rapid "run-off" from D_2 receptors; that is, there was rapid dissociation of the D_2 receptors (Kapur et al. 2000).

Like clozapine, quetiapine has strong binding at 5-hydroxytryptamine (serotonin) type 2 receptors (5-HT_2 receptors). This profile contrasts with its relatively weak affinity for other subclasses of the serotonin receptor family (Nemeroff et al. 2002). Quetiapine also has strong affinity for α_1-noradrenergic receptors. This antagonism may relate to its propensity to induce postural hypotension—especially during rapid dose titration. Additionally, quetiapine has strong antagonism at histamine type 1 (H_1) receptors. This most likely relates to its sedative effect. H_1 receptor antagonism also appears to be a key contributor to weight gain during quetiapine therapy (Kim et al. 2007).

Pharmacokinetics and Disposition

Quetiapine's absorption in the gastrointestinal tract is unaffected by food. With the tablet formulation, peak blood levels are achieved in about 2 hours, with effective plasma levels sustained for approximately 6 hours (DeVane and Nemeroff 2001). Although this provides the basis for the usual clinical regimen of twice-daily dosing, a short-term trial comparing once-daily dosing versus twice-daily dosing demonstrated that the two regimens were equivalent in terms of efficacy and tolerability (Chengappa et al. 2003b). A PET study (Mamo et al. 2008) found comparable plasma levels and D_2 receptor occupancy between the immediate-release (IR) and the extended-release (XR) formulation.

Quetiapine is metabolized by cytochrome P450 (CYP) 3A4 to inactive metabolites. Coadministration with drugs that alter CYP3A4 activity is likely to result in clinically significant interactions. For example, the anticonvulsants carbamazepine and phenytoin are CYP3A4 inducers, and in their presence quetiapine doses may need to be increased due to accelerated drug clearance (Potkin et al. 2002a, 2002b; Strakowski et al. 2002). Ritonavir, erythromycin, ketoconazole, and nefazodone are potent inhibitors of CYP3A4, and their concomitant use with quetiapine requires caution.

Clinical trials (Kahn et al. 2007; Lindenmayer et al. 2008) comparing the efficacy and tolerability of the XR formulation versus the regular IR formulation indicated that quetiapine XR given once daily (at dosages of 400–800 mg/day) was effective for the treatment of schizophrenia and on average was similar in efficacy and tolerability to treatment with quetiapine IR. Quetiapine is excreted in the kidneys and is not affected by gender or smoking status. The metabolism of quetiapine is reduced by approximately 30% with advancing age. Quetiapine is available only in tablet formulations; there are no liquid or intramuscular preparations.

Indications and Efficacy

Quetiapine in the XR and IR formulations is FDA approved for the following indications in adults: treatment of schizophrenia; acute treatment of manic or mixed episodes associated with bipolar I disorder, both as monotherapy and as an adjunct to lithium or divalproex; acute treatment of depressive episodes associated with bipolar I or II disorder; and maintenance treatment of bipolar I disorder as an adjunct to lithium or divalproex. The XR formulation is also approved for use as an adjunct to antidepressant therapy in the treatment of major depressive disorder in adults.

In addition, quetiapine is efficacious in the treatment of schizophrenia and bipolar disorder in pediatric populations (Barzman et al. 2006; DelBello et al. 2007; McConville et al. 2000). The IR formulation is FDA approved for the treatment of schizophrenia in adolescents (ages 13–17 years) and the acute treatment of manic or mixed episodes associated with bipolar I disorder in children and adolescents (ages 10–17 years).

There are also reports of quetiapine's efficacy in treating anxiety disorders, obsessive-compulsive disorder (OCD), and Parkinson's disease. These uses have not been approved by the FDA. The use of any medication (in this case quetiapine) in situations that are not FDA-approved indications is not recommended in clinical practice.

Schizophrenia

Registration and early trials of quetiapine (Arvanitis and Miller 1997; Borison et al. 1996; Copolov et al. 2000; King et al. 1998; Peuskens and Link 1997; Small et al. 1997) demonstrated that quetiapine is an efficacious antipsychotic for the treatment of schizophrenia. Short-term (6-week) trials compared quetiapine, haloperidol, and placebo using quetiapine at flexible daily dosages of ≤250 mg or ≤750 mg (Small et al. 1997) or fixed daily dosages of 75 mg, 150 mg, 300 mg, 600 mg, or 750 mg (Arvanitis and Miller 1997); the latter trial found that 300 mg/day was superior (but not statistically significantly so) to the lower and higher dosages and was the only dosage demonstrating efficacy for negative symptoms (Arvanitis and Miller 1997). These studies established a range of effective dosages for quetiapine and also suggested that dosages of ≥250 mg/day were superior to lower dosages.

Subsequent studies helped refine quetiapine dosing strategies. An 8-week fixed-dosage comparison trial of quetiapine at 600 mg/day versus haloperidol at 20 mg/day showed similar efficacy for the two drugs in patients who were "partial responders" to first-generation antipsychotics (FGAs) (Emsley et al. 2000). A study comparing a rapid titration strategy (beginning at 200 mg/day, increasing to 800 mg/day by day 4) with a more conventional dosing strategy (50 mg/day on day 1, up to 400 mg/day by day 5) showed similar efficacy and tolerability for the two strategies (Pae et al. 2007). Growing evidence from more recent studies (Honer et al. 2012; Lindenmayer et al. 2011) would discourage the use of very-high-dose quetiapine, and data are still lacking to indicate that dosages above 300–400 mg/day are more efficacious.

Most studies comparing quetiapine with either an FGA or another SGA have reported similar efficacy for the agents in treating schizophrenia (Emsley et al. 2000; Peuskens and Link 1997; Small et al. 1997). A 4-month open-label trial of quetiapine and risperidone showed overall comparability between the two agents (Mullen et al. 2001). An 8-week comparative trial of quetiapine (at an average dosage of 525 mg/day) and risperidone (at an average dosage of 5.2 mg/day) also found the drugs similar in efficacy (Zhong et al. 2006). Quetiapine-treated patients had fewer extrapyramidal side effects (EPS), lower prolactin levels, and fewer sexual side effects. Whereas weight gain was similar in both treatment groups, quetiapine was more sedating and was more frequently associated with dry mouth than was risperidone. A 6-month study comparing quetiapine and risperidone reported better efficacy for risperidone (Potkin et al. 2006), with quetiapine associated with more polypharmacy. A 6-month double-blind comparative trial of quetiapine and olanzapine (Kinon et al. 2006) reported that quetiapine-treated patients were less likely to complete the study, although relapse rates were comparable overall in the two treatment groups. More weight gain occurred in olanzapine recipients. As yet, no studies have directly compared quetiapine with aripiprazole, iloperidone, asenapine, or lurasidone in the treatment of schizophrenia.

The most extensive comparative evaluation of quetiapine and other SGAs comes from the Clinical Antipsychotic Trials of Intervention Effectiveness (CATIE). In the phase I study, more quetiapine-treated patients than olanzapine-treated patients had discontinued treatment by 18 months (78% vs. 64%), and a similar (not statistically significant) trend was seen in comparisons of quetiapine versus risperidone, ziprasidone, or perphenazine (Lieberman et al. 2005). In the phase II study, discontinuation rates favored clozapine and olanzapine over risperidone and quetiapine (McEvoy et al. 2006). The results from the tolerability pathways were mixed and showed similar efficacy for quetiapine versus other agents (Stroup et al. 2007). The findings relating to quetiapine's relative adverse-effects profile in this formative study are presented later in this chapter (see "Side Effects and Toxicology"). Another interesting analysis from the CATIE schizophrenia studies (Stroup et al. 2007) examined how those patients originally assigned to the perphenazine arm of the phase I study fared. In this analysis, switching to quetiapine was more efficacious than switching to any of the other agents. Much of the efficacy and tolerability differences among agents observed in the CATIE schizophrenia studies have been attributed to differential dosing profiles.

An analogous comparative trial of quetiapine, risperidone, and olanzapine was conducted with patients experiencing a first episode of psychosis—the Comparison of Atypicals in First Episode Psychosis (CAFÉ) study. Here, discontinuation rates were similar across drugs over the 1-year trial (McEvoy et al. 2007).

The use of quetiapine in patients with prodromal features of schizophrenia has not yet been studied. A small study of quetiapine in schizophrenia patients with comorbid substance abuse was inconclusive (Brunette et al. 2009).

Mood Disorders

There is evidence that quetiapine is an effective and well-tolerated antipsychotic for treating patients with bipolar mania and bipolar depression. Bowden et al. (2005) demonstrated that quetiapine was superior to placebo in the treatment of mania. In this multicenter study, significantly more patients treated with quetiapine than with placebo met criteria for response (greater than 50% decrease from baseline score on Young Mania Rating Scale) at 7, 21, and 84 days. Building on initial evidence for mood effects that was derived from observations on mood assessment items in the pivotal schizophrenia trials, the Quetiapine Experience with Safety and Tolerability (QUEST) study compared quetiapine with risperidone in a 4-month open-label, flexible-dose trial (Mullen et al. 2001). This study included patients with schizophrenia, schizoaffective disorder, bipolar disorder, and depression. At week 16, the mean dosage of quetiapine was 317 mg/day, and the mean dosage of risperidone was 4.5 mg/day. Mean improvement on the Hamilton Rating Scale for Depression was significantly greater in quetiapine recipients than in risperidone recipients.

Calabrese et al. (2005) and Thase et al. (2006) have studied quetiapine use in patients with bipolar depression. In an 8-week trial, Calabrese et al. (2005) compared two dosages of quetiapine (300 mg/day and 600 mg/day) versus placebo. Both dosages were efficacious, with improvements observed across the full range of depressive and anxiety symptoms. Fifty-eight percent of patients met a priori criteria for treatment response. Additionally, this antidepressant effect was observed with a once-daily dosage regimen. In a subsequent similar study of the same two dosages (300 mg/day and 600 mg/day; Thase et al. 2006), quetiapine was again compared with placebo in an 8-week trial in patients with bipolar depression. Again, both dosages of quetiapine showed efficacy across a broad range of depressive symptoms. These two studies led to FDA approval of quetiapine for treating bipolar depression.

Two large 8-week international multicenter studies—Efficacy of Monotherapy Seroquel in BipOLar DEpressioN (EMBOLDEN) I (Young et al. 2010) and II (McElroy et al. 2010)—compared quetiapine 300 and 600 mg/day against lithium 600–1,800 mg/day and placebo (EMBOLDEN I) or paroxetine 20 mg/day and placebo (EMBOLDEN II) in bipolar patients with a major depressive episode. In the first study (Young et al.

2010), quetiapine at both dosages, but not lithium, led to significant improvement in symptoms of depression and anxiety. Compared with patients receiving placebo, patients treated with quetiapine 300 and 600 mg/day showed significant improvement on the Sheehan Disability Scale. In the second study (McElroy et al. 2010), quetiapine 300 and 600 mg/day, but not paroxetine 20 mg/day, led to significant improvement in depressive and anxiety symptoms. Neither lithium nor paroxetine led to significant functional improvement over placebo in these studies. In both studies, a small subgroup of patients with rapid-cycling bipolar disorder failed to improve significantly from baseline with any of the drugs administered (quetiapine, lithium, or paroxetine).

In a long-term naturalistic study of quetiapine administered to 96 patients with bipolar disorder in a clinical setting, 38.5% of patients continued quetiapine for 328 days without addition of other psychotropics, whereas 22.9% of patients continued quetiapine for 613 days with addition of another psychotropic, most often for depression (Ketter et al. 2010). In a small double-blind, placebo-controlled pilot study of quetiapine 300–600 mg/day in depressed adolescents with bipolar disorder, quetiapine neither differentiated from placebo nor induced significant change in symptoms from baseline to endpoint on measures of depressive, anxiety, or manic symptoms or clinical global impressions of bipolar severity (DelBello et al. 2009).

Dorée et al. (2007) reported that in a pilot study ($n = 20$) quetiapine was an efficacious augmenting agent for antidepressant treatment in major depression. Anderson et al. (2009) also reported on quetiapine's efficacy as an adjunctive treatment for patients with refractory depression. Quetiapine XR monotherapy at a mean daily dose of 162.2 mg was shown to decrease symptoms of major depression at 8 weeks versus placebo (Bortnick et al. 2011). Cutler et al. (2009) reported that quetiapine XR 300 mg/day led to significantly higher rates of response and remission versus placebo in major depression, whereas quetiapine XR 150 mg/day had a significant effect only on response versus placebo. Quetiapine at dosages of 150–300 mg/day is now approved by the FDA as an adjunct to antidepressant treatment for a major depressive episode. In one of the studies leading to FDA approval of quetiapine XR for this indication, El-Khalili et al. (2010) demonstrated that quetiapine XR at 300 mg/day led to significant improvement in symptoms of depression from the first week of treatment when compared with placebo. In a review of registration studies for the major depression indication, McIntyre et al. (2009) concluded that quetiapine XR provides rapid and sustained relief of major depressive symptoms. Weisler et al. (2012) also reported substantial improvement in depressive symptoms in two 6-week clinical trials of quetiapine XR. Remission at 6 weeks was achieved by 23.5% of patients on 150 mg/day and by 28.8% of patients on 300 mg/day of quetiapine.

Anxiety Disorders

The sedative/calming effect of quetiapine was well described in a variety of product registration trials (Weiden et al. 2006; Chengappa et al. 2003a), and studies in bipolar I disorder and bipolar depression (Calabrese et al. 2005; Hirschfeld et al. 2006; Thase et al. 2006) demonstrated improvements in anxiety symptoms with quetiapine.

Quetiapine has been studied in the treatment of posttraumatic stress disorder (PTSD) (Ahearn et al. 2006; Byers et al. 2010; Hamner et al. 2003; Kozaric-Kovacic and Pivac 2007; Sokolski et al. 2003; Stathis and McKenna 2005). All but one of the studies (Stathis and McKenna 2005) involved quetiapine administered to veterans as an adjunctive agent added to selective serotonin reuptake inhibitors (SSRIs), other antidepressants, sedative-anxiolytics, or anticonvulsants. All were open-label studies, and with the exception of a retrospective chart review comparing quetiapine with prazosin

(Byers et al. 2010), none had a comparison group. The average quetiapine dosage used in these studies was 100–335 mg/day administered for 6–8 weeks. Quetiapine decreased symptoms of avoidance, hyperarousal, and recollection in the populations studied.

In a small 8-week study (Vaishnavi et al. 2007) of social phobia treatment, there was no significant difference in Brief Social Phobia Scale (BSPS) scores between the quetiapine and placebo groups, although people who took quetiapine did show a robust response as measured by Clinical Global Impression–Improvement Scale (CGI-I) scores.

Two small studies of quetiapine augmentation in patients with generalized anxiety disorder (GAD) who had not responded to antidepressant therapy (Katzman et al. 2008; Simon et al. 2008) yielded contradictory results. Quetiapine XR dosages of 50 mg/day and 150 mg/day were compared with paroxetine 20 mg/day and placebo in a large study of monotherapy for GAD (Bandelow et al. 2010). Quetiapine XR 50 mg/day and 150 mg/day separated from placebo and paroxetine in reducing Hamilton Anxiety Rating Scale (Ham-A) scores as early as 4 days into treatment. After 8 weeks of treatment, both quetiapine 150 mg/day and paroxetine 20 mg/day yielded higher anxiety remission rates (Ham-A score ≤7) compared with placebo. Weight gain greater than or equal to 7% of body weight was noted in a higher percentage of patients treated with quetiapine than of those treated with placebo. In a study reported by Katzman et al. (2011), 432 patients with GAD were randomly assigned to continue treatment long term with quetiapine XR or to switch to placebo after 12 weeks of open-label run-in and stabilization on quetiapine XR 50 mg, 150 mg, or 300 mg daily. Quetiapine XR significantly increased the time to occurrence of an anxiety event and decreased anxiety symptoms from randomization to the end of the study.

An analysis of the tolerability of quetiapine in patients with various disorders showed that patients with GAD, bipolar depression, or refractory major depression had significantly higher rates of discontinuation due to adverse effects versus placebo than did patients with schizophrenia or mania when treated with quetiapine XR dosages of ≥300 mg/day (Wang et al. 2011). In a systematic review and meta-analysis of all available trials of SGA medications, quetiapine was observed to have the most robust effect on anxiety symptoms (LaLonde and Van Lieshout 2011). The antianxiety effects of quetiapine were observed at lower dosages (typically 150 mg/day) than those used in schizophrenia studies, and the effects included overall improvement as well as remission. However, quetiapine was also associated with weight gain and high rates of medication discontinuation in these studies in anxiety disorder (LaLonde and Van Lieshout 2011). In three 8-week studies of quetiapine XR, Stein et al. (2011) reported rates of study discontinuation due to side effects of 13%, 16%, and 24% for quetiapine dosages of 50 mg/day, 150 mg/day, and 300 mg/day, respectively. In an 8-week placebo-controlled comparative trial of quetiapine XR and escitalopram, comparable improvements in anxiety symptoms, occurring early in the study, were observed between quetiapine and escitalopram (Merideth et al. 2012).

Several small studies of quetiapine augmentation (at dosages up to 400 mg/day) of SSRI pharmacotherapy in refractory OCD yielded contradictory results (Atmaca et al. 2002; Carey et al. 2005; Fineberg et al. 2005); although improvement in Yale-Brown Obsessive Compulsive Scale (Y-BOCS) scores was noted in patients treated with quetiapine, the response to quetiapine failed to differentiate from placebo. Quetiapine's efficacy as an augmenting agent with antidepressants in treatment-resistant OCD was recently reviewed in a meta-analysis of five double-blind, randomized controlled trials (RCTs) (Komossa et al. 2010). Adjunctive quetiapine was not superior to placebo in reducing Y-BOCS by 25% (the criterion for response in these studies), but it did reduce the Y-BOCS score significantly by the endpoint compared with placebo. A small case series also showed that adjunctive quetiapine response may be enduring (Dell'Osso et al. 2006).

At present, the FDA has not approved quetiapine for use in any anxiety disorders.

Other Conditions and Patient Populations

Quetiapine has also been used in elderly populations. In a 1-year open-label trial of quetiapine treatment in 151 elderly patients (mean age 76.8 years) with psychotic disorders (McManus et al. 1999), 52% of patients showed symptom improvement (as measured by a 20% or greater decline in Brief Psychiatric Rating Scale [BPRS] total score). Seventy percent of patients had some organic condition, predominantly Alzheimer's disease, with the remaining patients having a diagnosis of schizophrenia, schizoaffective disorder, or delusional disorder. Quetiapine was well tolerated at a mean dosage of 100 mg/day. A 10-week study comparing two dosages of quetiapine (100 mg/day and 200 mg/day) versus placebo in nursing home residents with dementia and agitation (Zhong et al. 2007) reported that only the 200 mg/day quetiapine dosage was efficacious in treating agitation. Quetiapine (100 mg/day) was also compared with risperidone (1.0 mg/day), olanzapine (5.5 mg/day), and placebo over 36 weeks in the CATIE Alzheimer's disease study (Schneider et al. 2006). Overall, no effect on the Alzheimer's Disease Cooperative Study–Clinical Global Impression of Change (ADCS-CGIC) scale was seen with any of the agents, and there were no differences between agents in time to discontinuation.

In contrast to the encouraging findings from open-label studies of quetiapine for Parkinson's-associated psychosis, four of five later double-blind RCTs (Kurlan et al. 2007; Ondo et al. 2005; Rabey et al. 2007; Shotbolt et al. 2009) found no benefit for quetiapine in this population. The single positive RCT (Fernandez et al. 2009) was small (N=16) and excluded patients with delusions, which appear to be more difficult to treat than hallucinations in Parkinson's disease (Shotbolt et al. 2010).

Agitation is a core aspect of several conditions. Currier et al. (2006) reported an interesting study of quetiapine in agitated patients in the emergency room. Here, Currier and colleagues reported that quetiapine could be used as an acute antiagitation agent if the dose titration is judicious. Postural hypotension was observed in this study. Other studies of quetiapine and agitation report benefits in treating hostility both in adults with schizophrenia (Chengappa et al. 2003a) or bipolar disorder (Buckley et al. 2007) and in children with hostile behaviors (Barzman et al. 2006; Findling et al. 2007).

Side Effects and Toxicology

To illustrate the profile of adverse effects typically seen with quetiapine, we have tabulated the results from an RCT of 8 weeks' duration (Zhong et al. 2006) (Table 18–1). Overall, quetiapine was well tolerated, with only 6% of patients discontinuing treatment due to adverse effects.

Somnolence is a common side effect of quetiapine that most likely relates to its antihistaminergic activity. Although somnolence occurs early in treatment and generally decreases over time, it may persist in some patients. It may also cause patients to stop taking their medication, because sedation is generally a poorly tolerated side effect. In the bipolar depression study by Calabrese et al. (2005), somnolence was observed in 24% of patients receiving quetiapine at a dosage of 300 mg/day and in 27% of patients receiving 600 mg/day. In the long-term study by Ketter et al. (2010), sedation was present in 19.8% of patients. Dizziness is another troublesome side effect, and it may be associated with postural hypotension, an effect that is of even greater concern. As with sedation, dizziness can sometimes cause discontinuation of quetiapine therapy.

TABLE 18–1. Comparative side-effect profile of quetiapine versus risperidone: adverse effects present in ≥5% of patients in an 8-week study

	Quetiapine (*N*=338; median dosage = 525 mg/day)	Risperidone (*N*=334; median dosage = 5.2 mg/day)	
Adverse effect	***N*** **(%)**	***N*** **(%)**	***P*** **value**[a]
Somnolence	89 (26.3)	66 (19.7)	0.044
Headache	51 (15.1)	56 (16.7)	0.599
Weight gain	48 (14.2)	45 (13.4)	0.824
Dizziness	48 (14.2)	32 (9.6)	0.0737
Dry mouth	41 (12.1)	17 (5.1)	<0.01
Dyspepsia	22 (6.5)	26 (7.8)	0.552
Nausea	21 (6.2)	22 (6.6)	0.876
Pain	21 (6.2)	24 (7.2)	0.536
Asthenia	17 (5.0)	14 (4.2)	0.714
Agitation	17 (5.0)	10 (3.0)	0.238
Pharyngitis	15 (4.4)	24 (7.2)	0.140
Akathisia	13 (3.8)	28 (8.4)	0.016
Vomiting	13 (3.8)	18 (5.4)	0.364
Dystonia	01 (0.3)	18 (5.4)	<0.001

[a]Fisher exact test, unadjusted.
Source. Adapted from Zhong et al. 2006.

There is major concern about antipsychotic-induced weight gain and metabolic disturbances (Allison et al. 1999; Newcomer 2005; Newcomer et al. 2002). Quetiapine is clearly associated with weight gain, although the weight gain effect is not as great as that seen with clozapine or olanzapine. On the other hand, the weight-effects profile of quetiapine is not as favorable as that of ziprasidone or aripiprazole (Newcomer 2005) or that of the newer agents asenapine and lurasidone (Merck 2012; Sunovion 2012).

In the 8-week comparative study by Zhong et al. (2006), weight gain that was clinically significant (a 7% increase above baseline weight) was observed in 10.4% of patients receiving quetiapine and in 10.5% of patients receiving risperidone. In the phase I CATIE study, quetiapine had a moderate effect on weight (and other aspects of the metabolic profile) compared with other agents (Lieberman et al. 2005). Those data are shown in Table 18–2. In the first-episode CAFÉ study, quetiapine had a less favorable weight-effects profile compared with olanzapine or risperidone. Eighty percent of patients taking quetiapine gained weight, compared with 50% of those taking olanzapine and 2% of those taking risperidone. Interestingly, females taking quetiapine were less likely than males to gain weight in this 1-year study of patients treated for their first episode of psychosis (Patel et al. 2009). It is also important to consider quetiapine's propensity to induce weight gain among bipolar patients (especially because these patients may also be

TABLE 18–2. Comparative metabolic profiles of antipsychotics in the phase I CATIE schizophrenia trial: change from baseline

	Olanzapine	Quetiapine	Perphenazine	Risperidone	Ziprasidone	P value
Weight gain >7%, *n*/total *N* (%)	92/307 (30)	49/305 (16)	29/243 (12)	42/300 (14)	12/161 (7)	<0.001
Weight change (lb), mean±SE	9.4±0.9	1.1±0.9	−2.0±1.10	0.8±0.9	−1.6±1.10	<0.001
Blood glucose change (mg/dL), exposure-adjusted mean±SE	13.7±2.50	7.5±2.5	5.4±2.8	6.6±2.5	2.9±3.4	0.59
Glycosylated Hb (%), exposure-adjusted mean±SE	0.40±0.07	0.04±0.08	0.09±0.09	0.07±0.08	0.11±0.09	0.01
Cholesterol (mg/dL), exposure-adjusted mean±SE	9.4±2.4	6.6±2.4	1.5±2.7	−1.3±2.40	−8.2±3.20	<0.001
Triglycerides (mg/dL), exposure-adjusted mean±SE	40.5±8.90	21.2±9.20	09.2±10.1	−2.4±9.10	−16.5±12.20	<0.001

Note. Hb = hemoglobin; SE = standard error.
P values for laboratory values and for the change in weight are based on ranked analysis of covariance with adjustment for whether patient had an exacerbation in the preceding 3 months and the duration of exposure to the study drug in phase I. Mean values for metabolic factors (other than weight change) were also adjusted for duration of exposure to study drug.

Source. Adapted from Lieberman et al. 2005.

taking lithium or valproic acid). In the 8-week EMBOLDEN I (Young et al. 2010) and II (McElroy et al. 2010) trials, weight gain of more than 7% body weight was present in 4.6% and 9%, respectively, of patients receiving quetiapine 300 mg/day versus 8.3% and 11.3%, respectively, of those receiving quetiapine 600 mg/day. In EMBOLDEN I and II, the average weight gains in quetiapine-treated patients were 0.6 kg and 1.1 kg, respectively, for the 300-mg/day groups and 0.8 kg and 1.7 kg, respectively, for the 600-mg/day groups.

In the bipolar depression study by Calabrese et al. (2005), the mean changes in glucose levels were 6 mg/dL and 3 mg/dL with quetiapine dosages of 600 mg/day and 300 mg/day, respectively. In the comparative study of quetiapine and risperidone in the treatment of schizophrenia (Zhong et al. 2006), the mean changes from baseline in fasting glucose levels were 1.8 mg/dL with quetiapine and 5.6 mg/dL with risperidone. The metabolic profile of quetiapine appeared moderate in the phase I CATIE schizophrenia study (see Table 18–2). Newcomer et al. (2009) conducted a euglycemic clamp study of quetiapine and found little evidence of insulin insensitivity. A recent meta-analysis by the Cochrane group involving head-to-head comparisons of SGAs (Komossa et al. 2010) found that quetiapine was associated with significantly greater cholesterol elevations than risperidone (mean difference 8.61 mg/dL) and ziprasidone (mean difference 16.01 mg/dL). In the CATIE I trial (Lieberman et al. 2005), which included patients with chronic schizophrenia, quetiapine led to a mean change from baseline fasting triglyceride levels of +19.2 mg/dL, whereas a mean change of +42.9 mg/dL was observed for olanzapine, +8.3 mg/dL for perphenazine, –2.6 mg/dL for risperidone, and –18.1 mg/dL for ziprasidone. In a population of young patients with early psychosis treated with quetiapine, olanzapine, or risperidone, the CAFÉ study (Patel et al. 2009) found that elevations in fasting triglyceride levels at 52 weeks were significantly greater in quetiapine-treated patients than in risperidone-treated patients (44.3 vs. 8.2 ng/mL, respectively). Overall, quetiapine appears to carry a risk of causing weight gain and other metabolic disturbances.

Quetiapine is associated with a low risk of raising prolactin levels (Hamner et al. 1996; Lieberman et al. 2005; Small et al. 1997; Zhong et al. 2006).

The low-EPS advantage of quetiapine is compelling and consistent across studies. In the Seroquel Patient Evaluation on Changing Treatment Relative to Usual Medication (SPECTRUM) switch study (Larmo et al. 2005), switching to quetiapine from haloperidol, olanzapine, or risperidone was associated with a robust reduction in EPS. This low propensity for EPS was also seen in the bipolar depression studies (Calabrese et al. 2005; Thase et al. 2006).

The potential of quetiapine to induce cataracts was studied in a pragmatic follow-up trial of patients (N=37; mean age 23 years) with first-episode psychosis that included regular slit-lamp ophthalmological examinations (Whitehorn et al. 2004). After exposure to quetiapine 500–600 mg/day for a mean of 22.4 months, none of the patients developed any ocular changes. Most clinicians do not obtain specialist eye examinations when prescribing quetiapine.

Abnormalities in thyroid hormone levels were observed in the large premarketing trials of quetiapine (Arvanitis and Miller 1997). A small RCT did find lower total thyroid hormone with quetiapine use, but not significant changes in free thyroxine (T_4) or thyroid-stimulating hormone (TSH) levels (Kelly and Conley 2005).

Quetiapine's prescribing information (AstraZeneca 2011a, 2011b) possesses a warning similar to that required in the prescribing information of many other antipsychotics concerning cardiovascular risks. The CATIE trial found no evidence of a heightened QTc risk with quetiapine relative to other SGAs and perphenazine (Lieberman et al. 2005). A curious and unsubstantiated claim is that quetiapine might have abuse potential (Pierre et al. 2005; Pinta and Taylor 2007). This observation merits further consideration and vigilance.

Overall, the adverse-effect profile of the XR formulation is similar to that of the IR formulation. As is the case with all SGAs, there is little information about the effects of quetiapine during pregnancy. A prospective study by McKenna et al. (2005) examined a sample of pregnant women in Canada, Israel, and England treated with SGAs, which was matched to a comparison group of pregnant women who were not exposed to these agents. Among them were 36 women treated with quetiapine. The pregnancy outcomes in the exposed and comparison groups were not significantly different, with the exceptions of the rate of low birth weight, which was 10% in exposed babies versus 2% in the comparison group ($P=0.05$), and the rate of therapeutic abortions, which was 9.9% in exposed women versus 1.3% in the comparison group ($P=0.003$). These findings suggest that atypical antipsychotics as a group are not associated with an increased risk for major malformations.

Conclusion

Quetiapine is now a well-established and widely prescribed antipsychotic. There is strong evidence for its efficacy in all of the current FDA-approved indications: the treatment of schizophrenia, acute bipolar mania, bipolar depression, and major depressive disorder. Quetiapine is also used extensively under circumstances not approved by the FDA (i.e., off-label use), and evidence for its efficacy in some of these uses has been reviewed in this chapter. Additional clinical trials of quetiapine are currently ongoing (www.clinicaltrials.gov).

References

Ahearn EP, Mussey M, Johnson C, et al: Quetiapine as an adjunctive treatment for post-traumatic stress disorder: an 8-week open-label study. Int Clin Psychopharmacol 21:29–33, 2006

Allison DB, Mentore JL, Heo M, et al: Antipsychotic-induced weight gain: a comprehensive research synthesis. Am J Psychiatry 156:1686–1696, 1999

Anderson IM, Sarsfield A, Haddad PM: Efficacy, safety and tolerability of quetiapine augmentation in treatment resistant depression: an open-label, pilot study. J Affect Disord 117:116–119, 2009

Arvanitis LA, Miller BG: Multiple fixed doses of "Seroquel" (quetiapine) in patients with acute exacerbation of schizophrenia: a comparison with haloperidol and placebo. The Seroquel Trial 13 Study Group. Biol Psychiatry 42:233–246, 1997

AstraZeneca Pharmaceuticals: Seroquel (quetiapine fumarate) tablets, full prescribing information. Revised December 2011a. Available at: http://www1.astrazeneca-us.com/pi/Seroquel.pdf. Accessed August 2012.

AstraZeneca Pharmaceuticals: Seroquel XR (quetiapine fumarate) extended-release tablets, full prescribing information. Revised December 2011b. Available at: http://www1.astrazeneca-us.com/pi/seroquelxr.pdf. Accessed August 2012.

Atmaca M, Kuloglu M, Tezcan E, et al: Quetiapine augmentation in patients with treatment resistant obsessive-compulsive disorder: a single-blind, placebo-controlled study. Int Clin Psychopharmacol 17:115–119, 2002

Bandelow B, Chouinard G, Bobes J, et al: Extended-release quetiapine fumarate (quetiapine XR): a once-daily monotherapy effective in generalized anxiety disorder: data from a randomized, double-blind, placebo- and active-controlled study. Int J Neuropsychopharmacol 13:305–320, 2010

Barzman DH, DelBello MP, Adler CM, et al: The efficacy and tolerability of quetiapine versus divalproex for the treatment of impulsivity and reactive aggression in adolescents with co-occurring bipolar disorder and disruptive behavior disorder(s). J Child Adolesc Psychopharmacol 16:665–670, 2006

Borison RL, Arvanitis LA, Miller BG: ICI 204,636, an atypical antipsychotic: efficacy and safety in a multicenter, placebo-controlled trial in patients with schizophrenia. US Seroquel Study Group. J Clin Psychopharmacol 16:158–169, 1996

Bortnick B, El-Khalili N, Banov M, et al: Efficacy and tolerability of extended release quetiapine fumarate (quetiapine XR) monotherapy in major depressive disorder: a placebo-controlled, randomized study. J Affect Disord 128:83–94, 2011

Bowden CL, Grunze H, Mullen J, et al: A randomized double-blind, placebo-controlled efficacy and safety study of quetiapine or lithium as monotherapy for mania in bipolar disorder. J Clin Psychiatry 66:111–121, 2005

Brunette MF, Dawson R, O'Keefe C, et al: An open label study of quetiapine in patients with schizophrenia and alcohol disorders. Mental Health and Substance Use: Dual Diagnosis 2(3):203–211, 2009

Buckley PF, Goldstein JM, Emsley RA: Efficacy and tolerability of quetiapine in poorly responsive, chronic schizophrenia. Schizophr Res 66:143–150, 2004

Buckley PF, Paulsson B, Brecher M: Treatment of agitation and aggression in bipolar mania: efficacy of quetiapine. J Affect Disord 100 (suppl 1): S33–S43, 2007

Byers MG, Allison KM, Wendel KS, et al: Prazosin versus quetiapine for nighttime posttraumatic stress disorder symptoms in veterans: an assessment of long-term comparative effectiveness and safety. J Clin Psychopharmacol 30:225–229, 2010

Calabrese JR, Keck PE Jr, Macfadden W, et al: A randomized, double-blind, placebo-controlled trial of quetiapine in the treatment of bipolar I or II depression. Am J Psychiatry 162:1351–1360, 2005

Carey PD, Vythilingum B, Seedat S, et al: Quetiapine augmentation of SRIs in treatment refractory obsessive-compulsive disorder: a double-blind, randomised, placebo-controlled study [ISRCTN 83050762]. BMC Psychiatry 5:5, 2005

Chengappa KN, Goldstein JM, Greenwood M, et al: A post hoc analysis of the impact on hostility and agitation of quetiapine and haloperidol among patients with schizophrenia. Clin Ther 25:530–541, 2003a

Chengappa KN, Parepally H, Brar JS, et al: A random-assignment, double-blind, clinical trial of once- vs twice-daily administration of quetiapine fumarate in patients with schizophrenia or schizoaffective disorder: a pilot study. Can J Psychiatry 48:187–194, 2003b

Copolov DL, Link CG, Kowalcyk B: A multicenter, double-blind randomized comparison of quetiapine (ICI 204,636, "Seroquel") and haloperidol in schizophrenia. Psychol Med 30:95–105, 2000

Currier GW, Trenton AJ, Walsh PG, et al: A pilot, open-label safety study of quetiapine for treatment of moderate psychotic agitation in the emergency setting. J Psychiatr Pract 12:223–228, 2006

Cutler AJ, Montgomery ST, Feifel D, et al: Extended release quetiapine fumarate monotherapy in major depressive disorder: a placebo- and duloxetine-controlled study. J Clin Psychiatry 70:526–539, 2009

DelBello MP, Adler CM, Whitsel RM, et al: A 12-week single-blind trial of quetiapine for the treatment of mood symptoms in adolescents at high risk for developing bipolar I disorder. J Clin Psychiatry 68:789–795, 2007

DelBello MP, Chang K, Welge JA, et al: A double-blind, placebo-controlled pilot study of quetiapine for depressed adolescents with bipolar disorder. Bipolar Disord 11:483–493, 2009

Dell'Osso B, Mundo E, Altamura AC: Quetiapine augmentation of selective serotonin reuptake inhibitors in treatment-resistant obsessive-compulsive disorder: a six-month follow-up case series. CNS Spectr 11:879–883, 2006

DeVane CL, Nemeroff CB: Clinical pharmacokinetics of quetiapine: an atypical antipsychotic. Clin Pharmacokinet 40:509–522, 2001

Dorée JP, Des Rosiers J, Lew V, et al: Quetiapine augmentation of treatment-resistant depression: a comparison with lithium. Curr Med Res Opin 23:333–341, 2007

El-Khalili N, Atkinson S, Joyce M, et al: Extended release quetiapine fumarate (quetiapine XR) as adjunctive therapy in major depressive disorder in patients in inadequate response to ongoing antidepressant treatment: a multicentre, randomized, double-blind, placebo-controlled study. Int J Neuropsychopharmacol 13:917–932, 2010

Emsley RA, Raniwalla J, Bailey PJ, et al: A comparison of the effects of quetiapine ("Seroquel") and haloperidol in schizophrenic patients with a history of and a demonstrated, partial response to conventional antipsychotic treatment. PRIZE Study Group. Int Clin Psychopharmacol 15:121–131, 2000

Fernandez HH, Okun MS, Rodriguez RL, et al: Quetiapine improves visual hallucinations in Parkinson disease but not through normalization of sleep architecture: results from a double-blind clinical-polysomnography study. Int J Neurosci 119:2196–2205, 2009

Findling RL, Reed MD, O'Riordan MA, et al: A 26-week open-label study of quetiapine in children with conduct disorder. J Child Adolesc Psychopharmacol 17:1–9, 2007

Fineberg N, Sivakumaran T, Roberts A: Adding quetiapine to SRI in treatment-resistant obsessive-compulsive disorder: a randomized controlled treatment study. Int Clin Psychopharmacol 20:223–226, 2005

Goldstein JM: Quetiapine fumarate (Seroquel): a new atypical antipsychotic. Drugs Today (Barc) 35:193–210, 1999

Hamner MB, Arvanitis LA, Miller BG, et al: Plasma prolactin in schizophrenia subjects treated with Seroquel (ICI 204, 636). Psychopharmacol Bull 32:107–110, 1996

Hamner MB, Deitsch SE, Brodrick PS, et al: Quetiapine treatment in patients with posttraumatic stress disorder: an open trial of adjunctive therapy. J Clin Psychopharmacol 23:15–20, 2003

Hirschfeld RM, Weisler RH, Raines SR: Quetiapine in the treatment of anxiety in patients with bipolar I or II depression: a secondary analysis from a randomized, double-blind, placebo-controlled study. J Clin Psychiatry 67:355–362, 2006

Honer WG, MacEwan GW, Gendron A, et al: A randomized, double-blind, placebo-controlled study of the safety and tolerability of high-dose quetiapine in patients with persistent symptoms of schizophrenia or schizoaffective disorder. STACK Study Group. J Clin Psychiatry 73:13–20, 2012

Kahn RS, Schulz SC, Palazov VD, et al: Efficacy and tolerability of once-daily extended release quetiapine fumarate in acute schizophrenia: a randomized, double-blind, placebo-controlled study. J Clin Psychiatry 68:832–842, 2007

Kapur S, Zipursky R, Jones C, et al: A positron emission tomography study of quetiapine in schizophrenia: a preliminary finding of an antipsychotic effect with only transiently high dopamine D2 receptor occupancy. Arch Gen Psychiatry 57:553–559, 2000

Katzman MA, Vermani, M, Jacobs L, et al: Quetiapine as an adjunctive pharmacotherapy for the treatment of non-remitting generalized anxiety disorder: a flexible-dose, open-label pilot trial. J Anxiety Disord 22:1480–1486, 2008

Katzman M, Brawman-Mintzer O, Reyes EB, et al: Extended release quetiapine fumarate (quetiapine XR) monotherapy as maintenance treatment for generalized anxiety disorder: a long-term, randomized, placebo-controlled trial. Int Clin Psychopharmacol 26:11–24, 2011

Kelly DL, Conley RR: Thyroid function in treatment-resistant schizophrenia patients treated with quetiapine, risperidone, or fluphenazine. J Clin Psychiatry 66:80–84, 2005

Ketter TA, Brooks JO III, Hoblyn JC, et al: Long-term effectiveness of quetiapine in bipolar disorder in a clinical setting. J Psychiatr Res 44:921–929, 2010

Kim SF, Huang AS, Snowman AM, et al: Antipsychotic drug-induced weight gain mediated by histamine H1 receptor-linked activation of hypothalamic AMP-kinase. Proc Natl Acad Sci U S A 104:3456–3459, 2007

King DJ, Link CG, Kowalcyk B: A comparison of bid and tid dose regimens of quetiapine (Seroquel) in the treatment of schizophrenia. Psychopharmacology (Berl) 137:139–146, 1998

Kinon BJ, Noordsy DL, Liu-Seifert H, et al: Randomized, double-blind 6-month comparison of olanzapine and quetiapine in patients with schizophrenia or schizoaffective disorder with prominent negative symptoms and poor functioning. J Clin Psychopharmacol 26:453–461, 2006

Komossa K, Depping AM, Meyer M, et al: Second-generation antipsychotics for obsessive compulsive disorder. Cochrane Database Syst Rev (12):CD008141, 2010

Kozaric-Kovacic D, Pivac N: Quetiapine treatment in an open trial in combat-related post-traumatic stress disorder with psychotic features. Int J Neuropsychopharmacol 10:253–261, 2007

Kurlan R, Cummings J, Raman R, et al: Quetiapine for agitation or psychosis in patients with dementia and parkinsonism. Neurology 68:1356–1363, 2007

LaLonde CD, Van Lieshout RJ: Treating generalized anxiety disorder with second generation antipsychotics: a systematic review and meta-analysis. J Clin Psychopharmacol 31:326–333, 2011

Larmo I, de Nayer A, Windhager E, et al: Efficacy and tolerability of quetiapine in patients with schizophrenia who switched from haloperidol, olanzapine or risperidone. Hum Psychopharmacol 20:573–581, 2005

Lieberman JA, Stroup TS, McEvoy JP, et al: Effectiveness of antipsychotic drugs in patients with chronic schizophrenia. N Engl J Med 353:1209–1223, 2005

Lindenmayer JP, Brown D, Liu S, et al: The efficacy and tolerability of once-daily extended release quetiapine fumarate in hospitalized patients with acute schizophrenia: a 6-week randomized, double-blind, placebo-controlled study. Psychopharmacol Bull 41:11–35, 2008

Lindenmayer JP, Citrome L, Khan A, et al: A randomized, double-blind, parallel-group, fixed-dose, clinical trial of quetiapine at 600 versus 1200 mg/d for patients with treatment-resistant schizophrenia or schizoaffective disorder. J Clin Psychopharmacol 31:160–168, 2011

Mamo DC, Uchida H, Vitcu I, et al: Quetiapine extended-release versus immediate-release formulation: a positron emission tomography study. J Clin Psychiatry 69:81–86, 2008

McConville BJ, Arvanitis LA, Thyrum PT, et al: Pharmacokinetics, tolerability, and clinical effectiveness of quetiapine fumarate: an open-label trial in adolescents with psychotic disorders. J Clin Psychiatry 61:252–260, 2000

McElroy SL, Weisler RH, Chang W, et al: A double-blind, placebo-controlled study of quetiapine and paroxetine as monotherapy in adults with bipolar depression (EMBOLDEN II). J Clin Psychiatry 71:163–174, 2010

McEvoy JP, Lieberman JA, Stroup TS, et al: Effectiveness of clozapine versus olanzapine, quetiapine, and risperidone in patients with chronic schizophrenia who did not respond to prior atypical antipsychotic treatment. Am J Psychiatry 163:600–610, 2006

McEvoy JP, Lieberman JA, Perkins DO, et al: Efficacy and tolerability of olanzapine, quetiapine, and risperidone in the treatment of early psychosis: a randomized, double-blind 52-week comparison. Am J Psychiatry 164:1050–1060, 2007

McIntyre RS, Muzlina DJ, Adams A, et al: Quetiapine XR efficacy and tolerability as monotherapy and as a adjunctive treatment to conventional antidepressants in the acute and maintenance treatment of major depressive disorder: a review of registration trials. Expert Opin Pharmacother 10:3061–3075, 2009

McKenna K, Koren G, Tetelbaum M, et al: Pregnancy outcome of women using atypical antipsychotic drugs: a prospective comparative study. J Clin Psychiatry 66:444–449, 2005

McManus DQ, Arvanitis LA, Kowalcyk BB: Quetiapine, a novel antipsychotic: experience in elderly patients with psychotic disorders. Seroquel Trial 48 Study Group. J Clin Psychiatry 60:292–298, 1999

Merck & Co.: Saphris (asenapine) sublingual tablets, full prescribing information. Revised May 2012. Available at: http://www.spfiles.com/pisaphrisv1.pdf. Accessed August 2012.

Merideth C, Cutler AJ, She F, et al: Efficacy and tolerability of extended release quetiapine fumarate monotherapy in the acute treatment of generalized anxiety disorder: a randomized, placebo controlled and active-controlled study. Int Clin Psychopharmacol 27:40–54, 2012

Möller H, Johnson S, Meulien D, et al: Once-daily quetiapine sustained release (SR) is effective and well tolerated in patients with schizophrenia switched from the same total daily dose of quetiapine immediate release (IR). Schizophr Bull 33:449, 2007

Mullen J, Jibson MD, Sweitzer D: A comparison of the relative safety, efficacy, and tolerability of quetiapine and risperidone in outpatients with schizophrenia and other psychotic disorders: the quetiapine experience with safety and tolerability (QUEST) study. Clin Ther 23:1839–1854, 2001

Nemeroff CB, Kinkead B, Goldstein J: Quetiapine: preclinical studies, pharmacokinetics, drug interactions, and dosing. J Clin Psychiatry 63 (suppl 13):5–11, 2002

Newcomer JW: Second-generation (atypical) antipsychotics and metabolic effects: a comprehensive literature review. CNS Drugs 19 (suppl 1): 1–93, 2005

Newcomer JW, Haupt DW, Fucetola R, et al: Abnormalities in glucose regulation during antipsychotic treatment of schizophrenia. Arch Gen Psychiatry 59:337–345, 2002

Newcomer JW, Ratner RE, Eriksson JW, et al: A 24-week multicenter, open-label, randomized study to compare changes in glucose metabolism in patients with schizophrenia receiving treatment with olanzapine, quetiapine and risperidone. J Clin Psychiatry 70:487–499, 2009

Ondo WG, Tintner R, Voung KD, et al: Double-blind, placebo-controlled, unforced titration parallel trial of quetiapine for dopaminergic-induced hallucinations in Parkinson's disease. Mov Disord 20:958–963, 2005

Pae CU, Kim JJ, Lee Cu, et al: Rapid versus conventional initiation of quetiapine in the treatment of schizophrenia: a randomized, parallel-group trial. J Clin Psychiatry 68:399–405, 2007

Patel JK, Buckley PF, Woolson S, et al: Metabolic profiles of second-generation antipsychotics in early psychosis: findings from the CAFÉ study. Schizophr Res 111:9–16, 2009

Peuskens J, Link CG: A comparison of quetiapine and chlorpromazine in the treatment of schizophrenia. Acta Psychiatr Scand 96:265–273, 1997

Peuskens JC, Trivedi JK, Malyarov S, et al: A randomized, placebo-controlled relapse-prevention study with once-daily quetiapine sustained release in patients with schizophrenia. Schizophr Bull 33:453, 2007

Pierre JM, Wirshing DA, Wirshing WC, et al: High-dose quetiapine in treatment refractory schizophrenia. Schizophr Res 73:373–375, 2005

Pinta ER, Taylor RE: Quetiapine addiction? Am J Psychiatry 164:174–175, 2007

Potkin SG, Thyrum PT, Alva G, et al: Effect of fluoxetine and imipramine on the pharmacokinetics and tolerability of the antipsychotic quetiapine. J Clin Psychopharmacol 22:174–182, 2002a

Potkin SG, Thyrum PT, Alva G, et al: The safety and pharmacokinetics of quetiapine when coadministered with haloperidol, risperidone, or thioridazine. J Clin Psychopharmacol 22:121–130, 2002b

Potkin SG, Gharabawi GM, Greenspan AJ, et al: A double-blind comparison of risperidone, quetiapine and placebo in patients with schizophrenia experiencing an acute exacerbation requiring hospitalization. Schizophr Res 85:254–265, 2006

Rabey JM, Prokhorov T, Miniovitz A, et al: Effect of quetiapine in psychotic Parkinson's disease patients: a double-blind labeled study of 3 months' duration. Mov Disord 22:313–318, 2007

Sacchetti E, Panariello A, Regini C, et al: Quetiapine in hospitalized patients with schizophrenia refractory to treatment with first-generation antipsychotics: a 4-week, flexible-dose, single-blind, exploratory, pilot trial. Schizophr Res 29:325–331, 2004

Schneider LS, Tariot PN, Dagerman KS, et al: Effectiveness of atypical antipsychotic drugs in patients with Alzheimer's disease. N Engl J Med 355:1525–1538, 2006

Shotbolt P, Samuel M, Fox C, et al: A randomized controlled trial of quetiapine for psychosis in Parkinson's disease. Neuropsychiatr Dis Treat 5:327–332, 2009

Shotbolt P, Samuel M, David A: Quetiapine in the treatment of psychosis in Parkinson's disease. Ther Adv Neurol Disord 3:339–350, 2010

Simon NM, Connor KM, LeBeau RT: Quetiapine augmentation of paroxetine CR for the treatment of refractory generalized anxiety disorder: preliminary findings. Psychopharmacology (Berl) 197:675–681, 2008

Small JG, Hirsch SR, Arvanitis LA, et al: Quetiapine in patients with schizophrenia: a high- and low-dose double-blind comparison with placebo. Arch Gen Psychiatry 54:549–557, 1997

Sokolski KN, Denson TF, Lee RT, et al: Quetiapine for treatment of refractory symptoms of combat-related post-traumatic stress disorder. Mil Med 168:486–489, 2003

Stathis SM, McKenna JG: A preliminary case series on the use of quetiapine for posttraumatic stress disorder in juveniles within a youth detention center. J Clin Psychopharmacol 25:539–544, 2005

Stein DJ, Bandelow B, Meridet C, et al: Efficacy and tolerability of extended release quetiapine fumarate (quetiapine XR) monotherapy in patients with generalized anxiety disorder: an analysis of pooled data from three 8-week placebo-controlled studies. Hum Psychopharmacol 26:614–628, 2011

Strakowski SM, Keck PE Jr, Wong YW, et al: The effect of multiple doses of cimetidine on the steady-state pharmacokinetics of quetiapine in men with selected psychotic disorders. J Clin Psychopharmacol 22:201–205, 2002

Stroup TS, Lieberman JA, McEvoy JP, et al: Effectiveness of olanzapine, quetiapine, and risperidone in patients with chronic schizophrenia after discontinuing perphenazine: a CATIE study. Am J Psychiatry 164:415–427, 2007

Sunovion Pharmaceuticals: Latuda (lurasidone hydrochloride) tablets, full prescribing information. Revised May 2012. Available at: http://www.latuda.com/LatudaPrescribingInformation.pdf. Accessed August 2012.

Thase ME, Macfadden W, Weisler RH, et al: Efficacy of quetiapine monotherapy in bipolar I and II depression: a double-blind, placebo-controlled study (the BOLDER II study). J Clin Psychopharmacol 26:600–609, 2006

Vaishnavi S, Alamy S, Zhang W: Quetiapine as monotherapy for social anxiety disorder: a placebo-controlled study. Prog Neuropsychopharmacol Biol Psychiatry 31:1464–1469, 2007

Wang Z, Kemp DE, Chan PK, et al: Comparisons of the tolerability and sensitivity of quetiapine-XR in the acute treatment of schizophrenia, bipolar mania, bipolar depression, major depressive disorder, and generalized anxiety disorder. Int J Neuropsychopharmacol 14:131–142, 2011

Weiden PJ, Young AH, Buckley PF: The art and science of switching of antipsychotic medications, part 1. J Clin Psychiatry 67(11):e15, 2006

Weisler RH, Montgomery SA, Earley WR, et al: Efficacy of extended release quetiapine fumarate monotherapy in patients with major depressive disorder: a pooled analysis of two 6-week, double-blind, placebo-controlled studies. Int Clin Psychopharmacol 27:27–39, 2012

Whitehorn D, Gallant J, Woodley H, et al: Quetiapine treatment in early psychosis: no evidence of cataracts. Schizophr Res 71:511–512, 2004

Young AH, McElroy SL, Bauer M, et al: A double-blind, placebo-controlled study of quetiapine and lithium monotherapy in adults in the acute phase of bipolar depression (EMBOLDEN I). J Clin Psychiatry 71:150–162, 2010

Zhong KX, Sweitzer DE, Hamer RM, et al: Comparison of quetiapine and risperidone in the treatment of schizophrenia: a randomized, double-blind, flexible-dose, 8-week study. J Clin Psychiatry 67:1093–1103, 2006

Zhong KX, Tariot PN, Mintzer J, et al: Quetiapine to treat agitation in dementia: a randomized, double-blind, placebo-controlled study. Curr Alzheimer Res 4:81–93, 2007

CHAPTER 19

Aripiprazole

Zafar A. Sharif, M.D.

Yvonne I. Cole, Ph.D.

Jeffrey A. Lieberman, M.D.

History and Discovery

Aripiprazole is a dihydroquinolinone antipsychotic agent. Chemically, it is unrelated to phenothiazine, butyrophenone, thienobenzodiazepine, or other antipsychotic agents. Pharmacologically, it exhibits a novel mechanism of action, combining partial agonist activity at dopamine$_2$ (D_2), dopamine$_3$ (D_3), and serotonin$_{1A}$ (5-HT_{1A}) receptors with antagonist activity at serotonin$_{2A}$ (5-HT_{2A}) and D_2 receptors (Burris et al. 2002; Jordan et al. 2002). Aripiprazole represents a significant innovation, following the introduction of typical (first-generation) and atypical (second-generation) antipsychotics, in the pharmacology of therapeutic agents for psychotic disorders.

Although effective in alleviating psychotic symptoms and preventing their recurrence, the typical agents are ineffective in up to 40% of patients with schizophrenia, lack efficacy against the negative symptoms and cognitive deficits of schizophrenia, and are associated with a considerable burden of extrapyramidal side effects (EPS).

The atypical antipsychotics are partially effective against negative as well as positive symptoms and are associated with fewer EPS compared with the conventional antipsychotics. Nevertheless, individual atypical agents are associated with side effects such as weight gain, hyperprolactinemia, QTc prolongation, and alterations in glucose and lipid levels (Allison et al. 1999; Glassman and Bigger 2001; Koro et al. 2002a, 2002b; McIntyre et al. 2001).

The development of aripiprazole was guided by prevailing hypotheses of the etiology of schizophrenia. The dopamine hypothesis (Seeman and Niznik 1990) proposes that abnormalities in dopaminergic neurotransmission in the brain cause the symptoms of schizophrenia and suggests that schizophrenia involves a biphasic disturbance in dopaminergic pathways (Davis et al. 1991; Pycock et al. 1980; Weinberger 1987). Underactivity of the mesocortical dopaminergic pathway leads to hypodopaminergic activity in the frontal cortex, whereas overactivity in the mesolimbic pathway causes increased dopaminergic neurotransmission. The latter is presumed to cause positive or psychotic symptoms, while the former is believed to underlie negative symptoms and cognitive impairment. Another influential hypothesis suggests that the activity of dopaminergic pathways is modulated by serotonergic neurons. In the striatum, serotonin release inhibits dopamine, while in the frontal cortex it has a modulatory effect on pyramidal neurons and can affect glutamate release.

Almost all typical and atypical antipsychotic agents behave as full D_2 antagonists. Their actions in the mesolimbic pathway would therefore be expected to benefit patients with schizophrenia by reducing positive symptoms. D_2 antagonism in the other dopaminergic pathways, however, would be expected to cause unwanted side effects, including exacerbation of negative symptoms (mesocortical pathways), EPS and tardive dyskinesia (nigrostriatal tract), and hyperprolactinemia (tuberoinfundibular pathway) (Figure 19–1).

The serotonin (5-HT) hypothesis may explain why the atypical agents, which have antagonist activity at 5-HT_{2A} receptors, are associated with fewer EPS and do not exacerbate (and, in fact, partially alleviate) negative symptoms and cognitive impairment (Leysen et al. 1993; Millan 2000; Rao and Möller 1994; Richelson 1999).

On the basis of aripiprazole's unique pharmacodynamic profile—partial agonist activity (rather than full antagonist activity) at both dopaminergic (D_2; Burris et al. 2002) and serotonergic (5-HT_{1A}; Jordan et al. 2002) receptors, and full antagonist activity at 5-HT_{2A} receptors (McQuade et al. 2002)—it was anticipated that aripiprazole treatment would be associated with a reduced burden of unwanted D_2 antagonist activity in the mesocortical, nigrostriatal, and tuberoinfundibular pathways—the activity associated with some of the side effects of typical and atypical antipsychotic agents (Figure 19–2).

Structure-Activity Relations

Aripiprazole is 7-[4-(4-[2,3-dichlorophenyl]-1-piperazinyl)butoxy]-3,4-dihydrocarbostyril, a dihydroquinolinone.

Pharmacological Profile

Aripiprazole exhibits potent partial agonist activity at D_2 (Burris et al. 2002) and 5-HT_{1A} (Jordan et al. 2002) receptors, together with potent antagonist activity at 5-HT_{2A} receptors. It also has high affinity for D_3 receptors; moderate affinity for dopamine$_4$ (D_4), serotonin$_{2C}$ (5-HT_{2C}), serotonin$_7$ (5-HT_7), α_1-adrenergic, and histamine$_1$ (H_1) receptors and the serotonin transporter (SERT); and negligible affinity for cholinergic muscarinic receptors (Table 19–1). The active metabolite of aripiprazole, dehydroaripiprazole, exhibits a similar affinity at D_2 receptors and has not been shown to have a pharmacological profile that is clinically significantly different from that of the parent compound.

Pharmacokinetics and Disposition

Aripiprazole is available for oral administration as tablets in strengths of 2, 5, 10, 15, 20, and 30 mg. The effective dose range is 10–30 mg/day for schizophrenia patients and 15–30 mg/day for bipolar I disorder patients. A rapidly disintegrating oral formulation of aripiprazole is available in 10-mg and 15-mg strengths. In addition, aripiprazole is available in a 1-mg/mL nonrefrigerated oral solution. Aripiprazole is taken once daily with or without food and is well absorbed after oral administration, with peak plasma concentrations occurring within 3–5 hours. Absolute

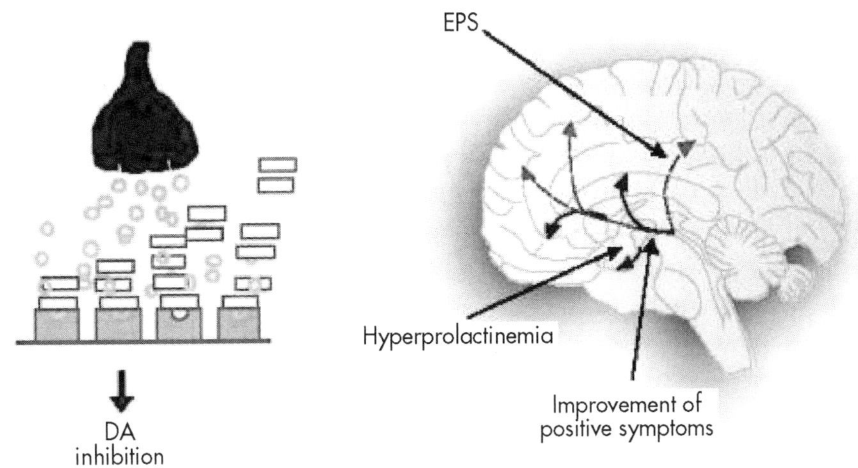

FIGURE 19–1. Conventional dopamine (DA) antagonist activity: effect on positive symptoms, extrapyramidal side effects (EPS), and prolactin levels.

oral bioavailability is 87%. An injectable form of aripiprazole for intramuscular (IM) use to provide rapid control of agitation in adults with schizophrenia or bipolar mania was approved by the U.S. Food and Drug Administration (FDA) in September 2006. Aripiprazole injection is available in single-dose, ready-to-use vials containing 9.75 mg aripiprazole in 1.3 mL of diluent (7.5 mg/mL); the recommended initial dose is 9.75 mg IM. Time to the peak plasma concentration is 1–3 hours after IM injection, and the absolute bioavailability of a 5-mg injection is 100%. The mean maximum concentration achieved after an IM dose is on average 19% higher than the maximum plasma concentration (C_{max}) of the oral tablet. Although the systemic exposure over 24 hours is generally similar for aripiprazole administered as an IM injection and as an oral tablet, the aripiprazole area under the curve (AUC) in the first 2 hours after an IM injection is 90% greater than the AUC after the same dose in a tablet (Otsuka Pharmaceutical 2012).

In plasma, aripiprazole and its major metabolite, dehydroaripiprazole, are both more than 99% bound to proteins, primarily albumin. Aripiprazole is extensively distributed outside the vascular system, and human studies demonstrating dose-dependent occupancy of D_2 receptors have confirmed that aripiprazole penetrates the brain. Elimination half-lives for aripiprazole and dehydroaripiprazole are 75 hours and 94 hours, respectively.

Aripiprazole is metabolized primarily in the liver. Two hepatic cytochrome P450 (CYP) enzymes, 2D6 and 3A4, catalyze dehydrogenation to dehydroaripiprazole. Therefore, coadministration with inducers or inhibitors of these CYP enzymes may require dosage adjustment of aripiprazole. The active metabolite accounts for 40% of drug exposure, but the predominant circulating moiety is the parent drug. Aripiprazole does not undergo direct glucuronidation and is not a substrate for the following CYP enzymes: 1A1, 1A2, 2A6, 2B6, 2C8, 2C9, 2C19, and 2E1. Interactions with inhibitors or inducers of these enzymes, or with chemicals related to cigarette smoke, are therefore unlikely to occur.

Mechanism of Action

Aripiprazole has partial agonist activity at D_2 receptors, a feature that distinguishes it

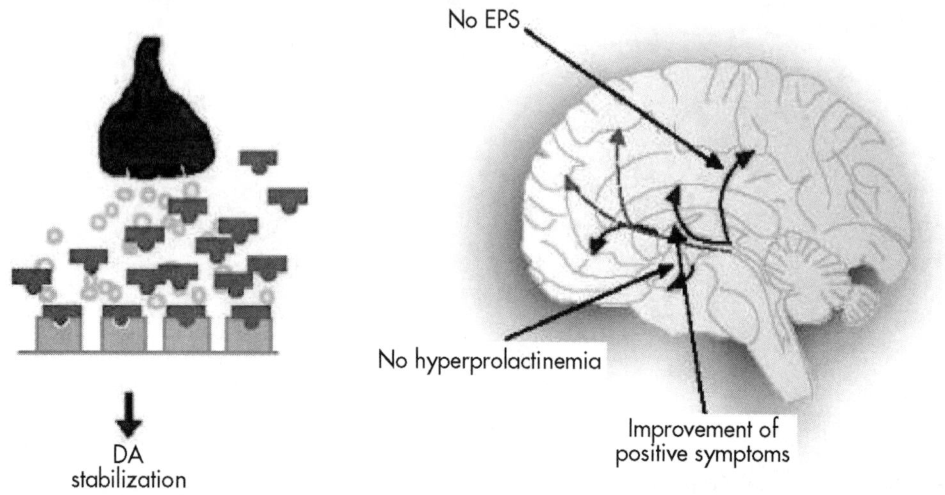

FIGURE 19–2. Dopamine (DA) partial agonist activity: effect on positive symptoms, extrapyramidal side effects (EPS), and prolactin levels.

from all other currently available antipsychotics. The activity of aripiprazole at D_2 receptors has been studied in animal models of schizophrenia (Kikuchi et al. 1995). In the intact rat with repetitive stereotyped behavior (stereotypy) induced by apomorphine, aripiprazole inhibits stereotypy and locomotion (Kikuchi et al. 1995). This agent may therefore be expected to inhibit hyperdopaminergic activity in the mesolimbic pathway of patients with schizophrenia and so, like other available agents, provide antipsychotic efficacy against the positive symptoms of schizophrenia. On the other hand, in animal models of hypodopaminergic activity, such as the reserpinized rat, aripiprazole has D_2 receptor agonist activity. Because aripiprazole may display either D_2 antagonist activity under hyperdopaminergic conditions or D_2 agonist activity under hypodopaminergic conditions, this agent may be less likely than other antipsychotics to cause excessive D_2 antagonism.

Aripiprazole may offer further therapeutic benefits through modulation of central serotonergic pathways. Preclinical studies showed that aripiprazole has antagonist activity at 5-HT_{2A} receptors (McQuade et al. 2002), a feature that has been associated with reductions in EPS (Meltzer 1999) and negative symptoms. In vitro studies also have shown that aripiprazole has partial agonist activity at 5-HT_{1A} receptors (Jordan et al. 2002), a feature that has been associated with improvement in negative, cognitive, depressive, and anxiety symptoms (Millan 2000).

The side effects of nausea/vomiting may be explained by the dopamine agonist effects of aripiprazole, whereas orthostatic hypotension and mild sedation/weight gain are likely related to its antagonist activity at α_1-adrenergic and H_1 receptors, respectively.

Indications and Efficacy

In the United States, aripiprazole is approved by the FDA for the following indications: treatment of schizophrenia in adults and in adolescents ages 13–17 years; acute treatment of manic or mixed episodes associated with bipolar I disorder as monotherapy and as an adjunct to lithium or valproate in adults and pediatric patients ages 10–17 years; maintenance treatment of manic or mixed episodes associated with bipolar I disorder as

TABLE 19–1. Receptor-binding profile of aripiprazole

RECEPTOR TYPE	**K_I (NM)**
Dopaminergic	
D_1	265
D_2[a]	0.34
D_3	0.8
D_4	44
D_5	95
Serotonergic	
$5\text{-}HT_{1A}$[b]	1.7
$5\text{-}HT_{2A}$	3.4
$5\text{-}HT_{2C}$	15
$5\text{-}HT_6$	214
$5\text{-}HT_7$	39
SERT	98
Histaminic	
H_1	61
Adrenergic	
α_1[c]	57
	IC_{50} (NM)
Muscarinic[c]	>1,000

Note. SERT = serotonin transporter.

Source. Adapted from McQuade RD, Burris KD, Jordan S, et al.: "Aripiprazole: A Dopamine-Serotonin System Stabilizer." *International Journal of Neuropsychopharmacology* 5 (Suppl 1):S176, 2002, with the following exceptions:

[a]Burris KD, Molski TF, Xu C, et al.: "Aripiprazole, A Novel Antipsychotic, Is a High Affinity Partial Agonist at Human Dopamine D_2 Receptors." *Journal of Pharmacology and Experimental Therapeutics* 302:381–389, 2002.

[b]Jordan S, Koprivica V, Chen R, et al.: "The Antipsychotic Aripiprazole Is a Potent, Partial Agonist at the Human $5\text{-}HT_{1A}$ Receptor." *European Journal of Pharmacology* 441:137–140, 2002.

[c]Abilify (Aripiprazole) Tablets: U.S. Full Prescribing Information. Tokyo, Japan, Otsuka Pharmaceutical Co, February 2012.

monotherapy and as an adjunct to lithium or valproate in adults; use as an adjunct to antidepressant treatment in adults with major depressive disorder who have had an inadequate response to antidepressant therapy; and treatment of irritability associated with autistic disorder in pediatric patients ages 6–17 years. Additionally, aripiprazole injection is indicated for the acute treatment of agitation associated with schizophrenia or bipolar disorder (manic or mixed) in adults (Otsuka Pharmaceutical 2012).

The efficacy of aripiprazole as a treatment for acute relapse of schizophrenia was demonstrated in four short-term (4-week) double-blind, placebo-controlled studies. Among these was a pivotal Phase III parallel-group multicenter study with four treatment arms comparing aripiprazole (15 or 30 mg/day) with placebo (Kane et al. 2002). Aripiprazole at either dose produced statistically significant improvements from baseline on standard psychometric scales by week 2. This trial suggests that at doses of 15 mg/day and 30 mg/day, aripiprazole provides effective symptom control in patients with acute relapse of schizophrenia.

In another short-term multicenter Phase III study involving acute relapse of schizophrenia or schizoaffective disorder (Potkin et al. 2003), patients were randomly assigned to aripiprazole 20 mg/day, aripiprazole 30 mg/day, risperidone 6 mg/day, or placebo for 4 weeks. Compared with placebo, aripiprazole at both doses and risperidone treatment produced statistically significant improvements in scores on standard scales designed to measure antipsychotic efficacy.

The antipsychotic efficacy of aripiprazole in acute relapse of schizophrenia was also demonstrated in two Phase II dose-ranging studies. Patients were randomly assigned to aripiprazole 2 mg, 10 mg, or 30 mg daily or haloperidol 10 mg/day (Daniel et al. 2000). All three doses of aripiprazole produced improvements in efficacy measures from baseline, and the 30-mg dose produced statistically significant improvement compared with placebo on all illness scores. Similarly, in a Phase II dose-titrating study, aripiprazole 5–30 mg/day was superior to placebo in improving Brief Psychiatric Rating Scale (BPRS)–Total, BPRS–Core, Clinical Global Impression–Severity (CGI-S), and Positive and Negative Syndrome Scale (PANSS)–Total scores (Petrie et al. 1997).

Results from the three 4-week fixed-dose studies discussed above were pooled for analysis with those of an additional 6-week placebo-controlled, fixed-dose study of aripiprazole at doses of 10, 15, and 20 mg/day (Lieberman et al. 2002). The pooled analysis involving 898 patients randomly assigned to aripiprazole showed that at all investigated doses greater than 2 mg/day, aripiprazole exhibited antipsychotic efficacy superior to placebo. Onset of efficacy was rapid, with improvement on psychometric scores detectable within 1 week of starting treatment. These pooled efficacy results demonstrate that doses of 10–30 mg/day represent an effective therapeutic range for aripiprazole treatment.

Two long-term double-blind, randomized, controlled multicenter trials yielded further confirmation of aripiprazole's efficacy. A 26-week placebo-controlled study in patients with chronic stable schizophrenia investigated the efficacy of aripiprazole 15 mg/day in relapse prevention (Pigott et al. 2003). Aripiprazole treatment significantly increased the time to relapse and resulted in significantly fewer relapses at endpoint compared with placebo (34% vs. 57%). From week 6 of therapy, PANSS–Total and PANSS positive subscale scores were significantly more improved with aripiprazole than with placebo.

In a 52-week study (Kasper et al. 2003), patients with acute relapse of schizophrenia were randomized to aripiprazole 30 mg/day or haloperidol 10 mg/day. Significantly more aripiprazole-treated patients were still taking the medication and were responding to treatment at weeks 8, 26, and 52 than were haloperidol-treated patients. Both treatments produced sustained improvements in the PANSS–Total and PANSS positive subscale scores from baseline. However, aripiprazole produced significantly greater improvements in negative and depressive symptoms at weeks 26 and 52 and was associated with significantly lower scores on all EPS assessments compared with haloperidol.

The efficacy of aripiprazole monotherapy in antipsychotic-resistant schizophrenia was evaluated in a 6-week double-blind, randomized trial in patients who had failed to improve in a prospective 4- to 6-week open trial with olanzapine or risperidone (Kane et al. 2007). Subjects were randomly assigned to aripiprazole (15–30 mg/day) or perphenazine (8–64 mg/day). After 6 weeks, there was no statistical difference between the two groups on efficacy measures. Compared with aripiprazole, perphenazine was associated with a higher rate of EPS and elevated serum prolactin.

The efficacy of aripiprazole in the treatment of schizophrenia in pediatric patients (ages 13–17 years) was evaluated in a 6-week placebo-controlled outpatient trial comparing two fixed doses of aripiprazole (10 mg/day or 30 mg/day) with placebo (Findling et al. 2008). Both aripiprazole doses showed statistically significant differences from placebo in reduction in PANSS–Total score; the 30 mg/day dose was not shown to be more efficacious than the 10 mg/day dose. Adverse events occurring in more than 5% of either aripiprazole group and with a combined incidence at least twice the rate for placebo were extrapyramidal disorder, somnolence, and tremor. Mean body weight changes were –0.8, 0.0, and +0.2 kg for placebo, aripiprazole 10 mg/day, and aripiprazole 30 mg/day, respectively.

The efficacy of aripiprazole in the treatment of acute manic episodes was established in two 3-week placebo-controlled trials in hospitalized patients who met DSM-IV (American Psychiatric Association 1994) criteria for bipolar I disorder with manic or mixed episodes (Keck et al. 2003; Sachs et al. 2006). Aripiprazole was superior to placebo in the reduction of Young Mania Rating Scale (YMRS) total score and Clinical Global Impression–Bipolar (CGI-BP) Severity of Illness score. In a third large randomized, double-blind trial (Vieta et al. 2005), aripiprazole was compared with haloperidol in the treatment of acute bipolar mania over a 12-week period. Significantly more patients remained in treatment and were classified as responders (>50% reduction in YMRS score from baseline) at week 12 for aripiprazole (49.7%) than for haloperidol (28.4%). EPS adverse events were more frequent with haloperidol than with aripiprazole (62.7% vs. 24.0%).

The efficacy of adjunctive aripiprazole with concomitant lithium or valproate in the treatment of manic or mixed episodes was established in a 6-week placebo-controlled study with a 2-week lead-in mood stabilizer monotherapy phase in adult patients who met DSM-IV criteria for bipolar I disorder. Adjunctive aripiprazole starting at 15 mg/day with concomitant lithium or valproate (in a therapeutic range of 0.6–1.0 mEq/L or 50–125 μg/mL, respectively) was superior to lithium or valproate with adjunctive placebo in the reduction of the YMRS total score and CGI-BP Severity of Illness score. Seventy-one percent of the patients coadministered valproate and 62% of the patients coadministered lithium were on 15 mg/day at the 6-week endpoint.

Aripiprazole monotherapy was also evaluated in the treatment of nonpsychotic depressive episodes associated with bipolar I disorder. The results of two identically designed 8-week randomized, double-blind, placebo-controlled multicenter studies were reported by Thase et al. (2008). The primary endpoint was mean change from baseline to week 8 (last observation carried forward [LOCF]) in the Montgomery-Åsberg Depression Rating Scale (MADRS) total score. Although statistically significant differences were observed during weeks 1–6, aripiprazole did not achieve statistical significance versus placebo at week 8 in either study in the change in MADRS total score.

To evaluate the long-term effectiveness of aripiprazole in delaying relapse in bipolar I disorder patients, a trial was conducted in patients meeting DSM-IV criteria for bipolar I disorder with a recent manic or mixed episode who had been stabilized on open-label aripiprazole and who had maintained a clinical response for at least 6 weeks (Keck et al. 2006). Aripiprazole-treated patients had significantly fewer relapses than placebo-treated patients (25% vs. 43%). Aripiprazole was superior to placebo in delaying the time to manic relapse but did not differ from placebo in delaying time to depressive relapse. Significant weight gain (≥7% increase from baseline) was seen in 13% of the aripiprazole patients and none of the placebo patients.

The efficacy of aripiprazole in the treatment of bipolar I disorder in pediatric patients (ages 10–17 years) was evaluated in a 4-week double-blind, placebo-controlled trial of outpatients who met DSM-IV criteria for bipolar I disorder manic or mixed episodes with or without psychotic features. The trial compared two fixed doses of aripiprazole (10 mg/day or 30 mg/day). Both doses of aripiprazole were superior to placebo in change from baseline to week 4 on the YMRS total score.

The efficacy of aripiprazole injection in controlling acute agitation was evaluated in three short-term (24-hour) randomized, double-blind, placebo-controlled studies in patients with schizophrenia (Andrezina et al. 2006; Tran-Johnson et al. 2007) and patients with bipolar disorder (manic or mixed) (Zimbroff et al. 2007). Aripiprazole injection was statistically superior to placebo (P<0.05) in all three studies, as measured with the PANSS Excited Component (PANSS EC). In the two studies in agitated patients with schizophrenia, injectable aripiprazole and IM haloperidol were both superior to placebo. In the study in agitated bipolar I disorder patients, aripiprazole injection and lorazepam injection were both superior to placebo.

De Deyn et al. (2005) compared the efficacy, safety, and tolerability of aripiprazole against placebo in patients with psychosis associated with Alzheimer's disease (AD) in a 10-week double-blind multicenter study. The initial aripiprazole dosage of 2 mg/day was titrated upward (to 5, 10, or 15 mg/day) according to efficacy and tolerability, and evaluations included the Neuropsychiatric Inventory (NPI) psychosis subscale and the BPRS. Aripiprazole-treated patients showed significantly greater improvements from baseline in BPRS psychosis subscale and BPRS–Core subscale scores at endpoint compared with placebo-treated patients.

In another double-blind, multicenter study (Mintzer et al. 2007), patients with psychosis associated with AD were randomized to placebo or aripiprazole, 2, 5, or 10 mg/day. Primary efficacy assessment was the mean change from baseline to week 10 on the Neuropsychiatric Inventory–Nursing Home (NPI-NH) version psychosis subscale score. Aripiprazole 10 mg/day showed significantly greater improvements than placebo. Aripiprazole 5 mg/day showed significant improvements versus placebo on BPRS and Cohen-Mansfield Agitation Inventory (CMAI) scores. Aripiprazole 2 mg/day was not efficacious. No antipsychotic is currently approved in the United States for treating the behavioral and psychotic symptoms that frequently accompany dementia, and all have a bolded warning based on increased mortality observed in patients with dementia-related psychosis treated with these agents.

Nickel et al. (2006) conducted a double-blind, placebo-controlled study in individuals meeting criteria for borderline personality disorder who were randomly assigned in a 1:1 ratio to 15 mg/day of aripiprazole or placebo for 8 weeks. Significant changes in scores on most scales of the Symptom Checklist (SCL-90-R), on the Hamilton Rating Scale for Depression (Ham-D), on the Hamilton Anxiety Scale (Ham-A), and on all scales of the State-Trait Anger Expression Inventory were observed in subjects treated with aripiprazole after 8 weeks. The improvements observed at 8 weeks of therapy were maintained at 18-month follow-up (Nickel et al. 2007).

Tiihonen et al. (2007) conducted a study in individuals meeting DSM-IV criteria for intravenous amphetamine dependence who were randomly assigned to receive aripiprazole (15 mg/day), slow-release methylphenidate (54 mg/day), or placebo for 20 weeks. The study was terminated prematurely because of the unexpected results of interim analysis. Contrary to the hypothesized result, patients who received aripiprazole treatment had significantly more amphetamine-positive urine samples than did patients in the placebo group, and patients who received methylphenidate had significantly fewer amphetamine-positive urine samples than patients who had received placebo. Studies in cocaine-abusing subjects are ongoing.

In a 12-week double-blind, placebo-controlled multicenter trial (Anton et al. 2008) evaluating the efficacy of aripiprazole in patients with alcohol dependence, aripiprazole did not differ from placebo on the study's primary efficacy measure, mean percentage of days abstinent.

The efficacy of aripiprazole in the adjunctive treatment of major depressive disorder was demonstrated in three short-term (6-week) placebo-controlled trials (Berman et al. 2007, 2009; Marcus et al. 2008). During prospective antidepressant treatment, patients received one of several antidepressants (escitalopram, fluoxetine, paroxetine controlled-release, sertraline, or venlafaxine extended-release), each with single-blind adjunctive placebo. Patients with incomplete response continued on the antidepressant and were randomly assigned to double-blind adjunctive placebo or adjunctive aripiprazole (2–15 mg/day with the potent CYP2D6 inhibitors fluoxetine or paroxetine; 2–20 mg/day with all other antidepressants). In all three trials, the mean change in MADRS total score was significantly greater with adjunctive aripiprazole than with adjunctive placebo. Akathisia and restlessness were significantly more frequent with adjunctive aripiprazole than adjunctive placebo.

Fava et al. (2012) evaluated the efficacy of low-dose aripiprazole added to antidepressant therapy in patients with major depressive disorder who had an inadequate response to prior antidepressant treatment. Two hundred twenty-five patients were randomly assigned to adjunctive treatment with aripiprazole 2 mg/day or placebo. The pooled, weighted response difference between aripiprazole 2 mg/day and placebo was 5.6% (P=0.18; NS); the difference on the MADRS was –1.51 (P= 0.065; NS). Importantly, there was no difference in the rate of akathisia with low-dose aripiprazole compared with placebo. Thus, a reasonable initial therapeutic approach may be to first try a low-dose (2 mg/day) augmentation of aripiprazole, in view of its better tolerability, and increase the dosage to 5 mg/day and, if necessary, to 10 or 15 mg/day in the face of continued nonresponse, given that the efficacy of the higher dosage range was supported by the robust evidence of three previous positive studies (Fava et al. 2012).

The efficacy of aripiprazole in the treatment of irritability associated with autistic disorder was established in two 8-week, placebo-controlled trials in children and adolescents (ages 6–17 years). Efficacy was evaluated with two assessment scales: the Aberrant Behavior Checklist (ABC) and the Clinical Global Impression–Improvement (CGI-I) scale. In one of the trials (Owen et al. 2009), pediatric patients with autistic disorder received daily doses of placebo or aripiprazole (2–15 mg, based on clinical response). Patients who received aripiprazole (at a mean daily dose of 8.6 mg at the end of 8-week treatment) demonstrated significantly improved scores on the ABC irritability (ABC-I) subscale and on the CGI-I scale compared with patients who received placebo. In the other trial (Marcus et al. 2009), three fixed dosages of aripiprazole (5, 10, or 15 mg/day) were compared with placebo. All three dosages of aripiprazole significantly improved scores on the ABC-I subscale compared with placebo.

Side Effects and Toxicology

A pooled analysis of safety and tolerability data from the five short-term studies (Marder et al. 2003; Stock et al. 2002) showed that aripiprazole treatment was well tolerated. The most commonly reported adverse events with aripiprazole were headache, insomnia, agitation, and anxiety. The incidence of adverse events was similar in the aripiprazole and placebo groups. The adverse-event profile of aripiprazole did not vary according to patient characteristics of age, gender, and race, and no deaths were reported during the short-term studies. Data from the four fixed-dose studies showed that somnolence was the only adverse event seen with aripiprazole that was possibly dose related. Objective rating scale assessments were used to measure changes in parkinsonian symptoms (Simpson-Angus Scale [SAS]), dyskinesias (Abnormal Involuntary Movement Scale [AIMS]), and akathisia (Barnes Akathisia Rating Scale [BAS]). SAS scores with aripiprazole did not differ significantly from those with placebo, whereas AIMS scores improved significantly from baseline with aripiprazole compared with placebo. Aripiprazole did not produce consistent dose-dependent changes in BAS scores. The rate of discontinuation due to adverse events was 7.3% (Otsuka Pharmaceutical 2012). According to the product labeling for aripiprazole in the United States, treatment-emergent adverse events reported with aripiprazole in short-term trials of patients with schizophrenia (up to 6 weeks) or bipolar disorder (up to 3 weeks) that occurred at an incidence greater than or equal to 10% and greater than placebo, respectively, included headache (30% vs. 25%), anxiety (20% vs. 17%), insomnia (19% vs. 14%), nausea (16% vs. 12%), vomiting (12% vs. 6%), dizziness (11% vs. 8%), constipation (11% vs. 7%), dyspepsia (10% vs. 8%), and akathisia (10% vs. 4%). A similar adverse-event profile was observed in a 26-week trial in schizophrenia except for a higher incidence of tremor (aripiprazole 8% vs. placebo 2%).

The most frequently reported adverse events with aripiprazole injection were headache (aripiprazole 12% vs. placebo 7%), nausea (aripiprazole 9% vs. placebo 3%), dizziness (aripiprazole 8% vs. placebo 5%), and somnolence (aripiprazole 7% vs. placebo 4%). In the three aripiprazole injection trials, the safety profile was comparable to that of placebo regarding the incidence of EPS, akathisia, or dystonia. The incidence of akathisia-related adverse events with aripiprazole injection was 2% (vs. 0% for placebo), while the incidence of dystonia with aripiprazole injection was less than 1% (vs. 0% for placebo). In addition, the incidence of QTc prolongation was also comparable between aripiprazole injection and placebo.

Minimal changes in mean body weight were observed with aripiprazole treatment in short-term studies (pooled data, +0.71 kg) (Marder et al. 2003) and long-term studies (26-week: –1.26 kg; 52-week: +1.05 kg) (Kasper et al. 2003; Pigott et al. 2003).

Olanzapine and aripiprazole were compared on their propensity to cause weight gain and other metabolic disturbances in a 26-week randomized, double-blind multicenter trial (McQuade et al. 2004). Statistically significant differences in mean weight change were observed between treatments beginning at week 1 and were sustained throughout the study. At week 26, there was a mean weight loss of 1.37 kg (3.04 lb) with aripiprazole compared with a mean weight gain of 4.23 kg (9.40 lb) with olanzapine among patients who remained on therapy ($P<0.001$). Changes in fasting plasma levels of total cholesterol, high-density lipoprotein cholesterol, and triglycerides were significantly different in the two treatment groups, with worsening of the lipid profile among patients treated with olanzapine.

Aripiprazole treatment was not associated with increases in prolactin levels during short- or long-term studies (in fact, prolactin levels were shown to be slightly decreased by aripiprazole).

Overall, aripiprazole treatment is associated with a low incidence of EPS-related symptoms (other than akathisia) and with minimal or no effects on weight gain, QTc interval, or circulating levels of cholesterol, glucose, and prolactin. Treatment with aripiprazole may reduce the burden of antipsychotic-associated side effects, which is expected to improve patient adherence and reduce the risk of acute relapse.

Drug-Drug Interactions

Aripiprazole is metabolized primarily by the hepatic cytochrome P450 enzymes 2D6 and 3A4, so it has the potential to interact with other substrates for these enzymes. Inducers of these enzymes may increase clearance and so lower blood levels of aripiprazole, whereas inhibitors of CYP3A4 or CYP2D6 may inhibit elimination and so increase blood levels of aripiprazole. In vivo studies showed decreased levels of aripiprazole and dehydroaripiprazole in the plasma when aripiprazole was coadministered with carbamazepine, a CYP3A4 inducer. The aripiprazole dose should therefore be increased when the drug is administered concomitantly with carbamazepine. In vivo studies coadministering aripiprazole and ketoconazole (a CYP3A4 inhibitor) or quinidine (a CYP2D6 inhibitor) suggest that the aripiprazole dose should be reduced when aripiprazole is administered with strong 3A4 or 2D6 inhibitors. Aripiprazole exhibits α_1-adrenergic receptor antagonist activity and so may enhance the effects of certain antihypertensive agents.

Conclusion

Aripiprazole is the first agent that is not a full D_2 antagonist to show rapid and sustained antipsychotic activity, and it may be considered the first partial dopamine agonist combined with 5-HT-stabilizing properties. Short-term and long-term clinical trials in adult and pediatric patients with schizophrenia and bipolar I disorder have demonstrated that aripiprazole combines sustained antipsychotic and mood-stabilizing efficacy with an excellent safety and tolerability profile. Additional augmentation trials have confirmed the utility of aripiprazole in alleviating depressive symptomatology in patients with major depressive disorder who have not achieved adequate symptom relief with antidepressants alone. In general, aripiprazole treatment is associated with a low liability for EPS, QTc interval prolongation, prolactin elevation, weight gain, or disturbances of glucose or lipid metabolism. This combination of efficacy, safety, and tolerability suggests that aripiprazole has the potential to improve treatment adherence and decrease relapse rates and so represents an important new option for both acute and long-term treatment of schizophrenia and bipolar I disorder and as an adjunct to antidepressants in major depressive disorder.

References

Allison DB, Mentore JL, Heo M, et al: Antipsychotic-induced weight gain: a comprehensive research synthesis. Am J Psychiatry 156:1686–1696, 1999

American Psychiatric Association: Diagnostic and Statistical Manual of Mental Disorders, 4th Edition. Washington, DC, American Psychiatric Association, 1994

Andrezina R, Josiassen RC, Marcus RN, et al: Intramuscular aripiprazole for the treatment of acute agitation in patients with schizophrenia or schizoaffective disorder: a double-blind, placebo-controlled comparison with intramuscular haloperidol. Psychopharmacology 188:281–292, 2006

Anton RF, Kranzler H, Breder C, et al: A randomized, multicenter, double-blind, placebo-controlled study of the efficacy and safety of aripiprazole for the treatment of alcohol dependence. J Clin Psychopharmacol 28:5–12, 2008

Berman RM, Marcus RN, Swanink R, et al: The efficacy and safety of aripiprazole as adjunctive therapy in major depressive disorder: a multicenter, randomized, double-blind, placebo-controlled study. J Clin Psychiatry 68:843–853, 2007

Berman RM, Fava M, Thase ME, et al: Aripiprazole augmentation in major depressive disorder: a double-blind, placebo-controlled study in patients with inadequate response to antidepressants. CNS Spectr 14:197–206, 2009

Burris KD, Molski TF, Xu C, et al: Aripiprazole, a novel antipsychotic, is a high affinity partial agonist at human dopamine D_2 receptors. J Pharmacol Exp Ther 302:381–389, 2002

Daniel DG, Saha AR, Ingenito G, et al: Aripiprazole, a novel antipsychotic: overview of a phase II study result (abstract). Int J Neuropsychopharmacol 3 (suppl):S157, 2000

Davis KL, Kahn RS, Ko G, et al: Dopamine in schizophrenia: a review and reconceptualization. Am J Psychiatry 148:1474–1486, 1991

De Deyn P, Jeste DV, Swanink R, et al: Aripiprazole for the treatment of psychosis in patients with Alzheimer's disease: a randomized, placebo-controlled study. J Clin Psychopharmacol 25:463–467, 2005

Fava M, Mischoulon D, Iosifescu D, et al: A double-blind, placebo-controlled study of aripiprazole adjunctive to antidepressant therapy among depressed outpatients with inadequate response to prior antidepressant therapy (ADAPT-A Study). Psychother Psychosom 81:87–97, 2012

Findling RL, Robb A, Nyilas M, et al: A multiple-center, randomized, double-blind, placebo-controlled study of oral aripiprazole for treatment of adolescents with schizophrenia. Am J Psychiatry 165:1432–1441, 2008

Glassman AH, Bigger JT Jr: Antipsychotic drugs: prolonged QTc interval, torsades de pointes, and sudden death. Am J Psychiatry 158:1774–1782, 2001

Jordan S, Koprivica V, Chen R, et al: The antipsychotic aripiprazole is a potent, partial agonist at the human 5-HT1A receptor. Eur J Pharmacol 441:137–140, 2002

Kane JM, Carson WH, Saha AR, et al: Efficacy and safety of aripiprazole and haloperidol vs placebo in patients with schizophrenia and schizoaffective disorder. J Clin Psychiatry 63:763–771, 2002

Kane JM, Meltzer HY, Carson WH Jr, et al: Aripiprazole for treatment-resistant schizophrenia: results of a multicenter, randomized, double-blind, comparison study versus perphenazine. J Clin Psychiatry 68:213–223, 2007

Kasper S, Lerman MN, McQuade RD, et al: Efficacy and safety of aripiprazole vs. haloperidol for long-term maintenance treatment following acute relapse of schizophrenia. Int J Neuropsychopharmacol 6:325–337, 2003

Keck PE Jr, Marcus R, Tourkodimitris S, et al: A placebo-controlled, double-blind study of the efficacy and safety of aripiprazole in patients with acute bipolar mania. Am J Psychiatry 160:1651–1658, 2003

Keck PE Jr, Calabrese JR, McQuade RD, et al: A randomized, double-blind, placebo-controlled 26-week trial of aripiprazole in recently manic patients with bipolar I disorder. J Clin Psychiatry 67:626–637, 2006

Kikuchi T, Tottori K, Uwahodo Y, et al: 7-{4-[4-(2,3-dichlorophenyl)-1-piperazinyl]butyloxy}-3,4-dihydro-2 (1H)-quinolinone (OPC-14597), a new putative antipsychotic drug with both presynaptic dopamine autoreceptor agonistic activity and postsynaptic D_2 receptor antagonist activity. J Pharmacol Exp Ther 274:329–336, 1995

Koro CE, Fedder DO, L'Italien GJ, et al: An assessment of the independent effects of olanzapine and risperidone exposure on the risk of hyperlipidemia in schizophrenic patients. Arch Gen Psychiatry 59:1021–1026, 2002a

Koro CE, Fedder DO, L'Italien GJ, et al: Assessment of independent effect of olanzapine and risperidone on risk of diabetes among patients with schizophrenia: population based nested case-control study. BMJ 325:243, 2002b

Leysen JE, Janssen PMF, Schotte A, et al: Interaction of antipsychotic drugs with neurotransmitter receptor sites in vitro and in vivo in relation to pharmacological and clinical role of 5-HT_2 receptors. Psychopharmacology (Berl) 112 (suppl):S40–S54, 1993

Lieberman J, Carson WH, Saha AR, et al: Meta-analysis of the efficacy of aripiprazole in schizophrenia. Int J Neuropsychopharmacol 5 (suppl): S186, 2002

Marcus RN, McQuade RD, Carson WH, et al: The efficacy and safety of aripiprazole as adjunctive therapy in major depressive disorder: a second multicenter, randomized, double-blind, placebo-controlled study. J Clin Psychopharmacol 28:156–165, 2008

Marcus RN, Owen R, Kamen L, et al: A placebo-controlled, fixed-dose study of aripiprazole in children and adolescents with irritability associated with autistic disorder. J Am Acad Child Adolesc Psychiatry 48:1110–1119, 2009

Marder SR, McQuade RD, Stock E, et al: Aripiprazole in the treatment of schizophrenia: safety and tolerability in short-term placebo-controlled trials. Schizophr Res 61:123–136, 2003

McIntyre RS, McCann SM, Kennedy SH: Antipsychotic metabolic effects: weight gain, diabetes mellitus, and lipid abnormalities. Can J Psychiatry 46:273–281, 2001

McQuade RD, Burris KD, Jordan S, et al: Aripiprazole: a dopamine-serotonin system stabilizer (abstract). Int J Neuropsychopharmacol 5 (suppl): S176, 2002

McQuade RD, Stock E, Marcus R, et al: A comparison of weight change during treatment with olanzapine or aripiprazole: results from a randomized, double-blind study. J Clin Psychiatry 65 (suppl):47–56, 2004

Meltzer HY: The role of serotonin in antipsychotic drug action. Neuropsychopharmacology 21 (suppl):106S–115S, 1999

Millan MJ: Improving the treatment of schizophrenia: focus on serotonin $(5\text{-HT})_{1A}$ receptors. J Pharmacol Exp Ther 295:853–861, 2000

Mintzer JE, Tune LE, Breder CD, et al: Aripiprazole for the treatment of psychoses in institutionalized patients with Alzheimer dementia: a multicenter, randomized, double-blind, placebo-controlled assessment of three fixed doses. Am J Geriatr Psychiatry 15:918–931, 2007

Nickel MK, Muehlbacher M, Nickel C, et al: Aripiprazole in the treatment of patients with borderline personality disorder: a double-blind, placebo-controlled study. Am J Psychiatry 163:833–838, 2006

Nickel MK, Loew TH, Gil FP: Aripiprazole in treatment of borderline patients, part II: an 18-month follow-up. Psychopharmacology 191:1023–1026, 2007

Otsuka Pharmaceutical: Abilify (Aripiprazole) tablets: U.S. full prescribing information. Revised February 2012. Available at: http://packageinserts.bms.com/pi/pi_abilify.pdf. Accessed September 16, 2012.

Owen R, Sikich L, Marcus RN, et al: Aripiprazole in the treatment of irritability in children and adolescents with autistic disorder. Pediatrics 124: 1533–1540, 2009

Petrie JL, Saha AR, McEvoy JP: Aripiprazole, a new novel atypical antipsychotic: phase II clinical trial result (abstract). Eur Neuropsychopharmacol 7 (suppl):S227, 1997

Pigott TA, Carson WH, Saha AR, et al: Aripiprazole for the prevention of relapse in stabilized patients with chronic schizophrenia: a placebo-controlled 26-week study. J Clin Psychiatry 64:1048–1056, 2003

Potkin SG, Saha AR, Kujawa MJ, et al: Aripiprazole, an antipsychotic with a novel mechanism of action, and risperidone vs placebo in patients with schizophrenia and schizoaffective disorder. Arch Gen Psychiatry 60:681–690, 2003

Pycock CJ, Kerwin RW, Carter CJ: Effect of lesion of cortical dopamine terminals on subcortical dopamine receptors in rats. Nature 286:74–76, 1980

Rao ML, Möller HJ: Biochemical findings of negative symptoms in schizophrenia and their positive relevance to pharmacologic treatment. Neuropsychobiology 30:160–164, 1994

Richelson E: Receptor pharmacology of neuroleptics: relation to clinical effects. J Clin Psychiatry 60 (suppl):5–14, 1999

Sachs G, Sanchez R, Marcus R, et al: Aripiprazole in the treatment of acute manic or mixed episodes in patients with bipolar I disorder: a 3-week placebo-controlled study. J Psychopharmacol 20:536–546, 2006

Seeman P, Niznik HB: Dopamine receptors and transporters in Parkinson's disease and schizophrenia. FASEB J 4:2737–2744, 1990

Stock E, Marder SR, Saha AR, et al: Safety and tolerability meta-analysis of aripiprazole in schizophrenia (abstract). Int J Neuropsychopharmacol 5 (suppl):S185, 2002

Thase ME, Jonas A, Khan A, et al: Aripiprazole monotherapy in nonpsychotic bipolar I depression: results of 2 randomized, placebo-controlled studies. J Clin Psychopharmacol 28:13–20, 2008

Tiihonen J, Kuoppasalmi K, Fohr J, et al: A comparison of aripiprazole, methylphenidate, and placebo for amphetamine dependence. Am J Psychiatry 164:160–162, 2007

Tran-Johnson TK, Sack DA, Marcus RN, et al: Efficacy and safety of intramuscular aripiprazole in patients with acute agitation: a randomized, double-blind, placebo-controlled trial. J Clin Psychiatry 68:111–119, 2007

Vieta E, Bourin M, Sanchez R, et al: Effectiveness of aripiprazole vs. haloperidol in acute bipolar mania: double-blind, randomised, comparative 12-week trial. Br J Psychiatry 187:235–242, 2005

Weinberger DR: Implications of normal brain development for the pathogenesis of schizophrenia. Arch Gen Psychiatry 44:660–669, 1987

Zimbroff DL, Marcus RN, Manos G, et al: Management of acute agitation in patients with bipolar disorder: efficacy and safety of intramuscular aripiprazole. J Clin Psychopharmacol 27:171–176, 2007

CHAPTER 20

Risperidone and Paliperidone

Michele Hill, M.R.C.Psych.

Donald C. Goff, M.D.

History and Discovery

A decade before clozapine was approved for marketing in the United States, Janssen Pharmaceuticals established a program to examine the potential role of serotonergic agents in schizophrenia. Early interest in serotonergic agents stemmed from preclinical literature demonstrating that both behavioral effects of dopamine agonists and haloperidol-induced catalepsy could be modulated by serotonin$_2$ (5-HT$_2$) antagonists; in addition, the early butyrophenone derivative pipamperone, which was observed to reduce agitation and improve social activity in patients with severe depression, was found to possess primarily 5-HT$_2$ antagonist activity (Ansoms et al. 1977; Leysen et al. 1978).

In 1981, Janssen Pharmaceuticals developed setoperone, a 5-HT$_2$ antagonist with weak dopamine$_2$ (D$_2$) antagonism that displayed antipsychotic effects and efficacy for negative symptoms in a preliminary open trial (Ceulemans et al. 1985). Janssen Pharmaceuticals additionally synthesized a selective 5-HT$_{2A}$ and 5-HT$_{2C}$ antagonist, ritanserin, which was shown to decrease extrapyramidal side effects (EPS) when combined with haloperidol in rat studies. Ritanserin also was active in animal models of anxiety (Colpaert and Meert 1985; Meert and Colpaert 1986) and partially ameliorated the behavioral effects of lysergic acid diethylamide (LSD) (Colpaert and Meert 1985). In placebo-controlled trials in patients with chronic schizophrenia, addition of ritanserin to first-generation antipsychotics (FGAs) improved negative symptoms and EPS (Bersani et al. 1990; Duinkerke et al. 1993; Gelders 1989; Reyntjens et al. 1986). Concluding that 5-HT$_2$ antagonism might improve efficacy of D$_2$ blockers, particularly for negative symptoms, and reduce EPS, but that it was not sufficiently effective as monotherapy, Paul Janssen and colleagues undertook development of risperidone, which combined potent 5-HT_{2A} and D_2 blockade.

After extensive preclinical characterization (Janssen et al. 1988), risperidone was first studied in clinical trials in 1986 and received U.S. Food and Drug Administration (FDA) approval for marketing in the United States in 1994. By the time risperidone became available to clinicians, the prominence of theories attributing 5-HT_2 enhancement of D_2 antagonism as a primary mechanism for clozapine's atypical properties (Meltzer et al. 1989), and the evidence from registration trials of reduced EPS and greater efficacy compared with high-dose haloperidol, resulted in considerable enthusiasm for the first of the "serotonin-dopamine antagonists." Risperidone was rapidly incorporated into clinical practice in the United States, where within 2 years it became the most frequently prescribed antipsychotic agent. In 2003, risperidone microspheres (Consta) received FDA approval as the first long-acting second-generation antipsychotic (SGA) designed for intramuscular (IM) injection. In December 2006, Janssen Pharmaceuticals introduced paliperidone (9-hydroxyrisperidone), the active metabolite of risperidone, formulated as an extended-release tablet marketed under the brand name Invega. Extended-release paliperidone is approved for the treatment of schizophrenia and schizoaffective disorder. A long-acting depot preparation, paliperidone palmitate (Sustenna), received FDA approval for schizophrenia in 2009 and was the first once-monthly depot formulation of an SGA to become available in the United States.

Pharmacological Profile

Risperidone, or 3-[2-(4-[6-fluoro-1,2-benzisoxazol-3-yl]-1-piperidinyl)ethyl]-6,7,8,9-tetrahydro-2-methyl-4H-pyrido[1,2-a]pyrimidin-4-one, is a benzisoxazole derivative characterized by very high affinity for 5-HT_{2A} and moderately high affinity for D_2, H_1, and α_1- and α_2-adrenergic receptors. In vitro, the affinity of risperidone for 5-HT_{2A} receptors is roughly 10- to 20-fold greater than for D_2 receptors (Leysen et al. 1994; Schotte et al. 1996); in vivo binding to rat striatal D_2 receptors occurs at a dose 10 times higher than does binding to 5-HT_{2A} receptors (Leysen et al. 1994). The affinity for 5-HT_{2A} receptors is more than 100-fold greater than for other serotonin receptor subtypes. The active metabolite 9-hydroxyrisperidone (paliperidone) has a similar receptor affinity profile, although paliperidone has lower affinity for α_1- and α_2-adrenergic receptors. Both risperidone and paliperidone display a high affinity for 5-HT_{2A} receptors in rat brain tissue and for cloned human receptors expressed in COS-7 cells (Leysen et al. 1994). Risperidone binds to 5-HT_{2A} receptors with approximately 20-fold greater affinity than clozapine and 170-fold greater affinity than haloperidol (Leysen et al. 1994).

The affinity of risperidone for D_2 receptors is approximately 50-fold greater than that of clozapine and approximately 20%–50% that of haloperidol (Leysen et al. 1994) (Table 20–1). Binding affinity for D_2 receptors was similar in rat mesolimbic and striatal tissue and in the long and short forms of cloned human D_2 receptors expressed in embryonic kidney cells (Leysen et al. 1993a). The affinities of risperidone and paliperidone for dopamine$_4$ (D_4) and D_1 receptors are similar to those of clozapine and haloperidol (Leysen et al. 1994). Risperidone and paliperidone have essentially no affinity for muscarinic acetylcholine receptors and modest histaminergic H_1 activity. Unlike haloperidol, risperidone does not bind to sigma sites (Leysen et al. 1994). However, compared with other agents, including paliperidone, risperidone has a relatively high affinity for α_2-adrenergic receptors that is substantially greater than that of clozapine or any FGA and that approaches the affinity of phentolamine (Richelson 1996). The affinity of risperidone for α_1-adrenergic receptors is roughly comparable to that of chlorpromazine and approximately 5 to 10 times greater than that of clozapine (Leysen et al. 1993b; Richelson 1996). The median effective dose (ED_{50}) of risperidone required to inhibit D_2-mediated apomorphine-induced stereotypies in rats is 0.5 mg/kg; at this dose, approximately 40% of D_2 receptors are occupied, as are 80% of 5-HT_{2A} receptors, 50% of H_1 receptors, 38% of α_1-adrenergic receptors, and 10% of α_2-adrenergic receptors (Leysen et al. 1994).

Several groups have studied the occupancy of D_2 and 5-HT_2 receptors in patients with schizophrenia, employing positron emission tomography (PET) or single-photon emission computed tomography (SPECT) ligand-binding techniques. Kapur et al. (1999) used PET to measure D_2 occupancy with ^{11}C-labeled raclopride and 5-HT_2 occupancy with ^{18}F-labeled setoperone in patients with chronic schizophrenia maintained on a stable clinician-determined dose of risperidone. The PET was performed 12–14 hours after the last dose of risperidone. Occupancy of D_2 receptors ranged from 63% to 89%; 50% occupancy was calculated to occur with a daily risperidone dose of 0.8 mg. Patients treated with risperidone (6 mg/day) exhibited a mean D_2 occupancy of 79%, which was consistent with the mean occupancy of 82% that was previously reported by Nyberg et al. (1999) and would be expected to exceed the putative threshold for EPS in some patients. A similar degree of D_2 occupancy was calculated to occur with olanzapine at approximately 30 mg daily (Kapur et al. 1999). A maximal 5-HT_2 occupancy of greater than 95% was achieved with risperidone at daily doses as low as 2–4 mg. In a small sample of patients treated biweekly for at least 10 weeks with risperidone microspheres (Consta), Remington et al. (2006) found that the 25-mg dose produced a mean D_2 occupancy of 54% (preinjection) and 71% (postinjection), whereas the 50-mg dose produced occupancy levels of 65% (preinjection) and 74% (postinjection). Arakawa et al. (2008) found a D_2 occupancy of 58% with paliperidone at 3 mg/day and 77% with 9 mg/day, consistent with clinical estimates that paliperidone is roughly half as potent as risperidone, perhaps due to reduced bioavailability (de Leon et al. 2010).

Preclinical characterization of risperidone in rats revealed more potent antiserotonergic activity, compared with ritanserin, in all tests (Janssen et al. 1988). For example, in reversal of tryptophan-induced effects in rats, risperidone was 6.4 times more potent than ritanserin for reversal of peripheral 5-HT_2-mediated effects and 2.4 times more potent for reversal of centrally mediated 5-HT_2 effects (Janssen et al. 1988). Risperidone was also found to completely block discrimination of LSD, in contrast to the partial attenuation observed with ritanserin (Meert et al. 1989). Although risperidone demonstrated activity in all dopamine-mediated tests, the dose-response pattern differed from that of haloperidol (Janssen et al. 1988). The two drugs were roughly equipotent for inhibition of certain dopamine effects, such as amphetamine-induced oxygen hyperconsumption, whereas the dose of risperidone necessary to cause pronounced catalepsy in rats was 18-fold higher than that of haloperidol (Janssen et al. 1988). Risperidone depressed vertical and horizontal activity in rats at a dose 2–3 times greater than that of haloperidol but required doses more than 30 times greater than those of haloperidol to depress small motor movements (Megens et al. 1988).

Pharmacokinetics and Disposition

Risperidone is rapidly absorbed after oral administration, with peak plasma levels achieved within 1 hour (Heykants et al. 1994). In early Phase I studies, risperidone demonstrated linear pharmacokinetics at dosages between 0.5 and 25 mg/day (Mesotten et al. 1989; Roose et al. 1988). After a single dose of the extended-release formulation of paliperidone (Invega), serum concen-

TABLE 20–1. Receptor-binding affinities (K_i values, in nM) of representative antipsychotics in cloned human receptors and rat brain

	Paliperidone	**Risperidone**	**Haloperidol**	**Clozapine**
Dopaminergic				
D_2[a]	4.8	5.9	2.2	190
D_1[a]	670	620	270	540
Serotonergic				
$5\text{-}HT_{2A}$[a]	1.0	0.52	200	9.6
$5\text{-}HT_{1A}$[a]	590	420	1,500	140
Adrenergic				
α_1[b]	4.0	2.3	19	23
α_2[b]	17	7.5	>5,000	160
H_1 histaminergic[a]	32	27	790	0.23
Muscarinic[b]	3,570	>5,000	4,670	34

[a]Cloned human receptor.
[b]Rat brain.
Source. Adapted from Schotte et al. 1996.

trations gradually increase until a maximum concentration is achieved approximately 24 hours after ingestion. Absorption of paliperidone is increased by approximately 50% when taken with a meal compared with the fasting state. Extended-release paliperidone also demonstrates dose-proportional pharmacokinetics within the recommended dosing range (3–12 mg/day). Because risperidone lacks a hydroxyl group to which an esther can be bound for a traditional oil-based depot preparation, polymer microsphere technology was used to produce a slow-release injectable formulation. Risperidone microspheres do not begin to release appreciable amounts of drug until 3 weeks after injection and continue to release drug for approximately 4 weeks, with maximal drug release occurring after about 5 weeks. Paliperidone palmitate is poorly soluble in water and dissolves slowly following IM injection, after which it is hydrolyzed to active paliperidone and absorbed into the systemic circulation. Systemic availability of paliperidone begins on day 1 and can last as long as 126 days after injection. Maximum blood levels are achieved a median of 13 days after injection. IM injection in the deltoid produces blood levels approximately 28% higher than those produced with gluteal injection. Risperidone is 90% plasma protein bound, whereas paliperidone is 74% plasma protein bound (Borison 1994). The absolute bioavailability of risperidone is about 100%; that of extended-release paliperidone is about 28%. Paliperidone may achieve relatively lower concentrations in the brain because of its higher affinity for the extruding P-glycoprotein transporter, which limits the amount of drug crossing the blood-brain barrier (de Leon et al. 2010).

Risperidone is metabolized by hydroxylation of the tetrahydropyridopyrimidinone ring at the seven and nine positions and by oxidative *N*-dealkylation (Mannens et al. 1993). The most important metabolite, 9-hydroxyrisperidone (paliperidone), accounts for up to 31% of the dose excreted in the urine. Because hydroxylation of risperidone is catalyzed by cytochrome P450 (CYP) 2D6, the half-life of the parent compound varies according to the relative activity of this enzyme. In extensive metabolizers, which include about 90% of Caucasians and as many as 99% of Asians, the half-life of risperidone is approximately 3 hours. Approximately 60% of paliperidone is excreted unchanged in the urine, and the remainder is metabolized by at least four different pathways (dealkylation, hydroxylation, dehydrogenation, and benzisoxazole scission), none of which accounts for more than 10% of the total. The terminal half-life of 9-hydroxyrisperidone (and of extended-release paliperidone) is 23 hours. Poor metabolizers metabolize risperidone primarily via oxidative pathways; the half-life may exceed 20 hours. In extensive metabolizers, radioactivity from ^{14}C-labeled risperidone is not detectable in plasma 24 hours after a single dose, whereas 9-hydroxyrisperidone accounts for 70%–80% of radioactivity. In poor metabolizers, risperidone is primarily responsible for radioactivity after 24 hours. In the U.S. multicenter registration trial, the correlations between risperidone dose and serum risperidone and 9-hydroxyrisperidone concentrations were 0.59 and 0.88, respectively (Anderson et al. 1993). Because of the longer half-life, paliperidone serum concentrations at steady state are approximately 5- to 10-fold higher than risperidone concentrations in 2D6 extensive metabolizers treated with risperidone (de Leon et al. 2010). However, in 2D6 poor metabolizers and patients concurrently taking 2D6 inhibitors, risperidone concentrations may be higher than paliperidone concentrations.

Mechanism of Action

As previously discussed, risperidone was developed specifically to exploit the apparent pharmacological advantages of combining 5-HT_2 antagonism with D_2 blockade. Selective 5-HT_{2A} antagonists administered alone have demonstrated activity in several animal models suggestive of antipsychotic effect, including blockade of both amphetamine- and phencyclidine (PCP)-induced locomotor activity (Schmidt et al. 1995). Dizocilpine-induced disruption of prepulse inhibition is also blocked by 5-HT_{2A} antagonists, suggesting that sensory gating deficits characteristic of schizophrenia and perhaps resulting from glutamatergic dysregulation might also benefit from the 5-HT_2 antagonism of risperidone (Varty et al. 1999). The disruption of prepulse inhibition by dizocilpine (MK-801, a noncompetitive N-methyl-D-aspartate [NMDA] antagonist) is attenuated by SGAs, but not by first-generation D_2 blockers (Geyer et al. 1990). From a study in which the selective 5-HT_{2A} antagonist M100907 was added to low-dose raclopride (a selective D_2 blocker), Wadenberg et al. (1998) concluded that 5-HT_{2A} antagonism facilitates D_2 antagonist blockade of conditioned avoidance, another behavioral model associated with antipsychotic efficacy, but does not block conditioned avoidance when administered alone.

One mechanism by which risperidone, paliperidone, and similar atypical agents might produce enhanced efficacy for negative symptoms and cognitive deficits and reduced risk for EPS is via 5-HT_{2A} receptor modulation of dopamine neuronal firing and cortical dopamine release. Prefrontal dopaminergic hypoactivity has been postulated to underlie negative symptoms and cognitive deficits in schizophrenia (Goff and Evins 1998); both clozapine and ritanserin have been shown to increase dopamine release in prefrontal cortex, whereas haloperidol does not (Busatto and Kerwin 1997). Following 21 days of administration, risperidone, but not haloperidol, continued to increase dopamine turnover in the dorsal striatum and prefrontal cortex (Stathis et al. 1996). Ritanserin has been shown to enhance midbrain dopamine cell firing by blocking a tonic inhibitory serotonin input (Ugedo et al. 1989). Ritanserin also normalized ventral tegmental dopamine neuron firing patterns in rats after hypofrontality was induced by experimental cooling of the frontal cortex (Svensson et al. 1989).

Svensson et al. (1995) have performed a series of elegant studies examining the impact of atypical antipsychotics on ventral tegmental dopamine firing patterns disrupted by glutamatergic NMDA receptor antagonists. In healthy human subjects, administration of the NMDA antagonist ketamine is widely regarded as a promising model for several clinical aspects of schizophrenia, including psychosis, negative symptoms, and cognitive deficits (Goff and Coyle 2001; Krystal et al. 1994). In rats, administration of the NMDA channel blockers dizocilpine or PCP increased burst firing of ventral tegmental dopamine neurons predominately projecting to limbic structures but reduced firing of mesocortical tract dopamine neurons and disrupted firing patterns. Administration of ritanserin or clozapine preferentially enhanced firing of dopamine neurons with cortical projections, and when added to a D_2 blocker, ritanserin increased dopamine release in prefrontal cortex. In addition to modulating ventral tegmental dopamine neuron firing, risperidone also blocks 5-HT_2 receptors on inhibitory γ-aminobutyric acid (GABA)-ergic interneurons, which could also influence activity of cortical pyramidal neurons that are regulated by these local inhibitory circuits (Gellman and Aghajanian 1994).

In placebo-controlled clinical trials, 5-HT_2 antagonists have reduced antipsychotic-induced parkinsonism and akathisia (Duinkerke et al. 1993; Poyurovsky et al. 1999). This effect may reflect 5-HT_{2A} antagonist effects on nigrostriatal dopamine release. When combined with haloperidol, selective 5-HT_2 antagonists increase dopamine metabolism in the striatum and prevent an increase in D_2 receptor density, thereby possibly reducing the effects of D_2 receptor blockade and dopamine supersensitivity (Saller et al. 1990). These agents do not affect dopamine metabolism in the absence of D_2 blockade.

The relative importance of 5-HT_2 antagonist activity in producing atypical characteristics is the subject of debate. As argued by Kapur and Seeman (2001) and Seeman (2002), most SGAs have dissociation constants for the D_2 receptor that are larger than the dissociation constant of dopamine. This "loose binding" to the D_2 receptor may allow displacement by endogenous dopamine and may contribute to a reduced liability for EPS and hyperprolactinemia. Unique among atypical agents, risperidone is "tightly bound" to the D_2 receptor, with a dissociation constant smaller than that of dopamine (Seeman 2002). A model for atypical antipsychotic mechanisms that emphasizes D_2 dissociation constants would predict that the apparent atypicality of risperidone, compared with that of haloperidol, reflects the reduced D_2 occupancy achieved by more favorable dosing rather than the intrinsic pharmacological characteristics of risperidone. According to some binding data, a comparable clinical dosage of haloperidol would be approximately 4 mg/day, rather than 20 mg/day as used in the North American multicenter registration trial (Kapur et al. 1999). Consistent with this view, benefits of risperidone for negative symptoms and EPS were less apparent when compared with lower doses of haloperidol or with lower-potency FGAs (see "Indications and Efficacy" section later in this chapter) than when compared with high-dose haloperidol (20 mg/day).

An additional mechanism possibly contributing to the enhanced efficacy of risperidone and paliperidone is their considerable α-adrenergic antagonism. In a placebo-controlled augmentation trial, Litman et al. (1996) demonstrated significant improvement in psychosis and negative symptoms with the α_2-adrenergic antagonist idazoxan when it was added to FGAs. Idazoxan has been shown to increase dopamine levels in the rat medial prefrontal cortex (Hertel et al. 1999). In aged rats (Haapalinna et al. 2000) and in patients with frontal dementias (Coull et al. 1996), α_2-adrenergic blockers have also been reported to improve cognitive functioning. Svensson et al. (1995) found that prazosin, an α_1 antagonist, inhibited both the behavioral activation and the increase in mesolimbic dopamine release produced by PCP or MK-801.

In summary, risperidone and paliperidone possess at least two mechanisms that may confer atypical characteristics. 5-HT_{2A} antagonism partially protects against D_2 antagonist–induced neurological side effects and may improve negative symptoms and cognitive functioning via modulation of mesocortical dopamine activity. In addition, blockade of adrenoceptors may further increase prefrontal cortical activity and could enhance antipsychotic efficacy by modulation of mesolimbic dopamine activity. Unlike other SGA agents, risperidone and paliperidone do not differ from FGAs in their dissociation constant for the D_2 receptor; this feature perhaps accounts for the risk of EPS at high doses, as well as their greater propensity to cause hyperprolactinemia.

Indications and Efficacy

Risperidone is approved by the FDA for the treatment of schizophrenia, bipolar mania, and irritability associated with autism. In August 2007, the indication for schizophrenia was extended to include adolescents ages 13–17 years, and the bipolar mania indication was extended to include children 10–17 years of age. The risperidone microsphere formulation (Consta long-acting injectable [LAI]) is approved for the treatment of schizophrenia and bipolar I disorder. Extended-release oral paliperidone (Invega) is approved for schizophrenia and schizoaffective disorder, and LAI paliperidone palmitate (Sustenna) is approved for the treatment of schizophrenia.

Schizophrenia

Clinical Trial Results for Risperidone

Eight-week trials. In the two North American registration trials (Chouinard et al. 1993; Marder and Meibach 1994), a total of 513 patients with chronic schizophrenia were randomly assigned to an 8-week double-blind, fixed-dose, placebo-controlled comparison of risperidone (2, 6, 10, or 16 mg/day) or haloperidol (20 mg/day). Risperidone dosages of 6, 10, and 16 mg/day produced significantly greater reductions, as compared with haloperidol, in each of the five domains of the Positive and Negative Syndrome Scale (PANSS), derived by principal-components analysis (Marder et al. 1997), and significantly higher response rates, defined as a 20% reduction in the PANSS total score. Effect sizes representing the difference in change scores between risperidone (6 mg/day) and haloperidol, although statistically significant, were uniformly small by Cohen's classification system (Cohen 1988): negative symptoms 0.31; positive symptoms 0.26; disorganized thoughts 0.22; uncontrolled hostility/excitement 0.29; and anxiety/depression 0.30 (Table 20–2). Severity of EPS was greater with haloperidol than with risperidone; further statistical analysis suggested that differences in EPS rates did not significantly influence the differences in PANSS subscale ratings (Marder et al. 1997). In fact, risperidone (10 and 16 mg/day) produced improvements in negative symptoms equivalent to those seen with risperidone (6 mg/day), despite increased EPS at the higher dosages of risperidone.

When risperidone (1, 4, 8, 12, and 16 mg/day) was compared with haloperidol (10 mg/day) in a large 8-week European trial involving 1,362 subjects with schizophrenia (Peuskens 1995), PANSS subscale change scores among risperidone-treated subjects indicated a preferential response to daily doses of 4 mg and 8 mg. However, neither the risperidone group taken as a whole nor individual risperidone doses achieved significantly better outcomes than haloperidol (10 mg/day) on any measure except for EPS, suggesting that the clinical superiority of risperidone over haloperidol in previous studies may have resulted from excessively high dosing of the comparator.

TABLE 20–2. Effect sizes on Positive and Negative Syndrome Scale (PANSS) symptom dimensions: North American trials (N=513)

	Adjusted mean change scores			Risperidone 6 mg/day	
	Placebo	Risperidone 6 mg/day	Haloperidol 20 mg/day	Effect size vs. placebo	Effect size vs. haloperidol
PANSS total	−3.8	−18.6	−5.1	0.53	0.31
Negative	0.2	−3.4	−0.1	0.27	0.26
Positive	0.9	−5.7	−2.3	0.48	0.22
Disorganized thought	0.1	−4.6	−0.2	0.43	0.24
Hostility/ excitement	0.2	−2.5	−0.1	0.47	0.29
Anxiety/ depression	−0.1	−2.5	−0.6	0.36	0.30

Source. Adapted from Marder et al. 1997.

CATIE. In the National Institute of Mental Health–funded Clinical Antipsychotic Trials of Intervention Effectiveness (CATIE; Stroup et al. 2003), 1,432 patients with chronic schizophrenia were randomly assigned to double-blind, flexibly dosed treatment for 18 months with risperidone, olanzapine, quetiapine, ziprasidone, or the FGA comparator perphenazine. Clinicians could adjust the dosage of each drug by prescribing 1–4 capsules daily; risperidone capsules contained 1.5 mg, and the mean daily dose administered in the study was 3.9 mg. Based on the primary outcome measure, time to all-cause discontinuation, risperidone was less effective than olanzapine (mean dosage 20 mg/day) and comparable in effectiveness to perphenazine, quetiapine, and ziprasidone (Lieberman et al. 2005). Although differences in rates of dropout due to intolerance did not reach statistical significance, risperidone consistently was the best-tolerated drug, particularly in subjects who had failed their first-assigned drug due to intolerance.

Maintenance treatment. Csernansky et al. (2002) randomly assigned 365 patients with stable schizophrenia or schizoaffective disorder to clinician-determined flexible dosing with risperidone or haloperidol for a minimum of 1 year. Kaplan-Meier estimates of the risk of relapse at the end of the study were 34% with risperidone, compared with 60% with haloperidol, a highly significant difference (P=0.001). The LAI risperidone microsphere formulation (Consta) at fixed doses of 25 mg, 50 mg, and 75 mg administered biweekly was superior in efficacy to placebo in a 12-week trial (Kane et al. 2003), but the 75-mg dose was not developed further due to an increased rate of EPS. In a 52-week maintenance study comparing fixed doses of risperidone microspheres administered every 2 weeks, the 25-mg dose was associated with a relapse rate of 21.6% and the 50-mg dose was associated with a 14.9% relapse rate (P=0.06) (Simpson et al. 2006). Comparisons of risperidone microspheres against oral SGAs have failed to demonstrate greater benefit with the LAI formulation. In 12-month randomized trials, the efficacy of risperidone microspheres was similar to that of oral risperidone (n=50; Bai et al. 2007), oral olanzapine (n=377; Keks et al. 2007), or clinician's choice of an oral antipsychotic other than clozapine ($n=369$; Rosenheck et al. 2011). By contrast, a nationwide cohort study using national databases in Norway found risperidone microspheres to be more effective in preventing readmission following a first hospitalization compared with oral risperidone and other oral antipsychotics with the exception of olanzapine and clozapine (Tiihonen et al. 2011). Because antipsychotic treatment in this naturalistic study was not randomized, conclusions are limited; nonetheless, the advantage found with depot formulations may reflect performance under typical clinical conditions.

Cognitive functioning in schizophrenia. Several early studies suggested that risperidone might enhance cognitive functioning, particularly verbal working memory, compared with haloperidol (Green et al. 1997; Harvey et al. 2005). A large double-blind trial that examined cognitive effects in 414 chronic schizophrenia patients treated for 52 weeks with risperidone (mean dosage 5.2 mg/day), olanzapine (12.3 mg/day), and haloperidol (8.2 mg/day) found no difference between treatments on the composite cognitive score, although risperidone and olanzapine were superior to haloperidol in a secondary analysis of completers (Keefe et al. 2006). When compared with low-dose haloperidol (mean dosage 5 mg/day), no cognitive advantage was found for risperidone (Green et al. 2002). In addition, in the CATIE, neither risperidone nor any other SGA demonstrated cognitive benefit compared with the FGA agent perphenazine (Keefe et al. 2007). A study in medication-naive patients found similar overall cognitive improvement with risperidone and olanzapine (Cuesta et al. 2009); however, another study of risperidone in medication-naive patients reported impairments of spatial working memory (Reilly et al. 2006) and procedural memory (Harris et al. 2009).

First-episode and treatment-refractory schizophrenia. Risperidone has been found to be well tolerated and effective in subgroups of patients with schizophrenia, including first-episode patients and elderly patients. In a 4-month double-blind trial comparing risperidone (mean dosage 3.9 mg/day) and olanzapine (mean dosage 11.8 mg/day) in 112 first-episode patients, both treatments were well tolerated, with an overall completion rate of 72% (Robinson et al. 2006). Response rates did not differ significantly between risperidone (54%) and olanzapine (44%), although patients who responded to risperidone were significantly more likely to retain their response. Experience in patients with treatment-resistant schizophrenia has been less consistent. In the U.S. multicenter registration study, Marder and Meibach (1994) found that patients who were presumed to have failed to respond to FGAs, on the basis of a history of hospitalization for at least 6 months prior to study entry, did not respond to haloperidol (20 mg/day) but did display significant response to risperidone (6 and 16 mg/day), compared with placebo. Wirshing et al. (1999) reported significant improvement with risperidone (6 mg/day), compared with haloperidol (15 mg/day), during a 4-week fixed-dose trial in 67 patients with schizophrenia and histories of treatment resistance. In contrast, Volavka et al. (2002) found no difference between high-dose risperidone (8–16 mg/day) and haloperidol (10–20 mg/day) in patients established by history to be treatment resistant to FGAs. In the CATIE, risperidone was more effective than quetiapine but did not differ from olanzapine and ziprasidone in patients who discontinued their first-assigned SGA medication due to lack of efficacy (Stroup et al. 2006). In contrast, patients who discontinued perphenazine (for any reason) subsequently did better on quetiapine or olanzapine than they did on risperidone (Stroup et al. 2007).

Clinical Trial Results for Paliperidone

In a 6-week trial in acutely ill schizophrenia patients, extended-release paliperidone (Invega) at dosages of 6, 9, and 12 mg/day was more effective than placebo (Kane et al.

2007), and in a flexibly dosed trial (9–15 mg/day), extended-release paliperidone significantly reduced relapse compared with placebo (Kramer et al. 2007). Combined results from three placebo-controlled trials including 1,326 acutely ill schizophrenia patients found significant improvement across a daily dose range of 3–15 mg (Meltzer et al. 2008). Three studies compared paliperidone with olanzapine 10 mg/day and found no difference in efficacy, but paliperidone was associated with more movement disorders and less weight gain (Nussbaum and Stroup 2008). LAI paliperidone palmitate treatment administered every 4 weeks has been demonstrated to be more effective than placebo (Hough et al. 2010; Kramer et al. 2010) and of similar efficacy to risperidone microspheres administered every 2 weeks (Pandina et al. 2011).

Affective Disorders

Six controlled trials of 3–4 weeks' duration that included a total of 1,343 patients have examined the efficacy of risperidone as monotherapy or in combination with a mood stabilizer for the acute treatment of bipolar mania (Rendell et al. 2006). As monotherapy and in combination, risperidone was more effective than placebo and similar in efficacy to haloperidol but produced more weight gain and fewer EPS (Rendell et al. 2006). In a placebo-controlled trial of open-label risperidone LAI microspheres in the maintenance treatment of bipolar I disorder, patients (n=303) with manic or mixed episodes who maintained response during a preceding 26-week period of risperidone following an initial 3-week period of oral risperidone were randomly allocated to placebo injections or continued treatment with risperidone LAI for up to 24 months. A switch to placebo injections significantly shortened the time to recurrence of manic episodes, but not depressive episodes (Quiroz et al. 2010).

Risperidone 1–2 mg/day was evaluated as an adjunct to antidepressant therapy in a 4-week placebo-controlled trial in 174 antidepressant-resistant patients with major depression recruited from 19 primary care and psychiatric centers (Mahmoud et al. 2007). Risperidone significantly lowered ratings of depressive symptoms compared with placebo. Remission rates were 25% with risperidone versus 11% with placebo (P=0.004). Risperidone was well tolerated, with an 81% completion rate (vs. 88% with placebo).

Autism

Risperidone was also studied in a large 8-week placebo-controlled trial in 101 children (ages 5–17 years) with autism accompanied by severe tantrums, aggression, or self-injurious behavior (McCracken et al. 2002). Flexible dosing with risperidone (range=0.5–3.5 mg/day; mean dosage=1.2 mg/day) resulted in a mean reduction of 57% in irritability, compared with a decrease of 14% in the placebo group, and the response rate was 69% with risperidone versus 12% with placebo. In a study of 32 children (ages 5–17 years) treated for 4 months with open-label risperidone (mean dosage 2 mg/day), those who continued treatment with risperidone during the second study arm, an 8-week double-blind substitution trial, had much lower relapse rates than patients switched to placebo (Research Units on Pediatric Psychopharmacology Autism Network 2005). Risperidone at a mean dosage of 2 mg/day was also found to be effective compared with placebo in a study of 31 adults with autism or pervasive developmental disorder (McDougle et al. 1998). In these studies, risperidone improved irritability and restricted, repetitive, and stereotyped behavioral problems associated with autism but was not effective for social or language deficits (McDougle et al. 2005). Risperidone at a dosage of 0.02–0.06 mg/kg was found to be well tolerated and effective for disruptive behaviors in children with low intelligence (intelligence quotient [IQ] between 36 and 84) in a 6-week placebo-controlled trial (Aman et al. 2002).

Other Disorders

Generalized Anxiety Disorder

In a 4-week placebo-controlled add-on trial of low-dose risperidone in 417 patients with persistence of generalized anxiety disorder symptoms despite 8 weeks of anxiolytic therapy, no benefit from risperidone was found in the primary analysis; however, risperidone was associated with greater improvement in patients with moderate or severe anxiety at baseline (Pandina et al. 2007). Risperidone was highly effective for obsessive-compulsive disorder symptoms in a 6-week placebo-controlled trial in 36 adults prospectively confirmed to be refractory to treatment with a selective serotonin reuptake inhibitor (McDougle et al. 2000). Symptoms of anxiety and depression also responded to risperidone compared with placebo. Fifty percent of risperidone-treated patients responded (mean dosage 2.2 mg/day), compared with none in the placebo group.

Alzheimer's Disease

In the CATIE–Alzheimer's Disease (CATIE-AD) study, risperidone had the longest time to discontinuation due to lack of effectiveness (27 weeks) of the agents studied; comparison results were 22 weeks for olanzapine, 9 weeks for quetiapine, and 9 weeks for placebo (Schneider et al. 2006). However, because of poor tolerability, none of the three antipsychotics differed from placebo on time to all-cause discontinuation.

Side Effects and Toxicology

Risperidone shares class warnings with other SGAs in the United States, including the risks of tardive dyskinesia, neuroleptic malignant syndrome, and hyperglycemia and diabetes, as well as the risk of increased mortality in elderly patients with dementia-related psychosis. However, risperidone generally has been very well tolerated in clinical trials. In the U.S. multicenter trial reported by Marder and Meibach (1994), only headache and dizziness were significantly more frequent with risperidone (6 mg/day) compared with placebo, whereas the group receiving risperidone (16 mg/day) treatment also reported more EPS and dyspepsia than did the group receiving placebo (Table 20–3). Fatigue, sedation, accommodation disturbances, orthostatic dizziness, palpitations or tachycardia, weight gain, diminished sexual desire, and erectile dysfunction displayed a statistically significant relationship to risperidone dose, although most were not significantly elevated compared with placebo. In a flexible-dose relapse prevention study reported by Csernansky et al. (2002), no side effects were more frequent with risperidone, compared with haloperidol, although risperidone produced significantly greater weight gain. In a flexibly dosed, placebo-controlled trial of risperidone for children with disruptive behavior, risperidone (mean dosage 1.2 mg/day) produced more somnolence, headache, vomiting, dyspepsia, weight gain, and prolactin elevation than did placebo; most side effects were rated mild to moderate and did not adversely affect compliance (Aman et al. 2002).

Metabolic Effects

Weight gain with risperidone is intermediate—that is, the degree of weight gain is between that associated with agents like molindone, amisulpride, and ziprasidone, which appear to be relatively weight neutral, and that associated with agents like clozapine, olanzapine, and low-potency phenothiazines (Rummel-Kluge et al. 2010; Sikich et al. 2008). In a meta-analysis of controlled trials, Allison et al. (1999), using a random effects model, estimated the mean weight gain at 10 weeks with risperidone to be 2.0 kg, compared with 0.5 kg with haloperidol, 3.5 kg with olanzapine, and 4.0 kg with clozapine. In the CATIE, in which risperidone had the lowest rate of discontinuation due to side effects, risperidone treatment was associated with a mean monthly weight gain of 0.4 lb,

TABLE 20–3. Side effects reported by patients with schizophrenia receiving placebo, risperidone, or haloperidol in the U.S. multicenter trial

	Percentage of patients			
	Placebo (N=66)	Risperidone 6 mg (N=64)	Risperidone 16 mg (N=64)	Haloperidol (N=66)
Insomnia	9.1	12.5	9.4	12.1
Agitation	7.6	10.9	12.5	16.7
Anxiety	1.5	7.8	4.7	1.5
Nervousness	1.5	6.3	1.6	0
Somnolence	0	3.1	9.4[a]	4.5
Extrapyramidal side effects	10.6	10.9	25.0[a]	25.8[a]
Headache	4.5	15.6[a]	9.4	7.6
Dizziness	0	9.4[a]	10.9[b]	0
Dyspepsia	4.5	9.4	6.3	4.5
Vomiting	1.5	6.3	6.3	3.0
Nausea	0	6.3	3.1	1.5
Constipation	0	1.6	6.3	1.5
Rhinitis	6.1	15.6	6.3	4.5
Coughing	1.5	9.4	3.1	3.0
Sinusitis	1.5	6.3	1.6	0
Fever	0	6.3	3.1	1.5
Tachycardia	0	4.7	6.3	1.5

[a]$P<0.05$ versus placebo.
[b]$P<0.01$ versus placebo.

Source. Adapted from Marder and Meibach 1994.

olanzapine with 2.0 lbs, and quetiapine with 0.5 lb; by contrast, perphenazine and ziprasidone were associated with a mean monthly weight *loss* of 0.2 lb and 0.3 lb, respectively (Lieberman et al. 2005). Although determining the risk for hyperglycemia is complex, and results of studies have not been completely consistent, it appears that risperidone does not produce insulin resistance to the degree associated with olanzapine and clozapine (American Diabetes Association et al. 2004; Henderson et al. 2006; Lieberman et al. 2005). A meta-analysis of head-to-head comparisons of SGAs found that risperidone produced more cholesterol elevation than aripiprazole and ziprasidone and less elevation than olanzapine and quetiapine (Rummel-Kluge et al. 2010). Metabolic side effects in children tend to be more severe than those in adults; for example, in one study of pediatric patients younger than 20 years, risperidone produced a mean weight gain of 5.3 kg (11.7 lb) over the 12-week treatment period (Correll et al. 2009). Metabolic side effects with paliperidone appear to be similar to those with risperidone.

High Dose and Overdose

Mesotten et al. (1989) reported the results of a safety trial involving 17 inpatients with psychosis in which, following a washout of previous medication, risperidone was started at 10 mg/day, and the dosage was then increased weekly by 5 mg/day to a maximum of 25 mg/day. Despite extremely high doses, sedation was the only prominent side effect. Although risperidone does not bind significantly to muscarinic cholinergic receptors, transient dry mouth, blurred vision, and urinary retention were observed in individual subjects. Palpitations occurred in 2 subjects. Heart rate significantly increased during the trial, and blood pressure slightly decreased; however; no cases of significant hypotension were reported. An endocrine battery, including plasma triiodothyronine, thyroid-stimulating hormone, growth hormone, prolactin, follicle-stimulating hormone, luteinizing hormone, and cortisol levels, was performed, and only prolactin was found to be affected. Reported overdoses with risperidone have generally been benign, with moderate QT prolongation and no serious cardiac complications (Brown et al. 1993; Lo Vecchio et al. 1996).

Extrapyramidal Side Effects

Significant reductions in EPS with risperidone, compared with high-dose haloperidol, were a consistent finding in the North American trials (Chouinard et al. 1993; Marder and Meibach 1994). Measurement of EPS in the placebo group was complicated because 25% of the subjects were taking depot antipsychotics prior to enrollment. Risperidone produced significantly fewer parkinsonian side effects than did haloperidol (20 mg/day), based on several measures, including self-report, change scores on the Extrapyramidal Symptom Rating Scale (ESRS), and use of anticholinergic medication. Patients receiving risperidone (2 and 6 mg/day) did not differ from the group receiving placebo in mean ratings of parkinsonism and in the use of anticholinergic medication. Parkinsonism change scores were significantly correlated with the risperidone dosage (r=0.94); however, risperidone (16 mg/day) was associated with fewer parkinsonian side effects than was haloperidol. Dystonia occurred in six of the patients treated with risperidone (1.7%) versus two of the patients treated with haloperidol (2.4%). Dystonia rates did not differ between treatment groups, and the rates did not exhibit a relationship to risperidone dosage.

In the large European multicenter trial, maximum ratings of parkinsonism, hyperkinesias, and dystonia were greater with haloperidol (10 mg/day) than with all dosages of risperidone (maximum of 12 mg/day), and anticholinergic dosing was accordingly higher in the group treated with haloperidol (Peuskens 1995). Similarly, in a flexible-dose comparison of risperidone (mean dosage 4.9 mg/day) and haloperidol (mean dosage 11.7 mg/day) for prevention of relapse, EPS rates and use of anticholinergic medication significantly favored the group taking risperidone (Csernansky et al. 2002). However, in a smaller double-blind, flexible-dose trial comparing risperidone (5–15 mg/day) and the moderate-potency FGA agent perphenazine (16–48 mg/day) in 107 patients, no difference in EPS rates was observed (Hoyberg et al. 1993), indicating that the potency of the comparator agent may in part determine the relative benefit of risperidone for EPS. Of interest, in a study of low-dose risperidone (mean dosage 1.2 mg/day) in children with behavioral disorders, ratings of EPS did not differ between risperidone and placebo (Aman et al. 2002). No differences in EPS ratings were found among any treatment groups in the CATIE (Lieberman et al. 2005), although discontinuation rates due to EPS significantly differed, with perphenazine producing the highest discontinuation rate (8%) and olanzapine (2%), risperidone (3%), and quetiapine (3%) producing the lowest.

The experience with tardive dyskinesia (TD) in patients treated with risperidone has been promising. Jeste et al. (1999) randomly treated 122 elderly patients with low-dose haloperidol (median daily dose 1 mg) versus risperidone (median daily dose 1 mg). The very high rates of treatment-emergent TD typically found in geriatric patients make this sample a sensitive assay for TD risk. After 9 months, treatment-emergent TD rates were 30% with haloperidol versus less than 5% with risperidone. Risperidone was also noted to decrease dyskinetic movements, compared with haloperidol, in a Canadian multicenter trial reported by Chouinard et al. (1993), and it was associated with a treatment-emergent TD rate of 0.6%, compared with a rate of 2.7% with haloperidol, in a relapse prevention trial reported by Csernansky et al. (2002).

Hyperprolactinemia

Unlike other SGA agents, risperidone and paliperidone substantially increase serum prolactin levels—in some studies, to a greater degree than does haloperidol (Kearns et al. 2000; Markianos et al. 1999)—although prolactin levels may decrease over time (Eberhard et al. 2007; Findling et al. 2003). The relationship between serum prolactin concentrations and clinical side effects remains somewhat unclear, however. Kleinberg et al. (1999) analyzed combined results from the North American and European multicenter registration trials, which included plasma prolactin concentrations from 841 patients and clinical ratings of symptoms associated with hyperprolactinemia from 1,884 patients. Mean prolactin levels significantly correlated with risperidone dosage; risperidone 6 mg/day produced elevations roughly comparable to those seen with haloperidol 20 mg/day and significantly higher than those seen with haloperidol 10 mg/day. The combined incidence of amenorrhea and galactorrhea in women, which varied between 8% and 12%, was similar for all dosages of risperidone and haloperidol (10 mg/day). Because symptom frequencies were available only for 14 women treated with placebo, comparisons with placebo were not informative. Sexual dysfunction or gynecomastia occurred in 15% of men treated with risperidone (4–6 mg/day), compared with 14% of men treated with haloperidol (10 mg/day) and 8% of men in the placebo group. Compared with placebo, ejaculatory dysfunction was significantly more frequent only in the group treated with risperidone (12–16 mg/day). Mean plasma prolactin levels were not significantly related to clinical side effects for either men or women. Decreased libido also did not differ between treatment groups and did not correlate with plasma prolactin levels. In the CATIE, prolactin levels increased by a mean of 15.4 ng/mL with risperidone, compared with a 0.4-ng/mL mean elevation with perphenazine and decreases of 4.5–9.3 ng/mL with the other SGAs (Lieberman et al. 2005). Despite having significantly higher serum prolactin concentrations, patients treated with risperidone did not report significantly higher rates of sexual dysfunction, gynecomastia, galactorrhea, or irregular menses.

Two reports of clinical trials with extended-release paliperidone have indicated low levels of prolactin-related side effects (1% and 4%) (Kane et al. 2007; Kramer et al. 2007). However, in the one publication that reported prolactin levels, substantial increases in mean plasma prolactin concentrations were observed (males: 17.4 ng/mL at baseline to 45.3 ng/mL at week 6; females: 38.0 ng/mL to 124.5 ng/mL) (Kane et al. 2007). In a 13-week comparison of paliperidone palmitate with risperidone microspheres, paliperidone palmitate was associated with moderately higher elevations from baseline in prolactin levels compared with risperidone (women: 21.8 vs. 15.6 ng/mL; men: 9.4 vs. 6.0 ng/mL) (Pandina et al. 2011). Two preliminary studies with risperidone found that plasma prolactin concentrations correlated with 9-hydroxyrisperidone (paliperidone) concentrations and not with risperidone concentrations (Melkersson 2006; Troost et al. 2007). The ratio of 9-hydroxyrisperidone levels to risperidone levels also correlated with prolactin concentration (Troost et al. 2007); in agreement with this finding, rapid metabolizers of CYP2D6 were found to have higher prolactin concentrations than poor metabolizers (Troost et al. 2007). Because of the difficulty in establishing dose equivalence between risperidone and paliperidone in clinical trials, it is not clear whether the two drugs differ in their potential to elevate prolactin. Additional studies are needed to compare prolactin elevations with the two drugs.

Cardiovascular Effects

Because of relatively high affinities for adrenoreceptors, risperidone would be expected to produce orthostatic hypotension. However, by following a 3- to 7-day dosage escalation schedule, initial postural hypotension and tachycardia have been avoided in clinical trials, with only rare cases of hypotension and syncope reported (Chouinard et al. 1993; Marder and Meibach 1994). Risperidone has very modest effects on cardiac conduction. No significant prolongation of the QTc interval was detected at dosages of up to 25 mg/day in early safety trials, and no relationship between QTc interval and risperidone dose was apparent (Mesotten et al. 1989). In the CATIE, risperidone was associated with the least QTc prolongation (mean 0.2 msec) and quetiapine with the most (mean 5.9 msec), although differences were not statistically significant (Lieberman et al. 2005). A mean QTc prolongation of 10 msec, measured after peak absorption of risperidone (16 mg/day), was found in a study comparing SGAs and FGAs, according to data filed with the FDA by Pfizer Inc. (Harrigan et al. 2004). In a retrospective cohort study of Medicaid enrollees in Tennessee, risperidone was associated with a 2.9-fold increase in rate of sudden cardiac death, compared with a 1.61-fold increase with haloperidol and a 3.67-fold increase with clozapine (Ray et al. 2009).

Drug-Drug Interactions

Because CYP2D6 status affects the half-life of risperidone and the relative ratio of risperidone to 9-hydroxyrisperidone in plasma, the total serum concentration of the "active moiety," or the sum of the concentrations of risperidone and 9-hydroxyrisperidone, may be significantly increased with addition of a CYP2D6 inhibitor (e.g., fluoxetine) in rapid metabolizers but not in poor metabolizers (Bondolfi et al. 2002; Spina et al. 2002). In one study of 9 patients treated with risperidone, addition of fluoxetine resulted in a 75% increase in blood levels of the active moiety (risperidone+9-hydroxyrisperidone); two patients developed parkinsonian side effects (Spina et al. 2002). Paliperidone plasma concentrations are not influenced by CYP2D6 status, nor are paliperidone plasma concentrations likely to be affected by drug-drug interactions. It has been hypothesized that the addition of a CYP2D6 inhibitor (e.g., fluoxetine) could decrease risperidone-induced prolactin elevation by increasing the ratio of risperidone to 9-hydroxyrisperidone (Troost et al. 2007) although this has not been rigorously tested.

Conclusion

Risperidone was the first antipsychotic agent developed specifically to exploit the clinical advantages of combined D_2 and 5-HT_{A2} antagonism. α-Adrenergic antagonism additionally may contribute to the antipsychotic and cognition-enhancing effects of risperidone. Risperidone's active metabolite, paliperidone, is pharmacologically quite similar to the parent drug and comprises roughly 80%–90% of the serum concentration of the active moiety (risperidone+paliperidone) in most patients treated with risperidone. Risperidone and paliperidone are generally quite well tolerated, producing moderate weight gain and mild sedation. Initial dosage titration is necessary to prevent orthostatic blood pressure changes and dizziness, although this may be less necessary with extended-release paliperidone. EPS are dose related and are typically less common with risperidone than with haloperidol but more common with risperidone compared with other SGAs. Risperidone and paliperidone markedly elevate prolactin levels, although the relationship between plasma prolactin concentrations and clinical symptoms is complex. The efficacy of risperidone was initially established in comparison with high-dose haloperidol, against which it was significantly more effective for all five symptom clusters derived from the PANSS. However, the magnitude of difference in effect size was not large for individual symptom clusters. In the CATIE, risperidone (at a mean daily dosage of 3.9 mg) did not differ from perphenazine in rates of discontinuation due to lack of effectiveness but was less effective than olanzapine (Lieberman et al. 2005). The risperidone microspheres product was the first FDA-approved SGA long-acting IM formulation, and paliperidone palmitate was the first SGA depot formulation that could be administered at an interval of every 4 weeks. However, superior efficacy in randomized maintenance trials has not been demonstrated for risperidone microspheres compared with oral antipsychotics. Overall, risperidone and paliperidone represent well-tolerated SGA agents with efficacy comparable to that of most other agents of their class.

References

Allison DB, Mentore JL, Heo M, et al: Antipsychotic-induced weight gain: a comprehensive research synthesis. Am J Psychiatry 156:1686–1696, 1999

Aman MG, De Smedt G, Derivan A, et al: Double-blind, placebo-controlled study of risperidone for the treatment of disruptive behaviors in children with subaverage intelligence. Am J Psychiatry 159:1337–1346, 2002

American Diabetes Association, American Psychiatric Association, American Association of Clinical Endocrinologists, et al: Consensus development conference on antipsychotic drugs and diabetes and obesity. Diabetes Care 27:596–601, 2004

Anderson CB, True JE, Ereshefsky L, et al: Risperidone dose, plasma levels, and response. Presentation at the 146th annual meeting of the American Psychiatric Association, San Francisco, CA, May 22–27, 1993

Ansoms C, Backer-Dierick GD, Vereecken JL: Sleep disorders in patients with severe mental depression: double-blind placebo-controlled evaluation of the value of pipamperone (Dipiperon). Acta Psychiatr Scand 55:116–122, 1977

Arakawa R, Ito H, Takano A, et al: Dose-finding study of paliperidone ER based on striatal and extrastriatal dopamine D2 receptor occupancy in patients with schizophrenia. Psychopharmacology (Berl) 197:229–235, 2008

Bai YM, Ting Chen T, Chen JY, et al: Equivalent switching dose from oral risperidone to risperidone long-acting injection: a 48-week randomized, prospective, single-blind pharmacokinetic study. J Clin Psychiatry 68:1218–1225, 2007

Bersani G, Grispini A, Marini S: 5-HT2 antagonist ritanserin in neuroleptic-induced parkinsonism: a double-blind comparison with orphenadrine and placebo. Clin Neuropharmacol 13:500–506, 1990

Bondolfi G, Eap CB, Bertschy G, et al: The effect of fluoxetine on the pharmacokinetics and safety of risperidone in psychotic patients. Pharmacopsychiatry 35:50–56, 2002

Borison RL: Risperidone: pharmacokinetics. J Clin Psychiatry 12:46–48, 1994

Brown K, Levy H, Brenner C, et al: Overdose of risperidone. Ann Emerg Med 22:1908–1910, 1993

Busatto FG, Kerwin RW: Perspectives on the role of serotonergic mechanisms in the pharmacology of schizophrenia. J Psychopharmacol 11:3–12, 1997

Ceulemans D, Gelders Y, Hoppenbrouwers M, et al: Effect of serotonin antagonism in schizophrenia: a pilot study with setoperone. Psychopharmacology (Berl) 85:329–332, 1985

Chouinard G, Jones B, Remington G, et al: A Canadian multicenter placebo-controlled study of fixed doses of risperidone and haloperidol in the treatment of chronic schizophrenic patients. J Clin Psychopharmacol 13:25–40, 1993

Cohen J: Statistical Power Analysis for the Behavioral Sciences, 2nd Edition. Hillsdale, NJ, Lawrence Erlbaum, 1988

Colpaert FC, Meert TF: Behavioral and 5-HT antagonist effects of ritanserin: pure and selective antagonist effects of LSD discrimination in the rat. Psychopharmacology 86:45–54, 1985

Correll CU, Manu P, Olshanskiy V, et al: Cardiometabolic risk of second-generation antipsychotic medications during first-time use in children and adolescents. JAMA 302:1765–1773, 2009; erratum in JAMA 302:2322, 2009

Coull JT, Sahakian BJ, Hodges JR: The alpha 2 antagonist idazoxan remediates certain attentional and executive dysfunction in patients with dementia of frontal type. Psychopharmacology (Berl) 123:239–249, 1996

Csernansky JG, Mahmoud R, Brenner R: A comparison of risperidone and haloperidol for the prevention of relapse in patients with schizophrenia. N Engl J Med 346:16–22, 2002

Cuesta MJ, Jalón EG, Campos MS, et al: Cognitive effectiveness of olanzapine and risperidone in first-episode psychosis. Br J Psychiatry 194:439–445, 2009

de Leon J, Wynn G, Sandson NB: The pharmacokinetics of paliperidone versus risperidone. Psychosomatics 51:80–88, 2010

Duinkerke SJ, Botter PA, Jansen AA, et al: Ritanserin, a selective 5-HT2/1C antagonist, and negative symptoms in schizophrenia: a placebo-controlled double blind trial. Br J Psychiatry 163:451–455, 1993

Eberhard J, Lindström E, Holstad M, et al: Prolactin level during 5 years of risperidone treatment in patients with psychotic disorders. Acta Psychiatr Scand 115:268–276, 2007

Findling RL, Kusumakar V, Daneman D, et al: Prolactin levels during long-term risperidone treatment in children and adolescents. J Clin Psychiatry 64:1362–1369, 2003

Gelders YG: Thymosthenic agents, a novel approach in the treatment of schizophrenia. Br J Psychiatry 155 (suppl 5):33–36, 1989

Gellman RL, Aghajanian GK: Serotonin 2 receptor-mediated excitation of interneurons in piriform cortex: antagonism by atypical antipsychotic drugs. Neuroscience 58:515–525, 1994

Geyer MA, Swerdlow NR, Mansbach RS, et al: Startle response models of sensorimotor gating, and habituation deficits in schizophrenia. Brain Res 25:485–498, 1990

Goff DC, Coyle JT: The emerging role of glutamate in the pathophysiology and treatment of schizophrenia. Am J Psychiatry 158:1367–1377, 2001

Goff D, Evins A: Negative symptoms in schizophrenia: neurobiological models and treatment response. Harv Rev Psychiatry 6:59–77, 1998

Green M, Marshall B, Wirshing W, et al: Does risperidone improve verbal working memory in treatment-resistant schizophrenia? Am J Psychiatry 154:799–804, 1997

Green MF, Marder SR, Glynn SM, et al: The neurocognitive effects of low-dose haloperidol: a two-year comparison with risperidone. Biol Psychiatry 51:972–978, 2002

Haapalinna A, Sirvio J, MacDonald E: The effects of a specific alpha(2)-adrenoceptor antagonist, atipamezole, on cognitive performance and brain neurochemistry in aged Fisher 344 rats. Eur J Pharmacol 387:141–150, 2000

Harrigan EP, Miceli JJ, Anziano R, et al: A randomized evaluation of the effects of six antipsychotic agents on QTc, in the absence and presence of metabolic inhibition. J Clin Psychopharmacol 24:62–69, 2004

Harris MS, Wiseman CL, Reilly JL, et al: Effects of risperidone on procedural learning in antipsychotic-naive first-episode schizophrenia. Neuropsychopharmacology 34:468–476, 2009

Harvey PD, Rabinowitz J, Eerdekens M, et al: Treatment of cognitive impairment in early psychosis: a comparison of risperidone and haloperidol in a large long-term trial. Am J Psychiatry 162:1888–1895, 2005

Henderson DC, Copeland PM, Borba CP, et al: Glucose metabolism in patients with schizophrenia treated with olanzapine or quetiapine: a frequently sampled intravenous glucose tolerance test and minimal model analysis. J Clin Psychiatry 67:789–797, 2006

Hertel P, Fagerquist M, Svensson TH: Enhanced cortical dopamine output and antipsychotic-like effects of raclopride by alpha2 adrenergic blockade. Science 286:105–107, 1999

Heykants J, Huang ML, Mannens G, et al: The pharmacokinetics of risperidone in humans: a summary. J Clin Psychiatry 55 (suppl):13–17, 1994

Hoyberg O, Fensbo C, Remvig J, et al: Risperidone versus perphenazine in the treatment of chronic schizophrenic patients with acute exacerbations. Acta Psychiatr Scand 88:395–402, 1993

Hough D, Gopal S, Vijapurkar U, et al: Paliperidone palmitate maintenance treatment in delaying the time-to-relapse in patients with schizophrenia: a randomized, double-blind, placebo-controlled study. Schizophr Res 116:107–117, 2010

Janssen PA, Niemegeers CJ, Awouters F, et al: Pharmacology of risperidone (R 64 766), a new antipsychotic with serotonin-S2 and dopamine D2-antagonist properties. J Pharmacol Exp Ther 244:685–693, 1988

Jeste DV, Lacro JP, Bailey A, et al: Lower incidence of tardive dyskinesia with risperidone compared to haloperidol in older patients. J Am Geriatr Soc 47:716–719, 1999

Kane JM, Eerdekens M, Lindenmayer JP, et al: Long-acting injectable risperidone: efficacy and safety of the first long-acting atypical antipsychotic. Am J Psychiatry 160:1125–1132, 2003

Kane J, Canas F, Kramer M, et al: Treatment of schizophrenia with paliperidone extended-release tablets: a 6-week placebo-controlled trial. Schizophr Res 90:147–161, 2007

Kapur S, Seeman P: Does fast dissociation from the dopamine D2 receptor explain the action of atypical antipsychotics? a new hypothesis. Am J Psychiatry 158:360–369, 2001

Kapur S, Zipursky R, Remington G: Clinical and theoretical implications of 5-HT2 and D2 occupancy of clozapine, risperidone and olanzapine in schizophrenia. Am J Psychiatry 156:286–293, 1999

Kearns A, Goff DC, Hayden D, et al: Risperidone-associated hyperprolactinemia. Endocr Pract 6:425–429, 2000

Keefe RS, Young CA, Rock SL, et al: One-year double-blind study of the neurocognitive efficacy of olanzapine, risperidone, and haloperidol in schizophrenia. Schizophr Res 81:1–15, 2006

Keefe RS, Bilder RM, Davis SM, et al: Neurocognitive effects of antipsychotic medications in patients with chronic schizophrenia in the CATIE Trial. Arch Gen Psychiatry 64:633–647, 2007

Keks NA, Ingham M, Khan A, et al: Long-acting injectable risperidone v. olanzapine tablets for schizophrenia or schizoaffective disorder. Randomised, controlled, open-label study. Br J Psychiatry 191:131–139, 2007

Kleinberg DL, Davis JM, deCoster R, et al: Prolactin levels and adverse events in patients treated with risperidone. J Clin Psychopharmacol 19: 57–61, 1999

Kramer M, Simpson G, Maciulis V, et al: Paliperidone extended-release tablets for prevention of symptom recurrence in patients with schizophrenia: a randomized, double-blind, placebo-controlled study. J Clin Psychopharmacol 27:6–14, 2007

Kramer M, Litman R, Hough D, et al: Paliperidone palmitate, a potential long-acting treatment for patients with schizophrenia. Results of a randomized, double-blind, placebo-controlled efficacy and safety study. Int J Neuropsychopharmacol 13:635–647, 2010

Krystal JH, Karper LP, Seibyl JP, et al: Subanesthetic effects of the noncompetitive NMDA antagonist, ketamine, in humans: psychotomimetic, perceptual, cognitive, and neuroendocrine responses. Arch Gen Psychiatry 51:199–214, 1994

Leysen JE, Niemegeers CJE, Tollenaere JP: Serotonergic component of neuroleptic receptors. Nature 272:168–171, 1978

Leysen JE, Gommeren W, Mertens J: Comparison of in vitro binding properties of a series of dopamine antagonists and agonists for cloned human dopamine D2S and D2L receptors and for D2 receptors in rat striatal and mesolimbic tissues, using [125I]2-iodospiperone. Psychopharmacology (Berl) 110:27–36, 1993a

Leysen JE, Janssen PM, Schotte A, et al: Interaction of antipsychotic drugs with neurotransmitter receptor sites in vitro and in vivo in relation to pharmacological and clinical effects: role of 5-HT2 receptors. Psychopharmacology (Berl) 112:S40–S54, 1993b

Leysen JE, Janssen PM, Megens AA, et al: Risperidone: a novel antipsychotic with balanced serotonin-dopamine antagonism, receptor occupancy profile, and pharmacologic activity. J Clin Psychiatry 55 (suppl 5):5–12, 1994

Lieberman JA, Stroup TS, McEvoy JP, et al: Effectiveness of antipsychotic drugs in patients with chronic schizophrenia. Clinical Antipsychotic Trials of Intervention Effectiveness (CATIE) Investigators. N Engl J Med 353:1209–1223, 2005

Litman RE, Su T-P, Potter WZ, et al: Idazozan and response to typical neuroleptics in treatment-resistant schizophrenia. Br J Psychiatry 168:571–579, 1996

Lo Vecchio FL, Hamilton RJ, Hoffman RJ: Risperidone overdose (letter). Am J Emerg Med 14:95–96, 1996

Mahmoud RA, Pandina GJ, Turkoz I, et al: Risperidone for treatment-refractory major depressive disorder: a randomized trial. Ann Intern Med 147:593–602, 2007

Mannens G, Huang M-L, Meuldermans W: Absorption, metabolism and excretion of risperidone in humans. Drug Metab Dispos 21:1134–1141, 1993

Marder SR, Meibach RC: Risperidone in the treatment of schizophrenia. Am J Psychiatry 151: 825–835, 1994

Marder S, Davis J, Chouinard G: The effects of risperidone on the five dimensions of schizophrenia derived by factor analysis: combined results of the North American trials. J Clin Psychiatry 58:538–546, 1997

Markianos M, Hatzimanolis J, Lykouras L: Gonadal axis hormones in male schizophrenic patients during treatment with haloperidol and after switch to risperidone. Psychopharmacology (Berl) 143:270–272, 1999

McCracken JT, McGough J, Shah B, et al: Risperidone in children with autism and serious behavioral problems. Research Units on Pediatric Psychopharmacology Autism Network. N Engl J Med 347:314–321, 2002

McDougle CJ, Holmes JP, Carlson DC, et al: A double-blind, placebo-controlled study of risperidone in adults with autistic disorder and other pervasive developmental disorders. Arch Gen Psychiatry 55:633–641, 1998

McDougle CJ, Epperson CN, Pelton GH, et al: A double-blind, placebo-controlled study of risperidone addition in serotonin reuptake inhibitor-refractory obsessive-compulsive disorder. Arch Gen Psychiatry 57:794–801, 2000

McDougle CJ, Scahill L, Aman MG, et al: Risperidone for the core symptom domains of autism: results from the study by the autism network of the research units on pediatric psychopharmacology. Am J Psychiatry 162:1142–1148, 2005

Meert TF, Colpaert FC: Effects of S2-antagonists in two conflict procedures that involve exploratory behavior. Psychopharmacology (Berl) 89:S23, 1986

Meert TF, de Haes P, Janssen PA: Risperidone (R 64 766), a potent and complete LSD antagonist in drug discrimination by rats. Psychopharmacology (Berl) 97:206–212, 1989

Megens AA, Awouters FHL, Niemegeers CJE: Differential effects of the new antipsychotic risperidone on large and small motor movements in rats: a comparison with haloperidol. Psychopharmacology (Berl) 95:493–496, 1988

Melkersson KI: Prolactin elevation of the antipsychotic risperidone is predominantly related to its 9-hydroxy metabolite. Hum Psychopharmacol 21:529–532, 2006

Meltzer HY, Bastani B, Ramirez L, et al: Clozapine: new research on efficacy and mechanism of action. Eur Arch Psychiatry Neurol Sci 238:332–339, 1989

Meltzer HY, Bobo WV, Nuamah IF, et al: Efficacy and tolerability of oral paliperidone extended-release tablets in the treatment of acute schizophrenia: pooled data from three 6-week, placebo-controlled studies. J Clin Psychiatry 69:817–829, 2008

Mesotten F, Suy E, Pietquin M, et al: Therapeutic effect and safety of increasing doses of risperidone (R 64766) in psychotic patients. Psychopharmacology (Berl) 99:445–449, 1989

Nussbaum AM, Stroup TS: Paliperidone for treatment of schizophrenia. Schizophr Bull 34:419–422, 2008

Nyberg S, Eriksson B, Oxenstierna G, et al: Suggested minimal effective dose of risperidone based on PET-measured D2 and 5-HT2A receptor occupancy in schizophrenic patients. Am J Psychiatry 156:869–875, 1999

Pandina GJ, Canuso CM, Turkoz I, et al: Adjunctive risperidone in the treatment of generalized anxiety disorder: a double-blind, prospective, placebo-controlled, randomized trial. Psychopharmacol Bull 40:41–57, 2007

Pandina G, Lane R, Gopal S, et al: A double-blind study of paliperidone palmitate and risperidone long-acting injectable in adults with schizophrenia. Prog Neuropsychopharmacol Biol Psychiatry 35:218–226, 2011

Peuskens J: Risperidone in the treatment of patients with chronic schizophrenia: a multi-national, multi-centre, double-blind, parallel-group study versus haloperidol. Br J Psychiatry 166: 712–726, 1995

Poyurovsky M, Shardorodsky M, Fuchs C, et al: Treatment of neuroleptic-induced akathisia with the 5-HT2 antagonist mianserin. Double-blind, placebo-controlled study. Br J Psychiatry 174:238–242, 1999

Quiroz JA, Yatham LN, Palumbo JM, et al: Risperidone long-acting injectable monotherapy in the maintenance treatment of bipolar I disorder. Biol Psychiatry 68:156–162, 2010

Ray WA, Chung CP, Murray KT, et al: Atypical antipsychotic drugs and the risk of sudden cardiac death. N Engl J Med 360:225–235, 2009; erratum in N Engl J Med 361:1814, 2009

Reilly JL, Harris MS, Keshavan MS, et al: Adverse effects of risperidone on spatial working memory in first-episode schizophrenia. Arch Gen Psychiatry 63:1189–1197, 2006

Remington G, Mamo D, Labelle A, et al: A PET study evaluating dopamine D2 receptor occupancy for long-acting injectable risperidone. Am J Psychiatry 163:396–401, 2006

Rendell JM, Gijsman HJ, Bauer MS, et al: Risperidone alone or in combination for acute mania. Cochrane Database Syst Rev (1):CD004043, 2006

Research Units on Pediatric Psychopharmacology Autism Network: Risperidone treatment of autistic disorder: longer-term benefits and blinded discontinuation after 6 months. Am J Psychiatry 162:1361–1369, 2005

Reyntjens A, Gelders YG, Hoppenbrouwers M, et al: Thymostenic effects of ritanserin (R55 667), a centrally active serotonin-S2 receptor blocker. Drug Dev Res 8:205–211, 1986

Richelson E: Preclinical pharmacology of neuroleptics: focus on new generation compounds. J Clin Psychiatry 57:S4–S11, 1996

Robinson DG, Woerner MG, Napolitano B, et al: Randomized comparison of olanzapine versus risperidone for the treatment of first-episode schizophrenia: 4-month outcomes. Am J Psychiatry 163:2096–2102, 2006

Roose K, Gelders YG, Heylen S: Risperidone (R64766) in psychotic patients: a first clinical therapeutic exploration. Acta Psychiatr Belg 88:233–241, 1988

Rosenheck RA, Krystal JH, Lew R, et al: Long-acting risperidone and oral antipsychotics in unstable schizophrenia. CSP555 Research Group. N Engl J Med 364:842–851, 2011

Rummel-Kluge C, Komossa K, Schwarz S, et al: Head-to-head comparisons of metabolic side effects of second generation antipsychotics in the treatment of schizophrenia: a systematic review and meta-analysis. Schizophr Res 123:225–233, 2010

Saller CF, Czupryna MJ, Salama AI: 5-HT2 receptor blockade by ICI 169,369 and other 5-HT2 antagonists modulates the effects of D-2 dopamine receptor blockade. J Pharmacol Exp Ther 253:1162–1170, 1990

Schmidt CJ, Sorensen SM, Kehne JH: The role of 5-HT2A receptors in antipsychotic activity. Life Sci 56:2209–2222, 1995

Schneider LS, Tariot PN, Dagerman KS, et al: Effectiveness of atypical antipsychotic drugs in patients with Alzheimer's disease. CATIE-AD Study Group. N Engl J Med 355:1525–1538, 2006

Schotte A, Janssen P, Gommeren W, et al: Risperidone compared with new and reference antipsychotic drugs: in vitro and in vivo receptor binding. Psychopharmacology (Berl) 124:57–73, 1996

Seeman P: Atypical antipsychotics: mechanism of action. Can J Psychiatry 47:27–38, 2002

Sikich L, Frazier JA, McClellan J, et al: Double-blind comparison of first- and second-generation antipsychotics in early-onset schizophrenia and schizo-affective disorder: findings from the treatment of early-onset schizophrenia spectrum disorders (TEOSS) study. Am J Psychiatry 165:1420–1431, 2008; erratum in Am J Psychiatry 165:1495, 2008

Simpson GM, Mahmoud RA, Lasser RA, et al: A 1-year double-blind study of 2 doses of long-acting risperidone in stable patients with schizophrenia or schizoaffective disorder. J Clin Psychiatry 67:1194–1203, 2006

Spina E, Avenoso A, Scordo MG, et al: Inhibition of risperidone metabolism by fluoxetine in patients with schizophrenia: a clinically relevant pharmacokinetic drug interaction. J Clin Psychopharmacol 22:419–423, 2002

Stathis P, Antoniou K, Papadopoulou-Daifotis Z, et al: Risperidone: a novel antipsychotic with many "atypical" properties? Psychopharmacology (Berl) 127:181–186, 1996

Stroup TS, McEvoy JP, Swartz MS, et al: The National Institute of Mental Health Clinical Antipsychotic Trials of Intervention Effectiveness (CATIE) project: schizophrenia trial design and protocol development. Schizophr Bull 29:15–31, 2003

Stroup TS, Lieberman JA, McEvoy JP, et al: Effectiveness of olanzapine, quetiapine, risperidone, and ziprasidone in patients with chronic schizophrenia following discontinuation of a previous atypical antipsychotic. Am J Psychiatry 163:611–622, 2006

Stroup TS, Lieberman JA, McEvoy JP, et al: Effectiveness of olanzapine, quetiapine, and risperidone in patients with chronic schizophrenia after discontinuing perphenazine: a CATIE study. Am J Psychiatry 164:415–427, 2007

Svensson TH, Tung C-S, Grenhoff J: The 5-HT2 antagonist ritanserin blocks the effect of prefrontal cortex inactivation on rat A10 dopamine neurons in vivo. Acta Physiol Scand 136:497–498, 1989

Svensson TH, Mathe JM, Andersson JL, et al: Mode of action of atypical neuroleptics in relation to the phencyclidine model of schizophrenia: role of 5-HT2 receptor and alpha1-adrenoreceptor antagonism. J Clin Psychopharmacol 15:S11–S18, 1995

Tiihonen J, Haukka J, Taylor M, et al: A nationwide cohort study of oral and depot antipsychotics after first hospitalization for schizophrenia. Am J Psychiatry 168:603–609, 2011; erratum in Am J Psychiatry 169:223, 2012

Troost PW, Lahuis BE, Hermans MH, et al: Prolactin release in children treated with risperidone: impact and role of CYP2D6 metabolism. J Clin Psychopharmacol 27:52–57, 2007

Ugedo L, Grenhoff J, Svensson TH: Ritanserin, a 5-HT2 receptor antagonist, activates midbrain dopamine neurons by blocking serotonergic inhibition. Psychopharmacology (Berl) 98:45–50, 1989

Varty GB, Bakshi VP, Geyer MA: M100907, a serotonin 5-HT2A receptor antagonist and putative antipsychotic, blocks dizocilpine-induced prepulse inhibition deficits in Sprague-Dawley and Wistar rats. Neuropsychopharmacology 20:311–321, 1999

Volavka J, Czobor P, Sheitman B, et al: Clozapine, olanzapine, risperidone, and haloperidol in the treatment of patients with chronic schizophrenia and schizoaffective disorder. Am J Psychiatry 159:255–262, 2002

Wadenberg ML, Hicks PB, Richter JT, et al: Enhancement of antipsychotic properties of raclopride in rats using the selective serotonin 2A receptor antagonist MDL 100907. Biol Psychiatry 44:508–515, 1998

Wirshing DA, Barringer DMJ, Green MF, et al: Risperidone in treatment-refractory schizophrenia. Am J Psychiatry 156:1374–1379, 1999

CHAPTER 21

Ziprasidone

John W. Newcomer, M.D.

Martin T. Strassnig, M.D.

History and Discovery

Ziprasidone (CP-88059) is an atypical, or *second-generation*, antipsychotic agent that has activity for treating positive, negative, cognitive, and affective symptoms of schizophrenia and schizoaffective disorder and for treating mania and mixed states in bipolar disorder, with limited adverse extrapyramidal, sedative, anticholinergic, and cardiometabolic effects. First approved in 2001, this antipsychotic was initially part of a new drug application for the treatment of psychotic disorders submitted to the U.S. Food and Drug Administration (FDA) in 1997. Because of concerns regarding an increase in the mean duration of the QT interval, an electrocardiographic measure of the ventricular depolarization and repolarization phases of cardiac conduction, the application was not initially approved. Further studies, designed in collaboration with the FDA, quantified the limited extent of the QTc interval lengthening effect seen with ziprasidone compared with that seen with other agents in wide use; these studies established the safety of ziprasidone with respect to cardiac conduction and a benchmark for the approach to evaluating drug effects on the QT interval that has subsequently been applied to other agents evaluated by the FDA. Ziprasidone has received regulatory approval and is available in over 90 countries.

Pharmacological Profile

Neuropharmacology and Receptor-Binding Profile

Ziprasidone, or 5-[2-[4-(1,2-benzisothiazol-3-yl)-1-piperazinyl]ethyl]-6-chloro-1,3-dihydro-2*H*-indol-2-one, is a novel benzisothiazolyl-piperazine antipsychotic.

Ziprasidone is a potent antagonist at dopamine type 2 (D_2) receptors but possesses inverse agonist activity at 5-hydroxytryptamine (serotonin) type 2A receptors (5-HT_{2A} receptors). D_2 receptor antagonism is thought to be a key mechanism explaining efficacy for the treatment of psychotic symptoms (Kapur and Remington 2001); positron emission tomography (PET) studies have shown that clinical antipsychotic response to ziprasidone is predicted by occupancy of at least 60% of striatal D_2 receptors. D_2 antagonism is also associated with potential liability for extrapyramidal side effects (EPS). However, ziprasidone also has inverse agonist activity at 5-HT_{2A} receptors, an effect that can disinhibit dopamine neurotransmission in the nigrostriatal, mesocortical, and tuberoinfundibular pathways (Kapur and Remington 1996; Schmidt et al. 2001). This effect suggests a mechanism for reduced liability for EPS compared with antipsychotics with unopposed D_2 antagonism and may contribute to therapeutic effects. Increased dopamine activity in the prefrontal cortex is linked to efficacy in improving the negative and cognitive symptoms of schizophrenia (Stahl and Shayegan 2003). Enhanced dopaminergic transmission in the tuberoinfundibular pathway minimizes the potential effect of D_2 receptor antagonism on prolactin secretion. Ziprasidone's relatively high in vitro 5-HT_{2A}/D_2 receptor affinity ratio, compared with that of other second-generation antipsychotics (SGAs), predicts low liability for EPS and potential therapeutic benefits for negative symptoms (Altar et al. 1986).

Ziprasidone exhibits antagonist activity at 5-HT_{1D} and 5-HT_{2C} receptors and unusual (among SGAs) agonist activity at 5-HT_{1A} receptors (see Table 21–1) (DeLeon et al. 2004; Schmidt et al. 2001). The 5-HT_{1A} affinity is comparable to that of buspirone, an agent with antidepressant and anxiolytic properties (Mazei et al. 2002), suggesting a mechanism that may contribute to beneficial effects on affective, cognitive, and negative symptoms in schizophrenia and schizoaffective disorder (Diaz-Mataix et al. 2005; Ichikawa et al. 2001; Millan 2000; Rollema et al. 2000; Sumiyoshi et al. 2003; Tauscher et al. 2002). Blockade of 5-HT_{2C} receptors disinhibits both dopamine and norepinephrine neurons in the cortex, an effect that could contribute to improvements in cognitive and affective abnormalities (Bremner et al. 2003; Bymaster et al. 2002; Mazei et al. 2002; Stahl 2003).

Although 5-HT_{2C} antagonist activity might predict weight gain liability, based largely on a 5-HT_{2C} knockout mouse model of obesity (Tecott et al. 1995), clinically significant predictive effects of 5-HT_{2C} antagonist activity on the relative weight gain risk associated with antipsychotic drugs have not been reliably detected (Kroeze et al. 2003), and the weight gain risk associated with ziprasidone is among the lowest of currently available antipsychotics (Allison et al. 1999b). Potent antagonism at 5-HT_{1D} receptors has been proposed to potentially mediate antidepressant and anxiolytic effects (Briley and Moret 1993; Zorn et al. 1998).

Another important feature of ziprasidone is its relatively high affinity for serotonin and norepinephrine transporters (Seeger et al. 1995; Tatsumi et al. 1999). In vitro, ziprasidone demonstrates dose-dependent reuptake inhibition of serotonin and norepinephrine transport, with effects ranging up to those of imipramine and amitriptyline (Schmidt et al. 2001), suggesting potential antidepressant activity. In vivo, the clinical significance of ziprasidone's monoaminergic reuptake inhibition may be limited by plasma protein binding or may be clinically relevant only at daily dosages higher than those currently approved. Monoaminergic reuptake inhibition is associated with hippocampal neurogenesis, suggesting potential value in countering the neuronal cell loss observed in both affective illness and schizophrenia (Arango et al. 2001; Duman 2004; Thome et al. 1998). Relevant to this activity, treatment with ziprasidone or risperidone is associated with an increase in cortical gray matter volume (Garver et al. 2005).

Ziprasidone has a low affinity for histaminergic$_1$ (H_1), muscarinic$_1$ (M_1), and α_1-noradrenergic receptors. Among the biogenic amine receptors, H_1 antagonist activity is the largest predictor of weight gain liability (Kroeze et al. 2003). H_1 antagonist activity also predicts sedative effects, which are potentially undesirable for patients aiming to maximize cognitive performance and social, occupational, and community engagement. Low affinity for α_1-adrenergic receptors predicts a lower likelihood of orthostatic hypotension and sedation with ziprasidone than with commonly used antipsychotics with potent α_1-adrenergic antagonist activity. Low affinity for M_1 receptors predicts a low risk for anticholinergic side effects such as dry mouth, blurry vision, urinary retention, constipation, confusion, and memory impairment.

Ziprasidone's complex neuropharmacology provides explanatory support for observed treatment effects on psychotic and affective symptoms of schizophrenia, schizoaffective disorder, and bipolar disorder and for the observed favorable tolerability profile with minimal EPS and minimal metabolic side effects (Stahl and Shayegan 2003).

Positron Emission Tomography Studies

An in vivo PET study (Mamo et al. 2004) examining the affinity of ziprasidone for D_2 and 5-HT_2 receptors observed that optimal D_2 receptor occupancy occurs at the high end of ziprasidone's initially recommended dosage range. In this study, the ziprasidone plasma concentration associated with 50% of maximal D_2 receptor occupancy was more than twice the plasma concentration associated with 50% of maximal 5-HT_2 receptor occupancy. Using an imaging protocol where 60% or greater D_2 dopamine receptor occupancy is generally predictive of antipsychotic activity, approximately 60% D_2 occupancy was observed in relation to plasma concentrations equivalent to those attained with a dosage at or above 120 mg/day. These results, consistent with clinical trial results discussed later in this chapter (see "Indications and Efficacy"), suggest that antipsychotic activity with ziprasidone is most commonly associated with dosages of 120 mg/day or greater (Figure 21–1).

Dosing Recommendations

In addition to the PET data described, evidence from clinical trials suggests that ziprasidone target dosages should be higher than those originally recommended. In the United States, it was initially recommended that ziprasidone treatment in patients with schizophrenia be initiated at a dosage of 20 mg twice daily and then titrated at no less than 2-day intervals to a maximal dosage of 80 mg twice daily (Pfizer Inc. 2008). In contrast, more recent FDA approval of ziprasidone for the treatment of bipolar mania includes a recommendation that treatment be initiated at 40 mg twice daily with a more rapid titration; on the second day of treatment, the dosage should be increased to 60 or 80 mg twice daily, with subsequent adjustment on the basis of tolerability and efficacy within a 40- to 80-mg twice-daily range.

Daily ziprasidone dosages of 120–160 mg are observed to be more effective than lower dosages in the treatment of acute schizophrenia (Kane et al. 2003) and bipolar disorders (Citrome et al. 2009b) in adults and also are associated with lower rates of medication discontinuation (Citrome et al. 2009c). A 6-month prospective, observational, naturalistic, uncontrolled study in Spain observed that dosages greater than 120 mg/day were associated with a lower risk of discontinuation for any cause (Arango et al. 2007). In an analysis of commercial and Medicare prescription databases, Citrome et al. (2009a) observed significantly lower discontinuation rates among schizophrenia and bipolar disorder patients receiving ziprasidone in the 120–160 mg/day dose range compared with those receiving ziprasidone at lower doses. Similarly, a European observational multicenter trial found that initial and overall underdosing of ziprasidone are associated with high discontinuation rates (Kudla et al. 2007), and a pooled analysis of both flexible-dose and fixed-dose studies (N=2,174) observed greater efficacy in patients who received an initial dosage of 80 mg/day compared with patients who received an initial dosage of 40 mg/day (Murray et al. 2004).

Finally, two large observational database analyses suggested that higher dosages of ziprasidone are associated with better treat-

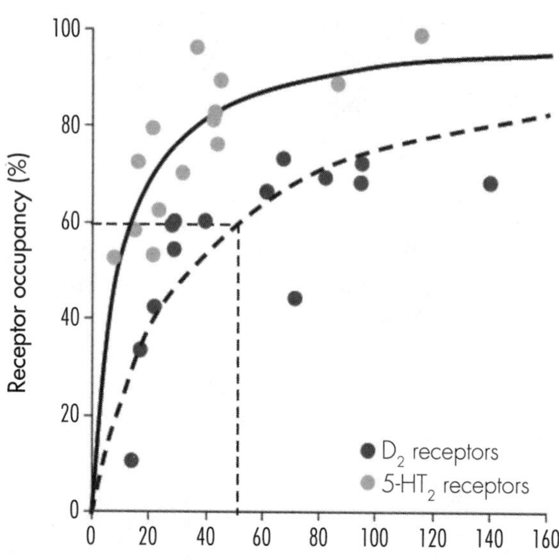

FIGURE 21–1. Relationship between dopamine$_2$ (D_2) and serotonin$_2$ (5-HT_2) receptor occupancy and ziprasidone plasma levels in 16 patients with schizophrenia or schizoaffective disorder receiving therapeutic dosages of ziprasidone.

Dotted straight lines represent minimal D_2 receptor occupancy and plasma concentration that would be expected to be associated with a clinical antipsychotic response, corresponding to a ziprasidone dosage of approximately 120 mg/day.

Source. Adapted from Mamo et al. 2004.

ment outcomes than lower dosages (Joyce et al. 2006; Mullins et al. 2006). Both studies used prescription refills as an indicator of prescription adherence. Joyce et al. (2006) examined records from more than 1,000 commercially insured patients with schizophrenia or schizoaffective disorder and concluded that an initial daily dosage of 120–160 mg was associated with a significantly lower risk of medication discontinuation at 6 months than an initial daily dosage of 60–80 mg. Mullins et al. (2006) evaluated more than 1,000 Medicaid recipients with schizophrenia and similarly concluded that patients receiving an initial dosage of 120–160 mg daily had lower rates of medication discontinuation than patients receiving 20–60 mg daily. Reported clinical experience with ziprasidone has also suggested the need for dosages greater than 160 mg/day in selected patients (Citrome et al. 2009a; Harvey and Bowie 2005; Nemeroff et al. 2005).

Taken together, results from receptor occupancy studies, clinical trials, and pharmacoepidemiological analyses support the conclusion that initiation and treatment with ziprasidone dosages greater than 120 mg/day, titrated rapidly, are more likely to be effective than lower dosages in the treatment of schizophrenia, schizoaffective disorder, and bipolar disorder.

Pharmacokinetics and Disposition

Absorption and Distribution

Based on evidence of enhanced absorption in the presence of food, it is recommended that oral ziprasidone be taken with meals of at least 500 kcal to avoid substantial reduction in drug absorption (Gandelman et al. 2009) that cannot be effectively compensated for by increased dose (Citrome 2009). Administration with food increases absorption by more than 50%, giving ziprasidone an oral bioavailability of approximately 60% (Pfizer Inc. 2008). Maximal plasma concentration (C_{max}) is achieved within 3.7–4.7 hours and reaches 45–139 μg/L in healthy volunteers receiving 20–60 mg twice daily, and steady-state serum concentrations occur within 1–3 days of twice-daily dosing (Hamelin et al. 1998; Miceli et al. 2000c). In contrast to oral administration, intramuscular administration of ziprasidone results in 100% bioavailability. A therapeutic plasma level is reached within 10 minutes, and C_{max} is achieved within 30 minutes of administration of a 20-mg dose (Pfizer Inc. 2008).

The mean apparent volume of distribution of ziprasidone is 1.5 L/kg (Pfizer Inc. 2008), which is lower than that of many other antipsychotic drugs. Given the wider potential for unwanted interactions with various intracellular targets that has been observed with lipophilic drugs having a high volume of distribution (Dwyer et al. 1999), this may be a favorable attribute for ziprasidone and other similar compounds. Ziprasidone is more than 99% bound to plasma proteins.

Metabolism and Elimination

Ziprasidone is extensively metabolized with a mean terminal elimination half-life of approximately 7 hours after oral administration within the recommended clinical dosage range (Pfizer Inc. 2008). The elimination half-life of intramuscular ziprasidone is less than 3 hours with a single dose (Brook et al. 2000). Ziprasidone is cleared primarily via three metabolic pathways to yield four major circulating metabolites. Elimination occurs primarily through hepatic metabolism, with less than one-third of metabolic clearance mediated via cytochrome P450 (CYP)–catalyzed oxidation and approximately two-thirds via reduction of the parent compound by aldehyde oxidase to dihydroziprasidone, which then undergoes S-methylation. The literature reports no commonly encountered clinically significant pharmacological inhibitors of aldehyde oxidase, suggesting limited real-world potential for drug-drug interactions that would alter the clinical activity of ziprasidone (Obach et al. 2004).

Additional secondary metabolic pathways include *N*-dealkylation (via CYP enzymes 3A4 and 1A2) and direct *S*-oxidation (via CYP3A4) (Beedham et al. 2003; Prakash et al. 2000). *S*-methyl-dihydroziprasidone is the only active metabolite, with lower D_2 receptor affinity and no significant binding to H_1, M_1, or α_1- and α_2-adrenergic receptors. A small amount of the parent compound is excreted unchanged in the urine (<1%) and feces (<4%).

There are no clinically significant age- or gender-related differences in the pharmacokinetics of oral ziprasidone (Pfizer Inc. 2008). Hepatic impairment might be expected to increase the area under the time-concentration curve (AUC). A multiple-dose study (Everson et al. 2000) comparing subjects with clinically significant (Child-Pugh Class A and B) cirrhosis versus healthy control subjects indicated that 12 hours after administration of ziprasidone, the AUC was 13% and 34% greater in subjects with Child-Pugh Class A and B cirrhosis, respectively, than in matched control subjects, suggesting that dose adjustments are generally not mandatory for patients with hepatic impairment. Impairment in renal function is unlikely to significantly alter the pharmacokinetics of oral ziprasidone, suggesting that ziprasidone would not be removed by hemodialysis (Pfizer Inc. 2008). Intramuscular ziprasidone has not been systematically evaluated in the elderly or in patients with hepatic or renal impairment. Intramuscular ziprasidone contains a cyclodextrin excipient that is cleared by renal filtration; thus, it should be administered with caution to patients with impaired renal function (Pfizer Inc. 2008).

Impact of Food on Pharmacokinetics

Pharmacokinetic studies have examined ziprasidone bioavailability under fasting conditions and after eating food with varying caloric and fat composition to better understand effects of food intake on drug availability (Gandelman et al. 2009; Lombardo et al. 2007). In an open-label, nonrandomized, six-way crossover study, healthy adults received single doses of ziprasidone under fasting conditions and then under fed conditions with a standard meal of 800–1,000 calories. Dose-proportional increases in ziprasidone AUC and C_{max} were observed under fed but not fasting conditions. C_{max} was significantly higher in fed states than in fasting states at doses of 40 mg (63% higher) and 80 mg (97% higher). Results from two additional open-label crossover studies further clarified the factors regulating drug bioavailability (Gandelman et al. 2009; Lombardo et al. 2007) and indicated that 1) medium-calorie meals (500 calories) are associated with ziprasidone exposure close to the exposure that can be achieved with high-calorie meals (1,000 calories) and nearly twice the exposure observed under fasting conditions, and 2) absorption is not significantly influenced by the fat content of the meal. These studies suggest that the administration of ziprasidone with even a low-fat meal of at least 500 calories provides linear pharmacokinetics and optimal absorption. In addition, the results suggest that total meal bulk sufficient to slow gastric and duodenal transit time (e.g., a bowl of oatmeal), rather than fat content or specific calorie counts, may be the key factor contributing to reliable dose-dependent drug absorption with meals.

Drug-Drug Interactions

A study of in vitro enzyme inhibition (Pfizer Inc. 2008) indicated that ziprasidone has little inhibitory effect on CYP1A2, CYP2C9, CYP2C19, CYP2D6, and CYP3A4 and is thus unlikely to interfere with the metabolism of other medications relying on these enzymes for clearance. In vivo studies indicated that ziprasidone has no effect on the pharmacokinetics of lithium, estrogen, progesterone, or dextromethorphan (Pfizer Inc. 2008). As noted above (in "Metabolism and Elimination" subsection), less than one-third of ziprasidone clearance is mediated by CYP-catalyzed oxidation, and based on this, one would not anticipate a substantial change in ziprasidone AUC during coadministration with CYP3A4 inhibitors or inducers. Aldehyde oxidase–mediated reduction constitutes the primary metabolic pathway for ziprasidone. As also noted above, currently no clinically significant pharmacological inhibitors of aldehyde oxidase are commonly encountered (Obach et al. 2004).

Consistent with this prediction, coadministration of ziprasidone with ketoconazole, a potent CYP3A4 inhibitor, results in only a modest increase in ziprasidone AUC (33%) and C_{max} (34%) (Miceli et al. 2000b), whereas coadministration with carbamazepine, an inducer of 3A4, results in modest reductions in ziprasidone AUC (44%) and C_{max} (39%) (Miceli et al. 2000a). Coadministration with CYP2D6 inhibitors has no effect on ziprasidone plasma levels. Coadministration of ziprasidone with lithium results in no significant change in steady-state lithium levels (Apseloff et al. 2000), and commonly used antacids and cimetidine do not significantly alter ziprasidone pharmacokinetics (Pfizer Inc. 2008).

Indications and Efficacy

Schizophrenia and Schizoaffective Disorder

Acute Treatment

Ziprasidone is indicated for the acute treatment of schizophrenia and schizoaffective disorder. Its efficacy in the treatment of hospitalized patients with acute schizophrenia or schizoaffective disorder has been demonstrated in a series of double-blind, placebo-controlled trials of 4–6 weeks' duration (Daniel et al. 1999; Kane 2003; Keck et al. 1998; Keck et al. 2001). Additional short-term (4- to 8-week) randomized, double-blind treatment studies using active antipsychotic comparator agents have indicated that ziprasidone has efficacy comparable to that of haloperidol, risperidone, and olanzapine for the treatment of positive symptoms and overall psychopathology (Addington et al. 2004; Goff et al. 1998; Simpson et al. 2004a). In a pooled analysis of four short-term placebo-controlled trials and three active-comparator trials, Murray et al. (2004) demonstrated that ziprasidone dosages of at least 120 mg/day, in comparison with lower dosages, are associated with a more rapid and favorable response in overall psychopathology as well as a lower discontinuation rate due to inadequate clinical response, suggesting the importance of rapid titration to at least 120 mg/day (Kane 2003; McCue et al. 2006).

Suboptimal dosing, inadequate titration regimens, and failure to administer ziprasidone with food may have negatively affected its performance in some clinical trials. Some clinical trials included efficacy analyses on dosages that would now be considered suboptimal (i.e., <120 mg/day), whereas other studies used prolonged titration of ziprasidone, only reaching a therapeutic dosage 1 week or more into the study. Clinical trials conducted before the release of pharmacokinetic data by Lombardo et al. (2007) may not have been designed to ensure that ziprasidone was administered with food for optimal oral absorption.

Ziprasidone has also been studied in the treatment of early psychosis and schizophrenia. Johnsen et al. (2010) consecutively randomized early psychosis patients admitted to the emergency ward to different SGAs, including ziprasidone, olanzapine, quetiapine, and risperidone. No clinically significant differences in effectiveness of the tested antipsychotics emerged after a 2-year follow-up period.

A series of meta-analyses has found no robust or consistent differences among the SGAs, either when comparing agents within the same class or when comparing SGAs with first-generation antipsychotics (FGAs) (Bagnall et al. 2003; Geddes et al. 2000; Leucht et al. 1999; Srisurapanont and Maneeton 1999; Tandon and Fleischhacker 2005). One meta-analysis of randomized, controlled trials by Davis et al. (2003) suggested that although some SGAs (i.e., clozapine, risperidone, olanzapine, and amisulpride) were significantly more efficacious than FGAs, ziprasidone was not. It is important to note that this meta-analysis excluded data relating to low dosages of other antipsychotics (olanzapine <11 mg/day and risperidone <4 mg/day) but included data on ziprasidone dosages as low as 80 mg/day. In addition, the Davis et al. meta-analysis included relatively few studies of ziprasidone (4 studies as compared with 31 studies of clozapine, 22 studies of risperidone, and 14 studies of olanzapine), leaving significance testing for this agent more vulnerable to issues associated with individual studies.

Using Medicaid claims data, Olfson et al. (2012) compared the effectiveness (as measured by rates of medication discontinuation and hospital admission) of commonly prescribed SGA medications in child and adolescent outpatients with schizophrenia or related disorders. Most youth (defined as 6–17 years of age) treated with quetiapine (70.7%), ziprasidone (73.3%), olanzapine (73.1%), risperidone (74.4%), or aripiprazole (76.5%) discontinued the medication within the first 180 days following medication initiation. Studies like these underscore both the comparable effectiveness among SGA agents and the high discontinuation rates associated with available treatments, the latter in part related to unwanted medication-induced adverse events. The favorable side-effect profile of ziprasidone recommends it as an important first-line option in the treatment of early psychosis.

Maintenance Therapy

The maintenance efficacy of ziprasidone in treating schizophrenia and schizoaffective disorder has been studied in a series of double-blind and open-label extension trials (Arato et al. 2002; Hirsch et al. 2002; Kane et al. 2003; Schooler 2003; Simpson et al. 2002, 2004b). These studies indicate that long-term therapy with ziprasidone maintains clinical response and is effective in preventing relapse.

Maintenance of effect. In two maintenance-of-effect studies, patients with schizophrenia or schizoaffective disorder who had previously demonstrated acute response to treatment (defined as a ≥20% decrease in Positive and Negative Syndrome Scale [PANSS] for schizophrenia total score and a Clinical Global Impression [CGI] Scale score of ≤2) were randomly assigned to receive either ziprasidone or a comparator antipsychotic agent for at least 26 weeks (Addington et al. 2009; Schooler 2003; Simpson et al. 2002, 2005). In both of these studies, the ziprasidone treatment groups demonstrated significant improvements from baseline in overall psychopathology, as measured by mean changes in symptom ratings using PANSS total, PANSS negative subscale, Brief Psychiatric Rating Scale–Depression Factor (BPRSd), and CGI–Severity (CGI-S) scores. These improvements were comparable to those seen in the olanzapine (Simpson et al. 2005) and risperidone (Addington et al. 2009) treatment groups.

Relapse prevention. To evaluate the efficacy of ziprasidone for relapse prevention, the Ziprasidone Extended Use in Schizophrenia study enrolled stable inpatients with chronic schizophrenia and randomly assigned participants to 1 year of treatment with ziprasidone 40 mg/day (n=72), 80 mg/day (n=68), or 160 mg/day (n=67) or placebo (n=71), with a planned primary Kaplan-Meier analysis of time to relapse (Arato et al. 2002). In this study, all three dosages of ziprasidone were superior to placebo in the prevention of relapse. In addition, a penultimate-observation-carried-forward analysis (in which the last visit prior to relapse is excluded) was performed to filter out clinical worsening associated with relapse that might otherwise obscure symptom response trends during the rest of maintenance therapy (O'Connor and Schooler 2003), which indicated that nonrelapsing patients treated with ziprasidone experienced modest symptomatic improvement during maintenance treatment. This study, like a number of other studies of other antipsychotic agents in schizophrenia patients, was limited by the relatively high level of attrition observed in all groups over the year of treatment.

Long-term response to treatment in symptomatic patients. A number of long-term double-blind trials designed to examine the efficacy of ziprasidone in symptomatic patients with schizophrenia have been performed (Breier et al. 2005; Hirsch et al. 2002; Kinon et al. 2006; Simpson et al. 2004a, 2005). Investigators (Hirsch et al. 2002) have compared the efficacy of ziprasidone (n=148) and haloperidol (n=153) in a 28-week double-blind trial of stable outpatients with schizophrenia with prominent negative symptoms. In this study, ziprasidone and haloperidol were similarly efficacious in reducing overall psychopathology, with an advantage for ziprasidone in the percentage of patients classified as negative symptom responders. Breier et al. (2005) conducted a 28-week study of ziprasidone and olanzapine in outpatients as well as inpatients (N=548) with active symptoms. In this study, olanzapine treatment was associated with greater improvement from baseline in total psychopathology scores (PANSS total, the primary efficacy measure) than ziprasidone and a higher rate of criterion-level response to treatment. Simpson et al. (2004a) conducted a 6-week double-blind, parallel-design flexible-dose comparison (N=269) of ziprasidone (n=136) and olanzapine ($n = 133$) where at least minimal responders (CGI-I score ≤2 or ≥20% reduction in PANSS total score) were enrolled in a 6-month double-blind continuation trial (Simpson et al. 2005). In both the 6-week and the 6-month analyses, no differences between the treatment groups were detected on any primary (e.g., Brief Psychiatric Rating Scale [BPRS] total, CGI severity) or secondary (e.g., PANSS total, CGI-I) measures.

Potkin et al. (2009) compared the effects of ziprasidone and haloperidol in a 196-week double-blind study using the Andreasen criteria for remission by longitudinal analysis. During the initial 40-week study, no differences in PANSS or Global Assessment of Functioning Scale (GAF) score changes between the two antipsychotics compared emerged. In a subsequent 3-year extension study, ziprasidone-treated subjects were more likely to achieve remission (51%) compared with haloperidol-treated subjects (40%). The PANSS total and GAF score trajectories favored the higher 80–160 mg/day ziprasidone dosage as opposed to lower dosages, and the superior outcome for ziprasidone versus haloperidol may in part be due to tolerability and adherence advantages.

Clinical effectiveness. There have been a number of effectiveness trials involving ziprasidone and using various definitions for *effectiveness*. The Clinical Antipsychotic Trials of Intervention Effectiveness (CATIE) studies, funded by the National Institute of Mental Health (NIMH), included a long-term, double-blind, randomized study of patients with schizophrenia ($N = 1{,}493$; Lieberman et al. 2005). Phase I of the CATIE schizophrenia study compared ziprasidone, olanzapine, quetiapine, risperidone, and perphenazine on a primary endpoint of time to discontinuation for lack of efficacy or for any cause. Because of the timing of its FDA approval, ziprasidone was added to the study after enrollment had begun for all other treatment arms; this resulted in a smaller sample size for the ziprasidone treatment arm and some limitations regarding conclusions about ziprasidone in phase I of the study.

The primary analysis for the phase I study detected significant differences in time to discontinuation across the treatment groups overall. The longest time to discontinuation was in the olanzapine group. In the total study sample, no significant differences were seen in the time to discontinuation between the ziprasidone and olanzapine treatment groups, nor between the ziprasidone group and other antipsychotic treatment groups.

Several considerations in this complex study are worth mentioning. Very few patients who entered the CATIE schizophrenia study were currently (i.e., prior to study entry) taking the relatively newly available medication, ziprasidone, compared with the number of patients taking the other antipsychotic medications in the trial. This resulted in a larger proportion of patients assigned to the ziprasidone treatment arm who were just starting to take a new medication and discontinuing their prior treatment. For example, 23% of subjects randomly assigned to olanzapine treatment were already receiving olanzapine monotherapy as their ongoing treatment, requiring no medication discontinuation or new drug initiation. Supplemental analysis of phase I CATIE data by Essock et al. (2006) indicated the overall importance, in terms of subsequent discontinuation rates, of whether randomized subjects were switching medications or whether the study randomization allowed them to continue receiving their prior treatment. A significantly higher rate of subsequent discontinuation was observed in patients who actually made a medication switch compared with those who were randomly assigned to stay with the same medication they had been taking prior to the trial. This effect of switching medications therefore favored treatment arms with a larger percentage of "nonswitchers" (i.e., olanzapine and risperidone recipients in the CATIE phase I study). In a reanalysis of phase I CATIE data that excluded those patients randomly assigned to continue taking the antipsychotic that they were already taking at baseline, Essock et al. (2006) found that differences between rates of discontinuation in the ziprasidone group and rates in the other antipsychotic groups were attenuated, and no statistically significant differences in the primary outcome measure were observed for any agent.

The Ziprasidone Experience in Schizophrenia in Germany/Austria (ZEISIG) study investigated the effectiveness of ziprasidone as measured by discontinuation rates and mean changes of the BPRS total in moderately ill and reasonably stable patients (N= 276) with schizophrenia or schizoaffective disorder (Kudla et al. 2007). Approximately 60% of subjects discontinued ziprasidone prematurely, most within the first 4 weeks of study treatment. In study completers, ziprasidone was associated with significant improvements in BPRS total score. The relatively high rate of discontinuation may be explained in part by the planned dosing strategy. In this study, ziprasidone use was initiated at a low dosage of 40 mg/day, which is now known to be associated with higher discontinuation rates and shorter durations of therapy compared with higher dosages (Joyce et al. 2006; Mullins et al. 2006). The maximal dosage allowed was 160 mg/day, which may be insufficient for some patients (Harvey and Bowie 2005; Nemeroff et al. 2005).

Arango et al. (2007), of the Ziprasidone in Spain Study Group, examined the effectiveness of ziprasidone (n=1,022 in the primary analysis sample) as measured by response rate (defined as a ≥30% reduction in the PANSS total score). Nearly half of the patients experienced the defined level of clinical response, and patients overall had significant and clinically relevant mean reductions in both the PANSS total score and the positive, negative, and general psychopathology subscale scores (effect sizes were 1.60, 1.83, 0.62, and 1.40, respectively). Ziprasidone dosages of greater than 120 mg/day were associated with a lower risk of discontinuation for any cause.

Diaz-Marsa et al. (2009) conducted a prospective, uncontrolled, naturalistic study to evaluate the effectiveness and tolerability of oral ziprasidone in psychiatric inpatients with an acute exacerbation of schizophrenia or schizoaffective disorder. Among the 196 patients enrolled, the mean dosage of ziprasidone at discharge was 186.3±67.7 mg/day. Progressive and statistically significant improvements in BPRS- and CGI-measured symptom severity were observed from the first week through discharge (after 23.4 ± 34.2 days). Changes from baseline to study endpoint were deemed clinically relevant, with reported effect sizes greater than d=0.8, indicating that the results are of notable clinical—not just statistical—significance.

The European First Episode Schizophrenia Trial (EUFEST; Kahn et al. 2008) included 49 sites in Europe and Israel and assessed 498 first-episode patients ages 18–40 years who had experienced psychosis for less than 2 years, had been exposed to antipsychotic drugs for less than 2 weeks during the preceding year, and had less than 6 weeks of total lifetime exposure to antipsychotic drugs. Participants were randomly assigned to haloperidol (which served as the FGA comparator) 1–4 mg/day, amisulpride 200–800 mg/day, olanzapine 5–20 mg/day, quetiapine 200–750 mg/day, or ziprasidone 40–160 mg/day and were followed up for 1 year. Analysis of all-cause treatment discontinuation revealed rates of 40% for haloperidol, 40% for amisulpride, 33% for olanzapine, 53% for quetiapine, and 45% for ziprasidone. Symptom reductions were similar in all groups, approximately 60%. In addition to efficacy considerations, tolerability differences—whether due to different pharmacological profiles or to patient preferences—should guide the clinician in choosing an appropriate first-line treatment.

Efficacy by Symptom Type

Efficacy for cognitive symptoms of schizophrenia. The effect of ziprasidone on cognitive function in schizophrenia patients was evaluated by a battery of cognitive tests included in a double-blind olanzapine comparator study that evaluated changes at 6 weeks and 6 months (Harvey et al. 2004, 2006a). Antipsychotic treatment with ziprasidone and with olanzapine both resulted in significant cognitive improvements from baseline in attention memory, working memory, motor speed, and executive functions, with olanzapine also associated with improvement in verbal fluency. Further improvements in both treatment groups were observed from the end of 6 weeks to the 6-month assessment time point on verbal learning, executive functioning, and verbal fluency, with no differences between treatment groups. It should be noted that despite these improvements, a substantial proportion of patients studied continued to experience clinically significant cognitive impairment posttreatment. Neuropsychological improvements in general are not related to clinical changes (Harvey et al. 2006b).

Data from the CATIE schizophrenia study indicate that treatment with all of the antipsychotics tested (i.e., ziprasidone, perphenazine, olanzapine, risperidone, and quetiapine) was associated with a small but significant improvement in neurocognition after 2 months of treatment, with no significant difference between ziprasidone and the other antipsychotics (Keefe et al. 2007). Neurocognitive improvement predicted a longer time to treatment discontinuation, independent of symptom improvement, in patients treated with quetiapine or ziprasidone.

Efficacy for affective symptoms. Ziprasidone has been hypothesized to be a promising treatment for affective disorders, based on its unique in vitro potency as a serotonin and norepinephrine reuptake inhibitor comparable to that of known antidepressants (see "Neuropharmacology and Receptor-Binding Profile" section above). Addressing the question of ziprasidone's potential antidepressant efficacy in schizophrenia patients with comorbid affective symptoms, data can be examined from randomized, double-blind, placebo-controlled clinical trials (Daniel et al. 1999; Keck et al. 1998; Keck et al. 2001) and from double-blind, head-to-head trials comparing ziprasidone to risperidone or olanzapine (Kane 2003). The results of placebo-controlled studies (Daniel et al. 1999; Keck et al. 1998) suggest that treatment of schizophrenia and schizoaffective disorder with ziprasidone is associated with significant improvement in comorbid depressive symptoms, based on intent-to-treat analyses, but sometimes only in the subset of patients with higher levels of baseline depression. The baseline severity of depressive symptoms in these studies tends to be relatively mild, so subgroups of patients with more pronounced comorbid depressive symptoms at baseline were also analyzed; the antidepressant effect of ziprasidone is larger than that of placebo in these analyses. In the two active-comparator studies, improvement in depression and anxiety symptoms in patients receiving ziprasidone was comparable to the improvement in olanzapine recipients but greater than the improvement in risperidone recipients. A smaller study (Kinon et al. 2006) compared the efficacy of olanzapine and ziprasidone over 24 weeks in the treatment of schizophrenia or schizoaffective disorder patients with prominent depressive symptoms. Both treatment groups had significant improvements in depressive symptoms for the first 8 weeks, with olanzapine-treated patients showing significantly greater improvements in depressive symptoms at study endpoint. However, the interpretation of this study is limited by that fact that a substantial number of patients (52.8% of $N=394$ at study entry) received concurrent treatment with nonstandardized antidepressants. These overall results provide preliminary evidence suggesting that ziprasidone, like some other antipsychotic agents, may be effective in treating comorbid depressive symptoms in patients with schizophrenia and schizoaffective disorder.

Efficacy for social deficits and improvement in quality of life. The NIMH CATIE study is the largest trial to date to have examined the effect of ziprasidone and other antipsychotics on psychosocial functioning in patients with schizophrenia (Swartz et al. 2007). This study employed the Quality of Life Scale, a widely used clinician-rated measurement (Heinrichs et al. 1984), to assess changes in social functioning, interpersonal relationships, vocational functioning, and psychological well-being. One-third of the patients in the phase I study antipsychotic treatment groups made modest improvements on the Quality of Life Scale from baseline to the 12-month endpoint (average effect size, 0.19 standard deviation units), with no significant differences between the agents.

The effect of ziprasidone on social functioning has also been evaluated using the prosocial subscale of the PANSS, including items related to active and passive social avoidance, emotional withdrawal, stereotypical thinking, and suspiciousness (Purnine et al. 2000). In three separate but related studies from one group, stable patients taking FGAs, olanzapine, or risperidone were switched to ziprasidone and followed for 6 weeks with ratings of safety, efficacy, and effectiveness (Weiden et al. 2003b). Six weeks of treatment with ziprasidone in all three prior-treatment groups resulted in significant improvement on the PANSS prosocial subscale (Loebel et al. 2004). The interpretation of results as being specific to ziprasidone use, rather than being simply an effect of extended, closely monitored treatment, is complicated by the absence of a control other than pretreatment baseline ratings.

Harvey et al. (2009) examined quality-of-life changes in community-dwelling patients with schizophrenia randomly assigned to either haloperidol ($n=47$) or ziprasidone ($n=139$) over a follow-up interval of up to 196 weeks. Long-term treatment with ziprasidone was associated with greater functional gains than treatment with haloperidol. Both treatment retention and functional gains favored ziprasidone in this long-term study, suggesting superior efficacy and tolerability, which may reflect back favorably on adherence rates. Post hoc analysis revealed the most significant quality-of-life improvements in the high-dose ziprasidone group (80–160 mg/day) (Stahl et al. 2010b), concordant with recent recommendations that higher doses of ziprasidone may be more effective than lower doses.

Treatment-Resistant Schizophrenia

Several studies have evaluated ziprasidone use in refractory schizophrenia, albeit using different criteria for "refractory." A 12-week double-blind comparison of ziprasidone and chlorpromazine ($N=306$ patients) defined treatment-resistant status as failure to achieve criterion-level response after 6 weeks of prospective treatment with haloperidol (Kane et al. 2005). The mean daily dose of ziprasidone at study endpoint was approximately 154 mg, compared with a mean daily chlorpromazine dose of approximately 744 mg. Treatment with ziprasidone produced significantly greater improvement at endpoint in PANSS negative subscale scores compared with chlorpromazine. In addition, ziprasidone treatment was associated with a 1.3-fold higher likelihood of achieving a 50% reduction in BPRS total score compared with chlorpromazine treatment. The Monitoring Oral Ziprasidone As Rescue Therapy (MOZART) study in neuroleptic-resistant/intolerant patients (Sacchetti et al. 2009), an 18-week randomized, flexible-dose, double-blind trial, evaluated ziprasidone as an alternative to clozapine in treatment-refractory schizophrenia. Patients had a history of resistance and/or intolerance to at least three acute cycles of different antipsychotic medications given at therapeutic doses with persistent PANSS total scores of at least 80. Patients were randomly assigned to receive ziprasidone 80–160 mg/day or clozapine 250–600 mg/day. A progressive and significant reduction from baseline in PANSS total score was observed from day 11 in both study arms, without between-drug differences and with similar rates of early discontinuation due to adverse events. Ziprasidone had a more tolerable metabolic profile in the short-term treatment.

A small amount of literature suggests that the addition of a second antipsychotic medication to clozapine in patients who do not respond or cannot tolerate standard doses of clozapine may provide additional benefits. In the context of safety concerns and increasing health care costs, there is currently limited empirical evidence for the efficacy and safety of such antipsychotic combinations (Kreyenbuhl et al. 2008). However, adjunctive treatment with ziprasidone or risperidone, for example, was found helpful in patients with refractory schizophrenia incompletely responsive to clozapine (Zink et al. 2009). Both adjunctive antipsychotics produced additional reductions of PANSS-measured positive and negative symptom scores after 6 weeks of treatment, and the intervention was well tolerated. Further investigations are needed before definitive recommendations can be made, and treatment resistance should be operationalized uniformly so as to facilitate comparative research.

Switching From Other Antipsychotics

The efficacy of ziprasidone has been found to be comparable to that of other SGAs and FGAs during both acute and maintenance treatment of schizophrenia and schizoaffective disorder. Evidence also points to the safety—particularly the cardiometabolic safety—of ziprasidone compared with other antipsychotics (see "Side Effects and Toxicology" section). These results support interest in switching from antipsychotic treatment with other agents to treatment with ziprasidone.

Several open-label, medication-switching studies evaluated strategies for switching from other antipsychotics to ziprasidone on measures of efficacy, safety, and tolerability, including the effect of different titration schedules on the outcome (Weiden et al. 2003b). In each study, patients were randomly assigned to one of three switching strategies to be completed in 1 week: 1) immediate discontinuation of the previous antipsychotic and immediate starting of ziprasidone the next day; 2) lowering the dose of the previous antipsychotic by half while simultaneously starting ziprasidone; or 3) overlapping the start of ziprasidone with the full dosage of the prior antipsychotic and then gradually reducing the prior antipsychotic dosage after 4 days of ziprasidone therapy.

For these switching strategies, the starting dosage of ziprasidone was 80 mg/day (40 mg twice daily), with subsequent dosage adjustments based on clinical judgment. In one study, patients taking high-potency FGAs such as haloperidol ($N = 108$) were switched to ziprasidone. In the second study, patients ($N = 58$) were switched from risperidone to ziprasidone. In the third study, patients ($N = 104$) were switched from olanzapine to ziprasidone. Discontinuation rates were low in all three studies, ranging from 2%–6% for lack of efficacy to 6%–9% for adverse events. In study completers, statistically significant improvements were observed on PANSS total, PANSS positive subscale, PANSS negative subscale, and BPRS total scores. Different switching strategies were not associated with a different likelihood of trial completion or different magnitude of clinical response.

Rossi et al. (2011) examined pooled data from 10 previously completed "switch" studies involving a total of 1,395 patients who were switched to ziprasidone. Switching from FGAs or other SGAs generally resulted in maintenance or improvement of efficacy across all studied symptom domains, including improvements in tolerability and acute and long-term benefits regarding cardiometabolic parameters. The recommended titration schedule was a "plateau cross-titration strategy," which the authors described as rapid up-titration of ziprasidone to a dose range of 60–80 mg administered twice daily with food. To facilitate the crossover and minimize patient discomfort, temporary coadministration of benzodizaepines, anticholinergics, or beta-blockers was recommended for management of potential rebound effects due to differences in pharmacological profiles of the pre-switch medications and ziprasidone.

The balance of the evidence from studies examining strategies for switching to ziprasidone favors rapid uptitration of ziprasidone to a comparatively higher dosage (up to 160 mg/day) combined with rapid discontinuation of the previous agent, including management of specific rebound effects, combined with close clinical monitoring during the switch. Predictable changes in tolerability (e.g., weight loss when switched from olanzapine, reduction in EPS when switched from haloperidol) are observed along with maintenance of efficacy.

Bipolar Disorder

Acute Mania

Ziprasidone has received regulatory approval (e.g., by the FDA) for the acute treatment of bipolar mania, with efficacy for acute mania demonstrated in two double-blind, placebo-controlled trials, each 3 weeks in duration, in patients with bipolar I disorder (Keck et al. 2003b; Potkin et al. 2005). In both studies, onset of action was rapid (within 48 hours) and sustained through 3 weeks of treatment in patients with bipolar mania or bipolar mixed states, with or without psychotic symptoms (results of Keck et al. [2003b] are shown in Figure 21–2). At endpoint, approximately half of the treated patients from both studies met response criteria for mania (≥50% reduction in Mania Rating Scale [MRS] scores).

A number of placebo-controlled trials evaluating the efficacy of short-term monotherapy with various antipsychotics, including haloperidol, ziprasidone, olanzapine, risperidone, quetiapine, and aripiprazole, have demonstrated comparable improvement in symptoms of mania (Bowden et al. 2005; Hirschfeld et al. 2004; Keck et al. 2003a, 2003b; Khanna et al. 2005; McIntyre et al. 2005; McQuade et al. 2003; Potkin et al. 2005; Sachs et al. 2006; Smulevich et al. 2005; Tohen et al. 1999, 2000; Vieta et al. 2010; Weisler et al. 2003). Two large meta-analyses of randomized, placebo-controlled trials have examined the relative efficacy of various SGAs for the adjunctive treatment of mania (Perlis et al. 2006; Scherk et al. 2007). Although the statistical results of the two meta-analyses are similar, the authors of each study interpreted the results somewhat differently. Perlis et al. (2006) concluded that add-on therapy with SGAs (ziprasidone, olanzapine, quetiapine, and risperidone) conferred an additional benefit over monotherapy with a traditional mood stabilizer in reducing manic symptoms, with no difference in efficacy among the drugs. Scherk et al. (2007) also concluded that SGAs as a group were significantly superior to placebo as adjunctive treatment for mania but that ziprasidone and other individual agents may not be significantly superior to placebo in the adjunctive treatment of manic symptoms. This conclusion is in contrast with results reported by Vieta et al. (2010) from a 12-week double-blind two-part study in 438 adults with bipolar-associated acute mania. In the first part, a 3-week period in which ziprasidone (80–160 mg/day) and placebo were compared with haloperidol (8–30 mg/day) as a reference standard, changes from baseline MRS scores for ziprasidone and haloperidol were superior to those for placebo beginning with day 2 of treatment until week 3. At week 3, response rates were 36.9%, 54.7%, and 20.5%, respectively, for ziprasidone, haloperidol, and placebo. In the 9-week extension phase to examine tolerability, during which ziprasidone replaced placebo, improvements were maintained for 96.3% of patients receiving haloperidol and 88.1% of those receiving ziprasidone, with ziprasidone demonstrating superior tolerability.

Finally, regulatory approvals for the individual agents have supported the efficacy and safety of a number of individual antipsychotics for the acute treatment of mania, including ziprasidone (which is also approved for the acute treatment of mixed states). Prospective head-to-head comparator trials like that of Vieta et al. (2010) may further clarify whether differences in efficacy suggested by some meta-analyses are clinically informative or merely related to limitations in study design or methodology (e.g., underdosing of ziprasidone or dosing without food).

Bipolar Depression

Preliminary results indicate that ziprasidone may be a viable treatment option in bipolar depression. For example, an 8-week open-label study investigating ziprasidone monotherapy for depressive symptoms in bipolar II patients ($n = 30$ completers) demonstrated effective attenuation of depression with a relatively low mean dosage of 58 mg/day (Liebowitz et al. 2009). The authors concluded that larger and controlled trials are required to confirm their findings.

Dysphoric Mania

Dysphoric mania is a common and often difficult-to-treat subset of bipolar mania that is associated with significant depressive symptoms. Data from a post hoc analysis of two similarly designed 3-week placebo-controlled trials (Stahl et al. 2010a) in acute bipolar mania that were pooled and analyzed indicated that ziprasidone significantly improved both depressive and manic mood symptoms in patients with dysphoric mania. Similar to the preliminary results obtained in bipolar depression, definitive conclusions await further prospective controlled trials.

Maintenance Treatment

Two 52-week open-label extension studies support the safety, tolerability, and sustained efficacy of ziprasidone as maintenance treatment for bipolar disorder (P.E. Keck et al. 2004, 2009; Weisler et al. 2004). P.E. Keck et al. (2004) reported that treatment with ziprasidone ($n = 127$; mean daily dosage, 123 mg) was associated with significantly lower MRS and CGI-S scores compared with baseline, beginning as early as the first week. Overall, improvements in manic symptoms achieved during acute treatment continued to consolidate during maintenance treatment with ziprasidone. During 52 weeks of treatment, only 6% of patients discontinued ziprasidone use due to relapse of mania. Similarly, only 4% of patients discontinued due to a clinical switch into depression. An important caveat regarding these results is the high rate of attrition observed by the end of 1 year, which is consistent with long-term studies involving other SGAs but still limits the full interpretation of results. Comparable results were observed in a separate extension study of adjunctive ziprasidone therapy (mean daily dosage 92.6 mg) by Weisler et al. (2004); this study reported a mean improvement from baseline in MRS scores at all points throughout the study (Patel and Keck 2006). Finally, subjects with DSM-IV bipolar I disorder achieving 8 or more consecutive weeks of stability with open-label ziprasidone (80–160 mg/day) and lithium or valproate were randomly assigned in a 6-month double-blind maintenance period to ziprasidone plus mood stabilizer or placebo plus mood stabilizer. The time to intervention for a mood episode was significantly longer for ziprasidone compared with placebo, and time to discontinuation for any reason was significantly longer for ziprasidone (Bowden et al. 2010), indicating that ziprasidone may be useful in lieu of a classic mood stabilizer for maintenance of euthymia in bipolar disorder.

Treatment-Resistant Depression

A series of uncontrolled studies have sparked interest in the efficacy of ziprasidone for treatment-resistant depression (Barbee et al. 2004; Jarema 2007; Papakostas et al. 2004). Papakostas et al. (2004) reported the results of a small study of 20 patients with major depression resistant to treatment with selective serotonin reuptake inhibitors (SSRIs). Open-

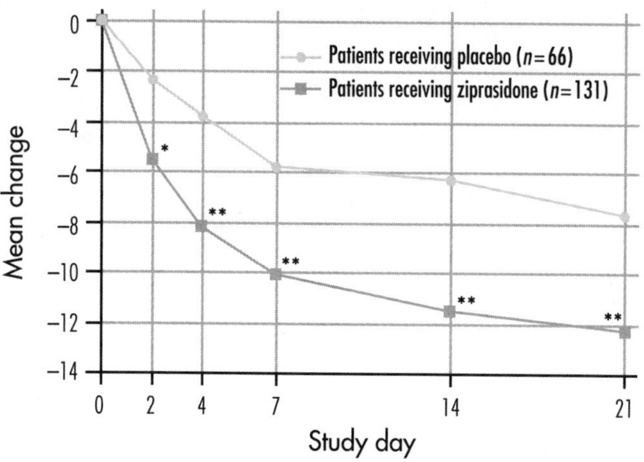

FIGURE 21–2. Effect of ziprasidone on mania: rating scale scores in patients with bipolar disorder receiving 21-day randomized treatment with ziprasidone or placebo.

*$P<0.003$ (F test), placebo-treated patients versus ziprasidone-treated patients.

**$P<0.001$ (F test), placebo-treated patients and ziprasidone-treated patients ($P<0.001$, F test).

Source. Adapted from Keck et al. 2003b.

label treatment with ziprasidone for 6 weeks, adjunctive to ongoing SSRI treatment, was evaluated with an intent-to-treat analysis that identified 10 treatment responders (defined as having a ≥50% decrease in depressive symptoms as measured by the Ham-D-17). Randomized studies are needed to evaluate the efficacy and safety of ziprasidone for patients with treatment-resistant depression.

Agitation

The efficacy of intramuscular ziprasidone for the treatment of agitated psychosis has been demonstrated in two randomized, double-blind trials (2 mg intramuscular vs. 20 mg or 10 mg intramuscular, respectively, with up to three more doses allowed as needed at 4-hour or 2-hour intervals, respectively), leading to regulatory approval by the FDA (Daniel et al. 2001; Lesem et al. 2001). Treatment with single 10- or 20-mg doses leads to rapid reductions in symptom severity, with most patients having remission of agitation within 1 hour of dosing. Treatment with intramuscular ziprasidone is associated with a relatively low rate of concomitant benzodiazepine use (<20%). Sequential use of intramuscular ziprasidone followed by oral ziprasidone for the treatment of acute psychotic agitation has demonstrated superior efficacy, compared with sequential use of intramuscular and oral haloperidol, in two 7-day randomized, open-label trials (Brook et al. 2000; Swift et al. 1998) as well as in a 6-week randomized, single-blind, flexible-dose study (Brook et al. 2005). Clinical improvement occurred more rapidly than with haloperidol in one study and as quickly as 30 minutes after the first intramuscular administration of ziprasidone (Swift et al. 1998). Cumulative data from these studies indicate that intramuscular ziprasidone can rapidly control agitation and psychotic symptoms and provide greater mean improvements in acute agitation than seen with intramuscular haloperidol (e.g., greater mean improvements in BPRS total score, agitation, and CGI-S score) (Brook 2003).

Pediatric Patients

Ziprasidone has been approved by the FDA as a second-line therapy for use in children and adolescents (10–17 years old) experiencing manic or mixed episodes associated with bipolar disorder (Kuehn 2009). FDA-approved use of ziprasidone is confined to patients who fulfill DSM-IV criteria for bipolar disorder. Results from randomized controlled trials of ziprasidone in children and adolescents (ages 10–17 years) with bipolar disorder (Versavel et al. 2005) and with bipolar disorder, schizophrenia, or schizoaffective disorder (DelBello et al. 2008) have been reported. In the former study, treatment with ziprasidone was associated with improvement in mania and overall psychopathology (Versavel et al. 2005). The latter study focused on safety and did not report any unexpected tolerability findings in this age population, using a starting dosage of 20 mg/day titrated to between 80 and 160 mg/day over 1–2 weeks for clinically determined optimal dosing (DelBello et al. 2008).

Side Effects and Toxicology

Ziprasidone has a favorable tolerability profile based on both short- and long-term clinical trials (Daniel 2003; Pfizer Inc. 2004). The four most common treatment-related adverse events associated with oral ziprasidone in short-term premarketing placebo-controlled trials for schizophrenia were somnolence (14%), EPS (14%), nausea (10%), and constipation (9%) (Pfizer Inc. 2008). In subsequent clinical trials, treatment with ziprasidone was associated with a low occurrence of adverse events, most of which were considered mild to moderate in severity (Arango et al. 2007; Arato et al. 2002; Lieberman 2007; Nemeroff et al. 2005; Weiden et al. 2002, 2003b). In addition to the comprehensive listing of potential adverse events available in the full U.S. prescribing information (USPI) (Pfizer Inc. 2008), published case reports offer accounts of various rare adverse events that may be associated with the use of ziprasidone (Akkaya et al. 2006; Kaufman et al. 2006; Miodownik et al. 2005; Murty et al. 2002; Villanueva et al. 2006). Intramuscular ziprasidone shows a favorable tolerability profile similar to that of oral ziprasidone. In premarketing trials of intramuscular ziprasidone, the most common side effects (those with an incidence of >5% and an incidence greater than that seen in placebo recipients) were somnolence (20%), headache (13%), and nausea (12%) (Pfizer Inc. 2008). Pooled data from clinical trials of intramuscular ziprasidone indicate that most treatment-related adverse events were mild to moderate in severity, with the most common side effects being headache, nausea, dizziness, insomnia, anxiety, and pain at the injection site (Daniel 2003; Zimbroff et al. 2002). Ziprasidone is considered a Category C drug in pregnancy. Although some specific developmental effects have been noted in animal studies at dosages ranging from 0.5 to 8.0 times the maximal recommended human dosage (Pfizer Inc. 2008), there are as yet no similar reports of such effects in humans. The reader is advised to consult the current USPI for a detailed listing of potential adverse drug effects identified in the regulatory approval process and postmarketing surveillance.

The FDA recently required the addition of black box warnings in the USPI regarding an increased risk of mortality associated with the use of both SGAs and FGAs in elderly patients with dementia-related psychosis. Observed causes of death have been varied, and the mechanism of any drug effect in schizophrenia remains uncertain (Pfizer Inc. 2008). In particular, it remains unclear to what extent these uncontrolled observations of increased mortality are due to specific drug effects or to the advanced medical risk characteristics of patients with dementia or delirium who tend to receive these medications (Farber et al. 2000; Rochon et al. 2008).

Retrospective analysis of intramuscular use of ziprasidone, olanzapine, or haloperidol in large matched cohorts of hospitalized patients did not indicate significant differences in mortality rates among the three cohorts (Holdridge et al. 2010).

Clinical experience with ziprasidone in the years following initial U.S. approval has suggested that a small subgroup of patients may experience insomnia or what has been characterized as *activation* or *akathisia* soon after initiation of treatment (Nemeroff et al. 2005). These presentations have been described as transient manifestations of anxiety, restlessness, insomnia, increased energy, or hypomania-like symptoms, occurring most commonly at what is now considered the lower end of the dosage range. Anecdotal reports suggest that starting dosages of 120 mg/day or greater and more rapid dose titration can substantially reduce the incidence of these clinical presentations (Weiden et al. 2002). These anecdotal clinical observations are consistent with controlled experimental evidence indicating that a significantly lower rate of discontinuation occurs in patients who begin ziprasidone therapy at higher dosages (120–160 mg/day) than in patients who receive initial dosages of 80 mg/day or less (Joyce et al. 2006). Several mechanisms may explain these observations. First, ziprasidone is less intrinsically sedating than many other antipsychotics in current use (e.g., due to less H_1 receptor antagonism), so that patients initiating ziprasidone treatment after months or years of receiving a more sedating therapy may experience initial difficulties adjusting to the new level of drug-related sedation. Second, as discussed above (see "Pharmacological Profile" and "Indications and Efficacy" sections earlier in chapter), many patients have been treated with ziprasidone at doses that were insufficient to achieve optimal D_2 receptor blocking, leading to undertreatment of the underlying illness compared with what might have been achieved with an appropriately dosed prior therapy.

Furthermore, ziprasidone underdosing with respect to D_2 receptor binding can produce a well-understood but unwanted pharmacodynamic situation with respect to the differential balance of 5-HT_{2C} receptor antagonism relative to D_2 receptor antagonism. As illustrated in Figure 21–1, using ziprasidone doses at the lower end of the clinical dosage range can allow 5-HT_2 receptors to reach 50% of maximal receptor occupancy or more, well before clinically significant levels of D_2 occupancy are achieved (Mamo et al. 2004). 5-HT_{2C} antagonist activity at this level disinhibits cortical monoaminergic neurotransmission (e.g., dopamine release), which, in the absence of sufficient D_2 blockade, may lead to clinically relevant excess monoaminergic neurotransmission (Bonaccorso et al. 2002; Pozzi et al. 2002). Clinicians commonly address these potential issues through appropriate dosing and through the transient targeted use of concomitant medication strategies (e.g., adjunctive benzodiazepine treatment) for relevant patients starting new treatment in the acute inpatient setting or for stable outpatients needing a smooth transition to new therapy.

Two other areas of potential adverse drug effects deserve further discussion: drug effects on risk for EPS and drug effects on cardiometabolic risk factors (e.g., changes in weight, plasma lipids, and glucose). These adverse-event domains are notable as areas of considerable clinical and research interest. For example, drug effects on EPS and cardiometabolic risk factors such as weight and plasma lipid level changes were the only side effect categories observed to contribute to differential rates of treatment discontinuation in the primary analysis of the NIMH-funded phase I CATIE study (Lieberman et al. 2005).

Extrapyramidal Side Effects

Short-term trials indicate that treatment with ziprasidone is associated with a larger incidence of EPS than treatment with placebo (Pfizer Inc. 2008; Potkin et al. 2005). In contrast, data from a 52-week trial (Arato et al. 2002) indicate that the incidence of abnormal movement disorders during treatment with ziprasidone is comparable to the incidence during placebo treatment. Other long-term studies suggest a low (<6%) incidence of treatment-related EPS (Arango et al. 2007; Kudla et al. 2007). Both active-comparator studies and medication-switching studies suggest that ziprasidone is associated with fewer EPS than risperidone (Addington et al. 2003, 2009; Weiden et al. 2003a, 2003b) or FGAs (Hirsch et al. 2002; Weiden et al. 2003a, 2003b). Comparing ziprasidone and olanzapine, a drug with intrinsic antimuscarinic activity as well as 5-HT_2 receptor antagonist activity, one direct comparison study indicates that treatment with olanzapine is associated with fewer EPS (Kinon et al. 2006), whereas two other direct comparison studies (Breier et al. 2005; Simpson et al. 2002) and one medication-switching study (Weiden et al. 2003b) have reported that both drugs exhibit a similar liability for EPS. With respect to akathisia, one comparison study indicates that less akathisia occurs with olanzapine use (Breier et al. 2005), whereas another study suggests no difference in akathisia rates with olanzapine versus ziprasidone (Kinon et al. 2006). Results from phase I and phase II of the large-scale CATIE trial suggest no significant differences among ziprasidone, perphenazine, olanzapine, quetiapine, and risperidone in the incidence of EPS and akathisia (Lieberman 2007; Lieberman et al. 2005; Stroup et al. 2006). However, the perphenazine arm in the CATIE study was restricted to patients who did not already have tardive dyskinesia, suggesting a possible selection bias toward patients less likely to experience EPS. Despite this advantage, the perphenazine group still had the highest rate of dropouts due to EPS. Investigating SGAs only, a recent meta-analysis (Rummel-Kluge et al. 2012) of 54 comparative clinical trials analyzed the use of antiparkinsonian medication as an indicator of treatment-related EPS. The authors reported that risperidone was associated with greater use of antiparkinsonian medication compared with clozapine, olanzapine, quetiapine, or ziprasidone. Ziprasidone was associated with more use of antiparkinsonian medication than olanzapine or quetiapine; however, the authors concluded that overall differences were small.

Intramuscular ziprasidone has been tolerated at dosages of up to 80 mg/day with a low liability for EPS (Daniel 2003; Daniel et al. 2001; Lesem et al. 2001). Both intramuscular ziprasidone use and sequential intramuscular/oral ziprasidone use are associated with a lower incidence of treatment-related movement disorders than intramuscular haloperidol use (Swift et al. 1998; Zimbroff et al. 2002) and sequential intramuscular/oral haloperidol use (Brook et al. 2000, 2005). Although the results of controlled experimental studies indicate a generally low risk of EPS with ziprasidone, there have been uncontrolled observational reports of EPS-related adverse events co-occurring with ziprasidone treatment and, in many cases, concomitant treatment with other agents (Dew and Hughes 2004; Duggal 2007; M.E. Keck et al. 2004; Mason et al. 2005; Papapetropoulos et al. 2005; Ramos et al. 2003; Rosenfield et al. 2007; Weinstein et al. 2006; Yumru et al. 2006; Ziegenbein et al. 2003).

Metabolic Adverse Events

Adverse medication effects on modifiable risk factors for cardiovascular disease and type 2 diabetes mellitus have become an important topic of clinical, research, and regulatory concern, based in part on the increased prevalence of these conditions and associated premature mortality in patients with major mental disorders (Brown 1997; Brown et al. 2000; Colton and Manderscheid 2006; Harris and Barraclough 1998; Hennekens et al. 2005; Joukamaa et al. 2001; Osby et al. 2000, 2001). Modifiable cardiometabolic risk factors include obesity, hyperglycemia, dyslipidemia, hypertension, and smoking, all prevalent conditions in patients with major mental disorders, with substantial evidence that primary and secondary prevention approaches are underutilized in these patients (Allison et al. 1999a; Brown et al. 2000; Druss and Rosenheck 1998; Druss et al. 2000, 2001; Frayne et al. 2005; Hippisley-Cox et al. 2007; McEvoy et al. 2005; Nasrallah et al. 2006; Newcomer and Hennekens 2007). In particular, use of recommended monitoring of changes in weight and in plasma glucose and lipid levels during antipsychotic treatment has heightened interest in cardiometabolic risk effects that may go undetected during the course of treatment (American Diabetes Association 2004; Morrato et al. 2008). All currently available antipsychotic medications are associated with a risk of weight gain, as well as potential adverse effects on plasma glucose and lipid levels, although there is substantial variability in the magnitude of these effects across individual agents (Casey et al. 2004; Eli Lilly 2008; "Eli Lilly updates label warning for Zyprexa" 2007; Newcomer 2005). Potential adverse treatment effects on body weight can increase the risk for cardiovascular disease and type 2 diabetes, commonly via adiposity-related increases in insulin resistance, dyslipidemia, and hyperglycemia (Fontaine et al. 2001; Haupt et al. 2007; Koro et al. 2002a, 2002b).

Treatment with ziprasidone is associated with a relatively low risk of clinically significant increases in body weight. An analysis of available studies with this agent and other antipsychotics, both FGAs and SGAs (Allison et al. 1999b), estimated a mean 0.04-kg weight gain over a 10-week treatment period with ziprasidone, identifying ziprasidone as having one of the lowest estimated effects on body weight of those analyzed. In a 6-week randomized controlled trial in patients with acute exacerbations of schizophrenia or schizoaffective disorder, treatment with ziprasidone 80 mg/day produced a median increase in body weight of 1 kg, compared with no change in median weight with ziprasidone 160 mg/day or placebo (Daniel et al. 1999). In a 28-week study of outpatients with schizophrenia, mean changes in body weight from baseline to endpoint were similar during treatment with ziprasidone (+0.31 kg) and haloperidol (+0.22 kg) (Hirsch et al. 2002). In a 28-week study comparing the effects of ziprasidone and olanzapine, ziprasidone-treated patients experienced a small decrease in mean body weight (–1.12 kg) compared with a statistically and clinically different 3.06-kg mean increase in body weight observed with olanzapine treatment (Hardy et al. 2003; Kinon et al. 2006). Reductions in body weight were also associated with ziprasidone treatment in the 1-year Ziprasidone Extended Use in Schizophrenia (ZEUS) study of patients with chronic, stable schizophrenia (Arato et al. 2002); this study reported mean decreases from baseline of 2.7 kg, 3.2 kg, and 2.9 kg reported with 40 mg/day, 80 mg/day, and 160 mg/day dosages of ziprasidone, respectively, compared with a 3.6-kg decrease observed with placebo treatment. Results from the phase I and phase IIT CATIE studies provide further confirmation that treatment with ziprasidone has a low intrinsic risk for producing clinically significant weight gain, with 6%–7% of ziprasidone recipients demonstrating a 7% or greater increase from baseline body weight compared with, for example, 27%–30% of olanzapine recipients (Lieberman 2007; Stroup et al. 2006). In the phase I CATIE study, ziprasidone treatment was associated with a mean reduction in body weight of 0.14 kg (0.3 lb) per month of treatment, compared with a mean increase of 0.91, 0.23, and 0.18 kg/month (2.0, 0.5, and 0.4 lb/month, respectively) during treatment with olanzapine, quetiapine, and risperidone, respectively, the other SGAs tested (Lieberman et al. 2005).

It is important to note that initial courses of treatment can clearly be associated with greater weight gain than subsequent courses of treatment (McEvoy et al. 2007). In addition, chronically treated patients switching treatment from a medication with greater weight gain liability to a medication with less weight gain liability are likely to lose body weight in relation to that medication change, an effect that likely underlies the mean reductions in weight noted in some of the trials with ziprasidone discussed above. The magnitude of change in body weight during treatment with ziprasidone varies as a function of the weight gain liability of the prior treatment: the greatest potential for weight loss is associated with switching from previous treatments with the greatest weight gain liability (Weiden et al. 2008). For example, 6 weeks of ziprasidone therapy was associated with statistically significant decreases in mean body weight from baseline in patients switched from olanzapine (–1.8 kg) and from risperidone (–0.9 kg), whereas patients switched from high-potency FGAs such as haloperidol experienced a small increase in weight (+0.3 kg) (Weiden et al. 2008). The 1-year extension of this medication-switching study indicated that weight loss was progressive and persistent throughout the 1-year period for patients who switched from olanzapine (–9.8 kg, or 10.3% of baseline body weight) and from risperidone (–6.9 kg, or 7.8% of baseline) (Figure 21–3; Weiden et al. 2008). Another study found significant decreases in weight in patients treated for 6 months with ziprasidone who were switched from olanzapine (–7.0 kg) and from risperidone (–2.2 kg) (Montes et al. 2006).

Ziprasidone's effects on plasma glucose and lipid levels are best understood as being a function of treatment-related changes in adiposity. Whereas some antipsychotics, such as clozapine and olanzapine, have been reported to produce adiposity-independent effects on insulin sensitivity and related changes in glucose and lipid metabolism, ziprasidone has demonstrated no similar adiposity-independent effects in this same experimental paradigm (Houseknecht et al. 2007). In general, increases in adiposity are associated with decreases in insulin sensitivity in individuals taking or not taking antipsychotic medications, with reduced insulin sensitivity leading to increased risk for hyperglycemia, dyslipidemia, and other adverse changes in cardiometabolic risk indicators (Haupt et al. 2007; Newcomer and Haupt 2006).

Both short- and long-term studies have shown minimal adverse effects of ziprasidone on glucose levels, plasma insulin levels, insulin resistance, or fasting and nonfasting lipid levels (Daniel et al. 1999; Glick et al. 2001; Rettenbacher et al. 2006; Simpson et al. 2004a, 2005), in contrast to the degree of adverse effects detected with some active comparators. For example, olanzapine treatment can produce statistically significant increases in fasting glucose and insulin levels (Glick et al. 2001; Hardy et al. 2003; Simpson et al. 2002, 2005). In the CATIE phase I study, ziprasidone treatment was associated with minimal drug exposure–adjusted mean increases in blood glucose (+2.9±3.4 mg/dL) and HbA_{1c} (+0.11±0.09%) and decreases in plasma triglycerides (–16.5±12.2 mg/dL) and total cholesterol (–8.2±3.2 mg/dL) (Lieberman 2007). In the CATIE phase IIT study, ziprasidone-treated patients showed minimal drug exposure–adjusted mean increases in blood glucose (+0.8±5.6 mg/dL) and HbA_{1c} (+0.46± 0.3%) and decreases in triglycerides (–3.5± 20.9 mg/dL) and total cholesterol (–10.7±5.1 mg/dL) (Stroup et al. 2006).

Similar to the effect of prior treatment conditions on changes in weight during treatment with ziprasidone, improvements in plasma lipid levels observed during ziprasidone treatment in the CATIE study can best be understood as the effect of switching from a previous treatment that is associated with larger adverse effects on lipid metabolism to a treatment with minimal adverse effects. Weiden et al. (2003a) noted that ziprasidone treatment was associated with significant decreases from baseline in both median nonfasting triglyceride levels and median nonfasting total cholesterol levels at the end of the 6-week treatment period in patients whose prior medication was olanzapine or risperidone, with minimal change following prior treatment with high-potency FGAs like haloperidol. Notably, the reductions in lipids observed in this study occurred within the first 6 weeks of initiating treatment with ziprasidone, with substantial reductions in total cholesterol (>20 mg/dL) and plasma triglycerides (78 mg/dL) in the patients previously treated with olanzapine. In the 12-month extension of this study, the

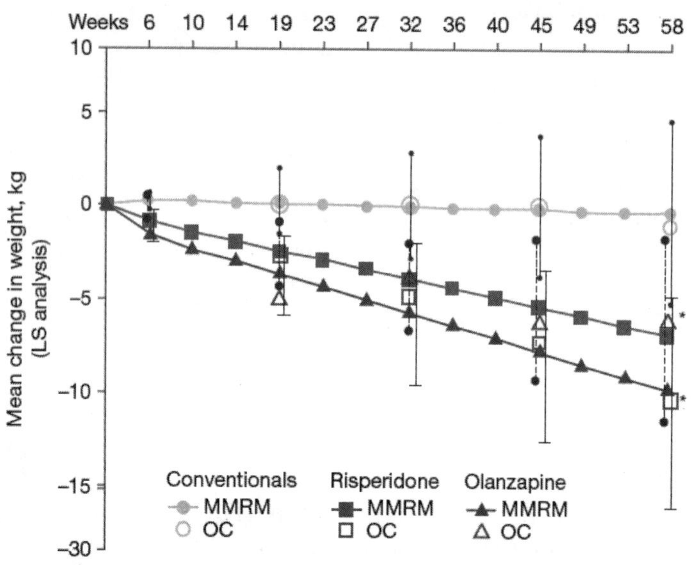

FIGURE 21–3. Time course of weight change over 58 weeks after switching to ziprasidone.

Previous treatments were conventional antipsychotics (line with circles; n=71), risperidone (line with squares; n=43), or olanzapine (line with triangles; n=71). Individual observed cases within each treatment group are also shown (circle = conventional agent: baseline weight, 198 lbs [90 kg]; square = risperidone: baseline weight, 194.9 lbs [88.6 kg]; triangle = olanzapine: baseline weight, 210.3 lbs [95.6 kg]).

LS = least-squares analysis; MMRM = mixed-model repeated-measures analysis; OC = observed case analysis.

*P<0.01 versus baseline (MMRM and OC).

Source. Adapted from Weiden PJ, Newcomer JW, Loebel AD, et al.: "Long-Term Changes in Weight and Plasma Lipids During Maintenance Treatment With Ziprasidone." *Neuropsychopharmacology* 33:985–994, 2008 (Figure 1, p. 988).

reductions achieved in the initial weeks following the switch from prior treatment were sustained during continued treatment with ziprasidone (Weiden et al. 2008).

Cardiac Conduction, Including Ventricular Depolarization and Repolarization

Some medications, including psychotropic medications, can increase the duration of the QTc interval (the QT interval corrected for heart rate). Basic research suggests plausible mechanisms by which an increase in the QTc interval could increase the risk of sudden cardiac death, and clinical investigations suggest that certain small subgroups of the general population may have an increased risk of sudden cardiac death, for example, those with a family history of congenital long-QT syndrome (>500 msec) and those who concomitantly use drugs that markedly increase the QTc interval (e.g., by >60 msec) via either pharmacokinetic or pharmacodynamic interactions (Montanez et al. 2004). This has understandably led to regulatory interest in drug effects on the QTc interval. It should be noted that epidemiological studies in the general population suggest that modest prolongations of the QTc interval are not a risk factor for cardiovascular mortality or sudden death, so any risk in the general population of modest QTc prolongations is likely to be small and difficult to detect reliably (Montanez et al. 2004). Compared with risks like obesity, hypercholesterolemia, diabetes, hypertension, physical inactivity, or cigarette smoking, each with well-characterized effects in the general population, modest QTc prolongations are not a comparable risk factor for cardiovascular mortality or sudden death in the general population.

With this background, thioridazine was required to add to its prescribing information a black box warning related to its QTc interval–prolonging effects, following decades of use. Other FGAs, including haloperidol, are also associated with some risk of QTc prolongation (Gury et al. 2000; O'Brien et al. 1999). Investigators (Glassman and Bigger 2001) have estimated the rate of occurrence of torsades de pointes with FGAs as "10–15 such events in 10,000 person-years of observation" (p. 1774). Ziprasidone, like certain other antipsychotic agents, can induce orthostatic hypotension, particularly early in treatment exposure, which can lead to transient tachycardia, dizziness, or syncope (Swainston Harrison and Scott 2006). However, tachycardia has been observed to be infrequent and as common in patients treated with ziprasidone as in those treated with placebo (Swainston Harrison and Scott 2006). Tachycardia and syncope related to hypotension are to be distinguished from ventricular arrhythmias that in rare cases can occur in relation to QTc prolongation.

Ziprasidone treatment has been demonstrated to result in a modestly increased risk of QTc prolongation (Pfizer Inc. 2008). This QTc prolongation at C_{max} (mean increase, >15 msec) is 9–14 msec greater than that seen with risperidone, olanzapine, quetiapine, or haloperidol but approximately 14 msec less than that seen with thioridazine. Unlike the case with thioridazine, the modest effect of ziprasidone on the QTc interval is not worsened by the presence of commonly encountered inhibitors of drug metabolism. In clinical trials of ziprasidone monotherapy that report QTc changes, in studies of high-dose intramuscular administration (Miceli et al. 2010), and in case reports of ziprasidone overdosing, there has been no evidence of any significant clinical sequelae such as torsades de pointes or sudden death (Arato et al. 2002; Arbuck 2005; Daniel 2003; Gomez-Criado et al. 2005; Harrigan et al. 2004; Insa Gómez and Gutiérrez Casares 2005; Levy et al. 2004; Lieberman 2007; Miceli et al. 2004; Montanez et al. 2004; Nemeroff et al. 2005; Tan et al. 2009; Taylor 2003; Weiden et al. 2002, 2003a). This is consistent with analyses of large population samples, which have failed to demonstrate any association between QTc duration and either cardiovascular or all-cause mortality (Goldberg et al. 1991).

The Ziprasidone Observational Study of Cardiac Outcomes (ZODIAC) was a large (>18,000 participants) international randomized trial designed to examine the risks of nonsuicide mortality and hospitalization associated with ziprasidone's use in routine medical practice settings (Strom et al. 2011). The main objective of ZODIAC was to evaluate nonsuicide mortality in the year following treatment initiation, which limited the study's ability to provide data on drug efficacy. Nevertheless, findings did not show an elevated risk of nonsuicide mortality for ziprasidone relative to olanzapine, and the study excluded a relative risk larger than 1.39 with a high probability. A total of 205 deaths occurred in the overall study population ($N = 18,154$). It should be noted that ZODIAC was not designed to measure electrocardiographic parameters or to examine the risk of rare cardiac events associated with lengthening of the QTc interval.

Rare cases of torsades de pointes have been reported in patients being treated with multiple medications including ziprasidone, but the incidence of these events appears to be below the known prevalence of torsades de pointes in community-based population samples (Heinrich et al. 2006). The USPI suggests that clinicians should nonetheless be cognizant of this potential risk and be aware of circumstances that may increase risk for the occurrence of torsades de pointes and/or sudden death in association with the use of any drugs that can prolong the QTc interval. Such circumstances include bradycardia, hypokalemia, or hypomagnesemia; concomitant use of other medications known to cause clinically significant QT prolongation (although an additive effect with ziprasidone has not been established); and presence of congenital long-QT syndrome. The USPI further states that ziprasidone should not be used in patients who have significant cardiovascular conditions, such as uncompensated heart failure or a cardiac arrhythmia, or in those who have had a recent acute myocardial infarction or persistent QTc measurements of greater than 500 msec, and the prudent clinician might consider employing the same caution with many other antipsychotic and psychotropic medications currently in use.

Conclusion

Ziprasidone was the fourth atypical antipsychotic following clozapine to become available in the United States. This agent has a unique pharmacological profile, with the highest 5-HT_{2A}/D_2 affinity ratio among currently available agents, potent serotonin and norepinephrine reuptake inhibition activity, agonist activity at 5-HT_{1A} receptors, and clinically relevant antagonist activity at various 5-HT_2 receptor subtypes. Ziprasidone has demonstrated rapid-onset and sustained efficacy for the treatment of schizophrenia, schizoaffective disorder, and bipolar mania, with promising evidence of favorable mood, cognitive, and prosocial effects. It is also available in an intramuscular formulation for the treatment of acute agitated psychoses, and it was approved for the use of bipolar mania in children and adolescents 10–17 years of age.

Ziprasidone has highly favorable safety and tolerability profiles with limited potential for drug-drug and drug-disease interactions, critical issues for a patient population that generally has a high burden of medical comorbidity and is commonly exposed to complex polypharmacy. The adverse-effect profile of ziprasidone is particularly noteworthy in areas that are key to safety and tolerability in patients with major mental disorders such as schizophrenia and bipolar disorder, including low drug-related risk for EPS and minimal effects on cardiometabolic risk factors like obesity and dyslipidemia.

References

Addington D, Pantelis C, Dineen M, et al: Ziprasidone vs risperidone in schizophrenia: 52 weeks' comparison. Poster presented at the annual meeting of the American Psychiatric Association, San Francisco, CA, May 17–22, 2003

Addington DE, Pantelis C, Dineen M, et al: Efficacy and tolerability of ziprasidone versus risperidone in patients with acute exacerbation of schizophrenia or schizoaffective disorder: an 8-week, double-blind, multicenter trial. J Clin Psychiatry 65:1624–1633, 2004

Addington DE, Labelle A, Kulkarni J, et al: A comparison of ziprasidone and risperidone in the long-term treatment of schizophrenia: a 44-week, double-blind, continuation study. Can J Psychiatry 54:46–54, 2009

Akkaya C, Sarandol A, Sivrioglu EY, et al: A patient using ziprasidone with polydipsia, seizure, hyponatremia and rhabdomyolysis. Prog Neuropsychopharmacol Biol Psychiatry 30:1535–1538, 2006

Allison DB, Fontaine KR, Heo M, et al: The distribution of body mass index among individuals with and without schizophrenia. J Clin Psychiatry 60:215–220, 1999a

Allison DB, Mentore JL, Heo M, et al: Antipsychotic-induced weight gain: a comprehensive research synthesis. Am J Psychiatry 156:1686–1696, 1999b

Altar CA, Wasley AM, Neale RF, et al: Typical and atypical antipsychotic occupancy of D2 and S2 receptors: an autoradiographic analysis in rat brain. Brain Res Bull 16:517–525, 1986

American Diabetes Association: Consensus development conference on antipsychotic drugs and obesity and diabetes. Diabetes Care 27:596–601, 2004

Apseloff G, Mullet D, Wilner KD, et al: The effects of ziprasidone on steady-state lithium levels and renal clearance of lithium. Br J Clin Pharmacol 49 (suppl 1):61S–64S, 2000

Arango C, Kirkpatrick B, Koenig J: At issue: stress, hippocampal neuronal turnover, and neuropsychiatric disorders. Schizophr Bull 27:477–480, 2001

Arango C, Gomez-Beneyto M, Brenlla J, et al: A 6-month prospective, observational, naturalistic, uncontrolled study to evaluate the effectiveness and tolerability of oral ziprasidone in patients with schizophrenia. Eur Neuropsychopharmacol 17:456–463, 2007

Arato M, O'Connor R, Meltzer HY: A 1-year, double-blind, placebo-controlled trial of ziprasidone 40, 80 and 160 mg/day in chronic schizophrenia: the Ziprasidone Extended Use in Schizophrenia (ZEUS) study. Int Clin Psychopharmacol 17:207–215, 2002

Arbuck DM: 12,800-mg ziprasidone overdose without significant ECG changes. Gen Hosp Psychiatry 27:222–223, 2005

Bagnall AM, Jones L, Ginnelly L, et al: A systematic review of atypical antipsychotic drugs in schizophrenia. Health Technol Assess 7:1–193, 2003

Barbee JG, Conrad EJ, Jamhour NJ: The effectiveness of olanzapine, risperidone, quetiapine, and ziprasidone as augmentation agents in treatment-resistant major depressive disorder. J Clin Psychiatry 65:975–981, 2004

Beedham C, Miceli JJ, Obach RS: Ziprasidone metabolism, aldehyde oxidase, and clinical implications. J Clin Psychopharmacol 23:229–232, 2003

Bonaccorso S, Meltzer HY, Li Z, et al: SR46349-B, a 5-HT(2A/2C) receptor antagonist, potentiates haloperidol-induced dopamine release in rat medial prefrontal cortex and nucleus accumbens. Neuropsychopharmacology 27:430–441, 2002

Bowden CL, Grunze H, Mullen J, et al: A randomized, double-blind, placebo-controlled efficacy and safety study of quetiapine or lithium as monotherapy for mania in bipolar disorder. J Clin Psychiatry 66:111–121, 2005

Bowden CL, Vieta E, Ice KS, et al: Ziprasidone plus a mood stabilizer in subjects with bipolar I disorder: a 6-month, randomized, placebo-controlled, double-blind trial. J Clin Psychiatry 71:130–137, 2010

Breier A, Berg PH, Thakore JH, et al: Olanzapine versus ziprasidone: results of a 28-week double-blind study in patients with schizophrenia. Am J Psychiatry 162:1879–1887, 2005

Bremner JD, Vythilingam M, Ng CK, et al: Regional brain metabolic correlates of alpha-methylparatyrosine-induced depressive symptoms: implications for the neural circuitry of depression. JAMA 289:3125–3134, 2003

Briley M, Moret C: Neurobiological mechanisms involved in antidepressant therapies. Clin Neuropharmacol 16:387–400, 1993

Brook S: Intramuscular ziprasidone: moving beyond the conventional in the treatment of acute agitation in schizophrenia. J Clin Psychiatry 64 (suppl 19):13–18, 2003

Brook S, Lucey JV, Gunn KP: Intramuscular ziprasidone compared with intramuscular haloperidol in the treatment of acute psychosis. Ziprasidone IM Study Group. J Clin Psychiatry 61:933–941, 2000

Brook S, Walden J, Benattia I, et al: Ziprasidone and haloperidol in the treatment of acute exacerbation of schizophrenia and schizoaffective disorder: comparison of intramuscular and oral formulations in a 6-week, randomized, blinded-assessment study. Psychopharmacology (Berl) 178:514–523, 2005

Brown S: Excess mortality of schizophrenia: a meta-analysis. Br J Psychiatry 171:502–508, 1997

Brown S, Inskip H, Barraclough B: Causes of the excess mortality of schizophrenia. Br J Psychiatry 177:212–217, 2000

Bymaster FP, Katner JS, Nelson DL, et al: Atomoxetine increases extracellular levels of norepinephrine and dopamine in prefrontal cortex of rat: a potential mechanism for efficacy in attention deficit/hyperactivity disorder. Neuropsychopharmacology 27:699–711, 2002

Casey DE, Haupt DW, Newcomer JW, et al: Antipsychotic-induced weight gain and metabolic abnormalities: implications for increased mortality in patients with schizophrenia. J Clin Psychiatry 65:4–18, 2004

Citrome L: Using oral ziprasidone effectively: the food effect and dose-response. Adv Ther 26:739–748, 2009

Citrome L, Jaffe A, Levine J: How dosing of ziprasidone in a state hospital system differs from product labeling. J Clin Psychiatry 70:975–982, 2009a

Citrome L, Reist C, Palmer L, et al: Impact of real-world ziprasidone dosing on treatment discontinuation rates in patients with schizophrenia or bipolar disorder. Schizophr Res 115:115–120, 2009b

Citrome L, Yang R, Glue P, et al: Effect of ziprasidone dose on all-cause discontinuation rates in acute schizophrenia and schizoaffective disorder: a post-hoc analysis of 4 fixed-dose randomized clinical trial. Schizophr Res 111:39–45, 2009c

Colton CW, Manderscheid RW: Congruencies in increased mortality rates, years of potential life lost, and causes of death among public mental health clients in eight states. Prev Chronic Dis 3:A42, 2006

Daniel DG: Tolerability of ziprasidone: an expanding perspective. J Clin Psychiatry 64 (suppl 19):40–49, 2003

Daniel DG, Zimbroff DL, Potkin SG, et al: Ziprasidone 80 mg/day and 160 mg/day in the acute exacerbation of schizophrenia and schizoaffective disorder: a 6-week placebo-controlled trial. Ziprasidone Study Group. Neuropsychopharmacology 20:491–505, 1999

Daniel DG, Potkin SG, Reeves KR, et al: Intramuscular (IM) ziprasidone 20 mg is effective in reducing acute agitation associated with psychosis: a double-blind, randomized trial. Psychopharmacology (Berl) 155:128–134, 2001

Davis JM, Chen N, Glick ID: A meta-analysis of the efficacy of second-generation antipsychotics. Arch Gen Psychiatry 60:553–564, 2003

DelBello MP, Versavel M, Ice K, et al: Tolerability of oral ziprasidone in children and adolescents with bipolar mania, schizophrenia, or schizoaffective disorder. J Child Adolesc Psychopharmacol 18:491–499, 2008

DeLeon A, Patel NC, Crismon ML: Aripiprazole: a comprehensive review of its pharmacology, clinical efficacy, and tolerability. Clin Ther 26:649–666, 2004

Dew RE, Hughes D: Acute dystonic reaction with moderate-dose ziprasidone. J Clin Psychopharmacol 24:563–564, 2004

Diaz-Marsa M, Sanchez S, Rico-Villademoros F, et al: Effectiveness and tolerability of oral ziprasidone in psychiatric inpatients with an acute exacerbation of schizophrenia or schizoaffective disorder: a multicenter, prospective, and naturalistic study. ZIP-IIG-79 Study Group. J Clin Psychiatry 70:509–517, 2009

Diaz-Mataix L, Scorza MC, Bortolozzi A, et al: Involvement of 5-HT1A receptors in prefrontal cortex in the modulation of dopaminergic activity: role in atypical antipsychotic action. J Neurosci 25:10831–10843, 2005

Druss BG, Rosenheck RA: Mental disorders and access to medical care in the United States. Am J Psychiatry 155:1775–1777, 1998

Druss BG, Bradford DW, Rosenheck RA, et al: Mental disorders and use of cardiovascular procedures after myocardial infarction. JAMA 283:506–511, 2000

Druss BG, Bradford WD, Rosenheck RA, et al: Quality of medical care and excess mortality in older patients with mental disorders. Arch Gen Psychiatry 58:565–572, 2001

Duggal HS: Ziprasidone-induced acute laryngeal dystonia. Prog Neuropsychopharmacol Biol Psychiatry 31:970; author reply 31:971, 2007

Duman RS: Depression: a case of neuronal life and death? Biol Psychiatry 56:140–145, 2004

Dwyer DS, Pinkofsky HB, Liu Y, et al: Antipsychotic drugs affect glucose uptake and the expression of glucose transporters in PC12 cells. Prog Neuropsychopharmacol Biol Psychiatry 23:69–80, 1999

Eli Lilly: Zyprexa (olanzapine tablets), Zyprexa (intramuscular olanzapine for injection), and Zyprexa Zydis (olanzapine orally disintegrating tablets), full prescribing information. August 2008. Available at: http://pi.lilly.com/us/zyprexa-pi.pdf. Accessed December 30, 2008.

Eli Lilly updates label warning for Zyprexa to better inform on side-effects. October 5, 2007. Available at: http://www.schizophrenia.com/sznews/archives/005617.html. Accessed December 30, 2008.

Essock SM, Covell NH, Davis SM, et al: Effectiveness of switching antipsychotic medications. Am J Psychiatry 163:2090–2095, 2006

Everson G, Lasseter KC, Anderson KE, et al: The pharmacokinetics of ziprasidone in subjects with normal and impaired hepatic function. Br J Clin Pharmacol 49 (suppl 1):21S–26S, 2000

Farber NB, Rubin EH, Newcomer JW, et al: Increased neocortical neurofibrillary tangle density in subjects with Alzheimer disease and psychosis. Arch Gen Psychiatry 57:1165–1173, 2000

Fontaine KR, Heo M, Harrigan EP, et al: Estimating the consequences of anti-psychotic induced weight gain on health and mortality rate. Psychiatry Res 101:277–288, 2001

Frayne SM, Halanych JH, Miller DR, et al: Disparities in diabetes care: impact of mental illness. Arch Intern Med 165:2631–2638, 2005

Gandelman K, Aldermman JA, Glue P, et al: The impact of calories and fat content of meals on oral ziprasidone absorption: a randomized, open-label, crossover trial. J Clin Psychiatry 70:58–62, 2009

Garver DL, Holcomb JA, Christensen JD: Cerebral cortical gray expansion associated with two second-generation antipsychotics. Biol Psychiatry 58:62–66, 2005

Geddes J, Freemantle N, Harrison P, et al: Atypical antipsychotics in the treatment of schizophrenia: systematic overview and meta-regression analysis. BMJ 321:1371–1376, 2000

Glassman AH, Bigger JT Jr: Antipsychotic drugs: prolonged QTc interval, torsade de pointes, and sudden death. Am J Psychiatry 158:1774–1782, 2001

Glick ID, Romano SJ, Simpson G, et al: Insulin resistance in olanzapine- and ziprasidone-treated patients: results of a double-blind, controlled 6-week trial. Paper presented at the annual meeting of the American Psychiatric Association, New Orleans, LA, May 5–10, 2001

Goff DC, Posever T, Herz L, et al: An exploratory haloperidol-controlled dose-finding study of ziprasidone in hospitalized patients with schizophrenia or schizoaffective disorder. J Clin Psychopharmacol 18:296–304, 1998

Goldberg RJ, Bengtson J, Chen ZY, et al: Duration of the QT interval and total and cardiovascular mortality in healthy persons (The Framingham Heart Study experience). Am J Cardiol 67:55–58, 1991

Gomez-Criado MS, Bernardo M, Florez T, et al: Ziprasidone overdose: cases recorded in the database of Pfizer-Spain and literature review. Pharmacotherapy 25:1660–1665, 2005

Gury C, Canceil O, Iaria P: Antipsychotic drugs and cardiovascular safety: current studies of prolonged QT interval and risk of ventricular arrhythmia [in French]. Encephale 26:62–72, 2000

Hamelin BA, Allard S, Laplante L, et al: The effect of timing of a standard meal on the pharmacokinetics and pharmacodynamics of the novel atypical antipsychotic agent ziprasidone. Pharmacotherapy 18:9–15, 1998

Hardy TA, Poole-Hoffmann V, Lu Y, et al: Fasting glucose and lipid changes in patients with schizophrenia treated with olanzapine or ziprasidone. Poster presented at the annual meeting of the American College of Neuropsychopharmacology, San Juan, PR, December 7–11, 2003

Harrigan EP, Miceli JJ, Anziano R, et al: A randomized evaluation of the effects of six antipsychotic agents on QTc, in the absence and presence of metabolic inhibition. J Clin Psychopharmacol 24:62–69, 2004

Harris EC, Barraclough B: Excess mortality of mental disorder. Br J Psychiatry 173:11–53, 1998

Harvey PD, Bowie CR: Ziprasidone: efficacy, tolerability, and emerging data on wide-ranging effectiveness. Expert Opin Pharmacother 6:337–346, 2005

Harvey PD, Siu CO, Romano S: Randomized, controlled, double-blind, multicenter comparison of the cognitive effects of ziprasidone versus olanzapine in acutely ill inpatients with schizophrenia or schizoaffective disorder. Psychopharmacology (Berl) 172:324–332, 2004

Harvey PD, Bowie CR, Loebel A: Neuropsychological normalization with long-term atypical antipsychotic treatment: results of a six-month randomized, double-blind comparison of ziprasidone vs. olanzapine. J Neuropsychiatry Clin Neurosci 18:54–63, 2006a

Harvey PD, Green MF, Bowie C, et al: The dimensions of clinical and cognitive change in schizophrenia: evidence for independence of improvements. Psychopharmacology (Berl) 187:356–363, 2006b

Harvey PD, Pappadopulos E, Lombardo I, et al: Reduction of functional disability with atypical antipsychotic treatment: a randomized long term comparison of ziprasidone and haloperidol. Schizophr Res 115:24–29, 2009

Haupt DW, Fahnestock PA, Flavin KA, et al: Adiposity and insulin sensitivity derived from intravenous glucose tolerance tests in antipsychotic-treated patients. Neuropsychopharmacology 32:2561–2569, 2007

Heinrich TW, Biblo LA, Schneider J: Torsades de pointes associated with ziprasidone. Psychosomatics 47:264–268, 2006

Heinrichs DW, Hanlon TE, Carpenter WT Jr: The Quality of Life Scale: an instrument for rating the schizophrenic deficit syndrome. Schizophr Bull 10:388–398, 1984

Hennekens CH, Hennekens AR, Hollar D, et al: Schizophrenia and increased risks of cardiovascular disease. Am Heart J 150:1115–1121, 2005

Hippisley-Cox J, Parker C, Coupland CA, et al: Inequalities in the primary care of coronary heart disease patients with serious mental health problems: a cross-sectional study. Heart 93:1256–1262, 2007

Hirsch SR, Kissling W, Bauml J, et al: A 28-week comparison of ziprasidone and haloperidol in outpatients with stable schizophrenia. J Clin Psychiatry 63:516–523, 2002

Hirschfeld RM, Keck PE Jr, Kramer M, et al: Rapid antimanic effect of risperidone monotherapy: a 3-week multicenter, double-blind, placebo-controlled trial. Am J Psychiatry 161:1057–1065, 2004

Holdridge KC, Sorsaburu S, Houston JP, et al: Characteristics and mortality among hospitalized patients treated with intramuscular antipsychotics: analysis of a United States hospital database. Curr Drug Saf 5:203–211, 2010

Houseknecht KL, Robertson AS, Zavadoski W, et al: Acute effects of atypical antipsychotics on whole-body insulin resistance in rats: implications for adverse metabolic effects. Neuropsychopharmacology 32:289–297, 2007

Ichikawa J, Ishii H, Bonaccorso S, et al: 5-HT(2A) and D(2) receptor blockade increases cortical DA release via 5-HT(1A) receptor activation: a possible mechanism of atypical antipsychotic-induced cortical dopamine release. J Neurochem 76:1521–1531, 2001

Insa Gómez FJ, Gutiérrez Casares JR: Ziprasidone overdose: cardiac safety. Actas Esp Psiquiatr 33:398–400, 2005

Jarema M: Atypical antipsychotics in the treatment of mood disorders. Curr Opin Psychiatry 20:23–29, 2007

Johnsen E, Kroken RA, Wentzel-Larsen T, et al: Effectiveness of second-generation antipsychotics: a naturalistic, randomized comparison of olanzapine, quetiapine, risperidone, and ziprasidone. BMC Psychiatry 10:26, 2010

Joukamaa M, Heliövaara M, Knekt P, et al: Mental disorders and cause-specific mortality. Br J Psychiatry 179:498–502, 2001

Joyce AT, Harrison DJ, Loebel AD, et al: Effect of initial ziprasidone dose on length of therapy in schizophrenia. Schizophr Res 83:285–292, 2006

Kahn RS, Fleischhacker WW, Boter H, et al: Effectiveness of antipsychotic drugs in first-episode schizophrenia and schizophreniform disorder: an open randomized clinical trial. EUFEST study group. Lancet 371:1085–1097, 2008

Kane JM: Oral ziprasidone in the treatment of schizophrenia: a review of short-term trials. J Clin Psychiatry 64 (suppl 19):19–25, 2003

Kane JM, Berg PH, Thakore J, et al: Olanzapine versus ziprasidone: results of the 28-week double-blind study in patients with schizophrenia (abstract). J Psychopharmacol 17:A50, 2003

Kane J, Khanna S, Giller E, et al: Ziprasidone's long-term efficacy in treatment-refractory schizophrenia. Poster presented at the International Congress on Schizophrenia Research, Savannah, GA, April 2–6, 2005

Kapur S, Remington G: Serotonin-dopamine interaction and its relevance to schizophrenia. Am J Psychiatry 153:466–476, 1996

Kapur S, Remington G: Dopamine D(2) receptors and their role in atypical antipsychotic action: still necessary and may even be sufficient. Biol Psychiatry 50:873–883, 2001

Kaufman KR, Stern L, Mohebati A, et al: Ziprasidone-induced priapism requiring surgical treatment. Eur Psychiatry 21:48–50, 2006

Keck ME, Müller MB, Binder EB, et al: Ziprasidone-related tardive dyskinesia. Am J Psychiatry 161:175–176, 2004

Keck P Jr, Buffenstein A, Ferguson J, et al: Ziprasidone 40 and 120 mg/day in the acute exacerbation of schizophrenia and schizoaffective disorder: a 4-week placebo-controlled trial. Psychopharmacology (Berl) 140:173–184, 1998

Keck PE Jr, Reeves KR, Harrigan EP: Ziprasidone in the short-term treatment of patients with schizoaffective disorder: results from two double-blind, placebo-controlled, multicenter studies. J Clin Psychopharmacol 21:27–35, 2001

Keck PE Jr, Marcus R, Tourkodimitris S, et al: A placebo-controlled, double-blind study of the efficacy and safety of aripiprazole in patients with acute bipolar mania. Am J Psychiatry 160: 1651–1658, 2003a

Keck PE Jr, Versiani M, Potkin S, et al: Ziprasidone in the treatment of acute bipolar mania: a three-week, placebo-controlled, double-blind, randomized trial. Am J Psychiatry 160:741–748, 2003b

Keck PE Jr, Potkin S, Warrington L, et al: Efficacy and safety of ziprasidone in bipolar disorder: short- and long-term data. Poster presented at the annual meeting of the American Psychiatric Association, New York, May 1–6, 2004

Keck PE, Versiani M, Warrington L, et al: Long-term safety and efficacy of ziprasidone in subpopulations of patients with bipolar mania. J Clin Psychiatry 70:844–851, 2009

Keefe RS, Bilder RM, Davis SM, et al: Neurocognitive effects of antipsychotic medications in patients with chronic schizophrenia in the CATIE trial. Arch Gen Psychiatry 64:633–647, 2007

Khanna S, Vieta E, Lyons B, et al: Risperidone in the treatment of acute mania: double-blind, placebo-controlled study. Br J Psychiatry 187:229–234, 2005

Kinon BJ, Lipkovich I, Edwards SB, et al: A 24-week randomized study of olanzapine versus ziprasidone in the treatment of schizophrenia or schizoaffective disorder in patients with prominent depressive symptoms. J Clin Psychopharmacol 26:157–162, 2006

Koro CE, Fedder DO, L'Italien GJ, et al: An assessment of the independent effects of olanzapine and risperidone exposure on the risk of hyperlipidemia in schizophrenic patients. Arch Gen Psychiatry 59:1021–1026, 2002a

Koro CE, Fedder DO, L'Italien GJ, et al: Assessment of independent effect of olanzapine and risperidone on risk of diabetes among patients with schizophrenia: population based nested case-control study. BMJ 325:243, 2002b

Kreyenbuhl J, Marcus SC, West JC, et al: Adding or switching antipsychotic medications in treatment-refractory schizophrenia. Focus 6:212–220, 2008

Kroeze WK, Hufeisen SJ, Popadak BA, et al: H1-histamine receptor affinity predicts short-term weight gain for typical and atypical antipsychotic drugs. Neuropsychopharmacology 28:519–526, 2003

Kudla D, Lambert M, Domin S, et al: Effectiveness, tolerability, and safety of ziprasidone in patients with schizophrenia or schizoaffective disorder: results of a multi-centre observational trial. Eur Psychiatry 22:195–202, 2007

Kuehn BM: FDA panel OKs 3 antipsychotic drugs for pediatric use, cautions against overuse. JAMA 302:833–834, 2009

Lesem MD, Zajecka JM, Swift RH, et al: Intramuscular ziprasidone, 2 mg versus 10 mg, in the short-term management of agitated psychotic patients. J Clin Psychiatry 62:12–18, 2001

Leucht S, Pitschel-Walz G, Abraham D, et al: Efficacy and extrapyramidal side-effects of the new antipsychotics olanzapine, quetiapine, risperidone, and sertindole compared to conventional antipsychotics and placebo: a meta-analysis of randomized controlled trials. Schizophr Res 35:51–68, 1999

Levy WO, Robichaux-Keene NR, Nunez C: No significant QTc interval changes with high-dose ziprasidone: a case series. J Psychiatr Pract 10: 227–232, 2004

Lieberman JA: Effectiveness of antipsychotic drugs in patients with chronic schizophrenia: efficacy, safety and cost outcomes of CATIE and other trials. J Clin Psychiatry 68:e04, 2007

Lieberman JA, Stroup TS, McEvoy JP, et al: Effectiveness of antipsychotic drugs in patients with chronic schizophrenia. N Engl J Med 353:1209–1223, 2005

Liebowitz MR, Salman E, Mech A, et al: Ziprasidone monotherapy in bipolar II depression: an open trial. J Affect Disord 118:205–208, 2009

Loebel A, Siu C, Romano S: Improvement in prosocial functioning after a switch to ziprasidone treatment. CNS Spectr 9:357–364, 2004

Lombardo I, Alderman J, Preskorn S, et al: Effect of food on absorption of ziprasidone. Abstract of poster presented at the International Congress on Schizophrenia Research, March 28–April 1, 2007, Colorado Springs, CO. Schizophr Bull 33:475–476, 2007

Mamo D, Kapur S, Shammi CM, et al: A PET study of dopamine D2 and serotonin 5-HT2 receptor occupancy in patients with schizophrenia treated with therapeutic doses of ziprasidone. Am J Psychiatry 161:818–825, 2004

Mason MN, Johnson CE, Piasecki M: Ziprasidone-induced acute dystonia. Am J Psychiatry 162: 625–626, 2005

Mazei MS, Pluto CP, Kirkbride B, et al: Effects of catecholamine uptake blockers in the caudate-putamen and subregions of the medial prefrontal cortex of the rat. Brain Res 936:58–67, 2002

McCue RE, Waheed R, Urcuyo L, et al: Comparative effectiveness of second-generation antipsychotics and haloperidol in acute schizophrenia. Br J Psychiatry 189:433–440, 2006

McEvoy JP, Meyer JM, Goff DC, et al: Prevalence of the metabolic syndrome in patients with schizophrenia: baseline results from the Clinical Antipsychotic Trials of Intervention Effectiveness (CATIE) schizophrenia trial and comparison with national estimates from NHANES III. Schizophr Res 80:19–32, 2005

McEvoy JP, Lieberman JA, Perkins DO, et al: Efficacy and tolerability of olanzapine, quetiapine, and risperidone in the treatment of early psychosis: a randomized, double-blind 52-week comparison. Am J Psychiatry 164:1050–1060, 2007

McIntyre RS, Brecher M, Paulsson B, et al: Quetiapine or haloperidol as monotherapy for bipolar mania—a 12-week, double-blind, randomised, parallel-group, placebo-controlled trial. Eur Neuropsychopharmacol 15:573–585, 2005

McQuade RD, Marcus R, Sanchez R: Aripiprazole vs placebo in acute mania: safety and tolerability pooled analysis. Poster presented at the International Conference on Bipolar Disorder, Pittsburgh, PA, June 12–14, 2003

Miceli JJ, Anziano RJ, Robarge L, et al: The effect of carbamazepine on the steady-state pharmacokinetics of ziprasidone in healthy volunteers. Br J Clin Pharmacol 49 (suppl 1):65S–70S, 2000a

Miceli JJ, Smith M, Robarge L, et al: The effects of ketoconazole on ziprasidone pharmacokinetics—a placebo-controlled crossover study in healthy volunteers. Br J Clin Pharmacol 49 (suppl 1):71S–76S, 2000b

Miceli JJ, Wilner KD, Hansen RA, et al: Single- and multiple-dose pharmacokinetics of ziprasidone under non-fasting conditions in healthy male volunteers. Br J Clin Pharmacol 49 (suppl 1): 5S–13S, 2000c

Miceli JJ, Murray S, Sallee FR, et al: Pharmacokinetic and pharmacodynamic QTc profile of oral ziprasidone in pediatric and adult subjects following single-dose administration. Poster presented at the annual meeting of the American Psychiatric Association, New York, May 1–6, 2004

Miceli JJ, Tensfeldt TG, Shiovitz T, et al: Effects of high-dose ziprasidone and haloperidol on the QTc interval after intramuscular administration: a randomized, single-blind, parallel-group study in patients with schizophrenia or schizoaffective disorder. Clin Ther 32:472–491, 2010

Millan MJ: Improving the treatment of schizophrenia: focus on serotonin (5-HT)(1A) receptors. J Pharmacol Exp Ther 295:853–861, 2000

Miodownik C, Hausmann M, Frolova K, et al: Lithium intoxication associated with intramuscular ziprasidone in schizoaffective patients. Clin Neuropharmacol 28:295–297, 2005

Montanez A, Ruskin JN, Hebert PR, et al: Prolonged QTc interval and risks of total and cardiovascular mortality and sudden death in the general population: a review and qualitative overview of the prospective cohort studies. Arch Intern Med 164:943–948, 2004

Montes JM, Rodriguez JL, Balbo E, et al: Improvement in antipsychotic-related metabolic disturbances in patients with schizophrenia switched to ziprasidone. Prog Neuropsychopharmacol Biol Psychiatry 31:383–388, 2006

Morrato EH, Newcomer JW, Allen RR, et al: Prevalence of baseline serum glucose and lipid testing in users of second-generation antipsychotic drugs: a retrospective, population-based study of Medicaid claims data. J Clin Psychiatry 69:316–322, 2008

Mullins CD, Shaya FT, Zito JM, et al: Effect of initial ziprasidone dose on treatment persistence in schizophrenia. Schizophr Res 83:277–284, 2006

Murray S, Mandel FS, Loebel A: Optimal initial dosing of ziprasidone: clinical trial data. Poster presented at the annual meeting of the American Psychiatric Association, New York, May 1–6, 2004

Murty RG, Mistry SG, Chacko RC: Neuroleptic malignant syndrome with ziprasidone. J Clin Psychopharmacol 22:624–626, 2002

Nasrallah HA, Meyer JM, Goff DC, et al: Low rates of treatment for hypertension, dyslipidemia and diabetes in schizophrenia: data from the CATIE schizophrenia trial sample at baseline. Schizophr Res 86:15–22, 2006

Nemeroff CB, Lieberman JA, Weiden PJ, et al: From clinical research to clinical practice: a 4-year review of ziprasidone. CNS Spectr 10 (suppl):s1–s20, 2005

Newcomer JW: Second-generation (atypical) antipsychotics and metabolic effects: a comprehensive literature review. CNS Drugs 19 (suppl 1): 1–93, 2005

Newcomer JW, Haupt DW: The metabolic effects of antipsychotic medications. Can J Psychiatry 51:480–491, 2006

Newcomer JW, Hennekens CH: Severe mental illness and risk of cardiovascular disease. JAMA 298:1794–1796, 2007

Obach RS, Huynh P, Allen MC, et al: Human liver aldehyde oxidase: inhibition by 239 drugs. J Clin Pharmacol 44:7–19, 2004

O'Brien JM, Rockwood RP, Suh KI: Haloperidol-induced torsade de pointes. Ann Pharmacother 33:1046–1050, 1999

O'Connor R, Schooler NR: Penultimate observation carried forward (POCF): a new approach to analysis of long-term symptom change in chronic relapsing conditions. Schizophr Res 60:319–320, 2003

Olfson M, Gerhard T, Huang C, et al: Comparative effectiveness of second-generation antipsychotic medications in early-onset schizophrenia. Schizophr Bull 38:845–853, 2012

Osby U, Correia N, Brandt L, et al: Mortality and causes of death in schizophrenia in Stockholm county, Sweden. Schizophr Res 45:21–28, 2000

Osby U, Brandt L, Correia N, et al: Excess mortality in bipolar and unipolar disorder in Sweden. Arch Gen Psychiatry 58:844–850, 2001

Papakostas GI, Petersen TJ, Nierenberg AA, et al: Ziprasidone augmentation of selective serotonin reuptake inhibitors (SSRIs) for SSRI-resistant major depressive disorder. J Clin Psychiatry 65:217–221, 2004

Papapetropoulos S, Wheeler S, Singer C: Tardive dystonia associated with ziprasidone. Am J Psychiatry 162:2191, 2005

Patel NC, Keck PE Jr: Ziprasidone: efficacy and safety in patients with bipolar disorder. Expert Rev Neurother 6:1129–1138, 2006

Perlis RH, Welge JA, Vornik LA, et al: Atypical antipsychotics in the treatment of mania: a meta-analysis of randomized, placebo-controlled trials. J Clin Psychiatry 67:509–516, 2006

Pfizer Inc.: Dear Healthcare Practitioner letter, August 2004. Available at: http://www.fda.gov/medwatch/SAFETY/2004/GeodonDearDoc.pdf. Accessed December 30, 2008.

Pfizer Inc.: Geodon (ziprasidone HCl) capsules and Geodon (ziprasidone mesylate) for injection, full prescribing information. June 2008

Potkin SG, Keck PE Jr, Segal S, et al: Ziprasidone in acute bipolar mania: a 21-day randomized, double-blind, placebo-controlled replication trial. J Clin Psychopharmacol 25:301–310, 2005

Potkin SG, Weiden PJ, Loebel AD, et al: Remission in schizophrenia: 196-week, double-blind treatment with ziprasidone vs. haloperidol. Int J Neurpsychopharmacol 12:1233–1248, 2009

Pozzi L, Acconcia S, Ceglia I, et al: Stimulation of 5-hydroxytryptamine (5-HT(2C)) receptors in the ventrotegmental area inhibits stress-induced but not basal dopamine release in the rat prefrontal cortex. J Neurochem 82:93–100, 2002

Prakash C, Kamel A, Cui D, et al: Identification of the major human liver cytochrome P450 isoform(s) responsible for the formation of the primary metabolites of ziprasidone and prediction of possible drug interactions. Br J Clin Pharmacol 49 (suppl 1):35S–42S, 2000

Purnine DM, Carey KB, Maisto SA, et al: Assessing positive and negative symptoms in outpatients with schizophrenia and mood disorders. J Nerv Ment Dis 188:653–661, 2000

Ramos AE, Shytle RD, Silver AA, et al: Ziprasidone-induced oculogyric crisis. J Am Acad Child Adolesc Psychiatry 42:1013–1014, 2003

Rettenbacher MA, Ebenbichler C, Hofer A, et al: Early changes of plasma lipids during treatment with atypical antipsychotics. Int Clin Psychopharmacol 21:369–372, 2006

Rochon PA, Normand SL, Gomes T, et al: Antipsychotic therapy and short-term serious events in older adults with dementia. Arch Intern Med 168:1090–1096, 2008

Rollema H, Lu Y, Schmidt AW, et al: 5-HT(1A) receptor activation contributes to ziprasidone-induced dopamine release in the rat prefrontal cortex. Biol Psychiatry 48:229–237, 2000

Rosenfield PJ, Girgis RR, Gil R: High-dose ziprasidone-induced acute dystonia. Prog Neuropsychopharmacol Biol Psychiatry 31:546–547, 2007

Rossi A, Canas F, Fagiolini A, et al: Switching among antipsychotics in everyday clinical practice: focus on ziprasidone. Postgrad Med 123:135–159, 2011

Rummel-Kluge C, Komossa K, Schwarz S, et al: Second-generation antipsychotic drugs and extrapyramidal side effects: a systematic review and meta-analysis of head-to-head comparisons. Schizophr Bull 38:167–177, 2012

Sacchetti E, Galluzzo A, Valsecchi P, et al: Ziprasidone vs clozapine in schizophrenia patients refractory to multiple antipsychotic treatments: the MOZART study. Schizophr Res 113:112–121, 2009

Sachs G, Sanchez R, Marcus R, et al: Aripiprazole in the treatment of acute manic or mixed episodes in patients with bipolar I disorder: a 3-week placebo-controlled study. J Psychopharmacol 20:536–546, 2006

Scherk H, Pajonk FG, Leucht S: Second-generation antipsychotic agents in the treatment of acute mania: a systematic review and meta-analysis of randomized controlled trials. Arch Gen Psychiatry 64:442–455, 2007

Schmidt AW, Lebel LA, Howard HR Jr, et al: Ziprasidone: a novel antipsychotic agent with a unique human receptor binding profile. Eur J Pharmacol 425:197–201, 2001

Schooler NR: Maintaining symptom control: review of ziprasidone long-term efficacy data. J Clin Psychiatry 64 (suppl 19):26–32, 2003

Seeger TF, Seymour PA, Schmidt AW, et al: Ziprasidone (CP-88,059): a new antipsychotic with combined dopamine and serotonin receptor antagonist activity. J Pharmacol Exp Ther 275: 101–113, 1995

Simpson G, Weiden P, Pigott TA, et al: Ziprasidone vs olanzapine in schizophrenia: 6-month continuation study. Eur Neuropsychopharmacol 12 (suppl):S310, 2002

Simpson GM, Glick ID, Weiden PJ, et al: Randomized, controlled, double-blind multicenter comparison of the efficacy and tolerability of ziprasidone and olanzapine in acutely ill inpatients with schizophrenia or schizoaffective disorder. Am J Psychiatry 161:1837–1847, 2004a

Simpson GM, Weiden PJ, Loebel A, et al: Ziprasidone: long-term post-switch efficacy in schizophrenia. Poster presented at the annual meeting of the American Psychiatric Association, New York, May 1–6, 2004b

Simpson GM, Weiden P, Pigott T, et al: Six-month, blinded, multicenter continuation study of ziprasidone versus olanzapine in schizophrenia. Am J Psychiatry 162:1535–1538, 2005

Smulevich AB, Khanna S, Eerdekens M, et al: Acute and continuation risperidone monotherapy in bipolar mania: a 3-week placebo-controlled trial followed by a 9-week double-blind trial of risperidone and haloperidol. Eur Neuropsychopharmacol 15:75–84, 2005

Srisurapanont M, Maneeton N: Comparison of the efficacy and acceptability of atypical antipsychotic drugs: a meta-analysis of randomized, placebo-controlled trials. J Med Assoc Thai 82:341–346, 1999

Stahl SM: Neurotransmission of cognition, part 2: selective NRIs are smart drugs: exploiting regionally selective actions on both dopamine and norepinephrine to enhance cognition. J Clin Psychiatry 64:110–111, 2003

Stahl SM, Shayegan DK: The psychopharmacology of ziprasidone: receptor-binding properties and real-world psychiatric practice. J Clin Psychiatry 64 (suppl 19):6–12, 2003

Stahl S, Lombardo I, Loebel A, et al: Efficacy of ziprasidone in dysphoric mania: polled analysis of two double-blind studies. J Affect Disord 122:39–45, 2010a

Stahl SM, Malla A, Newcomer JW, et al: A post hoc analysis of negative symptoms and psychosocial function in patients with schizophrenia: a 40-week randomized, double-blind study of ziprasidone versus haloperidol followed by a 3-year double-blind extension trial. J Clin Psychopharmacol 30:425–430, 2010b

Strom BL, Eng SM, Faich G, et al: Comparative mortality associated with ziprasidone and olanzapine in real-world use among 18,154 patients with schizophrenia: the Ziprasidone Observational Study of Cardiac Outcomes (ZODIAC). Am J Psychiatry 168:193–201, 2011

Stroup TS, Lieberman JA, McEvoy JP, et al: Effectiveness of olanzapine, quetiapine, risperidone, and ziprasidone in patients with chronic schizophrenia following discontinuation of a previous atypical antipsychotic. Am J Psychiatry 163:611–622, 2006

Sumiyoshi T, Jayathilake K, Meltzer HY: The effect of melperone, an atypical antipsychotic drug, on cognitive function in schizophrenia. Schizophr Res 59:7–16, 2003

Swainston Harrison T, Scott LJ: Ziprasidone: a review of its use in schizophrenia and schizoaffective disorder. CNS Drugs 20:1027–1052, 2006

Swartz MS, Perkins DO, Stroup TS, et al: Effects of antipsychotic medications on psychosocial functioning in patients with chronic schizophrenia: findings from the NIMH CATIE study. Am J Psychiatry 164:428–436, 2007

Swift RH, Harrigan EP, van Kammen DP: A comparison of fixed-dose intramuscular (IM) ziprasidone with flexible-dose IM haloperidol. Poster presented at the annual meeting of the American Psychiatric Association, Toronto, ON, Canada, May 30–June 4, 1998

Tan HH, Hoppe J, Heard K: A systematic review of cardiovascular effects after atypical antipsychotic medication overdose. Am J Emerg Med 27:607–616, 2009

Tandon R, Fleischhacker WW: Comparative efficacy of antipsychotics in the treatment of schizophrenia: a critical assessment. Schizophr Res 79:145–155, 2005

Tatsumi M, Jansen K, Blakely RD, et al: Pharmacological profile of neuroleptics at human monoamine transporters. Eur J Pharmacol 368:277–283, 1999

Tauscher J, Kapur S, Verhoeff NP, et al: Brain serotonin 5-HT(1A) receptor binding in schizophrenia measured by positron emission tomography and [11C]WAY-100635. Arch Gen Psychiatry 59:514–520, 2002

Taylor D: Ziprasidone in the management of schizophrenia: the QT interval issue in context. CNS Drugs 17:423–430, 2003

Tecott LH, Sun LM, Akana SF, et al: Eating disorder and epilepsy in mice lacking 5-HT2c serotonin receptors. Nature 374:542–546, 1995

Thome J, Foley P, Riederer P: Neurotrophic factors and the maldevelopmental hypothesis of schizophrenic psychoses: review article. J Neural Transm 105:85–100, 1998

Tohen M, Sanger TM, McElroy SL, et al: Olanzapine versus placebo in the treatment of acute mania. Olanzapine HGEH Study Group. Am J Psychiatry 156:702–709, 1999

Tohen M, Jacobs TG, Grundy SL, et al: Efficacy of olanzapine in acute bipolar mania: a double-blind, placebo-controlled study. The Olanzapine HGGW Study Group. Arch Gen Psychiatry 57:841–849, 2000

Versavel M, DelBello MP, Ice K, et al: Ziprasidone dosing study in pediatric patients with bipolar disorder, schizophrenia or schizoaffective disorder (abstract). Neuropsychopharmacology 30 (suppl):S122, 2005

Vieta E, Ramey T, Keller D, et al: Ziprasidone in the treatment of acute mania: a 12-week, placebo-controlled, haloperidol-referenced study. J Psychopharmacol 24:547–558, 2010

Villanueva N, Markham-Abedi C, McNeely C, et al: Probable association between ziprasidone and worsening hypertension. Pharmacotherapy 26:1352–1357, 2006

Weiden PJ, Iqbal N, Mendelowitz AJ, et al: Best clinical practice with ziprasidone: update after one year of experience. J Psychiatr Pract 8:81–97, 2002

Weiden PJ, Daniel DG, Simpson G, et al: Improvement in indices of health status in outpatients with schizophrenia switched to ziprasidone. J Clin Psychopharmacol 23:595–600, 2003a

Weiden PJ, Simpson GM, Potkin SG, et al: Effectiveness of switching to ziprasidone for stable but symptomatic outpatients with schizophrenia. J Clin Psychiatry 64:580–588, 2003b

Weiden PJ, Newcomer JW, Loebel AD, et al: Long-term changes in weight and plasma lipids during maintenance treatment with ziprasidone. Neuropsychopharmacology 33:985–994, 2008

Weinstein SK, Adler CM, Strakowski SM: Ziprasidone-induced acute dystonic reactions in patients with bipolar disorder. J Clin Psychiatry 67:327–328, 2006

Weisler R, Dunn J, English P: Ziprasidone in adjunctive treatment of acute bipolar mania: double-blind, placebo-controlled trial. Poster presented at the annual meeting of the Institute on Psychiatric Services, Boston, MA, October 29–November 2, 2003

Weisler R, Warrington L, Dunn J: Adjunctive ziprasidone in bipolar mania: short- and long-term data. Biol Psychiatry 55 (suppl):43S, 2004

Yumru M, Savas HA, Selek S, et al: Acute dystonia after initial doses of ziprasidone: a case report. Prog Neuropsychopharmacol Biol Psychiatry 30:745–747, 2006

Ziegenbein M, Schomerus G, Kropp S: Ziprasidone-induced Pisa syndrome after clozapine treatment. J Neuropsychiatry Clin Neurosci 15:458–459, 2003

Zimbroff DL, Brook S, Benattia I: Safety and tolerability of IM ziprasidone: review of clinical trial data. Poster presented at the annual meeting of the American Psychiatric Association, Philadelphia, PA, May 18–23, 2002

Zink M, Kuwilsky A, Krumm B, et al: Efficacy and tolerability of ziprasidone versus risperidone as augmentation in patients partially responsive to clozapine: a randomized controlled clinical trial. J Psychopharmacol 23:305–314, 2009

Zorn SH, Bebel LA, Schmidt AW, et al: Pharmacological and neurochemical studies with the new antipsychotic ziprasidone, in Interactive Monoaminergic Basis of Brain Disorders. Edited by Palomo T, Beninger R, Archer T. Madrid, Spain, Editorial Sintesis, 1998, pp 377–394

CHAPTER 22

Lurasidone

Philip D. Harvey, Ph.D.

Lurasidone (Latuda), the most recent addition to the atypical antipsychotic class, received U.S. Food and Drug Administration (FDA) approval for the treatment of schizophrenia in October 2010. As with all currently registered antipsychotic medications, lurasidone is a D_2 dopamine receptor antagonist. In addition, this compound is a full antagonist at the serotonin 2A ($5\text{-}HT_{2A}$) receptor, similar to other atypical antipsychotic medications. Lurasidone also has other receptor affinities that may contribute to additional beneficial or adverse effects. Because lurasidone is very new, its database is limited compared with other medications, and there are no published data yet available from systematic clinical trials aimed at conditions other than schizophrenia. Conference presentations have suggested that lurasidone may demonstrate efficacy for treatment-resistant depression, but those results have not been published.

In this chapter, I review the pharmacological properties and efficacy basis of lurasidone, the side effects and adverse events from the pivotal studies, and other features of the compound that may prove important in later studies as well as in the clinical applications of this agent. I also consider what, if anything, seems unique about lurasidone compared with other antipsychotic medications.

Pharmacological Properties

Receptor-Binding Profile

Lurasidone belongs to the chemical class of benzoisothiazol derivatives. The compound is a full antagonist at dopamine D_2 and serotonin $5\text{-}HT_{2A}$ receptors, which is similar to other atypical antipsychotics. Lurasidone also has high affinity for $5\text{-}HT_7$ receptors, with in vitro affinity for $5\text{-}HT_7$ being relatively higher than that shown by the drug for dopamine D_2 and $5\text{-}HT_{2A}$. Lurasidone is a partial agonist at $5\text{-}HT_{1A}$ receptors (Ishibashi et al. 2010). Lurasidone has moderate affinity for noradrenergic receptors. Lurasidone's minimal affinity for α_1-adrenergic receptors should be associated with reduced risk for orthostatic hypotension in comparison with compounds that have higher affinity for this receptor. Lurasidone appears to have weak affinity for $5\text{-}HT_{2C}$ receptors and no affinity for histamine H_1, a profile that should be associated with relatively low weight gain. Lurasidone lacks affinity for cholinergic M_1 receptors, which suggests reduced risk for cholinergic cognitive deficits and other side effects.

Pharmacokinetics and Dosing

Lurasidone is rapidly absorbed and reaches peak concentrations within 3 hours for a 40-mg dose. Steady state is reached within 7 days (Sunovion Pharmaceuticals 2012). The molecule is metabolized in the liver with the cytochrome P450 (CYP) 3A4 enzyme system, leading to the conclusion that lurasidone should not be used in the presence of strong inducers (e.g., rifampin) or inhibitors (e.g., ketoconazole) of CYP3A4. Lurasidone does show a food effect. A study examining food effects on lurasidone concentrations suggested that meals containing 350 calories or more, with either low or high fat content, led to a doubling of the bioavailability of lurasidone compared with dosing during fasting (Chiu et al. 2010).

The recommended starting dose of lurasidone is 40 mg once daily taken concurrently with at least 350 calories of food. Dosage adjustments to 160 mg/day are also currently approved. As noted above, lurasidone should not be administered to patients taking strong metabolic inducers or inhibitors of CYP3A4. There are no suggested dosage adjustments based on age, gender, ethnicity, or smoking, but individuals with renal or hepatic impairment should not be dosed at levels greater than 40 mg/day. Currently available formulations include 20-, 40-, and 80-mg tablets.

Lurasidone appears to require minimal adjustment and tinkering, as well as no titration period. Having a starting dose with substantial efficacy is a strong point for many patients. Food effects are an issue, given that optimal exposure requires the medication to be taken with at least 350 calories of food (with no minimum fat content specified); however, the lack of need for titration and minimal requirements for suitable meals will make it easier to apply this treatment to patients who may be challenged in their ability to adhere to complex regimens.

Efficacy and Tolerability

Pivotal Registration Trials

In the standard drug development program, lurasidone at daily doses of 40, 80, and 120 mg was compared against placebo across four different studies, only one of which (Meltzer et al. 2011) has been published. That study (Cucchiaro et al. 2010; Meltzer et al. 2011) included olanzapine 15 mg/day as an active comparator for assay sensitivity (other data based on conference presentations are reviewed by Citrome [2011a, 2011b]). Patients ranged in age from 18 to 74 years and were symptomatic with an acute exacerbation of psychosis. The dosage that most consistently separated from placebo was 80 mg/day, although 40 mg/day and 120 mg/day did as well in some trials. Lurasidone at 120 mg/day did not confer additional clinical benefit on the primary outcomes—improved scores on either the Positive and Negative Syndrome Scale (PANSS) or the Brief Psychiatric Rating Scale (BPRS)—across the different studies. However, recent clinical data submitted to the FDA led to an increase in the approved dosage for the medication to 160 mg/day.

Although the active comparator studies were not powered to detect changes between active treatments, in the olanzapine study (Cucchiaro et al. 2010; Meltzer et al. 2011) the improvement from baseline on the PANSS total score was 28.7 points for olanzapine, compared with 16 points for placebo at the endpoint assessment in a 6-week study. Lurasidone at 40 mg/day led to a 25.7-point improvement, and lurasidone at 120 mg/day led to a 23.6-point improvement. All of these active treatment changes separated from placebo.

Comparative Efficacy Studies

Two blinded and randomized studies have compared lurasidone with other agents. In the first (Potkin et al. 2011), lurasidone was compared with ziprasidone in a 3-week randomized trial in 301 patients with schizophrenia. Both treatments improved symptoms as measured by the PANSS, and there was no significant difference in endpoint PANSS scores. In the second study (Meltzer et al. 2011), lurasidone was compared with olanzapine in clinically unstable patients with schizophrenia who had been admitted to inpatient care. Both olanzapine and lurasidone were superior to placebo for clinical response. In addition, the weight gain with olanzapine was significantly greater than that with either lurasidone or placebo, whereas rates of akathisia were significantly higher in the lurasidone group compared with the other two groups.

Summary of Efficacy and Tolerability Data

The risk-benefit evaluation for lurasidone suggests a lower potential for metabolic consequences and QTc prolongation combined with a slightly higher risk of extrapyramidal side effects (EPS) and akathisia compared with some other atypical antipsychotic medications. Prolactin elevation appears to be minimal within the approved dosage range. Given our limited clinical experience with lurasidone, it may be premature to target an optimal patient for this medication; however, the reduced metabolic consequences of lurasidone would seem to be a very strong point. Patients who are extraordinarily vulnerable to EPS may require close monitoring. Although lurasidone's efficacy relative to other agents is impossible to assess at this time, findings from the one controlled trial conducted to date with an active comparator (olanzapine; Meltzer et al. 2011) yielded no suggestion of inferiority on the part of lurasidone.

Side Effects and Safety

Class Warnings

The typical class warnings are present on the lurasidone label, including the black box warning for increased stroke risk in elderly individuals and a variety of other class warnings regarding neuroleptic malignant syndrome, tardive dyskinesia, diabetes, hyperlipidemia, weight gain, glucose abnormalities, hyperprolactinemia, agranulocytosis, suicide, and seizures. Lurasidone has no warning for QTc alteration; a dedicated cardiac safety study (referenced in the package insert) found no evidence of QTc prolongation with lurasidone treatment.

Adverse-Event Reports

Because lurasidone lacks a substantial current clinical experience base, safety information is available only from the manufacturer's safety database. Dose-related adverse events that separated from placebo included somnolence, akathisia, and total scores on clinical ratings scales for EPS. Importantly, weight and metabolic parameters were only minimally affected in patients with schizophrenia in these clinical trials. While short-term changes in cholesterol, triglycerides, and glucose are likely due to transitions off medications with more substantial adverse profiles in these domains, the weight gain data are very noticeable.

Promising Features

Favorable Metabolic Profile

Lurasidone appears to have the promise of weight neutrality. Weight gain in the pooled 6-week studies across doses was 0.75 kg; in the pooled 12-month database from extension studies, patients lost an average of 0.71 kg. These statistics compare quite favorably with those of other antipsychotics in wide clinical use (see review by Citrome 2011b). It is important to note that special populations, outside the current label, may have greater weight gain risk than the typical patient with chronic schizophrenia in these trials. Nevertheless, the suggestion of no weight gain after a year's treatment, even for patients who may have gained weight with previous treatments, is quite promising.

Potential Cognitive Benefits

Compounds that interact with the 5-HT_7 receptor as their primary binding profile have historically being shown to have beneficial cognitive effects in animal models (Ballaz et al. 2007). Furthermore, partial agonist properties at the 5-HT_{1A} receptor have been postulated to have effects that could have potential benefit for the reduction of flat affect and related symptoms (Newman-Tancredi 2010). While acknowledging the challenges inherent in extrapolation from animal models, I will briefly review the evidence that 5-HT_7 blockade has potential cognitive benefit.

Research conducted with lurasidone by its developer has shown some basic science evidence of potential cognitive benefit. MK-801 is a glutamate receptor antagonist that is used to induce cognitive impairments quite similar to those seen in schizophrenia. Like other *N*-methyl-D-aspartate (NMDA) antagonists, MK-801 is capable of inducing deficits in memory and problem solving. Given that NMDA antagonists like ketamine and phencyclidine can induce a reliable analog of schizophrenia in healthy people (and exacerbate psychosis in patients with schizophrenia), such manipulations have more intrinsic validity than cholinergic manipulations such as scopolamine challenge. In rats, lurasidone has shown the potential to reverse MK-801–induced learning and memory deficits in the passive avoidance test (Ishiyama et al. 2007) and the Morris water maze (Enomoto et al. 2008). The Morris water maze task measures multiple memory parameters relevant to schizophrenia, including learning of new information, utilization of working memory, and short-term retention of previously acquired information.

Research utilizing cognitive impairments derived from animal models has notoriously failed to yield paradigms with adequate translational relevance to the specific cognitive domains affected in schizophrenia, particularly in terms of reliably predicting beneficial cognitive effects associated with pharmacological treatment (Harvey 2009). A possible reason for this failure may be that the adverse influences on human cognition of dopamine D_2 receptor antagonism associated with antipsychotic treatment may override the influences of a "secondary" receptor profile, preventing its beneficial effects from being realized (Harvey and McClure 2006). For instance, ziprasidone, a partial antagonist at the 5-HT_{1A} receptor, has never demonstrated cognitive superiority over antipsychotics that do not interact with that receptor (e.g., olanzapine; Harvey et al. 2004). Thus, clear evidence of cognitive enhancement in patients with schizophrenia treated with the medication of interest, compared with other treatments in similar populations, is the "bottom line" requirement for meaningful cognitive benefit.

Only one currently published study in patients with schizophrenia has addressed the issue of lurasidone's cognitive benefit compared with that of other antipsychotics (Harvey et al. 2011). Conducted during the early development phases of lurasidone, this study was a short-term double-blind, randomized head-to-head comparison of lurasidone versus ziprasidone in generally clinically stable outpatients with schizophrenia (Potkin et al. 2011). At the time of this study, no U.S. patients had ever been exposed to lurasidone. Patients were selected for being naive to treatment with ziprasidone as well. A 3-week randomized trial examined changes in performance on a neuropsychological assessment consisting of most of the tests in the widely used Measurement and Treatment Research to Improve Cognition in Schizophrenia (MATRICS) Consensus Cognitive Battery (MCCB; Nuechterlein et al. 2008) and an interview-based assessment of cognitive functioning, the Schizophrenia Cognition Rating Scale (SCoRS; Keefe et al. 2006), which allows detailed evaluation of both patient-reported and informant-reported cognitive functioning. Developed in response to the FDA's requirement that any study examining the cognitive benefits of a pharmacological treatment also show concurrent evidence of meaningfulness of benefit, the SCoRS consists of questions about the patient's ability to manage cognitively demanding, functionally relevant everyday tasks such as engaging in conversations, watching television, and using electronic devices.

The study found that lurasidone was associated with improvements on neuropsychological tests that were generally consistent with practice effects. There was one exception, processing speed, which improved more substantially and manifested relatively greater improvement with lurasidone than with ziprasidone (Harvey et al. 2011). However, improvements seen with lurasidone on the SCoRS were double the size of improvements on the neuropsychological assessments and nearly significantly larger than the improvements associated with ziprasidone. These results cannot be attributed to practice effects, given that the SCoRS is an interview, not a performance-based measure. Furthermore, the fact that the differential effects of lurasidone and ziprasidone were nearly significant ($P<0.06$) argues against a generalized bias effect, because the lurasidone effects were clearly larger.

Although these results clearly require replication, they suggest that any cognitive benefits of lurasidone are not attributable to 5-HT_{1A} receptor partial agonist effects, because those effects are common between the two compounds. At the same time, interview-based reports of functionally relevant cognitive processes and their treatment-related improvements clearly address a different element of cognitive functioning than do performance-based neurocognitive tests. Potential differential effects will need to be examined in detail in subsequent studies.

A particularly important issue to understand in regard to studies utilizing interview-based assessments of cognition is that patient self-reports have been found to be quite inaccurate. Overlaps between the reports of informants and patient self-reports are minimal, and correlations between patient self-reports and performance on neuropsychological assessments have been close to zero in several different studies using different self-report rating scales. Use of interview-based assessments requires contact with informants who are aware of the patient's performance. When reports from knowledgeable informants are included, ratings can be obtained that are meaningfully convergent with patient performance on cognitive tests.

Conclusion

Lurasidone is a new antipsychotic with some benefits compared with other available medications, including low weight-gain propensity and reduced risk for metabolic side effects. There is as yet very limited experience with this medication and sparse published data. None of the published data have been supported by sources other than the sponsor of the medication. We will watch this medication carefully to determine its benefit over time and its applicability to conditions other than schizophrenia, such as bipolar disorder and treatment-resistant depression.

References

Ballaz SJ, Akil H, Watson SJ. The 5-HT7 receptor: role in novel object discrimination and relation to novelty-seeking behavior. Neuroscience 149:192–202, 2007

Chiu YY, Preskorn S, Sarubbi D, et al: Effect of food on lurasidone absorption. Poster presented at the NCDEU Meeting, Boca Raton, FL, 14–17 June 2010

Citrome L: Lurasidone for schizophrenia: a brief review of a new second-generation antipsychotic. Clin Schizophr Relat Psychoses 4:251–257, 2011a

Citrome L: Lurasidone for schizophrenia: a review of the efficacy and safety profile for this newly approved second-generation antipsychotic. Int J Clin Pract 65:189–210, 2011b

Cucchiaro J, Silva R, Ogasa M, et al: Lurasidone in the treatment of acute schizophrenia: results of the double-blind, placebo-controlled PEARL 2 trial (abstract). Schizophr Res 117:493, 2010

Enomoto T, Ishibashi T, Tokuda K, et al: Lurasidone reverses MK-801-induced impairment of learning and memory in the Morris water maze and radial-arm maze tests in rats. Behav Brain Res 186:197–207, 2008

Harvey PD: Pharmacological cognitive enhancement. Neuropsychology Rev 19:324–335, 2009

Harvey PD, McClure MM: Pharmacological approaches to the management of cognitive dysfunction in schizophrenia. Drugs 66:1465–1473, 2006

Harvey PD, Siu C, Romano S: Randomized, controlled, double-blind, multicenter comparison of the cognitive effects of ziprasidone versus olanzapine in acutely ill inpatients with schizophrenia or schizoaffective disorder. Psychopharmacology 172:324–332, 2004

Harvey PD, Ogasa M, Cucchiaro J, et al: Performance and interview-based assessments of cognitive change in a randomized, double-blind comparison of lurasidone vs. ziprasidone. Schizophr Res 127:188–194, 2011

Ishibashi T, Horisawa T, Tokuda K, et al: Pharmacological profile of lurasidone, a novel antipsychotic agent with potent 5-hydroxytryptamine 7 (5-HT7) and 5-HT1A receptor activity. J Pharmacol Exp Ther 334:171–181, 2010

Ishiyama T, Tokuda K, Ishibashi T, et al: Lurasidone (SM-13496), a novel atypical antipsychotic drug, reverses MK-801-induced impairment of learning and memory in the rat passive-avoidance test. Eur J Pharmacol 572:160–170, 2007

Keefe RS, Poe M, Walker TM, et al: The Schizophrenia Cognition Rating Scale: an interview-based assessment and its relationship to cognition, real-world functioning, and functional capacity. Am J Psychiatry 163:426–432, 2006

Meltzer HY, Cucchiaro J, Silva R, et al: Lurasidone in the treatment of schizophrenia: a randomized, double-blind, placebo- and olanzapine-controlled study. Am J Psychiatry 168:957–967, 2011

Newman-Tancredi A: The importance of 5-HT1A receptor agonism in antipsychotic drug action: rationale and perspectives. Curr Opin Investig Drugs 11:802–812, 2010

Nuechterlein KH, Green MF, Kern RS, et al: The MATRICS Consensus Cognitive Battery, part 1: test selection, reliability, and validity. Am J Psychiatry 165:203–213, 2008

Potkin SG, Ogasa M, Cucchiaro J, et al: Double-blind comparison of the safety and efficacy of lurasidone and ziprasidone in clinically stable outpatients with schizophrenia or schizoaffective disorder. Schizophr Res 132:101–107, 2011

Sunovion Pharmaceuticals: Latuda (lurasidone HCl) tablets: prescribing information. Revised April 2012. Available at: http://www.latuda.com/LatudaPrescribingInformation.pdf. Accessed June 13, 2012.

CHAPTER 23

Asenapine

Leslie L. Citrome, M.D., M.P.H.

Eric D. Peselow, M.D.

Ira D. Glick, M.D.

History and Discovery

Asenapine as a sublingual tablet was initially approved by the U.S. Food and Drug Administration (FDA) in August 2009 for the treatment of acute schizophrenia and acute manic or mixed episodes associated with bipolar I disorder in adults. It was subsequently approved for maintenance treatment of schizophrenia and for adjunctive use with lithium or valproate in the treatment of acute manic or mixed episodes associated with bipolar I disorder (Merck 2011). In addition to the original unflavored formulation, a black cherry–flavored version of asenapine was brought to market in 2010.

Pharmacological Profile

The receptor-binding profile of asenapine is notable for high affinity (K_i [values in nM]) for several serotonin receptor subtypes, including 5-HT_{2C} (0.03), 5-HT_{2A} (0.06), 5-HT_7 (0.13), 5-HT_{2B} (0.16), and 5-HT_6 (0.25), as well as several dopamine receptor subtypes, including D_3 (0.42), D_2 (1.3), D_1 (1.4), and D_4 (1.1) (Merck 2011; Shahid et al. 2009). Asenapine also has high binding affinities to histamine H_1 (1.0) and to norepinephrine α_1 (1.2) and α_2 (1.2) receptors. Asenapine binds with somewhat lower affinity to serotonin 5-HT_5 (1.6), 5-HT_{1A} (2.5), and 5-HT_{1B} (4.0) receptors and histamine H_2 (6.2) receptors. Asenapine very weakly binds to muscarinic M_1 (8,128) receptors. Asenapine acts as an antagonist at all of the above receptors.

Asenapine has approximately 38 metabolites, none of them highly prevalent; these metabolites have little clinically relevant effects either because of their lower affinity for the relevant receptors or because of their inability to cross the blood-brain barrier (Citrome 2009; U.S. Food and Drug Administration 2009). Although the precise mechanism of action of asenapine in the treatment of schizophrenia is unknown, it is thought that antagonism at the dopamine D_2 and serotonin 5-HT_{2A} receptors mediates the drug's antipsychotic activity (Merck 2011). In studies using positron emission tomography, asenapine has demonstrated dose-dependent dopamine D_2 receptor occupancy (dose range 0.1–4.8 mg), with a significant correlation between D_2 occupancy and plasma concentration (U.S. Food and Drug Administration 2009); sublingual administration of 4.8 mg twice daily resulted in a mean D_2 occupancy of 79% approximately 3–6 hours after dosing.

Pharmacokinetics and Drug-Drug Interactions

Asenapine is the only commercially available antipsychotic that is absorbed primarily in the oral mucosa. It is formulated as a highly porous, rapid-dissolving tablet for sublingual administration, with a resulting bioavailability of approximately 35% (Schering-Plough 2009; U.S. Food and Drug Administration 2009). If the tablet is swallowed rather than allowed to orally dissolve, the drug's bioavailability is reduced to less than 2% because of high hepato-gastrointestinal first-pass metabolism (Merck 2011; U.S. Food and Drug Administration 2009). Patient instructions are to place the tablet under the tongue and to refrain from eating or drinking for 10 minutes after administration, because drinking water sooner than 10 minutes can result in reduced bioavailability of asenapine (Merck 2011).

Although asenapine was developed for sublingual administration, absorption will occur even if the tablet is placed elsewhere in the oral cavity, as was demonstrated in a study of healthy men who received single 5-mg doses of asenapine via sublingual, supralingual, and buccal routes (Gerrits et al. 2010). Drug exposure with buccal administration (i.e., "cheeking") as measured by plasma levels was almost 25% higher than that with sublingual administration, whereas exposure with supralingual administration was 6% lower. However, these differences in exposure by oral administration site are small in relation to the wide variability in asenapine's pharmacokinetics observed across the clinical studies used to obtain regulatory approval, where overall exposure varied by 37%, with a mean interindividual variability of 26% and a mean intraindividual variability of 26% (U.S. Food and Drug Administration 2009). Doubling the dose from 5 mg to 10 mg twice daily results in less than linear (1.7 times) increases in both the extent of exposure and the maximum concentration (Merck 2011).

Peak plasma levels occur 30–90 minutes after administration, partly explaining the recommendation for bid (twice daily) dosing (Merck 2011; Schering-Plough 2009; U.S. Food and Drug Administration 2009). Asenapine's mean terminal half-life is approximately 24 hours.

Asenapine is metabolized in the liver primarily through direct glucuronidation by UGT1A4 and oxidative metabolism by cytochrome P450 (CYP) isoenzymes (predominantly CYP1A2). Asenapine has a large volume of distribution and is highly bound (95%) to plasma proteins, including albumin and α_1-acid glycoprotein. Despite the fact that smoking can induce CYP1A2, concomitant smoking had no substantial effect on the pharmacokinetics of asenapine when tested in healthy male subjects (U.S. Food and Drug Administration 2009). Fluvoxamine, a potent CYP1A2 inhibitor, can increase exposure to asenapine by 29% and therefore should be coadministered with caution (Merck 2011).

Use of asenapine is not recommended in patients with severe hepatic impairment (Child-Pugh class C); asenapine exposures are on average 7 times higher in patients with severe impairment than in those with normal hepatic function. However, no dosage adjustment is required in patients with mild (Child-Pugh A) or moderate (Child-Pugh B) hepatic impairment. No dosage adjustment is required for patients with renal impairment.

Asenapine can inhibit CYP2D6, resulting in twofold increases in paroxetine concentrations (U.S. Food and Drug Administration 2009). The product label advises caution when coadministering asenapine with drugs that are both substrates and inhibitors of CYP2D6 (Merck 2011).

Indications and Efficacy

Approved Indications

Asenapine's efficacy in acute schizophrenia was tested in four pivotal short-term randomized, double-blind, placebo- and active comparator–controlled multicenter studies (Citrome 2011b). Two studies were accepted by the FDA as supportive of asenapine's efficacy in the acute treatment of schizophrenia in adults (Kane et al. 2010; Potkin et al. 2007). Asenapine's efficacy in the treatment of manic or mixed episodes of bipolar I disorder was supported in both of two completed Phase III randomized, placebo- and active comparator–controlled 3-week trials (McIntyre et al. 2009a, 2010a). Approximately 1 year after the initial approval of asenapine for these indications, the FDA approved asenapine for the maintenance treatment of schizophrenia (based on a double-blind, placebo-controlled multicenter clinical trial [Kane et al. 2011]) and for use as adjunctive therapy with either lithium or valproate in the acute treatment of manic or mixed episodes associated with bipolar I disorder (again based on a placebo-controlled trial [Calabrese et al. 2010]).

The recommended dose of asenapine for acute schizophrenia is 5 mg bid; that for bipolar manic or mixed episodes is 10 mg bid (5 mg bid if administered with lithium or valproate), based on the clinical trials used to obtain regulatory approval. Titration to these target doses is not necessary. In a modeling and simulation study (Friberg et al. 2009), asenapine doses of 5 and 10 mg bid had similar efficacy in the acute treatment of schizophrenia.

At present, asenapine is not approved for use in children or adolescents.

Schizophrenia

Short-Term Efficacy

In one of the two positive trials, 458 patients with acute schizophrenia were randomly assigned to fixed-dose treatment with asenapine at 5 mg bid, asenapine at 10 mg bid, placebo, or an active control for assay sensitivity (haloperidol at 4 mg bid) for 6 weeks (Kane et al. 2010). The primary efficacy endpoint was change from baseline in the Positive and Negative Syndrome Scale (PANSS; Kay et al. 1987) total score. On analyses of change in PANSS total score, asenapine at 5 mg bid and haloperidol were both superior to placebo, with statistically significant differences seen from day 21 onward. However, asenapine at 10 mg bid did not demonstrate an advantage over placebo, a finding that the authors suggested may have been due in part to the high placebo response rate in this trial. Rates of response—defined as a minimum reduction of 30% in the PANSS total score or a Clinical Global Impression–Improvement (CGI-I) score of 1 (very much improved) or 2 (much improved)—were 55% for asenapine 5 mg bid, 49% for asenapine 10 mg bid, 43% for haloperidol, and 33% for placebo, yielding numbers needed to treat (NNTs) (Citrome 2008) versus placebo of 5 for asenapine 5 mg bid, 7 for asenapine 10 mg bid, and 10 for haloperidol (Citrome 2011b).

In the second short-term acute schizophrenia trial that was considered positive and supportive of asenapine's efficacy, 182 patients were randomly assigned to asenapine 5 mg bid, placebo, or an active control for assay sensitivity (risperidone 3 mg bid) for 6 weeks (Potkin et al. 2007). The primary efficacy endpoint was change from baseline in the PANSS total score. Compared with placebo, asenapine produced significantly greater decreases in PANSS total scores from week 2 onward. Risperidone did not statistically significantly separate from placebo. Using the criterion of reduction in the PANSS total score of at least 30%, 38% of the patients in the asenapine group were rated as responders, compared with 39% of those in the risperidone group and 25% of those in the placebo group, yielding NNTs versus placebo of 8 for asenapine and 7 for risperidone (Citrome 2011b).

Two other 6-week acute schizophrenia trials were conducted (Citrome 2011b; U.S. Food and Drug Administration 2009). One trial was considered negative because asenapine at 5 or 10 mg bid failed to separate from placebo, whereas the active control (olanzapine at 15 mg/day) did. The other trial was considered a failed trial because neither asenapine at 5 or 10 mg bid nor the active control (olanzapine 10–20 mg/day) separated from placebo.

Longer-Term Efficacy

Asenapine's longer-term efficacy in schizophrenia was examined in a published 1-year double-blind study in 1,225 patients with schizophrenia or schizoaffective disorder. Patients were randomly assigned to receive asenapine (5 mg bid for the first week and then flexible dosing of 5 or 10 mg bid) or olanzapine (10 mg/day for the first week and then flexible dosing of 10 or 20 mg/day) (Schoemaker et al. 2010). There was no placebo arm. Rates of discontinuation because of insufficient therapeutic effect were 25.1% for asenapine and 14.5% for olanzapine (NNT = 10 for olanzapine vs. asenapine to avoid discontinuation because of insufficient therapeutic effect). Changes from baseline in PANSS total score were similar for asenapine and olanzapine at week 6 but showed a statistically significant difference in favor of olanzapine at endpoint (Last Observation Carried Forward). Among the patients who completed the entire year-long trial, changes in PANSS total score were similar for asenapine and olanzapine at week 6 and also at week 52. Completers were eligible to participate in an extension study in which clinical stability was further demonstrated (Schoemaker et al. 2012).

Asenapine's efficacy in the maintenance phase of schizophrenia was demonstrated in a published 26-week double-blind, placebo-controlled multicenter clinical trial (Kane et al. 2011). Patients were randomly assigned either to continue receiving asenapine or to receive placebo after having maintained stability on asenapine during the 26 weeks of open-label treatment immediately prior. Of the 700 enrolled patients who were treated with open-label asenapine, 386 met stability criteria and entered the double-blind phase. Times to relapse/impending relapse and to discontinuation for any reason were significantly longer with asenapine than with placebo. The incidence of relapse or impending relapse was 12.1% for asenapine and 47.4% for placebo (NNT = 3). Completion rates were 69.6% for asenapine and 37.5% for placebo (NNT = 4). The most commonly used dose of asenapine was 10 mg bid in both the open-label and the double-blind phases.

In two randomized, double-blind, 26-week studies and their respective 26-week extensions, Buchanan et al. (2012) tested the hypothesis that asenapine is superior to olanzapine for persistent negative symptoms of schizophrenia and assessed the comparative long-term efficacy and safety of the two agents. Approximately 1,000 subjects participated. In the two core studies, 26-week completion rates with asenapine were 64.7% and 49.6%, versus 80.4% and 63.8%, respectively, with olanzapine. In the two extension studies, completion rates were 84.3% and 66.3% with asenapine versus 89.0% and 80.9%, respectively, with olanzapine. Asenapine was not superior to olanzapine in change in the 16-item Negative Symptom Assessment Scale total score in either core study, but asenapine was superior to olanzapine at week 52 in one of the extension studies. Weight gain was consistently lower with asenapine. EPS-related adverse-event incidence was higher with asenapine, but Extrapyramidal Symptom Rating Scale–Abbreviated total score changes did not differ significantly between treatments.

Bipolar Disorder

In two identically designed 3-week acute studies of asenapine in the treatment of bipolar manic or mixed episodes (McIntyre et al. 2009a, 2010a), 977 subjects were randomly assigned to receive flexibly dosed asenapine

5–10 mg bid (starting dose 10 mg bid), olanzapine 5–20 mg/day (starting dose 15 mg/day), or placebo. The primary outcome measure for each of these studies was change from baseline in the Young-Mania Rating Scale (YMRS; Young et al. 1978) total score. In the first study (McIntyre et al. 2009a), YMRS total scores were statistically significantly improved from baseline to day 21 for asenapine and olanzapine compared with placebo. Sustained statistically significant improvement in the YMRS score compared with placebo was noted for asenapine and olanzapine from day 2 onward. Percentages of subjects meeting criteria for response (50% decrease from baseline YMRS total score) and remission (YMRS total score ≤12) were higher with asenapine (42.3% and 40.2%, respectively) than with placebo (25.2% and 22.3%, respectively), yielding NNTs for response and for remission versus placebo of 6. The NNT for response for olanzapine versus placebo was 5, and that for remission was 6.

In the second study (McIntyre et al. 2010a), YMRS total scores also were statistically significantly improved from baseline to day 21 for asenapine and olanzapine compared with placebo, with sustained statistically significant improvement in the YMRS total score versus placebo noted for asenapine and olanzapine from day 2 onward. In post hoc analyses, changes in YMRS total scores from baseline to day 21 were significantly greater for olanzapine than for asenapine with last observation carried forward analysis, but not with mixed model for repeated measures analysis. Rates of response (42.6%) and remission (35.5%) with asenapine did not differ significantly from those with placebo (34% and 30.9%, respectively), yielding NNTs of 12 and 22, respectively. Olanzapine was superior to placebo in rates of response (54.7%) and remission (46.3%), with NNTs for olanzapine versus placebo of 5 and 7, respectively, and for olanzapine versus asenapine of 9 and 10, respectively.

Asenapine's longer-term efficacy in patients with manic or mixed episodes of bipolar disorder was assessed in a 9-week extension (McIntyre et al. 2009b) to the above two studies, followed by an additional 40-week extension (McIntyre et al. 2010b). A total of 504 subjects received at least one dose of double-blind trial medication during the 9-week extension trial and included 181 subjects who were treated with asenapine and 229 who were treated with olanzapine from the feeder trials (and who continued on the same treatment in the extension). In addition, 94 subjects who were treated with placebo in the feeder trials were blindly allocated to receive asenapine 5–10 mg bid in the extension trial. The primary efficacy analysis demonstrated that asenapine was statistically noninferior to olanzapine as measured by the YMRS total score from baseline to day 84 for the observed case subjects who had 3 weeks of previous exposure to study medication. The proportions of participants who were YMRS responders and remitters were similar in the asenapine and olanzapine groups: the rates of response at last observation carried forward endpoint were 77% and 82% with asenapine and olanzapine, respectively, and the rates of remission were 75% and 79%, respectively. For the 218 patients who were subsequently enrolled for another 40 weeks of double-blinded treatment, maintenance of efficacy was observed for both asenapine and olanzapine, with no differences in response or remission rates.

Another study tested the efficacy of asenapine in the treatment of an acute manic or mixed episode when combined with lithium or divalproex over 12 weeks (Szegedi et al. 2012), and its findings supported this indication as approved by the FDA (Merck 2011). Adjunctive asenapine significantly improved mania versus placebo at week 3 (primary endpoint) and weeks 2–12. The YMRS response rates were similar at week 3 but significantly better with asenapine at week 12. The YMRS remission rates and changes from baseline on Clinical Global Impression for Bipolar Disorder for mania and overall illness were significantly better with asenapine at weeks 3 and 12. Patients completing the core study were eligible for a 40-week double-blind extension assessing safety and tolerability (Szegedi et al. 2012).

Side Effects and Toxicology

Common adverse reactions with asenapine observed in short-term trials (incidence ≥5% and twofold greater than placebo) were akathisia, oral hypoesthesia (numbness), and somnolence for patients with schizophrenia, and somnolence, dizziness, extrapyramidal symptoms (EPS) other than akathisia, and increased weight for patients with bipolar manic or mixed episodes (Merck 2011).

Somnolence is the single most common adverse event associated with asenapine treatment. The product label describes this effect as usually transient, with the highest incidence reported during the first week of treatment (Merck 2011). The highest rates of somnolence were observed in the short-term acute manic/mixed-episode bipolar trials (most common dosage = 10 mg bid), where somnolence was reported in 24% of patients receiving asenapine versus 6% of patients receiving placebo, for a number needed to harm (NNH) of 6; rates of reported somnolence in the short-term schizophrenia trials (dosage = 5 or 10 mg bid) were 13% for asenapine versus 7% for placebo, yielding an NNH of 17 (Citrome 2009). Comparisons of other antipsychotics against placebo on the outcome of somnolence in short-term acute trials of schizophrenia yielded a broad range of incidence rates, resulting in NNH values that ranged from 7 for olanzapine or quetiapine extended-release to a non–statistically significant 42 for paliperidone (Citrome and Nasrallah 2012). Although somnolence was frequently reported, somnolence/sedation led to discontinuation in only a small proportion (0.6%) of patients treated with asenapine (Merck 2011).

Dizziness can also occur and is attributable to asenapine's α_1-adrenergic antagonist activity; however, rates of syncope were observed to be low among patients in contrast to rates observed among healthy volunteers in the clinical pharmacology trials (U.S. Food and Drug Administration 2009). Asenapine has a dose-related association with EPS and akathisia, although the frequency of these events is substantially lower with asenapine than with haloperidol (Citrome 2009).

Unique to asenapine is the possibility of oral hypoesthesia, spontaneously reported as an adverse reaction in about 5% of the participants with acute schizophrenia in the clinical trials (Merck 2011). Directly asking patients about oral hypoesthesia may yield higher rates of this adverse effect, as was observed in a study that examined the effect of absorption site on the pharmacokinetics of asenapine in healthy male subjects (Gerrits et al. 2010). In this study, reported rates of oral paresthesias were 75.8%, 55.9%, and 45.7% for the sublingual, supralingual, and and buccal absorption sites, respectively.

Asenapine has a mild effect on QTc interval, similar to that seen with quetiapine (Chapel et al. 2009, 2011). Hypersensitivity reactions have been reported with asenapine, in some cases occurring after the first dose, and this risk is now highlighted in product labeling (Merck 2011).

Asenapine's effects on prolactin levels in the short-term schizophrenia and bipolar manic/mixed episode studies revealed no clinically relevant changes. In the 6-week acute schizophrenia trials, clinically relevant weight gain (≥7% over baseline) was observed in 4.9% of subjects receiving asenapine versus 2% of those receiving placebo. In the 3-week acute bipolar manic/mixed episode studies, clinically relevant weight gain was observed in 5.8% of subjects receiving asenapine versus 0.5% of those receiving placebo. In addition to a favorable weight-gain profile, asenapine has shown minimal effects on glucose-related laboratory parameters such as fasting glucose and fasting insulin (Schering-Plough 2009).

Of interest are longer-term safety and tolerability comparisons of asenapine with other antipsychotics. In a 1-year double-blind, randomized controlled trial comparing asenapine with olanzapine (Schoemaker et al. 2010), the incidence of treatment-emergent adverse events was 82% in both groups. Mean weight gain was 0.9 kg with asenapine and 4.2 kg with olanzapine. The proportion of patients experiencing clinically relevant weight gain (≥7%) was approximately 35% for olanzapine and approximately 15% for asenapine (olanzapine vs. asenapine, NNH=5). No notable changes or between-group differences were seen in measures of total cholesterol or glucose, but triglyceride levels rose substantially with olanzapine and declined slightly with asenapine. In the 2-year blinded extension study (Schoemaker et al. 2012), mean body weight during the extension did not change beyond the weight gain in the core study. In the core study, EPS reported as adverse events were more common with asenapine (18%) than with olanzapine (8%) (asenapine vs. olanzapine, NNH=10). The most commonly reported type of movement disorder in the asenapine and olanzapine groups was akathisia, with treatment-emergent rates of 10% for asenapine and 4% for olanzapine (asenapine vs. olanzapine, NNH= 17). In the 2-year blinded extension study, incidence rates of EPS-related adverse events that started during the extension were lower for both asenapine (4.5%) and olanzapine (3.3%) compared with those that started during the core study. Not many new cases of akathisia were reported during the extension period. There was little change in EPS severity during the extension of treatment.

Safety and tolerability outcomes are available from a 40-week extension to the acute bipolar trials (McIntyre et al. 2010b), where clinically relevant weight gain occurred in 21.9%, 39.2%, and 55.1% of patients in the placebo/asenapine, asenapine, and olanzapine groups, respectively. The NNH for clinically relevant weight gain for olanzapine versus asenapine was 7. The percentage of patients shifting to above a prespecified akathisia global rating scale threshold was higher in the asenapine group compared with the placebo/asenapine and olanzapine groups.

Conclusion

Asenapine's efficacy is evidenced both in short-term acute clinical trials and in longer-term studies. In the mind of the clinician, asenapine will likely be measured against other "metabolically friendly" second-generation antipsychotics such as ziprasidone, aripiprazole, iloperidone, and lurasidone (Citrome 2011a). Differences among these choices include dosing factors (daily versus twice-daily dosing, the need for dosage titration, special requirements for administration with or without food) as well as specific side-effect profiles. Relative efficacy rankings among these five agents (asenapine, ziprasidone, aripiprazole, iloperidone, and lurasidone) are not known and will require specifically designed and adequately powered head-to-head studies. Head-to-head comparisons with older second-generation antipsychotics such as quetiapine and risperidone would also be of interest.

Asenapine is unique in being the only antipsychotic that is absorbed primarily in the oral mucosa. Nonadherence by "cheeking" becomes moot. The possibility of oral hypoesthesia and dysgeusia (distorted or bad taste), a medication effect likely not experienced previously by the patient, necessitates advance warning.

In summary, asenapine's place in the treatment of schizophrenia and bipolar manic or mixed episodes is likely to be in patients for whom metabolic concerns are of import and in patients who would prefer a sublingual preparation. Substantial heterogeneity exists among the different antipsychotics and among individual patients (Volavka and Citrome 2009), so that asenapine has a legitimate place on a formulary.

Specific obstacles to the first-line use of asenapine are the recommendations for twice-daily versus once-daily administration and the recommendation to avoid food or liquids for 10 minutes after dosing. Cost may be a further impediment, given the availability of inexpensive generic versions of risperidone, quetiapine, and olanzapine in the United States, as well as other generic second-generation antipsychotics in other countries.

References

Buchanan RW, Panagides J, Zhao J, et al: Asenapine versus olanzapine in people with persistent negative symptoms of schizophrenia. J Clin Psychopharmacol 32:36–45, 2012

Calabrese J, Stet L, Kotari H, et al: Asenapine as adjunctive treatment for bipolar mania: a placebo-controlled 12-week study and 40-week extension (abstract no. PW01-28). Eur Psychiatry 25 (suppl 1):1447, 2010

Chapel S, Hutmacher MM, Haig G, et al: Exposure-response analysis in patients with schizophrenia to assess the effect of asenapine on QTc prolongation. J Clin Pharmacol 49:1297–1308, 2009

Chapel S, Hutmacher MM, Bockbrader H, et al. Comparison of QTc data analysis methods recommended by the ICH E14 guidance and exposure-response analysis: case study of a thorough QT study of asenapine. Clin Pharmacol Ther 89:75–80, 2011

Citrome L: Compelling or irrelevant? Using number needed to treat can help decide. Acta Psychiatr Scand 117:412–419, 2008

Citrome L: Asenapine for schizophrenia and bipolar disorder: a review of the efficacy and safety profile for this newly approved sublingually absorbed second-generation antipsychotic. Int J Clin Pract 63:1762–1784, 2009

Citrome L: Iloperidone, asenapine, and lurasidone: a brief overview of 3 new second-generation antipsychotics. Postgrad Med 123:153–162, 2011a

Citrome L: Role of sublingual asenapine in treatment of schizophrenia. Neuropsychiatr Dis Treat 7:325–339, 2011b

Citrome L, Nasrallah HA: On-label on the table: what the package insert informs us about the tolerability profile of oral atypical antipsychotics, and what it does not. Expert Opin Pharmacother 13:1599–1613, 2012

Friberg LE, De Greef R, Kerbusch T, et al: Modeling and simulation of the time course of asenapine exposure response and dropout patterns in acute schizophrenia. Clin Pharmacol Ther 86:84–91, 2009

Gerrits M, de Greef R, Peeters P: Effect of absorption site on the pharmacokinetics of sublingual asenapine in healthy male subjects. Biopharm Drug Dispos 31:351–357, 2010

Kane JM, Cohen M, Zhao J, et al: Efficacy and safety of asenapine in a placebo- and haloperidol-controlled trial in patients with acute exacerbation of schizophrenia. J Clin Psychopharmacol 30:106–115, 2010

Kane JM, Mackle M, Snow-Adami L, et al: A randomized placebo-controlled trial of asenapine for the prevention of relapse of schizophrenia after long-term treatment. J Clin Psychiatry 72:349–355, 2011

Kay SR, Fiszbein A, Opler LA: The positive and negative syndrome scale (PANSS) for schizophrenia. Schizophr Bull 13:261–276, 1987

McIntyre RS, Cohen M, Zhao J, et al: A 3-week, randomized, placebo-controlled trial of asenapine in the treatment of acute mania in bipolar mania and mixed states. Bipolar Disord 11:673–686, 2009a

McIntyre RS, Cohen M, Zhao J, et al: Asenapine versus olanzapine in acute mania: a double-blind extension study. Bipolar Disord 11:815–826, 2009b

McIntyre RS, Cohen M, Zhao J, et al: Asenapine in the treatment of acute mania in bipolar I disorder: a randomized, double-blind, placebo-controlled trial. J Affect Disord 122:27–38, 2010a

McIntyre RS, Cohen M, Zhao J, et al: Asenapine for long-term treatment of bipolar disorder: a double-blind 40-week extension study. J Affect Disord 126:358–365, 2010b

Merck & Co., Inc.: Saphris (asenapine) sublingual tablets. Product label, revised October 2011. Available at: http://www.spfiles.com/pisaphrisv1.pdf. Accessed October 12, 2011.

Potkin SG, Cohen M, Panagides J: Efficacy and tolerability of asenapine in acute schizophrenia: a placebo- and risperidone-controlled trial. J Clin Psychiatry 68:1492–1500, 2007

Schering-Plough Research Institute: Saphris (asenapine) Sublingual Tablets. Briefing Document (Background Package). 30 July 2009. Available at: http://www.fda.gov/downloads/AdvisoryCommittees/CommitteesMeetingMaterials/Drugs/PsychopharmacologicDrugsAdvisoryCommittee/UCM173876.pdf. Accessed October 12, 2011.

Schoemaker J, Naber D, Vrijland P, et al: Long-term assessment of asenapine vs. olanzapine in patients with schizophrenia or schizoaffective disorder. Pharmacopsychiatry 43:138–146, 2010

Schoemaker J, Stet L, Vrijland P, et al: Long-term efficacy and safety of asenapine or olanzapine in patients with schizophrenia or schizoaffective disorder: an extension study. Pharmacopsychiatry 45:196–203, 2012

Shahid M, Walker GB, Zorn SH, et al: Asenapine: a novel psychopharmacological agent with a unique human receptor signature. J Psychopharmacol 23:65–73, 2009

Szegedi A, Calabrese JR, Stet L, et al: Asenapine as adjunctive treatment for acute mania associated with bipolar disorder: results of a 12-week core study and 40-week extension. J Clin Psychopharmacol 32:46-55, 2012

U.S. Food and Drug Administration: Saphris (asenapine) Sublingual Tablets. Briefing Book. 30 July 2009. Available at: http://www.fda.gov/downloads/AdvisoryCommittees/CommitteesMeetingMaterials/Drugs/PsychopharmacologicDrugsAdvisoryCommittee/UCM173877.pdf. Accessed October 12, 2011.

Volavka J, Citrome L: Oral antipsychotics for the treatment of schizophrenia: heterogeneity in efficacy and tolerability should drive decision-making. Expert Opin Pharmacother 10:1917–1928, 2009

Young RC, Biggs JT, Ziegler VE, et al: A rating scale for mania: reliability, validity and sensitivity. Br J Psychiatry 133:429–435, 1978

CHAPTER 24

Iloperidone

Peter F. Buckley, M.D.

Adriana E. Foster, M.D.

Oliver Freudenreich, M.D.

Scott Van Sant, M.D.

History

Iloperidone was approved in 2009 by the U.S. Food and Drug Administration (FDA) for the treatment of schizophrenia. It meets the now generally appreciated profile of second-generation antipsychotics (SGAs), in that it has a complex pharmacology (with a predilection for dopamine and serotonin antagonism) and little propensity for extrapyramidal side effects (EPS) as well as efficacy against key symptoms of schizophrenia as shown in placebo-controlled clinical trials (Rado and Janicak 2010; Weiden 2012). The efficacy of iloperidone appears within the dosage range of 12–24 mg/day, with no clear advantage demonstrated at higher dosages. It is recommended that iloperidone be initiated and titrated upward with caution, largely due to the risk of dizziness and postural hypotension consequent to its antagonism of noradrenergic α_1 receptors. Clinical experience with the use of iloperidone is accruing. Comparative information for iloperidone in relation to other SGAs is limited at present (Tarazi and Stahl 2012). Additional clinical trials of iloperidone are ongoing (see www.clinicaltrials.gov).

Receptor Profile–Activity Relationship

Iloperidone is an SGA of the piperidinyl-benzisoxazole class. Other structurally similar benzisoxasole derivatives include risperidone and its metabolite paliperidone as well as ziprasidone. Iloperidone's chemistry and specific binding profile across multiple neuroreceptors are complex (Citrome 2010; Kalkman et al. 2003). In brief, like several other SGAs, iloperidone is a 5-HT_{2A-D2} antagonist. In addition, it has strong affinity for dopamine D_3 receptors, as well as a lesser (but still more pronounced compared with other SGAs) affinity at D_4 receptors. It also has affinity at both 5-HT_6 and 5-HT_7 receptors. Iloperidone is further distinguished by its antagonism of noradrenergic α_1 receptors. Beyond clozapine, the extent of iloperidone's α_1-receptor affinity exceeds that of all other SGAs. In contrast, iloperidone has low affinity for 5-HT_{1A} and histamine H_1 receptors. Collectively, this receptor affinity constellation may account for iloperidone's adverse-effect attributes of postural hypotension risk, prolactin-elevating capacity, modest weight-gain propensity, and mild sedative effects.

Pharmacokinetics and Disposition

Iloperidone is readily absorbed from the gastrointestinal tract and reaches peak plasma concentrations within approximately 2 hours after ingestion. Its absorption is slowed by food, but its bioavailability is unaffected; thus, it can be given either with or without food.

Iloperidone is extensively metabolized by the cytochrome P450 (CYP) enzyme system, particularly the 3A4 and 2D6 isoenzymes. The average half-life for iloperidone in "regular" (extensive) CYP2D6 metabolizers is approximately 24 hours. Clinicians need to be cautious when prescribing iloperidone concurrently with CYP2D6 and CYP3A4 enzyme inhibitors, including several antidepressant medications. It has been shown that a statistically significant greater proportion of iloperidone responders than of nonresponders have average plasma concentrations of ≥5 ng/mL, although plasma concentration of iloperidone is not available in clinical practices (Weiden 2012).

Iloperidone is currently available in tablet form. No liquid or short-term intramuscular formulations or long-acting injectable forms have been developed.

There is currently no clinical indication that the dosage of iloperidone should be adjusted to take account of age or gender, although it is also noteworthy that the potential for postural hypotension could be markedly higher in the elderly. Clinical studies of iloperidone in schizophrenia did not include sufficient numbers of patients 65 years and older to determine whether they respond differently than younger adult patients. Among more than 3,000 patients treated with iloperidone in these early registration trials, only 25 patients (0.5%) were ≥65 years old, and there were no patients ≥75 years old. Safety and effectiveness in pediatric patients have not yet been well studied; therefore, the drug should not be prescribed for children or adolescents. Additionally, the teratogenic risk of iloperidone is unknown. It is therefore advised that lactating women who are being treated with iloperidone refrain from breast-feeding their newborns. The most recent FDA recommendations regarding use of antipsychotics in pregnancy and neonatal periods also apply to iloperidone (see FDA MedWatch; www.fda.gov/Safety/MedWatch).

Indications and Efficacy

Iloperidone is FDA approved for the acute treatment of schizophrenia. There are no other indications for iloperidone under consideration by the FDA at the time of writing. However, the clinical trials program for this drug now includes investigative studies in mood disorders that are currently ongoing (see www.clinicaltrials.com).

Schizophrenia

Pivotal Clinical Trials

Iloperidone's FDA approval for the treatment of schizophrenia was predominantly based on four short-term placebo-controlled trials, highlighted in Table 24–1. In addition, one long-term trial has been published (Kane et al. 2008). An account of these studies is given below. A more complete review of drug development and initial trials in humans is provided elsewhere (Citrome 2010).

Potkin et al. (2008) described the 6-week double-blind period of the pivotal trials that evaluated iloperidone for treatment of schizophrenia. All of these trials included screening, a double-blind phase, and a long-term extension phase.

Study 1 enrolled patients ages 18–65 years with acute or subacute exacerbation of schizophrenia and schizoaffective disorder and Positive and Negative Syndrome Scale (PANSS) scores ≥60. One hundred twenty-one patients were randomly assigned to iloperidone 4 mg/day, 125 to iloperidone 8 mg/day, 124 to iloperidone 24 mg/day, 124 to haloperidol 15 mg/day, and 127 to placebo. After a screening and a 3-day placebo run-in period as well as a 7-day fixed-titration period, patients were maintained on study medication for 5 weeks. The primary objective was to determine the efficacy of iloperidone versus placebo. The primary efficacy variable was change in PANSS total score (PANSS-T) from baseline to endpoint (day 42 or last visit before discontinuation). While PANSS-T scores improved significantly from baseline for the iloperidone 12 mg/day (P=0.047) and haloperidol (P<0.001) groups, improvement for the combined iloperidone 8 mg/day and 12 mg/day groups was not significantly different from placebo. The all-reasons discontinuation rates were 57%, 64%, and 58% for iloperidone 4 mg/day, 8 mg/day, and 12 mg/day, respectively; 65% for haloperidol; and 69% for placebo.

In Study 2, patients selected according to the same inclusion criteria used in Study 1 were randomly assigned to iloperidone 4–8 mg/day (n=53; 52% discontinued the study before endpoint) or 10–16 mg/day (n=154; 44% discontinued), risperidone 4–8 mg (n=153; 42% discontinued), or placebo (n=156; 60% discontinued). The primary objective was again to determine the efficacy of iloperidone versus placebo. Both dosage ranges of iloperidone (4–8 mg/day and 10–16 mg/day) significantly changed symptom scores (measured with the Brief Psychiatric Rating Scale [BPRS]) from baseline compared with placebo.

In Study 3, iloperidone 12–16 mg/day (n=244; 46% discontinued), iloperidone 20–24 mg/day (n=145; 41% discontinued), risperidone 6–8 mg/day (n=157; 29% discontinued), or placebo (n=160; 46% discontinued) was administered to patients selected according to the same criteria described above. In this study the iloperidone 12–16 mg/day group failed to differentiate from placebo. A combined analysis of all three studies was done in order to eliminate the impact of early discontinuations in the initial 2 weeks of the studies, during which the drug reaches steady state. This analysis included all patients who remained on double-blind treatment for at least 2 weeks (n=1,553), and it showed that each iloperidone dosage range (4–8, 10–16, and 20–24 mg/day) differentiated significantly from placebo.

A 4-week double-blind study (Cutler et al. 2008) evaluated the efficacy of iloperidone 24 mg/day against placebo and ziprasidone 160 mg/day in patients with acute exacerbation of schizophrenia by measuring change from baseline in the PANSS-T score and the PANSS positive, negative, and general psychopathology scale scores; the Calgary Depression Scale for Schizophrenia (CDSS); and the Clinical Global Impression–Severity (CGI-S). Iloperidone significantly reduced PANSS-T scores at 4 weeks compared with placebo. Although both iloperidone and ziprasidone significantly improved negative and positive PANSS and CGI-S scores compared with placebo, none of the drugs improved PANSS general psychopathology scores significantly, nor did they affect CDSS scores.

Kane et al. (2008) reported on 473 of the patients who completed the 6-week double-blind phase of the three studies described above with at least 20% reduction in PANSS-T scores and a CGI score of less than 4 and who received at least one dose of long-term-phase medication. These patients were randomly assigned to iloperidone or haloperidol, and mean dosages at the end of 46 weeks of double-blind maintenance treatment were 12.5 mg/day for both drugs. The primary efficacy variable was relapse, defined as an increase in PANSS score of ≥25%. The difference in the time until relapse was not significant between the iloperidone and halo-

TABLE 24–1. Pivotal clinical trials of iloperidone efficacy in patients with schizophrenia and schizoaffective disorder

Study	*N* and diagnosis	Iloperidone and comparator drug dosages (mg/day)	Efficacy outcome measure	Symptom change from baseline to endpoint
Potkin et al. 2008 Three 6-week randomized, double-blind studies comparing ILO against PLA	1,943 patients with schizophrenia or schizoaffective disorder	*Study 1:* ILO 4, 8, 12; HAL 15; PLA *Study 2:* ILO 4–8, 10–16; RIS 4–8; PLA *Study 3:* ILO 12–16, 20–24; RIS 6–8; PLA	**Primary:** PANSS-T or PANSS-derived BPRS change from baseline to endpoint **Secondary:** PANSS-P, PANSS-N, PANSS-GP; BPRS change from baseline to each postbaseline assessment; CGI-S in Studies 2 and 3	*Study 1* • Changes in PANSS-T from baseline were significant with ILO 12 ($P=0.04$) and HAL 15 ($P<0.01$). • Combined ILO 8–12 was NS vs. PLA. • HAL vs. PLA was significant ($P<0.001$). *Studies 2 and 3* • ILO all dosages and RIS changed BPRS from baseline in Studies 2 and 3. • Compared with PLA, changes were significant with ILO 4–8 ($P=0.012$), 10–16 ($P=0.001$), and 20–24 ($P=0.01$) in Study 3. • ILO 12–16 vs. PLA was NS in Study 3. • RIS vs. PLA was significant in all studies ($P<0.001$). • All dosages ILO improved each variable vs. PLA except ILO 4–8 for PANSS-N in Study 2.
Potkin et al. 2008 Combined analysis of three studies	1,553 patients who remained in the studies at least 2 weeks			All dosages ILO as well as HAL and RIS were statistically significant vs. PLA ($P<0.05$).

TABLE 24–1. Pivotal clinical trials of iloperidone efficacy in patients with schizophrenia and schizoaffective disorder *(continued)*

Study	*N* and diagnosis	Iloperidone and comparator drug dosages (mg/day)	Efficacy outcome measure	Symptom change from baseline to endpoint
Kane et al. 2008 Long-term (46-week) double-blind maintenance phase after 6-week stabilization	473 patients with schizophrenia or schizoaffective disorder who had responded to ILO (*n*=371) or HAL (*n*=118) during stabilization phase (36.6% responded to ILO and 37.8% to HAL in the acute phase)	ILO 4–16; HAL 5–20 Mean dosage at end of maintenance = 12.5 for both drugs	**Primary:** time to relapse* **Secondary:** change from baseline to endpoint on PANSS, BPRS, and CGI-C	Difference in time to relapse between ILO (89.8 days) and HAL (101.8 days) was not significant. Relapse rate was 43.5% ILO vs. 41.2% HAL. Both groups improved; PANSS scores were not significantly different at endpoint between ILO and HAL.
Cutler et al. 2008 4-week 1-week titration 3-week double-blind treatment for acute exacerbation	593 patients with schizophrenia	ILO 24; ZIP 160; PLA	**Primary:** change from baseline in PANSS-T for ILO vs. PLA **Secondary:** change from baseline in BPRS, PANSS-P, PANSS-N, PANSS-GP, CGI-S, CGI-C, CDSS	ILO reduced PANSS-T significantly vs. PLA ($P<0.01$). ILO and ZIP significantly reduced all measures except PANSS-GP. ILO reduced PANSS-P, CGI-S, and CGI-C significantly vs. PLA. Neither ILO nor ZIP reduced CDSS significantly.

Note. HAL=haloperidol; ILO=iloperidone; PLA=placebo; RIS=risperidone.
PANSS-T=total; PANSS-P=positive symptoms; PANSS-N=negative symptoms; PANSS-GP=general psychopathology; CGI-S=severity; CGI-C=change.
*Relapse = 25% increase in PANSS-T scores; discontinuation due to lack of efficacy, hospitalization, or CGI increase by 2 points.

peridol groups—63.6% of both the iloperidone and haloperidol groups completed the long-term phase of the trial.

Pharmacogenetic Studies

Clinical trials of iloperidone also sought to establish the pharmacogenetic characteristics of iloperidone (Volpi et al. 2009a, 2009b) and explored the relationship between its efficacy and various candidate genes related to dopamine receptors, dopamine β-hydroxylase, the serotonin 1B ($5\text{-}HT_{1B}$) receptor, and the ciliary neurotrophic factor (CNTF). CNTF is a cytokine in the interleukin-6 cytokine family that suppresses noradrenergic and serotonergic function (Galter and Unsicker 1999). A null mutation in the CNTF gene leads to a non-G/G rs1800169 genotype, which does not produce functional protein and has been linked with an increased risk of psychosis (Thome et al. 1996). However, a meta-analysis including more than 1,000 patients and a similar number of control subjects (Lin and Tsai 2004) found no association between CNTF and schizophrenia.

Of 417 patients genotyped for CNTF, 279 received iloperidone and 138 received placebo in a 4-week randomized, placebo-controlled study (Lavedan et al. 2008). Iloperidone improved symptom scores significantly versus placebo in patients with an active CNTF gene, whereas patients with the CNTF null allele responded similarly to both iloperidone and placebo.

A whole-genome study of 407 patients from the same sample, of which 218 patients received iloperidone, identified six single-nucleotide polymorphisms (SNPs) associated with iloperidone efficacy (Volpi et al. 2009b). The loci identified included SNPs of the neuronal PAS domain protein 3 gene (*NPAS3*); the XK, Kell blood group complex subunit–related family, member 4 gene (*XKR4*); the tenascin-R gene (*TNR*); the glutamate receptor, ionotropic, AMPA 4 gene (*GRIA4*); the glial cell line–derived neurotrophic factor receptor alpha 2 gene (*GFRA2*); and the NUDT9P1 pseudogene located in the chromosomal region of the serotonin receptor 7 gene (*HTR7*). More than 75% of iloperidone-treated patients in the group with the optimal genotype combinations showed a ≥20% improvement, whereas only 37% of patients with other genotypes showed a ≥20% improvement.

Another whole-genome association study (Volpi et al. 2009a) was conducted in 183 patients with schizophrenia who received an electrocardiogram (ECG) on day 14 of treatment with iloperidone, after the drug established steady state. DNA polymorphisms associated with QT prolongation were found in six loci, including the *CERKL*, thought to be part of the ceramide pathway; the *SLCO3A1* gene, which encodes the organic anion-transporting polypeptide; genes involved in myocardial infarction (*PALLD*), cardiac structure and function (*BRUNOL4*), and cardiac development (*NRG3*); and SNP on *NUBPL* gene with unknown function. Each SNP defined two genotype groups associated with a low mean QT or a higher mean QT prolongation.

While these findings have drawn considerable interest from the field, the potential of iloperidone pharmacogenomics needs to be tested further in larger studies before this could be of clinical utility. Having said that, incorporation of pharmacogenetic testing into the regulatory registration trials of this drug represents an important new aspect of psychopharmacological drug development.

Other Indications

Little information is available on the use of iloperidone in patients with first-episode psychosis. Similarly, there are no studies to inform the use of iloperidone in patients with treatment-refractory schizophrenia. There is no information on the efficacy or tolerability of iloperidone in patients with comorbid substance abuse. Information on the use of iloperidone in other comorbid conditions and/or other primary psychiatric and neuropsychiatric disorders is scant. Accordingly, off-label use of this drug cannot be recommended.

Side Effects and Toxicology

The safety of iloperidone in short-term studies was examined in a pooled analysis of three Phase II short-term acute schizophrenia studies ($N = 1,943$) conducted between 1998 and 2002 (Potkin et al. 2008). A total of 1,912 patients received at least one dose of study medication and were included in this pooled analysis. The safety population included 440 patients on placebo, 463 on iloperidone 4–8 mg/day, 456 on iloperidone 10–16 mg/day, 125 on iloperidone 20–24 mg/day, 118 on haloperidol 15 mg/day, and 306 on risperidone 4–8 mg/day. The most common treatment-related adverse events associated with iloperidone across all three dosage groups were dizziness, dry mouth, somnolence, and dyspepsia (Table 24–2).

With respect to available data from long-term studies, three prospective multicenter studies—each with a 6-week stabilization period followed by a 46-week double-blind maintenance phase—inform our understanding of iloperidone's longer-term tolerability (see Table 24–2). Patients were randomly assigned to iloperidone 4–16 mg/day or haloperidol 5–20 mg/day. Of the 1,644 patients who were randomized and the 1,326 who completed the 6-week phase, 473 (iloperidone 359, haloperidol 114) were included in the long-term efficacy analysis and 489 (iloperidone 371, haloperidol 118) were included in the safety analysis. The most common adverse events reported for iloperidone were insomnia, anxiety, and headache.

In the pooled analysis of pivotal short-term trials comparing iloperidone, risperidone, and haloperidol, the overall rating of EPS on the Extrapyramidal Symptom Rating Scale (ESRS; Chouinard and Margolese 2005) demonstrated significant improvement from baseline to endpoint with all iloperidone dosages; by comparison, there was no significant change with risperidone and significant worsening with haloperidol. Akathisia items on the ESRS all showed significant improvement from baseline in the iloperidone 10–16 mg/day and 20–24 mg/day dosage ranges (Weiden et al. 2008). The low EPS profile of iloperidone is an advantage clinically, even in an era of predominantly SGA prescribing in which one's risk of EPS is much lower than heretofore (Weiden 2012). Moreover, the absence of a dose-related increase in EPS across dosage ranges in clinical trials of iloperidone is conspicuous and encouraging.

In view of its antagonism at α_1-noradrenergic receptors, iloperidone possesses the potential for autonomic side effects. In its clinical trials program, iloperidone was associated with decreases in supine and standing systolic and diastolic blood pressures in all dosage groups. Decreases in blood pressure were mostly observed within the first week of treatment and were generally not sustained. Orthostatic hypotension was observed more frequently in all active-treatment groups (iloperidone, risperidone, and haloperidol) than in the placebo group. Sustained orthostatic hypotension was observed in 0.4% ($n = 2$), 3.8% ($n = 17$), and 4.8% ($n = 6$) of patients receiving iloperidone 4–8 mg/day, 10–16 mg/day, and 20–24 mg/day, respectively. According to the product label, due to the risk of orthostatic hypotension, iloperidone should be titrated slowly, with a starting dosage of 1 mg twice daily, increasing to 2 mg, 4 mg, 6 mg, 8 mg, 10 mg, and 12 mg twice daily on days 2, 3, 4, 5, 6, and 7, respectively, to reach the 12–24 mg/day dosage range. Clinicians should therefore pay particular attention to dizziness early in treatment with iloperidone. It is also an important consideration to go even slower with initial titration in patients who may be at risk for postural hypotension (Weiden 2012).

One of the potential advantages of iloperidone could be its profile with respect to metabolic issues and weight gain (De Hert et al. 2012; Tarazi and Stahl 2012). Compared with patients receiving placebo, patients receiving iloperidone exhibited a small but statistically significant increase in weight across all dosages. For all patients complet-

TABLE 24–2. Safety profile of iloperidone in short- and long-term studies: adverse events occurring in at least 5% of patients in any active-treatment group

EVENT (%)	SHORT-TERM STUDIES[a]					LONG-TERM STUDIES[b]	
	ILO 4–8 MG/DAY (*n*=463)	ILO 10–16 MG/DAY (*n*=456)	ILO 20–24 MG/DAY (*n*=125)	HAL 15 MG/DAY (*n*=118)	RIS 4–8 MG/DAY (*n*=306)	ILO (*n*=371)	HAL (*n*=118)
Akathisia	3.7	1.5	4.8	13.6	6.9	3.8	14.4
Dizziness	12.1	10.3	23.2	5.1	7.2	5.1	4.2
EPS	5.4	4.8	4.0	20.3	9.5	0.8	5.9
Tremor	2.8	2.6	4.8	22.0	6.9	4.9	12.7
Dry mouth	5.2	7.9	10.4	2.5	2.9	*	*
Dyspepsia	7.8	5.5	4.8	11.0	5.9	*	*
Dystonia	0.9	0.9	0.8	11.9	2.6	*	*
Fatigue	4.3	4.6	6.4	7.6	1.6	*	*
Flatulence	1.9	1.3	1.6	5.1	2.3	*	*
Nasal congestion	4.8	5.0	5.6	1.7	2.6	*	*
Somnolence	5.0	5.7	8.0	6.8	5.9	*	*
Insomnia	*	*	*	*	*	18.1	16.9
Anxiety	*	*	*	*	*	10.8	11.0
Headache	*	*	*	*	*	6.2	4.2
Agitation	*	*	*	*	*	5.7	5.1
Muscle rigidity	*	*	*	*	*	4.0	12.7

TABLE 24–2. Safety profile of iloperidone in short- and long-term studies: adverse events occurring in at least 5% of patients in any active-treatment group *(continued)*

	Short-term studies[a]					Long-term studies[b]	
Event (%)	**ILO 4–8 mg/day (*n*=463)**	**ILO 10–16 mg/day (*n*=456)**	**ILO 20–24 mg/day (*n*=125)**	**HAL 15 mg/day (*n*=118)**	**RIS 4–8 mg/day (*n*=306)**	**ILO (*n*=371)**	**HAL (*n*=118)**
Restlessness	*	*	*	*	*	3.5	6.8
Constipation	*	*	*	*	*	2.2	5.1

Note. "Schizophrenia aggravated" and "psychosis aggravated" were listed as adverse events in the Kane et al. 2008 study but were not included in this table. EPS=extrapyramidal side effects; HAL=haloperidol; ILO=iloperidone; RIS=risperidone.

*Did not occur in at least 5% of comparators.

[a]Pooled analysis of 6-week studies.

[b]Long-term (46 weeks) maintenance treatment (mean dosage 12.5 mg/day at study end for both drugs).

Source. Adapted from Kane et al. 2008 and Weiden et al. 2008.

ing the respective studies, the mean weight gain was 2.4 kg in each iloperidone dosing group. Clinically significant weight gain (defined as ≥7% increase in body weight from baseline) occurred in 12.3% of all iloperidone groups (Weiden et al. 2008). The majority of the weight gain occurred within the first 6 weeks of the studies (6.4%). Long-term treatment with iloperidone also produced slight increases in total cholesterol, triglycerides, and glucose levels (Kane et al. 2008). Increased prolactin levels were not observed in the pooled analysis of the three 6-week trials. The product label, however, emphasizes findings from the 4-week iloperidone versus ziprasidone versus placebo trial, in which 26% of subjects receiving iloperidone versus 12% of those receiving placebo exhibited elevated plasma prolactin levels. Thus, the relatively more favorable weight and metabolic profiles of iloperidone constitute a distinction that might guide the selection and use of iloperidone in particular patient groups (Weiden 2012).

With respect to potentially life-threatening side effects, there was evidence of significant QT/ QTc interval prolongation across all iloperidone groups in the drug's pivotal study program, and this was a focus of review by the FDA. Specifically, the least square mean changes in QTc from baseline to endpoint in these studies were 2.9 msec, 3.9 msec, and 9.1 msec for iloperidone 4–8 mg/day, 10–16 mg/day, and 20–24 mg/day, respectively. It is noteworthy that no deaths or serious arrhythmias attributable to QT prolongation occurred in these studies (Weiden 2012; Weiden et al. 2008). According to the product label, iloperidone should be avoided in combination with other drugs that are known to prolong QTc, including Class Ia (e.g., quinidine, procainamide) or Class III (e.g., amiodarone, sotalol) antiarrhythmic medications, antipsychotic medications, antibiotics, or any other class of medications known to prolong the QTc interval. This prohibition makes sense, given iloperidone's metabolism through these cytochrome pathways. In addition, it is recommended that iloperidone be avoided in persons with congenital long-QT syndrome or cardiac arrhythmias. Similar to all other SGAs, iloperidone carries a black box warning regarding increased mortality in elderly patients with dementia-related psychosis. That said, iloperidone is not approved for the treatment of patients with dementia-related psychosis, and use in the elderly should be avoided pending future clinical trials.

Conclusion

Iloperidone is an FDA-approved antipsychotic for use in the treatment of schizophrenia. There remains much to be studied regarding its use in specific patient subgroups of psychotic patients. Its use in nonapproved areas of mood disorders is presently unknown. There is also a need for additional dose-finding studies to inform clinicians about the optimal use of this drug.

References

Citrome L: Iloperidone: chemistry, pharmacodynamics, pharmacokinetics and metabolism, clinical efficacy, safety and tolerability, regulatory affairs, and an opinion. Expert Opin Drug Metab Toxicol 6:1551–1564, 2010

Chouinard G, Margolese HC: Manual for the Extrapyramidal Symptom Rating Scale (ESRS). Schizophr Res 76:247–265, 2005

Cutler AJ, Kalali AH, Weiden PJ, et al: Four-week, double-blind, placebo- and ziprasidone-controlled trial of iloperidone in patients with acute exacerbations of schizophrenia. J Clin Psychopharmacol 28 (2 suppl 1):S20–S28, 2008

De Hert M, Yu W, Detraux J, et al: Body weight and metabolic adverse effects of asenapine, iloperidone, lurasidone and paliperidone in the treatment of schizophrenia and bipolar disorder: a systematic review and exploratory meta-analysis. CNS Drugs 26:733–759, 2012

Galter D, Unsicker K: Regulation of the transmitter phenotype of rostral and caudal groups of cultured serotonergic raphe neurons. Neuroscience 88:549–559, 1999

Kalkman HO, Feuerbach D, Lotscher E, et al: Functional characterization of the novel antipsychotic iloperidone at human D2, D3, alpha 2C, 5-HT6, and 5-HT1A receptors. Life Sci 73:1151–1159, 2003

Kane JM, Lauriello J, Laska E, et al: Long-term efficacy and safety of iloperidone: results from 3 clinical trials for the treatment of schizophrenia. J Clin Psychopharmacol 28 (2 suppl 1):S29–S35, 2008

Lavedan C, Volpi S, Polymeropoulos MH, et al: Effect of a ciliary neurotrophic factor polymorphism on schizophrenia symptom improvement in an iloperidone clinical trial. Pharmacogenomics 9:289–301, 2008

Lin PY, Tsai G: Meta-analyses of the association between genetic polymorphisms of neurotrophic factors and schizophrenia. Schizophr Res 71: 353–360, 2004

Potkin SG, Litman RE, Torres R, et al: Efficacy of iloperidone in the treatment of schizophrenia: initial phase 3 studies. J Clin Psychopharmacol 28 (2 suppl 1):S4–S11, 2008

Rado J, Janicak PG: Iloperidone for schizophrenia. Expert Opin Pharmacother 11:2087–2093, 2010

Tarazi FI, Stahl SM: Iloperidone, asenapine and lurasidone: a primer on their current status. Expert Opin Pharmacother 13:1911–1922, 2012

Thome J, Durany N, Harsanyi A, et al: A null mutation in the CNTF gene and schizophrenic psychoses. Neuroreport 7:1413–1416, 1996

Volpi S, Heaton C, Mack K, et al: Whole genome association study identifies polymorphisms associated with QT prolongation during iloperidone treatment of schizophrenia. Mol Psychiatry 14:1024–1031, 2009a

Volpi S, Potkin SG, Malhotra AK, et al: Applicability of a genetic signature for enhanced iloperidone efficacy in the treatment of schizophrenia. J Clin Psychiatry 70:801–809, 2009b

Weiden PJ: Iloperidone for the treatment of schizophrenia: an updated clinical review. Clin Schizophr Relat Psychoses 6:34–44, 2012

Weiden PJ, Cutler AJ, Polymeropoulos MH, et al: Safety profile of iloperidone: a pooled analysis of 6-week acute-phase pivotal trials. J Clin Psychopharmacol 28 (2 suppl 1):S12–S19, 2008

CHAPTER 25

Drugs to Treat Extrapyramidal Side Effects

Joseph K. Stanilla, M.D.

George M. Simpson, M.D.

Extrapyramidal Side Effects

History

The discovery of the therapeutic properties of chlorpromazine (Delay and Deniker 1952; Laborit et al. 1952) was soon followed by the description of its tendency to produce extrapyramidal side effects (EPS) that were indistinguishable from classical Parkinson's syndrome. A debate soon arose regarding the relationship between EPS and therapeutic efficacy, with some investigators suggesting that EPS were necessary for efficacy (Flügel 1953; Haase 1954).

Brooks (1956), on the other hand, suggested that "signs of parkinsonism heralded the particular effect being sought" (p. 1122) but that "the therapeutic effects were not dependent on extrapyramidal dysfunction. On the contrary, alleviation of such dysfunction, as soon as it occurred, sped the progress of recovery" (p. 1122).

Types

Four types of EPS have been delineated, and the treatment of each type should be individualized. *Acute dystonic reactions* (ADRs) are generally the first EPS to appear and are often the most dramatic (Angus and Simpson 1970b). *Dystonias* are involuntary sustained or spasmodic muscle contractions that cause abnormal twisting or rhythmical movements and/or postures. ADRs tend to occur suddenly and generally involve muscles of the head and neck (as in torticollis, facial grimacing, or oculogyric crisis). Nearly 90% of all ADRs occur within 4 days of antipsychotic initiation or dosage increase, and virtually 100% of all ADRs occur by day 10 (Singh et al. 1990; Sramek et al. 1986). Although tardive dystonia can occur after this period, movements occurring beyond this time frame are much less likely to be ADRs. Instead, other conditions, including seizures, need to be considered.

Akathisia is the second type of EPS to appear. Akathisia, meaning "inability to sit," consists of both an objective restless movement and a subjective feeling of restlessness that the patient experiences as the need to move. It may be difficult for a patient to explain the sensation of akathisia, and the diagnosis can be missed. At times, patients may display the classical movements of akathisia but without the subjective distress—a condition that has been termed *pseudoakathisia*, which may be a type of tardive syndrome (Barnes 1990).

The third type of EPS, *pseudoparkinsonism*, is virtually indistinguishable from classical Parkinson's syndrome. Symptoms of pseudoparkinsonism include a generalized slowing of movement (akinesia), masked facies, rigidity (including cogwheeling rigidity), resting tremor, and hypersalivation. Parkinson-like symptoms generally appear after a few weeks or more of antipsychotic treatment. Akinesia needs to be differentiated from both primary depression and the blunted affect of schizophrenia (Rifkin et al. 1975).

Tardive syndromes make up the fourth group of EPS. Tardive dyskinesia (TD), although clearly associated with the use of antipsychotic medications, was actually described prior to the advent of antipsychotics (Simpson 2000). TD consists of irregular stereotypical movements of the mouth, face, and tongue and choreoathetoid movements of the fingers, arms, legs, and trunk. It tends to appear after months to years of use of antipsychotic medications. Patients frequently have no awareness of the abnormal movements. The lack of awareness may be related to frontal lobe dysfunction (Sandyk et al. 1993).

Tardive dystonia, a variant of TD, also generally emerges months to years after treatment with antipsychotics (Burke et al. 1982). Unlike in ADRs, the movements associated with tardive dystonia tend to be persistent and more resistant to medical treatment (Kang et al. 1988).

Anticholinergic Medications

Trihexyphenidyl

History and Discovery

Antiparkinsonian medications are drugs that have primarily been used to treat EPS and include anticholinergic, antihistaminic, and dopaminergic agents (Table 25–1).

Trihexyphenidyl, a synthetic analog of atropine, was introduced as benzhexol hydrochloride in 1949. It was found to be effective in the treatment of Parkinson's disease in a study of 411 patients (Doshay et al. 1954). Thereafter, it was also used to treat neuroleptic-induced parkinsonism (NIP) (Rashkis and Smarr 1957). (The term *neuroleptic*, derived from Greek and meaning "to clasp the neuron," was introduced to describe chlorpromazine and the extrapyramidal effects that it produced [Delay et al. 1952].)

Structure-Activity Relations

Trihexyphenidyl, a tertiary-amine analog of atropine, is a competitive antagonist of acetylcholine and other muscarinic agonists that compete for a common binding site on muscarinic receptors (Yamamura and Snyder 1974). It exerts little blockade at nicotinic receptors (Timberlake et al. 1961). Trihexyphenidyl and all drugs in this class are referred to as anticholinergic, antimuscarinic, or atropine-like drugs. As a tertiary amine, trihexyphenidyl readily crosses the blood-brain barrier (Brown and Taylor 1996).

Pharmacological Profile

The pharmacological properties of trihexyphenidyl are qualitatively similar to those of atropine and other anticholinergic drugs, although trihexyphenidyl acts primarily centrally, with few peripheral effects and little sedation. In the eye, anticholinergic drugs block both the sphincter muscle of the iris, causing the pupil to dilate (mydriasis), and the ciliary muscle of the lens, preventing

TABLE 25–1. Pharmacological agents for the treatment of neuroleptic-induced parkinsonism and acute dystonic reactions

COMPOUND	RELATIVE EQUIVALENCE (MG)[a]	ROUTE	AVAILABILITY	DOSING	DOSAGE RANGE (MG/DAY)
Anticholinergic					
Trihexyphenidyl (Artane)	2	Oral	Tablets: 2, 5 mg Elixir: 2 mg/mL Sequels: 5 mg (sustained release)	qd–bid	2–30
Benztropine (Cogentin)	1	Oral	Tablets: 0.5, 1, 2 mg	qd–bid	1–12
		Injectable	Ampules: 1 mg/mL (2 mL)	Every 30 minutes (until symptom relief)	2–8
Biperiden (Akineton)	2	Oral Injectable	Tablets: 2 mg Ampules: 5 mg/mL (1 mL)	qd–tid Every 30 minutes (until symptom relief)	2–24 2–8
Procyclidine (Kemadrin)	2	Oral	Tablets: 5 mg (scored)	bid–tid	5–20
Antihistaminic					
Diphenhydramine (Benadryl)	50	Oral Injectable	Tablets: 25, 50 mg Ampules: 10 mg/mL (10, 30 mL), 50 mg/mL (10 mL)	bid–qd	50–200
Dopaminergic					
Amantadine (Symmetrel)	N/A	Oral	Tablets: 100 mg	qd–bid	100–300

Note. N/A = not applicable; qd = once daily; bid = twice daily; tid = three times daily.
[a]Adapted from Klett and Caffey 1972.

accommodation and causing cycloplegia. In the heart, anticholinergic drugs usually produce a mild tachycardia through vagal blockade at the sinoatrial node pacemaker, although a mild slowing can occur. In the gastrointestinal tract, anticholinergic drugs reduce gut motility and salivary and gastric secretions. Salivary secretion is particularly sensitive and can be completely abolished. In the respiratory system, anticholinergic agents reduce secretions and can produce mild bronchodilatation. Anticholinergics inhibit the activity of sweat glands and mildly decrease contractions in the urinary and biliary tracts (Brown and Taylor 1996).

Pharmacokinetics and Disposition

Peak concentration for trihexyphenidyl is reached 1–2 hours after oral administration, and its half-life is 10–12 hours (Cedarbaum and McDowell 1987). As a tertiary amine, trihexyphenidyl crosses the blood-brain barrier to enter the central nervous system (CNS).

Mechanism of Action

The presumed mechanism of action of trihexyphenidyl for treatment of EPS is the blockade of intrastriatal cholinergic activity, which is relatively increased, compared with nigrostriatal dopaminergic activity, which has become decreased by antipsychotic blockade. The blockade of cholinergic activity returns the system to its previous equilibrium.

Indications

Anticholinergic agents were reported to have been effective treatment for NIP from open empirical trials (Medina et al. 1962; Rashkis and Smarr 1957). Eventually, controlled trials were conducted, with most involving comparisons only with different anticholinergics and not with placebo. Despite the limited evidence of efficacy against placebo, anticholinergic agents became the mainstay of treatment for NIP, and they remain so today.

Trihexyphenidyl has U.S. Food and Drug Administration (FDA) approval for treatment of all forms of parkinsonism, including NIP. Daily doses of 5–30 mg have been used in studies of trihexyphenidyl in the treatment of Parkinson's disease and NIP. Much higher dosages (up to 75 mg/day) have been used for the treatment of primary dystonia. However, the benefits of high doses have been limited by the adverse effects on cognition and memory (Jabbari et al. 1989; Taylor et al. 1991). Side effects correlate with blood levels, but efficacy does not (Burke and Fahn 1985). The individual therapeutic dose must be determined empirically and can vary widely.

Side Effects and Toxicology

Peripheral side effects. The peripheral side effects of trihexyphenidyl result from parasympathetic muscarinic blockade, and they occur in a consistent hierarchy among different organs. They are qualitatively similar to the side effects of atropine and other anticholinergic drugs, but they are quantitatively less because of the reduced peripheral activity of trihexyphenidyl (Brown 1990).

Anticholinergic drugs initially depress salivary and bronchial secretions and sweat production. Reduced salivation leads to dry mouth and contributes to the high incidence of dental caries found among patients with chronic psychiatric problems (Winer and Bahn 1967). Treatment for this condition is unsatisfactory; relief obtained from chewing sugar-free gum or sucking on hard candy is limited by the need for constant use. Reduced sweating can contribute to heat prostration and heatstroke, particularly in warmer ambient temperatures.

The next physiological effects occur in the eyes and heart. Pupillary dilatation and inhibition of accommodation in the eye lead to photophobia and blurred vision. Attacks of acute glaucoma can occur in susceptible subjects with narrow-angle glaucoma, although this is relatively uncommon. Vagus nerve blockade leads to increased heart rate and is more apparent in patients with high vagal tone (usually younger males).

The next effects are inhibition of urinary bladder function and bowel motility, which can produce urinary retention, constipation, and obstipation. Sufficiently high doses of anticholinergics will inhibit gastric secretion and motility (Brown and Taylor 1996).

Central side effects. Memory disturbance is the most common central side effect of anticholinergic medications because memory is dependent on the cholinergic system

(Drachman 1977). Patients with underlying brain pathology are more susceptible to memory disturbance (Fayen et al. 1988). Patients with chronic psychiatric conditions often have a decreased ability to express themselves, making evaluation of memory more difficult; therefore, subtle memory changes can be missed or attributed to the underlying illness. Memory disturbances have been identified in patients with Parkinson's disease treated with anticholinergics (Yahr and Duvoisin 1968), even in some patients receiving only small doses (Stephens 1967). Patients receiving an antipsychotic and benztropine demonstrated significantly increased overall scores on the Wechsler Memory Scale when benztropine was withdrawn (Baker et al. 1983).

Anticholinergic toxicity produces restlessness, irritability, disorientation, hallucinations, and delirium. Elderly patients are at increased risk for both memory loss and toxic delirium, even at very low doses, because of the natural loss of cholinergic neurons with aging (Perry et al. 1977). Toxic doses can produce a clinical situation identical to atropine poisoning, including fixed dilated pupils, flushed face, sinus tachycardia, urinary retention, dry mouth, and fever. This condition can proceed to coma, cardiorespiratory collapse, and death.

Drug-Drug Interactions

There may be increased anticholinergic effects, including side effects, when trihexyphenidyl or any anticholinergic is combined with amantadine. Anticholinergic side effects are also much more likely to occur when drugs with anticholinergic properties are combined.

Anticholinergic effect on antipsychotic blood levels. Some investigators have suggested that anticholinergic medications can affect antipsychotic blood levels. However, a review of this subject suggests that the available data are too limited to reach a definite conclusion on this matter. The best studies indicate that anticholinergic drugs do not affect antipsychotic blood levels or, at most, that they lower these levels only transiently (McEvoy 1983).

Anticholinergic effect on antipsychotic activity. Haase and Janssen (1965) reported from open studies that when anticholinergic drugs are added to antipsychotic drugs given at the neuroleptic threshold, rigidity, hypokinesia, and therapeutic effects disappear but psychopathology worsens. (Haase [1954] postulated that the neuroleptic dose that produced minimal subclinical rigidity and hypokinesis [i.e., the "neuroleptic threshold"] was the minimal neuroleptic dose necessary for therapeutic antipsychotic effect and that it was manifested by micrographic handwriting changes.) Other studies have demonstrated no change or an improvement in scores of psychopathology with the addition of anticholinergics (Hanlon et al. 1966; Simpson et al. 1980).

Anticholinergic Abuse

Anticholinergic drugs may be abused for their euphoriant and hallucinogenic effects, and they may be combined with street drugs for enhanced effect (Crawshaw and Mullen 1984). Patients with a history of substance abuse are more likely to abuse anticholinergics (Wells et al. 1989). Cases of abuse have been reported with all anticholinergics, but trihexyphenidyl apparently is the anticholinergic most likely to be abused (MacVicar 1977). Theoretically, one anticholinergic should be as effective as another, although an idiosyncratic response is possible. The potential for abuse needs to be considered, particularly in patients with a history of substance abuse.

Benztropine

History and Discovery

Benztropine was synthesized by uniting the tropine portion of atropine with the benzhydryl portion of diphenhydramine hydrochloride. Benztropine was found to be effective in the treatment of 302 patients with Parkinson's disease (Doshay 1956). The best results in the control of rigidity, contracture, and tremor were obtained at doses of 1–4 mg once daily for older patients and 2–8 mg once daily for younger ones. Doses of 15–30 mg once daily caused excessive flaccidity in some patients, who became unable to lift their arms or raise their heads off the bed. Subsequently, benztropine was found to be effective for the treatment of NIP (Karn and Kasper 1959).

Structure-Activity Relations

Benztropine is a tertiary amine with activity similar to that of trihexyphenidyl. As a tertiary amine, benztropine enters the CNS.

Pharmacological Profile

Benztropine has the pharmacological properties of an anticholinergic and an antihistaminic; however, it produces less sedation (in experimental animals) than does diphenhydramine.

Pharmacokinetics and Disposition

Little is known about the pharmacokinetics of benztropine. A correlation between serum anticholinergic levels and the presence of EPS has been demonstrated (Tune and Coyle 1980). There is little correlation between the total daily dose of benztropine and the serum anticholinergic level, with the serum activity for a given dose varying 100-fold between subjects. When treated with increased doses of anticholinergics, patients with EPS demonstrate increased serum anticholinergic activity and decreased EPS. Relatively small increments in the oral dose of an anticholinergic drug can result in significant nonlinear increases in serum anticholinergic activity levels. Benztropine has a long-acting effect and can be given once or twice a day.

Mechanism of Action, Side Effects, and Drug-Drug Interactions

The mechanism of action and the drug interactions for benztropine are similar to those of trihexyphenidyl. The side effects of these two drugs are also similar, but the degree of sedation produced by benztropine may be less (Doshay 1956). Although not yet confirmed in double-blind studies, this reported difference in sedation might account for the fact that trihexyphenidyl is reportedly the anticholinergic drug more likely to be abused.

Indications

Benztropine has FDA approval for the treatment of all forms of parkinsonism, including NIP. Total daily doses of 1–8 mg have generally been used to treat NIP.

Biperiden

Biperiden is an analog of trihexyphenidyl that has greater peripheral anticholinergic activity than trihexyphenidyl and greater activity against nicotinic receptors (Timberlake et al. 1961). Biperiden is well absorbed from the gastrointestinal tract. Its metabolism, though not completely understood, involves hydroxylation in the liver. Its activity, pharmacological profile, and side effects are similar to those of other anticholinergics. It has FDA approval for use in the treatment of all forms of parkinsonism, including NIP. Total daily doses of 2–24 mg have been used in studies of biperiden for the treatment of parkinsonism and NIP.

Procyclidine

Procyclidine is an analog of trihexyphenidyl (Schwab and Chafetz 1955). Its activity, pharmacology, and side effects are similar to those of other anticholinergics. There is little information about its pharmacokinetics. Procyclidine has FDA approval for use in treating all forms of parkinsonism, including

NIP. Total daily doses of 5–30 mg have been used in studies of procyclidine for the treatment of parkinsonism and NIP.

Antihistaminic Medications

Diphenhydramine

History and Discovery

Antihistaminic agents have been used for the treatment of Parkinson's disease. Diphenhydramine, one of the first antihistamines developed and used clinically (Bovet 1950), has been the primary antihistamine studied in the treatment of EPS. Although some antihistamines may be effective, other antihistamines have not been systematically studied for the treatment of EPS.

Structure-Activity Relations

All drugs referred to as antihistamines are reversible competitive inhibitors of histamine at the histamine$_1$ (H_1) receptor. Some antihistamines also inhibit the action of acetylcholine at the muscarinic receptor. It is believed that central muscarinic blockade, rather than histaminic blockade, is responsible for the therapeutic effect of antihistamines for EPS. Ethanolamine antihistamines (diphenhydramine, dimenhydrinate, and carbinoxamine maleate) have the greatest anticholinergic activity, and ethylenediamine antihistamines have the least anticholinergic activity. Antihistamines such as terfenadine and astemizole have no anticholinergic activity, whereas many of the remaining antihistamines have very mild anticholinergic activity (Babe and Serafin 1996).

Pharmacological Profile

Antihistamines inhibit the constrictor action of histamine on respiratory smooth muscle. They restrict the vasoconstrictor and vasodilatory effects of histamine on vascular smooth muscle and block histamine-induced capillary permeability. Antihistamines with CNS activity are depressants, producing diminished alertness, slowed reaction times, and somnolence. They can also block motion sickness. Antihistaminic drugs with anticholinergic activity also possess mild antimuscarinic pharmacological properties similar to those of other atropine-like drugs (Babe and Serafin 1996).

Pharmacokinetics and Disposition

Diphenhydramine is well absorbed from the gastrointestinal tract. Peak concentrations occur 2–3 hours after oral administration. Its therapeutic effects usually last 4–6 hours, and it has a half-life of 3–9 hours. Diphenhydramine is widely distributed throughout the body, and as a tertiary amine, it enters the CNS. Age does not affect its pharmacokinetics. It undergoes demethylations in the liver and is then oxidized to carboxylic acid (Paton and Webster 1985).

Mechanism of Action

Diphenhydramine possesses some anticholinergic activity, which is believed to be the basis for its effect in diminishing EPS.

Indications

Diphenhydramine has FDA approval for parkinsonism, including NIP, in the elderly and for mild cases in other age groups. It is probably not as efficacious for treating EPS as are pure anticholinergic drugs, but it may be better tolerated in patients bothered by anticholinergic side effects, such as geriatric patients. Diphenhydramine also tends to be more sedating than anticholinergics, which can also be beneficial for some patients. The dosage generally ranges from 50 to 400 mg/day, given in divided doses.

Diphenhydramine also has indications for multiple other conditions that are unrelated to EPS.

Side Effects and Toxicology

The primary side effect of diphenhydramine is sedation. Although other antihistamines may cause gastrointestinal distress, diphenhydramine has a low incidence of such an effect. Drying of the mouth and respiratory passages can occur. In general, the toxic effects are similar to those of trihexyphenidyl and of other anticholinergics.

Drug-Drug Interactions

Diphenhydramine has no reported interactions with other drugs, but it has an additive depressant effect when used in combination with alcohol or with other CNS depressants.

Dopaminergic Medications

Amantadine

History and Discovery

Anticholinergic side effects and inadequate treatment response eventually led to the investigation of other agents to treat EPS. Initially, both methylphenidate and intravenous caffeine were investigated as treatments for NIP. Neither agent achieved general use, despite apparent efficacy (Brooks 1956; Freyhan 1959).

Amantadine is an antiviral agent that is effective against A2 (Asian) influenza (Wingfield et al. 1969). It was unexpectedly found to produce symptomatic improvement in patients with Parkinson's disease (Parkes et al. 1970; Schwab et al. 1969), and soon thereafter, it was reported to be effective for NIP (Kelly and Abuzzahab 1971).

Structure-Activity Relations

Amantadine is a water-soluble tricyclic amine. It binds to the M2 protein, a membrane protein that functions as an ion channel on the influenza A virus (Hay 1992). Its activity in reducing EPS is not known, although it has been shown to have activity at glutamate receptors (Stoof et al. 1992).

Pharmacological Profile

Amantadine is effective in preventing and treating illness from influenza A virus. It also reduces the symptoms of parkinsonism.

Pharmacokinetics and Disposition

In young healthy subjects, amantadine is slowly and well absorbed from the gastrointestinal tract, with unchanged oral bioavailability over the dose range of 50–300 mg. It reaches steady state in 4–7 days. Plasma concentrations (0.12–1.12 μg/mL) may have some correlation with improvement in EPS (Greenblatt et al. 1977; Pacifici et al. 1976). Amantadine has relatively constant blood levels and a long duration of action (Aoki et al. 1979) and is excreted unchanged by the kidneys. Its half-life for elimination is about 16 hours, which is prolonged in elderly patients and in patients with impaired renal function (Hayden et al. 1985).

Mechanism of Action

Amantadine inhibits viral replication by binding to the M2 protein on the viral membrane and inhibiting replication (Hay 1992). Its mechanism of action as an antiparkinsonian agent is less clear. It has no anticholinergic activity in tests on animals, being only 1/209,000th as potent as atropine (Grelak et al. 1970). It appears to cause the release of dopamine and other catecholamines from intraneuronal storage sites in an amphetamine-like mechanism. It has also been shown to have activity at glutamate receptors, which may contribute to its antiparkinsonian effect (Stoof et al. 1992). Amantadine has preferential selectivity for central catecholamine neurons (Grelak et al. 1970; Strömberg et al. 1970).

Indications

Amantadine has undergone more extensive investigation than have anticholinergic agents with regard to the efficacy of EPS. Most studies, though not all, found amantadine to be equal in efficacy to benztropine or biperiden in the treatment of parkinsonism (DiMascio et al. 1976; Fann and Lake 1976; Konig et al. 1996; Silver et al. 1995; Stenson et al. 1976). Some studies found amantadine to be more effective than benztropine (Merrick and Schmitt 1973) or effective for EPS that are refractory to benztropine (Gelenberg 1978). However, other studies found that amantadine was inferior to benztropine (Kelly et al. 1974), no more effective than placebo (Mindham et al. 1972), or unable to control EPS when used to replace an anticholinergic agent (McEvoy et al. 1987). The varying results can be attributed to differing methodologies and patient populations.

The conclusion that can be drawn from these studies is that amantadine is an effective drug for treating parkinsonism but that there are no clear data to support its use prior to using anticholinergic agents. Most of the studies were of short duration, and in patients with Parkinson's disease, amantadine appears to lose efficacy after several weeks (Mawdsley et al. 1972; Schwab et al. 1972). Similar studies evaluating the long-term efficacy of amantadine have not been conducted for EPS.

Amantadine has also been evaluated for the treatment of akathisia, but in only a small number of patients. The conclusion from these studies is that amantadine is probably not effective for treating akathisia (Fleischhacker et al. 1990).

Amantadine has FDA approval for the treatment of NIP and Parkinson's disease/ syndrome, as well as for the treatment and prophylaxis of influenza A respiratory illness. Dosages of 100–300 mg/day are used for the treatment of NIP, and plasma concentrations may have some correlation with improvement.

Side Effects and Toxicology

At dosages of 100–300 mg/day, amantadine does not produce adverse effects as readily as do anticholinergic medications. Side effects of amantadine result from CNS stimulation, with symptoms including irritability, tremor, dysarthria, ataxia, vertigo, agitation, reduced concentration, hallucinations, and delirium (Postma and Tilburg 1975). Hallucinations are often visual. Side effects are more likely to occur in elderly patients and in patients with reduced renal function (Borison 1979; Ing et al. 1979). Toxic effects are directly related to elevated amantadine serum levels (>1.5 μg/mL). Resolution of toxic symptoms is dependent on renal clearance and may require dialysis in extreme cases, although less than 5% of amantadine is removed through dialysis.

Patients with congestive heart failure or peripheral edema should be monitored because of amantadine's ability to increase the availability of catecholamines. Long-term use of amantadine may produce livedo reticularis in the lower extremities from the local release of catecholamines and resulting vasoconstriction (Cedarbaum and Schleifer 1990). Amantadine should be used with caution in patients with seizures because of possible increased seizure activity. Amantadine is embryotoxic and teratogenic in animals, but there are no well-controlled studies in women regarding teratogenicity.

Drug-Drug Interactions

There are no reported interactions between amantadine and other drugs. There may be increased anticholinergic side effects when amantadine is used in combination with an anticholinergic agent.

Beta-Adrenergic Receptor Antagonists

History and Discovery

Propranolol was reported to be effective for the treatment of restless legs syndrome (Ekbom syndrome; Ekbom 1965), which resembles the physical movements of akathisia (Strang 1967). Later it was reported to be effective in the treatment of neuroleptic-induced akathisia (Kulik and Wilbur 1983; Lipinski et al. 1983). Subsequently, other β-blockers have also been investigated for the treatment of akathisia.

Structure-Activity Relations

Competitive β-adrenergic receptor antagonism is the property common to all β-blockers. β-Blockers are distinguished by the additional properties of their relative affinity for β_1 and β_2 receptors (selectivity), lipid solubility, intrinsic β-adrenergic receptor *agonist* activity, blockade of β receptors, capacity to induce vasodilation, and general pharmacokinetic properties (Hoffman and Lefkowitz 1996). β-Blockers with high lipid solubility readily cross the blood-brain barrier.

Pharmacological Profile

The major pharmacological effects of β-blockers involve the cardiovascular system. β-Blockers slow the heart rate and decrease cardiac contractility; however, these effects are modest in a normal heart. In the lung, they can cause bronchospasm, although, again, there is little effect in normal lungs. They block glycogenolysis, preventing production of glucose during hypoglycemia (Hoffman and Lefkowitz 1996). β-Blockers affect lipid metabolism by preventing release of free fatty acids while elevating triglycerides (Miller 1987). In the CNS, they produce fatigue, sleep disturbance (insomnia and nightmares), and CNS depression (see Drayer 1987; Gengo et al. 1987).

Pharmacokinetics and Disposition

All β-blockers, except atenolol and nadolol, are well absorbed from the gastrointestinal tract (McDevitt 1987). All β-blockers undergo metabolism in the liver. Propranolol and metoprolol undergo significant first-pass effect, with bioavailability as low as 25%. Large interindividual variation (as much as 20-fold) leads to wide variation in clinically therapeutic doses (Hoffman and Lefkowitz 1996). Metabolites appear to have limited β-receptor antagonistic activity. The degree to which a particular β-blocker enters the CNS is related directly to its lipid solubility (see Table 25–2).

Mechanism of Action

The exact mechanism of action of β-blockers in the treatment of EPS is unclear. The existence of a noradrenergic pathway from the locus coeruleus to the limbic system has been proposed as a modulator involved in symptoms of TD, akathisia, and tremor (Wilbur et al. 1988). It appears that lipid solubility and the corresponding ability to enter the CNS are the most important factors determining the efficacy of a β-blocker in treating akathisia and perhaps other types of EPS (Adler et al. 1991).

Indications

β-Blockers have FDA approval primarily for cardiovascular indications, and propranolol is also indicated for familial essential tremor, but there are no FDA-approved indications for the treatment of any type of EPS.

β-Blockers have been studied primarily for the treatment of akathisia. Both nonselective (β_1 and β_2 antagonism) and selective (β_1 antagonism) β-blockers have been reported to be efficacious. The studies have generally been for short periods of time, involving small numbers of patients who were often receiving varying combinations of additional antiparkinsonian agents or benzodiazepines to which β-blockers had been added (Fleischhacker et al. 1990). From these studies, it is difficult to draw any firm conclusions, but β-blockers probably have some efficacy in the treatment of akathisia. The maximum benefit for propranolol occurred at 5 days (Fleischhacker et al. 1990). Betaxolol may be the β-blocker of choice in patients with lung disease and smokers because of its β_1 selectivity at lower dosages (5–10 mg/day).

In addition to essential tremor, β-blockers have also been reported to be beneficial for the tremor of Parkinson's disease (Foster

TABLE 25–2. Characteristics of β-blockers investigated in the treatment of akathisia

COMPOUND	BETA$_1$ BLOCKADE	BETA$_2$ BLOCKADE	LIPID SOLUBILITY	EFFECTIVE FOR EPS	DOSAGE RANGE (MG/DAY)
Propranolol (Inderal)	++	++	++++	Yes	20–120
Nadolol (Corgard)	++	++	+	Yes	40–80
Metoprolol (Lopressor)	++	0 at low doses; + at high doses	++	Yes	~300
Pindolol (Visken)	++	++	++	Yes	5
Atenolol (Tenormin)	++	0	0	No	50–100
Betaxolol (Kerlone)	++	0	+++	Yes	5–20
Sotalol (Betapace)	++	++	0	No	40–80

Note. EPS = extrapyramidal side effects; 0 = insignificant; + = low; ++ = moderate; +++ = high; ++++ = very high.

Source. Adapted from Hoffman and Lefkowitz 1996.

et al. 1984) and lithium-induced tremor (Gelenberg and Jefferson 1995). However, for neuroleptic-induced tremor, propranolol was found to be not any better than placebo (Metzer et al. 1993), which could be an indication of a difference in etiologies for the different tremors.

Side Effects and Toxicology

The side effects of β-blockers result from β receptor blockade. β_2 blockade of bronchial smooth muscle produces bronchospasm. Individuals with normal lung function are unlikely to be affected, but smokers and others with lung disease can develop serious breathing difficulties. β-Blockers can contribute to heart failure in susceptible individuals, such as those with compensated heart failure, acute myocardial infarction, or cardiomegaly. Abrupt cessation of β-blockers can also exacerbate coronary heart disease in susceptible patients, producing angina or, potentially, myocardial infarction (see Hoffman and Lefkowitz 1996 for details).

In individuals with normal heart function, bradycardia produced by β-blockers is insignificant; however, in patients with conduction defects or when combined with other drugs that impair cardiac conduction, β-blockers can contribute to serious conduction problems.

β-Blockers can block the tachycardia associated with hypoglycemia, eliminating this warning sign in patients with diabetes. β_2 blockade also can inhibit glycogenolysis and glucose mobilization, interfering with recovery from hypoglycemia (Hoffman and Lefkowitz 1996).

β-Blockers can impair exercise performance and produce fatigue, insomnia, and major depression. However, the development of major depression probably only occurs in individuals with a predisposition to developing depression.

Drug-Drug Interactions

β-Blockers can have significant interactions with other drugs. Chlorpromazine in combination with propranolol may increase the blood levels of both drugs. Additive effects on cardiac conduction and blood pressure can occur when β-blockers are combined with drugs having similar effects (e.g., calcium channel blockers). Phenytoin, phenobarbital, and rifampin increase the clearance of propranolol. Cimetidine increases propranolol blood levels by decreasing hepatic metabolism. Theophylline clearance is reduced by propranolol. Aluminum salts (antacids), cholestyramine, and colestipol may reduce the absorption of β-blockers (Hoffman and Lefkowitz 1996).

Benzodiazepines

History and Discovery

Diazepam was initially shown to be effective in the treatment of restless legs syndrome (Ekbom syndrome), which resembles the physical movements of akathisia (Ekbom 1965). Subsequently, diazepam, lorazepam, and clonazepam were reported to be beneficial for neuroleptic-induced akathisia (Adler et al. 1985; Donlon 1973; Kutcher et al. 1987). Clonazepam has also been reported to be beneficial for drug-induced dystonia (O'Flanagan 1975) and TD (Thaker et al. 1987).

Mechanism of Action

All benzodiazepines promote the binding of γ-aminobutyric acid (GABA) to $GABA_A$ receptors, magnifying the effects of GABA. The mechanism of action regarding improvement of EPS is unknown, but it may be related to the augmentation of inhibitory GABAergic effect (Hobbs et al. 1996). For a complete discussion of the properties of benzodiazepines, see Chapter 13.

Indications

Benzodiazepines have FDA approval for their use in treating anxiety disorders, agoraphobia, insomnia, management of alcohol withdrawal, anesthetic premedication, seizure disorders, and skeletal muscle relaxation; however, there is no approval for its use in treating any type of EPS. As noted above, a few initial reports have indicated that benzodiazepines are beneficial for the treatment of akathisia. Other studies have also reported similar benefit (Bartels et al. 1987; Braude et al. 1983; Gagrat et al. 1978; Horiguchi and Nishimatsu 1992; Kutcher et al. 1989; Pujalte et al. 1994).

Clonazepam has also been reported to be effective in the treatment of TD (Bobruff et al. 1981; Thaker et al. 1990). Doses of 1–10 mg were used in the first study, although the optimal dosage was found to be 4 mg/day, with many patients unable to tolerate higher dosages. In the second study, dosages of 2–4.5 mg/day were used, and tolerance developed after 5–8 months.

Although some of the studies were limited by short duration and by the small number of subjects also receiving other antiparkinsonian agents, the overall conclusion was that benzodiazepines probably have some efficacy in the treatment of akathisia and TD. However, the potential problems associated with the chronic use of benzodiazepines (i.e., tolerance and abuse) need to be kept in mind.

Lorazepam (intermediate-acting) and clonazepam (long-acting) are the two primary benzodiazepines that have been studied in the treatment of EPS. Because of its long duration of action, clonazepam can often be given once a day. Lorazepam has the advantage of having no active metabolites, which eliminates potential side effects and toxicity.

Botulinum Toxin

History and Discovery

Botulinum toxin, produced by *Clostridium botulinum*, causes botulism when ingested. The first clinical use of the toxin was in the treatment of childhood strabismus (Scott

1980). The first focal dystonia treated was blepharospasm (Elston 1988). Botulinum toxin has been subsequently used to treat a number of other conditions associated with excessive muscle activity, including neuroleptic-induced dystonias (Hughes 1994).

Structure-Activity Relations

There are seven immunologically distinct botulinum toxins (Simpson 1981). Type A is the primary type used clinically (Hambleton 1992). Type F and possibly type B also have clinical utility, but they have much shorter durations of action (≤3 weeks, compared with ≥3 months for type A) (Borodic et al. 1996). The toxin is quantified by bioassay and is expressed as mouse units, which refers to the dose that is lethal to 50% of animals following intraperitoneal injection (Quinn and Hallet 1989).

Pharmacological Profile

Botulinum toxin binds to cholinergic motor nerve terminals, preventing release of acetylcholine and producing a functionally denervated muscle. The prevention of acetylcholine release occurs within a few hours, but the clinical effect does not occur for 1–3 days. The innervation gradually becomes restored, although the number or size of active muscle fibers is reduced (Odergren et al. 1994).

Pharmacokinetics and Disposition

After binding to the presynaptic nerve terminal, the toxin is taken into the nerve cell and is metabolized. When antibodies are present, the toxin is metabolized by immunological processes.

Mechanism of Action

Botulinum toxin acts presynaptically to prevent the release of acetylcholine at the neuromuscular junction. This produces a functional chemical denervation and paralysis of the muscle. When botulinum toxin is used clinically, the aim is to reduce the excessive muscle activity without producing significant weakness (Hughes 1994).

Indications

The FDA has approved the use of botulinum toxin for strabismus, blepharospasm, and other facial nerve disorders (see Jankovic and Brin 1991). Botulinum toxin has been used to treat focal neuroleptic-induced dystonias that may occur as part of TD, including laryngeal dystonia (Blitzer and Brin 1991) and refractory torticollis (Kaufman 1994). For laryngeal dystonia, the toxin is injected percutaneously through the cricothyroid membrane into the thyroarytenoid muscle bilaterally. The response rate is 80%–90%, and the effect lasts 3–4 months and sometimes longer. Botulinum treatment of tardive cervical dystonia has been found to be effective; the observed improvement is similar to the improvement seen in the treatment of idiopathic cervical dystonia, although patients with tardive cervical dystonia required higher doses (Brashear et al. 1998).

Side Effects and Toxicology

The major potential side effect of botulinum toxin is focal weakness in the muscle group injected—an effect that is usually dose dependent. This effect is generally temporary, given the mechanism of action. Transient weakness can occur through diffusion of the toxin into surrounding noninjected muscles (Hughes 1994).

Antibodies to the toxin can occur and thus can prevent a therapeutic response, particularly during subsequent treatments. The two main factors that apparently contribute to the development of antibodies are early age at first treatment with the toxin and total cumulative dose (Jankovic and Schwartz 1995). Some patients with antibodies will respond to other botulinum serotypes, such as type F (Greene and Fahn 1993). Local skin reactions can also occur. Some degree of muscle atrophy is apparent in injected muscles (Hughes 1994). Reinnervation usually takes place over the course of 3–4 months (Odergren et al. 1994).

There are no known contraindications. Because the effect on the fetus is unknown, use of the toxin is not recommended during pregnancy. In conditions in which there are neuromuscular junction disorders, such as myasthenia gravis, patients could theoretically experience increased weakness. The long-term effects are unknown (Hughes 1994).

Drug-Drug Interactions

There are no known interactions of botulinum toxin with other drugs.

Vitamin E (Alpha-Tocopherol)

History and Discovery

Vitamin E was proposed as a treatment for TD after it was noted that a neurotoxin in rats induced an irreversible movement disorder and axonal damage similar to that caused by vitamin E deficiency. It was proposed that chronic antipsychotic use might produce free radicals, which would contribute to neurological damage and TD, and that the antioxidant effect of vitamin E could attenuate the damage (Cadet et al. 1986).

Side Effects and Toxicology

Side effects are minimal when vitamin E is given orally. High levels of vitamin E can exacerbate bleeding abnormalities that are associated with vitamin K deficiency. Dosages of up to 3,200 mg/day in studies for other conditions have been used without significant adverse effects (Kappus and Diplock 1992). The only known drug interactions are with vitamin K (when it is being given for a deficiency) and bleeding abnormalities and possibly with oral anticoagulants. High doses of vitamin E can exacerbate the coagulation abnormalities in both cases and therefore are contraindicated (Kappus and Diplock 1992).

Indications

The only known indication for vitamin E is treatment of vitamin E deficiency, which almost always results from malabsorption syndromes or abnormal transport, such as with abetalipoproteinemia (Bieri and Farrell 1976).

Early studies of vitamin E treatment of TD demonstrated a range of results from general benefit (Adler et al. 1993; Dabiri et al. 1994; Lohr et al. 1988) to benefit only in subjects with TD of less than 5 years' duration (Egan et al. 1992; Lohr and Caligiuri 1996) to no benefit (Schmidt et al. 1991; Shriqui et al. 1992). Subsequently, a major double-blind study comparing vitamin E with placebo found that vitamin E was no more beneficial than placebo (Adler et al. 1999). There were no significant effects of vitamin E on total scores or subscale scores for the Abnormal Involuntary Movement Scale (AIMS; Guy 1976), on electromechanical measures of dyskinesia, or on scores for four other scales measuring dyskinesia. The authors concluded that there was no evidence for efficacy of vitamin E in the treatment of TD (Adler et al. 1999).

The use of vitamin E supplementation is not without risk. A meta-analysis of high-dosage vitamin E supplementation trials showed a statistically significant relationship between vitamin E dosage and all-cause mortality, with increased risk of dosages greater than 150 IU/day (Miller et al. 2005). Given the lack the data demonstrating consistent effectiveness for TD, we do not recommend that vitamin E be used for this purpose.

Treatment of Extrapyramidal Side Effects

Acute Dystonic Reactions

Intramuscular anticholinergics are the treatment of choice for ADRs. Benztropine 2 mg or diphenhydramine 50–100 mg generally will produce complete resolution within 20–30 minutes, with a second dose repeated after 30 minutes if there is not a complete recovery. Benztropine has been shown to resolve ADRs in less time than diphenhydramine (Lee 1979). Starting a standing dose of an antiparkinsonian agent afterward is generally not necessary. ADRs do not recur, unless large doses of high-potency antipsychotics are being used or unless the dose is increased. A more complete discussion of prophylaxis is given below.

Parkinsonism and Akathisia

The initial steps in treatment of parkinsonism (Table 25–3) and of akathisia (referred to here as EPS) are identical: evaluating the dose and type of antipsychotic. It has been shown that an increase in dose beyond the neuroleptic threshold will not produce any greater therapeutic benefit but will increase EPS (Angus and Simpson 1970a; Baldessarini et al. 1988; McEvoy et al. 1991). It has also been demonstrated that EPS frequently can be eliminated with a reduction in dosage or a change to a lower-potency antipsychotic (Braude et al. 1983; Stratas et al. 1963).

If this approach does not resolve EPS or if a lower-potency antipsychotic cannot be substituted, the addition of an anticholinergic drug is the next step. Maximum therapeutic response occurs in 3–10 days, with more severe EPS taking a longer time to respond (DiMascio et al. 1976; Fann and Lake 1976). The anticholinergic dose should be increased until EPS are alleviated or until an unacceptable degree of anticholinergic side effects is obtained. Akathisia frequently does not respond as well to anticholinergic medications and amantadine as do parkinsonism and ADRs (DiMascio et al. 1976). Akathisia is more likely to be responsive to anticholinergic agents if symptoms of parkinsonism are also present (Fleischhacker et al. 1990).

If EPS remain uncontrolled, amantadine can be either added to the regimen or substituted as a single agent. The next step would be the addition of a benzodiazepine or a β-blocker, although there are fewer data supporting both of these treatments.

In the case of severe EPS, the antipsychotic should be temporarily stopped, because severe EPS may be a risk factor for the development of neuroleptic malignant syndrome (Levinson and Simpson 1986).

Additional drugs have been studied or suggested as treatments for akathisia. The data supporting the use of amantadine for the treatment of akathisia are limited. Clonidine has been studied in a small number of patients, but its benefit was limited by sedation and hypotension (Fleischhacker et al. 1990). Sodium valproate was reported to have had no significant effect on akathisia and was found to increase parkinsonism (Friis et al. 1983).

Atypical Antipsychotics for Treatment of Parkinsonism and Akathisia

Patients treated with clozapine were found to have significantly less parkinsonism than patients treated with the combination of chlorpromazine and an antiparkinsonian agent (benztropine) (Kane et al. 1988). The prevalence and incidence of akathisia have also been shown to be less in patients treated with clozapine than in patients treated with typical antipsychotics (Chengappa et al. 1994; Kurz et al. 1995; Stanilla et al. 1995). Subsequently, the new atypical antipsychotics (risperidone, olanzapine, quetiapine, ziprasidone, and aripiprazole) have also been shown to produce less EPS than haloperidol.

At lower doses, risperidone usually does not produce significant parkinsonism, but unlike clozapine, it can produce significant parkinsonism at higher doses (Chouinard et al. 1993). In initial studies comparing risperidone with haloperidol, the extrapyramidal scores for patients receiving risperidone were not significantly different from the scores of patients receiving placebo at 6 mg once daily. Risperidone can cause ADRs, and patients with severe EPS at baseline were more likely

TABLE 25–3. Treatment of parkinsonism

Step	Action
1	Reduce dose of antipsychotic, if clinically possible.
2	Substitute a lower-potency antipsychotic, or carry out step 8.
3	Add an anticholinergic agent.
4	Titrate anticholinergic to maximum dose tolerable.
5	Add amantadine in combination with anticholinergic or as a single agent.
6	Add a benzodiazepine or a β-blocker.
7	In severe cases of extrapyramidal side effects, stop antipsychotic temporarily and repeat process, beginning with step 3.
8	Substitute antipsychotic with atypical antipsychotic or clozapine.

to develop EPS when treated with risperidone (Simpson and Lindenmayer 1997). Olanzapine has also been shown to have an antipsychotic effect comparable to that of haloperidol while producing less dystonia, parkinsonism, and akathisia (Tollefson et al. 1997). The reduced incidence of EPS was observed across the entire therapeutic dosage range of 5–24 mg/day.

Quetiapine has been found to have antipsychotic activity comparable to that of haloperidol at dosages ranging from 150 to 750 mg/day while producing parkinsonism at a level similar to that produced by placebo across the entire dosage range (Arvanitis and Miller 1997; Small et al. 1997). For most patients, there were no significant changes in AIMS scores at baseline and in scores at the end of a 6-week period of treatment.

A double-blind, dose-ranging trial comparing ziprasidone with haloperidol found comparable antipsychotic effect at higher dosages of ziprasidone. Concomitant benztropine use at any time during the study was less frequent with the highest dosage (160 mg/day) of ziprasidone (15%) than with haloperidol (53%) (Goff et al. 1998). Studies of ziprasidone found no significant differences in baseline-to-endpoint mean changes in Simpson-Angus Scale (Simpson and Angus 1970) and AIMS scores with placebo or ziprasidone (40–160 mg/day) (Keck et al. 2001).

Aripiprazole was found to be comparable to risperidone in antipsychotic effect while producing EPS comparable to those seen with placebo (Kane et al. 2002; Potkin et al. 2003).

Extended-release paliperidone was found to have an incidence of EPS nearly comparable to that of placebo (7% vs. 3%) at a dosage range of 3–15 mg/day (Kramer et al. 2007).

Asenapine was evaluated in a 6-week double-blind trial of 458 patients with acute schizophrenia. Patients were given asenapine (5 mg bid or 10 mg bid), haloperidol (4 mg bid), or placebo. The incidence of EPS was found to be 15% and 18%, respectively, for the two dosages of asenapine; 34% for haloperidol; and 10% for placebo (Kane et al. 2010). In a study of 488 patients with manic or mixed episodes of bipolar disorder, patients receiving asenapine (5–10 mg bid) were compared with those receiving olanzapine (5–20 mg/day) and placebo. The incidence of EPS was found to be 10.3% for asenapine, 6.8% for olanzapine, and 3.1% for placebo (McIntyre et al. 2010).

Lurasidone was compared with placebo in a 6-week double-blind study of 180 patients with acute schizophrenia. Patients receiving lurasidone 80 mg/day were found to have no clinically significant differences in objective measures of EPS compared with patients receiving placebo (Nakamura et al. 2009).

The efficacy and safety of iloperidone were evaluated from the pooled results of three double-blind studies of 1,912 patients with schizophrenia. Patients received iloperidone (4–24 mg/day), haloperidol (15 mg/day), risperidone (4–8 mg/day), or placebo. The incidences of akathisia and EPS were lower with iloperidone than with risperidone and haloperidol and were generally similar to incidences with placebo (Potkin et al. 2008).

In general, the novel antipsychotics have a reduced incidence of EPS compared with high-potency typical antipsychotics. Data from the Clinical Antipsychotic Trials of Intervention Effectiveness (CATIE) studies showed that there was no clinically significant difference in the incidence of parkinsonian symptoms and akathisia between the atypical agents and a moderate-potency typical agent, perphenazine. Although a statistically significantly greater number of perphenazine-treated subjects than of atypical-treated subjects discontinued treatment because of EPS (8% vs. 2%–4%), the EPS incidence was low and of limited clinical significance (Miller et al. 2005).

In the past, if a patient receiving a typical antipsychotic developed severe parkinsonism or akathisia and did not respond to antiparkinsonian treatment, the recommended strategy was to switch to an atypical antipsychotic. Now the recommendation can be made to consider the use of a less potent typical antipsychotic as one of the options for treatment, along with possibly changing to an atypical.

For patients with severe refractory EPS who have not responded to standard treatments, the use of clozapine specifically to treat the EPS is indicated (Casey 1989). This is particularly true for akathisia, given its significant negative correlation with the outcome of schizophrenia. This is also true for patients who do not have any psychotic symptoms, if the EPS are judged to be severe enough to be disabling or potentially life-threatening, such as laryngeal dystonia.

Tardive Dyskinesia and Tardive Dystonia

Historically, TD has been refractory to treatment, which explains the large number of drugs employed in attempts to alleviate the condition. Treatments investigated have included, but are not limited to, noradrenergic antagonists (propranolol and clonidine), antagonists of dopamine and other catecholamines, dopamine agonists, catecholamine-depleting drugs (reserpine and tetrabenazine), GABAergic drugs, cholinergic drugs (deanol, choline, and lecithin), catecholaminergic drugs (Kane et al. 1992), calcium channel blockers (Cates et al. 1993), and selective monoamine oxidase inhibitors (selegiline) (Goff et al. 1993). Based on the investigations of the above drugs, the American Psychiatric Association Task Force on Tardive Dyskinesia concluded that there is no consistently effective treatment for TD (Kane et al. 1992).

There are inherent difficulties in evaluating the effects of any treatment for TD. These include the variability of clinical raters (Bergen et al. 1984), the variability of placebo response (Sommer et al. 1994), and the diurnal and longitudinal variability of TD (Hyde et al. 1995; Stanilla et al. 1996). The degree of improvement needs to be greater than the sum of the above variations in order to demonstrate an actual benefit.

The first step in evaluating TD is to determine the type of antipsychotic agent that is being used. If a typical antipsychotic is necessary, it is important to use the lowest dose possible (Simpson 2000). Second, if anticholinergic antiparkinsonian medications are being used, the patient should be gradually weaned from these medications and the medications then discontinued. In contrast to their effect on other extrapyramidal movements, anticholinergic medications will make TD movements worse (see Greil et al. 1984; Jeste and Wyatt 1982).

Some drugs have been shown to have some benefit in the treatment of TD, but they have limitations. Clonazepam has been reported to reduce the movements of TD for up to 9 months, although tolerance to the benefits developed (Thaker et al. 1990). Additional limitations are the inherent problems associated with chronic use of a benzodiazepine. Botulinum toxin is beneficial for treating localized tardive dystonias, particularly laryngeal and cervical dystonias (Hughes 1994). The injections need to be repeated every 3–6 months, and botulinum toxin is not a general treatment for TD. Vitamin E has not consistently been shown to be beneficial in all studies, and a large long-term double-blind study found no benefit for vitamin E compared with placebo (Adler et al. 1999).

Tardive dystonia also tends to be resistant to treatment; however, unlike TD, it may respond to anticholinergic medications (Wojcik et al. 1991) and to reserpine (Kang et al. 1988).

Atypical Antipsychotics for Treatment of Tardive Dyskinesia and Tardive Dystonia

Clozapine has been shown to decrease the symptoms of TD (Simpson and Varga 1974; Simpson et al. 1978), with the greatest improvement occurring in cases of severe TD and tardive dystonia (Lieberman et al. 1991). These findings have been replicated and suggest that clozapine is unlikely to cause TD (Chengappa et al. 1994; Kane et al. 1993). The disadvantages to clozapine are the potential side effects of agranulocytosis and seizures and the need for regular blood monitoring.

More data demonstrating the potential benefit of the other novel antipsychotics in the prevention and treatment of TD are being reported. In a prospective double-blind study of patients with schizophrenia being treated with either olanzapine or haloperidol and followed for up to 2.6 years, there was a significantly decreased risk for the development of TD with olanzapine. The 1-year risk was 0.52% for olanzapine and 7.45% for haloperidol (Beasley et al. 1999).

A prospective study examined the incidence of emergent dyskinesia in middle-aged to elderly patients (mean age 66 years) being treated with haloperidol and low-dose risperidone (mean total daily dose of 1 mg). The patients treated with risperidone were significantly less likely to develop TD (Jeste et al. 1999). A double-blind prospective study comparing 397 stable patients with schizophrenia who were switched to either risperidone or haloperidol and followed for at least a year found that only 1 of the patients receiving risperidone developed dyskinetic movements, compared with 5 of the patients receiving haloperidol (Csernansky et al. 2002).

The data regarding the long-term effect of atypical antipsychotics on TD are more limited; however, any drug that is less likely to produce EPS is probably less likely to produce TD.

The best treatment for TD is prevention. Of the 1,460 subjects involved in the CATIE study, Miller et al. (2005) found 212 to have probable TD by Schooler-Kane criteria. They found that subjects with TD were older, had a longer duration of receiving antipsychotic medications, and were more likely to have been receiving a conventional antipsychotic and an anticholinergic agent. They also found that substance abuse significantly predicted TD, as well as subjects with higher ratings of psychopathology, parkinsonian symptoms, and akathisia (Miller et al. 2005).

Patients with TD who are taking typical antipsychotics are candidates for switching to an atypical antipsychotic. In the case of severe TD or dystonia that has been unresponsive to other treatment, the use of clozapine is indicated (Simpson 2000).

Prophylaxis of Extrapyramidal Side Effects

Prophylactic use of antiparkinsonian agents to prevent EPS is a common but not completely accepted practice. Most controlled prospective studies regarding prophylactic use of antiparkinsonian medication have shown that prophylaxis can be beneficial for certain patients who are at high risk but that it is *not* beneficial in routine use across all patient groups (Hanlon et al. 1966; Sramek et al. 1986). Studies that have demonstrated a greater general benefit across all groups have involved the use of very high doses of antipsychotics. Several retrospective studies have also demonstrated that there is a limited need for prophylaxis of EPS (Swett et al. 1977). The retrospective studies that demonstrated a greater benefit from prophylaxis also involved the use of high antipsychotic dosages (Keepers et al. 1983; Stern and Anderson 1979). The prophylactic use of antiparkinsonian medication is not routinely indicated for all patients but should be reserved for those patients at high risk of developing ADRs.

Table 25–4 summarizes the risk factors for developing ADRs, which include younger age (<35 years), higher doses of antipsychotic, higher potency of antipsychotic, intramuscular route of delivery, (possibly) male gender (Sramek et al. 1986), and a history of ADRs from a similar antipsychotic (Keepers and Casey 1991). The use of cocaine has also been suggested as a possible risk factor (van Harten et al. 1998).

Dosages that have been used for prophylaxis are 1–4 mg/day for benztropine, 5–15 mg/day for trihexyphenidyl, and 75–150 mg/day for diphenhydramine, although the dose required to achieve prophylaxis is highly variable for each individual and can only be determined by trial and error (Moleman et al. 1982; Sramek et al. 1986). Serious anticholinergic side effects, such as acute urinary retention or paralytic ileus, can occur even in a young patient; therefore, high doses of anticholinergics cannot be used with impunity, even for short periods.

Prophylactic anticholinergics for ADRs need only be used for a limited time because 85%–90% of ADRs occur within the first 4 days of treatment, and the incidence drops to nearly zero after 10 days (Keepers et al. 1983; Singh et al. 1990; Sramek et al. 1986). After 10 days, anticholinergics can be weaned slowly while the patient is being observed for development of parkinsonism or akathisia.

TABLE 25–4. Risk factors leading to acute dystonic reactions

High-potency antipsychotics
Haloperidol
Fluphenazine
Trifluoperazine
High dose
Younger age (<35 years of age)[a]
Intramuscular route of delivery
Previous dystonic reaction to similar antipsychotic and dose
Male sex?

[a]Approaches 100% at ages <20 years.

Depot Antipsychotics

In patients receiving depot antipsychotics, prophylactic anticholinergics also only need to be used for patients at high risk of developing ADRs (Idzorek 1976). However, the onset and characterization of EPS may be different in people receiving depot antipsychotics, including more bizarre dystonic reactions (Simpson 1970). The buildup of antipsychotic levels with depot antipsychotics can lead to the development of EPS at later stages of treatment; therefore, an ongoing evaluation is necessary. Some patients receiving fluphenazine decanoate were found to experience EPS only between days 3 and 10 following injection (McClelland et al. 1974).

Withdrawal of Prophylactic Agents

Studies examining withdrawal of antiparkinsonian agents have demonstrated that not all subjects redevelop EPS, a serendipitous finding noted when only 20% of patients withdrawn from benztropine in preparation for a trial of a new antiparkinsonian agent developed recurrent parkinsonian symptoms. This led to the suggestion that antiparkinsonian agents should be withdrawn after 2 months and that their use should only be resumed in patients who develop EPS again (Cahan and Parrish 1960).

Subsequently, other withdrawal studies have been conducted that revealed wide-ranging rates of EPS recurrence. Differences in rates of recurrence are related to the varying methodologies involved in the studies, including methods of rating and the initial reason for treatment with anticholinergics—prophylaxis or active treatment (Ananth et al. 1970). The types, dosages, and combinations of antipsychotics used—the same factors that contribute to the initial development of EPS—have also been major factors in determining recurrence rates (Baker et al. 1983; McClelland et al. 1974).

Almost all anticholinergic withdrawal studies have involved abrupt withdrawal of the anticholinergic medications. Abrupt, compared with gradual, withdrawal is more likely to result in a return of EPS. Gradual withdrawal studies have demonstrated that a large percentage (up to 90%) of patients can be completely withdrawn from anticholinergic medications without developing EPS, while the remaining patients can have their EPS controlled with a considerably reduced dose (Double et al. 1993; Ungvari et al. 1999).

Patients are more likely to develop EPS on withdrawal of antiparkinsonian agents if the risk factors for developing EPS are present. If these risk factors are minimized, the rate of EPS recurrence is lowered.

In patients who experience a recurrence of EPS, the EPS generally reappear within 2 weeks and control is easily reestablished (Klett and Caffey 1972). Patients respond rapidly and often require smaller doses of antiparkinsonian medications for control while continuing to take the same dose of antipsychotic (McClelland et al. 1974).

Conclusion

The unique properties of chlorpromazine and other similarly active agents in ameliorating psychotic symptoms and producing parkinsonian side effects were described in the early 1950s by French psychiatrists. Theories soon arose regarding the relationship between these two properties. The recognition of the benefits of reducing Parkinson-like side effects led to investigations of methods to reduce EPS and to the development of instruments to measure EPS.

The debate regarding the routine and prophylactic use of antiparkinsonian agents has continued since that time. It appears that prophylactic antiparkinsonian agents need to be used in some situations, but probably with less frequency and for briefer periods of time than has generally been the practice. The trend toward the use of lower dosages of antipsychotics should also lead to a decreased need for the use of antiparkinsonian agents.

Finally, the advent of atypical antipsychotic agents has opened a new chapter in both the treatment and prevention of EPS and suggests that, in the future, EPS will be less of a problem than they have been in the past.

A summary of an American Psychiatric Association Task Force report on TD suggested that a "deliberate and sustained effort must be made to maintain patients on the lowest effective amount of drug and to keep the treatment regimen as simple as possible" (Baldessarini et al. 1980, p. 1168) and to discontinue anticholinergic drugs as soon as possible. Apart from a greater emphasis on avoiding the initial use of antiparkinsonian agents, this statement remains valid.

References

Adler L, Angrist B, Peselow E, et al: Efficacy of propranolol in neuroleptic-induced akathisia. J Clin Psychopharmacol 5:164–166, 1985

Adler LA, Angrist B, Weinreb H, et al: Studies on the time course and efficacy of β-blockers in neuroleptic-induced akathisia and the akathisia of idiopathic Parkinson's disease. Psychopharmacol Bull 27:107–111, 1991

Adler LA, Peselow E, Rotrosen J, et al: Vitamin E treatment of tardive dyskinesia. Am J Psychiatry 150:1405–1407, 1993

Adler LA, Rotrosen J, Edson R, et al: Vitamin E treatment for tardive dyskinesia. Veterans Affairs Cooperative Study #394 Study Group. Arch Gen Psychiatry 56:836–841, 1999

Ananth JV, Horodesky S, Lehmann HE, et al: Effect of withdrawal of antiparkinsonian medication on chronically hospitalized psychiatric patients. Laval Med 41:934–938, 1970

Angus JW, Simpson GM: Handwriting changes and response to drugs—a controlled study. Acta Psychiatr Scand Suppl 21:28–37, 1970a

Angus JW, Simpson GM: Hysteria and drug-induced dystonia. Acta Psychiatr Scand Suppl 21:52–58, 1970b

Aoki FY, Sitar DS, Ogilvie RI: Amantadine kinetics in healthy young subjects after long-term dosing. Clin Pharmacol Ther 26:729–736, 1979

Arvanitis LA, Miller BG: Multiple fixed doses of "Seroquel" (quetiapine) in patients with acute exacerbation of schizophrenia: a comparison with haloperidol and placebo. The Seroquel Trial 13 Study Group. Biol Psychiatry 42:233–246, 1997

Babe KS, Serafin WE: Histamine, bradykinin, and their antagonists, in Goodman and Gilman's The Pharmacological Basis of Therapeutics, 9th Edition. Edited by Hardman JG, Limbird LE, Molinoff PB, et al. New York, McGraw-Hill, 1996, pp 581–600

Baker LA, Cheng LY, Amara IB: The withdrawal of benztropine mesylate in chronic schizophrenic patients. Br J Psychiatry 143:584–590, 1983

Baldessarini RJ, Cole JO, Davis JM, et al: Tardive dyskinesia: summary of a task force report of the American Psychiatric Association. Am J Psychiatry 137:1163–1172, 1980

Baldessarini RJ, Cohen BM, Teicher MH: Significance of neuroleptic dose and plasma level in the pharmacological treatment of psychoses. Arch Gen Psychiatry 45:79–91, 1988

Barnes TR: Movement disorder associated with antipsychotic drugs: the tardive syndromes. Int Rev Psychiatry 2:355–366, 1990

Bartels M, Heide K, Mann K, et al: Treatment of akathisia with lorazepam: an open clinical trial. Pharmacopsychiatry 20:51–53, 1987

Beasley CM, Dellva MA, Tamura RN, et al: Randomised double-blind comparison of the incidence of tardive dyskinesia in patients with schizophrenia during long-term treatment with olanzapine or haloperidol. Br J Psychiatry 174:23–30, 1999

Bergen JA, Griffiths DA, Rey JM, et al: Tardive dyskinesia: fluctuating patient or fluctuating rater. Br J Psychiatry 144:498–502, 1984

Bieri JG, Farrell PM: Vitamin E. Vitam Horm 34:31–75, 1976

Blitzer A, Brin MF: Laryngeal dystonia: a series with botulinum toxin therapy. Ann Otol Rhinol Laryngol 100:85–89, 1991

Bobruff A, Gardos G, Tarsy D, et al: Clonazepam and phenobarbital in tardive dyskinesia. Am J Psychiatry 138:189–193, 1981

Borison RL: Amantadine-induced psychosis in a geriatric patient with renal disease. Am J Psychiatry 136:111–112, 1979

Borodic G, Johnson E, Goodnough M, et al: Botulinum toxin therapy, immunologic resistance, and problems with available materials. Neurology 46:26–29, 1996

Bovet D: Introduction to antihistamine agents and antergan derivatives. Ann N Y Acad Sci 50: 1089–1126, 1950

Brashear A, Ambrosius WT, Eckert GJ, et al: Comparison of treatment of tardive dystonia and idiopathic cervical dystonia with botulinum toxin type A. Mov Disord 13:158–161, 1998

Braude WM, Barnes TR, Gore SM: Clinical characteristics of akathisia: a systematic investigation of acute psychiatric inpatient admissions. Br J Psychiatry 143:139–150, 1983

Brooks GW: Experience with use of chlorpromazine and reserpine in psychiatry with special reference to the significance and management of extrapyramidal dysfunction. N Engl J Med 254:1119–1123, 1956

Brown JH: Atropine, scopolamine, and related antimuscarinic drugs, in Goodman and Gilman's The Pharmacological Basis of Therapeutics, 8th Edition. Edited by Gilman AG, Rall TW, Nies AS, et al. New York, Pergamon, 1990, pp 150–165

Brown JH, Taylor P: Muscarinic receptor agonists and antagonists, in Goodman and Gilman's The Pharmacological Basis of Therapeutics, 9th Edition. Edited by Hardman JG, Limbird LE, Molinoff PB, et al. New York, McGraw-Hill, 1996, pp 141–160

Burke RE, Fahn S: Serum trihexyphenidyl levels in the treatment of torsion dystonia. Neurology 35:1066–1069, 1985

Burke RE, Fahn S, Jankovic J, et al: Tardive dystonia: late-onset and persistent dystonia caused by antipsychotic drugs. Neurology 32:1335–1346, 1982

Cadet JL, Lohr J, Jeste D: Free radicals and tardive dyskinesia (letter). Trends Neurosci 9:107–108, 1986

Cahan RB, Parrish DD: Reversibility of drug-induced parkinsonism. Am J Psychiatry 116:1022–1023, 1960

Casey DE: Clozapine: neuroleptic-induced EPS and tardive dyskinesia. Psychopharmacology (Berl) 99:S47–S53, 1989

Cates M, Lusk K, Wells BG: Are calcium-channel blockers effective in the treatment of tardive dyskinesia? Ann Pharmacother 27:191–196, 1993

Cedarbaum JM, McDowell FH: Sixteen-year follow-up of 100 patients begun on levodopa in 1968: emerging problems, in Advances in Neurology, Vol 45: Parkinson's Disease. Edited by Yahr MD, Bergmann KJ. New York, Raven, 1987, pp 469–472

Cedarbaum JM, Schleifer LS: Drugs for Parkinson's disease, spasticity, and acute muscle spasms, in Goodman and Gilman's The Pharmacological Basis of Therapeutics, 8th Edition. Edited by Gilman AG, Rall TW, Nies AS, et al. New York, Pergamon, 1990, pp 463–484

Chengappa KN, Shelton MD, Baker RW, et al: The prevalence of akathisia in patients receiving stable doses of clozapine. J Clin Psychiatry 55: 142–145, 1994

Chouinard G, Jones B, Remington G, et al: A Canadian multicenter placebo-controlled study of fixed doses of risperidone and haloperidol in the treatment of chronic schizophrenic patients (erratum appears in J Clin Psychopharmacol 13:149, 1993). J Clin Psychopharmacol 13:25–40, 1993 (Erratum appears in Am J Psychiatry 158:1759, 2001)

Crawshaw JA, Mullen PE: A study of benzhexol abuse. Br J Psychiatry 145:300–303, 1984

Csernansky JG, Mahmoud R, Brenner R: A comparison of risperidone and haloperidol for the prevention of relapse in patients with schizophrenia. N Engl J Med 346:16–22, 2002

Dabiri LM, Pasta D, Darby JK, et al: Effectiveness of vitamin E for treatment of long-term tardive dyskinesia. Am J Psychiatry 151:925–926, 1994

Delay J, Deniker P: [Thirty-eight cases of psychoses treated with a long and continued course of 4560 RP. The Congress of the French Language for Alienists and Neurologists, Luxembourg, 21–27 July 1952.] Paris, Masson et Cie, 1952, pp 503–513

Delay J, Deniker P, Harl JM: [Therapeutic method derived from hiberno-therapy in excitation and agitation states.] Annales Medico-Psychologiques (Paris) 110:267–273, 1952

DiMascio A, Bernardo DL, Greenblatt DJ, et al: A controlled trial of amantadine in drug-induced extrapyramidal disorders. Arch Gen Psychiatry 33:599–602, 1976

Donlon PT: The therapeutic use of diazepam for akathisia. Psychosomatics 14:222–225, 1973

Doshay LJ: Five-year study of benztropine (Cogentin) methanesulfonate: outcome in three hundred two cases of paralysis agitans. JAMA 162: 1031–1034, 1956

Doshay LJ, Constable K, Zier A: Five year follow-up of treatment with trihexyphenidyl (Artane): outcome in four hundred and eleven cases of paralysis agitans. JAMA 154:1334–1336, 1954

Double DB, Warren GC, Evans M, et al: Efficacy of maintenance use of anticholinergic agents. Acta Psychiatr Scand 88:381–384, 1993

Drachman DA: Memory and cognitive function in man: does the cholinergic system have a specific role? Neurology 27:783–790, 1977

Drayer DE: Lipophilicity, hydrophilicity, and the central nervous system side effects of beta blockers. Pharmacotherapy 7:87–91, 1987

Egan MF, Hyde TM, Albers GW, et al: Treatment of tardive dyskinesia with vitamin E. Am J Psychiatry 149:773–777, 1992

Ekbom KA: [Restless legs]. Swed Med J 62:2376–2378, 1965

Elston J: Botulinum toxin treatment of blepharospasm. Adv Neurol 50:579–581, 1988

Fann WE, Lake CR: Amantadine versus trihexyphenidyl in the treatment of neuroleptic-induced parkinsonism. Am J Psychiatry 133:940–943, 1976

Fayen M, Goldman MB, Moulthrop MA, et al: Differential memory function with dopaminergic versus anticholinergic treatment of drug-induced extrapyramidal symptoms. Am J Psychiatry 145: 483–486, 1988

Fleischhacker WW, Roth SD, Kane JM: The pharmacologic treatment of neuroleptic-induced akathisia. J Clin Psychopharmacol 10:12–21, 1990

Flügel F: [Clinical observations on the effect of the phenothiazine derivative megaphen on psychic disorders in children.] Med Klin 48:1027–1029, 1953

Foster NL, Newman RP, LeWitt, et al: Peripheral beta-adrenergic blockade treatment of parkinsonian tremor. Ann Neurol 16:505–508, 1984

Freyhan FA: Therapeutic implications of differential effects of new phenothiazine compounds. Am J Psychiatry 115:577–585, 1959

Friis T, Christensen TR, Gerlach J: Sodium valproate and biperiden in neuroleptic-induced akathisia, parkinsonism and hyperkinesia: a double-blind crossover study with placebo. Acta Psychiatr Scand 67:178–187, 1983

Gagrat D, Hamilton J, Belmaker RH: Intravenous diazepam in the treatment of neuroleptic-induced acute dystonia and akathisia. Am J Psychiatry 135:1232–1233, 1978

Gelenberg AJ: Amantadine in the treatment of benztropine refractory extrapyramidal disorders induced by antipsychotic drugs. Curr Ther Res Clin Exp 23:375–380, 1978

Gelenberg AJ, Jefferson JW: Lithium tremor. J Clin Psychiatry 56:283–287, 1995

Gengo FM, Huntoon L, McHugh WB: Lipid-soluble and water-soluble beta-blockers: comparison of the central nervous system depressant effect. Arch Intern Med 147:39–43, 1987

Goff DC, Renshaw PF, Sarid-Segal O, et al: A placebo-controlled trial of selegiline (L-deprenyl) in the treatment of tardive dyskinesia. Biol Psychiatry 33:700–706, 1993

Goff DC, Posever T, Herz L, et al: An exploratory haloperidol-controlled dose-finding study of ziprasidone in hospitalized patients with schizophrenia or schizoaffective disorder. J Clin Psychopharmacol 18:296–304, 1998

Greenblatt DJ, DiMascio A, Harmatz JS, et al: Pharmacokinetics and clinical effects of amantadine in drug-induced extrapyramidal symptoms. J Clin Pharmacol 17:704–708, 1977

Greene PE, Fahn S: Use of botulinum toxin type F injections to treat torticollis in patients with immunity to botulinum toxin type A. Mov Disord 8:479–483, 1993

Greil W, Haag H, Rossnagl G, et al: Effect of anticholinergics on tardive dyskinesia: a controlled discontinuation study. Br J Psychiatry 145:304–310, 1984

Grelak RP, Clark R, Stump JM, et al: Amantadine-dopamine interaction: possible mode of action in parkinsonism. Science 169:203–204, 1970

Guy W: ECDEU Assessment Manual for Psychopharmacology, Revised Edition. Washington, DC, U.S. Department of Health, Education, and Welfare, 1976

Haase HJ: [The presentation and meaning of the psychomotor Parkinson syndrome during long-term treatment with megaphen, also known as Largactil.] Nervenarzt 25:486–492, 1954

Haase HJ, Janssen PAJ: The Action of Neuroleptic Drugs. Chicago, IL, Year Book Medical, 1965

Hambleton P: Clostridium botulinum toxins: a general review of involvement in disease, structure, mode of action and preparation for clinical use. J Neurol 239:16–20, 1992

Hanlon TE, Schoenrich C, Freinek W, et al: Perphenazine-benztropine mesylate treatment of newly admitted psychiatric patients. Psychopharmacologia 9:328–339, 1966

Hay AJ: The action of amantadine against influenza A viruses: inhibition of the M2 ion channel protein. Semin Virol 3:21–30, 1992

Hayden FG, Minocha A, Spyker DA, et al: Comparative single dose pharmacokinetics of amantadine hydrochloride and rimantadine hydrochloride in young and elderly adults. Antimicrob Agents Chemother 28:216–221, 1985

Hobbs WR, Rall TW, Verdoorn TA: Hypnotics and sedatives; ethanol, in Goodman and Gilman's The Pharmacological Basis of Therapeutics, 9th Edition. Edited by Hardman JG, Limbird LE, Molinoff PB, et al. New York, McGraw-Hill, 1996, pp 361–396

Hoffman BB, Lefkowitz RJ: Catecholamines, sympathomimetic drugs, and adrenergic receptor antagonists, in Goodman and Gilman's The Pharmacological Basis of Therapeutics, 9th Edition. Edited by Hardman JG, Limbird LE, Molinoff PB, et al. New York, McGraw-Hill, 1996, pp 199–248

Horiguchi J, Nishimatsu O: Usefulness of antiparkinsonian drugs during neuroleptic treatment and the effect of clonazepam on akathisia and parkinsonism occurred after antiparkinsonian drug withdrawal: a double-blind study. Jpn J Psychiatry Neurol 46:733–739, 1992

Hughes AJ: Botulinum toxin in clinical practice. Drugs 48:888–893, 1994

Hyde TM, Egan MF, Brown RJ, et al: Diurnal variation in tardive dyskinesia. Psychiatry Res 56:53–57, 1995

Idzorek S: Antiparkinsonian agents and fluphenazine decanoate. Am J Psychiatry 133:80–82, 1976

Ing TS, Daugirdas JT, Soung LS, et al: Toxic effects of amantadine in patients with renal failure. CMAJ 120:695–698, 1979

Jabbari B, Scherokman B, Gunderson CH, et al: Treatment of movement disorders with trihexyphenidyl. Mov Disord 4:202–212, 1989

Jankovic J, Brin MF: Therapeutic uses of botulinum toxin. N Engl J Med 324:1186–1194, 1991

Jankovic J, Schwartz K: Response and immunoresistance to botulinum toxin injections. Neurology 45:1743–1746, 1995

Jeste DV, Wyatt RJ: Therapeutic strategies against tardive dyskinesia: two decades of experience. Arch Gen Psychiatry 39:803–816, 1982

Jeste DV, Lacro JP, Bailey A, et al: Lower incidence of tardive dyskinesia with risperidone compared with haloperidol in older patients. J Am Geriatr Soc 47:716–719, 1999

Kane J, Honigfeld G, Singer J, et al: Clozapine for the treatment-resistant schizophrenic, double-blind comparison with chlorpromazine. Arch Gen Psychiatry 45:789–796, 1988

Kane JM, Jeste DV, Barnes TR, et al: Treatment of tardive dyskinesia, in Tardive Dyskinesia: A Task Force Report of the American Psychiatric Association. Washington, DC, American Psychiatric Association, 1992, pp 103–120

Kane JM, Werner MG, Pollack S, et al: Does clozapine cause tardive dyskinesia? J Clin Psychiatry 54:327–330, 1993

Kane JM, Carson WH, Saha AR, et al: Efficacy and safety of aripiprazole and haloperidol versus placebo in patients with schizophrenia and schizoaffective disorder. J Clin Psychiatry 63:763–771, 2002

Kane JM, Cohen M, Zhao J, et al: Efficacy and safety of asenapine in a placebo- and haloperidol-controlled trial in patients with acute exacerbation of schizophrenia. J Clin Psychopharmacol 30:106–115, 2010

Kang UJ, Burke RE, Fahn S: Tardive dystonia. Adv Neurol 50:415–429, 1988

Kappus H, Diplock AT: Tolerance and safety of vitamin E: a toxicological position report. Free Radic Biol Med 13:55–74, 1992

Karn WN, Kasper S: Pharmacologically induced Parkinsonlike signs as index of the therapeutic potential. Dis Nerv Syst 20:119–122, 1959

Kaufman DM: Use of botulinum toxin injections for spasmodic torticollis of tardive dystonia. J Neuropsychiatry Clin Neurosci 6:50–53, 1994

Keck PE Jr, Reeves KR, Harrigan EP: Ziprasidone in the short-term treatment of patients with schizoaffective disorder: results from two double-blind, placebo-controlled multicenter studies. J Clin Psychopharmacology 21:27–35, 2001

Keepers GA, Casey DE: Use of neuroleptic-induced extrapyramidal symptoms to predict future vulnerability to side effects. Am J Psychiatry 148: 85–89, 1991

Keepers GA, Clappison VJ, Casey DE: Initial anticholinergic prophylaxis for neuroleptic-induced extrapyramidal syndromes. Arch Gen Psychiatry 40:1113–1117, 1983

Kelly JT, Abuzzahab FS: The antiparkinson properties of amantadine in drug-induced parkinsonism. J Clin Pharmacol 11:211–214, 1971

Kelly JT, Zimmermann RL, Abuzzahab FS Sr, et al: A double-blind study of amantadine hydrochloride versus benztropine mesylate in drug-induced parkinsonism. Pharmacology 12:65–73, 1974

Klett CJ, Caffey E: Evaluating the long-term need for antiparkinsonian drugs by chronic schizophrenics. Arch Gen Psychiatry 26:374–379, 1972

Konig P, Chwatal K, Havelec L, et al: Amantadine versus biperiden: a double-blind study of treatment efficacy in neuroleptic extrapyramidal movement disorders. Neuropsychobiology 33: 80–84, 1996

Kramer M, Simpson, GM, Maciulis V, et al: Paliperidone extended-release tablets for prevention of symptom recurrence in patients with schizophrenia: a randomized, double-blind, placebo-controlled study. J Clin Psychopharmacol 27:6–14, 2007

Kulik AV, Wilbur R: Case report of propranolol (Inderal) pharmacotherapy for neuroleptic-induced akathisia and tremor. Prog Neuropsychopharmacol Biol Psychiatry 7:223–225, 1983

Kurz M, Hummer M, Oberbauer H, et al: Extrapyramidal side effects of clozapine and haloperidol. Psychopharmacology (Berl) 118:52–56, 1995

Kutcher SP, Mackenzie S, Galarraga W, et al: Clonazepam treatment of adolescents with neuroleptic-induced akathisia (letter). Am J Psychiatry 144:823–824, 1987

Kutcher S, Williamson P, MacKenzie S, et al: Successful clonazepam treatment of neuroleptic-induced akathisia in older adolescents and young adults: a double-blind, placebo-controlled study. J Clin Psychopharmacol 9:403–406, 1989

Laborit H, Huguenard P, Alluaume R: [A new vegetative stabilizer (4560 RP).] Presse Med 60:206–208, 1952

Lee A-S: Treatment of drug-induced dystonic reactions. JACEP 8:453–457, 1979

Levinson DF, Simpson GM: Neuroleptic-induced extrapyramidal symptoms with fever: heterogeneity of the "neuroleptic malignant syndrome." Arch Gen Psychiatry 43:839–848, 1986

Lieberman JA, Saltz BL, Johns CA, et al: The effects of clozapine on tardive dyskinesia. Br J Psychiatry 158:503–510, 1991

Lipinski JF, Zubenko GS, Barreira P, et al: Propranolol in the treatment of neuroleptic-induced akathisia. Lancet 1:685–686, 1983

Lohr JB, Caligiuri MP: A double-blind placebo-controlled study of vitamin E treatment of tardive dyskinesia. J Clin Psychiatry 57:167–173, 1996

Lohr JB, Cadet JL, Lohr MA, et al: Vitamin E in the treatment of tardive dyskinesia: the possible involvement of free radical mechanisms. Schizophr Bull 14:291–296, 1988

MacVicar K: Abuse of antiparkinsonian drugs by psychiatric patients. Am J Psychiatry 134:809–811, 1977

Mawdsley C, Williams IR, Pullar IA, et al: Treatment of parkinsonism by amantadine and levodopa. Clin Pharmacol Ther 13:575–583, 1972

McClelland HA, Blessed G, Bhate S, et al: The abrupt withdrawal of antiparkinsonian drugs in schizophrenic patients. Br J Psychiatry 124:151–159, 1974

McDevitt DG: Comparison of pharmacokinetic properties of beta-adrenoceptor blocking drugs. Eur Heart J 8 (suppl M):9–14, 1987

McEvoy JP: The clinical use of anticholinergic drugs as treatment for extrapyramidal side effects of neuroleptic drugs. J Clin Psychopharmacol 3:288–302, 1983

McEvoy JP, McCue M, Freter S: Replacement of chronically administered anticholinergic drugs by amantadine in outpatient management of chronic schizophrenia. Clin Ther 9:429–433, 1987

McEvoy JP, Hogarty GE, Steingard S: Optimal dose of neuroleptic in acute schizophrenia: a controlled study of the neuroleptic threshold and higher haloperidol dose. Arch Gen Psychiatry 48:739–745, 1991

McIntyre RS, Cohen M, Zhao J, et al: Asenapine in the treatment of acute mania in bipolar I disorder: a randomized, double-blind, placebo-controlled trial. J Affect Disord 122:27–38, 2010

Medina C, Kramer MD, Kurland AA: Biperiden in the treatment of phenothiazine-induced extrapyramidal reactions. JAMA 182:1127–1129, 1962

Merrick EM, Schmitt P: A controlled study of the clinical effects of amantadine hydrochloride (Symmetrel). Curr Ther Res Clin Exp 15:552–558,1973

Metzer WS, Paige SR, Newton JE: Inefficacy of propranolol in attenuation of drug-induced parkinsonian tremor. Mov Disord 8:43–46, 1993

Miller DD, McEvoy JP, Davis SM, et al: Clinical correlates of tardive dyskinesia in schizophrenia: baseline data from the CATIE schizophrenia trial. Schizophr Res 80:33–43, 2005

Miller ER, Pastor-Barriuso R, Dalal D, et al: Meta-analysis: high-dosage vitamin E supplementation may increase all-cause mortality. Ann Intern Med 142:37–46, 2005

Miller NE: Effects of adrenoceptor-blocking drugs on plasma lipoprotein concentrations. Am J Cardiol 60:17E–23E, 1987

Mindham RHS, Gaind R, Anstee BH, et al: Comparison of amantadine, orphenadrine, and placebo in the control of phenothiazine-induced parkinsonism. Psychol Med 2:406–413, 1972

Moleman P, Schmitz PJM, Ladee GA: Extrapyramidal side effects and oral haloperidol: an analysis of explanatory patient and treatment characteristics. J Clin Psychiatry 43:492–496, 1982

Nakamura M, Ogasa M, Guarino J, et al: Lurasidone in the treatment of acute schizophrenia: a double-blind, placebo-controlled trial. J Clin Psychiatry 70:829–836, 2009

Odergren T, Tollback A, Borg J: Electromyographic single motor unit potentials after repeated botulinum toxin treatments in cervical dystonia. Electroencephalogr Clin Neurophysiol 93:325–329, 1994

O'Flanagan PM: Clonazepam in the treatment of drug-induced dyskinesia. BMJ 1(5952):269–270, 1975

Pacifici GM, Nardini M, Ferrari P, et al: Effect of amantadine on drug-induced parkinsonism: relationship between plasma levels and effect. Br J Clin Pharmacol 3:883–889, 1976

Parkes JD, Zilkha KJ, Calver DM, et al: Controlled trial of amantadine hydrochloride in Parkinson's disease. Lancet 1(7641):259–262, 1970

Paton DM, Webster DR: Clinical pharmacokinetics of H1 receptor antagonists (the antihistamines). Clin Pharmacokinet 10:477–497, 1985

Perry EK, Perry RH, Blessed G, et al: Necropsy evidence of central cholinergic deficits in senile dementia (letter). Lancet 1(8004):189, 1977

Postma JU, Tilburg VW: Visual hallucinations and delirium during treatment with amantadine (Symmetrel). J Am Geriatr Soc 23:212–215, 1975

Potkin SG, Saha AR, Kujawa MJ, et al: Aripiprazole, an antipsychotic with a novel mechanism of action, and risperidone vs placebo in patients with schizophrenia and schizoaffective disorder. Arch Gen Psychiatry 60:681–690, 2003

Potkin SG, Litman RE, Torres R, et al: Efficacy of iloperidone in the treatment of schizophrenia: initial phase 3 studies. J Clin Psychopharmacol 28 (suppl 1):S4–S11, 2008

Pujalte D, Bottaï T, Huë B, et al: A double-blind comparison of clonazepam and placebo in the treatment of neuroleptic-induced akathisia. Clin Neuropharmacol 17:236–242, 1994

Quinn N, Hallet M: Dose standardisation of botulinum toxin (letter) (erratum appears in Lancet 1[8646]:1092, 1989). Lancet 1(8644):964, 1989

Rashkis HA, Smarr ER: Protection against reserpine-induced "Parkinsonism" (clinical note). Am J Psychiatry 113:1116, 1957

Rifkin A, Quitkin F, Klein DF: Akinesia, a poorly recognized drug-induced extrapyramidal behavioral disorder. Arch Gen Psychiatry 32:672–674, 1975

Sandyk R, Kay SR, Awerbuch GI: Subjective awareness of abnormal involuntary movements in schizophrenia. Int J Neurosci 69:1–20, 1993

Schmidt M, Meister P, Baumann P: Treatment of tardive dyskinesias with vitamin E. Eur Psychiatry 6:201–207, 1991

Schwab RS, Chafetz ME: Kemadrin in the treatment of parkinsonism. Neurology 5:273–277, 1955

Schwab RS, England AC, Poskanzer DC, et al: Amantadine in the treatment of Parkinson's disease. JAMA 208:1160–1170, 1969

Schwab RS, Poskanzer DC, England AC Jr, et al: Amantadine in Parkinson's disease: review of more than two years' experience. JAMA 222: 792–795, 1972

Scott AB: Botulinum toxin injections into extra ocular muscles as an alternative to strabismus surgery. Ophthalmology 87:1044–1049, 1980

Shriqui CL, Bradwejn J, Annable L, et al: Vitamin E in the treatment of tardive dyskinesia: a double-blind placebo-controlled study. Am J Psychiatry 149:391–393, 1992

Silver H, Geraisy N, Schwartz M: No difference in the effect of biperiden and amantadine on parkinsonian- and tardive dyskinesia-type involuntary movements: a double-blind crossover, placebo-controlled study in medicated chronic schizophrenic patients (erratum appears in J Clin Psychiatry 56:435, 1995). J Clin Psychiatry 56:167–170, 1995

Simpson GM: Long-acting antipsychotic agents and extrapyramidal side effects. Dis Nerv Syst 31 (suppl):12–14, 1970

Simpson GM: The treatment of tardive dyskinesia and tardive dystonia. J Clin Psychiatry 61 (suppl 4):39–44, 2000

Simpson GM, Angus JWS: A rating scale for extrapyramidal side effects. Acta Psychiatr Scand 212:11–19, 1970

Simpson GM, Lindermayer JP: Extrapyramidal symptoms in patients treated with risperidone. J Clin Psychopharmacol 17:194–201, 1997

Simpson GM, Varga E: Clozapine—a new antipsychotic agent. Curr Ther Res 18:679–868, 1974

Simpson GM, Lee JH, Shrivastava RK: Clozapine in tardive dyskinesia. Psychopharmacologia 56:75–80, 1978

Simpson GM, Cooper TB, Bark N, et al: Effect of antiparkinsonian medications on plasma levels of chlorpromazine. Arch Gen Psychiatry 37:205–208, 1980

Simpson LL: The origin, structure, and pharmacologic activity of botulinum toxin. Pharmacol Rev 33:155–188, 1981

Singh H, Levinson DF, Simpson GM, et al: Acute dystonia during fixed-dose neuroleptic treatment. J Clin Psychopharmacol 10:389–396, 1990

Small JG, Hirsch SR, Arvanitis LA, et al: Quetiapine in patients with schizophrenia: a high- and low-dose double-blind comparison with placebo. Arch Gen Psychiatry 54:549–557, 1997

Sommer BR, Cohen BM, Satlin A, et al: Changes in tardive dyskinesia symptoms in elderly patients treated with ganglioside GM1 or placebo. J Geriatr Psychiatry Neurol 7:234–237, 1994

Sramek JJ, Simpson GM, Morrison RL, et al: Anticholinergic agents for prophylaxis of neuroleptic-induced dystonic reactions: a prospective study. J Clin Psychiatry 47:305–309, 1986

Stanilla JK, Nair C, de Leon J, et al: Clozapine does not produce akathisia or parkinsonism. Poster presented at the 34th annual meeting of the American College of Neuropsychopharmacology, San Juan, Puerto Rico, December 11–15, 1995

Stanilla JK, Büchel C, Alarcon J, et al: Diurnal and weekly variation of tardive dyskinesia measured by digital image processing. Psychopharmacology (Berl) 124:373–376, 1996

Stenson RL, Donlon PT, Meyer JE: Comparison of benztropine mesylate and amantadine HCL in neuroleptic-induced extrapyramidal symptoms. Compr Psychiatry 17:763–768, 1976

Stephens DA: Psychotoxic effects of benzhexol hydrochloride (Artane). Br J Psychiatry 113:213–218, 1967

Stern TA, Anderson WH: Benztropine prophylaxis of dystonic reactions. Psychopharmacologia 61:261–262, 1979

Stoof JC, Booij J, Drukarch B: Amantadine as N-methyl-D-aspartic acid receptor antagonist: new possibilities for therapeutic applications? Clin Neurol Neurosurg 94:S4–S6, 1992

Strang RR: The syndrome of restless legs. Med J Aust 24:1211–1213, 1967

Stratas NE, Phillips RD, Walker PA, et al: A study of drug induced parkinsonism. Dis Nerv Syst 24:180, 1963

Strömberg U, Svensson TH, Waldeck B: On the mode of action of amantadine. J Pharm Pharmacol 22:959–962, 1970

Swett C, Cole JO, Shapiro S, et al: Extrapyramidal side effects in chlorpromazine recipients. Arch Gen Psychiatry 34:942–943, 1977

Taylor AE, Lang AE, Saint-Cyr JA, et al: Cognitive processes in idiopathic dystonia treated with high-dose anticholinergic therapy: implications for treatment strategies. Clin Neuropharmacol 14:62–77, 1991

Thaker GK, Tamminga CA, Alphs LD, et al: Brain gamma-aminobutyric acid abnormality in tardive dyskinesia: reduction in cerebrospinal fluid GABA levels and therapeutic response to GABA agonist treatment. Arch Gen Psychiatry 44:522–529, 1987

Thaker GK, Nguyen JA, Strauss ME, et al: Clonazepam treatment of tardive dyskinesia: a practical GABAmimetic strategy. Am J Psychiatry 147:445–451, 1990

Timberlake WH, Schwab RS, England AC Jr: Biperiden (Akineton) in parkinsonism. Arch Neurol 5:560–564, 1961

Tollefson GD, Beasley CM Jr, Tran PV, et al: Olanzapine versus haloperidol in the treatment of schizophrenia and schizoaffective and schizophreniform disorders: results of an international collaborative trial. Arch Gen Psychiatry 54:457–465, 1997

Tune L, Coyle JT: Serum levels of anticholinergic drugs in treatment of acute extrapyramidal side effects. Arch Gen Psychiatry 37:293–297, 1980

Ungvari GS, Chiu HF, Lam LC, et al: Gradual withdrawal of long-term anticholinergic antiparkinson medication in Chinese patients with chronic schizophrenia. J Clin Psychopharmacol 19:141–148, 1999

van Harten PN, van Trier JC, Horwitz EH, et al: Cocaine as a risk factor for neuroleptic-induced acute dystonia. J Clin Psychiatry 59:128–130, 1998

Wells BG, Marken PA, Rickman LA, et al: Characterizing anticholinergic abuse in community mental health. J Clin Psychopharmacol 9:431–435, 1989

Wilbur R, Kulik FA, Kulik AV: Noradrenergic effects in tardive dyskinesia, akathisia and pseudoparkinsonism via the limbic system and basal ganglia. Prog Neuropsychopharmacol Biol Psychiatry 12:849–864, 1988

Winer JA, Bahn S: Loss of teeth with antidepressant drug therapy. Arch Gen Psychiatry 16:239–240, 1967

Wingfield WL, Pollack D, Grunert RR: Therapeutic efficacy of amantadine HCl and rimantadine HCl in naturally occurring influenza A2 respiratory illness in man. N Engl J Med 281:579–584, 1969

Wojcik JD, Falk WE, Fink JS, et al: A review of 32 cases of tardive dystonia (see comments). Am J Psychiatry 148:1055–1059, 1991

Yahr MD, Duvoisin RC: Medical therapy of parkinsonism. Mod Treat 5:283–300, 1968

Yamamura HI, Snyder SH: Muscarinic cholinergic receptor binding in the longitudinal muscle of the guinea pig ileum with [3H]quinuclidinyl benzilate. Mol Pharmacol 10:861–867, 1974

Drugs for Treatment of Bipolar Disorder

CHAPTER 26

Lithium

Jamie M. Dupuy, M.D.
Curtis W. Wittmann, M.D.
Erika F. H. Saunders, M.D.
Alan J. Gelenberg, M.D.
Marlene P. Freeman, M.D.

History and Discovery

After noting the sedating properties of lithium in animals, Cade (1949) first described the successful treatment of mania with lithium salts. The U.S. Food and Drug Administration (FDA) approved lithium for use in treating acute mania in 1970 and for the prophylaxis of bipolar disorder 4 years later (Jefferson and Greist 1977). However, lithium did not come onto the market easily in the United States. Pharmaceutical companies were reluctant to produce this inexpensive drug that they could not patent (Kline 1973). Lithium is a highly cost-effective treatment for bipolar disorder (Chisholm et al. 2005). In contrast to many medications for bipolar disorder, lithium is available generically and is relatively inexpensive. Several medications have been proven effective for bipolar disorder since the introduction of lithium, including anticonvulsants and second-generation (atypical) antipsychotics; however, lithium is still widely used today and is an effective and inexpensive treatment.

Structure-Activity Relations

Lithium is the lightest alkali metal and a monovalent cation, and it shares some properties with sodium, potassium, and calcium (Baldessarini 1996; Ward et al. 1994). It is the third element of the periodic table. Substitution or competition with other cations may contribute to its effects (Ward et al. 1994).

Pharmacological Profile

Lithium is minimally protein bound, does not undergo biotransformation, and is renally eliminated (Kilts 2000). The narrow therapeutic index necessitates careful drug monitoring. Lithium appears to affect multiple neurotransmitter systems and affects second-messenger systems such as cyclic adenosine monophosphate (cAMP) and cyclic guanosine monophosphate (cGMP) (Ward et al. 1994).

Pharmacokinetics and Disposition

Lithium is available in multiple preparations, including lithium carbonate tablets and capsules, lithium citrate, and slow-release forms (Jefferson et al. 1983). Lithium is absorbed from the gastrointestinal tract and renally excreted unchanged in approximately 24 hours (Baldessarini and Tarazi 2001). Peak plasma concentrations are reached within 1–2 hours with rapid-release preparations and 4–5 hours after sustained-release formulations (Finley et al. 1995). Lithium is not protein bound and is evenly distributed in total body water space (Jermain et al. 1991). Lithium excretion is controlled by osmotic factors and is a function of renal sufficiency (Birch et al. 1980). Steady-state concentrations are achieved within 4–5 days (Keck and McElroy 2002).

Mechanism of Action

Despite extensive research, the exact mechanism of action of lithium as a mood stabilizer has yet to be elucidated. Multiple theories, based on animal models and on limited studies in humans, have been proposed; those with the most compelling evidence are reviewed here. A unifying theory posits that lithium's mechanism of action may be related to its neurotrophic and neuroprotective effects (Quiroz et al. 2010). In addition to its effects on inositol phospholipids, glycogen synthase kinase, and protein kinase C, lithium activates cyclic adenosine monophosphate response element binding and increases brain-derived neurotrophic factor, mechanisms that are also suggestive of a role for neurotrophic effects (Quiroz et al. 2010).

Inositol Depletion

There has been much focus on the role of the inositol cycle in the clinical effects of lithium. Lithium is a noncompetitive inhibitor of inositol monophosphatase, depleting free inositol within 5 days of treatment initiation (Berridge et al. 1989). These changes last for 3–4 weeks after lithium's discontinuation (Moore et al. 1997). Depletion of free inositol can lead to effects on neurotransmitter and second-messenger systems linked to the inositol cycle. For example, adrenergic, serotonergic, and cholinergic receptor subtypes are coupled to the cycle via G proteins, and the cycle in turn regulates protein kinase C action, which appears to be influenced by lithium treatment in mania (Hahn et al. 2005).

Of note, depression is associated with low cerebrospinal fluid inositol levels in humans (Barkai et al. 1978). Exogenous inositol can alleviate depression (Levine et al. 1993, 1995) and panic attacks (Benjamin et al. 1995). Belmaker et al. (1996) suggested a complex "pendulum" relationship between inositol and lithium, which may be a basis for understanding lithium's antimanic and antidepressant effects.

Glycogen Synthase Kinase Inhibition

Lithium inhibits glycogen synthase kinase–3 (GSK-3) (Klein and Melton 1996; Li et al. 2007). Valproic acid also inhibits GSK-3, making this theory attractive because it involves a common mechanism in two known mood stabilizers (G. Chen et al. 1999). GSK-3 is an inhibitor of the Wnt protein signaling pathway, which affects neuronal signal transduction. Lithium thus would be predicted to mimic Wnt signaling (Phiel and Klein 2001). Wnt signaling stimulates a cascade of events that leads to stimulation of protein kinase C activity (Grahame-Smith 1998; Williams and Harwood 2000). Thus, lithium's actions on both the inositol cycle and the GSK-3 signaling pathway lead to a common effect on protein kinase C.

Lithium's Effects on Neurotransmitter Systems

Perhaps because of its effects on second-messenger systems, lithium brings about changes in all of the major neurotransmitter systems in the brain. Chronic administration of lithium in mice increases and stabilizes glutamate uptake. This could, in part, explain lithium's antimanic effect because it results in overall reduction of an excitatory neurotransmitter (Dixon and Hokin 1998). Lithium also normalizes low cerebrospinal fluid γ-aminobutyric acid levels in bipolar subjects (see Berrettini et al. 1983, 1986).

Lithium enhances norepinephrine and serotonin function in the central nervous system, which could explain its antidepressant effects (Price et al. 1990; Schildkraut et al. 1969; Stern et al. 1969). Of particular interest is lithium's confirmed antagonistic action at serotonin$_{1A}$ (5-HT$_{1A}$) and serotonin$_{1B}$ (5-HT$_{1B}$) autoreceptors (Haddjeri et al. 2000; Massot et al. 1999); such action would increase serotonin availability in the synaptic cleft (Shaldubina et al. 2001). Clinically, 5-HT$_{1A}$ may be involved in alleviation of depression, and 5-HT$_{1B}$ receptors may play a role in the regulation of sleep, sensorimotor inhibition, and locomotor activity (Monti et al. 1995; Sipes and Geyer 1996).

Indications and Efficacy

Bipolar Disorder

Acute Mania

Cade (1949) first published data on the efficacy of lithium in mania more than half a century ago. As we begin the twenty-first century, lithium remains one of the most efficacious treatments for bipolar disorder.

Lithium versus placebo. Lithium is more efficacious than placebo for acute mania (Bowden et al. 1994, 2005; Goodwin et al. 1969; Maggs 1963; Schou et al. 1954; Stokes et al. 1971). Analysis of response rates in randomized trials indicates that lithium was at least somewhat efficacious in the treatment of mania in 87 of 124 patients (70%) (Keck et al. 2000).

Lithium versus antipsychotics. Early studies with lithium established its antimanic efficacy relative to first-generation (typical) antipsychotics. A study by Prien et al. (1972) comparing lithium against chlorpromazine found that although chlorpromazine was more effective in reducing manic symptoms in severely ill patients, lithium also reduced symptoms while causing fewer side effects.

A review of studies by Goodwin and Zis (1979) found lithium to be efficacious in at least 70% of patients, as defined by remission or marked improvement. In a 3-week double-blind study of lithium, haloperidol, and their combination for acute mania, patients who received haloperidol or haloperidol plus lithium had more significant improvement than did those who received lithium alone (Garfinkel et al. 1980). The combination of lithium and haloperidol was as well tolerated as haloperidol alone. More recently, Segal et al. (1998) reported that inpatients with acute mania responded equally well to lithium, haloperidol, and risperidone.

Lithium has also been studied in comparison with atypical (second-generation) antipsychotic medications. However, many of these trials were focused on assessing the efficacy of the antipsychotic in a noninferiority approach rather than on demonstrating significant differences between the medications. For example, in a direct comparison with lithium, olanzapine produced greater improvement in manic symptoms over 4 weeks, but it also produced more weight gain (Niufan et al. 2008). By and large, antipsychotics appear to work faster than lithium but carry higher risks for weight gain and other metabolic effects.

Lithium versus anticonvulsants. Double-blind, randomized studies suggest that carbamazepine and lithium are equally effective in the treatment of acute mania (Lerer et al. 1987; Small et al. 1991). In a direct comparison of lithium and divalproex, Bowden et al. (1994) demonstrated a similar advantage for both agents over placebo, with lithium and divalproex each achieving response in about 48% of patients over 3 weeks. A 12-week study of patients randomly assigned to open treatment with lithium or divalproex yielded additional evidence of the two agents' comparable efficacy over a longer-than-usual study period (Bowden et al. 2008). In a meta-analysis of the efficacy of lithium, valproate, and carbamazepine in mania, no significant differences in efficacy were found among the three agents (Emilien et al. 1996). Only some of the included studies were placebo controlled. Anticonvulsants were generally better tolerated than lithium. Neurological abnormalities may predict a better response to anticonvulsants than to lithium in mania. Patients with electroencephalogram abnormalities are more likely to respond to valproate than to lithium (Reeves et al. 2001).

Mixed mania—the co-occurrence of mania with depression—may predict a poorer response to lithium. Freeman et al. (1992), in a direct comparison of lithium and valproate, showed that a favorable response to valproate was associated with high pretreatment depressive symptom scores. To further investigate the relation between co-occurring depressive symptoms and treatment response in acute mania, Swann et al. (1997) designed a parallel-group study of lithium versus divalproex and analyzed outcomes relative to the presence of a mixed affective state. They found that pretreatment depressive symptoms during acute mania were associated with a poorer response to lithium and a better response to divalproex.

Bipolar Depression

Lithium is considered a first-line treatment for acute bipolar depression (Compton and Nemeroff 2000). Goodwin and Jamison (1990) analyzed the placebo-controlled trials that have been completed in bipolar depression and found that 79% of bipolar patients had either a complete or a partial response to lithium. Placebo-controlled trials showing the efficacy of lithium in bipolar depression include those by Baron et al. (1975), Donnelly et al. (1978), Fieve et al. (1968), Goodwin et al. (1969, 1972), Greenspan et al. (1970), Mendels (1975), and Noyes et al. (1974). These studies generally were small (involving between 3 and 40 patients [Goodwin et al. 1972]).

A more recent study in 802 patients compared response over 8 weeks of treatment with lithium, quetiapine (300 or 600 mg), or placebo (Young et al. 2010). In this study, lithium failed to separate significantly from placebo on the main efficacy measure (Montgomery-Åsberg Depression Rating Scale [MADRS] score); however, the study was powered to show an effect of quetiapine, and the mean serum level in lithium-treated subjects was low (0.6 mmol/L).

In 2004, an expert consensus report recommended lithium as monotherapy for mild to moderate depression in bipolar I disorder and as a component of an initial medication regimen in severe nonpsychotic and psychotic depression (Keck et al. 2004).

Rapid Cycling

In 1974, Dunner and Fieve observed that bipolar patients who failed to respond to long-term lithium prophylaxis were more likely to have had four or more mood episodes in a year, giving rise to the belief that lithium is not effective in treating rapid cycling. However, subsequent studies have shown that rapid cyclers do poorly with most available treatments and that treatment with lithium does improve the burden of illness. In a study examining the effect of lithium treatment among 29 patients with rapid-cycling bipolar disorder, Dunner et al. (1977) found that patients who had received lithium for at least 1 year had a higher percentage of "well time" relative to baseline and experienced reductions in the severity and duration of episodes. Wehr et al. (1988) analyzed retrospective and prospective data for 51 patients with rapid-cycling affective disorder, showing that even among patients with continuous rapid cycling, the manic phases were abbreviated and attenuated. A long-term prospective study of open-label treatment with lithium found a higher rate of recurrence among rapid cyclers versus non–rapid cyclers but similar improvement in symptoms and morbidity (measured as percentage of time ill, episode frequency, and time to recurrence) (Baldessarini et al. 2000). Finally, a meta-analysis of clinical studies comparing subjects with rapid-cycling and non-rapid-cycling bipolar disorder showed that although lithium was less effective in preventing recurrence among rapid cyclers, it did have beneficial effects on severity and duration of episodes (Kupka et al. 2003).

Prophylaxis and Maintenance

Prophylactic or maintenance therapy is often considered after the resolution of an acute mood episode. Lithium is the best-studied drug for this indication. Tondo et al. (2001) found lithium effective in long-term use (more than 1 year) in decreasing frequency of mood episodes and "time ill" in patients with bipolar I and bipolar II disorders. Benefits of lithium treatment were not significantly different among patients with psychotic or mixed episodes, rapid cycling, or more classic forms. There was no decrease in efficacy with long-term use. Despite the evidence for efficacy, Kulhara et al. (1999) found that only 24% of the patients followed in a lithium clinic were free of mood episodes while receiving lithium prophylaxis (average duration of monitoring = 11 years). Noncompliance and/or subtherapeutic lithium serum levels (<0.4 mEq/L), high number of psychosocial stressors, higher number of depressive episodes before lithium treatment, and poor social support predicted poorer response to lithium prophylaxis. In contrast, starting lithium early in the course of illness predicted a better response to treatment (P<0.001), after polarity, sex, age at onset, duration of illness, and duration of lithium prophylaxis were accounted for (Franchini et al. 1999).

In a comparison of lithium, divalproex, and placebo in a 1-year treatment study of patients with bipolar I disorder after recovery from an index manic episode, Bowden et al. (2000) found that median times to 50% survival without mood episode were 40 weeks for divalproex, 24 weeks for lithium, and 28 weeks for placebo, although the differences were not statistically significant. Patients who received divalproex remained in treatment significantly longer than did those who received lithium.

The recent Bipolar Affective Disorder: Lithium/Anticonvulsant Evaluation (BALANCE) study examined the effects of lithium monotherapy, valproate monotherapy, or lithium-plus-valproate combination therapy for relapse prevention in a large international trial (BALANCE investigators et al. 2010). More than 300 patients with bipolar I disorder initially completed a "run-in" phase during which they took both lithium and valproate. Of those who tolerated the combination, a subsequent randomization phase assigned subjects to lithium alone, valproate alone, or continued combination treatment for up to 2 years of follow-up. The primary outcome was time to new intervention (either medication change or hospitalization) for an emerging affective episode. The study results clearly showed that the combination of lithium and valproate was superior to valproate alone and also suggested that lithium monotherapy was superior to valproate monotherapy. The apparent discrepancy between the latter finding and the conclusions of Bowden et al. (2000) described above may reflect differences in the population studied and the outcome measures used; alternatively, the valproate dose in BALANCE may have been suboptimal for preventing acute mania.

In patients with mixed or manic episodes who responded to cotreatment with lithium and olanzapine, investigators conducted a double-blind, randomized maintenance trial of lithium versus olanzapine (Tohen et al. 2005). Recurrence rates were similar between groups, with 38.8% of patients on lithium and 30.0% of those on olanzapine experiencing relapse, with similar prophylaxis for depressive episodes between treatments and some advantage for prevention of mania and mixed episodes with olanzapine.

Maintenance dosing. Once-daily dosing of lithium at bedtime yields higher brain-to-serum ratios of lithium levels than twice-daily dosing schedules (Soares et al. 2001). Investigators have observed substantial variation in brain lithium levels among individuals with similar serum lithium levels (Gonzalez et al. 1993). In a study evaluating maintenance treatment with lithium at dosages resulting in low (0.4–0.6 mmol/L) versus standard (0.8–1.0 mmol/L) serum levels, Gelenberg et al. (1989) found that the risk of relapse was 2.6 times higher in patients randomly assigned to maintenance lithium at the lower serum level. However, in a reanalysis of the data (Perlis et al. 2002), the higher relapse rate observed with the lower serum level was found to be associated with the abrupt reduction in lithium dosage that occurred following randomization in patients who were switched from the standard range to the low range. Thus, an abrupt reduction in lithium dosage may negatively impact the course of illness.

Unipolar Depression

Analysis of five controlled trials of lithium augmentation for unipolar depression found significant improvement in 56%–96% of patients (Austin et al. 1991; Heit and Nemeroff 1998; Heninger et al. 1983; Kantor et al. 1986; Schopf et al. 1989; Stein and Bernadt 1993; Zusky et al. 1988). In treatment-refractory depression, open-label data support the addition of lithium to antidepressants, including tricyclics, trazodone, and selective serotonin reuptake inhibitors (SSRIs) (De Montigny et al. 1981, 1983, 1985; Dinan 1993; Fontaine et al. 1991; Price et al. 1986). Double-blind studies support the use of lithium for augmentation of tricyclics, monoamine oxidase inhibitors (MAOIs), trazodone, and SSRIs (Baumann et al. 1996; Fava et al. 1994; Heninger et al. 1983; Joffe et al. 1993; Kantor et al. 1986; Katona et al. 1995; Nierenberg et al. 2006; Schopf et al. 1989; Zusky et al. 1988). In the large Sequenced Treatment Alternatives to Relieve Depression (STAR*D) multisite trial, 15.9% of subjects who did not experience remission with citalopram monotherapy and another medication trial experienced remission after the addition of lithium (Nierenberg et al. 2006).

Time of onset of lithium action as an adjunct to antidepressants remains unclear. Also, new studies are needed to determine the appropriate duration of treatment with lithium augmentation and the appropriate serum lithium levels (Heit and Nemeroff 1998).

Suicide: Is Lithium Protective?

Up to 50% of bipolar patients attempt suicide (Compton and Nemeroff 2000). In an analysis of studies of lithium treatment (Schou 1998), patients treated with lithium had a lower overall mortality rate than bipolar patients in general and did not have a significantly higher suicide rate than the general population. Tondo et al. (1997) reviewed studies of the use of lithium in the treatment of major mood disorders; these included 28 studies that involved more than 17,000 patients. Risks of completed and attempted suicides were 8.6-fold higher in patients who were not given lithium compared with those who were. In meta-analyses of studies of lithium treatment in major mood disorders, Tondo et al. (2001), Baldessarini et al. (2006), and Guzzetta et al. (2007) found significantly lower suicide risk for subjects who were receiving treatment with lithium. Methodological problems exist in the studies that have examined lithium and suicide risk, and large-scale prospective studies are needed to inform treatment decisions (Gelenberg 2001). In the first randomized, placebo-controlled trial investigating the effect of adjunctive lithium treatment in prevention of suicidal behavior, which was conducted by Lauterbach et al. (2008), survival analysis showed no significant difference in suicidal acts between lithium- and placebo-treated groups. However, post hoc analysis showed that all completed suicides occurred in the placebo group, suggesting that lithium may be effective in reducing the risk of completed suicide.

Use in Special Populations

Children and Adolescents

Lithium is FDA approved for the treatment of bipolar disorder in adolescents and has been shown to be significantly more efficacious than placebo for both bipolar disorder and substance abuse, but not for major depression (Geller et al. 1998a, 1998b; Ryan et al. 1999). Lithium has a large effect size in the open-label treatment of acute mania or mixed episodes in children and adolescents (Kowatch et al. 2000) and of bipolar depression in adolescents with bipolar I disorder (Patel et al. 2006). Lithium and divalproex showed a similar time to relapse in a randomized, double-blind maintenance trial of lithium versus divalproex in children 5–17 years of age (Findling et al. 2005). After weight and serum lithium levels are controlled for, younger age is associated with more side effects (Campbell et al. 1991).

The Elderly

In a retrospective trial, significantly more patients 55 years or older improved with lithium than with valproate, especially in cases of classic mania, whereas the two drugs had similar results when considering only the cases of mixed mania (S.T. Chen et al. 1999). The therapeutic range for elderly patients was similar to that for younger adults: ≥0.8 mmol/L.

Medical comorbidity may be a consideration in elderly patients. Volume depletion, use of nonsteroidal anti-inflammatory drugs, and use of thiazide diuretics can increase lithium levels (Stoudemire et al. 1990). Also, patients with kidney disease receiving hemodialysis do not eliminate lithium other than through dialysis. Lithium should only be given after a dialysis treatment and need not be given daily (Stoudemire et al. 1990).

Lithium appears to have neuroprotective effects, decreasing oxidative damage, and could play a role in the prevention of neurocognitive decline in aging and the prevention of Alzheimer's disease (Bachmann et al. 2005; Chen et al. 2000; Cui et al. 2007; Engle et al. 2006; Phiel et al. 2003; Shao et al. 2005; Su et al. 2004; Tsaltas et al. 2007; Yoshida et al. 2006). A Denmark study that followed more than 4,800 patients with newly diagnosed bipolar disorder over 10 years found that long-term treatment with lithium, but not with other psychopharmacological agents, was associated with a reduced risk of subsequent dementia (Kessing et al. 2010).

Pregnant/Lactating Women

The risks and benefits of lithium treatment must be carefully assessed in the context of pregnancy and breast-feeding. Data suggest that lithium exposure during pregnancy is less harmful than experts believed in past decades (Cohen et al. 1994). In fact, although the overall risk of Ebstein's anomaly—a rare cardiac malformation with an incidence of 1 per 20,000 live births—may be higher with lithium use (relative risk of 10–20 compared with the general population) than without, the prevalence associated with first-trimester lithium exposure is 0.05%–0.1% (Cohen and Rosenbaum 1998). This risk is substantially lower than the risk of neural tube defects associated with some anticonvulsants used for mood stabilization. Overall, lithium is not a high-risk teratogen.

Although lithium is today considered a first-line treatment of bipolar disorder during pregnancy, many women wish to discontinue psychotropic medications during pregnancy. In a longitudinal study of 89 women with bipolar disorder who continued or discontinued mood stabilizer treatment during pregnancy, Viguera et al. (2007b) reported an overall risk of recurrence of 71%. Risk of recurrence was twofold greater in women who discontinued mood stabilizer treatment, and time to recurrence was 11 times shorter if the mood stabilizer was discontinued abruptly instead of gradually. Risk of recurrence was 1.6 times higher in women using a mood stabilizer other than lithium (Viguera et al. 2007b). In an earlier study of rates of relapse after lithium discontinuation in pregnant and nonpregnant women with bipolar disorder, Viguera et al. (2000) found that rates of relapse were initially similar in the two groups but increased sharply in pregnant women during the postpartum period (70% vs. 24% in nonpregnant patients matched for time after discontinuation) (Viguera et al. 2000). This high risk of recurrence has prompted experts in the field to recommend postpartum prophylactic treatment with a mood stabilizer for women with bipolar disorder (Cohen et al. 1995).

Lithium is known to be passed on to breast-feeding infants and is found in breast milk and infant serum. For this reason, and also because of a small number of case reports of adverse effects to breast-feeding infants of mothers taking lithium, the American Academy of Pediatrics (AAP) had previously considered lithium use to be contraindicated in breast-feeding women (Chaudron and Jefferson 2000). However, the AAP now classifies lithium in the category of medications that should be used with caution in breast-feeding due to reports of adverse events (American Academy of Pediatrics Committee on Drugs 2001). In a recent study of 10 mother-baby pairs, serum lithium levels in the babies ranged from 0.09 to 0.3 mEq/L (mean 0.16 mEq/L). Transient elevations in infant thyroid-stimulating hormone, blood urea nitrogen, and creatinine levels were observed without evident long-term effects (Viguera et al. 2007a). The study authors concluded that breast-feeding in the context of lithium therapy may be considered reasonable for a healthy infant when the mother's bipolar disorder is clinically stable, lithium monotherapy or a simple medication regimen is being used, and the pediatrician supports breast-feeding while the mother is being treated with lithium.

Side Effects and Toxicology

Laboratory Monitoring

Before lithium therapy is started, medical history should be obtained, as well as baseline renal laboratory tests (blood urea nitrogen, creatinine level), thyroid function tests, and an electrocardiogram for patients older than 40 years (American Psychiatric Association 2002). The American Psychiatric Association practice guideline suggests that renal function should be assessed every 2–3 months and thyroid function tested once or twice during the first 6 months of treatment. After the first 6 months, renal laboratory tests and thyroid function tests should be monitored every 6–12 months or whenever clinically indicated (American Psychiatric Association 2002).

Side Effects

Cognitive side effects and weight gain have been reported to be the most disturbing side effects experienced in patients receiving lithium maintenance treatment, whereas self-reported noncompliance was mostly associated with lithium's effects on cognition and coordination (Gitlin et al. 1989). Weight gain may be a greater risk for patients who are obese before commencement of lithium treatment, compared with normal-weight individuals (Bowden et al. 2006). A minority (27.8%) of patients with excessive levels of lithium (≥1.5 mmol/L) manifested symptoms of toxicity when hospitalized (Webb et al. 2001). Women and the elderly were most likely to have excessive levels.

Neurotoxicity

Neurotoxicity, delirium, and encephalopathy have been reported with lithium use. Specific populations have been noted to be at higher risk. Also, certain circumstances such as concomitant electroconvulsive therapy or other psychotropics—especially typical antipsychotics—have been implicated in increasing the risk of such adverse effects of lithium treatment.

Neurotoxic reactions are potentially irreversible. Permanent neurological deficits have been reported after episodes of lithium intoxication (Apte and Langston 1983; Donaldson and Cuningham 1983). These have included deficits in recent memory, ataxia, and movement disorders. Early hemodialysis may help prevent permanent sequelae. Donaldson and Cuningham (1983) also reported persistent neurological sequelae of lithium toxicity involving multiple sites within the nervous system. Himmelhoch et al. (1980) found a greater incidence of neurotoxicity secondary to lithium treatment in the elderly. Stoll et al. (1996) reported a case series in which seven patients who experienced lithium-associated cognitive deficits improved when switched to treatment with divalproex sodium.

Tremor

A fine postural tremor affects between 4% and 65% of the patients who receive lithium (Gelenberg and Jefferson 1995). The tremor may decrease with time; a severe tremor may indicate toxicity. Elimination of caffeine may actually worsen tremor because renal lithium clearance can be reduced with reduction of caffeine intake (Jefferson 1988). Lithium tremor, which resembles essential tremor, may worsen with age.

Thyroid Function

In a chart review of 135 patients who received maintenance treatment with lithium, 38% were found to have abnormal thyroid function tests (thyroid-stimulating hormone and/or free thyroxine index), with an association between these laboratory abnormalities and length of time on lithium (Fagiolini et al. 2006). In another retrospective study of 209 patients who received lithium, Kirov (1998) found that 14.9% of the females and 3.4% of the males developed hypothyroidism. Female patients and patients older than 50 years were more likely to develop hypothyroidism. Other reports suggested that subclinical hypothyroidism is more frequent (Lombardi et al. 1993). A family history of thyroid disease may lead to earlier onset of hypothyroidism that occurs with lithium use (Kusalic and Engelsmann 1999).

Renal Complications

Lithium has multiple renal effects, including those that occur early in treatment and those that occur with chronic use. Lithium can induce tubular dysfunction early in treatment, with reduced urinary concentrating capacity occurring over the first 8 weeks of treatment. Nephrogenic diabetes insipidus occurs in 20%–40% of patients on lithium (Stone 1999). These effects may be partially mediated by lithium's action on water and sodium channels in the kidney (Grunfeld and Rossier 2009); thus, there has been renewed interest in using amiloride, a sodium channel–blocking diuretic, to attempt to modify lithium's toxicity.

Another important renal effect of lithium is chronic kidney disease, which tends to occur after 10–20 years of lithium administration (Presne et al. 2003). The clearest risk factor is length of lithium use; however, additional possible risk factors are older age, previous episodes of lithium toxicity, and presence of comorbid disorders. The potential for chronic renal disease is the reason that close laboratory monitoring is required in patients on long-term lithium. The decision of whether to stop lithium in the setting of renal impairment must be made collaboratively by the patient, the psychiatrist, and the nephrologist. Chronic kidney disease can progress to renal failure even after lithium is stopped; however, it appears that there may be a benefit if a change is made with mild or moderate renal dysfunction (Grunfeld and Rossier 2009).

Cardiac Changes

Lithium intoxication has been reported to cause cardiac alterations, including sinus bradycardia and sinus node dysfunction (Steckler 1994). Sinus node dysfunction is more prevalent in patients who have been taking lithium for at least a year when compared with age-matched control subjects, although clinically significant dysfunction is uncommon (Rosenqvist et al. 1993). Also, cases of atrioventricular block in patients with therapeutic lithium levels have been reported (Martin and Piascik 1985). Electrocardiographic T-wave changes, as well as ventricular irritability, may occur (Mitchell and Mackenzie 1982). In patients with clinical indications for lithium use, cardiovascular disease does not preclude the possibility of lithium use. Dosage adjustment and frequent cardiac monitoring are essential for the safe use of lithium in patients with cardiac disease (Tilkian et al. 1976). Because of the risk of sinus node dysfunction and other cardiac effects, careful monitoring of the pulse and electrocardiographic monitoring are recommended in patients older than 50 years (Roose et al. 1979).

Drug-Drug Interactions

Lithium and Other Mood Stabilizers

Lithium and Anticonvulsants

Lithium is commonly used in combination with other mood stabilizers, and although such combinations can be synergistic, polypharmacy may introduce an increased risk of adverse reactions (Freeman and Stoll 1998; Lenox et al. 1996). The combination of lithium and valproate is often used in refractory mania. Interactions may include additive side effects, such as sedation, tremor, or weight gain, but the pharmacokinetics of lithium are not altered by the addition of valproate (Granneman et al. 1996). Lithium and carbamazepine also have been combined for bipolar disorder refractory to lithium alone, but this combination may increase risk for neurotoxicity (Chaudhry and Waters 1983; Frances et al. 1996; Kishimoto 1992; Shukla et al. 1984, 1985; Small et al. 1995). Neurotoxic and other adverse reactions have been associated with the concomitant administration of lithium with calcium channel blockers (Dubovsky et al. 1987; Finley et al. 1995; Helmuth et al. 1989; Wright and Jarrett 1991).

Lithium and Antipsychotics

Although many investigators have reported safe and efficacious results from combining lithium and typical antipsychotics (Baastrup et al. 1976; Bigelow et al. 1981; Carman et al. 1981; Garfinkel et al. 1980; Goldney and Spence 1986), neurotoxicity and even tardive dyskinesia can occur (Cohen and Cohen 1974; Dinan and Kohen 1989; Mani et al. 1996; Mann et al. 1983; Miller et al. 1986; Perenyi et al. 1983, 1984; Spring 1979; Spring and Frankel 1981). Goodwin and Jamison (1990) recommended that when incorporating a typical antipsychotic into a regimen of lithium therapy, the antipsychotic should be used in lower doses and the lithium levels should be maintained below 1.0 mEq/L.

The use of lithium with atypical antipsychotics also may result in adverse reactions. Use of clozapine and lithium may cause diabetic ketoacidosis, neuroleptic malignant syndrome, and neurological side effects (Blake et al. 1992; Garcia et al. 1994; Lemus et al. 1989; Peterson and Byrd 1996; Pope et al. 1986). Some investigators have reported safe and effective use of risperidone and lithium (Ghaemi et al. 1997; Tohen et al. 1996), although adverse effects, including fever, increased white blood cell counts and creatine phosphokinase levels, and delirium, also have been reported (Chen and Cardasis 1996; Swanson et al. 1995). Preliminary data suggest that the combination of lithium and olanzapine is efficacious and well tolerated in acute mania (Madhusoodanan et al. 2000; Sanger et al. 2001). Gabapentin is also used adjunctively in the treatment of bipolar disorder, and because gabapentin has no known drug interactions, it is likely safe with lithium use (Frye et al. 1998; Vollmer et al. 1986). Benzodiazepines are not especially problematic when used with lithium (Adler 1986; Modell et al. 1985; Sachs et al. 1990a, 1990b).

Lithium and Antidepressants

Lithium is often used concomitantly with antidepressants in the treatment of bipolar depression and refractory unipolar depression. Serotonin syndrome—a constellation of mental status and behavioral changes (either agitation or sedation), motor symptoms (restlessness, weakness, hyperreflexia, or ataxia), and autonomic dysfunction (nausea and/or vomiting, dizziness, sweating, fever) (Lejoyeux et al. 1994)—has been reported with the use of lithium and serotonergic antidepressants (Fagiolini et al. 2001; Karle and Bjorndal 1995; Mekler and Woggon 1997; Muly et al. 1993; Ohman and Spigset 1993; Sobanski et al. 1997).

Lithium and Nonpsychotropic Medications

When lithium is used with concurrent nonsteroidal anti-inflammatory drugs, signs and symptoms of toxicity and lithium levels must be monitored more carefully because nonsteroidal anti-inflammatory drugs increase the risk of toxicity (Johnson et al. 1993). Because lithium excretion relies on renal clearance, diuretic medications may affect lithium levels, depending on their site of action. Thiazide diuretics trigger a compensatory increase in reabsorption in the proximal tubule and lead to elevations in lithium levels, whereas loop diuretics do not promote lithium reabsorption and do not greatly affect lithium levels (Finley et al. 1995). Osmotic diuretics enhance lithium excretion and may serve to counteract lithium toxicity, and either no change or a slight increase in lithium levels has been reported with potassium-sparing diuretics. Angiotensin-converting enzyme inhibitors may raise lithium levels (DasGupta et al. 1992; Finley et al. 1996). Serum lithium levels may increase in the context of sodium restriction (Bennett 1997).

Conclusion

Lithium is an important option in the evidence-based rational treatment of bipolar disorder. Bipolar disorder is a mental illness that affects between 1% and 5% of the population (Akiskal et al. 2000). Bipolar disorder causes significant morbidity and mortality, and the diagnosis of bipolar disorder carries a high risk for suicide. Of patients with bipolar disorder, 25%–50% attempt suicide and an estimated 19% complete suicide (Goodwin and Jamison 1990).

Lithium has been shown to be effective for acute mania and bipolar depression and as a prophylactic treatment for bipolar disorder. Some data suggest that conditions such as comorbid neurological illness and mixed episodes favor other mood stabilizers rather than lithium. Evidence also suggests that lithium can play a role in the treatment of refractory unipolar depression in patients at risk for suicide. Lithium may be less risky than anticonvulsants in pregnancy. We seek new treatments in our field and hope that they will be more efficacious and better tolerated than our "old" medications. At present, lithium remains an important treatment option.

References

Adler LW: Mixed bipolar disorder responsive to lithium and clonazepam. J Clin Psychiatry 47:49–50, 1986

Akiskal HS, Bourgeois ML, Angst J, et al: Re-evaluating the prevalence of and diagnostic composition within the broad clinical spectrum of bipolar disorders. J Affect Disord 59 (suppl):S5–S30, 2000

American Academy of Pediatrics Committee on Drugs: Transfer of drugs and other chemicals into human milk. Pediatrics 108:776–789, 2001

American Psychiatric Association: Practice guideline for the treatment of patients with bipolar disorder (revision). Am J Psychiatry 159 (suppl):1–50, 2002

Apte SN, Langston JW: Permanent neurological deficits due to lithium toxicity. Ann Neurol 13:453–455, 1983

Austin MPV, Souza FGM, Goodwin GM: Lithium augmentation in antidepressant-resistant patients: a quantitative analysis. Br J Psychiatry 159:510–514, 1991

Baastrup PC, Hollnagel P, Sorensen R, et al: Adverse reactions in treatment with lithium carbonate and haloperidol. JAMA 236:2645–2646, 1976

Bachmann RF, Schloesser RJ, Gould TD, et al: Mood stabilizers target cellular plasticity and resilience cascades: implications for the development of novel therapeutics. Mol Neurobiol 32:173–202, 2005

BALANCE investigators and collaborators, Geddes JR, Goodwin GM, Rendell J, et al: Lithium plus valproate combination therapy versus monotherapy for relapse prevention in bipolar I disorder (BALANCE): a randomised open-label trial. Lancet 375:385–395, 2010

Baldessarini RJ: Drugs and the treatment of psychiatric disorders: depression and mania, in Goodman and Gilman's The Pharmacological Basis of Therapeutics, 9th Edition. Edited by Hardman JG, Limbird LE. New York, McGraw-Hill, 1996, pp 431–459

Baldessarini RJ, Tarazi FI: Drugs and the treatment of psychiatric disorders: psychosis and mania, in Goodman and Gilman's The Pharmacological Basis of Therapeutics, 10th Edition. Edited by Hardman JG, Limbird LE. New York, McGraw-Hill, 2001, pp 485–520

Baldessarini RJ, Tondo L, Floris G, et al: Effects of rapid cycling on response to lithium maintenance treatment in 360 bipolar I and II disorder patients. J Affect Disord 61:13–22, 2000

Baldessarini RJ, Tondo L, Davis P, et al: Decreased risk of suicides and attempts during long-term lithium treatment: a meta-analytic review. Bipolar Disord 5:625–639, 2006

Barkai IA, Dunner DL, Gross HA, et al: Reduced myo-inositol levels in cerebrospinal fluid from patients with affective disorder. Biol Psychiatry 13:65–72, 1978

Baron M, Gerson ES, Rudy V, et al: Lithium carbonate response in depression: prediction by unipolar/bipolar illness, average-evoked response, catechol-O-methyl transferase, and family history. Arch Gen Psychiatry 32:1107–1111, 1975

Baumann P, Nil R, Souche A, et al: A double-blind, placebo-controlled study of citalopram with and without lithium in the treatment of therapy-resistant depressive patients: a clinical, pharmacokinetic, and pharmacogenetic investigation. J Clin Psychopharmacol 16:307–314, 1996

Belmaker RH, Bersudsky Y, Agam G, et al: How does lithium work on manic depression? Clinical and psychological correlates of the inositol theory. Annu Rev Med 47:47–56, 1996

Benjamin J, Levine J, Fux M, et al: Inositol treatment for panic disorder: a double-blind placebo-controlled crossover trial. Am J Psychiatry 152:1084–1086, 1995

Bennett WM: Drug interactions and consequences of sodium restriction. Am J Clin Nutr 65:678–681, 1997

Berrettini WH, Nurnberger JI Jr, Hare T, et al: Reduced plasma and CSF γ-aminobutyric acid in affective illness: effect of lithium carbonate. Biol Psychiatry 18:185–194, 1983

Berrettini WH, Nurnberger JI Jr, Hare T, et al: CSF GABA in euthymic manic-depressive patients and controls. Biol Psychiatry 21:842–844, 1986

Berridge MJ, Downes CP, Hanley RR: Neural and developmental action of lithium: a unifying hypothesis. Cell 59:411–419, 1989

Bigelow LB, Weinberger DR, Wyatt RJ: Synergism of combined lithium-neuroleptic therapy: a double-blind, placebo-controlled case study. Am J Psychiatry 138:81–83, 1981

Birch NJ, Greenfield AA, Hullin RP: Pharmacodynamic aspects of long-term prophylactic lithium. Int Pharmacopsychiatry 15:91–98, 1980

Blake LM, Marks RC, Luchins DJ: Reversible neurologic symptoms with clozapine and lithium. J Clin Psychopharmacol 12:297–299, 1992

Bowden CL, Brugger AM, Swann AC, et al: Efficacy of divalproex vs lithium and placebo in the treatment of mania. The Depakote Mania Study Group. JAMA 271:918–924, 1994 (erratum in JAMA 271:1830, 1994)

Bowden CL, Calabrese JR, McElroy SL, et al: A randomized, placebo-controlled 12-month trial of divalproex and lithium in treatment of outpatients with bipolar I disorder. Arch Gen Psychiatry 57:481–489, 2000

Bowden CL, Grunze H, Mullen J, et al: A randomized, double-blind, placebo-controlled efficacy and safety study of quetiapine or lithium as monotherapy for mania in bipolar disorder. J Clin Psychiatry 66:111–121, 2005

Bowden CL, Calabrese JR, Ketter KA, et al: Impact of lamotrigine and lithium on weight in obese and nonobese patients with bipolar I disorder. Am J Psychiatry 163:1199–1201, 2006

Bowden C, Gogus A, Grunze H, et al: A 12-week, open, randomized trial comparing sodium valproate to lithium in patients with bipolar I disorder suffering from a manic episode. Int Clin Psychopharmacol 23:254–262, 2008

Cade JF: Lithium salts in the treatment of psychotic excitement. Med J Aust 36:349–352, 1949

Campbell M, Silva RR, Kafantaris V, et al: Predictors of side effects associated with lithium administration in children. Psychopharmacol Bull 27:373–380, 1991

Carman JS, Bigelow LB, Wyatt RJ: Lithium combined with neuroleptics in chronic schizophrenic and schizoaffective patients. J Clin Psychiatry 42:124–128, 1981

Chaudhry RP, Waters BG: Lithium and carbamazepine interaction: possible neurotoxicity. J Clin Psychiatry 44:30–31, 1983

Chaudron LH, Jefferson JW: Mood stabilizers during breastfeeding: a review. J Clin Psychiatry 61:79–90, 2000

Chen B, Cardasis W: Delirium induced by lithium and risperidone combination. Am J Psychiatry 153:1233–1234, 1996

Chen G, Huang LD, Jiang YM, et al: The mood stabilizing agent valproate inhibits the activity of glycogen synthase kinase 3. J Neurochem 72: 1327–1330, 1999

Chen G, Rajkowska G, Du F, et al: Enhancement of hippocampal neurogenesis by lithium. J Neurochem 75:1729–1734, 2000

Chen ST, Altshuler LL, Melnyk KA, et al: Efficacy of lithium vs valproate in the treatment of mania in the elderly: a retrospective study. J Clin Psychiatry 60:181–186, 1999

Chisholm D, van Ommeren M, Ayuso-Mateos JL, et al: Cost-effectiveness of clinical interventions for reducing the global burden of bipolar disorder. Br J Psychiatry 187:559–567, 2005

Cohen LS, Rosenbaum JF: Psychotropic drug use during pregnancy: weighing the risks. J Clin Psychiatry 59:18–28, 1998

Cohen LS, Friedman JM, Jefferson JW, et al: A reevaluation of risk of in utero exposure to lithium. JAMA 271:146–150, 1994

Cohen LS, Sichel DA, Robertson LM, et al: Postpartum prophylaxis for women with bipolar disorder. Am J Psychiatry 152:1641–1645, 1995

Cohen WJ, Cohen NH: Lithium carbonate, haloperidol, and irreversible brain damage. JAMA 230:1283–1287, 1974

Compton MT, Nemeroff CB: The treatment of bipolar depression. J Clin Psychiatry 61 (suppl): 57–67, 2000

Cui J, Shao L, Young LT, et al: Role of glutathione in neuroprotective effects of mood stabilizing drugs lithium and valproate. Neuroscience 144:1447–1453, 2007

DasGupta K, Jefferson JW, Kobak KA, et al: The effect of enalapril on serum lithium levels in healthy men. J Clin Psychiatry 53:398–400, 1992

De Montigny C, Grunberg F, Mayer A, et al: Lithium induces rapid relief of depression in tricyclic antidepressant drug non-responders. Br J Psychiatry 138:252–256, 1981

De Montigny C, Cournoyer G, Morissette R, et al: Lithium carbonate addition in tricyclic antidepressant-resistant unipolar depression: correlations with the neurobiologic actions of tricyclic antidepressant drugs and lithium ion on the serotonin system. Arch Gen Psychiatry 40:11327–11334, 1983

De Montigny C, Elie R, Caille G: Rapid response to the addition of lithium in iprindole-resistant unipolar depression: a pilot study. Am J Psychiatry 142:220–223, 1985

Dinan T: Lithium augmentation in sertraline-resistant depression: a preliminary dose-response study. Acta Psychiatr Scand 88:300–301, 1993

Dinan T, Kohen D: Tardive dyskinesia in bipolar affective disorder: relationship to lithium therapy. Br J Psychiatry 155:55–57, 1989

Dixon JF, Hokin LE: Lithium acutely inhibits and chronically up-regulates and stabilizes glutamate uptake by presynaptic nerve endings in mouse cerebral cortex. Proc Natl Acad Sci U S A 95:8363–8368, 1998

Donaldson IM, Cuningham J: Persisting neurologic sequela of lithium carbonate therapy. Arch Neurol 40:747–751, 1983

Donnelly EF, Goodwin FK, Waldman IN, et al: Prediction of antidepressant responses to lithium. Am J Psychiatry 135:552–556, 1978

Dubovsky SL, Franks RD, Allen S: Verapamil: a new antimanic drug with potential interactions with lithium. J Clin Psychiatry 48:371–372, 1987

Dunner DL, Fieve RR: Clinical factors in lithium prophylaxis failure. Arch Gen Psychiatry 30:229–233, 1974

Dunner DL, Patrick V, Fieve RR: Rapid cycling manic depressive patients. Compr Psychiatry 18:561–566, 1977

Emilien G, Maloteau JM, Seghers A, et al: Lithium compared to valproic acid and carbamazepine in the treatment of mania: a statistical meta-analysis. Eur Neuropsychopharmacol 6:245–252, 1996

Engle T, Goni-Oliver P, Lucas JJ, et al: Chronic lithium administration to FTDP-17 tau and GSK-3beta overexpressing mice prevents tau hyperphosphorylation and neurofibrillary tangle formation, but pre-formed neurofibrillary tangles do not revert. J Neurochem 99:1445–1455, 2006

Fagiolini A, Buysse DJ, Frank E, et al: Tolerability of combined treatment with lithium and paroxetine in patients with bipolar disorder and depression. J Clin Psychopharmacol 21:474–478, 2001

Fagiolini A, Kupfer DJ, Scott J, et al: Hypothyroidism in patients with bipolar I disorder treated primarily with lithium. Epidemiol Psichiatr Soc 15:123–127, 2006

Fava M, Rosenbaum JF, McGrath PJ, et al: Lithium and tricyclic augmentation of fluoxetine treatment for resistant major depression: a double-blind, controlled study. Am J Psychiatry 151: 1372–1374, 1994

Fieve RR, Platman SR, Plutchik RR: The use of lithium in affective disorders, I: acute endogenous depression. Am J Psychiatry 125:79–83, 1968

Findling RL, McNamara NK, Youngstrom EA, et al: Double-blind 18-month trial of lithium versus divalproex maintenance treatment in pediatric bipolar disorder. J Am Acad Child Adolesc Psychiatry 44:409–417, 2005

Finley P, Warner M, Peabody C: Clinical relevance of drug interactions with lithium. Clin Pharmacokinet 29:172–191, 1995

Finley PR, O'Brien JG, Coleman RW: Lithium and angiotensin-converting enzyme inhibitors: evaluation of a potential interaction. J Clin Psychopharmacol 16:68–71, 1996

Fontaine R, Ontiveros A, Elie R, et al: Lithium carbonate augmentation of desipramine and fluoxetine in refractory depression. Biol Psychiatry 29:946–948, 1991

Frances A, Docherty JP, Kahn DA: Treatment of bipolar disorder. J Clin Psychiatry 57 (suppl):5–58, 1996

Franchini L, Zanardi R, Smeraldi E, et al: Early onset of lithium prophylaxis as a predictor of good long-term outcome. Eur Arch Psychiatry Clin Neurosci 249:227–230, 1999

Freeman MP, Stoll AL: Mood stabilizers in combination: a review of safety and efficacy. Am J Psychiatry 155:12–21, 1998

Freeman TW, Clothier JL, Pazzaglia P, et al: A double-blind comparison of valproate and lithium in the treatment of acute mania. Am J Psychiatry 149:108–111, 1992

Frye MA, Kimbrell TA, Dunn RT, et al: Gabapentin does not alter single-dose lithium pharmacokinetics. J Clin Psychopharmacol 18:461–464, 1998

Garcia G, Crismon M, Dorson P: Seizures in two patients after the addition of lithium to a clozapine regimen. J Clin Psychopharmacol 14:426–428, 1994

Garfinkel PE, Stancer HC, Persad E: A comparison of haloperidol, lithium carbonate and their combination in the treatment of mania. J Affect Disord 2:279–288, 1980

Gelenberg AJ: Can lithium help to prevent suicide? (editorial). Acta Psychiatr Scand 104:161, 2001

Gelenberg AJ, Jefferson JW: Lithium tremor. J Clin Psychiatry 56:283–287, 1995

Gelenberg AJ, Kane JM, Keller MB, et al: Comparison of standard and low serum levels of lithium for maintenance treatment of bipolar disorder. N Engl J Med 321:1489–1493, 1989

Geller B, Cooper TB, Sun K, et al: Double-blind and placebo-controlled study of lithium for adolescent bipolar disorders with secondary substance dependency. J Am Acad Child Adolesc Psychiatry 37:171–178, 1998a

Geller B, Cooper TB, Zimerman B, et al: Lithium for prepubertal depressed children with family history predictors of future bipolarity: a double-blind, placebo-controlled study. J Affect Disord 51:165–175, 1998b

Ghaemi SN, Sachs GS, Baldassano CF, et al: Acute treatment of bipolar disorder with adjunctive risperidone in outpatients. Can J Psychiatry 42:196–199, 1997

Gitlin MJ, Cochran SD, Jamison KR: Maintenance lithium treatment: side effects and compliance. J Clin Psychiatry 50:127–131, 1989

Goldney RD, Spence ND: Safety of the combination of lithium and neuroleptic drugs. Am J Psychiatry 143:882–884, 1986

Gonzalez RG, Guimaraes AR, Sachs GS, et al: Measurement of human brain lithium in vivo by MR spectroscopy. Am J Neuroradiol 14:1027–1037, 1993

Goodwin FK, Jamison KR: Manic Depressive Illness. New York, Oxford University Press, 1990

Goodwin FK, Zis AP: Lithium in the treatment of mania: comparisons with neuroleptics. Arch Gen Psychiatry 36:840–844, 1979

Goodwin FK, Murphy DL, Bunny WF: Lithium carbonate treatment in depression and mania: a longitudinal double-blind study. Arch Gen Psychiatry 21:486–496, 1969

Goodwin FK, Murphy DL, Dunner DL, et al: Lithium response in unipolar versus bipolar depression. Am J Psychiatry 129:44–47, 1972

Grahame-Smith DG: Disorder of synaptic homeostasis as a cause of depression and a target for treatment, in Antidepressant Therapy at the Dawn of the Third Millennium. Edited by Briley M, Montgomery S. London, Martin Dunitz, 1998, pp 111–140

Granneman GR, Schneck DW, Cavanaugh JH, et al: Pharmacokinetic interactions and side effects resulting from concomitant administration of lithium and divalproex sodium. J Clin Psychiatry 57:204–206, 1996

Greenspan K, Schildkraut JJ, Gordon EK, et al: Catecholamine metabolism in affective disorders, III: MHPG and other catecholamine metabolites in patients treated with lithium carbonate. J Psychiatr Res 7:171–182, 1970

Grunfeld JP, Rossier BC: Lithium nephrotoxicity revisited. Nat Rev Nephrol 5:270–276, 2009

Guzzetta F, Tondo L, Centorrino F, et al: Lithium treatment reduces suicide risk in recurrent major depressive disorder. J Clin Psychiatry 68:380–383, 2007

Haddjeri N, Szabo ST, De Montigny C, et al: Increased tonic activation of rat forebrain 5-HT(1A) receptors by lithium addition to antidepressant treatments. Neuropsychopharmacology 22:346–356, 2000

Hahn CG, Umapathy, Wang HY, et al: Lithium and valproic acid treatments reduce PKC activation and receptor–G protein coupling in platelets of bipolar manic patients. J Psychiatr Res 39:355–363, 2005

Heit S, Nemeroff CB: Lithium augmentation of antidepressants in treatment-refractory depression. J Clin Psychiatry 59 (suppl):28–33, 1998

Helmuth D, Ljaljevic Z, Ramirez L, et al: Choreoathetosis induced by verapamil and lithium treatment. J Clin Psychopharmacol 9:454–455, 1989

Heninger GR, Charney DS, Sternberg DE: Lithium carbonate augmentation of antidepressant treatment. Arch Gen Psychiatry 40:1335–1342, 1983

Himmelhoch JM, Neil JK, May SJ, et al: Age, dementia, dyskinesias, and lithium response. Am J Psychiatry 137:941–945, 1980

Jefferson JW: Lithium tremor and caffeine intake: two cases of drinking less and shaking more. J Clin Psychiatry 49:72–73, 1988

Jefferson JW, Greist JH: Primer of Lithium Therapy. Baltimore, MD, Williams & Wilkins, 1977

Jefferson JW, Greist JH, Ackerman DL: Lithium Encyclopedia for Clinical Practice. Washington, DC, American Psychiatric Press, 1983

Jermain DM, Crismon ML, Martin ES III: Population pharmacokinetics of lithium. Clin Pharm 10:376–381, 1991

Joffe RT, Singer W, Levitt AJ, et al: A placebo-controlled comparison of lithium and triiodothyronine augmentation of tricyclic antidepressants in unipolar refractory depression. Arch Gen Psychiatry 50:387–393, 1993

Johnson AG, Seideman P, Day RO: Adverse drug interactions with nonsteroidal anti-inflammatory drugs (NSAIDs): recognition, management and avoidance. Drug Saf 8:99–127, 1993

Kantor D, McNevin S, Leichner P, et al: The benefit of lithium carbonate adjunct in refractory depression. Am J Psychiatry 31:416–418, 1986

Karle J, Bjorndal F: Serotonergic syndrome in combination therapy with lithium and fluoxetine. Ugeskr Laeger 157:1204–1205, 1995

Katona CLE, Abou-Saleh MT, Harrison DA, et al: Placebo-controlled study of lithium augmentation of fluoxetine and lofepramine. Br J Psychiatry 166:80–86, 1995

Keck PE Jr, McElroy SL: Clinical pharmacodynamics and pharmacokinetics of antimanic and mood-stabilizing medications. J Clin Psychiatry 63 (suppl):3–11, 2002

Keck PE Jr, Mendlwicz J, Calabrese JR, et al: A review of randomized, controlled clinical trials in acute mania. J Affect Disord 59:S31–S37, 2000

Keck PE Jr, Perlis RH, Otto MW, et al: The Expert Consensus Guidelines: treatment of bipolar disorder 2004. Postgrad Med Special Report (December):1–120, 2004

Kessing LV, Forman JL, Anderson PK: Does lithium protect against dementia? Bipolar Disord 12:87–94, 2010

Kilts CD: In vivo imaging of the pharmacodynamics and pharmacokinetics of lithium. J Clin Psychiatry 61:41–46, 2000

Kirov G: Thyroid disorders in lithium-treated patients. J Affect Disord 50:33–40, 1998

Kishimoto A: The treatment of affective disorder with carbamazepine: prophylactic synergism of lithium and carbamazepine combination. Prog Neuropsychopharmacol Biol Psychiatry 16:483–493, 1992

Klein PS, Melton DA: A molecular mechanism for the effect of lithium on development. Proc Natl Acad Sci U S A 93:8455–8459, 1996

Kline NS: A narrative account of lithium usage in psychiatry, in Lithium: Its Role in Psychiatric Research and Treatment. Edited by Gershon S, Shopsin B. New York, Plenum, 1973, pp 5–24

Kowatch RA, Suppes T, Carmody TJ, et al: Effect size of lithium, divalproex sodium, and carbamazepine in children and adolescents with bipolar disorder. J Am Acad Child Adolesc Psychiatry 39:713–720, 2000

Kulhara P, Basu D, Mattoo SK, et al: Lithium prophylaxis of recurrent bipolar affective disorder: long-term outcome and its psychosocial correlates. J Affect Disord 54:87–96, 1999

Kupka RW, Luckenbaugh MA, Post RM, et al: Rapid and non-rapid cycling bipolar disorder: a meta-analysis of clinical studies. J Clin Psychiatry 64:1483–1494, 2003

Kusalic M, Engelsmann F: Effect of lithium maintenance therapy on thyroid and parathyroid function. J Psychiatry Neurosci 24:227–233, 1999

Lauterbach E, Felber W, Muller-Oerlinghausen B, et al: Adjunctive lithium treatment in the prevention of suicidal behaviour in depressive disorders: a randomised, placebo-controlled, 1-year trial. Acta Psychiatr Scand 118:469–479, 2008

Lejoyeux M, Ades J, Rouillon F: Serotonin syndrome: incidence, symptoms and treatment. CNS Drugs 2:132–143, 1994

Lemus C, Lieberman J, Johns C: Myoclonus during treatment with clozapine and lithium: the role of serotonin. Hillside J Clin Psychiatry 11:127–130, 1989

Lenox RH, McNamara RK, Watterson JM, et al: Myristoylated alanine-rich C kinase substrate (MARCKS): a molecular target for the therapeutic action of mood stabilizers in the brain? J Clin Psychiatry 57 (suppl):23–31, 1996

Lerer B, Moore N, Meyendorff E, et al: Carbamazepine versus lithium in mania: a double-blind study. J Clin Psychiatry 48:89–93, 1987

Levine J, Gonsalves M, Babur I, et al: Inositol 6 g daily may be effective in depression but not in schizophrenia. Hum Psychopharmacol 8:49–53, 1993

Levine J, Barak Y, Gonsalves M, et al: A double-blind controlled trial of inositol treatment in depression. Am J Psychiatry 152:792–794, 1995

Li X, Friedman AB, Zhu W, et al: Lithium regulates glycogen synthase kinase-3beta in human peripheral blood mononuclear cells: implication in the treatment of bipolar disorder. Biol Psychiatry 61:216–222, 2007

Lombardi G, Panza N, Biondi B, et al: Effects of lithium treatment on hypothalamic-pituitary-thyroid axis: a longitudinal study. J Endocrinol Invest 16:259–263, 1993

Madhusoodanan S, Brenner R, Suresh P, et al: Efficacy and tolerability of olanzapine in elderly patients with psychotic disorders: a prospective study. Ann Clin Psychiatry 12:11–18, 2000

Maggs R: Treatment of manic illness with lithium carbonate. Br J Psychiatry 109:56–65, 1963

Mani J, Tandel S, Shah P, et al: Prolonged neurological sequelae after combination treatment with lithium and antipsychotic drugs. J Neurol Neurosurg Psychiatry 60:350–351, 1996

Mann SC, Greenstein RA, Eilers R: Early onset of severe dyskinesia following lithium-haloperidol treatment. Am J Psychiatry 140:1385–1386, 1983

Martin CA, Piascik MT: First-degree A-V block in patients on lithium carbonate. Can J Psychiatry 30:114–116, 1985

Massot O, Rousselle JC, Fillion MP, et al: 5-HT1B receptors: a novel target for lithium: possible involvement in mood disorders. Neuropsychopharmacology 21:533–541, 1999

Mekler G, Woggon B: A case of serotonin syndrome caused by venlafaxine and lithium. Pharmacopsychiatry 30:272–273, 1997

Mendels J: Lithium in the treatment of depressive states, in Lithium Research and Therapy. Edited by Johnson FN. New York, Academic Press, 1975, pp 43–62

Miller F, Menninger J, Whitcup S: Lithium-neuroleptic neurotoxicity in the elderly bipolar patient. J Clin Psychopharmacol 6:176–178, 1986

Mitchell JE, Mackenzie TB: Cardiac effects of lithium therapy in man: a review. J Clin Psychiatry 43:47–51, 1982

Modell JG, Lenox RH, Weiner S: Inpatient clinical trial of lorazepam for the management of manic agitation. J Clin Psychopharmacol 5:109–113, 1985

Monti JM, Monti D, Jantos H, et al: Effects of selective activation of the 5-HT1B receptor with CP-94,253 on sleep and wakefulness in the rat. Neuropharmacology 34:1647–1651, 1995

Moore GJ, Bebchuk JM, Manji HK: Proton MRS in manic depressive illness: monitoring of lithium induced modulation of brain myo-inositol. Soc Neurosci 23:335–336, 1997

Muly EC, McDonald W, Steffens D, et al: Serotonin syndrome produced by a combination of fluoxetine and lithium. Am J Psychiatry 150:1565, 1993

Nierenberg AA, Fava M, Trivedi MH, et al: A comparison of lithium and T3 augmentation following two failed medication treatments for depression: a STAR*D report. Am J Psychiatry 163:1519–1530, 2006

Niufan G, Tohen M, Qiuqing A, et al: Olanzapine versus lithium in the acute treatment of bipolar mania: a double-blind, randomized, controlled trial. J Affect Disord 105:101–108, 2008

Noyes R Jr, Dempsey GM, Blum A, et al: Lithium treatment of depression. Compr Psychiatry 15:187–193, 1974

Ohman R, Spigset O: Serotonin syndrome induced by fluvoxamine–lithium interaction. Pharmacopsychiatry 26:263–264, 1993

Patel NC, DelBello MP, Bryan HS, et al: Open-label lithium for the treatment of adolescents with bipolar depression. J Am Acad Child Adolesc Psychiatry 45:289–297, 2006

Perenyi A, Rihmer Z, Banki C: Parkinsonian symptoms with lithium, lithium-neuroleptic, and lithium-antidepressant treatment. J Affect Disord 5:171–177, 1983

Perenyi A, Szucs R, Frecska E: Tardive dyskinesia in patients receiving lithium maintenance therapy. Biol Psychiatry 19:1573–1578, 1984

Perlis RH, Sachs GS, Lafer B, et al: Effect of abrupt change from standard to low serum levels of lithium: a reanalysis of double-blind lithium maintenance data. Am J Psychiatry 159:1155–1159, 2002

Peterson GA, Byrd SL: Diabetic ketoacidosis from clozapine and lithium cotreatment. Am J Psychiatry 153:737–738, 1996

Phiel CJ, Klein PS: Molecular targets of lithium action. Annu Rev Pharmacol Toxicol 41:789–813, 2001

Phiel CJ, Wilson CA, Lee VM, et al: GSK-3alpha regulates production of Alzheimer's disease amyloid-beta peptides. Nature 423:435–439, 2003

Pope HG Jr, Cole JO, Choras PT, et al: Apparent neuroleptic malignant syndrome with clozapine and lithium. J Nerv Ment Dis 174:493–495, 1986

Presne C, Fakhouri F, Noel LH, et al: Lithium-induced nephropathy: rate of progression and prognostic factors. Kidney Int 64:585–592, 2003

Price LH, Charney DX, Heninger GR: Variability of response to lithium augmentation in refractory depression. Am J Psychiatry 143:1387–1392, 1986

Price LH, Charney DS, Delgado PL, et al: Lithium and serotonin function: implications for the serotonin hypothesis of depression. Psychopharmacology (Berl) 100:3–12, 1990

Prien RF, Caffey EM Jr, Klett CJ: Comparison of lithium carbonate and chlorpromazine in the treatment of mania. Report of the Veterans Administration and National Institute of Mental Health Collaborative Study Group. Arch Gen Psychiatry 26:146–153, 1972

Quiroz JA, Machado-Vieira R, Zarate CA Jr, et al: Novel insights into lithium's mechanism of action: neurotrophic and neuroprotective effects. Neuropsychobiology 62:50–60, 2010

Reeves RR, Struve FA, Patrick G: Does EEG predict response to valproate versus lithium in patients with mania? Ann Clin Psychiatry 13:69–73, 2001

Roose SP, Nurnberger JI, Dunner DL, et al: Cardiac sinus node dysfunction during lithium treatment. Am J Psychiatry 136:804–806, 1979

Rosenqvist M, Bergfeldt L, Aili H, et al: Sinus node dysfunction during long-term lithium treatment. Br Heart J 70:371–375, 1993

Ryan ND, Bhatara VS, Perel JM: Mood stabilizers in children and adolescents. J Am Acad Child Adolesc Psychiatry 38:529–536, 1999

Sachs GS, Rosenbaum JF, Jones L: Adjunctive clonazepam for maintenance treatment of bipolar affective disorder. J Clin Psychopharmacol 10:42–47, 1990a

Sachs GS, Weilburg JB, Rosenbaum JF: Clonazepam vs neuroleptics as adjuncts to lithium maintenance. Psychopharmacol Bull 26:137–143, 1990b

Sanger TM, Grundy SL, Gibson PJ, et al: Long-term olanzapine therapy in the treatment of bipolar I disorder: an open-label continuation phase study. J Clin Psychiatry 62:273–281, 2001

Schildkraut JJ, Logue MA, Dodge GA: The effect of lithium salts on the turnover and metabolism of norepinephrine in the rat brain. Psychopharmacologia 14:135–141, 1969

Schopf J, Baumann P, Lemarchand T, et al: Treatment of endogenous depressions resistant to tricyclic antidepressants of related drugs by lithium addition: results of a placebo-controlled double-blind study. Pharmacopsychiatry 22:183–187, 1989

Schou M: The effect of prophylactic lithium treatment on mortality and suicidal behavior: a review for clinicians. J Affect Disord 50:253–259, 1998

Schou M, Juel-Nielson N, Stromgren E: The treatment of manic psychoses by administration of lithium salts. J Neurol Neurosurg Psychiatry 17:250–260, 1954

Segal J, Berk M, Brook S: Risperidone compared with both lithium and haloperidol in mania: a double-blind randomized controlled trial. Clin Neuropharmacol 21:176–180, 1998

Shaldubina A, Agam G, Belmaker RH: The mechanism of lithium action: state of the art, ten years later. Prog Neuropsychopharmacol Biol Psychiatry 25:855–866, 2001

Shao L, Young RT, Wang JF: Chronic treatment with mood stabilizers lithium and valproate prevents excitotoxicity by inhibiting oxidative stress in rat cerebral cortical cells. Biol Psychiatry 58:879–884, 2005

Shukla S, Godwin CD, Long LEB, et al: Lithium-carbamazepine neurotoxicity and risk factors. Am J Psychiatry 141:1604–1606, 1984

Shukla S, Cook BL, Miller MG: Lithium-carbamazepine versus lithium-neuroleptic prophylaxis in bipolar illness. J Affect Disord 9:219–222, 1985

Sipes TE, Geyer MA: Functional behavioral homology between rat 5-HT1B and guinea pig 5-HT1D receptors in the modulation of prepulse inhibition of startle. Psychopharmacology 122:231–237, 1996

Small JG, Klapper MH, Milstein V, et al: Carbamazepine compared with lithium in the treatment of mania. Arch Gen Psychiatry 48:915–921, 1991

Small JG, Klapper MH, Marhenke JD, et al: Lithium combined with carbamazepine in the treatment of mania. Psychopharmacol Bull 31:265–272, 1995

Soares JC, Boada F, Spencer S, et al: Brain lithium concentrations in bipolar disorder patients: preliminary (7)Li magnetic resonance studies at 3 T. Biol Psychiatry 49:437–443, 2001

Sobanski T, Bagli M, Laux G, et al: Serotonin syndrome after lithium add-on medication to paroxetine. Pharmacopsychiatry 30:106–107, 1997

Spring G: Neurotoxicity with combined use of lithium and thioridazine. J Clin Psychiatry 40:135–138, 1979

Spring G, Frankel M: New data on lithium and haloperidol incompatibility. Am J Psychiatry 138:818–821, 1981

Steckler TL: Lithium- and carbamazepine-associated sinus node dysfunction: nine-year experience in a psychiatric hospital. J Clin Psychopharmacol 14:336–339, 1994

Stein G, Bernadt B: Lithium augmentation therapy in tricyclic-resistant depression. Br J Psychiatry 162:634–640, 1993

Stern DN, Fieve RR, Neff NH, et al: The effect of lithium chloride administration on brain and heart norepinephrine turnover rates. Psychopharmacologia 14:315–322, 1969

Stokes PE, Shamoian CA, Stoll PM, et al: Efficacy of lithium as acute treatment of manic depressive illness. Lancet 1:1319–1325, 1971

Stoll AL, Locke CA, Vuckovic A, et al: Lithium-associated cognitive and functional deficits reduced by a switch to divalproex sodium: a case series. J Clin Psychiatry 57:356–359, 1996

Stone KA: Lithium-induced nephrogenic diabetes insipidus. J Am Board Fam Pract 12:43–47, 1999

Stoudemire A, Moran MG, Fogel BS: Psychotropic drug use in the medically ill. Psychosomatics 21:377–391, 1990

Su Y, Ryder J, Li B, et al: Lithium, a common drug for bipolar disorder treatment, regulates amyloid-beta precursor protein processing. Biochemistry 43:6899–6908, 2004

Swann AC, Bowden CL, Morris D, et al: Depression during mania: treatment response to lithium or divalproex. Arch Gen Psychiatry 54:37–42, 1997

Swanson CL Jr, Price WA, McEvoy JP: Effects of concomitant risperidone and lithium treatment (letter). Am J Psychiatry 152:1096, 1995

Tilkian AG, Schroeder JS, Kao JJ, et al: The cardiovascular effects of lithium in man: a review of the literature. Am J Med 61:665–670, 1976

Tohen M, Zarate CA Jr, Centorrino F, et al: Risperidone in the treatment of mania. J Clin Psychiatry 57:249–253, 1996

Tohen M, Greil W, Calabrese JR, et al: Olanzapine versus lithium in the maintenance treatment of bipolar disorder: a 12-month, randomized, double-blind, controlled clinical trial. Am J Psychiatry 162:1281–1290, 2005

Tondo L, Jamison KR, Baldessarini RJ: Effect of lithium maintenance on suicidal behavior in major mood disorders. Ann N Y Acad Sci 836:339–351, 1997

Tondo L, Hennen J, Baldessarini RJ: Lower suicide risk with long-term lithium treatment in major affective illness: a meta-analysis. Acta Psychiatr Scand 104:163–172, 2001

Tsaltas E, Kontis D, Boulougouris V, et al: Enhancing effects of chronic lithium on memory in the rat. Behav Brain Res 177:51–60, 2007

Viguera AC, Nonacs R, Cohen LS, et al: Risk of recurrence of bipolar disorder in pregnant and nonpregnant women after discontinuing lithium maintenance. Am J Psychiatry 157:179–184, 2000

Viguera AC, Newport DJ, Ritchie J, et al: Lithium in breastmilk and nursing infants: clinical implications. Am J Psychiatry 164:342–345, 2007a

Viguera AC, Whitfield T, Baldessarini RJ, et al: Risk of recurrence in women with bipolar disorder during pregnancy: prospective study of mood stabilizer discontinuation. Am J Psychiatry 164:1817–1823, 2007b

Vollmer KO, Von Hodenberg A, Kolle EU: Pharmacokinetics and metabolism of gabapentin in rat, dog, and man. Arzneimittelforschung 36:830–839, 1986

Ward ME, Musa MN, Bailey L: Clinical pharmacokinetics of lithium. J Clin Pharmacol 34:280–285, 1994

Webb A, Solomon DA, Ryan C: Lithium levels and toxicity among hospitalized patients. Psychiatr Serv 52:229–231, 2001

Wehr TA, Sack DA, Rosenthal NE, et al: Rapid cycling affective disorder: contributing factors and treatment responses in 51 patients. Am J Psychiatry 145:179–184, 1988

Williams RS, Harwood AJ: Lithium therapy and signal transduction. Trends Pharmacol Sci 21:61–64, 2000

Wright B, Jarrett D: Lithium and calcium channel blockers: possible neurotoxicity. Biol Psychiatry 30:635–636, 1991

Yoshida S, Maeda M, Kaku S, et al: Lithium inhibits stress-induced changes in tau phosphorylation in the mouse hippocampus. J Neural Transm 113:1803–1814, 2006

Young AH, McElroy SL, Bauer M, et al: A double-blind, placebo-controlled study of quetiapine and lithium monotherapy in adults in the acute phase of bipolar depression (EMBOLDEN I). J Clin Psychiatry 71:150–162, 2010

Zusky PM, Biederman J, Rosenbaum JF, et al: Adjunct low dose lithium carbonate in lithium-resistant depression: a placebo-controlled study. J Clin Psychopharmacol 8:120–124, 1988

CHAPTER 27

Valproate

Charles L. Bowden, M.D.

History and Discovery

Valproate was the first mood stabilizer to be studied as an alternative to lithium (Lambert et al. 1966). An enteric-coated formulation, divalproex sodium, was approved in the United States for the treatment of mania in 1995. An extended-release formulation of divalproex was approved for migraine in 2001 and for mania in 2006. Valproate, either as divalproex or as other formulations, is now approved worldwide for the treatment of mania.

Pharmacological Profile

Valproic acid (dipropylacetic acid) is an eight-carbon, branched-chain carboxylic acid that is structurally distinct from other antiepileptic and psychotropic compounds (Bocci and Beretta 1976; Levy 1984). Its three-dimensional structure overlays that of naturally occurring fatty acids (e.g., oleic and linolenic acids). Valproate binds in a saturable fashion to the neuronal membrane sites to which these longer-chain fatty acids attach. Some of valproate's molecular mechanisms are likely a consequence of this physiochemical property.

Pharmacokinetics and Disposition

The bioavailability of valproate approaches 100% with all preparations (Wilder 1992). With the exception of divalproex sodium, all preparations taken orally are rapidly absorbed. Sodium valproate and valproic acid attain peak serum concentrations within 2 hours. Divalproex sodium reaches peak serum concentrations within 3–8 hours. The extended-release (ER) form of divalproex sodium has an earlier onset of absorption than the regular-release tablets and approximately a 20% smaller difference in trough and peak serum levels than regular-release divalproex (Figure 27–1).

Valproate is highly protein bound, predominantly to serum albumin and proportional to the albumin concentration. Although patients with low levels of albumin have a higher fraction of unbound drug, the steady-state level of total drug is not altered. Only the unbound drug crosses the blood-brain barrier and is bioactive. Thus, when valproate is displaced from protein-binding sites through drug interactions, the total drug concentration may not change; however, the pharmacologically active unbound drug does

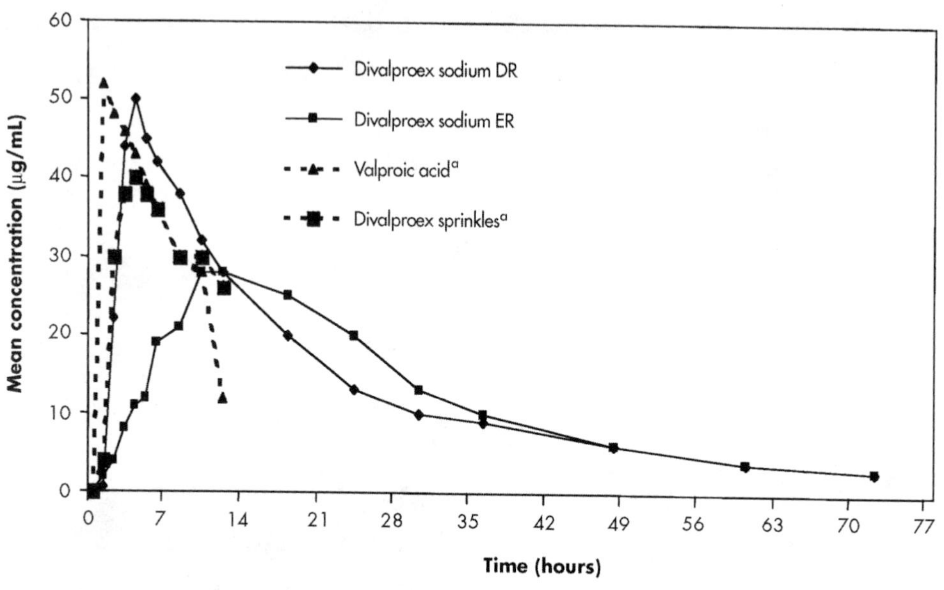

FIGURE 27–1. Mean plasma valproate concentrations with different formulations.
[a]Data derived from different studies after 500-mg doses.
DR = delayed-release; ER = extended-release.
Source. Abbott Laboratories, data on file.

increase and may produce signs and symptoms of toxicity. Moreover, when the plasma concentration of valproate rises in response to increased dosing, the amount of unbound (active) valproate increases disproportionately and is metabolized, with an apparent increase in clearance of total drug, yielding lower-than-expected total plasma concentrations (Levy 1984; Wilder 1992) (Figure 27–2). In addition, protein binding of valproate is increased by low-fat diets and decreased by high-fat diets. Because of lower serum protein levels, women and elderly patients will generally have a higher proportion of the active free moiety.

The concentration range required for good clinical effect in mania is approximately 45 to 125 μg/mL (Bowden et al. 1996). Patients who tolerate higher serum levels—up to around 125 μg/mL—may experience greater improvement (Allen et al. 2006). One open report suggested that patients with bipolar II conditions and cyclothymia may

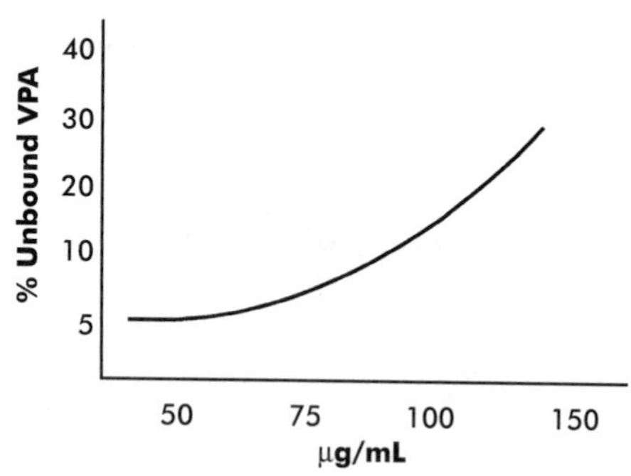

FIGURE 27–2. Total valproate (VPA) concentrations.

As the total concentration of VPA increases, protein-binding sites become saturated, and the percentage of unbound to bound VPA increases.

Source. Reprinted from Wilder BJ: "Pharmacokinetics of Valproate and Carbamazepine." *Journal of Clinical Psychopharmacology* 12 (1, suppl):64S–68S, 1992. Used with permission.

respond to serum valproate concentrations of less than 50 µg/mL (Jacobsen 1993). In maintenance treatment, patients whose serum valproate levels were maintained between 75 and 99 µg/mL had superior outcomes compared with patients whose serum levels were either lower or higher than this range (Keck et al. 2005). Valproate is metabolized in the liver primarily through glucuronidation.

Treatment with valproate for bipolar disorder is usually begun at a dosage of 15–20 mg/kg/day. The drug can be "orally loaded" at 20–30 mg/kg/day in patients with acute mania to induce a more rapid response. The dosage of valproate is increased according to the patient's response and side effects, usually by 250–500 mg/day every 1–3 days, to serum concentrations of 45–125 µg/mL. Of note, sedation, increased appetite, and reductions in white blood counts and platelet counts all become more frequent at serum concentrations above 100 µg/mL (Bowden et al. 2000).

Mechanism of Action

Valproate stimulates extracellular signal-regulated kinase (ERK) and indirectly inhibits glycogen synthase kinase 3 (GSK-3) (Cournoyer and Desrosiers 2009). Valproate stimulates the activity of bcl-2, a neuroprotective substance (Gray et al. 2003). Valproate inhibits histone deacetylase, and many of its subcellular effects (e.g., increasing brain-derived neurotrophic factor) are likely a consequence of this action (Harwood and Agam 2003; Perova et al. 2010).

Indications and Efficacy

Acute Mania in Bipolar Disorder

In a placebo-controlled study, patients with more severe manic symptoms experienced greater benefits from valproate versus placebo than did patients with milder manic symptomatology (Bowden et al. 2006). In this study, the antimanic response to valproate occurred as early as 5 days following initiation of treatment.

Valproate has been studied in adjunctive regimens with various antipsychotics, with findings consistently pointing to greater efficacy for combination treatment versus monotherapy (Bowden 2011; Marcus et al. 2011; Muller-Oerlinghausen et al. 2000; Tohen et al. 2002; Yatham et al. 2003). A 3-week double-blind, placebo-controlled study (Sachs et al. 2002) evaluated the efficacy of risperidone or haloperidol in combination with a mood stabilizer in two groups of bipolar patients: 1) patients who had received treatment with either valproate or lithium at an adequate dosage for at least 2 weeks and were still manic (in which case they were randomly assigned to add-on treatment with risperidone, haloperidol, or placebo) and 2) patients who were manic but had not yet received mood stabilizer treatment (in which case either lithium or valproate was started concurrently with randomization to the add-on treatment). Patients who started mood stabilizer treatment on entering the study showed no advantage from the add-on antipsychotic, whereas patients who were already receiving valproate or lithium but still symptomatic at study entry *did* demonstrate an advantage from the combination treatment (Sachs et al. 2002). These findings suggest that in most circumstances, combination therapy should be limited to patients who fail to respond to a relatively short period of adequate monotherapy treatment.

Few studies of any manic agent have addressed its effectiveness in hypomania, which is more common than manic episodes, even in diagnostically bipolar I patients. In an 8-week randomized, double-blind, placebo-controlled study in outpatient hypomanic bipolar spectrum patients with Young Mania Rating Scale (YMRS) scores between 10 and 20, divalproex ER was significantly more effective than placebo in reducing hypomanic/mild manic symptoms (P=0.024) and nonsignificantly more effective in improving depression (McElroy et al. 2010).

Acute Depression in Bipolar Disorder

An 8-week randomized, placebo-controlled, blinded study reported that divalproex-treated subjects experienced significantly greater improvement than placebo-treated patients in both depressive and anxious symptomatology, based on Hamilton Rating Scale for Depression (Ham-D) and Hamilton Anxiety Scale (Ham-A) scores (Davis et al. 2005). In a 6-week randomized, blinded study in bipolar depression, divalproex was superior to placebo, with primary improvement noted on core mood symptoms rather than on anxiety or insomnia (Ghaemi et al. 2007). Smith et al. (2010) conducted a meta-analysis of these and two other small randomized, blinded studies in acute bipolar depression and reported a significant reduction in depression scale scores for valproate compared with placebo (standardized mean difference = –0.35, range = –0.69 to –0.02). Tolerability was good, but improvement of anxiety was modest and nonsignificant. Valproate has also demonstrated significant prophylactic benefit in reducing risk of relapse into depression, both as monotherapy and as an adjunct to selective serotonin reuptake inhibitor (SSRI) treatment. In a 1-year randomized, double-blind study of bipolar patients who were initially manic, divalproex was more effective than lithium or placebo in delaying time to clinical depression (Gyulai et al. 2003). In those subjects who developed depression, divalproex plus paroxetine or sertraline was superior to either antidepressant alone in treatment of the depression (Gyulai et al. 2003). Ketter et al. (2011) calculated a number needed to treat (NNT) for depression prevention for divalproex of 11; by comparison, an NNT of 49 was calculated for lithium, 15 for lamotrigine, 12 for olanzapine, and 64 for aripiprazole (Ketter et al. 2011).

Maintenance Treatment of Bipolar Disorder

One large double-blind, placebo-controlled maintenance study of valproate monotherapy has been published (Bowden et al. 2000). Patients who recovered with open treatment with either divalproex or lithium were randomly assigned to maintenance treatment with divalproex, lithium, or placebo. The divalproex group did not differ significantly from the placebo group in time to any mood episode ($P=0.06$), in part because the rate of relapse into mania with placebo was lower than anticipated. On secondary outcome measures, divalproex was superior to placebo, with lower rates of discontinuation for either any recurrent mood episode or a depressive episode (Bowden 2004). Divalproex was superior to lithium on some comparisons, including longer duration of successful prophylaxis in the study and less deterioration in depressive symptom scores. Among the subset of patients treated with divalproex in the open acute phase, those subsequently randomized to divalproex had significantly longer times to recurrence of any mood episode ($P=0.05$) or a depressive episode ($P=0.03$), and the proportion of patients who completed the 1-year study without developing either a manic or a depressive episode was significantly higher for divalproex than for placebo (41% vs. 13%; $P=0.01$). This is the only study published to date that has allowed a statistical test of the relationship between acute-episode response to treatment and maintenance treatment outcomes (Bowden et al. 2000). A post hoc review of the study employing relative risk analysis found that patients treated with divalproex were significantly less likely than those treated with placebo to have prematurely left the study because of a mood episode (relative risk [RR]=0.63, 95% confidence interval [CI]= 0.44–0.90) (Bowden 2004). A post hoc analysis of time to any mood episode or early discontinuation for any reason, a measure of effectiveness that has been incorporated in more recent maintenance studies in bipolar disorder, indicated a significant advantage for divalproex over lithium ($P>0.004$) (Bowden 2003a).

A comparison of valproate and lithium in a randomized, blinded trial of rapid-cycling patients reported that only one-quarter of patients enrolled met criteria for an acute bimodal response to either drug, with fewer than 25% of those randomized retaining benefits without relapse for the 20-month maintenance period. The results indicate that monotherapy regimens with either valproate or lithium are unlikely to be effective in any more than a small minority of rapid-cycling patients (Calabrese et al. 2005).

Over the past decade, more studies employing enriched designs in adjunctive treatment have been conducted for all drugs. Such studies are more likely to yield superiority for the adjunctive regimen, because the only patients eligible are ones who have failed to respond to monotherapy regimens. Most of these studies have added atypical antipsychotics—or, in one case, lamotrigine—to regimens of valproate or lithium. Despite the design inequality, the designs have the merit of following a common pattern of clinical practice. In all of these studies, valproate has been adequately tolerated along with the added drug. In most adjunctive design studies, no separate analysis of the results for valproate and lithium has been reported. In a study of adjunctive ziprasidone or placebo added for patients who continued to display manic symptoms while taking valproate or lithium, the adjunctive regimen was superior to continued lithium monotherapy, whereas the outcome of valproate monotherapy was equal to that of valproate plus ziprasidone (Bowden 2011).

A 12-week randomized, blinded comparison of valproate and olanzapine showed equivalent efficacy in mania for the two treatments (Zajecka et al. 2002). A 47-week study of the two drugs reported low rates of completion for both treatments (15% vs. 16%), with earlier symptomatic remission with olanzapine but equivalent efficacy for the two drugs over the remaining portion of the study (Tohen et al. 2003). For both drugs, patients who were in remission at the end of week 3 of treatment were significantly more likely to complete the 47-week trial than were those not in remission (divalproex: 26.2% vs. 11.1%; olanzapine: 20.3% vs. 10.6%; $P=0.001$). This finding indicates that acute treatment response to a drug (either valproate or olanzapine) during a manic episode is predictive of effective treatment with the same drug in maintenance therapy. In both studies, weight gain was greater with olanzapine than with divalproex, and divalproex was associated with a significant reduction in cholesterol levels, compared with an increase in cholesterol levels with olanzapine (Tohen et al. 2003; Zajecka et al. 2002).

Mania Secondary to Head Trauma or Organic Brain Syndromes

Evidence suggesting that secondary or complicated mania responds well to valproate is mixed. In an open study of 56 valproate-treated patients with mania, response was associated with the presence of nonparoxysmal abnormalities on the electroencephalogram but not with neurological soft signs or abnormalities on computed axial tomography scans of brain (McElroy et al. 1988). Findings suggested that responders were more likely to have experienced a closed-head injury antedating the onset of their affective symptoms (Pope et al. 1988). Furthermore, case reports described successful valproate treatment of organic brain syndromes with affective features (Kahn et al. 1988) and mental retardation in patients with bipolar disorder or bipolar symptoms (Kastner et al. 1990; Sovner 1989).

Bipolar Disorder in Children and Adolescents

Few adequately powered and designed studies have been conducted in pediatric bipolar disorder. Findings from the first placebo-controlled trial of divalproex in bipolar youth (ages 10–17 years) were recently published (Wagner et al. 2009). Divalproex was not significantly superior to placebo, and side effects were similar for divalproex and placebo.

In the only blinded, randomized study to compare two medications in young adolescent patients with bipolar disorder, risperidone compared with valproate showed somewhat earlier onset of improvement and resulted in a higher proportion of patients responding by the end of the 6-week trial (Pavuluri et al. 2010). This study lacked a placebo control group.

Attention-deficit/hyperactivity disorder (ADHD) symptoms are commonly intertwined with specific symptoms of bipolar disorder in youth. A pragmatic study of 40 patients between the ages of 6 and 17 years with bipolar I (77%) or bipolar II (23%) disorder, YMRS scores ≥14, and ADHD symptomatology were first treated with divalproex. Thirty-two subjects achieved ≥50% improvement in YMRS scores, but only 3 showed improvement in ADHD symptoms. Mixed amphetamines or placebo were then added for the 30 subjects who entered the placebo crossover phase. Amphetamines plus divalproex were superior to divalproex alone in improving ADHD symptoms. Both regimens were well tolerated, and no patient had worsening of manic symptoms (Scheffer et al. 2005).

One double-blind, randomized, placebo-controlled study has been conducted in youth ages 8–10 years who met criteria for oppositional defiant disorder or conduct disorder and had experienced temper and mood lability but did not meet the full criteria for bipolar disorder. By the end of phase 1, 8 of 10 patients who received divalproex had responded, compared with none on placebo. Of the 15 patients who completed both phases, 12 had superior responses to divalproex (Donovan et al. 2000).

Agitation and Clinical Decline in Elderly Patients With Dementia

Patients with dementia are most frequently institutionalized for agitation and behavioral disturbances. In a randomized, blinded study of 56 nursing home patients with agitation and dementia treated with either placebo or individualized doses of divalproex, the drug-placebo difference in Brief Psychiatric Rating Scale Agitation scores significantly favored divalproex. Side effects occurred in 68% of the divalproex group versus 33% of the placebo group and were generally rated as mild (Porsteinsson et al. 2001). Six weeks of open continuation treatment resulted in further improvement of agitation. Serum levels were above 40 μg/mL in both the acute blinded phase and the open continuation phase (Porsteinsson et al. 2003). Patients with dementia should generally be treated with valproate dosages below 1,000 mg/day for adequate tolerability (Profenno et al. 2005). A small randomized, placebo-controlled study of valproate in the treatment of aggression in dementia failed to find any difference between valproate and placebo, although the fixed dosage used (valproate 480 mg/day) may have been inadequate (Sival et al. 2002).

Valproate was also studied for possible delay or prevention of illness progression in 313 nursing home residents with moderate Alzheimer's disease who had not yet experienced agitation or psychosis. Time to emergence of clinically significant agitation or psychosis did not differ between valproate and placebo groups, and valproate was associated with serious adverse effects in the patients (Tariot et al. 2011). Taken in the aggregate, these studies suggest that whereas valproate at relatively low dosages can improve dementia-related agitation in some patients, valproate has no utility in slowing or preventing disease progression in Alzheimer's dementia.

Impulsivity, Irritability, and Aggression

Valproate has been reported to be effective in reducing irritability and aggression among diverse patient populations, including individuals with autism spectrum disorders or personality disorders. In a 12-week double-blind study of children and adolescents with autism spectrum disorders, irritability measures were significantly improved with divalproex compared with placebo. Overall, 62% of divalproex subjects versus 9% of placebo subjects (odds ratio: 16.7) were responders (Hollander et al. 2010). In a randomized, placebo-controlled, double-blind study, 249 patients with Cluster B personality disorders, intermittent explosive disorder, or posttraumatic stress disorder were treated for 12 weeks with divalproex or placebo. Divalproex did not differ from placebo among all subjects, but among the 96 Cluster B patients, aggression and irritability scores were improved significantly over the course of the study (Hollander et al. 2003).

Cotherapy in Schizophrenia

The use of valproate among patients with schizophrenia has increased, with one report indicating that over one-third received valproate during hospitalization (Citrome et al. 2000). A 4-week randomized, double-blind study of 242 schizophrenic patients who received risperidone or olanzapine alone, or divalproex plus the antipsychotic drug, indicated significantly greater improvement in Positive and Negative Syndrome Scale (PANSS)–Total and PANSS positive symptom subscale scores among combination therapy patients from day 3 through day 21, but not at day 28. Platelet count was lower with combination therapy. Cholesterol levels increased with olanzapine or risperidone, compared with the significantly lower levels seen with antipsychotic plus divalproex. Weight gain did not differ between olanzapine and divalproex plus olanzapine; weight gain was greater with divalproex plus risperidone (7.5 lbs) than with risperidone (4.2 lbs) (Casey et al. 2003).

Bipolar Disorder With Alcoholism

Bipolar disorder is often associated with substance use disorders, particularly alcoholism. In the largest prospective, blinded, placebo-controlled study, 59 bipolar I patients with alcohol dependence were treated with lithium carbonate and psychosocial interventions for 24 weeks, with half randomly assigned to receive adjunctive valproate. The addition of valproate was associated with significantly fewer heavy drinking days, fewer drinks per heavy drinking day, and fewer drinks per drinking day. Higher serum valproate concentrations were correlated with improved alcohol use outcomes. Both manic and depressive symptoms improved equivalently (Salloum et al. 2005).

In a 12-week double-blind, placebo-controlled trial, divalproex was associated with a significantly smaller percentage of individuals relapsing to heavy drinking, but there were no significant differences in other alcohol-related outcomes. There were significantly greater decreases in irritability in the divalproex-treated group but no significant between-group differences on measures of impulsivity (Brady et al. 2002).

Predictors of Positive Response to Valproate Versus Lithium

Mixed Mania

Patients treated with divalproex who had mixed manic presentations had greater improvement in manic symptoms with divalproex than with lithium treatment in two randomized studies, one of which was placebo controlled (Bowden 1995; Freeman et al. 1992; Swann et al. 1997). Patients with mixed manic or pure manic symptoms who received divalproex had equivalent improvement, thereby indicating a lack of differential effectiveness of divalproex for the two subtypes (Swann et al. 1997). By contrast, during maintenance treatment, patients with mixed mania had equivalent responses to divalproex or lithium, with evidence of higher adverse effects as a function of illness features of mixed mania, compared with rates of adverse effects in patients with euphoric mania (Bowden et al. 2005). The results suggest that mixed manic states require more complex regimens than monotherapies for effective long-term management.

High Lifetime Number of Episodes

Divalproex was significantly more effective than lithium among manic patients with more than 10 episodes of illness (Swann et al. 1999) or more than 2 depressive episodes (Swann et al. 2000).

Side Effects and Toxicology

Valproate has been extensively used over several decades; thus, its adverse-effect profile is well characterized (DeVane 2003; Prevey et al. 1996). Patients treated for epilepsy are more likely to experience adverse events than patients treated for migraine or mania, consequent to generally higher doses of valproate and more complex drug regimens in epilepsy. In a large 1-year placebo-controlled study in bipolar disorder, tremor and reported weight gain were the only symptoms more commonly seen with divalproex than with placebo (DeVane 2003).

Gastrointestinal Effects

Common gastrointestinal effects include nausea, vomiting, diarrhea, dyspepsia, and anorexia. These are dose dependent, are usually encountered at the start of treatment, and are often transient (DeVane 2003). Immediate-release formulations of valproic acid are more likely to cause adverse events compared with the ER and enteric-coated formulations (Horn and Cunanan 2003; Zarate et al. 2000).

Tremor

Tremor consequent to valproate resembles benign essential tremor and may respond to a reduction in dosage. ER or enteric-coated formulations may lessen the frequency of tremor (Wilder 1992; Zarate et al. 1999).

Sedation

Mild sedation is common at the initiation of treatment. This adverse effect is dose dependent and may be minimized by dosage reduction, slower titration, use of ER formulations, and taking all medication at bedtime.

Pancreatitis

Valproate is associated with infrequent onset of idiosyncratic acute pancreatitis. In clinical trials, rates of amylase elevation with valproate were similar to those with placebo (Pellock et al. 2002), suggesting that precautionary amylase levels offer little benefit in predicting pancreatitis. Therefore, clinicians should routinely assess clinical presentation to identify possible signs of pancreatitis.

Hematological Effects

Leukopenia and thrombocytopenia are directly related to higher valproate serum level, usually ≥ 100 μg/mL (Acharya and Bussel 1996; Bowden et al. 2000). Thrombocytopenia is usually mild and rarely associated with bleeding complications. Management consists of dosage reduction. Platelet counts below 75,000/mm^3 should also be regularly reassessed, since levels below this are more often associated with bruising or bleeding (Zarate et al. 1999).

Hepatotoxicity

None of the longer-term studies of the past decade has found evidence of hepatic dysfunction or significant worsening of hepatic indices in valproate-treated patients as compared with results seen in placebo-treated or comparator-treated patients (Bowden et al. 2000; Tohen et al. 2002; Zajecka et al. 2002).

The risk of liver toxicity is largely limited to patients younger than 2 years of age, whose hepatic function is still immature. In long-term study of divalproex, full-dosage regimens for 1 year were associated with improvements in laboratory indices of hepatic function, and no hepatotoxicity was reported in the 187 patients treated with divalproex (Bowden et al. 2000). Similar results were reported in a 47-week study of divalproex in bipolar disorder (Tohen et al. 2003).

A risk factor for the development of hepatotoxicity is the concomitant administration of other anticonvulsants such as carbamazepine, which cause induction of enzymes involved in the metabolism of valproate, leading to increased concentrations of an active and hepatotoxic metabolite, 2-propyl-4-pentenoic acid.

Weight Gain

Weight gain of 3–24 lbs is seen in 3%–20% of patients treated with valproic acid over a time course that has ranged from 3 to 12 months (Bowden 2003b). Weight gain has been consistently less with valproate than with olanzapine in comparison studies (1.22 kg vs. 2.79 kg) (Tohen et al. 2003; Zajecka et al. 2002). Valproate serum levels greater than 125 μg/mL are more likely to cause weight gain than those below this level (Bowden 2000). If increased appetite and weight gain occur, valproate dosage should be lowered so long as clinical effectiveness is maintained; alternatively, valproate should be discontinued and replaced by a regimen without risks of weight gain.

Cognitive Effects

Valproate has infrequent adverse effects on cognitive functioning, and it improves cognition in some patients (Prevey et al. 1996). In a 20-week randomized, observer-blinded, parallel-group trial, the addition of valproate to carbamazepine resulted in improvement on short-term verbal memory (Aldenkamp et al. 2000). No adverse cognitive effects with the use of valproate were seen in a group of elderly patients (mean age = 77 years) (Craig and Tallis 1994).

Lipid Profile Effects

Several studies indicate that valproate significantly reduces total and low-density lipoprotein (LDL) cholesterol levels and increases high-density lipoprotein (HDL) cholesterol levels in long-term treatment (Geller et al. 2012) and that it protects against the adverse effects of some antipsychotic drugs on lipid function (Bowden et al. 2000; Casey et al. 2003; Tohen et al. 2003). A 3-week study in mania indicated reductions in cholesterol, HDL, and LDL compared with placebo and reported the effect to be limited to those subjects who had total cholesterol levels of ≥200 mg/dL at study entry (Bowden et al. 2006).

Polycystic Ovarian Syndrome

The prevalence of menstrual disturbances in women with bipolar disorder is higher than that in the general population. A cross-sectional study of women found evidence of a higher rate of polycystic ovarian syndrome (PCOS) in subjects who reported valproate as a component of their prior treatment regimen (Joffe et al. 2006). A study of 10 lithium-treated, 10 valproate-treated, and 2 carbamazepine-treated women with bipolar disorder found a high frequency of menstrual dysfunction in all groups. Hormonal assessment of estrone, luteinizing hormone, follicle-stimulating hormone, testosterone, and dehydroepiandrosterone (DHEA) yielded no abnormal values in any patient (Rasgon et al. 2000). Obesity may be a mechanistic pathway whereby valproate (and potentially other drugs) predisposes women to PCOS. It is advisable to treat weight gain as a risk factor for possible development of PCOS and intervene as needed to avoid clinically significant weight gain.

Hair Loss

Hair loss may occur early in treatment and is usually transient. Frequency of hair loss may be greater in women than in men (Lajee and Parsonage 1980). Dosage reduction and separation of valproate dosing from meals can be helpful in controlling this effect; supplemental zinc and selenium ingestion via multivitamin tablets may also be useful.

Use During Pregnancy and Lactation

Teratogenic and Developmental Effects

Valproate is associated with an increased incidence of birth defects, including neural tube defects, craniofacial anomalies, limb abnormalities, and cardiovascular anomalies, if infants are exposed to valproic acid in the first 10 weeks of gestation (Kinrys et al. 2003; Samren et al. 1997). Neural tube defects, the most serious of the congenital anomalies, occur in 1%–4% of such infants. Prenatal exposure to valproate prior to the closure of the neural tube, during the fourth week of gestation, leads to a prevalence of spina bifida in 1%–2% of infants, a 10–20 times greater rate than in the general population (Kinrys et al. 2003). Most of the available data involved patients with epilepsy, who are generally treated with higher doses of valproate than the doses employed for bipolar disorder and migraine and who are often concurrently treated with other teratogenic anticonvulsants (Bowden 2003b). The risk of malformations is increased with higher dosages and higher serum levels of valproate, as well as with concomitant use of other anticonvulsants (due to higher concentration of 2-propyl-4-pentenoic acid, a teratogenic agent); is possibly decreased with supplemental folic acid; and is definitely reduced with lower dosages of valproate (Bowden 2003b). The inhibitory effect of valproate on histone deacetylase, linked to Wnt signaling, which is involved in cell division, is a plausible mechanism by which teratogenic effects could develop.

Because alternative treatment strategies lacking teratogenic risk may work to effectively manage bipolar symptoms, valproate should generally be discontinued if conception is desired and during the early course of pregnancy if it occurs.

Cognitive effects of prenatal exposure to valproate have been found. When assessed at age 3 years, children who had experienced fetal exposure to valproate had IQ scores 6–9 points lower than those of children who had fetal exposure to lamotrigine, carbamazepine, or phenytoin (Meador et al. 2009).

Breast-Feeding

Valproate is minimally present in breast milk. Piontek et al. (2000) reported that among six mother-infant pairs, serum valproate levels in the infants ranged from 0.9% to 2.3% of the mother's serum levels, with absolute serum levels of 0.7–1.56 μg/mL. The valproate concentration in an infant was 1.5% of the maternal concentration (Wisner and Perel 1998).

Overdose

Regarding overdose, recovery from coma has occurred with serum valproate concentrations of greater than 2,000 μg/mL. In addition, serum valproate concentrations have been reduced by hemodialysis and hemoperfusion, and valproate-induced coma has been reversed with naloxone (Rimmer and Richens 1985).

Drug-Drug Interactions

Because valproate is highly protein bound and extensively metabolized by the liver, a number of potential drug-drug interactions may occur with other protein-bound or metabolized drugs (Fogel 1988; Rimmer and

Richens 1985). Thus, free fraction concentrations of valproate in serum can be increased and valproate toxicity can be precipitated by coadministration of other highly protein-bound drugs (e.g., aspirin) that can displace valproate from its protein-binding sites.

The competitive inhibition by valproate of excretion of lamotrigine via glucuronidation requires that lamotrigine be started at a lower dosage, usually 25 mg every other day, and increased more cautiously. Steady-state dosage of lamotrigine used with valproate is also generally lower, but not in all patients.

Conclusion

The broad spectrum of efficacy in bipolar spectrum disorders and generally good tolerability of valproate make it a foundation of treatment for many patients with bipolar disorders. For optimal results, most patients should be treated with the formulation that permits single daily dosing and has the lowest peak-to-trough serum level, which in the United States currently is divalproex ER. Although onset of action of valproate is prompt with loading-dose strategies, given the paramount importance of tolerability and adherence by bipolar patients to long-term treatment regimens, gradual dosage increase is preferable for all but severely manic states.

During maintenance treatment, it is often important to reduce dosage if adverse effects persist. Valproate alleviates and is prophylactic principally for manic symptoms, although prophylactic benefits for depression are now relatively well established. A history of many episodes or current irritability may be a particularly strong indicator of a favorable response to valproate. Although some patients may have acute and sustained remission with valproate monotherapy, many patients are more effectively treated with combinations, including other mood stabilizers and adjunctive medications. All current medications with established or putative roles in bipolar disorder can be combined with valproate.

References

Acharya S, Bussel JB: Hematologic toxicity of sodium valproate. J Pediatr Neurol 14:303–307, 1996

Aldenkamp AP, Baker G, Mulder OG, et al: A multicenter, randomized clinical study to evaluate the effect on cognitive function of topiramate compared with valproate as add-on therapy to carbamazepine in patients with partial-onset seizures. Epilepsia 41:1167–1178, 2000

Allen MH, Hirschfeld RM, Wozniak PJ, et al: Linear relationship of valproate serum concentration to response and optimal serum levels for acute mania. Am J Psychiatry 163:272–275, 2006

Bocci U, Beretta G: Esperienze sugli alcoolisti e tossicomania con dipropilacetate di sodio. Lavoro Neuropsichiatrico 58:51–61, 1976

Bowden CL: Predictors of response to divalproex and lithium. J Clin Psychiatry 56:25–30, 1995

Bowden CL: Valproate in mania, in Bipolar Medications: Mechanisms of Action. Edited by Manji HK, Bowden CL, Belmaker RH. Washington, DC, American Psychiatric Press, 2000, pp 357–365

Bowden CL: Acute and maintenance treatment with mood stabilizers. Int J Neuropsychopharmacol 6:269–275, 2003a

Bowden CL: Valproate. Bipolar Disord 5:189–202, 2003b

Bowden CL: Relationship of acute mania symptomatology to maintenance treatment response. Curr Psychiatry Rep 6:473–477, 2004

Bowden CL: The role of ziprasidone in adjunctive use with lithium or valproate in maintenance treatment of bipolar disorder. Neuropsychiatr Dis Treat 7:87–92, 2011

Bowden CL, McElroy SL: History of the development of valproate for treatment of bipolar disorder. J Clin Psychiatry 56:3–5, 1995

Bowden CL, Janicak PG, Orsulak P, et al: Relation of serum valproate concentration to response in mania. Am J Psychiatry 153:765–770, 1996

Bowden CL, Calabrese JR, McElroy SL, et al: A randomized, placebo-controlled 12-month trial of divalproex and lithium in treatment of outpatients with bipolar I disorder. Divalproex Maintenance Study Group. Arch Gen Psychiatry 57:481–489, 2000

Bowden CL, Collins MA, McElroy SL, et al: Relationship of mania symptomatology to maintenance treatment response with divalproex, lithium or placebo. Neuropsychopharmacology 30:323–330, 2005

Bowden CL, Swann AC, Calabrese JR, et al: A randomized, placebo-controlled, multicenter study of valproex sodium extended release in the treatment of acute mania. J Clin Psychiatry 67:1501–1510, 2006

Brady KT, Myrick H, Henderson S, et al: The use of divalproex in alcohol relapse prevention: a pilot study. Drug Alcohol Depend 67:323–330, 2002

Calabrese JR, Shelton MD, Rapport DJ, et al: A 20-month, double-blind, maintenance trial of lithium versus divalproex in rapid-cycling bipolar disorder. Am J Psychiatry 162:2152–2161, 2005

Casey DE, Daniel DG, Wassef AA, et al: Effect of divalproex combined with olanzapine or risperidone in patients with an acute exacerbation of schizophrenia. Neuropsychopharmacology 28:182–192, 2003

Citrome L, Levine J, Allingham B: Changes in use of valproate and other mood stabilizers for patients with schizophrenia from 1994 to 1998. Psychiatr Serv 51:634–638, 2000

Cournoyer P, Desrosiers RR: Valproic acid enhances protein L-isoaspartylmethyltransferase expression by stimulating extracellular signal-regulated kinase signaling pathway. Neuropharmacology 56:839–848, 2009

Craig I, Tallis R: Impact of valproate and phenytoin on cognitive function in elderly patients: results of a single-blind randomized comparative study. Epilepsia 35:381–390, 1994

Davis LL, Bartolucci A, Petty F: Divalproex in the treatment of bipolar depression: a placebo-controlled study. J Affect Disord 85:259–266, 2005

DeVane CL: Pharmacokinetics, drug interactions and tolerability of valproate. Psychopharmacol Bull 37 (suppl):25–42, 2003

Donovan SJ, Stewart JW, Nunes EV, et al: Divalproex treatment for youth with explosive temper and mood lability: a double-blind, placebo-controlled crossover design. Am J Psychiatry 157:818–820, 2000

Fogel BS: Combining anticonvulsants with conventional psychopharmacologic agents, in Use of Anticonvulsants in Psychiatry: Recent Advances. Edited by McElroy SL, Pope HG Jr. Clifton, NJ, Oxford Health Care, 1988, pp 77–94

Freeman TW, Clothier JL, Pazzaglia P, et al: A double-blind comparison of valproate and lithium in the treatment of acute mania. Am J Psychiatry 149:108–111, 1992

Geller B, Luby JL, Joshi P, et al: A randomized controlled trial of risperidone, lithium, or divalproex sodium for initial treatment of bipolar I disorder, manic or mixed phase, in children and adolescents. Arch Gen Psychiatry 69:515–528, 2012

Ghaemi NS, Gilmer WS, Goldberg JF, et al. Divalproex in the treatment of acute bipolar depression: a preliminary double-blind, randomized, placebo-controlled pilot study. J Clin Psychiatry 68:1840–1844, 2007

Gray NA, Zhou R, Du J, et al: The use of mood stabilizers as plasticity enhancers in the treatment of neuropsychiatric disorders. J Clin Psychiatry 64 (suppl):3–17, 2003

Gyulai L, Bowden CL, McElroy SL, et al: Maintenance efficacy of divalproex in the prevention of bipolar depression. Neuropsychopharmacology 28:1374–1382, 2003

Harwood AJ, Agam G: Search for a common mechanism of mood stabilizers. Biochem Pharmacol 66:179–189, 2003

Hollander E, Tracy KA, Swann AC, et al: Divalproex in the treatment of impulsive aggression: efficacy in Cluster B personality disorders. Neuropsychopharmacology 28:1186–1197, 2003

Hollander E, Chaplin W, Soorya L, et al: Divalproex sodium vs placebo for the treatment of irritability in children and adolescents with autism spectrum disorders. Neuropsychopharmacology 35:990–998, 2010

Horn RL, Cunanan C: Safety and efficacy of switching psychiatric patients from a delayed-release to an extended-release formulation of divalproex sodium. J Clin Psychopharmacol 23:176–181, 2003

Jacobsen FM: Low dose valproate: a new treatment for cyclothymia, mild rapid cycling disorders, and premenstrual syndrome. J Clin Psychiatry 54:229–234, 1993

Joffe H, Cohen LS, Suppes T, et al: Valproate is associated with new-onset oligoamenorrhea with hyperandrogenism in women with bipolar disorder. Biol Psychiatry 59:1078–1086, 2006

Kahn D, Stevenson E, Douglas CJ: Effect of sodium valproate in three patients with organic brain syndromes. Am J Psychiatry 145:1010–1011, 1988

Kastner T, Friedman DL, Plummer AT, et al: Valproic acid for the treatment of children with mental retardation and mood symptomatology. Pediatrics 86:467–472, 1990

Keck PE Jr, Bowden CL, Meinhold JM, et al: Relationship between serum valproate and lithium levels and efficacy and tolerability in bipolar maintenance therapy. Int J Psychiatry Clin Pract 9:271–277, 2005

Ketter TA, Citrome L, Wang PW, et al: Treatments for bipolar disorder: can number needed to treat/harm help inform clinical decisions? Acta Psychiatr Scand 123:175–189, 2011

Kinrys G, Pollack MH, Simon NM, et al: Valproic acid for the treatment of social anxiety disorder. Int Clin Psychopharmacol 18:169–172, 2003

Lajee HCK, Parsonage MJ: Unwanted effects of sodium valproate in the treatment of adult patients with epilepsy, in The Place of Sodium Valproate in the Treatment of Epilepsy. Edited by Parsonage NJ, Caldwell ADS. London, Royal Society of Medicine, 1980, pp 141–158

Lambert PA, Cavaz G, Borselli S, et al: Action neuropsychotrope d'un nouvel anti-epileptique: le depamide. Ann Med Psychol 1:707–710, 1966

Levy MN: Cardiac sympathetic-parasympathetic interactions. Fed Proc 43:2598–2602, 1984

Marcus R, Khan A, Rollin L, et al: Efficacy of aripiprazole adjunctive to lithium or valproate in the long-term treatment of patients with bipolar I disorder with an inadequate response to lithium or valproate monotherapy: a multicenter, double-blind, randomized study. Bipolar Disord 13:133–144, 2011

Meador KJ, Baker GA, Browning N, et al: Cognitive function at 3 years of age after fetal exposure to antiepileptic drugs. N Engl J Med 360:1597–1605, 2009

McElroy SL, Pope HG Jr, Keck PE Jr: Treatment of psychiatric disorders with valproate: a series of 73 cases. Psychiatrie Psychobiologie 3:81–85, 1988

McElroy SL, Martens BE, Creech RS, et al: Randomized, double-blind, placebo-controlled study of divalproex extended release loading monotherapy in ambulatory bipolar spectrum disorder patients with moderate-to-severe hypomania or mild mania. J Clin Psychiatry 71:557–565, 2010

Muller-Oerlinghausen B, Retzow A, Henn FA, et al: Valproate as an adjunct to neuroleptic medication for the treatment of acute episodes of mania: a prospective, randomized, double-blind, placebo-controlled, multicenter study. European Valproate Mania Study Group. J Clin Psychopharmacol 20:195–203, 2000

Pavuluri MN, Henry DB, Findling RL, et al: Double-blind randomized trial of risperidone versus divalproex in pediatric bipolar disorder. Bipolar Disord 12:593–605, 2010

Pellock JM, Wilder BJ, Deaton R, et al: Acute pancreatitis coincident with valproate use: a critical review. Epilepsia 43:1421–1424, 2002

Perova T, Kwan M, Li PP, et al: Differential modulation of intracellular Ca2+ responses in B lymphoblasts by mood stabilizers. Int J Neuropsychopharmacol 13:693–702, 2010

Piontek CM, Baab S, Peindl KS, et al: Serum valproate levels in 6 breastfeeding mother-infant pairs. J Clin Psychiatry 61:170–172, 2000

Pope HG Jr, McElroy SL, Satlin A, et al: Head injury, bipolar disorder, and response to valproate. Compr Psychiatry 29:34–38, 1988

Porsteinsson AP, Tariot PN, Erb R, et al: Placebo-controlled study of divalproex sodium for agitation in dementia. Am J Geriatr Psychiatry 9:58–66, 2001

Porsteinsson AP, Tariot PN, Jakimovich LJ, et al: Valproate therapy for agitation in dementia. Am J Geriatr Psychiatry 11:434–440, 2003

Prevey ML, Delaney RC, Cramer JA, et al: Effect of valproate on cognitive functioning: comparison with carbamazepine. The Department of Veteran Affairs Epilepsy Cooperative Study 264 Group. Arch Neurol 53:1008–1016, 1996

Profenno LA, Jakimovich L, Holt CJ, et al: A randomized, double-blind, placebo-controlled pilot trial of safety and tolerability of two doses of divalproex sodium in outpatients with probable Alzheimer's disease. Curr Alzheimer Res 2:553–558, 2005

Rasgon NL, Altshuler LL, Gudeman D, et al: Medication status and polycystic ovary syndrome in women with bipolar disorder: a preliminary report. J Clin Psychiatry 61:173–178, 2000

Rimmer E, Richens A: An update on sodium valproate. Pharmacotherapy 5:171–184, 1985

Sachs GS, Grossman F, Ghaemi SN, et al: Combination of a mood stabilizer with risperidone or haloperidol for treatment of acute mania: a double-blind, placebo-controlled comparison of efficacy and safety. Am J Psychiatry 159:1146–1154, 2002

Salloum IM, Cornelius JR, Daley DC, et al: Efficacy of valproate maintenance in patients with bipolar disorder and alcoholism: a double-blind placebo-controlled study. Arch Gen Psychiatry 62:37–45, 2005

Samren EB, Duijn CM, Koch S, et al: Maternal use of antiepileptic drugs and the risk of major congenital malformations: a joint European prospective study of human teratogens associated with maternal epilepsy. Epilepsia 38:981–990, 1997

Scheffer RE, Kowatch RA, Carmody T, et al: Randomized, placebo-controlled trial of mixed amphetamine salts for symptoms of comorbid ADHD in pediatric bipolar disorder after mood stabilization with divalproex sodium. Am J Psychiatry 162:58–64, 2005

Sival RC, Haffmans PM, Jansen PA, et al: Sodium valproate in the treatment of aggressive behavior in patients with dementia: a randomized placebo controlled clinical trial. Int J Geriatr Psychiatry 17:579–585, 2002

Smith LA, Cornelius VR, Azorin JM, et al: Valproate for the treatment of acute bipolar depression: systematic review and meta-analysis. J Affect Disord 122:1–9, 2010

Sovner R: The use of valproate in the treatment of mentally retarded persons with typical and atypical bipolar disorders. J Clin Psychiatry 50:40–43, 1989

Swann AC, Bowden CL, Morris D, et al: Depression during mania: treatment response to lithium or divalproex. Arch Gen Psychiatry 54:37–42, 1997

Swann AC, Bowden CL, Calabrese JR, et al: Differential effect of number of previous episodes of affective disorder on response to lithium or divalproex in acute mania. Am J Psychiatry 156:1264–1266, 1999

Swann AC, Bowden CL, Calabrese JR, et al: Mania: differential effects of previous depressive and manic episodes on response to treatment. Acta Psychiatr Scand 101:444–451, 2000

Tariot PN, Schneider LS, Cummings J, et al: Chronic divalproex sodium to attenuate agitation and clinical progression of Alzheimer disease. Arch Gen Psychiatry 68:853–861, 2011

Tohen M, Chengappa KN, Suppes T, et al: Efficacy of olanzapine in combination with valproate or lithium in the treatment of mania in patients partially nonresponsive to valproate or lithium monotherapy. Arch Gen Psychiatry 59:62–69, 2002

Tohen M, Ketter TA, Zarate CA: Olanzapine versus divalproex sodium for the treatment of acute mania and maintenance of remission: a 47 week study. Am J Psychiatry 160:1263–1271, 2003

Wagner KD, Redden L, Kowatch RA, et al: A double-blind, randomized, placebo-controlled trial of divalproex extended-release in the treatment of bipolar disorder in children and adolescents. J Am Acad Child Adolesc Psychiatry 48:519–532, 2009

Wilder BJ: Pharmacokinetics of valproate and carbamazepine. J Clin Psychopharmacol 12 (suppl): 64S–68S, 1992

Wisner KL, Perel JM: Serum levels of valproate and carbamazepine in breastfeeding mother-infant pairs. J Clin Psychopharmacol 18:167–169, 1998

Yatham LN, Grossman F, Augustyns I, et al: Mood stabilisers plus risperidone or placebo in the treatment of acute mania. International, double-blind, randomised controlled trial. Br J Psychiatry 182:141–147, 2003 (Erratum appears in Br J Psychiatry 182:369, 2003)

Zajecka J, Weisler R, Sachs G, et al: A comparison of the efficacy, safety and tolerability of divalproex sodium and olanzapine in the treatment of bipolar disorder. J Clin Psychiatry 63:1148–1155, 2002

Zarate CA Jr, Tohen M, Narendram R, et al: The adverse effect profile and efficacy of divalproex sodium compared with valproic acid: a pharmacoepidemiology study. J Clin Psychiatry 60:232–236, 1999

Zarate CA Jr, Tohen M, Narendran R, et al: The adverse effect profile and efficacy of divalproex sodium compared with valproic acid: a pharmacoepidemiology study. J Clin Psychiatry 60:232–236, 2000

CHAPTER 28

Carbamazepine and Oxcarbazepine

Terence A. Ketter, M.D.

Po W. Wang, M.D.

Robert M. Post, M.D.

Pharmacotherapy of bipolar disorder is a complex and rapidly evolving field. The development of new treatments has helped to refine concepts of illness subtypes and generated important new management options. Although the mood stabilizers—the first-line agents lithium, valproate, and lamotrigine and the alternative agents carbamazepine (CBZ) and oxcarbazepine (OXC)—are considered the primary medications for bipolar disorder, antipsychotics, antidepressants, anxiolytics, and a new generation of anticonvulsants are commonly combined with mood stabilizers in clinical settings (American Psychiatric Association 2002).

In this chapter, we review the preclinical and clinical pharmacology of CBZ and its analog OXC. In the past, CBZ was considered an alternative to lithium and valproate rather than a first-line intervention in the treatment of bipolar disorder (American Psychiatric Association 2002) in view of methodological limitations of early studies of efficacy in bipolar disorder, complexity of use because of adverse effects and drug-drug interactions, and lack of a U.S. Food and Drug Administration (FDA) indication for the treatment of bipolar disorder. However, evidence of the efficacy of a proprietary CBZ extended-release formulation (Equetro) in two randomized, double-blind, placebo-controlled, parallel-group studies in bipolar disorder patients (Weisler et al. 2004, 2005) addressed methodological concerns and led to this formulation's receiving an indication for the treatment of acute manic and mixed episodes in patients with bipolar disorder. CBZ's low propensity to cause the weight gain and metabolic problems seen with some other agents may lead clinicians to reassess its role in the management of patients with bipolar disorder (Ketter 2010).

History and Discovery

CBZ, as one of the initial alternatives to lithium and older antipsychotics, has played an important role in the development of therapeutic interventions for bipolar disorder. CBZ was developed in 1957 by J.R. Geigy AG in Europe, and its efficacy in epilepsy and paroxysmal pain was appreciated by the 1960s and in bipolar disorder by the early 1970s. CBZ was approved for the treatment of epilepsy in adults in 1974.

In the 1970s, acute mania was managed primarily with lithium and first-generation antipsychotics. Lithium proved dramatically effective in classic euphoric mania but had limitations, which included the need for initial titration and a clinically significant response latency. In addition, lithium proved less effective in patients with mixed or dysphoric mania, rapid cycling, greater numbers of previous episodes, mood-incongruent delusions, or concurrent substance abuse than in those with classic bipolar disorder (Ketter and Wang 2002). The response latency and spectrum of efficacy limitations of lithium resulted in the common practice of concurrently administering first-generation antipsychotics in acute mania.

Limitations of lithium and first-generation antipsychotics led investigators to explore other treatment options for bipolar disorder. On the basis of early reports of favorable psychotropic profiles in epilepsy patients and preliminary observations in mood disorders, systematic investigations of CBZ commenced (Ballenger and Post 1978). CBZ was used off-label for bipolar disorder in the 1980s and early 1990s. The CBZ analog OXC was anecdotally reported as useful in bipolar disorder in the 1980s (Müller and Stoll 1984) but was not marketed in the United States for the treatment of epilepsy until 2000.

Because of economic concerns such as patent protection limitations and the high cost of obtaining FDA approval, a CBZ indication for bipolar disorder was not initially sought in the United States but was obtained from agencies in several other countries. Divalproex, a well-tolerated proprietary valproate formulation, received FDA approval for the treatment of acute mania in 1995, and its use overtook that of CBZ and even lithium by the late 1990s. Divalproex's efficacy in acute mania was considered better established than that of CBZ, because the pivotal trials for obtaining the divalproex mania indication were conducted with contemporary randomized, parallel, double-blind, placebo-controlled paradigms (Bowden et al. 1994; Pope et al. 1991), whereas early controlled CBZ studies in bipolar disorder used alternative (e.g., active comparator and on-off-on) designs, as described later in this chapter (see section "Indications and Efficacy"). Despite the limitations in the controlled maintenance data for both drugs, CBZ and divalproex were considered mood stabilizers along with lithium.

Evidence of the efficacy of a proprietary CBZ extended-release formulation (Equetro) in two randomized, double-blind, placebo-controlled studies (Weisler et al. 2004, 2005) led to an FDA indication in late 2004 for this CBZ formulation in the treatment of acute manic and mixed episodes in patients with bipolar disorder.

OXC was approved for the treatment of epilepsy in the United States in 2000, in the setting of the development of several new anticonvulsants in the 1990s. The new anticonvulsants appear to have heterogeneous psychotropic profiles (Ketter et al. 2003), with only OXC thus far showing benefit in some controlled (albeit small) trials in acute mania (Emrich 1990) and lamotrigine in the prophylaxis of and (to a lesser extent) acute treatment of bipolar depression. Economic concerns such as patent protection limitations and the high cost of obtaining FDA approval were substantial barriers to seeking an OXC indication for acute mania in the United States. Because of its greater ease of use, OXC was considered by some to be an important alternative to CBZ (American Psychiatric Association 2002).

Licarbazepine, the active monohydroxy metabolite of OXC, was initially assessed by Novartis for treatment of acute mania rather than epilepsy. However, as of mid-2012, three randomized controlled licarbazepine acute mania trials (on clinicaltrials.gov) had not been published. In 2009, the European Medicines Agency approved eslicarbazepine acetate, a prodrug for the S-enantiomer of licarbazepine (Zebinix; BIAL-Portela & Ca, S.A.), for the treatment of epilepsy. However, in 2010, a new drug application for eslicarbazepine (Stedesa; submitted by Sepracor, now Sunovion, under license from BIAL-Portela & Ca, S.A.) for epilepsy failed to obtain FDA approval. As of midyear 2012, randomized controlled eslicarbazepine acetate trials accessed on clinicaltrials.gov included studies in epilepsy, postherpetic neuralgia, neuropathic pain, and diabetic neuropathic pain, but not bipolar disorder.

Structure-Activity Relations

CBZ is an iminostilbine derivative with a dibenzazepine nucleus. CBZ's tricyclic nucleus appears to relate more to local anesthetic and antihistaminic actions than to anticonvulsant actions. In contrast, the carbamyl (carboxamide) group at position 5 appears related to substantial anticonvulsant effects. CBZ's 5-carboxamide substituent, in contrast to the 5-aryl substituent of imipramine, appears to account for CBZ's markedly different effects compared with those of imipramine, as described below (see section "Mechanisms of Action"). OXC differs structurally from CBZ only in that it has a ketone substitution at the 10,11 position, and as noted below, the bulk of the evidence thus far suggests that this structural similarity is paralleled by a mechanistic similarity.

Pharmacological Profile

CBZ and OXC have a preclinical anticonvulsant profile similar to that of phenytoin and less broad than that of valproate or lamotrigine. Thus, CBZ and OXC, like phenytoin, valproate, and lamotrigine, are effective in the maximal electroshock model of generalized tonic and/or clonic seizures, and like phenytoin but unlike valproate and lamotrigine, they are not effective in the pentylenetetrazole model of absence seizures. CBZ and OXC, like phenytoin, valproate, and lamotrigine, are effective in blocking seizures resulting from amygdala kindling (a model of partial seizures). However, CBZ and OXC, like phenytoin and lamotrigine but unlike valproate, fail to block kindling development (a model of epileptogenesis).

As expected from their preclinical profiles, CBZ and OXC, like phenytoin, valproate, and lamotrigine, are effective in partial seizures with and without secondary generalization, and like phenytoin but unlike valproate and lamotrigine, they are ineffective in absence seizures. CBZ and OXC also have analgesic effects and thus are effective in trigeminal neuralgia.

Pharmacokinetics and Disposition

Carbamazepine

CBZ is available in the United States in a proprietary immediate-release formulation (Tegretol) marketed for epilepsy by Novartis Pharmaceuticals Corporation in suspension (100 mg/5 mL), chewable tablets (100 mg), nonchewable tablets (200 mg), and extended-release (Tegretol XR) tablets (100-, 200-, and 400-mg) (Physicians' Desk Reference 2012). An additional proprietary extended-release formulation marketed for epilepsy as Carbatrol (by Shire US Inc.) and for bipolar disorder as Equetro (by Validus Pharmaceuticals) is available in 100-, 200-, and

300-mg capsules (Physicians' Desk Reference 2012). Intramuscular and depot formulations are not available. CBZ is also available in generic immediate-release and extended-release formulations. Differences have been observed in the bioavailability of proprietary and generic formulations (Meyer et al. 1992).

CBZ is extensively metabolized, with only about 3% excreted unchanged in the urine. The main metabolic pathway of CBZ (to its active 10,11-epoxide, CBZ-E) appears to be mediated primarily by cytochrome P450 (CYP) 3A3/4 (Kerr et al. 1994). This pathway accounts for about 40% of CBZ disposition and an even greater proportion in patients with induced metabolism (presumably via CYP3A3/4 induction) (Faigle and Feldmann 1995). With enzyme induction, formation of CBZ-E triples, its subsequent transformation to the inactive diol (CBZ-D) doubles, and thus the ratio of CBZ-E to CBZ increases.

CBZ has erratic absorption and a bioavailability of about 80%. CBZ should not be exposed to humidity, because this can cause solidification and decrease bioavailability. It is about 75% bound to plasma proteins and has a moderate volume of distribution (about 1 L/kg). Before autoinduction of the epoxide pathway, the half-life of CBZ is about 24 hours, and the clearance is about 25 mL/minute. However, after autoinduction (2–4 weeks into therapy), the half-life falls to about 8 hours, and clearance rises to about 75 mL/minute. This may require dosage adjustment to maintain adequate blood concentrations and therapeutic effects. The active CBZ-E metabolite has a half-life of about 6 hours and is converted to an inactive diol (CBZ-D) by epoxide hydrolase. The extended-release CBZ formulations available in the United States given twice a day yield steady-state CBZ concentrations similar to those seen with the immediate-release formulation given four times a day.

In the treatment of acute mania, two divergent clinical needs influence the rate of dosage titration. First, there is a pressing need for rapid control of the manic syndrome, which suggests that faster titration to higher doses could provide more rapid attainment of sufficient serum concentrations, potentially yielding quicker onset not only of nonspecific sedation but also of specific antimanic effects. On the other hand, there is a need to not excessively burden patients with the increased adverse effects associated with overly rapid escalation of CBZ dosage. Such adverse effects include neurotoxicity (sedation, diplopia, and ataxia) and gastrointestinal disturbances that not only can complicate acute management but also may lead patients to develop negative perceptions about the adverse effects of CBZ that later interfere with their adherence to prophylactic therapy. Thus, although a loading-dose strategy may be tolerated and effective in the treatment of mania with valproate, the potential for neurotoxic adverse effects limits such an approach with CBZ.

Nonetheless, in the inpatient therapy of mania, CBZ is commonly started at 400–800 mg/day in divided doses, with the dosage increased as tolerated (by 200 mg/day every 1–4 days) to provide clinical efficacy. Titration of dosage against adverse effects is more important than blood concentrations, which usually reach between 4 and 12 μg/mL, and there does not appear to be a close blood concentration–efficacy relationship for CBZ in treating either seizure or mood disorders. Usual dosages are 800–1,600 mg/day given in up to three or four divided doses with the immediate-release formulation. Sustained-release formulations permit two divided doses per day, and most mood disorder patients may even be able to take the entire daily dose at bedtime. Although this strategy is convenient, it may not be feasible in some individuals because of neurotoxicity at peak serum concentrations, which occurs about 4–8 hours after ingesting CBZ. CBZ has fairly rapid onset of antimanic efficacy, in some comparisons similar to that of neuroleptics. Thus, lack of clinical improvement after 7–10 days may be an indication that augmentation or alternative strategies should be considered.

In outpatients, CBZ is generally titrated more slowly, starting at 200 mg/day and increasing (as necessary and tolerated) by 200 mg/day every 4–7 days to 600–1,600 mg/day. Starting with 50 mg (half of a chewable 100-mg tablet) at bedtime and increasing the dosage by 50 mg every 4 days may yield better tolerability. Moreover, doses of CBZ initially associated with adverse effects during the first 2 weeks of therapy may be readily used after 1 month of therapy, once autoinduction of CBZ metabolism has reduced serum CBZ concentrations (Cereghino 1975) and accommodation and tolerance to adverse effects such as sedation have occurred.

It is common practice to gradually increase CBZ dosage as tolerated, monitoring both adverse effects and clinical efficacy, until adequate therapeutic efficacy is achieved, adverse effects supervene, or serum concentrations exceed 12 μg/mL. The 4- to 12-μg/mL serum CBZ concentration range used in epilepsy may be considered a broad target, and CBZ serum concentrations may be used as checks for pharmacokinetic problems. CBZ dosages and serum concentrations are commonly in the higher portion of this range for acute mania therapy and in the lower portion of the range for acute bipolar depression therapy, adjunctive therapy, and bipolar maintenance therapy. The active CBZ-E metabolite can yield therapeutic and adverse effects similar to those of CBZ but is not detectable in conventional CBZ assays. Thus, the unwary clinician may misinterpret the significance of therapeutic or adverse effects associated with low or moderate serum CBZ concentrations.

In responders, a dose-response relationship may be evident, so that slowly increasing CBZ doses to maximize response in the absence of significant adverse effects is a clinically useful strategy. However, if there is no hint of therapeutic response at moderate doses, it is unlikely that pushing to very high doses will be beneficial.

Oxcarbazepine

OXC is available in the United States as a proprietary product (Trileptal) manufactured by Novartis Pharmaceuticals Corporation as a generic medication and is produced in a 300-mg/5-mL suspension and in 150-, 300-, and 600-mg tablets (Physicians' Desk Reference 2012). Sustained-release, intramuscular, and depot formulations are not available.

OXC is 96% absorbed, and the modest effect of food on OXC kinetics does not appear to be of therapeutic consequence. OXC is 60% bound to plasma proteins. OXC is rapidly reduced to an active monohydroxy derivative (MHD; also called licarbazepine) by cytosol arylketone reductase. The MHD is 40% bound to plasma proteins, has a moderate volume of distribution (about 0.8 L/kg), and has a half-life of about 9 hours. OXC is eliminated primarily in the form of MHD (70%) and MHD glucuronide conjugates (20%), with small portions (10%) in the form of OXC glucuronide conjugates and CBZ-D. OXC does not cause autoinduction and yields substantially less heteroinduction than does CBZ. Thus, as described later in this chapter (see section "Drug-Drug Interactions"), medication interactions are less problematic with OXC than with CBZ.

OXC is typically started at 150 mg/day and increased each second day by 150 mg/day, to a target of about 1,200–1,600 mg/day in two or three divided doses. OXC dosage may be further increased (as necessary and tolerated) up to about 2,400 mg/day. Equipotent doses of OXC range from 1.2 to 1.5 times the CBZ dose. OXC serum concentrations in the treatment of epilepsy commonly range from 13 to 35 μg/mL. For bipolar disorder, OXC, like CBZ, is titrated to clinical desired effect as tolerated, with the serum concentration range used in epilepsy considered a broad target and with OXC serum concentrations considered checks for pharmacokinetic problems.

Mechanisms of Action

CBZ and OXC have not only structural but also mechanistic similarities. However, these agents have such a diversity of biochemical effects that linking these mechanisms to their varying clinical actions presents a considerable challenge.

Carbamazepine

Although CBZ has a tricyclic structure like imipramine's, the two agents have markedly different neurochemical, hepatic, and clinical effects. Thus, CBZ, unlike imipramine, lacks major effects on monoamine reuptake or high affinity for histaminergic or cholinergic receptors and, unlike many antidepressants, fails to downregulate β-adrenergic receptors. Also, CBZ, unlike antipsychotics, does not block dopamine receptors. However, CBZ has a wide range of other cellular and intracellular effects, some but not all of which overlap those of other mood stabilizers.

One potentially useful way of considering CBZ's diverse mechanisms is from the perspective of onset of action (Post 1988). Thus, CBZ cellular actions with acute onset that might parallel the time course of clinical anticonvulsant effects include decreasing sodium influx and glutamate release, increasing potassium conductance, and acting on peripheral benzodiazepine and α_2-adrenergic receptors. Acute gamma-aminobutyric acid type B ($GABA_B$) receptor actions like those of baclofen may relate to the rapid onset of clinical analgesic effects. Acute or subchronic actions such as increasing striatal cholinergic neurotransmission; decreasing adenylate cyclase activity stimulated by dopamine, norepinephrine, and serotonin; and decreasing turnover of dopamine, norepinephrine, and GABA may be pertinent to clinical antimanic effects. Finally, actions requiring chronic administration may be most closely related to clinical antidepressant effects. These include increasing serum and urinary free cortisol, free tryptophan, substance P sensitivity, and adenosine A_1 receptors and decreasing cerebrospinal somatostatin-like immunoreactivity.

Oxcarbazepine

Less is known about OXC mechanisms than about CBZ mechanisms. The bulk of the evidence thus far suggests that OXC's structural similarity to CBZ is paralleled by mechanistic similarity (Ambrosio et al. 2002). For example, OXC, like CBZ, appears to decrease sodium and calcium influx, glutamate release (Ambrosio et al. 2001), and serum thyroxine (T_4) concentrations (Isojarvi et al. 2001); increase potassium conductance and dopaminergic neurotransmission; and block adenosine A_1 receptors. However, there may be some mechanistic dissociations, particularly given OXC's and CBZ's marked differences in degree of hepatic enzyme induction. For example, OXC appears to be a less potent modulator of voltage-gated calcium channels compared with CBZ. The general OXC-CBZ mechanistic overlap is consistent with the hypothesis that OXC and CBZ have similar effects in bipolar disorder, which is consistent with preliminary clinical observations but remains to be established in large controlled clinical studies.

Indications and Efficacy

Seizure Disorders and Trigeminal Neuralgia

In the United States, CBZ is approved by the FDA as monotherapy for the treatment of trigeminal neuralgia and complex partial, generalized tonic-clonic, and mixed seizure disorders (Physicians' Desk Reference 2012). OXC is approved for the treatment of partial seizures as monotherapy in adults and children older than 4 years and as adjunctive therapy in adults and children older than 2 years (Physicians' Desk Reference 2012). CBZ and OXC appear to have overlapping anticonvulsant effects, with similar efficacy in patients with newly diagnosed epilepsy. However, there may be dissociations. For example, switching to OXC may be effective in patients with inadequate responses or intolerable adverse effects with CBZ (Beydoun et al. 2000; Van Parys and Meinardi 1994). Historically, both CBZ and OXC lacked FDA bipolar indications and were generally considered alternative agents in the management of bipolar disorder (American Psychiatric Association 2002). However, FDA approval in late 2004 of a proprietary CBZ beaded extended-release capsule formulation (Equetro) for the treatment of acute manic and mixed episodes in patients with bipolar disorder may eventually lead to a reconsideration of the roles of both of these agents in the treatment of bipolar disorder.

Acute Mania

Twenty-four controlled studies have investigated CBZ and OXC efficacy in acute mania (Table 28–1) (Ballenger and Post 1978; Brown et al. 1989; Emrich 1990; Emrich et al. 1985; Gangadhar et al. 1987; Goncalves and Stoll 1985; Grossi et al. 1984; Kakkar et al. 2009; Klein et al. 1984; Lenzi et al. 1986; Lerer et al. 1987; Lusznat et al. 1988; Möller et al. 1989; Müller and Stoll 1984; Okuma et al. 1979, 1989, 1990; Post et al. 1987; Small et al. 1991; Stoll et al. 1986; Wagner et al. 2006; Weisler et al. 2004, 2005; Zhang et al. 2007). In these studies, there is more compelling evidence for CBZ efficacy (18 studies including 594 patients receiving CBZ) than for OXC efficacy (6 studies including 149 patients receiving OXC).

Two trials, which found a proprietary CBZ beaded extended-release capsule formulation (Equetro) superior to placebo, are of particular interest because they used a randomized, double-blind, placebo-controlled paradigm (Weisler et al. 2004, 2005) and yielded an FDA indication for the treatment of acute manic and mixed episodes in patients with bipolar disorder.

These reports are consistent with multiple earlier studies using placebo-drug-placebo, active-comparator (lithium or neuroleptics), and adjunctive (compared with placebo, lithium, or neuroleptics added to lithium or neuroleptics) designs. Thus, across studies that used diverse paradigms (see Table 28–1), overall antimanic response rates were generally comparable to those seen with lithium or neuroleptics (Ketter 2010). Taken together, this collection of clinical trials provides substantial evidence for the acute antimanic efficacy of CBZ and preliminary evidence for the acute antimanic efficacy of OXC. For CBZ, this current body of existing data appears greater than that initially considered by the FDA in approving lithium for the treatment of acute mania. However, for OXC, the evidence remains preliminary because of important sample size and design limitations. OXC may be less effective than CBZ in severe mania.

Improvement appears to occur across the entire manic syndrome and does not seem to be due to nonspecific sedative properties, in that patients often show dramatic clinical improvement in the absence of marked sedation. Because CBZ and OXC are frequently used in combination with other medications in the acute treatment of mania, knowledge of CBZ's extensive and OXC's more limited drug-drug interactions (as described later in this chapter) is often required to achieve optimal outcomes.

Acute Depression

There are few controlled data regarding the acute antidepressant effects of CBZ and no published controlled studies of the antidepressant effects of OXC. Although CBZ appears to have weaker antidepressant than antimanic properties, some evidence suggests that it may provide antidepressant benefit in about one-third of treatment-resistant patients (Neumann et al. 1984; Post et al. 1986; Small 1990), and in a Chinese study, CBZ yielded a response rate closer to two-thirds in non-treatment-resistant patients (Zhang et al. 2007). However, most of these studies are limited by the use of small samples of heterogeneous (both bipolar and unipolar) and highly treatment-resistant patients. Nevertheless, studies have provided evidence of individual responsiveness in at least a subgroup of depressed bipolar patients.

Prophylaxis

Findings from a series of 18 double-blind, randomized, open randomized, or otherwise par-

TABLE 28–1. Carbamazepine (CBZ) and oxcarbazepine (OXC) in acute mania: 24 double-blind studies

Study	Design	CBZ/OXC (*N*)	Comparator (*N*)	Duration (days)	CBZ/OXC response	Comparator response
Weisler et al. 2004	CBZ vs. PBO	101	103	21	42%	22%
Weisler et al. 2005	CBZ vs. PBO	122	117	21	61%	29%
Zhang et al. 2007	CBZ vs. PBO	41	21	84	88%	57%
Wagner et al. 2006	OXC vs. PBO	55	55	42	42%	26%
Ballenger and Post 1978; Post et al. 1987	PBO–CBZ–PBO	19	—	11–56	63%	Frequent relapse
Emrich et al. 1985	PBO–OXC–PBO	7	—	Varied	67%	—
Klein et al. 1984	CBZ vs. PBO adjunct (HAL)	14	13	35	71%	54%
Müller and Stoll 1984; Goncalves and Stoll 1985	CBZ vs. PBO adjunct (HAL)	6	6	21	CBZ>PBO	—
Gangadhar et al. 1987	CBZ vs. PBO adjunct (Li)	5	5	28	CBZ>PBO	—
Möller et al. 1989	CBZ vs. PBO adjunct (HAL)	11	9	21	CBZ=PBO	—
Okuma et al. 1989	CBZ vs. PBO adjunct (NL)	82	80	28	48%	30%
Okuma et al. 1979	CBZ vs. NL (CPZ)	32	28	21–35	66%	54%
Grossi et al. 1984	CBZ vs. NL (CPZ)	18	19	21	67%	76%
Emrich 1990	OXC vs. NL (HAL)	19	19	14	OXC=HAL	—
Stoll et al. 1986	CBZ vs. NL (HAL) adjunct (CPZ)	14	18	21	86%	67%
Brown et al. 1989	CBZ vs. NL (HAL) adjunct (CPZ)	8	9	28	75%	33%
Müller and Stoll 1984	OXC vs. NL (HAL) adjunct (HAL)	10	10	14	OXC=HAL	—

TABLE 28–1. Carbamazepine (CBZ) and oxcarbazepine (OXC) in acute mania: 24 double-blind studies *(continued)*

Study	Design	CBZ/OXC (*N*)	Comparator (*N*)	Duration (days)	CBZ/OXC response	Comparator response
Lerer et al. 1987	CBZ vs. Li	14	14	28	29%	79%
Small et al. 1991	CBZ vs. Li	24	24	56	33%	33%
Emrich 1990	OXC vs. Li	28	24	14	OXC=Li	—
Kakkar et al. 2009	OXC vs. DVPX	30	30	84	OXC=DVPX	—
Lenzi et al. 1986	CBZ vs. Li adjunct (CPZ)	11	11	19	73%	73%
Lusznat et al. 1988	CBZ vs. Li adjunct (CPZ, HAL)	22	22	42	CBZ=Li	—
Okuma et al. 1990	CBZ vs. Li adjunct (NL)	50	51	28	62%	59%
Total		**743**	**688**			
Response rates[a]	CBZ/OXC monotherapy				55% (237/433)	
	NL monotherapy					64% (30/47)
	Li monotherapy					50% (19/38)
	PBO monotherapy					28% (83/296)
Response rates[a]	CBZ/OXC adjunctive				59% (106/179)	
	NL adjunctive					56% (15/27)
	Li adjunctive					61% (38/62)
	PBO adjunctive					33% (31/93)

Note. CBZ=carbamazepine; CPZ=chlorpromazine; DVPX=divalproex; HAL=haloperidol; Li=lithium; NL=neuroleptic; NS=not stated; OXC=oxcarbazepine; PBO=placebo.

[a]Weighted means of patients with response data.

tially controlled studies (Ballenger and Post 1978; Bellaire et al. 1988; Berky et al. 1998; Cabrera et al. 1986; Coxhead et al. 1992; Denicoff et al. 1997; Di Costanzo and Schifano 1991; Elphick et al. 1988; Greil et al. 1997; Hartong et al. 2003; Kishimoto and Okuma 1985; Lusznat et al. 1988; Mosolov 1991; Okuma et al. 1981; Placidi et al. 1986; Post et al. 1983; Vieta et al. 2008; Watkins et al. 1987; Wildgrube 1990) have examined CBZ and OXC prophylaxis in bipolar disorder (Table 28–2). The 15 CBZ trials are consistent with a very substantial uncontrolled literature suggesting that CBZ may be effective in preventing bipolar manic and depressive episodes when administered as long-term prophylaxis, either alone or in combination with lithium, in patients who previously had not responded to lithium. Indeed, five reviews of different subsets of studies included in Table 28–2 broadly indicated that CBZ and lithium monotherapy had comparable prophylactic effects in bipolar disorder patients (Ceron-Litvoc et al. 2009; Dardennes et al. 1995; Davis et al. 1999; Hirschfeld and Kasper 2004; Smith et al. 2007). CBZ may have equal *prophylactic* efficacy as an antidepressant and an antimanic, in contrast to its less potent *acute* antidepressant versus antimanic effects. By contrast, data regarding the prophylactic efficacy of OXC in controlling mood episodes in patients with bipolar disorder are far more limited (Cabrera et al. 1986; Vieta et al. 2008; Wildgrube 1990). Indeed, a 2008 Cochrane review concluded that the available evidence base was insufficient to provide guidance on the use of OXC in maintenance treatment of bipolar disorder (Vasudev et al. 2008).

In one study, the overall analysis suggested that maintenance treatment was more effective with lithium than with CBZ (Greil et al. 1997), but subsequent analysis revealed subgroup differences. Thus, maintenance treatment was more effective with lithium than with CBZ in patients with "classic" bipolar disorder (bipolar I disorder with no mood-incongruent delusions or comorbidity) but tended to be more effective with CBZ than with lithium in patients with "nonclassic" bipolar disorder (bipolar II disorder, bipolar disorder not otherwise specified, bipolar disorder with mood-incongruent delusions or comorbidity) (Greil et al. 1998).

In another study, maintenance treatment appeared to be more effective with lithium than with CBZ in patients with no more than 6 months' prior exposure to either agent (Hartong et al. 2003). However, this advantage was offset by more early discontinuations in the lithium group, so that similar proportions (about one-third) of lithium-treated and CBZ-treated patients completed 2 years with no episode. Patients on lithium compared to CBZ tended to have a somewhat greater risk of episodes in the first 3 months and markedly less risk of episodes after the first 3 months, with a recurrence risk of only 10% per year with lithium after the first 3 months. Patients on CBZ had a more consistent rate of relapse/recurrence of about 40% per year.

Some CBZ prophylaxis trials have been criticized due to methodological limitations (Murphy et al. 1989), but such difficulties are common in maintenance studies. For example, apparently due in part to methodological limitations, divalproex and lithium failed to separate from placebo on the primary efficacy measure in a 1-year maintenance study (Bowden et al. 2000). Taken together, the randomized, placebo-controlled, placebo-drug-placebo, and lithium comparator studies and trials in patients with rapid-cycling or lithium-resistant illness constitute substantial evidence for the efficacy of CBZ (Prien and Gelenberg 1989). CBZ may be effective in some individuals with valproate-resistant illness (Post et al. 1984), and the CBZ plus valproate combination may be effective in patients who show little or no response to either agent alone (Keck et al. 1992; Ketter et al. 1992).

In a retrospective study, although 22 of 34 (65%) patients with treatment-resistant bipolar disorder responded to primarily adjunctive open CBZ acutely, when patients were assessed 3–4 years later, only 7 of 34 (21%) and 2 of 34 (6%) were considered probable and clear responders, respectively (Frankenburg et al. 1988). Post and colleagues (Post and Weiss 2010; Post et al. 1990) have suggested that loss of CBZ prophylactic efficacy over time may be related to a unique form of contingent tolerance. In these instances, the optimal algorithm for recapturing CBZ response has not been determined. However, techniques such as switching to another treatment regimen with a different mechanism of action or returning later to CBZ (after a period of not taking CBZ) are worth considering, based on case reports and anecdotal observations. Systematic clinical trials are required to better determine the efficacy of these and other approaches for recapturing CBZ response.

Response Predictors

Predictors of CBZ and OXC response have not been adequately elucidated. CBZ appears to be effective in patients with a history of lithium unresponsiveness or intolerance (Okuma et al. 1979; Post et al. 1987). Nonclassic bipolar disorder (Greil et al. 1998; Small et al. 1991) and stable or decreasing episode frequency (Post et al. 1990) have been reported to be associated with CBZ response. Studies have indicated that patients with a history of affective illness in first-degree relatives may have preferential responses to lithium, whereas the converse may be the case for CBZ (Ballenger and Post 1978; Post et al. 1987). Himmelhoch and colleagues (Himmelhoch 1987; Himmelhoch and Garfinkel 1986) have suggested that patients with comorbid neurological or substance abuse problems and inadequate lithium responses might respond to CBZ or valproate.

There are varying reports with respect to the relationships between CBZ response and dysphoric manic presentations (Lusznat et al. 1988; Post et al. 1989) and illness severity (Post et al. 1987; Small et al. 1991). Although several investigators have suggested that psychosensory symptoms (which have been hypothesized to be due to limbic dysfunction) may indicate preferential response to CBZ and other anticonvulsants, such a relationship has not been observed in acute therapy, and the relationship to prophylactic response remains to be delineated.

Antidepressant responses to CBZ may be seen in patients with more severe depression, more discrete depressive episodes, less chronicity, and greater decreases in serum T_4 concentrations with CBZ (Post et al. 1986, 1991).

Although the initial studies of Post et al. (1987) and Okuma et al. (1981; Okuma 1983) indicated that some rapid-cycling patients were responsive to CBZ, other investigators found less robust results (Dilsaver et al. 1993; Joyce 1988). As with lithium, later studies by Okuma (1993) reported a lower CBZ maintenance response rate in rapid-cycling compared with non-rapid-cycling illness. However, even these rapid-cycling patients had a CBZ response rate (40%) that was higher than the rates reported for other agents in other studies. Denicoff et al. (1997) also observed that patients with a history of rapid cycling had a lower CBZ maintenance response rate compared with those without such a history (19% vs. 54%).

Side Effects and Toxicology

Baseline evaluation of bipolar disorder patients includes not only psychosocial assessment but also general medical evaluation, in view of the risk of medical processes, which could confound diagnosis or influence management decisions, and the risk of adverse effects, which may occur with treatment. Assessment commonly includes history; physical examination; complete blood count with differential and platelets; renal, hepatic, and thyroid function; toxicology; pregnancy tests; and other chemistries and electrocardiogram as clinically indicated (American Psychiatric Association 2002). Such evaluation provides baseline values for parameters that influence decisions about choice of

TABLE 28–2. Carbamazepine (CBZ) and oxcarbazepine (OXC) in prophylaxis of bipolar disorder: 18 controlled or quasi-controlled studies

Study	Design	CBZ (*N*)	Comparator (*N*)	Duration (years)	CBZ/OXC response	Comparator response
Okuma et al. 1981	CBZ vs. PBO (B, R)	12	10	1	60%	22%
Ballenger and Post 1978; Post et al. 1983b	CBZ vs. PBO (B, M)	7	7	1.7	86%	—
Placidi et al. 1986	CBZ vs. Li (B, R)	20	16	≤3	67%	67%
Watkins et al. 1987	CBZ vs. Li (B, R)	19	18	1.5	84%	83%
Lusznat et al. 1988	CBZ vs. Li (B, R)	16	15	≤1	56%	29%
Coxhead et al. 1992	CBZ vs. Li (B, R)	13	15	1	54%	47%
Bellaire et al. 1988	CBZ vs. Li (R)	46	52	1	CBZ=Li	—
Greil et al. 1997	CBZ vs. Li (R)	70	74	2.5	45%	65%
Berky et al. 1998	CBZ vs. Li (R)	84	84	1	CBZ=Li	—
Hartong et al. 2003	CBZ vs. Li (R)	50	44	2	58%	73%
Di Costanzo and Schifano 1991	CBZ+Li vs. Li (R)	8	8	≤5	CBZ+Li>Li	—
Mosolov 1991	CBZ vs. Li (R?)	30	30	≥1	73%	70%
Cabrera et al. 1986	OXC vs. Li (R)	4	6	≤22	75%	100%
Elphick et al. 1988	CBZ vs. Li (B, C)	8	11	0.75	38%	73%
Denicoff et al. 1997	CBZ vs. Li (B, C)	46	50	1	33%	55%
Kishimoto and Okuma 1985	CBZ vs. Li (C)	18	18	≥2	CBZ>Li	—

TABLE 28–2. Carbamazepine (CBZ) and oxcarbazepine (OXC) in prophylaxis of bipolar disorder: 18 controlled or quasi-controlled studies

Study	Design	CBZ (*N*)	Comparator (*N*)	Duration (years)	CBZ/OXC response	Comparator response
Wildgrube 1990	OXC vs. Li (NR)	8	7	≤33	33%	67%
Vieta et al. 2008	OXC vs. PBO adjunct (B, R)	26	29	1	50%	34%
Total		**485**	**486**			
Response rates[a]	CBZ/OXC				54% (178/329)	
	Li					64% (185/286)
	PBO					32% (12/38)

Note. B = blind; C = crossover; CBZ = carbamazepine; Li = lithium; M = mirror image; NR = not randomized; OXC = oxcarbazepine; PBO = placebo; R = randomized.
[a]Weighted means of patients with response data.

medication and intensity of clinical and laboratory monitoring.

Carbamazepine

CBZ adverse effects appear to have substantial impact on the utility of CBZ in the treatment of bipolar disorder. Adverse effects requiring discontinuation may occur more commonly with CBZ than with other drugs, particularly during acute therapy if CBZ is rapidly introduced. However, some patients may tolerate CBZ better than other agents, particularly during longer-term treatment, as CBZ appears to have a low propensity to cause adverse effects such as weight gain and metabolic disturbance that can limit the utility of some other agents (Ketter 2010).

CBZ has several common dose-related adverse effects that can generally be minimized by attention to drug-drug interactions and gradual titration of dosage or reversed by decreasing dosage. At high dosages, patients can develop neurotoxicity with sedation, ataxia, diplopia, and nystagmus, particularly early in therapy before autoinduction and the development of some tolerance to CBZ's central nervous system adverse effects occur. However, in contrast to neuroleptic treatment, CBZ therapy is not associated with extrapyramidal adverse effects. Because there is wide interindividual variation in susceptibility to adverse effects at any given concentration, it is most useful clinically to titrate doses against each patient's adverse-effects threshold rather than targeting a fixed dosage or serum concentration range.

Dizziness, ataxia, or diplopia emerging 1–2 hours after an individual dose is often a sign that the adverse-effects threshold has been exceeded and that dosage redistribution (spreading out the dose or giving more of the dosage at bedtime) or dosage reduction may be required. Use of extended-release formulations can also attenuate CBZ peak serum concentrations, enhancing tolerability.

CBZ therapy is associated with common and benign—as well as rare and serious—adverse events. A mild rash occurs in about 1 in 10 patients, with the slight possibility that this usually benign phenomenon may herald a more malignant Stevens-Johnson syndrome. Similarly, a benign white cell suppression is common, but the risk of agranulocytosis or aplastic anemia—seen at rates of about 16 and 48 cases per million patient-years, respectively—warrants concern (Physicians' Desk Reference 2012). Thus, increased monitoring and particular care are needed if clinical or laboratory evidence suggests hematological, dermatological, or hepatic abnormalities.

In view of the risk of rare but serious decreases in blood counts, which prompted a black box warning in the CBZ prescribing information, it is important to alert patients to seek immediate medical evaluation if they develop signs and symptoms of possible hematological reactions, such as fever, sore throat, oral ulcers, petechiae, and easy bruising or bleeding. In general, CBZ should be discontinued if the white blood cell count falls below 3,000/mm^3 or the absolute neutrophil count falls below 1,000–1,500/mm^3. In the instance of benign leukopenia, the addition of lithium can increase the neutrophil count back toward normal (Kramlinger and Post 1990), but this strategy is not likely to be helpful for the suppression of red cells or platelets, which is likely to be indicative of a more problematic process.

The risk of serious rash may be 10 times as high in some Asian countries and has been strongly linked to the HLA-B*1502 allele (Physicians' Desk Reference 2012). Thus, the U.S. prescribing information includes a black box warning that Asians should be genetically tested and, if found to be HLA-B*1502 positive, should not be treated with CBZ unless the benefit clearly outweighs the risk. A 12-fold increased risk of a hypersensitivity syndrome has also been linked to the HLA-A*3101 allele in whites of Northern European descent (McCormack et al. 2011). In view of the risk of rare but serious rashes, it is important to alert patients to seek medical evaluation if they develop a rash. In particular, rash presenting with systemic illness or involvement of the eyes, mouth, or bladder (dysuria) constitutes a medical emergency, and CBZ should be discontinued immediately and the patient assessed emergently. For more benign presentations, CBZ is generally discontinued, as there is little ability to predict which rashes will progress to more severe, potentially life-threatening problems. However, in rare instances of resistance to all medications except CBZ, a repeat trial of CBZ with a course of prednisone may be well tolerated (Murphy et al. 1991; Vick 1983). If there is evidence of systemic allergy, fever, or malaise, prednisone is less likely to be helpful. A substantial number of patients with CBZ-induced rashes may not develop a rash on reexposure (even without prednisone coverage), but if a rash again develops, it usually appears more rapidly than in the first occurrence. Only 25%–30% of the patients who develop a rash while taking CBZ also develop a rash (cross-sensitivity) with OXC.

CBZ, in common with OXC and nine other anticonvulsants, may increase the risk of suicidality (suicidal behavior or ideation) (Physicians' Desk Reference 2012). In controlled trials, anticonvulsants compared to placebo increased suicidality risk from 0.57% to 0.85% (1.5-fold relative and 0.29% absolute increase) for psychiatric patients (Physicians' Desk Reference 2012).

Due to the risk of rare hepatitis, patients should be advised to seek medical evaluation immediately if they develop malaise, abdominal pain, or other marked gastrointestinal symptoms. In general, CBZ (like other anticonvulsants) is discontinued if liver function tests exceed three times the upper limit of the normal range.

CBZ may affect cardiac conduction and should be used with caution in patients with cardiac disorders such as heart block. A baseline electrocardiogram is worth considering if the patient has a positive cardiac history.

Conservative laboratory monitoring during CBZ therapy includes baseline studies and reevaluation of complete blood count, differential, platelets, and hepatic indices initially at 2, 4, 6, and 8 weeks and then every 3 months (American Psychiatric Association 1994, 2002). Most of the serious hematological reactions occur in the first 3 months of therapy (Tohen et al. 1995). In clinical practice, less focus is placed on scheduled monitoring; instead, monitoring as clinically indicated (e.g., when a patient becomes ill with a fever) is emphasized. Serum CBZ concentrations are typically assessed at steady state and then as clinically indicated (e.g., by inefficacy or adverse effects).

Dividing or reducing doses, moving doses in relation to mealtimes, and changing formulations can attenuate CBZ-induced gastrointestinal disturbances. CBZ suspension may have more proximal absorption and thus exacerbate upper gastrointestinal (nausea and vomiting) or attenuate lower gastrointestinal (diarrhea) adverse effects. The reverse holds for extended-release preparations.

Weight gain and obesity are important clinical concerns in the management of patients with bipolar disorder. Medications and the hyperphagia, hypersomnia, and anergy commonly seen in bipolar depression can contribute to this important obstacle to optimal outcomes. CBZ is less likely than lithium (Coxhead et al. 1992; Denicoff et al. 1997) or valproate (Mattson et al. 1992) to yield weight gain. Given its relatively favorable effect on weight, CBZ may provide an important alternative to other mood stabilizers for patients who struggle with weight gain and obesity. Cholesterol should be checked periodically in patients at high risk, given that CBZ can increase levels by about 20 points.

CBZ can induce hyponatremia that may be tolerated well by some younger patients but can be particularly problematic in the elderly. If confusion develops in an elderly patient, serum sodium should be assessed. In rare instances, water intoxication and seizures can occur. In some cases, hyponatremia can be effectively counteracted with the addition of lithium or the antibiotic demeclocycline (Ringel and Brick 1986).

CBZ appears to reduce serum concentrations of both female and male sex hormones (Verrotti et al. 2011) and, like several other anticonvulsants, may adversely affect bone density (Verrotti et al. 2010).

CBZ is teratogenic (FDA Category D) and is associated with low birth weight, craniofacial deformities, digital hypoplasia, and (in approximately 1%–3% of exposures) spina bifida (Jones et al. 1989; Rosa 1991). For the latter, folate supplementation may attenuate the risk, and fetal ultrasound studies may allow early detection. In rare patients with severe mood disorders, clinicians may determine in consultation with a gynecologist that the benefits of treating with CBZ outweigh the risks in comparison with other treatment options (Sitland-Marken et al. 1989). In one study of children born to women with epilepsy, in utero exposure to CBZ or valproate, but not to lamotrigine, had a detrimental effect on child neurodevelopment (Cummings et al. 2011), although CBZ appears less likely than valproate to cause major developmental delay.

CBZ is present in breast milk at concentrations about half those present in maternal blood but may not accumulate in fetal blood (Froescher et al. 1984; Kuhnz et al. 1983; Pynnönen et al. 1977; Shimoyama et al. 2000). Clinicians may prefer to avoid the putative risks of exposing infants to CBZ in breast milk (Frey et al. 2002) and discourage breast-feeding in women taking CBZ (Physicians' Desk Reference 2012).

Oxcarbazepine

Adverse effects may limit the use of OXC, as with CBZ. However, OXC may have tolerability advantages over CBZ, perhaps in part related to the absence of the CBZ-E metabolite.

OXC appears to have less potential for neurotoxicity and rash compared with CBZ. About 75% of patients who develop a rash from CBZ will tolerate OXC. Of importance, OXC, unlike CBZ, has not shown sufficient risks of serious rashes and blood dyscrasias to warrant black box warnings for these problems, and its prescribing information lacks recommendations for routine tissue typing in Asians and for hematological monitoring.

As noted earlier, the U.S. prescribing information for OXC (in common with that for CBZ and nine other anticonvulsants) now includes a class warning regarding increased risk of suicidality.

OXC, like CBZ, may produce transaminase elevations and gastrointestinal adverse effects but is associated with less weight gain than valproate (Rattya et al. 1999).

Hyponatremia occurs with OXC (Friis et al. 1993) and may be the main adverse effect that occurs more commonly than with CBZ. However, clinically significant hyponatremia is less common than asymptomatic hyponatremia.

OXC, like CBZ and several other anticonvulsants, may adversely affect bone density (Verrotti et al. 2010).

In comparison with CBZ, OXC has less impact on blood concentrations of thyroid and sex hormones, likely because of its less marked hepatic enzyme induction. Importantly, as noted below (see "Drug-Drug Interactions"), OXC induction of female hormone metabolism is sufficient to decrease the efficacy of hormonal contraceptives (Fattore et al. 1999; Klosterskov Jensen et al. 1992).

OXC, in contrast to CBZ, has not to date been associated with congenital malformations in humans (FDA Pregnancy Category C). This could be merely related to fewer OXC exposures. However, the absence of the CBZ-E metabolite could render OXC less teratogenic; in mice, CBZ-E (but not OXC) yielded two- to fourfold increases in malformations compared with placebo (Bennett et al. 1996). As with CBZ, in rare patients with severe mood disorders, clinicians may determine in consultation with a gynecologist that the benefits of treating with OXC outweigh the risks in comparison with other treatment options.

OXC is present in breast milk, and as with CBZ, clinicians may prefer to avoid the putative risks of exposing infants to OXC in breast milk and discourage breast-feeding in women taking OXC (Physicians' Desk Reference 2012).

Drug-Drug Interactions

Combination therapy is common in bipolar disorder, with up to two-thirds of patients receiving more than one medication (Kupfer et al. 2002). Patients with treatment-resistant illness may require a stepped-care approach and appear to be receiving increasingly complex medication regimens (Frye et al. 2000). CBZ and, to a lesser extent, OXC have clinically significant drug-drug interactions, which increase the complexity of managing patients with bipolar disorder.

Carbamazepine

The pharmacokinetic properties of CBZ are typical of older enzyme-inducing anticonvulsants used by neurologists but atypical among medications prescribed by psychiatrists and necessitate special care when treating patients concurrently with other medications (Ketter et al. 1991a, 1991b). Three major principles appear to contribute importantly to CBZ drug-drug interactions:

1. **CBZ is a robust inducer of catabolic enzymes (including CYP3A3/4) and decreases the serum concentrations of many medications, including CBZ itself (Table 28–3).** CBZ induces not only CYP3A3/4 and conjugation but also presumably other cytochrome P450 isoforms that remain to be characterized. Thus, CBZ decreases the serum concentrations not only of CBZ itself (autoinduction) but also of many other medications (heteroinduction). CBZ-induced decreases in serum concentrations of certain concurrent medications can render them ineffective (see Table 28–3). Moreover, if CBZ is discontinued (or in some instances, if replaced with OXC), serum concentrations of these other medications can increase, potentially leading to adverse effects.
2. **CBZ metabolism (which is primarily by CYP3A3/4) can be inhibited by certain enzyme inhibitors, yielding increases in serum CBZ concentrations and CBZ intoxication (Table 28–4).** Autoinduction makes CBZ particularly vulnerable to the effects of enzyme inhibitors. Thus, a variety of agents that inhibit CYP3A3/4 can yield increased serum CBZ concentrations and intoxication (see Table 28–4).
3. **CBZ has an active epoxide (CBZ-E) metabolite.** Valproate inhibits epoxide hydrolase, yielding increased serum CBZ-E (but not CBZ) concentrations and intoxication (see Table 28–4). Free CBZ may also increase because of valproate-induced displacement of CBZ protein binding.

Knowledge of CBZ drug-drug interactions is crucial in effective management, and patients should be instructed to consult their pharmacist when prescribed other medications by other physicians. Advances in molecular pharmacology have characterized the specific cytochrome P450 isoforms responsible for metabolism of various medications. This may allow clinicians to anticipate and avoid pharmacokinetic drug-drug interactions and thus provide more effective combination pharmacotherapies. Below, we review CBZ drug interactions with other medications, with agents of particular interest in the management of mood disorders indicated in **boldface** type. The reader interested in detailed reviews of CBZ drug-drug interactions may find these in other articles (Ketter et al. 1991a, 1991b).

Interactions With Mood Stabilizers

The combination of CBZ plus lithium is frequently used in bipolar disorder and may provide additive or synergistic antimanic (Kramlinger and Post 1989a) and antidepressant

TABLE 28–3. Drugs whose serum concentrations are DECREASED by carbamazepine (and oxcarbazepine)

Antidepressants
- Bupropion
- Citalopram
- Mirtazapine
- Sertraline
- Tricyclics
- Vilazodone (?)

Antipsychotics
- Aripiprazole
- Chlorpromazine (?)
- Clozapine
- Fluphenazine (?)
- Haloperidol
- Iloperidone (?)
- Lurasidone (?)
- Olanzapine
- Quetiapine
- Risperidone
- Thiothixene (?)
- Ziprasidone (?)

Anxiolytics/sedatives
- ***Alprazolam*** (?)
- Buspirone
- ***Clonazepam***
- Eszopiclone (?)
- Midazolam

Stimulants
- Armodafinil
- Modafinil

Anticonvulsants
- Carbamazepine
- Ethosuximide
- Felbamate
- ***Lamotrigine***
- Levetiracetam (?)
- Oxcarbazepine
- Phenytoin
- Primidone
- Tiagabine
- Topiramate
- Valproate
- Zonisamide

Analgesics
- Alfentanil
- ***Buprenorphine***
- Fentanyl (?)
- Levobupivacaine
- Methadone
- Tramadol

Anticoagulants
- Warfarin

Anti-infectives
- Caspofungin
- Delavirdine
- Doxycycline
- Praziquantel
- Protease inhibitors

Dihydropyridine CCBs
- ***Felodipine***
- Nimodipine

Immunosuppressants
- Cyclosporine (?)
- Sirolimus
- Tacrolimus

Muscle relaxants
- Atracurium
- Cisatracurium
- Doxacurium
- Mivacurium
- Pancuronium
- Pipercuronium
- Rocuronium
- Vecuronium

Steroids
- Dexamethasone
- ***Hormonal contraceptives***
- Mifepristone
- Prednisolone

Others
- ***Paclitaxel***
- Quinidine
- ***Repaglinide***
- Theophylline (?)
- Thyroid hormones

Note. ***Boldface italic*** type indicates that serum concentration of the medication may decrease to a clinically significant extent not only with carbamazepine but also with oxcarbazepine, hindering efficacy of the agent. CCBs = calcium channel blockers; (?) = Unclear clinical significance.

TABLE 28–4. Drugs that INCREASE serum concentrations of carbamazepine (but not oxcarbazepine)

Antidepressants	**Calcium channel blockers**
Fluoxetine	Diltiazem
Fluvoxamine	Verapamil
Nefazodone	
	Hypolipidemics
Anti-infectives	Gemfibrozil
Isoniazid	Nicotinamide
Quinupristin/dalfopristin	
	Others
Azole antifungals	Acetazolamide
Fluconazole	Cimetidine
Itraconazole	Danazol
Ketoconazole	Grapefruit juice
	Omeprazole
Macrolide antibiotics	d-Propoxyphene
Clarithromycin	Ritonavir
Erythromycin	Ticlopidine (?)
Troleandomycin	Valproate (increases CBZ-E)

Note. CBZ-E=carbamazepine-10,11-epoxide; (?)=Unclear clinical significance.

(Kramlinger and Post 1989b) effects. The combination is generally well tolerated, with merely additive neurotoxicity (McGinness et al. 1990), which can be minimized by gradual dosage escalation. Pharmacokinetic interactions between these drugs do not occur, because lithium is excreted by the kidney, with no hepatic metabolism. Adverse effects of lithium and CBZ can be either additive or complementary, so that combination therapy decreases the serum concentrations of thyroid hormones in an additive fashion (Kramlinger and Post 1990), whereas lithium-induced increases in leukocytes and neutrophils override the common benign decreases in these indices seen with CBZ (Kramlinger and Post 1990). However, there is no evidence that lithium can alter the course of the rare severe bone marrow suppression caused by CBZ (Joffe and Post 1989). Also, the diuretic effect of lithium overrides the antidiuretic effect of CBZ. Thus, CBZ will not reverse lithium-induced diabetes insipidus, but lithium attenuates CBZ-induced hyponatremia.

Reports suggest that the CBZ plus **valproate** combination not only is tolerated but also may show psychotropic synergy (Keck et al. 1992; Ketter et al. 1992; Tohen et al. 1994). However, the effective use of these two medications together requires a thorough knowledge of their drug interactions, which can be simplified into the general principle that usual doses of CBZ should be reduced. Valproate inhibits CBZ metabolism (Macphee et al. 1988) and also displaces CBZ from plasma proteins, increasing the free CBZ fraction that is active and available to be metabolized (Macphee et al. 1988; Moreland et al. 1984). Depending on which effect predominates, total serum CBZ concentrations can rise, fall, or remain unchanged. Valproate inhibits epoxide hydrolase, increasing the serum CBZ-E concentration, at times without altering the total serum CBZ concentration (Brodie et al. 1983; Rambeck et al. 1987).

Thus, these interactions can potentially confound clinicians, because patients can have neurotoxicity due to elevated serum CBZ-E or free CBZ concentrations despite having therapeutic serum total CBZ concentrations (Kutt et al. 1985). CBZ decreases serum valproate concentrations (Kondo et al. 1990), and its discontinuation can yield increased serum valproate concentrations and toxicity (Jann et al. 1988). Although fatal hepatitis in infants treated with combinations of valproate with other anticonvulsants is of great concern (Scheffner et al. 1988), the risk of combined therapy is much lower in adults.

As a general rule, clinicians should clinically monitor patients receiving the CBZ plus valproate combination for adverse effects and consider decreasing the CBZ dose in advance (because of the expected displacement of CBZ from plasma proteins and increase in CBZ-E) and possibly increasing the valproate dose (because of expected CBZ-induced decrements in valproate).

CBZ increases **lamotrigine** metabolism and approximately halves blood lamotrigine concentrations. Thus, lamotrigine doses can be doubled with this combination. In addition, CBZ combined with lamotrigine may have additive neurotoxicity, probably due to a pharmacodynamic interaction. CBZ even appears to affect **OXC** metabolism; in patients with epilepsy, CBZ yielded decreased serum MHD concentrations.

Interactions With Antidepressants

Antidepressants are commonly combined with mood stabilizers in the treatment of bipolar disorder. Because CBZ can increase metabolism of some antidepressants, and because some antidepressants can inhibit CBZ metabolism, dosage adjustments may be necessary in combination therapy.

Fluoxetine, fluvoxamine, and **nefazodone** may increase CBZ concentrations, possibly by inhibition of CYP3A4. In addition, parkinsonian symptoms have been reported after addition of fluoxetine to CBZ (Gernaat et al. 1991). In contrast, sertraline, paroxetine, citalopram, and mirtazapine do not appear to alter CBZ metabolism. CBZ appears to decrease serum concentrations of racemic **citalopram,** including those of the active enantiomer **escitalopram** (Steinacher et al. 2002). CBZ also appears to induce the metabolism of **mirtazapine, mianserin** (Eap et al. 1999), **sertraline,** nefazodone, most likely **vilazodone** (Physicians' Desk Reference 2012), and to some extent trazodone. The combination of CBZ with mirtazapine is also of potential concern given that mirtazapine has been associated with rare agranulocytosis.

Patients receiving CBZ and **bupropion** have extremely low serum bupropion concentrations and high hydroxybupropion (metabolite) concentrations (Ketter et al. 1995a). Because hydroxybupropion is active, the clinical impact of this dramatic decrease in the bupropion-to-hydroxybupropion ratio is probably not problematic, and the combination of CBZ and bupropion may often be effective and well tolerated.

CBZ may increase rather than decrease serum levels of transdermal selegiline and its metabolites (Physicians' Desk Reference 2012). Although theoretical grounds have been stated for concern about combining CBZ with monoamine oxidase inhibitors (MAOIs) (Physicians' Desk Reference 2012; Thweatt 1986), case reports and a series of 10 patients (Ketter et al. 1995b) suggest that the addition of phenelzine or tranylcypromine to CBZ may be well tolerated, does not affect CBZ pharmacokinetics, and may provide relief of resistant depressive symptoms in some patients. However, the antituberculosis drug isoniazid, which is also an MAOI, increases CBZ levels.

CBZ appears to induce the metabolism of **tricyclic antidepressants (TCAs),** including amitriptyline, nortriptyline, imipramine, desipramine, doxepin, and clomipramine, so if patients fail to respond to standard doses of TCAs, TCA and metabolite concentrations should be checked.

Interactions With Antipsychotics

Combinations of antipsychotics with mood stabilizers are commonly required in treatment of severe mania (American Psychiatric Association 2002) and are increasingly used in bipolar maintenance treatment (Ketter 2010; Physicians' Desk Reference 2012). CBZ can on occasion be used effectively in combination with antipsychotics, although clinicians need to be aware of potential drug-drug interactions with some antipsychotics that can undermine the benefits of such combinations.

CBZ increases **haloperidol** metabolism, dramatically lowering its blood concentrations. Some patients show improvement in psychiatric status or experience fewer neuroleptic adverse effects during combination treatment, while others show deterioration in psychiatric status (Jann et al. 1989; Kahn et al. 1990). Neurotoxicity possibly related to receiving the combination of CBZ and haloperidol has been very rarely reported (Brayley and Yellowlees 1987). There is weaker evidence that CBZ may increase the metabolism of other first-generation antipsychotic agents, including fluphenazine, chlorpromazine, and thiothixene, but not thioridazine, and that loxapine, chlorpromazine, and amoxapine may increase CBZ-E concentrations. Also, animal studies suggest that promazine, chlorpromazine, perazine, chlorprothixene, and flupenthixol may increase CBZ concentrations. In view of the above, serum antipsychotic medication concentrations should be checked if patients fail to respond to standard dosages of antipsychotic agents during combination therapy with CBZ.

Combination of **clozapine** with CBZ is not recommended in view of the hypothetical possibility of synergistic bone marrow suppression (Physicians' Desk Reference 2012). However, these drugs have been used in combination in some European centers, one of which reported that CBZ decreases clozapine concentrations (Raitasuo et al. 1993). Thus, clinicians wishing to combine a psychotropic anticonvulsant with clozapine should consider valproate, lamotrigine, or another anticonvulsant rather than CBZ, except under unusual circumstances.

CBZ increases the metabolism of **olanzapine, risperidone, quetiapine, aripiprazole,** most likely **lurasidone,** possibly **iloperidone,** and to a limited extent **ziprasidone.** Thus, CBZ-related decreases in serum antipsychotic concentrations may have contributed to a reported lack of benefit in acute mania patients when risperidone (Yatham et al. 2003) or olanzapine (Tohen et al. 2008) was added to CBZ.

Interactions With Anxiolytics and Sedatives

Although in general CBZ can be used effectively with **benzodiazepines,** CBZ may decrease serum concentrations of clonazepam and alprazolam. On the other hand, clonazepam and clobazam (Goggin and Callaghan 1985; Munoz et al. 1990) appear to have variable effects on CBZ metabolism. Of interest, CBZ may be effective in ameliorating benzodiazepine withdrawal symptoms (Ries et al. 1989).

Interactions With Stimulants

Methylphenidate metabolism entails deesterification by nonmicrosomal hydrolytic esterases rather than P450 oxidation and is thus not expected to be generally affected by CBZ, although individual case reports suggest that in some patients, CBZ could decrease methylphenidate serum concentrations. In contrast, modafinil and armodafinil are CYP3A4 substrates, raising greater concern regarding the possibility that potent inducers such as CBZ could decrease serum concentrations of these agents.

Interactions With Calcium Channel Blockers

Of clear clinical importance, elevated serum CBZ concentrations and neurotoxicity have been reported during concurrent treatment with the nondihydropyridines **verapamil** and **diltiazem,** but not the dihydropyridines nifedipine and nimodipine. These observations are consistent with the finding that verapamil and diltiazem, but not nifedipine, inhibit the hepatic oxidative metabolism of various drugs. Preliminary observations also indicate that the dihydropyridine nimodipine may not substantially influence CBZ kinetics and that the addition of CBZ to nimodipine may yield therapeutic synergy (Pazzaglia et al. 1993, 1998).

Enzyme-inducing anticonvulsants such as CBZ appear to decrease serum concentrations of **dihydropyridines** such as nimodipine and felodipine.

Interactions With Substances of Abuse

Although ethanol and CBZ do not have pharmacokinetic interactions, CBZ attenuates alcohol withdrawal symptoms (Malcolm et al. 1989), a potentially useful property given the risk of alcohol abuse in bipolar disorder patients. Combination therapy with disulfiram and CBZ is well tolerated and does not cause clinically significant changes in serum CBZ and CBZ-E concentrations.

Tobacco smoking does not alter CBZ metabolism, and CBZ does not alter caffeine pharmacokinetics.

Preliminary clinical studies suggested that CBZ attenuated acute cocaine effects and seizures and possibly cocaine craving, but later controlled studies generally failed to support these observations.

Interactions With Nonpsychotropic Drugs

Drug-drug interactions between CBZ and other (nonpsychotropic) drugs are also of substantial clinical importance. CBZ induces metabolism of diverse medications, raising the possibility of undermining the efficacy of steroids such as **hormonal contraceptives,** dexamethasone, prednisolone, and mifepristone; the anticonvulsants **CBZ** (autoinduction), ethosuximide, felbamate, **lamotrigine, OXC,** phenytoin, primidone, tiagabine, **topiramate, valproate,** and **zonisamide; methylxanthines** such as theophylline and aminophylline; antibiotics such as **doxycycline;** antivirals such as **protease inhibitors;** the antihelmintic **praziquantel; neuromuscular blockers** such as pancuronium, vecuronium, and doxacurium; analgesics such as **methadone; immunosuppressants** such as sirolimus and tacrolimus; and the anticoagulants **warfarin** and possibly dicumarol (see Table 28–3). Concerns have been raised that CBZ may induce metabolism of additional CYP3A4 substrates such as the anti-HIV agents delavirdine and etravirine, the azole antifungal voriconazole, the antineoplastic pazopanib, and the antianginal agent ranolazine.

A variety of medications can increase serum CBZ concentrations, yielding clinical toxicity; these include **isoniazid, azole antifungals** such as ketoconazole, **macrolide antibiotics** such as erythromycin and clarithromycin, **protease inhibitors** such as ritonavir and nelfinavir, **quinine, hypolipidemics** such as gemfibrozil and nicotinamide, and the carbonic anhydrase inhibitor **acetazolamide** (see Table 28–4). In addition, other medications, such as phenytoin, phenobarbital, primidone, methsuximide, felbamate, cisplatin, and doxorubicin, may decrease serum CBZ levels, potentially yielding inefficacy.

Oxcarbazepine

In contrast to CBZ, OXC has fewer clinically significant drug-drug interactions. Differences in three major areas appear to contribute importantly to differences between OXC and CBZ drug-drug interactions:

1. **OXC is only a modest to moderate enzyme (CYP3A4) inducer and produces clinically significant decreases in serum concentrations of some medications (see Table 28–3).** Although the extent of OXC induction of metabolism of other

drugs is commonly clinically insignificant, it is clinically significant for some medications (e.g., hormonal contraceptives), compromising their efficacy (Fattore et al. 1999) and requiring higher doses. Thus, serum concentrations of some of the medications listed (in ***boldface italic*** type) in Table 28–3 may decrease to a clinically significant degree with OXC, hindering the efficacy of those agents. In contrast, induction of metabolism is more limited for valproate and lamotrigine, yielding more modest clinical impact on clearance of these drugs. In some instances, OXC induction is substantially less robust than CBZ induction, so that switching from OXC to CBZ (or vice versa) will make adjustments of doses of other medications necessary.

2. **OXC metabolism (which is primarily by arylketone reductase) generally is not susceptible to enzyme inhibitors.** The absence of autoinduction and the robust actions of cytosol reductases that mediate conversion to MHD appear to render OXC metabolism not susceptible to the common phenomenon of inhibition by other agents seen with CBZ. Thus, the medications listed in Table 28–4 that can elevate serum CBZ concentrations and yield neurotoxicity do NOT appear to have such interactions with OXC.
3. **OXC has an active (MHD) metabolite.** However, MHD metabolism, unlike CBZ-E catabolism, is not inhibited by valproate, presumably due to the lack of involvement of epoxide hydrolase in MHD disposition. Thus, coadministration of valproate does NOT yield toxicity related to increased MHD.

Interactions With Mood Stabilizers

OXC, in contrast to CBZ, does not induce valproate metabolism, and OXC appears to have a more modest effect on **lamotrigine** metabolism. **CBZ** induces OXC metabolism, yielding decreased serum MHD concentrations.

Interactions With Antidepressants

OXC, in contrast to CBZ, may not robustly induce citalopram metabolism.

Interactions With Antipsychotics

OXC, unlike CBZ, may not robustly induce antipsychotic metabolism.

Interactions With Anxiolytics and Sedatives

OXC may decrease serum concentrations of **benzodiazepines.**

Interactions With Calcium Channel Blockers

OXC appears to decrease serum concentrations of **dihydropyridine** calcium channel blockers (which are CYP3A4 substrates) to some extent.

Interactions With Nonpsychotropic Drugs

OXC, compared with CBZ, also appears to have fewer interactions with nonpsychotropic drugs. Thus, neither the CYP3A4 inhibitor erythromycin nor the heteroinhibitor cimetidine appears to alter OXC pharmacokinetics in healthy volunteers. Also, OXC does not appear to robustly induce warfarin metabolism.

However, as noted earlier in this chapter, OXC appears to have a clinically significant interaction with **hormonal contraceptives;** in healthy female volunteers, OXC appeared to decrease ethinylestradiol and levonorgestrel derived from hormonal contraceptives by up to about 50% (Fattore et al. 1999; Klosterskov Jensen et al. 1992).

OXC, like CBZ, may decrease serum concentrations of the analgesic buprenorphine, the anticancer agent paclitaxel, and the antidiabetic agent repaglinide. In addition, the anticonvulsants **CBZ,** phenytoin, phenobarbital, and primidone may induce OXC metabolism. Finally, OXC can increase serum phenytoin concentrations, presumably by inhibiting the activity of CYP2C19.

Conclusion

In the past, because of lack of an FDA indication, complexity of use, and methodological concerns regarding earlier efficacy studies, CBZ was generally considered an alternative rather than a first-line intervention in bipolar disorder. However, the approval of a proprietary CBZ beaded extended-release capsule formulation (Equetro) for the treatment of acute manic and mixed episodes in patients with bipolar disorder and the low propensity of CBZ to cause weight gain and metabolic problems seen with some other agents may lead clinicians to reassess its role in the management of patients with bipolar disorder (Ketter 2010).

OXC, compared with CBZ, has more limited evidence of efficacy in bipolar disorder but has enhanced tolerability and fewer drug-drug interactions. For example, with CBZ (but not OXC), common benign leukopenia is difficult to distinguish from what may be a harbinger of the very rare but serious aplastic anemia, and patients and caregivers need to monitor carefully for symptoms of this adverse effect. In addition, CBZ (and to a lesser extent OXC) in combination therapy induces metabolism of other drugs, sometimes undermining their efficacy unless doses are adjusted. Also, other drugs (such as erythromycin or verapamil) can inhibit CBZ (but not OXC) metabolism, causing CBZ toxicity. Instructing patients to alert their other caregivers and pharmacists that they are receiving CBZ may help avoid drug interactions. Informing patients of several of the common interactions can further assist in the warning process, as other practitioners may inadvertently introduce commonly used drugs such as erythromycin with the attendant risk of CBZ toxicity.

CBZ and OXC are important treatment options for bipolar disorder patients who experience inadequate responses to or unacceptable adverse effects with lithium and valproate. Awareness of CBZ and OXC pharmacology and potential drug-drug interactions will provide clinicians with the opportunity to enhance outcomes when managing bipolar disorder with these agents.

References

Ambrosio AF, Silva AP, Malva JO, et al: Inhibition of glutamate release by BIA 2-093 and BIA 2-024, two novel derivatives of carbamazepine, due to blockade of sodium but not calcium channels. Biochem Pharmacol 61:1271–1275, 2001

Ambrosio AF, Soares-Da-Silva P, Carvalho CM, et al: Mechanisms of action of carbamazepine and its derivatives, oxcarbazepine, BIA 2-093, and BIA 2-024. Neurochem Res 27:121–130, 2002

American Psychiatric Association: Practice guideline for the treatment of patients with bipolar disorder. Am J Psychiatry 151:1–36, 1994

American Psychiatric Association: Practice guideline for the treatment of patients with bipolar disorder (revision). Am J Psychiatry 159:1–50, 2002

Ballenger JC, Post RM: Therapeutic effects of carbamazepine in affective illness: a preliminary report. Comm Psychopharmacol 2:159–175, 1978

Bellaire W, Demish K, Stoll KD: Carbamazepine versus lithium in prophylaxis of recurrent affective disorder (abstract). Psychopharmacology (Berl) 96:287, 1988

Bennett GD, Amore BM, Finnell RH, et al: Teratogenicity of carbamazepine-10,11-epoxide and oxcarbazepine in the SWV mouse. J Pharmacol Exp Ther 279:1237–1242, 1996

Berky M, Wolf C, Kovacs G: Carbamazepine versus lithium in bipolar affective disorders [abstract P174]. Eur Arch Psychiatry Clin Neurosci 248:S119, 1998

Beydoun A, Sachdeo RC, Rosenfeld WE, et al: Oxcarbazepine monotherapy for partial-onset seizures: a multicenter, double-blind, clinical trial. Neurology 54:2245–2251, 2000

Bowden CL, Brugger AM, Swann AC, et al: Efficacy of divalproex vs lithium and placebo in the treatment of mania. The Depakote Mania Study Group. JAMA 271:918–924, 1994

Bowden CL, Calabrese JR, McElroy SL, et al: A randomized, placebo-controlled 12-month trial of divalproex and lithium in treatment of outpatients with bipolar I disorder. Divalproex Maintenance Study Group [see comments]. Arch Gen Psychiatry 57:481–489, 2000

Brayley J, Yellowlees P: An interaction between haloperidol and carbamazepine in a patient with cerebral palsy. Aust N Z J Psychiatry 21: 605–607, 1987

Brodie MJ, Forrest G, Rapeport WG: Carbamazepine 10,11 epoxide concentrations in epileptics on carbamazepine alone and in combination with other anticonvulsants. Br J Clin Pharmacol 16:747–749, 1983

Brown D, Silverstone T, Cookson J: Carbamazepine compared to haloperidol in acute mania. Int Clin Psychopharmacol 4:229–238, 1989

Cabrera JF, Muhlbauer HD, Schley J, et al: Long-term randomized clinical trial of oxcarbazepine vs lithium in bipolar and schizoaffective disorders: preliminary results. Pharmacopsychiatry 19:282–283, 1986

Cereghino JJ: Serum carbamazepine concentration and clinical control, in Advances in Neurology. Edited by Penry JK, Daly DD. New York, Raven, 1975, pp 309–330

Ceron-Litvoc D, Soares BG, Gedde J, et al: Comparison of carbamazepine and lithium in treatment of bipolar disorder: a systematic review of randomized controlled trials. Hum Psychopharmacol 24:19–28, 2009

Coxhead N, Silverstone T, Cookson J: Carbamazepine versus lithium in the prophylaxis of bipolar affective disorder. Acta Psychiatr Scand 85:114–118, 1992

Cummings C, Stewart M, Stevenson M, et al: Neurodevelopment of children exposed in utero to lamotrigine, sodium valproate and carbamazepine. Arch Dis Child 96:643–647, 2011

Dardennes R, Even C, Bange F, et al: Comparison of carbamazepine and lithium in the prophylaxis of bipolar disorders: a meta-analysis. Br J Psychiatry 166:378–381, 1995

Davis JM, Janicak PG, Hogan DM: Mood stabilizers in the prevention of recurrent affective disorders: a meta-analysis. Acta Psychiatr Scand 100:406–417, 1999

Denicoff K, Smith-Jackson E, Disney E, et al: Comparative prophylactic efficacy of lithium, carbamazepine, and the combination in bipolar disorder. J Clin Psychiatry 58:470–478, 1997

Di Costanzo E, Schifano F: Lithium alone or in combination with carbamazepine for the treatment of rapid-cycling bipolar affective disorder. Acta Psychiatr Scand 83:456–459, 1991

Dilsaver SC, Swann AC, Shoaib AM, et al: The manic syndrome: factors which may predict a patient's response to lithium, carbamazepine and valproate. J Psychiatry Neurosci 18:61–66, 1993

Eap CB, Yasui N, Kaneko S, et al: Effects of carbamazepine coadministration on plasma concentrations of the enantiomers of mianserin and of its metabolites. Ther Drug Monit 21:166–170, 1999

Elphick M, Lyons F, Cowen PJ: Low tolerability of carbamazepine in psychiatric patients may restrict its clinical usefulness. J Psychopharmacol 2:1–4, 1988

Emrich HM: Studies with (Trileptal) oxcarbazepine in acute mania. Int Clin Psychopharmacol 5:83–88, 1990

Emrich HM, Dose M, von Zerssen D: The use of sodium valproate, carbamazepine and oxcarbazepine in patients with affective disorders. J Affect Disord 8:243–250, 1985

Faigle JW, Feldmann KF: Carbamazepine: chemistry and biotransformation, in Antiepileptic Drugs, 4th Edition. Edited by Levy RH, Mattson RH, Meldrum BS. New York, Raven, 1995, pp 499–513

Fattore C, Cipolla G, Gatti G, et al: Induction of ethinylestradiol and levonorgestrel metabolism by oxcarbazepine in healthy women. Epilepsia 40:783–787, 1999

Frankenburg FR, Tohen M, Cohen BM, et al: Long-term response to carbamazepine: a retrospective study. J Clin Psychopharmacol 8:130–132, 1988

Frey B, Braegger CP, Ghelfi D: Neonatal cholestatic hepatitis from carbamazepine exposure during pregnancy and breast feeding. Ann Pharmacother 36:644–647, 2002

Friis ML, Kristensen O, Boas J, et al: Therapeutic experiences with 947 epileptic out-patients in oxcarbazepine treatment. Acta Neurol Scand 87:224–227, 1993

Froescher W, Eichelbaum M, Niesen M, et al: Carbamazepine levels in breast milk. Ther Drug Monit 6:266–271, 1984

Frye MA, Ketter TA, Leverich GS, et al: The increasing use of polypharmacotherapy for refractory mood disorders: 22 years of study. J Clin Psychiatry 61:9–15, 2000

Gangadhar BN, Desai NG, Channabasavanna SM: Potentiation of lithium with carbamazepine in acute mania. Indian J Psychiatry 29:73–75, 1987

Gernaat HB, Van de Woude J, Touw DJ: Fluoxetine and parkinsonism in patients taking carbamazepine (letter). Am J Psychiatry 148:1604–1605, 1991

Goggin T, Callaghan N: Blood levels of clobazam and its metabolites and therapeutic effect, in Clobazam: Human Psychopharmacology and Clinical Applications (International Congress and Symposium Series, No 74). Edited by Hindmarch I, Stonier PD, Trimble MR. London, Royal Society of Medicine, 1985, pp 149–153

Goncalves N, Stoll KD: [Carbamazepine in manic syndromes: a controlled double-blind study.] Nervenarzt 56:43–47, 1985

Greil W, Ludwig-Mayerhofer W, Erazo N, et al: Lithium versus carbamazepine in the maintenance treatment of bipolar disorders—a randomised study. J Affect Disord 43:151–161, 1997

Greil W, Kleindienst N, Erazo N, et al: Differential response to lithium and carbamazepine in the prophylaxis of bipolar disorder. J Clin Psychopharmacol 18:455–460, 1998

Grossi E, Sacchetti E, Vita A, et al: Carbamazepine versus chlorpromazine in mania: a double-blind trial, in Anticonvulsants in Affective Disorders. Edited by Emrich HM, Okuma T, Müller AA. Amsterdam, Excerpta Medica, 1984, pp 177–187

Hartong EG, Moleman P, Hoogduin CA, et al: Prophylactic efficacy of lithium versus carbamazepine in treatment-naive bipolar patients. J Clin Psychiatry 64:144–151, 2003

Himmelhoch JM: Cerebral dysrhythmia, substance abuse, and the nature of secondary affective illness. Psychiatric Annals 17:710–727, 1987

Himmelhoch JM, Garfinkel ME: Sources of lithium resistance in mixed mania. Psychopharmacol Bull 22:613–620, 1986

Hirschfeld RM, Kasper S: A review of the evidence for carbamazepine and oxcarbazepine in the treatment of bipolar disorder. Int J Neuropsychopharmacol 7:507–522, 2004

Isojarvi JI, Turkka J, Pakarinen AJ, et al: Thyroid function in men taking carbamazepine, oxcarbazepine, or valproate for epilepsy. Epilepsia 42:930–934, 2001

Jann MW, Fidone GS, Israel MK, et al: Increased valproate serum concentrations upon carbamazepine cessation. Epilepsia 29:578–581, 1988

Jann MW, Fidone GS, Hernandez JM, et al: Clinical implications of increased antipsychotic plasma concentrations upon anticonvulsant cessation. Psychiatry Res 28:153–159, 1989

Joffe RT, Post RM: Lithium and carbamazepine-induced agranulocytosis (letter). Am J Psychiatry 146:404, 1989

Jones KL, Lacro RV, Johnson KA, et al: Pattern of malformations in the children of women treated with carbamazepine during pregnancy. N Engl J Med 320:1661–1666, 1989

Joyce PR: Carbamazepine in rapid cycling bipolar affective disorder. Int Clin Psychopharmacol 3:123–129, 1988

Kahn EM, Schulz SC, Perel JM, et al: Change in haloperidol level due to carbamazepine—a complicating factor in combined medication for schizophrenia. J Clin Psychopharmacol 10:54–57, 1990

Kakkar AK, Rehan HS, Unni KE, et al: Comparative efficacy and safety of oxcarbazepine versus divalproex sodium in the treatment of acute mania: a pilot study. Eur Psychiatry 24:178–182, 2009

Keck P Jr, McElroy SL, Vuckovic A, et al: Combined valproate and carbamazepine treatment of bipolar disorder. J Neuropsychiatry Clin Neurosci 4:319–322, 1992

Kerr BM, Thummel KE, Wurden CJ, et al: Human liver carbamazepine metabolism: role of CYP3A4 and CYP2C8 in 10,11-epoxide formation. Biochem Pharmacol 47:1969–1979, 1994

Ketter TA: Handbook of Diagnosis and Treatment of Bipolar Disorder. Washington, DC, American Psychiatric Publishing, 2010

Ketter TA, Wang PW: Predictors of treatment response in bipolar disorders: evidence from clinical and brain imaging studies. J Clin Psychiatry 63:21–25, 2002

Ketter TA, Post RM, Worthington K: Principles of clinically important drug interactions with carbamazepine, part I. J Clin Psychopharmacol 11:198–203, 1991a

Ketter TA, Post RM, Worthington K: Principles of clinically important drug interactions with carbamazepine, part II. J Clin Psychopharmacol 11:306–313, 1991b

Ketter TA, Pazzaglia PJ, Post RM: Synergy of carbamazepine and valproic acid in affective illness: case report and review of the literature. J Clin Psychopharmacol 12:276–281, 1992

Ketter TA, Jenkins JB, Schroeder DH, et al: Carbamazepine but not valproate induces bupropion metabolism. J Clin Psychopharmacol 15:327–333, 1995a

Ketter TA, Post RM, Parekh PI, et al: Addition of monoamine oxidase inhibitors to carbamazepine: preliminary evidence of safety and antidepressant efficacy in treatment-resistant depression. J Clin Psychiatry 56:471–475, 1995b

Ketter TA, Wang PW, Becker OV, et al: The diverse roles of anticonvulsants in bipolar disorders. Ann Clin Psychiatry 15:95–108, 2003

Kishimoto A, Okuma T: Antimanic and prophylactic effects of carbamazepine in affective disorders (abstract 506.4), in 4th World Congress of Biological Psychiatry, September 8–13, 1985, p 363

Klein E, Bental E, Lerer B, et al: Carbamazepine and haloperidol v placebo and haloperidol in excited psychoses: a controlled study. Arch Gen Psychiatry 41:165–170, 1984

Klosterskov Jensen P, Saano V, Haring P, et al: Possible interaction between oxcarbazepine and an oral contraceptive. Epilepsia 33:1149–1152, 1992

Kondo T, Otani K, Hirano T, et al: The effects of phenytoin and carbamazepine on serum concentrations of mono-unsaturated metabolites of valproic acid. Br J Clin Pharmacol 29:116–119, 1990

Kramlinger KG, Post RM: Adding lithium carbonate to carbamazepine: antimanic efficacy in treatment-resistant mania. Acta Psychiatr Scand 79:378–385, 1989a

Kramlinger KG, Post RM: The addition of lithium to carbamazepine: antidepressant efficacy in treatment-resistant depression. Arch Gen Psychiatry 46:794–800, 1989b

Kramlinger KG, Post RM: Addition of lithium carbonate to carbamazepine: hematological and thyroid effects. Am J Psychiatry 147:615–620, 1990

Kuhnz W, Jager-Roman E, Rating D, et al: Carbamazepine and carbamazepine-10,11-epoxide during pregnancy and postnatal period in epileptic mother and their nursed infants: pharmacokinetics and clinical effects. Pediatric Pharmacology (New York) 3:199–208, 1983

Kupfer DJ, Frank E, Grochocinski VJ, et al: Demographic and clinical characteristics of individuals in a bipolar disorder case registry. J Clin Psychiatry 63:120–125, 2002

Kutt H, Solomon G, Peterson H, et al: Accumulation of carbamazepine epoxide caused by valproate contributing to intoxication syndromes. Neurology 35:286–287, 1985

Lenzi A, Lazzerini F, Grossi E, et al: Use of carbamazepine in acute psychosis: a controlled study. J Int Med Res 14:78–84, 1986

Lerer B, Moore N, Meyendorff E, et al: Carbamazepine versus lithium in mania: a double-blind study. J Clin Psychiatry 48:89–93, 1987

Lusznat RM, Murphy DP, Nunn CM: Carbamazepine vs lithium in the treatment and prophylaxis of mania. Br J Psychiatry 153:198–204, 1988

Macphee GJ, Mitchell JR, Wiseman L, et al: Effect of sodium valproate on carbamazepine disposition and psychomotor profile in man. Br J Clin Pharmacol 25:59–66, 1988

Malcolm R, Ballenger JC, Sturgis ET, et al: Double-blind controlled trial comparing carbamazepine to oxazepam treatment of alcohol withdrawal. Am J Psychiatry 146:617–621, 1989

Mattson RH, Cramer JA, Collins JF: A comparison of valproate with carbamazepine for the treatment of complex partial seizures and secondarily generalized tonic-clonic seizures in adults. The Department of Veterans Affairs Epilepsy Cooperative Study No. 264 Group. N Engl J Med 327:765–771, 1992

McCormack M, Alfirevic A, Bourgeois S, et al: HLA-A*3101 and carbamazepine-induced hypersensitivity reactions in Europeans. N Engl J Med 364:1134–1143, 2011

McGinness J, Kishimoto A, Hollister LE: Avoiding neurotoxicity with lithium-carbamazepine combinations. Psychopharmacol Bull 26:181–184, 1990

Meyer MC, Straughn AB, Jarvi EJ, et al: The bioinequivalence of carbamazepine tablets with a history of clinical failures. Pharm Res 9:1612–1616, 1992

Möller HJ, Kissling W, Riehl T, et al: Double-blind evaluation of the antimanic properties of carbamazepine as a comedication to haloperidol. Prog Neuropsychopharmacol Biol Psychiatry 13:127–136, 1989

Moreland TA, Chang SL, Levy RH: Mechanisms of interaction between sodium valproate and carbamazepine in the rhesus monkey and in the isolated perfused rat liver, in Metabolism of Antiepileptic Drugs. Edited by Levy RH, Pitlick WH, Eichelbaum M, et al. New York, Raven, 1984, pp 53–60

Mosolov SN: [Comparative effectiveness of preventive use of lithium carbonate, carbamazepine and sodium valproate in affective and schizoaffective psychoses]. Zh Nevrol Psikhiatr Im S S Korsakova 91:78–83, 1991

Müller AA, Stoll KD: Carbamazepine and oxcarbazepine in the treatment of manic syndromes: studies in Germany, in Anticonvulsants in Affective Disorders. Edited by Emrich HM, Okuma T, Müller AA. Amsterdam, Excerpta Medica, 1984, pp 139–147

Munoz JJ, De Salamanca RE, Diaz-Obregon C, et al: The effect of clobazam on steady state plasma concentrations of carbamazepine and its metabolites. Br J Clin Pharmacol 29:763–765, 1990

Murphy DJ, Gannon MA, McGennis A: Carbamazepine in bipolar affective disorder (letter). Lancet 2(8672):1151–1152, 1989

Murphy JM, Mashman J, Miller JD, et al: Suppression of carbamazepine-induced rash with prednisone. Neurology 41:144–145, 1991

Neumann J, Seidel K, Wunderlich HP: Comparative studies of the effect of carbamazepine and trimipramine in depression, in Anticonvulsants in Affective Disorders. Edited by Emrich HM, Okuma T, Müller AA. Amsterdam, Excerpta Medica, 1984, pp 160–166

Okuma T: Therapeutic and prophylactic effects of carbamazepine in bipolar disorders. Psychiatr Clin North Am 6:157–174, 1983

Okuma T: Effects of carbamazepine and lithium on affective disorders. Neuropsychobiology 27:138–145, 1993

Okuma T, Inanaga K, Otsuki S, et al: Comparison of the antimanic efficacy of carbamazepine and chlorpromazine: a double-blind controlled study. Psychopharmacology 66:211–217, 1979

Okuma T, Inanaga K, Otsuki S, et al: A preliminary double-blind study on the efficacy of carbamazepine in prophylaxis of manic-depressive illness. Psychopharmacology (Berl) 73:95–96, 1981

Okuma T, Yamashita I, Takahashi R, et al: A double-blind study of adjunctive carbamazepine versus placebo on excited states of schizophrenic and schizoaffective disorders. Acta Psychiatr Scand 80:250–259, 1989

Okuma T, Yamashita I, Takahashi R, et al: Comparison of the antimanic efficacy of carbamazepine and lithium carbonate by double-blind controlled study. Pharmacopsychiatry 23:143–150, 1990

Pazzaglia PJ, Post RM, Ketter TA, et al: Preliminary controlled trial of nimodipine in ultra-rapid cycling affective dysregulation. Psychiatry Res 49:257–272, 1993

Pazzaglia PJ, Post RM, Ketter TA, et al: Nimodipine monotherapy and carbamazepine augmentation in patients with refractory recurrent affective illness. J Clin Psychopharmacol 18:404–413, 1998

Physicians' Desk Reference: Physicians' Desk Reference, 66th Edition. Montvale, NJ, Thomson Healthcare, 2012

Placidi GF, Lenzi A, Lazzerini F, et al: The comparative efficacy and safety of carbamazepine versus lithium: a randomized, double-blind 3-year trial in 83 patients. J Clin Psychiatry 47:490–494, 1986

Pope HG Jr, McElroy SL, Keck PE Jr, et al: Valproate in the treatment of acute mania: a placebo-controlled study. Arch Gen Psychiatry 48:62–68, 1991

Post RM: Time course of clinical effects of carbamazepine: implications for mechanisms of action. J Clin Psychiatry 49:35–48, 1988

Post RM, Weiss SR: Tolerance to the prophylactic effects of carbamazepine and related mood stabilizers in the treatment of bipolar disorders. CNS Neurosci Ther 18:256–271, 2010

Post RM, Uhde TW, Ballenger JC, et al: Prophylactic efficacy of carbamazepine in manic-depressive illness. Am J Psychiatry 140:1602–1604, 1983

Post RM, Berrettini W, Uhde TW, et al: Selective response to the anticonvulsant carbamazepine in manic-depressive illness: a case study. J Clin Psychopharmacol 4:178–185, 1984

Post RM, Uhde TW, Roy-Byrne PP, et al: Antidepressant effects of carbamazepine. Am J Psychiatry 143:29–34, 1986

Post RM, Uhde TW, Roy-Byrne PP, et al: Correlates of antimanic response to carbamazepine. Psychiatry Res 21:71–83, 1987

Post RM, Rubinow DR, Uhde TW, et al: Dysphoric mania: clinical and biological correlates. Arch Gen Psychiatry 46:353–358, 1989

Post RM, Leverich GS, Rosoff AS, et al: Carbamazepine prophylaxis in refractory affective disorders: a focus on long-term follow-up. J Clin Psychopharmacol 10:318–327, 1990

Post RM, Altshuler LL, Ketter TA, et al: Antiepileptic drugs in affective illness: clinical and theoretical implications. Adv Neurol 55:239–277, 1991

Prien RF, Gelenberg AJ: Alternatives to lithium for preventive treatment of bipolar disorder. Am J Psychiatry 146:840–848, 1989

Pynnönen S, Kanto J, Sillanpaa M, et al: Carbamazepine: placental transport, tissue concentrations in foetus and newborn, and level in milk. Acta Pharmacol Toxicol (Copenh) 41:244–253, 1977

Raitasuo V, Lehtovaara R, Huttunen MO: Carbamazepine and plasma levels of clozapine (letter). Am J Psychiatry 150:169, 1993

Rambeck B, May T, Juergens U: Serum concentrations of carbamazepine and its epoxide and diol metabolites in epileptic patients: the influence of dose and comedication. Ther Drug Monit 9:298–303, 1987

Rattya J, Vainionpaa L, Knip M, et al: The effects of valproate, carbamazepine, and oxcarbazepine on growth and sexual maturation in girls with epilepsy. Pediatrics 103:588–593, 1999

Ries RK, Roy-Byrne PP, Ward NG, et al: Carbamazepine treatment for benzodiazepine withdrawal. Am J Psychiatry 146:536–537, 1989

Ringel RA, Brick JF: Perspective on carbamazepine-induced water intoxication: reversal by demeclocycline. Neurology 36:1506–1507, 1986

Rosa FM: Spina bifida in infants of women treated with carbamazepine during pregnancy. N Engl J Med 324:674–677, 1991

Scheffner D, Konig S, Rauterberg-Ruland I, et al: Fatal liver failure in 16 children with valproate therapy. Epilepsia 29:530–542, 1988

Shimoyama R, Ohkubo T, Sugawara K: Monitoring of carbamazepine and carbamazepine 10,11-epoxide in breast milk and plasma by high-performance liquid chromatography. Ann Clin Biochem 37:210–215, 2000

Sitland-Marken PA, Rickman LA, Wells BG, et al: Pharmacologic management of acute mania in pregnancy. J Clin Psychopharmacol 9:78–87, 1989

Small JG: Anticonvulsants in affective disorders. Psychopharmacol Bull 26:25–36, 1990

Small JG, Klapper MH, Milstein V, et al: Carbamazepine compared with lithium in the treatment of mania. Arch Gen Psychiatry 48:915–921, 1991

Smith LA, Cornelius V, Warnock A, et al: Effectiveness of mood stabilizers and antipsychotics in the maintenance phase of bipolar disorder: a systematic review of randomized controlled trials. Bipolar Disord 9:394–412, 2007

Steinacher L, Vandel P, Zullino DF, et al: Carbamazepine augmentation in depressive patients non-responding to citalopram: a pharmacokinetic and clinical pilot study. Eur Neuropsychopharmacol 12:255–260, 2002

Stoll KD, Bisson HE, Fischer E, et al: Carbamazepine versus haloperidol in manic syndromes—first report of a multicentric study in Germany, in Biological Psychiatry 1985. Edited by Shagass C. Amsterdam, Elsevier, 1986, pp 332–334

Thweatt RE: Carbamazepine/MAOI interaction (letter). Psychosomatics 27:538, 1986

Tohen M, Castillo J, Pope H Jr, et al: Concomitant use of valproate and carbamazepine in bipolar and schizoaffective disorders. J Clin Psychopharmacol 14:67–70, 1994

Tohen M, Castillo J, Baldessarini RJ, et al: Blood dyscrasias with carbamazepine and valproate: a pharmacoepidemiological study of 2,228 patients at risk. Am J Psychiatry 152:413–418, 1995

Tohen M, Bowden CL, Smulevich AB, et al: Olanzapine plus carbamazepine vs carbamazepine alone in treating manic episodes. Br J Psychiatry 192:135–143, 2008

Van Parys JA, Meinardi H: Survey of 260 epileptic patients treated with oxcarbazepine (Trileptal) on a named-patient basis. Epilepsy Res 19:79–85, 1994

Vasudev A, Macritchie K, Watson S, et al: Oxcarbazepine in the maintenance treatment of bipolar disorder. Cochrane Database Syst Rev (1):CD005171, 2008

Verrotti A, Coppola G, Parisi P, et al: Bone and calcium metabolism and antiepileptic drugs. Clin Neurol Neurosurg 112:1–10, 2010

Verrotti A, D'Egidio C, Mohn A, et al: Antiepileptic drugs, sex hormones, and PCOS. Epilepsia 52:199–211, 2011

Vick NA: Suppression of carbamazepine-induced skin rash with prednisone (letter). N Engl J Med 309:1193–1194, 1983

Vieta E, Cruz N, Garcia-Campayo J, et al: A double-blind, randomized, placebo-controlled prophylaxis trial of oxcarbazepine as adjunctive treatment to lithium in the long-term treatment of bipolar I and II disorder. Int J Neuropsychopharmacol 11:445–452, 2008

Wagner KD, Kowatch RA, Emslie GJ, et al: A double-blind, randomized, placebo-controlled trial of oxcarbazepine in the treatment of bipolar disorder in children and adolescents. Am J Psychiatry 163:1179–1186, 2006

Watkins SE, Callender K, Thomas DR, et al: The effect of carbamazepine and lithium on remission from affective illness. Br J Psychiatry 150:180–182, 1987

Weisler RH, Kalali AH, Ketter TA: A multicenter, randomized, double-blind, placebo-controlled trial of extended-release carbamazepine capsules as monotherapy for bipolar disorder patients with manic or mixed episodes. J Clin Psychiatry 65:478–484, 2004

Weisler RH, Keck PE Jr, Swann AC, et al: Extended-release carbamazepine capsules as monotherapy for acute mania in bipolar disorder: a multicenter, randomized, double-blind, placebo-controlled trial. J Clin Psychiatry 66:323–330, 2005

Wildgrube C: Case studies on prophylactic long-term effects of oxcarbazepine in recurrent affective disorders. Int Clin Psychopharmacol 5:89S–94S, 1990

Yatham LN, Grossman F, Augustyns I, et al: Mood stabilisers plus risperidone or placebo in the treatment of acute mania. International, double-blind, randomised controlled trial. Br J Psychiatry 182:141–147, 2003

Zhang ZJ, Kang WH, Tan QR, et al: Adjunctive herbal medicine with carbamazepine for bipolar disorders: a double-blind, randomized, placebo-controlled study. J Psychiatr Res 41:360–369, 2007

CHAPTER 29

Gabapentin and Pregabalin

Mark A. Frye, M.D.

Katherine Marshall Moore, M.D.

Gabapentin

Early observations of enhanced general well-being in epileptic patients treated with anticonvulsants, as well as various early hypotheses of kindling and sensitization proposed as models of affective illness progression (Weiss and Post 1998), have promoted controlled investigations of anticonvulsant drugs as potential mood-stabilizing agents.

Gabapentin is U.S. Food and Drug Administration (FDA) approved for the adjunctive treatment of complex partial epilepsy with and without generalization and for the management of postherpetic neuralgia in adults. A retrospective review of five placebo-controlled trials of gabapentin in more than 700 patients with refractory partial seizure disorder additionally supported the concept of improvement in general well-being, prompting controlled investigation of the drug in primary psychiatric conditions (Dimond et al. 1996).

Pharmacological Profile and Mechanism of Action

The mechanism of gabapentin's anticonvulsant and psychotropic actions is not fully understood. Gabapentin was originally developed as a γ-aminobutyric (GABA) analog. As reviewed by Taylor et al. (1998), GABA is the major inhibitory neurotransmitter in the cerebral cortex. Preclinical studies have suggested that gabapentin increases brain and intracellular GABA by an amino acid active transporter at the blood-brain barrier and multiple enzymatic regulatory mechanisms, respectively. In vitro, gabapentin increases the activity of glutamic acid decarboxylase, the enzyme that converts glutamate to GABA (Taylor et al. 1992). Conversely, gabapentin has been shown to inhibit GABA-transaminase (GABA-T), the enzyme primarily responsible for GABA catabolism (Loscher et al. 1991). Glutamate metabolism is also modulated by gabapentin. In vitro, gabapentin inhibits branched-chain amino acid aminotransferase (BCAA-T), an enzyme responsible for glutamate synthesis (Hutson et al. 1998), and activates glutamate dehydrogenase, an enzyme primarily involved in glutamate catabolism (Goldlust et al. 1995).

These enzymatic regulatory mechanisms that suggest an increased synthesis and decreased degradation of GABA are clinically relevant. Several, but not all, studies have reported decreased levels of cerebrospinal fluid (Gerner et al. 1996; Gold et al. 1980; Roy et al. 1991), plasma (Petty et al. 1990), and magnetic resonance (MR) spectroscopic GABA (Sanacora et al. 1999) in patients with affective illness in comparison with healthy control subjects. Furthermore, increased MR spectroscopic occipital GABA concentrations have been reported with serotonin reuptake inhibitor treatment in depressed patients (Sanacora et al. 2002) and gabapentin treatment in patients with complex partial epilepsy (Petroff et al. 1996).

Gabapentin has also been shown to bind to the α_2 subunit receptor of brain voltage-dependent calcium channels, which may relate to the subsequent inhibition of monoaminergic transmission (Schlicker et al. 1985). There is no known direct activity at the dopamine, serotonin, benzodiazepine, or histamine receptors. However, gabapentin has been reported to increase whole-blood levels of serotonin in healthy control subjects (Rao et al. 1988).

Pharmacokinetics and Disposition

All bioavailability, distribution, and elimination parameters are based on the gabapentin molecule itself, as there is no active metabolite. Gabapentin exhibits nonlinear bioavailability most likely related to an active saturable L-amino acid transport carrier present in gut and blood-brain barrier (McLean 1999). There is no evidence of plasma protein binding, hepatic metabolism, or cytochrome P450 (CYP) autoinduction. Elimination half-life is 6–8 hours, with a recommended three-times-a-day dosing strategy. Gabapentin is eliminated from systemic circulation unchanged by renal excretion. Patients with compromised renal function will show evidence of reduced gabapentin clearance.

Indications and Efficacy

Epilepsy

Gabapentin currently is FDA approved as an adjunctive treatment for partial seizures with and without secondary generalization in adults with epilepsy (Physicians' Desk Reference 2006). This indication was based on controlled evaluations of gabapentin at daily doses of 600–1,800 mg. Additional research has reported efficacy and tolerability for gabapentin monotherapy at daily dosages up to 4,800 mg in patients with refractory epilepsy (Beydoun et al. 1998). There is no established therapeutic plasma level for seizure control. Gabapentin has a highly desirable side-effect profile. Only mild side effects (sedation, dizziness, and ataxia) have been commonly reported.

Nonepilepsy Neurological Conditions

Neuropathic pain. On the basis of two placebo-controlled studies (Rice et al. 2001; Rowbotham et al. 1998), gabapentin has received FDA approval for use in the management of postherpetic neuralgia in adults. Gabapentin has also been systemically evaluated in diabetic neuropathy (Backonja et al. 1998).

The initial postherpetic neuralgia (Rowbotham et al. 1998) and diabetic neuropathy (Backonja et al. 1998) studies were randomized, double-blind, placebo-controlled, parallel-group multicenter investigations with three phases of evaluation. The first phase identified the subject population (patients with diabetic neuropathy of 1–5 years' duration [Backonja et al. 1998] or postherpetic neuralgia of 3 months' duration [Rowbotham et al. 1998]). The 8-week double-blind phases consisted of a 4-week step titration (week 1, 900 mg; week 2, 1,800 mg; week 3, 2,400 mg; and week 4, 3,600 mg) and a 4-week fixed-dose period wherein the dose that was effective and tolerable from the titration phase was held constant. There were no differences in demographics or rates of dropout because of inefficacy or adverse events between the gabapentin group and the placebo group.

Among the 229 postherpetic neuralgia patients (Rowbotham et al. 1998), greater pain reduction occurred with gabapentin, noted as early as week 2 and maintained throughout the entire study period. Similarly, secondary measures of mood such as depression, anger-hostility, fatigue-inertia, and physical functioning were more effectively treated with gabapentin than with placebo. Eighty-three percent of the gabapentin group was maintained on the 2,400-mg daily dose, and 65% were maintained on the 3,600-mg daily dose.

Among the 165 diabetic neuropathy patients (Backonja et al. 1998), greater pain reduction (as measured with an 11-point Likert scale) occurred with gabapentin than with placebo; this difference was statistically significant as early as week 2 of the blind titration phase and remained significant for the duration of the 8-week study. Significant reductions in sleep interference related to pain were also reported, as well as improved quality of life. Gabapentin appeared to be well tolerated, as 67% of the patient group maintained a maximum dose of 3,600 mg.

Finally, a 7-week placebo-controlled study evaluated gabapentin (1,800 or 2,400 mg/day in three divided doses) in 334 patients with postherpetic neuralgia (Rice et al. 2001). Pain was significantly reduced with both gabapentin doses, with similar improvements in sleep. The improvement in pain score was noted as early as week 1 and was maintained throughout the study.

Movement disorders. Controlled investigations of gabapentin have been conducted in several movement disorders. These studies, albeit controlled, were much smaller than the neuropathic pain studies mentioned in the prior section but included amyotrophic lateral sclerosis (ALS) (Miller et al. 1996), essential tremor (Ondo et al. 2000; Pahwa et al. 1998), and parkinsonism (Olson et al. 1997).

In a study of 152 patients with ALS, patients were randomly assigned to a 2,400-mg daily dose of gabapentin or placebo for 6 months. Decline in muscle strength, the primary outcome measure, was slower in the gabapentin-treated patients than in the placebo-treated patients (Miller et al. 1996).

Controlled studies of gabapentin for essential tremor have reported mixed results. The first 2-week controlled study showed no difference between gabapentin 1,800 mg/day and placebo for treatment of essential tremor (Pahwa et al. 1998). A second 6-week controlled study evaluating two gabapentin dosages—1,800 mg/day and 3,600 mg/day—in patients with essential tremor found significant improvements in self-report scores, observed tremor scores, and activities of daily living scores in patients who were randomly assigned to gabapentin compared with patients who received placebo (Ondo et al. 2000).

In a 1-month double-blind, placebo-controlled evaluation of gabapentin in 19 patients with advanced parkinsonism, gabapentin at a mean daily total dose of 1,200 mg was superior to placebo in reducing rigidity, bradykinesia, and tremor, as measured by the United Parkinson's Disease Rating Scale (Olson et al. 1997). The rigidity and bradykinesia improvements were independent of tremor improvement.

Migraine headache. The comorbidity of migraine headache disorder and bipolar disorder is highly prevalent and clinically significant (Mahmood et al. 1999). Anticonvulsants, because of their mood-stabilizing and migraine prophylactic properties, appear to be ideal in this patient population. Mathew et al. (2001) suggested that gabapentin is an effective agent for migraine prophylaxis. One hundred forty-three patients with migraine (with and without aura) participated in this three-phase controlled evaluation of gabapentin. Phase 1 was a 4-week single-blind placebo period during which baseline migraine headache frequency was established. Phase 2 was a 4-week double-blind, placebo-controlled, flexible-dose titration period during which patients received gabapentin dosages of up to 2,400 mg/day. Phase 3 was an 8-week double-blind, placebo-controlled period during which the dosage of gabapentin was held constant. Patients randomly assigned to 2,400 mg/day gabapentin had significant reductions in migraine attacks in comparison with placebo-treated patients. Dropout rates were higher with gabapentin and were primarily related to drowsiness and somnolence.

Anxiety Disorders

Gabapentin exhibits a dose-dependent anxiolytic response in animal models (Singh et al. 1996). Open-trial investigations have reported positive results with add-on gabapentin in the treatment of generalized anxiety disorder (Pollack et al. 1998), panic disorder (Pollack et al. 1998), and refractory obsessive-compulsive disorder (Cora-Locatelli et al. 1998). Two controlled investigations of gabapentin in social phobia (Pande et al. 1999) and panic disorder (Pande et al. 2000b) suggest anxiolytic activity.

Pande et al. (1999) investigated gabapentin in a 14-week randomized, double-blind, placebo-controlled two-site study of 69 outpatients with DSM-IV (American Psychiatric Association 1994)–confirmed social phobia. All patients were required to have a score of 50 or higher on the Liebowitz Social Anxiety Scale (LSAS) at baseline. Reduction in the LSAS score served as the primary outcome measure. In intent-to-treat analysis, gabapentin was more effective than placebo in reducing social anxiety symptoms. The dosage range for gabapentin was 900–3,600 mg/day, with 56% of patients responding to and tolerating the maximum daily dosage of 3,600 mg. Dizziness and dry mouth were significantly more common in patients treated with gabapentin.

The second study was an 8-week randomized, placebo-controlled six-site monotherapy study of 103 patients with DSM-IV-confirmed panic disorder with or without agoraphobia (Pande et al. 2000b). Gabapentin was dosed flexibly between 600 and 3,600 mg/day. The primary outcome measure was a decrease in the Panic and Agoraphobia Scale (PAS) score. There were no differences in dropout rate. In the intent-to-treat analysis, no difference in PAS score reduction was seen between patients randomly assigned to gabapentin and those given placebo. In a post hoc stratification between high (≥20) and low (<20) PAS symptom severity, patients with high symptom severity randomly assigned to gabapentin had a greater baseline-to-endpoint decrease in the PAS score than did those randomly assigned to placebo. Somnolence, headache, dizziness, infection, asthenia, and ataxia were more common in gabapentin-treated patients.

Bipolar Disorder

Numerous case reports and open trials of gabapentin as a mood stabilizer, encompassing more than 400 patients with a pooled response rate between 65% and 70%, have been reviewed elsewhere (Frye et al. 2000; Yatham et al. 2002).

One double-blind, placebo-controlled outpatient study evaluated add-on gabapentin for the treatment of bipolar I disorder with manic, hypomanic, or mixed symptoms (Pande et al. 2000a). The first phase of the study involved a 2-week single-blind, placebo lead-in wherein doses of the subject's primary mood stabilizer (lithium or valproate) could be adjusted to maximal clinical benefit and minimum threshold of therapeutic level (i.e., lithium level of 0.5 mmol/L, valproate level >50 μg/mL). The second phase of the study was a 10-week double-blind phase in which subjects were randomly assigned to gabapentin—dosed flexibly between 600 and 3,600 mg/day (three-times-a-day dosing)—or placebo. In the intent-to-treat population, 117 subjects were randomized; no differences in demographic profile or dropout rate were found between the two groups. The primary outcome measure—total decreased score on the Young Mania Rating Scale—was significantly different between groups in favor of add-on placebo. In a post hoc analysis, lithium adjustments in the single-blind, placebo lead-in phase were made more frequently in the placebo group than in the gabapentin group; most of these adjustments (9 of 12; 75%) consisted of a dosage increase. This fact suggests either a strong placebo response or the effect of maximizing lithium blood levels to achieve a greater antimanic response. Of the gabapentin-treated patients who had drug levels measured, nearly 20% had plasma gabapentin levels that were undetectable.

The second controlled study was a 6-week double-blind, placebo-controlled crossover comparative trial of gabapentin monotherapy, lamotrigine monotherapy, and placebo in 35 inpatients with refractory mood disorder (Frye et al. 2000; Obrocea et al. 2002). In the preliminary analysis (Frye et al. 2000) and final analysis (Obrocea et al. 2002), gabapentin demonstrated no better treatment response than placebo in a group of patients with highly refractory bipolar (primarily rapid-cycling) disorder.

There appears to be a marked contrast between the pooled results of the uncontrolled observations (generally positive) and the results of the controlled studies (generally negative). The important limitations of the controlled investigations include placebo response versus maximized lithium response in the placebo group, lack of rigorous compliance assessment, and use of a monotherapy study design in a cohort of patients with primarily rapid-cycling, treatment-refractory illness.

Substance Abuse and Withdrawal

Mood-stabilizing anticonvulsants such as divalproex sodium and carbamazepine are possible treatments for alcohol-abusing bipolar patients (Malcolm et al. 2001). Gabapentin has been shown to decrease excitability and convulsions in animal models of alcohol withdrawal (Watson et al. 1997). The lack of hepatic metabolism, CYP enzyme induction, protein binding, and addictive potential makes gabapentin a potentially useful compound in this patient population.

The potential of gabapentin for treating alcohol withdrawal was considered after initial positive reports emerged (Bozikas et al. 2002). One study demonstrated a similar efficacy to phenobarbital in treating alcohol withdrawal (Mariani et al. 2006), although another controlled trial did not substantiate gabapentin's benefit over placebo (Bonnet et al. 2003). In a post hoc analysis (Bonnet et al. 2007), there was a significant increase in the Profile of Mood States (POMS) vigor subscore in the gabapentin group versus the placebo group; this was particularly robust in patients with comorbid mild depression.

Despite the conflicting results for gabapentin's efficacy in alcohol withdrawal, there is increasing recognition of its therapeutic benefit for the sleep disturbance component of alcohol withdrawal syndrome. Low-dose gabapentin (mean dose = 900 mg) in the treatment of alcohol withdrawal, in comparison with trazodone, was associated with greater improvement in sleep problems, as assessed with the Sleep Problems Questionnaire (Karam-Hage and Brower 2003). In addition, gabapentin, in comparison with lorazepam, was associated with significant reductions in self-reported sleep disturbances and daytime sleepiness (Malcolm et al. 2007).

One 4-week placebo-controlled, randomized, double-blind study evaluated gabapentin in alcohol abuse relapse prevention (Furieri and Nakamura-Palacios 2007). After detoxification, 60 alcohol-dependent men who had been consuming, on average, 17 drinks per day for the preceding 3 months were randomly assigned to gabapentin (300 mg twice daily) or placebo. The gabapentin group showed significant reductions in number of drinks per day, percentage of heavy drinking days, and craving for alcohol (specifically automaticity of drinking) as well as increases in percentage of days abstinent. More recently, the addition of gabapentin to naltrexone was reported to significantly improve drinking outcomes compared with naltrexone alone or placebo in a study of 150 alcohol-dependent subjects (Anton et al. 2011).

Finally, in a proof-of-concept randomized controlled study in 50 treatment-seeking outpatients with cannabis dependence, gabapentin at 1,200 mg/day was significantly more effective than placebo in reducing cannabis use and decreasing withdrawal symptoms (Mason et al. 2012).

Side Effects and Toxicology

Gabapentin has a highly desirable side-effect profile that has been remarkably consistent among the controlled studies of diverse disease states. Sedation, drowsiness, and dizziness always have been reported, and ataxia, dry mouth, infection, and asthenia have been reported in at least one placebo-controlled study.

Adverse events caused by gabapentin have been few but have important psychiatric implications. Gabapentin-induced hypomania and mania have been reported (Lewke et al. 1999; Short and Cooke 1995). The controlled mania study did not report data on percentage of the patients with exacerbation of mania secondary to gabapentin treatment (Pande et al. 2000a). Gabapentin also has been associated with aggression, both in pediatric epilepsy (Wolf et al. 1996) and in adult mania (Pinninti and Mahajan 2001).

Gabapentin has a broad therapeutic index and appears to be safe in overdose. The broadness of the therapeutic index is most likely related to its nonlinear bioavailability secondary to a saturable transport carrier (McLean 1999).

Drug-Drug Interactions

Given its lack of hepatic metabolism, CYP autoinduction, and minimal plasma protein binding, gabapentin has been shown not to affect levels of anticonvulsant drugs; similarly, gabapentin pharmacokinetics were unchanged with hepatically metabolized anticonvulsants (Physicians' Desk Reference 2006). Gabapentin's renal excretion, however, does pose potential risk when the drug is used concomitantly with lithium.

Although the therapeutic index with gabapentin is large, that is not the case with lithium. In a single 600-mg lithium dose pharmacokinetic study, there was no difference in maximal lithium concentration (Li C_{max}), time to reach C_{max}, or area under the curve in 13 patients receiving steady-state gabapentin (mean dose = 3,645.15 ± 931.5 mg) compared with those receiving steady-state placebo (Frye et al. 1998). It is important to emphasize that this study was in a patient population with normal renal function; cases of reversible renal impairment associated with gabapentin have been reported (Grunze et al. 1998).

Summary for Gabapentin

Controlled studies of gabapentin clearly have suggested its efficacy in several medical conditions, including complex partial epilepsy, postherpetic neuropathy, diabetic neuropathy, and migraine prophylaxis. Conclusions are less clear, either because of positive controlled studies of a small sample size or because of negative studies in alcohol abuse/dependence relapse prevention, ALS, essential tremor, parkinsonism, social phobia, and panic disorder. Gabapentin's role as a mood stabilizer is not clearly established. Gabapentin has a favorable pharmacokinetic profile, with particular advantage in patients with compromised hepatic function. Its minimal drug-drug interactions, low risk of toxicity, and favorable side-effect profile make it a useful addition to the pharmacopoeia.

Pregabalin

Pregabalin is an anticonvulsant drug approved by the FDA for the adjunctive treatment of partial-onset seizures in adults. It is also approved for the treatment of neuropathic pain associated with diabetic peripheral neuropathy, postherpetic neuralgia, and fibromyalgia. Like many of the newer anticonvulsant agents, pregabalin has been evaluated in carefully controlled studies for possible utility in neurological and psychiatric conditions other than primary epilepsy.

Pharmacological Profile and Mechanism of Action

Pregabalin, like gabapentin, is a structural analog of the inhibitory neurotransmitter GABA. Pregabalin had greater potency than gabapentin in preclinical models of epilepsy, pain, and anxiety (Hamandi and Sander 2006). Although pregabalin is a GABA structural analog, it has no clinically significant effect at either the $GABA_A$ or $GABA_B$ receptor and is not converted metabolically into GABA or a GABA agonist (Kavoussi 2006). Furthermore, pregabalin does not bind to any serotonergic, dopaminergic, or glutamatergic receptors. It does bind to the $\alpha_2\delta$ subunit of the presynaptic voltage-gated calcium channel, producing a decrease in excitatory neurotransmitter release (Dooley et al. 2002; Kavoussi 2006). In contrast to other GABA reuptake inhibitory anticonvulsants (e.g., tiagabine) or anticonvulsants that modulate enzymatic activity related to GABA production (e.g., vigabatrin), pregabalin does not have any direct GABA reuptake–inhibitory effects or GABA transaminase–inhibiting effects.

Pharmacokinetics and Disposition

Pregabalin exhibits linear pharmacokinetics and is not associated with any significant protein binding or hepatic metabolism. Its oral bioavailability is greater than 90% and independent of dose. Steady-state plasma levels are generally achieved within 24–48 hours. Administration with food has no clinically significant effect on the extent of absorption or on elimination. The elimination half-life of the drug is approximately 6.5 hours (Montgomery 2006). Because it is highly lipophilic and does not bind to plasma protein, pregabalin readily crosses the blood-brain barrier. Pregabalin is primarily renally excreted and has no active metabolites. Dosage adjustment is required in patients with renal impairment. Pregabalin does not induce or inhibit CYP enzymes, nor do CYP enzyme inhibitors alter its pharmacokinetics as a consequence.

Indications and Efficacy

Epilepsy

Several placebo-controlled studies have evaluated pregabalin in the treatment of patients with refractory partial epilepsy (Elger et al. 2005; Hamandi and Sander 2006). Response rates for pregabalin dosed at 600 mg/day were similar to those reported in other trials of antiepileptic drugs in refractory epilepsy. The study by Elger et al. (2005) showed that pregabalin administered in either fixed or flexible doses was highly effective and generally well tolerated as add-on therapy for partial seizures with or without secondary generalization.

Nonepilepsy Neurological Conditions

Postherpetic neuralgia. Four placebo-controlled studies have evaluated pregabalin for postherpetic neuropathic pain (Dworkin et al. 2003; Freynhagen et al. 2005; Sabatowski et al. 2004; Van Seventer et al. 2006). The first study (Dworkin et al. 2003) was an 8-week parallel-group, double-blind, placebo-controlled, randomized multicenter trial of patients with postherpetic neuralgia, who received either pregabalin 600 mg/day (300 mg/day if there was reduced creatinine clearance) or placebo. At study endpoint, there was a significant decrease in mean pain scores for patients treated with pregabalin compared with placebo. The superior pain relief with pregabalin was identified as early as day 2 and was maintained throughout the 8 weeks of double-blind treatment. In a second study (Freynhagen et al. 2005), patients with chronic postherpetic neuralgia or diabetic peripheral neuropathy were randomly assigned to placebo, flexible-dose pregabalin titrated upward to a maximum dosage of 600 mg/day, or fixed-dose pregabalin at 300 mg/day for the first week followed by 600 mg/day for the remaining 11 weeks. Both flexible- and fixed-dose pregabalin significantly reduced endpoint mean pain scores and were significantly superior to placebo in improving pain-related sleep interference. In a third study, Van Seventer et al. (2006) evaluated pregabalin (150, 300, or 600 mg/day in bid dosing) or placebo in 370 patients with postherpetic neuralgia. Pregabalin provided significant dose-proportional pain relief at endpoint, different from placebo. Sleep interference in all pregabalin groups was significantly improved at endpoint. Similar results were obtained in the Sabatowski et al. (2004) study, which reported improvement in sleep and mood disturbance in patients treated with pregabalin. In total, these four studies showed benefit in pain reduction, sleep improvement, and mood associated with pregabalin treatment. The most common side effects were dizziness, peripheral edema, weight gain, and somnolence.

Diabetic peripheral neuropathy. Freeman et al. (2008) conducted a pooled analysis of data from seven published randomized, placebo-controlled trials encompassing 400 patients with diabetic peripheral neuropathy. The primary outcome measure was change from baseline to endpoint in mean pain score from patients' daily pain diaries. With three-times-daily administration, all pregabalin dosages (150, 300, and 600 mg/day) significantly reduced pain and pain-related sleep interference in comparison with placebo. With twice-daily administration, only the 600-mg/day dosage showed efficacy. Pregabalin's pain-reducing and sleep-improving properties appeared to be positively correlated with dose, with the greatest effect observed in patients treated with 600 mg/day.

Fibromyalgia

Pregabalin is the first medication to receive an FDA indication for the treatment of fibromyalgia. Fibromyalgia is a common chronic pain disorder characterized by widespread, diffuse musculoskeletal pain and tenderness frequently accompanied by significant psychiatric comorbidity, including fatigue, sleep disturbance, and mood and anxiety disorders. Classifications of disease severity for fibromyalgia have been published by the American College of Rheumatology (Wolfe et al. 1990). Prevalence estimates for fibromyalgia are 2% of the U.S. population, with rates higher in adult women than in men (Arnold et al. 2007).

Two placebo-controlled acute-treatment studies (Crofford et al. 2005; Mease et al. 2008) and one placebo-controlled relapse prevention study (Crofford et al. 2008) have evaluated pregabalin in the treatment of patients with fibromyalgia. In the first, an 8-week double-blind, randomized, placebo-controlled study of pregabalin (150, 300, and 450 mg/day) versus placebo, the 450-mg daily dose significantly reduced the average severity of pain in comparison with placebo (Crofford et al. 2005). Sleep improvement was noted at both the 300- and the 450-mg daily dosages. Dizziness and somnolence were the most frequent adverse events. Arnold et al. (2007), in recognition of the large overlap of psychiatric comorbidity in fibromyalgia, conducted a post hoc analysis of the Crofford et al. (2005) study to assess symptoms of anxiety and depression and their impact on pregabalin treatment. Of 529 patients who had enrolled in pregabalin treatment for fibromyalgia, significantly more patients endorsed anxiety symptoms (71%) than endorsed depressive symptoms (56%). Improvement in pain symptoms with pregabalin versus placebo did not depend on baseline anxiety or depression; in fact, 75% of the pain reduction was not explained by improvements in mood and/or anxiety.

The second 13-week double-blind, placebo-controlled multicenter study randomly assigned 748 patients with fibromyalgia to receive either placebo or pregabalin dosages of 300, 450, or 600 mg/day (twice-daily dosing) (Mease et al. 2008). The primary outcome measure was symptomatic relief of pain associated with fibromyalgia, as measured by a mean pain score from an 11-point numeric rating scale (0 = no pain; 10 = worst possible pain) from patients' daily diaries. Patients in all pregabalin groups showed statistically significant improvement in endpoint mean pain scores as well as in sleep.

Finally, the 6-month double-blind, placebo-controlled Fibromyalgia Relapse Evaluation and Efficacy for Durability Of Meaningful Relief (FREEDOM) study evaluated pregabalin in nearly 600 patients with fibromyalgia (Crofford et al. 2008). This study included an initial 6-week open-label phase followed by a 26-week double-blind treatment with ongoing pregabalin or blind substitution to placebo. The primary outcome measure was time to loss of therapeutic response, defined as less than 30% reduction in pain or worsening of symptoms of fibromyalgia. Time to loss of therapeutic response was significantly greater for the pregabalin group than for the placebo group, with Kaplan-Meier estimates of time to event showing that half of the placebo group had relapsed by day 19, whereas half of the pregabalin group had still not lost response by trial end.

These three placebo-controlled studies in patients with fibromyalgia in the acute or relapse prevention phase mark a substantial advance in clinical trial design of novel uses of anticonvulsants and represent a milestone in the first FDA-approved treatment for fibromyalgia.

Anxiety Disorders

Generalized anxiety disorder. Findings from four placebo-controlled studies contributed to the approval of pregabalin in Europe for generalized anxiety disorder (Montgomery et al. 2006; Pande et al. 2003; Pohl et al. 2005; Rickels et al. 2005). In the first study (Pande et al. 2003), 276 patients with generalized anxiety disorder were randomly assigned to pregabalin 150 or 600 mg/day, lorazepam 6 mg/day, or placebo. The 6-week trial included a 1-week placebo lead-in, 4 weeks of blind treatment, and a 1-week taper. The primary efficacy outcome measure was the endpoint Hamilton Anxiety Scale (Ham-A) score. The mean baseline-to-endpoint decrease in Ham-A total score in all three active-treatment groups (pregabalin 150 mg/day, pregabalin 600 mg/day, and lorazepam 6 mg/day) was significantly greater than the decrease in the placebo group. Percentages of subjects who met a secondary outcome measure, a reduction of 50% or greater in the Ham-A score, were significantly higher in the pregabalin 600-mg/day group (46%) and the lorazepam group (61%) than in the placebo group (27%). There were no significant differences in response rates by either definition between patients receiving pregabalin 150 mg/day and patients receiving placebo.

In the second study by Pohl et al. (2005), twice-daily versus three-times-daily dosing of pregabalin was evaluated in a 6-week double-blind, placebo-controlled study. In this study, 250 patients with generalized anxiety disorder were randomly assigned to pregabalin 100 mg twice daily, 200 mg twice daily, 150 mg three times daily, or placebo. Mean improvement in the Ham-A total score was significantly greater with pregabalin at all doses than with placebo. Pairwise comparisons of twice-daily versus three-times-daily dosing found no significant differences in outcome. All three pregabalin groups showed significantly greater improvement in comparison with placebo at endpoint.

In the third study by Rickels et al. (2005), 454 patients with generalized anxiety disorder were randomly assigned in a 4-week design to pregabalin 300 mg/day, 450 mg/day, or 600 mg/day; alprazolam 1.5 mg/day; or placebo.

The primary outcome measure was change from baseline to endpoint in the total Ham-A score. In comparison with the placebo group, all treatment groups showed significantly greater reductions in mean Ham-A total score at last-observation-carried-forward (LOCF) analysis. A significantly higher proportion of patients in the pregabalin (all dosages) and alprazolam groups than in the placebo group met the endpoint response criterion of 50% or greater reduction in Ham-A total score. The response rate for the 300-mg/day pregabalin group (61%) was significantly higher than that for the alprazolam group (43%).

In the only pregabalin study with an active antidepressant comparator, Montgomery et al. (2006) randomly assigned 421 patients with generalized anxiety disorder to 6 weeks of double-blind treatment with pregabalin (400 or 600 mg/day), venlafaxine (75 mg/day), or placebo. The primary outcome measure was change in the Ham-A total score from baseline to LOCF analysis. Pregabalin (both dosages) and venlafaxine produced significantly greater improvement in the Ham-A total score than did placebo. Patients receiving pregabalin 400 mg/day experienced significant improvement in all primary and secondary outcome measures in comparison with those receiving placebo. Rates of discontinuation associated with adverse events were highest in the venlafaxine group (20.4%), followed by the pregabalin 600 mg/day (13.6%), pregabalin 400 mg/day (6.2%), and placebo (9.9%) groups.

Other trials have followed in the wake of these earlier studies, and a recent meta-analysis of seven trials still points to pregabalin's greater efficacy versus placebo in generalized anxiety disorder, although the effect sizes are relatively small (approximately 0.35 for psychic anxiety symptoms) (Boschen 2011). Pregabalin has also been reported to be an effective adjunctive treatment in patients with suboptimal response to selective serotonin reuptake inhibitor or serotonin–norepinephrine reuptake inhibitor monotherapy (Rickels et al. 2012).

Social anxiety disorder. In a study by Pande et al. (2004), 135 patients with social anxiety disorder were randomly assigned to 10 weeks of double-blind treatment with either pregabalin (low dose: 150 mg/day; high dose: 600 mg/day) or placebo. The primary outcome measure was change from baseline to endpoint in the LSAS total score. Patients randomly assigned to pregabalin 600 mg/day showed significant decreases in LSAS total score compared with those receiving placebo. Significant differences between high-dose pregabalin and placebo were also noted on several secondary measures, including the LSAS subscales total fear, avoidance, social fear, and social avoidance. Low-dose pregabalin (150 mg/day) was not significantly better than placebo. Somnolence and dizziness were the most frequently reported adverse events. In a more recent study in 329 patients, pregabalin at 600 mg/day—but not at 300 mg/day or 450 mg/day—separated from placebo (Feltner et al. 2011), a result consistent with the finding of Pande et al. (2004) that a daily dosage of 600 mg was required for efficacy in this disorder. Finally, a long-term study in 153 patients who had responded to an initial course of pregabalin therapy indicated that 450 mg/day was effective as a maintenance treatment in the disorder (Greist et al. 2011).

Substance Abuse and Withdrawal

As previously noted, pregabalin has no hepatic metabolism and is excreted essentially unchanged in the urine. This pharmacokinetic profile is ideal for patients with alcohol abuse or dependence who have elevated transaminases but need safe, efficacious treatment for symptoms of alcohol withdrawal. One preclinical study highlighted the potential use of pregabalin and its anticonvulsant, analgesic, anxiolytic properties in a mouse model of alcohol dependence (Becker et al. 2006). Controlled clinical studies of pregabalin in alcohol-dependent patients are encouraged. A recent study in patients with generalized anxiety disorder indicated that pregabalin was helpful in weaning patients off long-term benzodiazepine therapy (Hadley et al. 2012).

Side Effects and Toxicology

In general, the side effects commonly occurring with pregabalin treatment have been mild and not associated with a severity sufficient to warrant drug discontinuation. The most frequently reported symptoms have been dizziness, sedation, dry mouth, edema, blurred vision, weight gain, and concentration difficulty. In controlled clinical trials with pregabalin, significant weight gain (a gain of 7% or more over baseline) was observed in 9% of patients treated with pregabalin, compared with 2% of patients treated with placebo. Pregabalin treatment does not appear to be associated with significant changes in heart rate, blood pressure, respirations, or electrocardiogram measures. Peripheral edema has occurred in a small percentage of patients, but only in rare circumstances has it been identified as severe.

Available preclinical and clinical data suggest that pregabalin has very low abuse liability and is unlikely to produce significant physical dependence. There have been postmarketing reports of angioedema and hypersensitivity in patients treated with pregabalin (Pfizer 2006).

Drug-Drug Interactions

Pregabalin does not induce or inhibit CYP enzymes, nor do CYP enzyme inhibitors alter its pharmacokinetics as a consequence. Therefore, hepatic and CYP drug-drug interactions are not relevant when pregabalin is part of a complex polypharmacotherapy regimen. Because of the drug's renal elimination, dosage adjustment is required for patients with renal impairment. To date, no pharmacokinetic drug-drug interactions have been identified. There is some literature to suggest that there can be an additive cognitive impairment when pregabalin is taken in conjunction with oxycodone and that pregabalin may potentiate the effects of lorazepam and alcohol (Pfizer 2006).

Summary for Pregabalin

Controlled studies of pregabalin clearly have suggested its efficacy in complex partial epilepsy, postherpetic neuropathy, diabetic neuropathy, fibromyalgia, generalized anxiety disorder, and social anxiety disorder. Like gabapentin, pregabalin has a favorable pharmacokinetic profile, with particular advantages in patients with compromised hepatic function. Its minimal drug-drug interactions, low risk of toxicity, and favorable side-effect profile make it a useful addition to the pharmacopoeia.

Conclusion

There is increasing interest in the use of anticonvulsant drugs in mood and anxiety disorders. Controlled studies are needed to further assess specific patient populations and disease states that can benefit from these agents.

References

American Psychiatric Association: Diagnostic and Statistical Manual of Mental Disorders, 4th Edition. Washington, DC, American Psychiatric Association, 1994

Anton RF, Myrick H, Wright TM, et al: Gabapentin combined with naltrexone for the treatment of alcohol dependence. Am J Psychiatry 168:709–717, 2011

Arnold LM, Crofford LJ, Martin SA, et al: The effect of anxiety and depression on improvements in pain in a randomized, controlled trial of pregabalin for treatment of fibromyalgia. Pain Medicine 8:633–638, 2007

Backonja M, Beydoun A, Edwards KR, et al: Gabapentin for the symptomatic treatment of painful neuropathy in patients with diabetes mellitus. JAMA 280:1831–1836, 1998

Becker HC, Myrick H, Veatch LM: Pregabalin is effective against behavioral and electrographic seizures during alcohol withdrawal. Alcohol Alcohol 4:399–406, 2006

Beydoun A, Fakhoury T, Nasreddine W, et al: Conversion to high dose gabapentin monotherapy in patients with medically refractory partial epilepsy. Epilepsia 39:188–193, 1998

Bonnet U, Banger M, Leweke FM, et al: Treatment of acute alcohol withdrawal with gabapentin: results from a controlled two-center trial. J Clin Psychopharmacol 23:514–519, 2003

Bonnet U, Specka M, Leweke FM, et al: Gabapentin's acute effect on mood profile—a controlled study on patients with alcohol withdrawal. Prog Neuropsychopharmacol Biol Psychiatry 31:434–438, 2007

Boschen MJ: A meta-analysis of the efficacy of pregabalin in the treatment of generalized anxiety disorder. Can J Psychiatry 56:558–566, 2011

Bozikas V, Petrikis P, Gamvrula K, et al: Treatment of alcohol withdrawal with gabapentin. Prog Neuropsychopharmacol Biol Psychiatry 26:197–199, 2002

Cora-Locatelli G, Greenburg BD, Martin JD, et al: Gabapentin augmentation for fluoxetine-treated patients with obsessive-compulsive disorder. J Clin Psychiatry 59:480–481, 1998

Crofford LJ, Rowbotham MC, Mease PJ, et al: Pregabalin for the treatment of fibromyalgia syndrome: results of a randomized, double-blind, placebo-controlled trial. Pregabalin 1008–105 Study Group. Arthritis Rheum 52:1264–1273, 2005

Crofford LJ, Mease PJ, Simpson SL, et al: Fibromyalgia Relapse Evaluation and Efficacy for Durability Of Meaningful Relief (FREEDOM): a 6-month, double-blind, placebo-controlled trial with pregabalin. Pain 136:419–431, 2008

Dimond KR, Pande AC, Lamoreaux L, et al: Effect of gabapentin (Neurontin) on mood and well-being in patients with epilepsy. Prog Neuropsychopharmacol Biol Psychiatry 20:407–417, 1996

Dooley DJ, Donovan CM, Meder WP, et al: Preferential action of gabapentin and pregabalin at P/Q-type voltage-sensitive calcium channels: inhibition of K+-evoked [3H]-norepinephrine release from rat neocortical slices. Synapse 45:171–190, 2002

Dworkin RH, Corbin AE, Young JP, et al: Pregabalin for the treatment of postherpetic neuralgia: a randomized, placebo-controlled trial. Neurology 60:1274–1283, 2003

Elger CE, Brodie MJ, Anhut H, et al: Pregabalin add-on treatment in patients with partial seizures: a novel evaluation of flexible-dose and fixed-dose treatment in a double-blind, placebo-controlled study. Epilepsia 46:1926–1935, 2005

Feltner DE, Liu-Dumaw M, Schweizer E, et al: Efficacy of pregabalin in generalized social anxiety disorder: results of a double-blind, placebo-controlled, fixed dose study. Int Clin Psychopharmacol 26:213–220, 2011

Freeman R, Durso-Decruz E, Emir B: Efficacy, safety, and tolerability of pregabalin treatment of painful diabetic peripheral neuropathy: findings from 7 randomized controlled trials across a range of doses. Diabetes Care 31:1448–1454, 2008

Freynhagen R, Strojek K, Griesing T, et al: Efficacy of pregabalin in neuropathic pain evaluated in a 12-week randomized, double-blind, multicentre, placebo-controlled trial of flexible and fixed dose regimens. Pain 115:254–263, 2005

Frye MA, Kimbrell TA, Dunn RT, et al: Gabapentin does not alter single-dose lithium pharmacokinetics. J Clin Psychopharmacol 18:461–464, 1998

Frye MA, Ketter TA, Kimbrell TA, et al: A placebo-controlled study of lamotrigine and gabapentin monotherapy in refractory mood disorders. J Clin Psychopharmacol 20:607–614, 2000

Furieri FA, Nakamura-Palacios EM: Gabapentin reduces alcohol consumption and craving: a randomized, double-blind, placebo-controlled trial. J Clin Psychiatry 11:1691–1700, 2007

Gerner RH, Fairbanks L, Anderson GM, et al: Plasma levels of GABA and panic disorder. Psychiatry Res 63:223–225, 1996

Gold BI, Bowers MB, Roth RH, et al: GABA levels in CSF of patients with psychiatric disorders. Am J Psychiatry 137:362–364, 1980

Goldlust A, Su T, Welty DF, et al: Effects of the anticonvulsant drug gabapentin on enzymes in the metabolic pathways of glutamate and GABA. Epilepsy Res 22:1–11, 1995

Greist JH, Liu-Dumaw M, Schweizer E, et al: Efficacy of pregabalin in preventing relapse in patients with generalized social anxiety disorder: results of a double-blind, placebo-controlled 26-week study. Int Clin Psychopharmacol 26:243–251, 2011

Grunze H, Dittert S, Bungert M, et al: Renal impairment as a possible side effect of gabapentin: a single case report. Neuropsychobiology 38:198–199, 1998

Hadley SJ, Mandel FS, Schweizer E: Switching from long-term benzodiazepine therapy to pregabalin in patients with generalized anxiety disorder: a double-blind, placebo-controlled trial. J Psychopharmacol 26:461–470, 2012

Hamandi K, Sander JW: Pregabalin: a new antiepileptic drug for refractory epilepsy. Seizure 15:73–78, 2006

Hutson SM, Berkich D, Drown P, et al: Role of branched-chain aminotransferase isoenzymes and gabapentin in neurotransmitter metabolism. J Neurochem 71:863–874, 1998

Karam-Hage M, Brower KJ: Open pilot study of gabapentin versus trazodone to treatment insomnia in alcoholic outpatients. Psychiatry Clin Neurosci 57:542–544, 2003

Kavoussi R: Pregabalin: from molecule to medicine. Eur Neuropsychopharmacol 16:S128–S133, 2006

Leweke FM, Bauer J, Elger CE: Manic episode due to gabapentin treatment. Br J Psychiatry 175:291, 1999

Loscher W, Honack D, Taylor CP: Gabapentin increased aminooxyacetic acid-induced GABA accumulation in several regions of rat brain. Neurosci Lett 128:150–154, 1991

Mahmood T, Romans S, Silverstone T: Prevalence of migraine in bipolar disorder. J Affect Disord 99:239–241, 1999

Malcolm R, Myrick H, Brady KT, et al: Update on anticonvulsants for the treatment of alcohol withdrawal. Am J Addict 10 (suppl):16–23, 2001

Malcolm R, Myrick LH, Veatch LM, et al: Self-reported sleep, sleepiness, and repeated alcohol withdrawals: a randomized, double blind, controlled comparison of lorazepam vs gabapentin. J Clin Sleep Med 3:24–32, 2007

Mariani JJ, Rosenthal RN, Tross S, et al: A randomized, open-label, controlled trial of gabapentin and phenobarbital in the treatment of alcohol withdrawal. Am J Addict 15:76–84, 2006

Mason BJ, Crean R, Goodell V, et al: A proof-of-concept randomized controlled study of gabapentin: effects on cannabis use, withdrawal and executive function deficits in cannabis-dependent adults. Neuropsychopharmacology 37:1689–1698, 2012

Mathew NT, Rapoport A, Saper J, et al: Efficacy of gabapentin in migraine prophylaxis. Headache 41:119–128, 2001

McLean MJ: Gabapentin in the management of convulsive disorders. Epilepsia 40 (suppl 6): S39–S50, 1999

Mease PJ, Russell J, Arnold LM, et al: A randomized, double-blind, placebo-controlled phase III trial of pregabalin in the treatment of patients with fibromyalgia. J Rheumatol 35:502–514, 2008

Miller RG, Moore D, Young LA, et al: Placebo-controlled trial of gabapentin in patients with ALS. Neurology 47:1383–1388, 1996

Montgomery SA: Pregabalin for the treatment of generalised anxiety disorder. Expert Opin Pharmacother 7:2139–2154, 2006

Montgomery SA, Tobias K, Zornberg GL, et al: Efficacy and safety of pregabalin in the treatment of generalized anxiety disorder: a 6-week, multicenter, randomized, double-blind, placebo-controlled comparison of pregabalin and venlafaxine. J Clin Psychiatry 67:771–782, 2006

Obrocea GV, Dunn RM, Frye MA, et al: Clinical predictors of response to lamotrigine and gabapentin monotherapy in refractory affective disorders. Biol Psychiatry 51:253–260, 2002

Olson W, Gruenthal M, Muller ME, et al: Gabapentin for parkinsonism: a double-blind, placebo-controlled, cross-over trial. Am J Med 102:60–66, 1997

Ondo W, Hunter C, Vuong KD, et al: Gabapentin for essential tremor: a multiple-dose, double-blind, placebo controlled trial. Mov Disord 15:678–682, 2000

Pahwa R, Lyons K, Hubble JP, et al: Double-blind controlled trial of gabapentin in essential tremor. Mov Disord 13:465–467, 1998

Pande AC, Davidson JR, Jefferson JW, et al: Treatment of social phobia with gabapentin: a placebo-controlled study. J Clin Psychopharmacol 19:341–348, 1999

Pande AC, Crockatt JG, Janney CA, et al: Gabapentin in bipolar disorder: a placebo-controlled trial of adjunctive therapy. Gabapentin Bipolar Disorder Study Group. Bipolar Disord 2 (3 pt 2):249–255, 2000a

Pande AC, Pollack MH, Crockatt J, et al: Placebo-controlled study of gabapentin treatment of panic disorder. J Clin Psychopharmacol 20:467–471, 2000b

Pande AC, Crockatt JG, Feltner DE, et al: Pregabalin in generalized anxiety disorder: a placebo-controlled trial. Am J Psychiatry 160:533–540, 2003

Pande AC, Feltner DE, Jefferson JW, et al: Efficacy of the novel anxiolytic pregabalin in social anxiety disorder: a placebo-controlled, multicenter study. J Clin Psychopharmacol 24:141–149, 2004

Petroff OA, Rothman Dl, Behar KL, et al: The effect of gabapentin on brain gamma-aminobutyric acid in patients with epilepsy. Ann Neurol 39:95–99, 1996

Petty F, Kraemer GL, Dunnam D, et al: Plasma GABA in mood disorders. Psychopharmacol Bull 26:157–161, 1990

Pfizer: Lyrica (pregabalin) tablets: prescribing information. New York, Pfizer, 2006

Physicians' Desk Reference, 60th Edition. Montvale, NJ, Medical Economics Company, 2006

Pinninti NR, Mahajan DS: Gabapentin-associated aggression. J Neuropsychiatry Clin Neurosci 13:424–429, 2001

Pohl RB, Feltner DE, Rieve RR, et al: Efficacy of pregabalin in the treatment of generalized anxiety disorder: double-blind, placebo-controlled comparison of BPI versus TID dosing. J Clin Psychopharmacol 25:151–158, 2005

Pollack MH, Matthews M, Scott EL: Gabapentin as a potential treatment for anxiety disorders. Am J Psychiatry 155:992–993, 1998

Rao ML, Clarenbach P, Vahlensieck M, et al: Gabapentin augments whole blood serotonin in healthy young men. J Neural Transm 73:129–134, 1988

Rice AS, Maton S, Postherpetic Neuralgia Study Group: Gabapentin in postherpetic neuralgia: a randomised, double blind, placebo controlled study. Pain 94:215–224, 2001

Rickels K, Pollack MH, Feltner DE, et al: Pregabalin for treatment of generalized anxiety disorder: a 4-week, multicenter, double-blind, placebo-controlled trial of pregabalin and alprazolam. Arch Gen Psychiatry 62:1022–1030, 2005

Rickels K, Shiovitz TM, Ramey TS, et al: Adjunctive therapy with pregabalin in generalized anxiety disorder patients with partial response to SSRI or SNRI treatment. Int Clin Psychopharmacol 27:142–150, 2012

Rowbotham M, Harden N, Stacey B, et al: Gabapentin for the treatment of postherpetic neuralgia. JAMA 280:1837–1842, 1998

Roy A, Dejong J, Ferraro T: CSF GABA in depressed patients and normal controls. Psychol Med 21:613–618, 1991

Sabatowski R, Gálvez R, Cherry DA, et al: Pregabalin reduces pain and improves sleep and mood disturbances in patients with post-herpetic neuralgia: results of a randomised, placebo-controlled clinical trial. Pain 109:26–35, 2004

Sanacora G, Mason GF, Rothman DL, et al: Reduced cortical gamma-aminobutyric acid levels in depressed patients determined by proton magnetic resonance spectroscopy. Arch Gen Psychiatry 56:1043–1047, 1999

Sanacora G, Mason GF, Rothman DL, et al: Increased occipital cortex GABA concentrations in depressed patients after therapy with selective serotonin reuptake inhibitors. Am J Psychiatry 159:663–665, 2002

Schlicker E, Reimann W, Gothert M: Gabapentin decreases monoamine release without affecting acetylcholine release in the brain. Arzneimittelforschung 35:1347–1349, 1985

Short C, Cooke L: Hypomania induced by gabapentin. Br J Psychiatry 166:679–680, 1995

Singh L, Field MJ, Ferris P, et al: The antiepileptic agent gabapentin (Neurontin) processes anxiolytic-like and antinociceptive actions that are reversed by D-serine. Psychopharmacology 127:1–9, 1996

Taylor CP, Vartanian MG, Andruszkiewicz R, et al: 3-Alkyl GABA and 3-alkylglutamic acid analogues: two new classes of anticonvulsants agents. Epilepsy Res 11:103–110, 1992

Taylor CP, Gee NS, Su TZ, et al: A summary of mechanistic hypotheses of gabapentin pharmacology. Epilepsy Res 29:233–249, 1998

Van Seventer R, Feister HA, Young JP, et al: Efficacy and tolerability of twice-daily pregabalin for treating pain and related sleep interference in postherpetic neuralgia: a 13-week randomized trial. Curr Med Res Opin 222:375–384, 2006

Watson WP, Robinson E, Little HJ: The novel anticonvulsant gabapentin protects against both convulsant and anxiogenic aspects of the ethanol withdrawal syndrome. Neuropsychopharmacology 36:1369–1375, 1997

Weiss SR, Post RM: Kindling: separate vs shared mechanisms in affective disorders and epilepsy. Neuropsychobiology 38:167–180, 1998

Wolf SM, Shinnar S, Kang H, et al: Gabapentin toxicity in children manifesting as behavioral changes. Epilepsia 36:1203–1205, 1996

Wolfe F, Smythe HA, Yunus MB, et al: The American College of Rheumatology 1990 Criteria for the Classification of Fibromyalgia: report of the Multicenter Criteria Committee. Arthritis Rheum 33:160–172, 1990

Yatham LN, Kusumakar V, Calabrese JR, et al: Third generation anticonvulsants in bipolar disorder: a review of efficacy and summary of clinical recommendations. J Clin Psychiatry 63:275–283, 2002

CHAPTER 30

Lamotrigine

David E. Kemp, M.D., M.S.
Marc L. van der Loos, M.D., Ph.D.
Keming Gao, M.D., Ph.D.
Joseph R. Calabrese, M.D.

History and Discovery

During the clinical development of lamotrigine as a treatment for intractable seizures, improved mood in lamotrigine-treated patients was anecdotally reported (Jawad et al. 1989; Smith et al. 1993). In 1993, the addition of lamotrigine to an existing antiepileptic drug (AED) regimen was evaluated in a small study of 81 patients with epilepsy (Smith et al. 1993). Lamotrigine-treated patients reported significantly higher levels of happiness and an improvement in perceived internal locus of control. There was no correlation between perceived happiness and changes in seizure frequency or severity. Thus, it was preliminarily concluded that lamotrigine may have an effect on mood independent of its antiepileptic effect.

Mechanism of Action and Pharmacokinetics

Lamotrigine (3,5-diamino-6-[2,3-dichlorophenyl]-1,2,4-triazine, $C_9H_7Cl_2N_5$) is an AED of the phenyltriazine class; it is chemically unrelated to hepatic enzyme inducers (e.g., carbamazepine) and enzyme inhibitors (e.g., valproic acid). Lamotrigine has not been shown to inhibit the reuptake of norepinephrine, dopamine, or serotonin. Although it exerts inhibitory effects at the serotonin$_3$ (5-HT_3) receptor, this activity is weak and unlikely to contribute to its therapeutic profile. Lamotrigine does not exhibit high binding affinity to adrenergic (α_1, α_2, β), dopamine (D_1, D_2), γ-aminobutyric acid (GABA), histamine (H_1), opioid (κ or σ), or muscarinic (M_1, M_2) acetylcholine receptors. Lamotrigine inhibits use-dependent sodium channels, allowing continued normal depolarizations while suppressing paroxysmal burst firing encountered in seizures and hypoxic insult.

The inhibition of voltage-activated sodium channels (Xie and Hagan 1998) may best characterize lamotrigine's mechanism of action. In addition to inhibitory activity on sodium channels, there is also evidence for antagonistic action by lamotrigine on N-type calcium channels (Stefani et al. 1996; von Wegerer et al. 1997).

Antiglutamatergic action is an additional means by which lamotrigine may affect mood. Presynaptic inhibition of voltage- and use-sensitive sodium channels, calcium channels, and potassium channels (Grunze et al. 1998) is believed to result in decreased release of the excitatory amino acid glutamate. The reduction of glutamate may occur through suppression of postsynaptic α-amino-3-hydroxy-5-methyl-4-isoxazolepropionic acid (AMPA) receptors (Lee et al. 2008). Interestingly, one of the most replicated susceptibility genes for bipolar disorder (*ANK3*) codes for a protein that regulates the assembly of voltage-gated sodium channels (Schulze et al. 2009). These genetic findings, coupled with the action of lamotrigine on sodium and calcium channels, suggest that channelopathies may be involved in the pathophysiology of bipolar disorder.

Oral lamotrigine is rapidly absorbed with negligible first-pass metabolism. Peak plasma concentrations are reached in approximately 2–4 hours, and its half-life is approximately 25 hours (GlaxoSmithKline 2011). Lamotrigine is approximately 55% bound to plasma proteins and is unlikely to significantly interact with drugs that are highly protein bound. Metabolism is primarily achieved by competitive glucuronic acid conjugation. At steady-state concentrations, the pharmacokinetics of lamotrigine are linear within a dosage range of 100–700 mg/day (Leach et al. 1995). The clearance of lamotrigine is reduced in the setting of renal insufficiency and hepatic disease.

During pregnancy, clinically significant perturbations in lamotrigine levels can occur. The rate of lamotrigine clearance increases during each trimester, reaching a peak of 330% of baseline clearance by week 32 gestational age (Pennell et al. 2004). Plasma levels are noted to rapidly return to normal during the first few postpartum weeks.

Indications and Efficacy

In 2003, lamotrigine was granted approval by the U.S. Food and Drug Administration (FDA) for use in the maintenance treatment of bipolar I disorder to delay the time to recurrence of new mood episodes. Lamotrigine is also indicated for adjunctive antiepileptic therapy in adults with partial seizures, for generalized seizures secondary to Lennox-Gastaut syndrome, and for adjunctive use in primary and generalized tonic-clonic seizures in adults and pediatric patients (≥2 years of age).

Maintenance Therapy in Bipolar I Disorder

Two large randomized, double-blind, parallel-group, placebo-controlled multicenter studies led to the approval of lamotrigine as a maintenance therapy in bipolar I disorder (Bowden et al. 2003; Calabrese et al. 2003). Both of these paired studies included a screening phase of up to 2 weeks; an 8- to 16-week open-label phase during which lamotrigine was initiated as adjunctive or monotherapy and other psychotropic drugs were discontinued; and an 18-month double-blind phase during which patients received lamotrigine, lithium, or placebo as maintenance therapy. The primary efficacy variable in both studies was time to intervention for any mood episode. One of the studies (Bowden et al. 2003) evaluated subjects who were or had recently been in a manic, hypomanic, or mixed state. The other study (Calabrese et al. 2003) examined subjects who were or had recently been depressed.

Both lamotrigine and lithium were superior to placebo on time to intervention for any mood episode ($P = 0.018$ for previously manic; $P = 0.029$ for previously depressed). Lamotrigine, but not lithium, was superior to placebo at prolonging the time to a depressive episode ($P = 0.015$ for previously manic; $P = 0.047$ for previously depressed). Lithium, but not lamotrigine, was superior to placebo at prolonging the time to a manic, hypomanic, or mixed episode ($P = 0.006$ for previously manic; $P = 0.026$ for previously depressed).

A pooled analysis of these two clinical trials found lithium and lamotrigine to be statistically superior to placebo at prolonging the time to intervention for a manic, hypomanic, or mixed episode ($P = 0.034$ for lamotrigine vs. placebo; $P \leq 0.001$ for lithium vs. placebo) (Goodwin et al. 2004). However, lamotrigine, but not lithium, remained the only compound that was superior to placebo at prolonging the time to intervention for a depressive episode ($P = 0.009$ for lamotrigine vs. placebo; $P = 0.120$ for lithium vs. placebo).

In the interpretation of maintenance-phase data, it is important to distinguish between efficacy in relapse prevention and pure prophylactic efficacy (Ghaemi et al. 2004). Mood episodes of the same polarity as the index episode that occur during the initial 2 months following recovery are generally regarded as *relapses*. Alternatively, mood episodes that occur beyond this phase during the period of remission are regarded as *recurrences*. To test the pure maintenance efficacy of lamotrigine, Calabrese et al. (2006) conducted a post hoc analysis of the two double-blind 18-month maintenance trials that compared lamotrigine and lithium against placebo. In their analysis, all subjects were excluded who experienced a relapse to a mood episode of the same polarity as the index episode within 90 or 180 days of randomization. Both lamotrigine and lithium were found to be more effective than placebo at delaying the time to intervention for a mood episode ($P = 0.02$ for lamotrigine; $P = 0.010$ for lithium). Similar results were found when patients who relapsed to a mood episode of the same polarity as their index episode within 180 days of randomization were excluded, suggesting that lamotrigine and lithium possess true maintenance efficacy.

Acute Monotherapy and Adjunctive Therapy in Bipolar Depression

A series of double-blind, placebo-controlled multicenter studies was completed to replicate and extend preliminary open-label prospective findings suggesting moderate to marked efficacy in bipolar depression, hypomania, and mixed states (Calabrese et al. 1999a). The first study in this series evaluated the efficacy and safety of two doses of lamotrigine compared with placebo in the acute treatment of a major depressive episode in 195 patients with bipolar I disorder (Calabrese et al. 1999b). Outpatients received lamotrigine (50 or 200 mg/day) or placebo as monotherapy for 7 weeks. Psychiatric evaluations, including the Hamilton Rating Scale for Depression (Ham-D), the Montgomery-Åsberg Depression Rating Scale (MADRS), the Mania Rating Scale (MRS), and the Severity of Illness and Improvement subscales of the Clinical Global Impression Scale (CGI-S and CGI-I, respectively), were completed at 4 days and then weekly. Lamotrigine at a dosage of 200 mg/day demonstrated significant antidepressant efficacy on the MADRS, Ham-D Item 1, CGI-S, and CGI-I compared with placebo. However, lamotrigine did not separate from placebo on the overall Ham-D score, which was selected as the a priori primary outcome measure.

Although there is expert consensus that lamotrigine is effective for acute bipolar depression and confirmation from one adequately powered placebo-controlled trial (Calabrese et al. 1999b), there have been four randomized, parallel-group, placebo-controlled monotherapy trials in which lamotrigine failed to separate from placebo, probably due to a high placebo response rate

(40%–50%) (Calabrese et al. 2008). In none of the four studies were significant improvements over placebo observed on the 17- and 31-item Ham-D, the MADRS, the CGI-S, or the CGI-I.

To clarify the effects of lamotrigine in acute bipolar depression, Geddes et al. (2009) conducted a systematic meta-analysis of individual patient data from 1,072 participants in five randomized controlled trials comparing lamotrigine with placebo. The pooled analysis showed that more patients treated with lamotrigine than with placebo responded on both the Ham-D and the MADRS (P=0.002). However, the advantage of lamotrigine over placebo was larger in more severely depressed patients.

Despite the modest effect sizes when lamotrigine is prescribed as monotherapy, the Canadian Network for Mood and Anxiety Treatments and the International Society for Bipolar Disorders collaborative guidelines recommend lamotrigine as a first-line agent for the treatment of acute bipolar depression (Yatham et al. 2009). However, lamotrigine may have even greater utility as an add-on to lithium in bipolar depressed patients who have shown insufficient response to lithium (van der Loos et al. 2009). Although negative controlled studies now outweigh positive studies of lamotrigine administered as monotherapy for bipolar depression, the negative findings in individual trials may be more a reflection of the patient composition than a property of the drug itself, given the lack of a comparator arm to determine assay sensitivity and the relatively high rates of placebo response (Grunze et al. 2010). Because of lamotrigine's greater efficacy in patients who are more severely ill (Geddes et al. 2009) and patients with treatment-refractory depression (Nierenberg et al. 2006), the guidelines established by the World Federation of Societies of Biological Psychiatry assigned a grade 3 recommendation to lamotrigine, reflective of category B evidence and limited positive evidence from controlled studies (Grunze et al. 2010).

Additional Efficacy Considerations

Calabrese et al. (2000) conducted a maintenance study with lamotrigine in rapid-cycling bipolar disorder. The difference between the treatment groups in time to additional pharmacotherapy for a developing or fully developed mood episode did not achieve statistical significance. However, overall survival time in the study (i.e., time to dropout for any reason) was significantly different between the treatment groups in favor of lamotrigine (P=0.036). When patients with bipolar I and II subtypes were compared, lamotrigine-treated bipolar II disorder patients demonstrated a significantly longer median survival of 17 weeks compared with a median of 7 weeks for placebo-treated patients (P=0.015).

To date, only two compounds are FDA approved for the treatment of acute bipolar depression: an olanzapine-fluoxetine combination (OFC) and quetiapine. To compare efficacy with an established agent for managing bipolar depression, a head-to-head randomized, double-blind, parallel-group study of lamotrigine and OFC was conducted over 7 weeks in patients with bipolar I disorder in an acute depressive phase (Brown et al. 2006). The study randomly assigned 410 subjects to either lamotrigine (titrated to 200 mg/day; n=205) or OFC (6/25, 6/50, 12/25, or 12/50 mg/day; n=205). Overall response and remission rates were comparable between the active agents, although differences did emerge in regard to tolerability profiles. Adverse-event rates of suicidal and self-injurious behavior were more common among patients treated with lamotrigine (3.4%) compared with OFC (0.5%; P=0.037). On the other hand, significant differences in mean change from baseline to endpoint for clinically relevant laboratory and physiological parameters favored treatment with lamotrigine, including measures such as hemoglobin A1c, prolactin, total cholesterol, high-density lipoprotein cholesterol, low-density lipoprotein cholesterol, triglycerides, and body weight.

An add-on trial comparing lamotrigine with placebo in the treatment of bipolar I and II depression has also been conducted (van der Loos et al. 2009). All patients were required to be taking lithium maintained at a therapeutic blood level (0.6–1.2 mmol/L) prior to random assignment to lamotrigine (n=64) or placebo (n=60). Subjects were treated for 8 weeks and assessed for response using the MADRS (primary outcome measure) and the CGI Scale–Bipolar Version (CGI-BP; Spearing et al. 1997). The change from baseline to endpoint on the MADRS was significantly greater in lamotrigine-treated subjects (15.4) compared with those receiving placebo (11.0; P=0.02). A higher percentage of patients responded (>50% reduction in MADRS score) to add-on lamotrigine (51.6%) compared with placebo (31.7%; P=0.030), although no difference was observed in the CGI-BP response rate (64.1% for lamotrigine vs. 48.3% for placebo; P=0.10). After open-label addition of paroxetine for another 8 weeks in nonresponders, further improvement in the lithium-plus-placebo group outweighed the improvement in the lithium-plus-lamotrigine group (van der Loos et al. 2010). However, this effect was not statistically significant as measured by the change in MADRS scores from baseline to week 16 between lithium plus lamotrigine (plus paroxetine in nonresponders) versus lithium plus placebo (plus paroxetine in nonresponders) (–17.91 vs. –15.40; P= 0.25). After 16 weeks, all responders in both groups were followed for up to 68 weeks or until a relapse or recurrence of a depressive or manic episode occurred. Time to relapse or recurrence was longer for the lamotrigine group (median time 10.0 months [confidence interval 1.1–18.8]) versus the placebo group (3.5 months [confidence interval: 0.7–7.0]) (van der Loos et al. 2011).

Another study compared adjunctive lamotrigine against placebo in patients with rapid-cycling bipolar depression who had failed to respond to prospective treatment with lithium and valproate. A unique aspect of this study was that all participants met criteria for a recent substance use disorder. Although the double-blind study phase was underpowered (n=36), lamotrigine was numerically but not statistically superior to placebo in reducing depression severity, as measured by the baseline-to-endpoint change in MADRS total score (Wang et al. 2010).

Lamotrigine does not appear to possess acute antimanic activity. Two placebo-controlled trials have been conducted in patients with bipolar I disorder experiencing an acute manic or mixed episode, including a 3-week monotherapy trial and a 6-week add-on trial (Bowden et al. 2000). In both studies, lamotrigine failed to separate from placebo on the primary outcome measure of change in symptom severity on the MRS.

Dosing and Drug-Drug Interactions

The recommended dosing schedule for lamotrigine in adults involves initiating therapy with 25 mg daily for the first 14 days and then advancing to 50 mg daily for the third and fourth weeks of treatment. During the fifth week of treatment, lamotrigine can be increased to 100 mg daily, followed by titration to 200 mg daily during the sixth and seventh weeks of treatment. When lamotrigine is added to valproate in adult patients, the recommended titration schedule begins at 25 mg every other day for 14 days, advances to 25 mg daily for 14 days, and then increases by 50 mg daily beginning each of the fifth and sixth weeks of treatment, reaching a target dose of 100 mg daily. Titration of adjunctive lamotrigine in the presence of an enzyme-inducing AED begins at 50 mg daily for 14 days, advances to 100 mg daily (divided doses) for 14 days, to a target dosage of 400 mg daily. There are no published data supporting greater efficacy of lamotrigine in the treatment of bipolar disorder at dosages greater than 200 mg/day in the absence of an enzyme inducer. Additionally, there is no clear association between serum levels of lamotrigine and measures of affective response.

Lamotrigine is not known to inhibit the activity of the cytochrome P450 2D6 enzyme. However, the addition of adjunctive lamotrigine to enzyme inducers such as carbamazepine, phenytoin, primidone, and phenobarbital decreases lamotrigine plasma concentrations by approximately 40%–50% (Hahn et al. 2004). The inducing effect of oxcarbazepine is approximately half that of carbamazepine (Weintraub et al. 2005). Because lamotrigine is nearly exclusively metabolized by glucuronidation, the introduction of adjunctive valproate (an enzyme inhibitor) results in immediate and successful competition for metabolism, with resultant increases in half-life.

Evidence has emerged that oral contraceptives containing estrogen have the potential to decrease serum concentrations of lamotrigine by up to 64% (Sabers et al. 2001, 2003). During the long-term treatment of bipolar disorder, use of ethinyl estradiol–containing compounds may require an increase in the maintenance dose of lamotrigine by as much as twofold over the recommended target maintenance dose. Conversely, stopping estrogen-containing oral contraceptives, including during the "pill-free" week, may increase lamotrigine levels to a clinically significant range.

Side Effects and Toxicity

In controlled monotherapy trials of lamotrigine in the treatment of mood disorders, the drug has been associated with headache, changes in sleep habits, nausea, and dizziness (Bowden et al. 2004). Although the prevalence of rash in mood disorder randomized trials did not exceed that of placebo, rash is generally recognized as the side effect most likely to significantly complicate lamotrigine's clinical use. More recently, the rare occurrence of aseptic meningitis has been reported in association with lamotrigine (Boot 2009; Kilfoyle et al. 2005; Lam et al. 2010). Clinical manifestations have included meningismus, photophobia, headache, vomiting, and fever. Symptoms have been reported to occur within 1 day to 1½ months following initiation of treatment. In several cases, sudden and severe symptoms of meningitis have occurred within minutes of reintroducing lamotrigine. In most cases of drug-induced aseptic meningitis, complete recovery typically occurs once the offending agent has been discontinued (Moris and Garcia-Monco 1999).

In early epilepsy trials, rash led to hospitalization and treatment discontinuation or Stevens-Johnson syndrome in 0.3% of adults treated with lamotrigine (Calabrese et al. 2002). The annual incidence of serious drug-based skin reactions associated with lamotrigine was highest in 1993 (4.2%) but steadily declined and had stabilized by 1998 (0.02%). This is likely attributable to the manufacturer's dosage revision in 1994, which advised a more protracted titration schedule (Calabrese et al. 2002; Messenheimer et al. 1998). It is well documented that the risk of rash is heightened in children younger than 12 years, by coadministration of valproic acid, or by exceeding the recommended initial dosage or rate of dosage escalation of lamotrigine.

The most common lamotrigine-associated rash is an exanthematic maculopapular or morbilliform eruption that is benign. However, a clinically similar eruption may be associated with more rare and serious systemic hypersensitivity reactions (Guberman et al. 1999). Thus, all patients who develop a rash during the first few months of lamotrigine therapy should be instructed to hold the next dose and immediately seek medical consultation. The greatest risk of rash appears to be during the first 8 weeks of treatment. A rash during the first 5 days of therapy is usually due to a nondrug cause. Because immune tolerance to lamotrigine is lost following interruption of dosage for more than 1 week, patients should be instructed to resume lamotrigine at the prior initial start-up dose and to gradually titrate upward whenever therapy has been interrupted for more than a few days.

In comparison with other agents used in the management of bipolar disorder, a distinctive feature of lamotrigine is its weight-neutral tolerability profile (Sachs et al. 2006). A post hoc analysis revealed that nonobese patients taking lamotrigine are unlikely to experience a change in weight. However, obese patients are significantly more likely to lose weight with lamotrigine and to gain weight with lithium (Bowden et al. 2006).

Use During Pregnancy

Lamotrigine may represent an option for women with bipolar disorder during pregnancy due to its favorable tolerability profile and maintenance effects against bipolar depression. An observational study by Newport et al. (2008) examined risk of illness recurrence in pregnant women with stable bipolar disorder who continued lamotrigine treatment during pregnancy ($n = 10$) versus those who discontinued mood stabilizer therapy during pregnancy ($n = 16$). The risk of illness recurrence was 3.3 times lower when lamotrigine was continued (30.0% recurrence [3/10] vs. 100% recurrence [16/16] when patients discontinued mood stabilizers; $P < 0.0001$), suggesting that lamotrigine may provide protective effects in pregnancy.

In newborns of mothers receiving lamotrigine, extensive placental transfer of drug has been found to occur, with umbilical cord concentrations approaching those of maternal serum (Ohman et al. 2000). Nursing infants demonstrate plasma lamotrigine concentrations approximately 23%–50% of maternal levels.

Potential adverse effects in the developing fetus of mothers receiving lamotrigine have been suggested by data collected as part of international pregnancy registries (Cunnington and Tennis 2004; Holmes et al. 2006). As with any mood stabilizer, lamotrigine use during pregnancy represents an inherent dilemma for clinicians and expectant mothers, who must balance the risks associated with untreated bipolar disorder with the potential for occurrence of major congenital malformations. During treatment with valproate or carbamazepine, neural tube defects are estimated to occur in 1%–5% of neonates after first-trimester exposure. The risk for malformations with newer antiepileptic drugs, including lamotrigine, is less well characterized. Preliminary data from the North American Antiepileptic Drug Pregnancy Registry suggest a possible association between first-trimester exposure to lamotrigine monotherapy and cleft lip and/or cleft palate (Holmes et al. 2006). However, an International Lamotrigine Pregnancy Registry, maintained by GlaxoSmithKline since 1992, recorded a total of 14 congenital malformations among 414 outcomes (2.9%) involving a first-trimester monotherapy exposure (Cunnington and Tennis 2004). This is similar to the background risk of 2%–3% for congenital malformations in the general population. A recent analysis from an Australian pregnancy registry found no statistically significant difference between the risk of fetal malformations among women exposed to lamotrigine monotherapy during pregnancy and the risk among pregnant women with epilepsy taking no antiepileptic drugs (Vajda et al. 2010). Expert guidelines conclude that there is likely a relationship between the total dosage of lamotrigine taken by a woman during pregnancy and the risk of a major congenital malformation in her offspring. Thus, limiting the dosage during the first trimester should be considered (Harden et al. 2009). Lamotrigine is listed as Pregnancy Category C in terms of teratogenic effects.

Conclusion

The mechanism by which lamotrigine achieves its therapeutic effect in the treatment of bipolar disorder is unknown. However, its discovery has provided investigators with a novel AED for empirical validation in the routine treatment of bipolar disorder. Although initial results from trials of lamotrigine in the treatment of mania were unfavorable, subsequent maintenance studies have provided compelling data to show that lamotrigine prevents the recurrence of mood episodes and displays antidepressant efficacy, albeit most convincingly for the prophylaxis against depression in contrast to the acute diminution of depression. Even with its ability to stabilize mood from below baseline, lamotrigine appears to have a switch rate to mania or hypomania that is similar to treatment with placebo. Lamotrigine's neutral effects on body weight and favorable side-effect profile make it appealing for use in patients who have comorbid metabolic syndrome or those in whom other treatments have resulted in poor tolerability. At present, lamotrigine remains the only AED mood stabilizer with more established efficacy in the depressed illness phase than in mania or hypomania.

References

Boot B: Recurrent lamotrigine-induced aseptic meningitis. Epilepsia 50:968–969, 2009

Bowden CL, Calabrese JR, Ascher J, et al: Spectrum of efficacy of lamotrigine in bipolar disorder: overview of double-blind, placebo-controlled studies. Presented at the American College of Neuropsychopharmacology (ACNP) Annual Meeting, San Juan, PR, December 2000

Bowden CL, Calabrese JR, Sachs G, et al: A placebo-controlled 18-month trial of lamotrigine and lithium maintenance treatment in recently manic or hypomanic patients with bipolar I disorder. Arch Gen Psychiatry 60:392–400, 2003

Bowden CL, Asnis GM, Ginsberg LD, et al: Safety and tolerability of lamotrigine for bipolar disorder. Drug Saf 27:173–184, 2004

Bowden CL, Calabrese JR, Ketter TA, et al: Impact of lamotrigine and lithium on weight in obese and nonobese patients with bipolar I disorder. Am J Psychiatry 163:1199–1201, 2006

Brown EB, McElroy SL, Keck PE Jr, et al: A 7-week, randomized, double-blind trial of olanzapine/fluoxetine combination versus lamotrigine in the treatment of bipolar I depression. J Clin Psychiatry 67:1025–1033, 2006

Calabrese JR, Bowden CL, McElroy SL, et al: Spectrum of activity of lamotrigine in treatment-refractory bipolar disorder. Am J Psychiatry 156:1019–1023, 1999a

Calabrese JR, Bowden CL, Sachs GS, et al: A double-blind placebo-controlled study of lamotrigine monotherapy in outpatients with bipolar I depression. J Clin Psychiatry 60:79–88, 1999b

Calabrese JR, Suppes T, Bowden C, et al: A double-blind, placebo-controlled, prophylaxis study of lamotrigine in rapid-cycling bipolar disorder. J Clin Psychiatry 61:841–850, 2000

Calabrese JR, Sullivan JR, Bowden CL, et al: Rash in multicenter trials of lamotrigine in mood disorders: clinical relevance and management. J Clin Psychiatry 63:1012–1019, 2002

Calabrese JR, Bowden CL, Sachs G, et al: A placebo-controlled 18-month trial of lamotrigine and lithium maintenance treatment in recently depressed patients with bipolar I disorder. J Clin Psychiatry 64:1013–1024, 2003

Calabrese JR, Goldberg JF, Ketter TA, et al: Recurrence in bipolar I disorder: a post hoc analysis excluding relapses in two double-blind maintenance studies. Biol Psychiatry 59:1061–1064, 2006

Calabrese JR, Huffman RF, White RL, et al: Lamotrigine in the acute treatment of bipolar depression: results of five double-blind, placebo-controlled clinical trials. Bipolar Disord 10:323–333, 2008

Cunnington M, Tennis P: International Lamotrigine Pregnancy Registry Scientific Advisory Committee: Lamotrigine and the risk of malformations in pregnancy. Neurology 64:955–960, 2004

Geddes JR, Calabrese JR, Goodwin GM: Lamotrigine for treatment of bipolar depression: an independent meta-analysis and meta-regression of individual patient data from 5 randomized trials. Br J Psychiatry 194:4–9, 2009

Ghaemi SN, Pardo RB, Hsu DJ: Strategies for preventing the recurrence of bipolar disorder. J Clin Psychiatry 65 (suppl):16–23, 2004

GlaxoSmithKline: Lamictal (lamotrigine) prescribing information. Research Triangle Park, NC, GlaxoSmithKline, December 2011. Available at: http://us.gsk.com/products/assets/us_lamictal.pdf. Accessed April 13, 2012.

Goodwin GM, Bowden CL, Calabrese JR, et al: A pooled analysis of 2 placebo-controlled 18-month trials of lamotrigine and lithium maintenance in bipolar I disorder. J Clin Psychiatry 65:432–441, 2004

Grunze H, von Wegerer J, Greene RW, et al: Modulation of calcium and potassium currents by lamotrigine. Neuropsychobiology 38:131–138, 1998

Grunze H, Vieta E, Goodwin GM, et al: The World Federation of Societies of Biological Psychiatry (WFSBP) Guidelines for the Biological Treatment of Bipolar Disorders: update 2010 on the treatment of acute bipolar depression. World J Biol Psychiatry 11:81–109, 2010

Guberman A, Besag F, Brodie M, et al: Lamotrigine-associated rash: risk/benefit considerations in adults and children. Epilepsia 40:985–991, 1999

Hahn CG, Gyulai L, Baldassano CF, et al: The current understanding of lamotrigine as a mood stabilizer. J Clin Psychiatry 65:791–804, 2004

Harden CL, Meador KJ, Pennell PB: Practice parameter update: management issues for women with epilepsy—focus on pregnancy (an evidence-based review): teratogenesis and perinatal outcomes: report of the Quality Standards Subcommittee and Therapeutics and Technology Assessment Subcommittee of the American Academy of Neurology and American Epilepsy Society. Neurology 73:133–141, 2009

Holmes LB, Wyszynski DF, Baldwin EJ, et al: Increased risk for nonsyndromic cleft palate among infants exposed to lamotrigine during pregnancy. Birth Defects Res A Clin Mol Teratol 76:318, 2006

Jawad S, Richens A, Goodwin G, et al: Controlled trial of lamotrigine (Lamictal) for refractory partial seizures. Epilepsia 30:656–663, 1989

Kilfoyle DH, Anderson NE, Wallis WE: Recurrent severe aseptic meningitis after exposure to lamotrigine in a patient with systemic lupus erythematosus. Epilepsia 46:327–328, 2005

Lam GM, Edelson DP, Whelan CT: Lamotrigine: an unusual etiology for aseptic meningitis. Neurologist 16:35–36, 2010

Leach MJ, Lees G, Riddall DR: Lamotrigine: mechanisms of action, in Antiepileptic Drugs, 4th Edition. Edited by Levy RH, Mattson RH, Meldrum BS. New York, Raven, 1995, pp 861–869

Lee CY, Fu WM, Chen CC, et al: Lamotrigine inhibits postsynaptic AMPA receptor and glutamate release in the dentate gyrus. Epilepsia 49:888–897, 2008

Messenheimer JA, Mullens EL, Giorgi L, et al: Safety review of adult clinical trial experience with lamotrigine. Drug Saf 18:281–296, 1998

Moris G, Garcia-Monco JC: The challenge of drug-induced aseptic meningitis. Arch Intern Med 159:1185–1194, 1999

Newport DJ, Stowe ZN, Viguera AC, et al: Lamotrigine in bipolar disorder: efficacy during pregnancy. Bipolar Disord 10:432–436, 2008

Nierenberg AA, Ostacher MJ, Calabrese JR, et al: Treatment-resistant bipolar depression: a STEP-BD equipoise randomized effectiveness trial of antidepressant augmentation with lamotrigine, inositol, or risperidone. Am J Psychiatry 163: 210–216, 2006

Ohman I, Vitols S, Tomson T: Lamotrigine in pregnancy: pharmacokinetics during delivery, in the neonate, and during lactation. Epilepsia 41:709–713, 2000

Pennell PB, Newport DJ, Stowe ZN, et al: The impact of pregnancy and childbirth on the metabolism of lamotrigine. Neurology 62:292–295, 2004

Sabers A, Buchholt J, Uldall P, et al: Lamotrigine plasma levels reduced by oral contraceptives. Epilepsy Res 47:151–154, 2001

Sabers A, Ohman I, Christensen J, et al: Oral contraceptives reduce lamotrigine plasma levels. Neurology 26:570–571, 2003

Sachs G, Bowden CL, Calabrese JR, et al: Effects of lamotrigine and lithium on body weight during maintenance treatment of bipolar I disorder. Bipolar Disord 8:175–181, 2006

Schulze TG, Detera-Wadleigh SD, Akula N, et al: Two variants in Ankyrin 3 (ANK3) are independent genetic risk factors for bipolar disorder. Mol Psychiatry 14:487–491, 2009

Smith D, Chadwick D, Baker G, et al: Seizure severity and the quality of life. Epilepsia 34 (suppl): S31–S35, 1993

Spearing MK, Post RM, Leverich GS, et al: Modification of the Clinical Global Impressions (CGI) Scale for use in bipolar illness (BP): the CGI-BP. Psychiatry Res 73:159–171, 1997

Stefani A, Spadoni F, Sinischali A, et al: Lamotrigine inhibits Ca2+ currents in cortical neurons: functional implications. Eur J Pharmacol 307:113–116, 1996

Vajda FJ, Graham JE, Hitchcock AA, et al: Is lamotrigine a significant human teratogen? Observations from the Australian Pregnancy Register. Seizure 19:558–561, 2010 van der Loos ML, Mulder PG, Hartong EG, et al: Efficacy and safety of lamotrigine as add-on treatment to lithium in bipolar depression: a multicenter, double-blind, placebo-controlled trial. J Clin Psychiatry 70:223–231, 2009

van der Loos ML, Mulder P, Hartong EG, et al: Efficacy and safety of two treatment algorithms in bipolar depression consisting of a combination of lithium, lamotrigine or placebo and paroxetine. Acta Psychiatr Scand 122:246–254, 2010

van der Loos ML, Mulder P, Hartong EG, et al: Long-term outcome of bipolar depressed patients receiving lamotrigine as add-on to lithium with the possibility of the addition of paroxetine in nonresponders: a randomized, placebo-controlled trial with a novel design. Bipolar Disord 13:111–117, 2011

von Wegerer J, Hesslinger B, Berger M, et al: A calcium antagonistic effect of the new antiepileptic drug lamotrigine. Eur Neuropsychopharmacol 7:77–78, 1997

Wang Z, Gao K, Kemp DE, et al: Lamotrigine adjunctive therapy to lithium and divalproex in depressed patients with rapid cycling bipolar disorder and a recent substance use disorder: a 12-week, double-blind, placebo-controlled pilot study. Psychopharmacol Bull 43:5–21, 2010

Weintraub D, Buchsbaum R, Resor SR Jr, et al: Effect of antiepileptic drug comedication on lamotrigine clearance. Arch Neurol 62:1432–1436, 2005

Xie X, Hagan RM: Cellular and molecular actions of lamotrigine: possible mechanisms of efficacy in bipolar disorder. Neuropsychobiology 38:119–130, 1998

Yatham LN, Kennedy SH, Schaffer A, et al: Canadian Network for Mood and Anxiety Treatments (CANMAT) and International Society for Bipolar Disorders (ISBD) collaborative update of CANMAT guidelines for the management of patients with bipolar disorder: update 2009. Bipolar Disord 11:225–255, 2009

CHAPTER 31

Topiramate

Susan L. McElroy, M.D.
Paul E. Keck Jr., M.D.

History and Discovery

Topiramate was approved by the U.S. Food and Drug Administration (FDA) for the treatment of epilepsy in 1996 and for migraine prevention in 2004. Reports appearing in the late 1990s of the drug having potential beneficial effects in bipolar disorder led Johnson & Johnson Pharmaceutical Research and Development (PRD), the discoverer and manufacturer of topiramate, to conduct a large clinical study program of topiramate in the treatment of acute bipolar mania (McElroy and Keck 2004). Controlled trials of the drug in bipolar adults with manic symptoms failed to demonstrate significant separation between the topiramate and placebo groups (Chengappa et al. 2006; Kushner et al. 2006). However, topiramate has been shown in placebo-controlled trials to be efficacious in several neuropsychiatric conditions often comorbid with bipolar disorder, including binge-eating disorder (BED), bulimia nervosa, alcohol dependence, borderline personality disorder (BPD), psychotropic-associated weight gain, and obesity, in addition to migraine headache.

Pharmacological Profile

Topiramate has multiple pharmacological properties that may contribute to its anticonvulsant and neuropsychiatric effects (Langtry et al. 1997; Rho and Sankar 1999; Rosenfeld 1997; Shank et al. 2000; White 2002, 2005; White et al. 2007). First, topiramate inhibits voltage-gated sodium channels in a voltage-sensitive, use-dependent manner and thus suppresses action potentials associated with sustained repetitive cell firing (Kawasaki et al. 1998; Shank et al. 2000). Second, topiramate increases brain γ-aminobutyric acid (GABA) levels, possibly by activating a site on the $GABA_A$ receptor, thereby enhancing the inhibitory chloride ion influx mediated by the $GABA_A$ receptor and potentiating GABA-evoked currents (Kuzniecky et al. 1998;

Petroff et al. 2001; Simeone et al. 2006). Because this action is not blocked by the benzodiazepine antagonist flumazenil, it is thought that topiramate exerts this effect via an interaction with the $GABA_A$ receptor that is not modulated by benzodiazepines (White et al. 2000).

Third, topiramate antagonizes glutamate receptors of the α-amino-3-hydroxy-5-methyl-4-isoxazole-propionic acid (AMPA)/kainate subtype and may selectively inhibit glutamate receptor 5 ($GluR_5$) kainate receptors (Kaminski et al. 2004). It has essentially no effect on glutamate *N*-methyl-D-aspartate (NMDA) receptors. AMPA/kainate receptors mediate fast excitatory postsynaptic potentials responsible for excitatory neurotransmission; blockade of kainate-evoked currents decreases neuronal excitability.

Fourth, topiramate negatively modulates high-voltage-activated calcium channels (Zhang et al. 2000). Of note, Shank et al. (2000) proposed that topiramate's combined effects on voltage-activated sodium channels, $GABA_A$ receptors, AMPA/kainate receptors, and high-voltage-activated calcium channels are unique as compared with those of other antiepileptic drugs. Indeed, Schiffer et al. (2001) found that pretreatment with topiramate inhibited nicotine-induced increases in mesolimbic extracellular dopamine and norepinephrine, but not serotonin. They hypothesized that this property was a result of the drug's ability to affect both GABAergic and glutamatergic function.

Fifth, topiramate weakly inhibits some carbonic anhydrase isoenzymes, including subtypes II and VI. Carbonic anhydrase is essential for the generation of $GABA_A$-mediated depolarizing responses. By inhibiting carbonic anhydrase, topiramate has been shown to reversibly reduce the $GABA_A$-mediated depolarizing responses evoked by either synaptic stimulation or pressure application of GABA (but not to modify $GABA_A$-mediated hyperpolarizing postsynaptic potentials) (Herrero et al. 2002).

Finally, topiramate has a number of other properties. These include an interaction with glycine receptor channels (Mohammadi et al. 2005), effects on mitochondrial permeability (Kudin et al. 2004), and antikindling properties in some animal models (Wauguier and Zhou 1996).

Pharmacokinetics and Disposition

Topiramate has a favorable pharmacokinetic profile (Bialer et al. 2004; Doose and Streeter 2002; Langtry et al. 1997; Rosenfeld 1997; Shank et al. 2000). It is rapidly and almost completely absorbed after oral administration, with bioavailability estimated to be about 80%. Peak plasma concentrations are reached within 2–4 hours. Plasma concentration increases in proportion to dose over the pharmacologically relevant dose range. Topiramate is minimally protein bound (9%–17%).

Topiramate is minimally metabolized by the liver in the absence of hepatic enzyme–inducing drugs. It inhibits cytochrome P450 (CYP) enzyme 2C19 but not other hepatic CYP enzymes. Topiramate is excreted mostly unchanged (approximately 70%) in the urine. The nonrenal (hepatic) clearance of topiramate increases two- to threefold when the drug is administered with hepatic enzyme–inducing drugs such as carbamazepine and phenytoin. Six minor metabolites have been identified (Shank et al. 2000).

Topiramate's elimination half-life is 19–25 hours, with linear pharmacokinetics in the dose range of 100–1,200 mg. The pharmacokinetics of topiramate in children are similar to those in adults, except that clearance is 50% higher, resulting in 33% lower plasma concentrations. Moderate or severe renal failure is associated with reduced renal clearance and increased elimination half-life of topiramate. Moderate or severe liver impairment is associated with clinically insignificant increased plasma concentrations of the drug.

Mechanism of Action

Although the mechanism of topiramate's anticonvulsant action is unknown, it has been hypothesized to be due to some combination of the drug's multiple pharmacological properties (Rho and Sankar 1999; Shank et al. 2000; White 2002, 2005; White et al. 2007). For example, the drug's anticonvulsant profile, as well as its benefits in substance use and eating disorders, has been hypothesized to be due to its dual actions on the GABAergic and glutamatergic systems (Johnson et al. 2003, 2005; McElroy et al. 2003, 2007; Rho and Sankar 1999; Schiffer et al. 2001).

Indications and Efficacy

FDA-Approved Indications

Topiramate is indicated by the FDA as initial monotherapy in patients 10 years of age and older with partial-onset or primary generalized tonic-clonic seizures; as adjunctive therapy for adults and pediatric patients ages 2–16 years with partial-onset seizures or primary generalized tonic-clonic seizures; and in patients 2 years of age and older with seizures associated with Lennox-Gastaut syndrome (van Passel et al. 2006). Topiramate is also indicated for the prophylaxis of migraine headache in adults (Brandes 2005; Bussone et al. 2006).

Other Indications

Topiramate is not approved by the FDA for use in the treatment of any psychiatric disorder. Because the drug was widely used off-label in the treatment of bipolar disorder after it came to market (see subsection "Bipolar Disorder" below), Johnson & Johnson PRD, the discoverer of topiramate, conducted a large study program of topiramate in adults with acute bipolar mania. These placebo-controlled studies failed to demonstrate a significant benefit of topiramate over placebo on the Young Mania Rating Scale (YMRS) (Chengappa et al. 2001a; Kushner et al. 2006; McElroy and Keck 2004). In contrast, findings from randomized, placebo-controlled trials suggest that topiramate may be effective in BED, bulimia nervosa, alcohol dependence, psychotropic-induced weight gain, and obesity.

Bipolar Disorder

Five randomized, placebo-controlled studies have shown that topiramate monotherapy is not efficacious in the short-term treatment of acute manic or mixed episodes in adults with bipolar I disorder (Kushner et al. 2006; McElroy and Keck 2004). All five studies used week 3 as the primary endpoint; in addition, three studies had a week 12 secondary endpoint, two studies had lithium comparator groups, and all trials measured weight as a secondary outcome. In each trial, the primary efficacy outcome—the change from baseline to week 3 in the YMRS score—failed to show a statistically significant separation between topiramate and placebo. There was also no drug-versus-placebo separation in the three trials with week 12 data. By contrast, in the two trials in which lithium was used, lithium did show statistical superiority to placebo.

Similarly, in the only placebo-controlled study of adjunctive topiramate in bipolar disorder, 287 outpatients experiencing a manic or mixed episode (by DSM-IV [American Psychiatric Association 1994] criteria) and a YMRS score ≥18 while taking therapeutic levels of valproate or lithium showed similar reductions (40%) in baseline YMRS scores for both topiramate and placebo after 12 weeks (Chengappa et al. 2006). In the only placebo-controlled study of topiramate in pediatric bipolar I disorder, 56 children and adolescents (6–17 years) experiencing a manic or mixed episode were randomly assigned to topiramate or placebo for 4 weeks (DelBello et al. 2005). Initially designed to enroll approximately 230 subjects, the study was prematurely discontinued when the adult mania trials were negative. Decrease in mean YMRS score from baseline to final visit using last observation carried forward (LOCF) analysis was not statistically different between treatment groups. However, a post hoc repeated-measures linear regression model of the primary efficacy analysis showed a statistically significant difference in the slopes of the linear mean profiles (P=0.003).

No placebo-controlled study of topiramate has yet been done in acute bipolar depression. Results from an 8-week single-blind comparison trial in which 36 outpatient adults with bipolar depression were randomly assigned to receive either topiramate (mean dosage=176 mg/day; range=50–300 mg/day) or bupropion sustained release (SR) (mean dosage=250 mg/day; range=100–400 mg/day) suggested that the drug might have antidepressant properties in some bipolar patients (McIntyre et al. 2002). The percentage of patients meeting a priori response criteria (50% or greater decrease from baseline in mean total score on the 17-item Hamilton Rating Scale for Depression [Ham-D]) was significant for both topiramate (56%) and bupropion SR (59%).

A number of open-label reports have described the successful topiramate treatment of various comorbid psychiatric or general medical disorders in bipolar patients. Comorbid psychiatric conditions in which improvement was seen included alcohol abuse; anxiety disorders such as obsessive-compulsive disorder (OCD) and posttraumatic stress disorder (PTSD); eating disorders such as bulimia nervosa, BED, and anorexia nervosa; impulse-control disorders; and catatonia (Barzman and DelBello 2006; Guille and Sachs 2002; Huguelet and Morand-Collomb 2005; McDaniel et al. 2006; McElroy et al. 2008; Shapira et al. 2000). Comorbid general medical conditions in which improvement was seen included obesity, psychotropic-induced weight gain, type 2 diabetes mellitus, tremor, and Tourette's disorder (Chengappa et al. 2001b; Guille and Sachs 2002; McIntyre et al. 2005; Vieta et al. 2002).

Depressive Disorders

In the only controlled study of topiramate in a depressive disorder, 64 females with DSM-IV recurrent major depressive disorder were randomly assigned to topiramate or placebo for 10 weeks (C. Nickel et al. 2005a). Topiramate was superior to placebo in reducing depressive and anger symptoms. All subjects tolerated topiramate well, and there were no suicidal events.

Psychotic Disorders

Four randomized, placebo-controlled studies of topiramate targeting psychopathology in psychotic disorders have been conducted. Three of these studies were in schizophrenia. In the first, 26 patients with treatment-resistant schizophrenia had topiramate (gradually increased to 300 mg/day) or placebo added to their ongoing antipsychotic regimens over two 12-week crossover treatment periods (Tiihonen et al. 2005). In the intent-to-treat analysis, topiramate was superior to placebo in reducing general psychopathological symptoms as assessed by the Positive and Negative Syndrome Scale (PANSS), but no significant improvement was observed in positive or negative symptoms. In the second study, topiramate up to 300 mg/day or placebo was added to the clozapine regimens of 32 patients with schizophrenia for 56 days (Afshar et al. 2009). At day 56, total PANSS values, as well as scores for all three subscales (negative symptoms, positive symptoms, and general psychopathology), were significantly improved with topiramate compared with placebo. In the third study, 43 patients with treatment-resistant schizophrenia receiving clozapine were given topiramate up to 200 mg/day or placebo for 24 weeks (Muscatello et al. 2011). Topiramate was associated with a significant reduction in bizarre behavior as assessed on the Scale for the Assessment of Positive Symptoms (P<0.002). No significant improvement in positive, negative, affective, or overall clinical symptomatology was otherwise seen with topiramate.

In the fourth study, 48 patients with schizoaffective disorder, bipolar type, were randomly assigned in a 2:1 ratio (favoring topiramate) to 8 weeks of double-blind treatment with topiramate (100–400 mg/day) or placebo (Chengappa et al. 2007). Patients who had achieved ≥20% decrease from baseline in their PANSS total scores were given the opportunity to continue for an additional 8 weeks of double-blind treatment. Adjunctive topiramate (nearly 275 mg/day) did not show increased efficacy relative to placebo on the PANSS (the primary outcome measure) or on any of the secondary outcome measures. There are several case reports of the successful use of topiramate to treat catatonia in patients with chronic psychotic disorders (McDaniel et al. 2006).

Eating Disorders

Five positive randomized, placebo-controlled studies in 640 subjects with bulimia nervosa (n=2 studies, 99 subjects) or BED (n=3 studies, 541 subjects) have shown that topiramate reduces binge eating. In the first study in bulimia nervosa, a 10-week trial in 69 subjects, topiramate (median dosage = 100 mg/day; range = 25–400 mg/day) was superior to placebo in reducing the frequency of binge and purge days (days during which at least one binge-eating or purging episode occurred; P= 0.004) (Hedges et al. 2003; Hoopes et al. 2003). Binge-eating/purging remission rates were 32% for topiramate and 6% for placebo (P=NS). Dropout rates were 34% for topiramate and 47% for placebo. In the second study, 60 subjects with DSM-IV bulimia nervosa received 10 weeks of topiramate (titrated to 250 mg/day in the sixth week) (n=30) or placebo (n=30) (C. Nickel et al. 2005b). Topiramate was associated with significant decreases in binge/purge frequency (defined as a >50% reduction; 37% for topiramate and 3% for placebo), body weight (difference in weight loss between the 2 groups = 3.8 kg), and all of the SF-36 Health Survey scales (all Ps<0.001).

In the first controlled study in BED, 61 subjects with DSM-IV BED and obesity received topiramate or placebo for 14 weeks (McElroy et al. 2003). Topiramate was significantly superior to placebo in reducing binge frequency, as well as global severity of illness, obsessive-compulsive features of binge-eating symptoms, body weight, and body mass index (BMI). The dropout rate, however, was high—14 (47%) subjects receiving topiramate and 12 (39%) subjects receiving placebo failed to complete the trial.

The second controlled study of topiramate in BED was a multicenter trial in which subjects with DSM-IV BED and ≥3 binge-eating days per week, a BMI ranging from 30 kg/m^2 to 50 kg/m^2, and no current psychiatric disorders or substance abuse were randomly assigned to topiramate or placebo for 16 weeks (McElroy et al. 2007). Of 407 subjects enrolled, 13 failed to meet inclusion criteria; 195 topiramate and 199 placebo subjects were therefore evaluated for efficacy. Topiramate significantly reduced binge-eating days per week, binge episodes per week, weight, and BMI compared with placebo (all Ps<0.001). The drug also significantly decreased measures of obsessive-compulsive symptoms, impulsivity, hunger, and disability. Fifty-eight percent of topiramate-treated subjects achieved remission compared with 29% of placebo-treated subjects (P<0.001). Discontinuation rates were 30% in each group; adverse events were the most common reason for topiramate discontinuation (16%; placebo, 8%).

The third controlled study of topiramate in BED was another multicenter trial in which 73 patients with BED and obesity were randomly assigned to 19 sessions of cognitive-behavioral therapy in conjunction with topiramate or placebo for 21 weeks (Claudino et al. 2007). Compared with patients given placebo, patients given topiramate showed a significantly greater rate of reduction in weight, the primary outcome measure, over the course of treatment (P<0.001). Topiramate recipients also showed a significant weight loss (−6.8 kg) relative to placebo recipients (−0.9 kg). A greater percentage of topiramate-treated patients (31 of 37) than of placebo-treated patients (22 of 36) attained remission of binge eating ($P=0.03$). There was no difference between groups in completion rates, although one topiramate recipient withdrew because of an adverse effect.

In open studies, topiramate has also been reported to have long-term therapeutic effects in BED with obesity; to reduce symptoms of BED, bulimia nervosa, and anorexia nervosa with comorbid mood disorders; and to reduce nocturnal eating and overweight in patients with night-eating syndrome and sleep-related eating disorders (Guille and Sachs 2002; McElroy et al. 2008; Winkelman 2006). However, there is a report of topiramate possibly triggering a recurrent episode of anorexia nervosa in a woman with epilepsy and several reports of eating disorder patients misusing the drug to lose weight (McElroy et al. 2008).

Substance Use Disorders

Four randomized, placebo-controlled studies suggest that topiramate may have therapeutic effects in alcohol, cocaine, and nicotine dependence. Two studies examined topiramate in alcohol dependence. In the first, 150 subjects with alcohol dependence were randomly assigned to topiramate (up to 300 mg/day) or placebo for 12 weeks (Johnson et al. 2003). All subjects received compliance enhancement therapy. At study end, subjects receiving topiramate, compared with those on placebo, had significantly fewer drinks per day ($P=0.0006$), fewer drinks per drinking day ($P=0.0009$), fewer heavy drinking days ($P=0.0003$), more days abstinent ($P=0.0003$), and a log plasma gamma-glutamyl transferase (GGT) ratio of 0.07 (–0.11 to –0.02) less ($P=0.0046$). Craving was also significantly more improved with topiramate than with placebo. In the second study, 371 subjects were randomly assigned to topiramate (up to 300 mg) or placebo, along with a weekly compliance enhancement intervention, at 16 sites for 14 weeks (Johnson et al. 2007). Topiramate was significantly superior to placebo in reducing the percentage of heavy drinking days and other drinking outcomes such as drinks per drinking day, increasing the percentage of days abstinent, and improving the log plasma GGT ratio (all $Ps \leq 0.002$).

In the study in cocaine dependence, 40 subjects were randomly assigned to topiramate (titrated gradually over 8 weeks to 200 mg/day) or placebo for 13 weeks (Kampman et al. 2004). Topiramate-treated subjects were more likely to be abstinent from cocaine after week 8 compared with placebo-treated subjects ($P=0.01$). They were also more likely to achieve 3 weeks of continuous abstinence from cocaine ($P=0.05$).

In the first of two controlled studies in smoking cessation, topiramate was superior to placebo in 94 subjects with comorbid alcohol dependence (Johnson et al. 2005). This study was a subgroup analysis of the first controlled study of topiramate in alcohol dependence (Johnson et al. 2003). In the second study, the drug was superior to placebo for smoking cessation in male ($n=38$), but not female ($n=49$), subjects ($n=90$) who had no associated psychopathology (Anthenelli et al. 2008).

There have also been case reports of the successful use of topiramate in opiate and benzodiazepine withdrawal, but these uses will need to be evaluated in placebo-controlled trials (Michopoulos et al. 2006; Zullino et al. 2004).

Anxiety Disorders

Topiramate has been evaluated in two placebo-controlled studies in PTSD. In the first, 38 civilian patients with PTSD were randomly assigned to flexible doses of topiramate alone (median dosage = 150 mg/day) or placebo for 12 weeks (Tucker et al. 2007). No significant difference was found on the primary efficacy measure, the total Clinician-Administered PTSD Scale (CAPS) score. However, significant or near-significant effects were found in favor of topiramate on the eight-item Treatment Outcome PTSD scale (TOP-8) (decrease in overall severity 68% vs. 42%; $P=0.025$) and endpoint Clinical Global Impression Scale—Improvement (CGI-I) scores (1.9 ± 1.2 vs. 2.6 ± 1.1; $P=0.055$). In the second study, 40 male veterans with chronic PTSD, most of whom were receiving antidepressants, were given topiramate up to 200 mg/day or placebo for 7 weeks (Lindley et al. 2007). No significant difference was found on the CAPS, CGI–Severity (CGI-S), or Patient Global Impression–Improvement Scales (PGI-I).

One study has evaluated adjunctive topiramate (mean endpoint dosage 179 mg/day) versus placebo in 36 adult patients with obsessive-compulsive disorder receiving selective serotonin reuptake inhibitors (Berlin et al. 2011). Topiramate significantly reduced the compulsion subscale score ($P=0.014$) of the Yale-Brown Obsessive Compulsive Scale (Y-BOCS), but not the obsession subscale score or the total score.

Borderline Personality Disorder

Three placebo-controlled studies, all conducted by the same group, have evaluated topiramate in DSM-IV-defined BPD. In the first, 29 female subjects were randomly assigned in a 2:1 ratio to topiramate or placebo for 8 weeks (M.K. Nickel et al. 2004). Topiramate dosage was increased to 250 mg/day over 6 weeks. At study end, significant improvement on four subscales of the STAXI (state–anger, trait–anger, anger–out, and anger–control) was observed for topiramate compared with placebo. In the second study, 42 male subjects with BPD received topiramate or placebo for 8 weeks (M.K. Nickel et al. 2005a). Similar to the study in females, significant improvement on the same four subscales on the STAXI was found for topiramate compared with placebo. In the third study, 56 women with BPD received topiramate or placebo for 10 weeks (Loew et al. 2006). Topiramate was titrated to 200 mg/day over 6 weeks and then held constant. Topiramate was superior to placebo on the somatization, interpersonal sensitivity, anxiety, hostility, phobic anxiety, and Global Severity Index subscales of the Symptom Checklist–90 (SCL-90-R) (all $Ps<0.001$); all eight scales of the SF-36 Health Survey (all $Ps<0.01$); and four of eight scales of the Inventory of Interpersonal Problems (all $Ps<0.001$). In all three studies, topiramate was well tolerated, and there were no psychotic or suicidal adverse events.

Psychotropic-Associated Weight Gain

Four placebo-controlled studies suggest that topiramate reduces antipsychotic-related weight gain in patients with psychotic or mood disorders. In one study, 66 inpatients with schizophrenia receiving antipsychotic medication and "carrying excess weight" were randomly assigned to topiramate 100 mg/day, topiramate 200 mg/day, or placebo for 12 weeks (Ko et al. 2005). Body weight, BMI, and waist and hip circumferences decreased significantly in the topiramate 200 mg/day group compared with the topiramate 100 mg/day and placebo groups. Scores on the CGI-S and the Brief Psychiatric Rating Scale (BPRS) were also significantly decreased, but the decreases were not thought to be clinically meaningful. In another study, 43 women with mood or psychotic disorders who had gained weight while receiving olanzapine were given topiramate or placebo for 10 weeks (M.K. Nickel et al. 2005b). Weight loss was significantly greater (by 5.6 kg) in the topiramate group. Topiramate-treated subjects also experienced significantly greater improvement in measures of health-related quality of life and psychological impairment.

In the third study, adjunctive topiramate was ineffective for manic symptoms in bipolar I manic or mixed patients receiving lithium or valproate but was associated with significantly greater reductions in body weight compared with placebo (−2.5 vs. 0.2 kg, respectively; $P<0.001$) and BMI (−0.84 vs. 0.07 kg/m^2, respectively; $P<0.001$) (Chengappa et al. 2006). In the fourth study, adjunctive topiramate was evaluated for the prevention of olanzapine-related weight gain (Narula et al. 2010). In a 12-week trial, 72 patients with schizophrenia were randomly assigned to receive olanzapine plus topiramate 100 mg or olanzapine plus placebo. Whereas topiramate augmentation was associated with statistically significant weight loss, placebo-augmented olanzapine was associated with significant weight gain ($P=0.05$ between-group difference). Topiramate augmentation was also associated with significantly greater improvement in several metabolic variables, systolic and diastolic blood pressure, and PANSS general psychopathology and total scores.

Obesity

Nine randomized, placebo-controlled trials have evaluated topiramate (Astrup et al. 2004; Bray et al. 2003; Eliasson et al. 2007; Stenlöf et al. 2007; Tonstad et al. 2005; Toplak et al. 2007; Tremblay et al. 2007; Wilding et al. 2004) or a controlled-release (CR) formulation of topiramate (Rosenstock et al. 2007) for weight loss in subjects with obesity. In all nine studies, topiramate was superior to placebo for weight loss at all dosages (range 64–400 mg/day) and at all endpoints (range 28 weeks–1 year) evaluated. The four long-term studies (duration 40 weeks to 1 year) found that topiramate was associated with weight loss that increased up to 1 year without plateauing (Astrup et al. 2004; Eliasson et al. 2007; Stenlöf et al. 2007; Wilding et al. 2004). In a study in obese subjects with comorbid hypertension, there were significant decreases in diastolic, but not systolic, blood pressure in the two groups receiving topiramate compared with the placebo group (Tonstad et al. 2005). In four studies of topiramate in obese subjects with comorbid type 2 diabetes, topiramate-treated subjects showed significant decreases in glycosylated hemoglobin (Hb_{A1c}) compared with placebo-treated subjects (Eliasson et al. 2007; Rosenstock et al. 2007; Stenlöf et al. 2007; Toplak et al. 2007).

Side Effects and Toxicology

The side-effect profile of topiramate may vary with the patient's illness, mood state, and concomitant medications. The most common side effects of topiramate in the initial dose-ranging studies in patients with epilepsy when used in combination with other antiepileptic drugs at dosages of 200–1,000 mg/day were related to the central nervous system and included dizziness, somnolence, psychomotor slowing, nervousness, paresthesias, ataxia, difficulty with memory, difficulty with concentration or attention, confusion, and speech disorders or related speech problems (Langtry et al. 1997; Shorvon 1996). Other side effects were nystagmus, depression, nausea, diplopia, abnormal vision, anorexia, language problems, and tremor. When used as monotherapy in patients with epilepsy, the most common side effects were dizziness, anxiety, paresthesias, insomnia, somnolence, myalgia, anorexia, nausea, dyspepsia, and diarrhea. The most common side effects of topiramate in the large registration trials for migraine headache (which used total daily doses of 50, 100, and 200 mg) were paresthesias, fatigue, memory difficulties, concentration/attention problems, and mood problems (Bussone et al. 2006). In the monotherapy trials in adult mania, paresthesias, decreased appetite, dry mouth, and weight loss were more common with topiramate than placebo (Kushner et al. 2006). In the obesity trials, events related to the central or peripheral nervous system or to psychiatric disorders were most commonly reported (Rosenstock et al. 2007). These included paresthesias; fatigue; difficulty with attention, concentration, and/or memory; taste perversion; and anorexia. Overall, paresthesias and cognitive complaints are the most troublesome adverse events (van Passel et al. 2006). A meta-analysis suggested that a dose-response relationship exists for dizziness, cognitive impairment, and fatigue (Zaccara et al. 2008).

The central nervous system and gastrointestinal effects of topiramate are usually mild to moderate in severity and often decrease or resolve with time or dosage reduction (Meador et al. 2003; Shorvon 1996). Also, they may be minimized by slow titration of topiramate dosage (Biton et al. 2001). However, topiramate may be associated with more cognitive impairment than some of the other new antiepileptic drugs (Martin et al. 1999; Meador et al. 2003).

Infrequent but serious side effects of topiramate include nephrolithiasis, an ocular syndrome of acute myopia with secondary angle-closure glaucoma, oligohydrosis and hyperthermia, and metabolic acidosis (van Passel et al. 2006). The incidence of nephrolithiasis has been estimated to be 1.5% (Shorvon 1996). In the epilepsy trials, more than 75% of the patients who developed renal stones elected to continue treatment with topiramate (Reife et al. 2000). Nephrolithiasis is thought to be related to topiramate exerting carbonic anhydrase inhibition in the kidney (Welch et al. 2006).

The secondary angle-closure glaucoma associated with topiramate is characterized by acute onset of bilateral blurred vision and ocular pain (Fraunfelder and Fraunfelder 2004; Fraunfelder et al. 2004). Ophthalmological findings include bilateral myopia, conjunctival hyperemia, anterior chamber shallowing, and increased intraocular pressure. Most cases have occurred within 1 month of topiramate initiation and fully resolve with drug discontinuation. Peripheral iridectomy and laser iridotomy are not effective. The syndrome has been attributed to sulfamate-induced ciliary body edema.

There were no clinically relevant changes in hepatic, renal, or hematological parameters in the registration trials of topiramate, and laboratory monitoring was initially thought not to be required (Reife et al. 2000; Sachdeo and Karia 2002). In addition, no treatment-related changes in physical or neurological examinations (except body weight loss), in electrocardiograms, or in ophthalmological or audiometric test results were noted. However, as a carbonic anhydrase inhibitor, topiramate reduces serum bicarbonate levels, and it is believed that this is the mechanism underlying reports of reversible metabolic acidosis in some patients (Sachdeo and Karia 2002; van Passel et al. 2006; Welch et al. 2006). It is now recommended that baseline and periodic serum bicarbonate levels be measured in patients receiving topiramate. A growing concern is the psychiatric adverse-event profile of antiepileptic drugs in patients with epilepsy, including whether such drugs cause suicidality and psychosis. Although some data suggest that a subgroup of epilepsy patients may be susceptible to such psychiatric adverse events, other data indicate that topiramate may be associated with depression in epilepsy patients, especially during rapid titration (Mula and Sander 2007). There are also isolated reports of topiramate's induction of mood and anxiety symptoms in psychiatric patients (Damsa et al. 2006; Klufas and Thompson 2001). Moreover, one obesity study reported eight (6.2%) suicidal-related events occurring in topiramate-treated subjects versus none in placebo-treated subjects (Rosenstock et al. 2007).

Topiramate can cause fetal harm when given to pregnant women. Prenatal exposure to topiramate is associated with an increased risk of oral clefts (Hunt et al. 2008).

Drug-Drug Interactions

The clearance of topiramate can be increased by the coadministration of hepatic enzyme–inducing drugs (Bialer et al. 2004; Gidal 2002; Langtry et al. 1997; Rosenfeld et al. 1997; van Passel et al. 2006). Thus, carbamazepine and phenytoin may substantially decrease topiramate levels. Conversely, topiramate has mild enzyme-inducing properties and may enhance metabolism of ethinyl estradiol. Available data suggest that at topiramate dosages of 200 mg/day or lower, this induction is insignificant, but at dosages greater than 200 mg/day, induction becomes dose dependent and occurs to a great extent (Bialer et al. 2004). Women taking combination oral contraceptive agents therefore need to be counseled about this potential interaction.

Although there have been reports of topiramate causing increased lithium levels (Abraham and Owen 2004), this effect appears to be rarely clinically significant (Bialer et al. 2004).

References

Abraham G, Owen J: Topiramate can cause lithium toxicity. J Clin Psychopharmacol 24:565–567, 2004

Afshar H, Roohafza H, Mousavi G, et al: Topiramate add-on treatment in schizophrenia: a randomised, double-blind, placebo-controlled clinical trial. J Psychopharmacol 23:157–162, 2009

American Psychiatric Association: Diagnostic and Statistical Manual of Mental Disorders, 4th Edition. Washington, DC, American Psychiatric Association, 1994

Anthenelli RM, Blom TJ, McElroy SL, et al: Preliminary evidence for gender-specific effects of topiramate as a potential aid to smoking cessation. Addiction 103:687–694, 2008

Astrup A, Caterson I, Zelissen P, et al: Topiramate: long-term maintenance of weight loss induced by low-calorie diet in obese subjects. Obes Res 12:1658–1669, 2004

Barzman DH, DelBello MP: Topiramate for co-occurring bipolar disorder and disruptive behavior disorders (letter). Am J Psychiatry 163:1451–1452, 2006

Berlin HA, Koran LM, Jenike MA, et al: Double-blind, placebo-controlled trial of topiramate augmentation in treatment-resistant obsessive-compulsive disorder. J Clin Psychiatry 72:716–721, 2011

Bialer M, Doose DR, Murthy B, et al: Pharmacokinetic interactions of topiramate. Clin Pharmacokinet 43:763–780, 2004

Biton V, Edwards KR, Montouris GD, et al: Topiramate titration and tolerability. Ann Pharmacother 35:173–179, 2001

Brandes JL: Practical use of topiramate for migraine prevention. Headache Suppl 1:S66–S73, 2005

Bray GA, Hollander P, Klein S, et al: A 6-month randomized, placebo-controlled, dose-ranging trial of topiramate for weight loss in obesity. Obes Res 11:722–733, 2003

Bussone G, Usai S, D'Amico D: Topiramate in migraine prophylaxis: data from a pooled analysis and open-label extension study. Neurol Sci 27 (suppl 2):159–163, 2006

Chengappa KN, Gershon S, Levine J: The evolving role of topiramate among other mood stabilizers in the management of bipolar disorder. Bipolar Disord 3:215–232, 2001a

Chengappa [Roy Chengappa] KN, Levine J, Rathore D, et al: Long-term effects of topiramate on bipolar mood instability, weight change and glycemic control: a case-series. Eur Psychiatry 16: 186–190, 2001b

Chengappa [Roy Chengappa] KN, Schwarzman LK, Hulihan JF, et al: Adjunctive topiramate therapy in patients receiving a mood stabilizer for bipolar I disorder: a randomized, placebo-controlled trial. J Clin Psychiatry 67:1698–1706, 2006

Chengappa [Roy Chengappa] KN, Kupfer DJ, Parepally H, et al: A placebo-controlled, random-assignment, parallel-group pilot study of adjunctive topiramate for patients with schizoaffective disorder, bipolar type. Bipolar Disord 9:609–617, 2007

Claudino AM, de Oliveira IR, Appolinario JC, et al: Double-blind, randomized, placebo-controlled trial of topiramate plus cognitive-behavior therapy in binge-eating disorder. J Clin Psychiatry 68:1324–1332, 2007

Damsa C, Warczyk S, Cailhol L, et al: Panic attacks associated with topiramate. J Clin Psychiatry 67:326–327, 2006

DelBello MP, Findling RL, Kushner S, et al: A pilot controlled trial of topiramate for mania in children and adolescents with bipolar disorder. J Am Acad Child Adolesc Psychiatry 44:539–547, 2005

Doose DR, Streeter AJ: Topiramate: chemistry, biotransformation, and pharmacokinetics, in Antiepileptic Drugs, 5th Edition. Edited by Levy RH, Mattson RH, Meldrum BS, et al. Philadelphia, PA, Lippincott Williams & Wilkins, 2002, pp 727–734

Eliasson B, Gudbjörnsdottir S, Cederholm J, et al: Weight loss and metabolic effects of topiramate in overweight and obese type 2 diabetic patients: randomized double-blind placebo-controlled trial. Int J Obes (Lond) 31:1140–1147, 2007

Fraunfelder FW, Fraunfelder FT: Adverse ocular drug reactions recently identified by the National Registry of Drug-Induced Ocular Side Effects. Ophthalmology 111:1275–1279, 2004

Fraunfelder FW, Fraunfelder FT, Keates EU: Topiramate-associated acute, bilateral, secondary angle-closure glaucoma. Ophthalmology 111:109–111, 2004

Gidal BE: Topiramate: drug interactions, in Antiepileptic Drugs, 5th Edition. Edited by Levy RH, Mattson RH, Meldrum BS, et al. Philadelphia, PA, Lippincott Williams & Wilkins, 2002, pp 735–739

Guille C, Sachs G: Clinical outcome of adjunctive topiramate treatment in a sample of refractory bipolar patients with comorbid conditions. Prog Neuropsychopharmacol Biol Psychiatry 26:1035–1039, 2002

Hedges DW, Reimherr FW, Hoopes SP, et al: Treatment of bulimia nervosa with topiramate in a randomized, double-blind, placebo-controlled trial, part 2: improvement in psychiatric measures. J Clin Psychiatry 64:1449–1454, 2003

Herrero AL, Del Olmo N, González-Escalada JR, et al: Two new actions of topiramate: inhibition of depolarizing GABAA-mediated responses and activation of a potassium conductance. Neuropharmacology 42:210–220, 2002

Hoopes SP, Reimherr FW, Hedges DW, et al: Part I: Topiramate in the treatment of bulimia nervosa: a randomized, double-blind, placebo-controlled trial. J Clin Psychiatry 64:1335–1341, 2003

Huguelet P, Morand-Collomb S: Effect of topiramate augmentation on two patients suffering from schizophrenia or bipolar disorder with comorbid alcohol abuse. Pharmacol Res 52:392–394, 2005

Hunt S, Russell A, Smithson WH, et al: Topiramate in pregnancy: preliminary experience from the UK Epilepsy and Pregnancy Register. Neurology 71:272–276, 2008

Johnson BA, Ait-Daoud N, Bowden CL, et al: Oral topiramate for treatment of alcohol dependence: a randomized controlled trial. Lancet 361:1677–1685, 2003

Johnson BA, Ait-Daoud N, Akhtar FZ, et al: Use of oral topiramate to promote smoking abstinence among alcohol-dependent smokers: a randomized controlled trial. Arch Intern Med 165:1600–1605, 2005

Johnson BA, Rosenthal N, Capece JA, et al: Topiramate for treating alcohol dependence: a randomized controlled trial. JAMA 298:1641–1651, 2007

Kaminski RM, Banerjee M, Rogawski MA: Topiramate selectively protects against seizures induced by ATPA, a GluR5 kainate receptor agonist. Neuropharmacology 46:1097–1104, 2004

Kampman KM, Pettinati H, Lynch KG, et al: A pilot trial of topiramate for the treatment of cocaine dependence. Drug Alcohol Depend 75:233–240, 2004

Kawasaki H, Tancredi V, D'Arcangelo G, et al: Multiple actions of the novel anticonvulsant drug topiramate in the rat subiculum in vitro. Brain Res 807:125–134, 1998

Klufas A, Thompson D: Topiramate-induced depression (letter). Am J Psychiatry 158:1736, 2001

Ko YH, Joe SH, Jung IK, et al: Topiramate as an adjuvant treatment with atypical antipsychotics in schizophrenic patients experiencing weight gain. Clin Neuropharmacol 28:169–175, 2005

Kudin AP, Debska-Vielhaber G, Vielhaber S, et al: The mechanism of neuroprotection by topiramate in an animal model of epilepsy. Epilepsia 45:1478–1487, 2004

Kushner SF, Khan A, Lane R, et al: Topiramate monotherapy in the management of acute mania: results of four double-blind placebo-controlled trials. Bipolar Disord 8:15–27, 2006

Kuzniecky R, Hetherington H, Ho S, et al: Topiramate increases cerebral GABA in healthy humans. Neurology 51:627–629, 1998

Langtry HD, Gillis JC, Davis R: Topiramate: a review of its pharmacodynamic and pharmacokinetic properties and clinical efficacy in the management of epilepsy. Drugs 54:752–773, 1997

Lindley SE, Carlson EB, Hill K: A randomized, double-blind, placebo-controlled trial of augmentation topiramate for chronic combat-related posttraumatic stress disorder. J Clin Psychopharmacol 27:677–681, 2007

Loew TH, Nickel MK, Muehlbacher M, et al: Topiramate treatment for women with borderline personality disorder: a double-blind, placebo-controlled study. J Clin Psychopharmacol 26: 61–66, 2006

Martin R, Kuzniecky R, Ho S, et al: Cognitive effects of topiramate, gabapentin, and lamotrigine in healthy young adults. Neurology 52:321–327, 1999

McDaniel WW, Spiegel DR, Sahota AK: Topiramate effect in catatonia: a case series. J Neuropsychiatry Clin Neurosci 18:234–238, 2006

McElroy SL, Keck PE Jr: Topiramate, in American Psychiatric Publishing Textbook of Psychopharmacology, 3rd Edition. Edited by Schatzberg AF, Nemeroff CB. Washington, DC, American Psychiatric Publishing, 2004, pp 627–636

McElroy SL, Arnold LA, Shapira AN, et al: Topiramate in the treatment of binge eating disorder associated with obesity: a randomized, placebo controlled trial (erratum appears in Am J Psychiatry 160:612, 2003). Am J Psychiatry 160:255–261, 2003

McElroy SL, Hudson JI, Capece JA, et al: Topiramate for the treatment of binge eating disorder associated with obesity: a placebo-controlled study. Biol Psychiatry 61:1039–1048, 2007

McElroy SL, Guerdjikova A, Keck PE Jr, et al: Antiepileptic drugs in obesity, psychotropic-associated weight gain, and eating disorders, in Antiepileptic Drugs to Treat Psychiatric Disorders. Edited by McElroy SL, Keck PE Jr, Post RM. New York, Informa Healthcare, 2008, pp 283–309

McIntyre RS, Mancini DA, McCann S, et al: Topiramate versus bupropion SR when added to mood stabilizer therapy for the depressive phase of bipolar disorder: a preliminary single-blind study. Bipolar Disord 4:207–213, 2002

McIntyre RS, Riccardelli R, Binder C, et al: Open-label adjunctive topiramate in the treatment of unstable bipolar disorder. Can J Psychiatry 50: 415–422, 2005

Meador KJ, Loring DW, Hulihan JF, et al: Differential cognitive and behavioral effects of topiramate and valproate. Neurology 60:1483–1488, 2003

Michopoulos I, Douzenis A, Christodoulou C, et al: Topiramate use in alprazolam addiction. World J Biol Psychiatry 7:265–267, 2006

Mohammadi B, Krampfl K, Cetinkaya C, et al: Interaction of topiramate with glycine receptor channels. Pharmacol Res 51:587–592, 2005

Mula M, Sander JW: Negative effects of antiepileptic drugs on mood in patients with epilepsy. Drug Saf 30:555–567, 2007

Muscatello M, Bruno A, Pandolfo G, et al: Topiramate augmentation of clozapine in schizophrenia: a double-blind, placebo-controlled study. J Psychopharmacol 25:667–674, 2011

Narula PK, Rehan HS, Unni KE, et al: Topiramate for prevention of olanzapine associated weight gain and metabolic dysfunction in schizophrenia: a double-blind, placebo-controlled trial. Schizophr Res 118:218–223, 2010

Nickel C, Lahmann C, Tritt K, et al: Topiramate in the treatment of depressive and anger symptoms in female depressive patient: a randomized, double-blind, placebo-controlled study. J Affect Disord 87:243–252, 2005a

Nickel C, Tritt K, Muehlbacher M, et al: Topiramate treatment in bulimia nervosa patients: a randomized, double-blind, placebo-controlled trial. Int J Eat Disord 38:295–300, 2005b

Nickel MK, Nickel C, Mitterlehner FO, et al: Topiramate treatment of aggression in female borderline personality disorder patients: a double-blind, placebo-controlled study. J Clin Psychiatry 65:1515–1519, 2004

Nickel MK, Nickel C, Kaplan P, et al: Treatment of aggression with topiramate in male borderline patients: a double-blind, placebo-controlled study. Biol Psychiatry 57:495–499, 2005a

Nickel MK, Nickel C, Muehlbacher M, et al: Influence of topiramate on olanzapine-related adiposity in women: a random, double-blind, placebo-controlled study. J Clin Psychopharmacol 25:211–217, 2005b

Petroff OA, Hyder F, Rothman DL, et al: Topiramate rapidly raises brain GABA in epilepsy patients. Epilepsia 42:543–548, 2001

Reife R, Pledger G, Wu S-C: Topiramate as add-on therapy: pooled analysis of randomized controlled trials in adults. Epilepsia 41 (suppl 1): S66–S71, 2000

Rho JM, Sankar R: The pharmacologic basis of antiepileptic drug action. Epilepsia 40:1471–1483, 1999

Rosenfeld WE: Topiramate: a review of preclinical, pharmacokinetic, and clinical data. Clin Ther 19:1294–1308, 1997

Rosenfeld WE, Doose DR, Walker SA, et al: Effect of topiramate on the pharmacokinetics of an oral contraceptive containing norethindrone and ethinyl estradiol in patients with epilepsy. Epilepsia 38:317–323, 1997

Rosenstock J, Hollander P, Gadde KM, et al: A randomized, double-blind, placebo-controlled multicenter study to assess the efficacy and safety of topiramate controlled-release in the treatment of obese, type 2 diabetic patients. Diabetes Care 30:1480–1486, 2007

Sachdeo RC, Karia RM: Topiramate: adverse effects, in Antiepileptic Drugs, 5th Edition. Edited by Levy RH, Mattson RH, Meldrum BS, et al. Philadelphia, PA, Lippincott Williams & Wilkins, 2002, pp 760–764

Schiffer WK, Gerasimov MR, Marsteller DA, et al: Topiramate selectively attenuates nicotine induced increases in monoamine release. Synapse 42:196–198, 2001

Shank RP, Gardocki JF, Streeter AJ, et al: An overview of the preclinical aspects of topiramate: pharmacology, pharmacokinetics, and mechanism of action. Epilepsia 41 (suppl 1):S3–S9, 2000

Shapira NA, Goldsmith TD, McElroy SL: Treatment of binge-eating disorder with topiramate: a clinical case series. J Clin Psychiatry 61:368–372, 2000

Shorvon SD: Safety of topiramate: adverse events and relationships to dosing. Epilepsia 37 (suppl 2): S18–S22, 1996

Simeone TA, Wilcox KS, White HS: Subunit selectivity of topiramate modulation of heteromeric GABA(A) receptors. Neuropharmacology 50: 845–857, 2006

Stenlöf K, Rössner S, Vercruysse F, et al: Topiramate in the treatment of obese subjects with drug-naive type 2 diabetes. Diabetes Obes Metab 9: 360–368, 2007

Tiihonen J, Halonen P, Wahlbeck K, et al: Topiramate add-on in treatment-resistant schizophrenia: a randomized, double-blind, placebo-controlled, crossover trial. J Clin Psychiatry 66:1012–1015, 2005

Tonstad S, Tykarski A, Weissgarten J, et al: Efficacy and safety of topiramate in the treatment of obese subjects with essential hypertension. Am J Cardiol 96:243–251, 2005

Toplak H, Hamann A, Moore R, et al: Efficacy and safety of topiramate in combination with metformin in the treatment of obese subjects with type 2 diabetes: a randomized, double-blind, placebo-controlled study. Int J Obesity 31:138–146, 2007

Tremblay A, Chaput J-P, Bérubé S, et al: The effect of topiramate on energy balance in obese men: a 6-month double-blind randomized placebo-controlled study with a 6-month open-label extension. Eur J Clin Pharmacol 63:123–134, 2007

Tucker P, Trautman RP, Wyatt DB, et al: Efficacy and safety of topiramate monotherapy in civilian posttraumatic stress disorder: a randomized, double-blind, placebo-controlled study. J Clin Psychiatry 68:201–206, 2007

van Passel L, Arif H, Hirsch LJ: Topiramate for the treatment of epilepsy and other nervous system disorders. Expert Rev Neurother 6:19–31, 2006

Vieta E, Torrent C, Garcia-Ribas G, et al: Use of topiramate in treatment-resistant bipolar spectrum disorders. J Clin Psychopharmacol 22:431–435, 2002

Wauguier A, Zhou S: Topiramate: a potent anticonvulsant in the amygdala-kindled rat. Epilepsy Res 24:73–77, 1996

Welch BJ, Graybeal D, Moe OW, et al: Biochemical and stone-risk profiles with topiramate treatment. Am J Kidney Dis 48:555–563, 2006

White HS: Topiramate: mechanisms of action, in Antiepileptic Drugs, 5th Edition. Edited by Levy RH, Mattson RH, Meldrum BS, et al. Philadelphia, PA, Lippincott Williams & Wilkins, 2002, pp 719–726

White HS: Molecular pharmacology of topiramate: managing seizures and preventing migraine. Headache 45 (suppl 1):S48–S56, 2005

White HS, Brown SD, Woodhead JH, et al: Topiramate modulates GABA-evoked currents in murine cortical neurons by a nonbenzodiazepine mechanism. Epilepsia 41 (suppl 1):S17–S20, 2000

White HS, Smith MD, Wilcox KS: Mechanisms of action of antiepileptic drugs. Int Rev Neurobiol 81:85–110, 2007

Wilding J, Gaal L, Rissanan A, et al: A randomized double-blind placebo-controlled study of the long-term efficacy and safety of topiramate in the treatment of obese subjects. Int J Obes Relat Metab Disord 28:1399–1410, 2004

Winkelman JW: Efficacy and tolerability of open-label topiramate in the treatment of sleep-related eating disorder: a retrospective case series. J Clin Psychiatry 67:1729–1734, 2006

Zaccara G, Gangemi PE, Cincotta M: Central nervous system adverse effects of new antiepileptic drugs. A meta-analysis of placebo-controlled studies. Seizure 17:405–421, 2008

Zhang X, Velumian AA, Jones OT, et al: Modulation of high voltage-activated calcium channels in dentate granule cells by topiramate. Epilepsia 41 (suppl 1):S52–S60, 2000

Zullino DF, Krenz S, Zimmerman G, et al: Topiramate in opiate withdrawal—comparison with clonidine and with carbamazepine/mianserin. Subst Abus 25:27–33, 2004

Other Agents

CHAPTER 32

Cognitive Enhancers

Frank W. Brown, M.D.

Disruption of cholinergic neurotransmission and excitatory amino acids is correlated with the development of cognitive impairment and, specifically, Alzheimer's disease (Mesulam 2004). Multiple mechanisms exist that may account for the progression of cognitive impairment, including those related to cholinesterase, N-methyl-D-aspartate (NMDA), vascular disease, and oxidative damage (Aisen and Davis 1994; Bartus et al. 1982; Behl 1999; Behl et al. 1992; Jick et al. 2000; Kalaria et al. 1996; Selkoe 2000; Terry and Buccafusco 2003; Wolozin et al. 2000). An outcome of the disruption of many neurotransmitter systems, cognitive impairment may occur at any time during the disease process as synaptic plasticity becomes impaired, degrading the efficiency of neuronal transmission (Malik et al. 2007). It is intuitive that the earliest intervention prior to irreversible disease progression is optimal. Currently, it is unknown when the irreversible disease processes begin; no specific markers have been identified that could guide clinicians to initiate prophylactic treatment prior to the development of cognitive or behavioral manifestations.

Cognitive enhancer is a general term that denotes a pharmacological or nutraceutical intervention that improves cognitive functioning in an impaired or normal brain by reversing or delaying underlying neuropathological changes within the brain or by modulating the existing neurochemistry to facilitate a desired performance differential. The molecular pathogenesis of cognitive impairment is not fully understood; thus, an ideal pharmacological agent has been difficult to develop. No single agent developed to date is ideally suited for this task; however, several agents have shown beneficial results. In this chapter, I review the established and the most promising potential cognitive enhancers.

Cholinesterase-Related Therapies

Impairment of cholinergic neurotransmission, especially in the hippocampus and cerebral cortex, has been clearly established over the last 35 years as a significant factor in the clinical signs of cognitive impairment, including those of Alzheimer's disease (Davies and Maloney 1976; Mesulam 2004; Whitehouse et al. 1982). Butyrylcholinesterase

(BChE) and acetylcholinesterase (AChE) are the two main types of cholinesterase present in the brain. The development of AChE inhibitors (AChEIs) to increase acetylcholine levels in the brain for enhanced synaptic transmission has been successful, with marginal positive clinical outcomes to date (Birks 2006; Thompson et al. 2004). Four AChEIs have been marketed in the United States for cognitive therapy: tacrine, donepezil, rivastigmine, and galantamine. These pharmaceuticals are primarily for symptomatic relief and have limited current value in stopping or reversing the disease process, although research into subtle neurotrophic and neuroprotective effects of these agents proceeds (Murphy et al. 2006). A significant number of AChEI nonresponders exist (Jones 2003). Improvements in cognitive functioning have been shown with AChEIs without major differences in their efficacy (Birks 2006; Seltzer 2006; Thompson et al. 2004). The major side effects of AChEIs are gastrointestinal.

Recommendations

Tacrine is no longer recommended for routine clinical use. Donepezil, rivastigmine, and galantamine are recommended with or without other cognitive enhancers (e.g., memantine). Tolerability is improved by slow dosage titration. All cholinesterase inhibitors have significant potential for side effects; it is difficult to determine whether one AChEI has a significantly better side-effect profile than another AChEI, given individual patients' variability. Switching AChEIs can be a reasonable treatment strategy if lack of efficacy or tolerability is an issue.

Donepezil

Donepezil, a piperidine-based, reversible, noncompetitive AChEI with a plasma half-life of about 70 hours, was approved for the treatment of mild to moderate Alzheimer's disease in the United States in 1996 and for severe Alzheimer's disease in 2006. Donepezil is given once daily in 5-mg, 10-mg, or 23-mg doses; 5-mg therapy is only slightly less effective than 10-mg therapy and can be an appropriate regimen, especially when tolerability is an issue (Birks and Harvey 2006). The 23-mg dose is generally initiated after a patient has been stable for at least 3 months on the 10-mg dose.

Donepezil has shown benefit in treating mild, moderate, and severe Alzheimer's disease (Birks and Harvey 2006; Wallin et al. 2007) and has been studied for efficacy in patients with mild cognitive impairment (Chen et al. 2006; Seltzer 2007). A meta-analysis of pooled data on the use of donepezil indicated that caution is warranted in its use to treat mild cognitive impairment due to modest treatment effects with significant side effects (Birks and Flicker 2006).

Rivastigmine

Rivastigmine, a carbamyl derivative, is a slowly reversible AChEI and butyrylcholinesterase inhibitor (BChEI) with an elimination half-life of about 2 hours. It was approved in 2000 for use in the United States and is indicated for the treatment of mild to moderate dementia of Alzheimer's disease and Parkinson's disease. Rivastigmine inhibits the G1 isoenzyme of AChE selectively up to four times more potently than it does the G4 isoenzyme (Enz et al. 1993). This unique compound with its BChEI properties has been postulated to be of greater benefit than other AChEIs in the treatment of Alzheimer's disease because BChE activity increases in the hippocampus and cortex while AChE activity diminishes (Tasker et al. 2005); to date, this has not been conclusively shown to be of clinical significance. However, as a therapy involving multiple target receptor sites, this agent does have a theoretical advantage over single-target approaches. A rivastigmine skin patch received U.S. Food and Drug Administration approval in 2007; gastrointestinal side effects are reduced in frequency with this drug delivery system. An oral solution is also available.

Rivastigmine is initiated at 1.5 mg taken twice daily; the dosage is increased by 1.5 mg every 2 weeks to a daily maximum of 6–12 mg divided into two doses. Transdermal therapy is initiated at one 4.6-mg skin patch applied daily for at least 4 weeks, at which time the dosage may be increased to the 9.5-mg daily patch.

Galantamine

Galantamine hydrobromide, a tertiary alkaloid, is a specific, competitive, and reversible AChEI with a plasma half-life of 6–8 hours that was first marketed in the United States in 2001 as a treatment for mild to moderate dementia of Alzheimer's disease. Galantamine is unique in that it modulates neuronal nicotinic receptors (Coyle and Kershaw 2001). Whether this nicotinic receptor modulation imparts any significant clinical benefit in disease modification remains unknown. The optimal dosage range is 16–24 mg/day. The extended-release galantamine formulation for once-daily dosing has similar efficacy and side effects as the twice-daily dosing formulation. An oral suspension is available as well. Pooled data from trials in patients with mild cognitive impairment have shown significantly higher rates of death due to bronchial carcinoma/sudden death, cerebrovascular disorder/syncope, myocardial infarction, and suicide in the galantamine treatment groups (Cusi et al. 2007; Loy and Schneider 2006); follow-up studies are under way to clarify these findings. One double-blind, placebo-controlled trial of galantamine with antipsychotic medication in the treatment of subjects with schizophrenia did not show significant benefit, although there was a trend toward improvement in several cognitive domains (Lee et al. 2007).

Other Agents

Physostigmine, a reversible inhibitor of BChE and AChE, is poorly tolerated due to multiple gastrointestinal side effects, especially nausea and vomiting, and has a very short half-life.

Huperzine alpha (more commonly known as huperzine A) is sold in the United States as a dietary supplement for cognitive enhancement and is a slow, reversible inhibitor of AChE. Huperzine A is believed to have neuroprotective effects by reducing neuronal cell death caused by glutamate (Ved et al. 1997). The combination of other AChEIs with huperzine A may exacerbate gastrointestinal side effects; patients' usage of this over-the-counter supplement should be monitored, especially if other AChEIs are considered for treatment.

Metrifonate, a long-acting irreversible cholinesterase inhibitor, was tested in clinical trials, but further development was discontinued after a higher-than-expected incidence of neuromuscular dysfunction and respiratory paralysis was found.

Selective and nonselective neuronal nicotinic receptor agonists have shown statistically significant cognitive enhancement in young, healthy subjects and mixed results in subjects with Alzheimer's disease (Dunbar et al. 2007; Newhouse et al. 1997; Potter et al. 1999; Sunderland et al. 1988). The use of selective neuronal nicotinic receptor agonists is an intuitive combination therapy with AChEIs for cognitive enhancement; research continues in this developing area.

N-Methyl-D-Aspartate–Related Therapies

Glutamate is an agonist of kainate, NMDA, and α-amino-3-hydroxy-5-methyl-4-isoxazole propionic acid (AMPA) receptors. Neuronal plasticity of memory and learning is influenced by glutamate's direct modulation of the NMDA postsynaptic receptor; glutamate acts as an excitatory neurotransmitter activating the NMDA receptor. Glutamate excess results in neurotoxicity, affecting cognitive functioning (Koch et al. 2005).

Recommendations

Memantine appears to reduce the level of cognitive impairment in patients with moderate to severe Alzheimer's disease. Memantine in combination with an AChEI is an appropriate consideration for improvement in cognition and behavior.

Memantine

Memantine is a noncompetitive NMDA receptor antagonist approved in the United States for treating moderate to severe Alzheimer's disease. The NMDA receptor modulates memory function. Memantine may prevent neurotoxicity due to its low-affinity antagonism of glutamate, which has been linked to neurodegeneration and excitotoxicity (Lipton and Rosenberg 1994). Memantine has been shown to be effective in reducing the level of cognitive impairment in patients with moderate to severe Alzheimer's disease (Bullock 2006; Reisberg et al. 2003). Memantine is available in tablets and as an oral solution; dosing should be adjusted for patients with moderate or severe renal impairment. It is recommended that memantine be initiated at a dosage of 5 mg/day for 1 week, increasing weekly by 5 mg/day up to a target dosage of 20 mg/day. Memantine is generally given in twice-daily doses, although the elimination half-life ranges from 60 to 80 hours.

Memantine Combination Therapy

Memantine in combination with an AChEI has been shown to improve cognitive domains significantly and to ameliorate symptoms of behavioral dyscontrol (agitation/aggression, eating/appetite, irritability/lability) (Cummings et al. 2006; Tariot et al. 2004). Given the disruption of multiple neurotransmitter systems and pathways in Alzheimer's disease and other cognitive disorders, the use of adjunctive cognition-enhancing medications is understandable (Grossberg et al. 2006). The specific neurobiological deficit(s) that may be affected by a pharmacological or nutraceutical intervention should be considered.

Vascular and Inflammation-Related Therapies

Major known modifiable risk factors for vascular cognitive impairment (with or without dementia) include diabetes mellitus, hypertension, cardiac ischemia, atrial fibrillation, smoking, hyperlipidemia, and peripheral vascular disease (Desmond et al. 1993; Rockwood et al. 1997). Controversial risk factors include hyperhomocysteinemia. Established vascular therapeutic interventions have included low-dose aspirin and other antiplatelet agents, anticoagulation agents, antihypertensives, aggressive management of diabetes mellitus, carotid endarterectomy for selected patients, and treatment of hyperlipidemia. There is a significant overlap of patients with vascular cognitive impairment and those with Alzheimer's disease (Gearing et al. 1995; O'Brien 1994). Cholinergic receptors (muscarinic and nicotinic) are known modulators of cerebral blood flow (Schwarz et al. 1999; Zhang et al. 1998). Ischemia-induced NMDA stimulation may further cognitive impairment.

A meta-analysis of four randomized, placebo-controlled studies of AChEIs to treat vascular dementia—two with donepezil and two with galantamine—showed statistically significant cognitive enhancement even though the treatment effect was less than what has been observed in Alzheimer's disease patients (Birks and Flicker 2007). In addition, the authors analyzed pooled results from memantine studies and found statistically significant improvement of cognitive functioning with memantine treatment in patients with vascular impairment similar to that seen with the AChEIs (Birks and Flicker 2007). A Cochrane review indicated that donepezil in doses of either 5 mg or 10 mg improves both functional ability and cognitive symptoms in patients with mild to moderate vascular cognitive impairment; donepezil was well tolerated in this analysis (Malouf and Birks 2004). A Cochrane review of the use of galantamine to treat vascular cognitive impairment showed statistically significant results in terms of cognition and executive function with galantamine versus placebo in one study but not in a second study that had fewer subjects; gastrointestinal side effects were noted to be higher in galantamine recipients (Craig and Birks 2006).

Recommendations

AChEIs appear to have a valid role in the treatment of vascular cognitive impairment. Combination therapy is an important consideration, especially with other known vascular risk modifiers including aspirin, other nonsteroidal anti-inflammatory drugs (NSAIDs), and cytidine 5′-diphosphocholine (CDP-choline). Randomized controlled trials do not currently support the use of aspirin or other NSAIDs for the treatment of vascular cognitive impairment. The active use of statins for the prevention and treatment of vascular cognitive impairment is currently not well supported by the literature; however, research with statins remains very active in this pursuit. Aspirin remains a cornerstone first-line intervention for decreasing potential cardiovascular comorbidity; aspirin may have a future role as a combination therapy with cognitive enhancers.

Other Therapies

Antioxidant-related treatment for cognitive impairment remains poorly supported by placebo-controlled, double-blind studies. Ginkgo biloba could be classified within several potential treatment categories, including antioxidants, nutraceuticals, cholinergic agents, and vasodilators; most studies have shown only marginal benefit for this agent. Vitamin E (including tocopherols and tocotrienols), vitamin C, and carotenoids have antioxidant properties; however, reports of benefit in treating patients with cognitive impairment are mixed. Although antioxidants may have potential as a combination therapy modality, further research is required before endorsing specific treatment recommendations with current antioxidants.

Various other agents have been tested and studied for their potential to improve cognitive impairment; these include secretase inhibitors, tramiprosate, modafinil, hormone replacement therapy, nutraceuticals (*Rubia cordifolia*, *Salvia lavandulaefolia*, *Rosmarinus officinalis*, and *Melissa officinalis*), dehydro-3-epiandrosterone (DHEA), aniracetam, piracetam, and unifiram. Currently, no recommendations can be made for use of any of these agents as monotherapy or combination therapy.

Antiamyloid immunization may provide one of the greatest opportunities to prevent amyloid-β deposition. Immunization strategies generally focus on active or passive immunization and direct central nervous system delivery of anti–amyloid-β antibodies. Active immunization with β-amyloid antibodies can reduce plaque formation (Lemere et al. 2006; Solomon 2006). Passive immunization with monoclonal antibodies or preparations of immunoconjugates shows promise for treating cognitive impairment due to Alzheimer's disease and may be safer than active immunization (Geylis and Steinitz 2006; Solomon 2007). Active and passive immunization may cause microhemorrhages, and further research continues to seek safer vaccines.

Conclusion

The molecular pathogenesis of nerve cell death remains elusive, especially as it relates to the onset and progression of cognitive impairment. Alzheimer's disease and other types of cognitive impairment represent a wide spectrum of neurosystem dysfunction, and no single treatment modality yet found is sufficient to address the global apoptosis and degeneration that occur. Due to the multiple types of neurochemical and substructure dysfunction occurring in cognitive impairment, multiple-drug interventions will likely be required (Siskou et al. 2007; Sunderland et al. 1992).

Future studies will explore second-messenger modulation, inhibition of the synthesis of amyloid-β using a mimic of the prion protein to inhibit β-secretase cleavage of the amyloid precursor protein, amyloid plaque sheet breakers, AMPA receptor modulators, and the role of σ_1-receptor agonists and selective neuronal nicotinic receptor agonists (Parkin et al. 2007; Rose et al. 2005; Sarter 2006). Currently, the AChEIs and memantine are appropriate choices for slowing the progression of cognitive impairment. Several other promising agents are likely to become available within the next decade.

References

Aisen PS, Davis KL: Inflammatory mechanisms in Alzheimer's disease: implications for therapy. Am J Psychiatry 151:1105–1113, 1994

Bartus RT, Dean RL, Beer B, et al: The cholinergic hypothesis of geriatric memory dysfunction. Science 217:408–414, 1982

Behl C: Vitamin E and other antioxidants in neuroprotection. Int J Vitam Nutr Res 69:213–219, 1999

Behl C, Davis J, Cole GM, et al: Vitamin E protects nerve cells from a-beta protein toxicity. Biochem Biophys Res Commun 186:944–950, 1992

Birks J: Cholinesterase inhibitors for Alzheimer's disease. Cochrane Database Syst Rev (1): CD005593, 2006

Birks J, Flicker L: Donepezil for mild cognitive impairment. Cochrane Database Syst Rev (3): CD006104, 2006

Birks J, Flicker L: Investigational treatment for vascular cognitive impairment. Expert Opin Investig Drugs 16:647–658, 2007

Birks J, Harvey RJ: Donepezil for dementia due to Alzheimer's disease. Cochrane Database Syst Rev (1):CD001190, 2006

Bullock R: Efficacy and safety of memantine in moderate-to-severe Alzheimer disease: the evidence to date. Alzheimer Dis Assoc Disord 20:23–29, 2006

Chen X, Magnotta VA, Duff K, et al: Donepezil effects on cerebral blood flow in older adults with mild cognitive deficits. J Neuropsychiatry Clin Neurosci 18:178–185, 2006

Coyle J, Kershaw P: Galantamine, a cholinesterase inhibitor that allosterically modulates nicotinic receptors: effects on the course of Alzheimer's disease. Biol Psychiatry 49:289–299, 2001

Craig D, Birks J: Galantamine for vascular cognitive impairment. Cochrane Database Syst Rev (1): CD004746, 2006

Cummings JL, Schneider E, Tariot PN, et al: Behavioral effects of memantine in Alzheimer disease patients receiving donepezil treatment. Neurology 67:57–63, 2006

Cusi C, Cantisani T, Celani M, et al: Galantamine for Alzheimer's disease and mild cognitive impairment. Neuroepidemiology 28:116–117, 2007

Davies P, Maloney AFJ: Selective loss of central cholinergic neurons in Alzheimer's disease (letter). Lancet 2:1403, 1976

Desmond DW, Tatemichi TK, Paik M, et al: Risk factors for cerebrovascular disease as correlates of cognitive function in a stroke-free cohort. Arch Neurol 50:162–166, 1993

Dunbar G, Boeijinga PH, Demazieres A, et al: Effects of TC-1734 (AZD3480), a selective neuronal nicotinic receptor agonist, on cognitive performance and the EEG of young healthy male volunteers. Psychopharmacology (Berl) 191:919–929, 2007

Enz A, Amstutz R, Boddeke H, et al: Brain selective inhibition of acetylcholinesterase: a novel approach to therapy for Alzheimer's disease. Prog Brain Res 98:431–438, 1993

Gearing M, Mirra SS, Hedreen JC, et al: The Consortium to Establish a Registry for Alzheimer's Disease (CERAD): part X: neuropathology confirmation of the clinical diagnosis of Alzheimer's disease. Neurology 45:461–466, 1995

Geylis V, Steinitz M: Immunotherapy of Alzheimer's disease (AD): from murine models to anti-amyloid beta (Abeta) human monoclonal antibodies. Autoimmun Rev 5:33–39, 2006

Grossberg GT, Edwards KR, Zhao Q: Rationale for combination therapy with galantamine and memantine in Alzheimer's disease. J Clin Pharmacol 46:17S–26S, 2006

Jick H, Zornberg GL, Jick SS, et al: Statins and the risk of dementia. Lancet 356:1627–1631, 2000

Jones RW: Have cholinergic therapies reached their clinical boundary in Alzheimer's disease? Int J Geriatr Psychiatry 18:S7–S13, 2003

Kalaria RN, Cohen DL, Premkumar DR: Cellular aspects of the inflammatory response in Alzheimer's disease. Neurodegeneration 5:497–503, 1996

Koch HJ, Uyanik G, Fischer-Barnicol D: Memantine: a therapeutic approach in treating Alzheimer's and vascular dementia. Curr Drug Targets CNS Neurol Disord 4:499–506, 2005

Lee SW, Lee JG, Lee BJ, et al: A 12-week, double-blind, placebo-controlled trial of galantamine adjunctive treatment to conventional antipsychotics for the cognitive impairments in chronic schizophrenia. Int Clin Psychopharmacol 22: 63–68, 2007

Lemere CA, Maier M, Jiang L, et al: Amyloid-beta immunotherapy for the prevention and treatment of Alzheimer disease: lessons from mice, monkeys, and humans. Rejuvenation Res 9:77–84, 2006

Lipton SA, Rosenberg PA: Excitatory amino acids as a final common pathway for neurologic disorders. N Engl J Med 330:613–622, 1994

Loy C, Schneider L: Galantamine for Alzheimer's disease and mild cognitive impairment. Cochrane Database Syst Rev (1):CD001747, 2006

Malik R, Sangwan A, Saihgal R, et al: Towards better brain management: nootropics. Curr Med Chem 14:123–131, 2007

Malouf R, Birks J: Donepezil for vascular cognitive impairment. Cochrane Database Syst Rev (1): CD004395, 2004

Mesulam M: The cholinergic lesion of Alzheimer's disease: pivotal factor or side show? Learn Mem 11:43–49, 2004

Murphy KJ, Foley AG, O'Connell AW, et al: Chronic exposure of rats to cognition enhancing drugs produces a neuroplastic response identical to that obtained by complex environment rearing. Neuropsychopharmacology 31:90–100, 2006

Newhouse PA, Potter A, Levin ED: Nicotinic system involvement in Alzheimer's and Parkinson's diseases: implications for therapeutics. Drugs Aging 11:206–228, 1997

O'Brien MD: How does cerebrovascular disease cause dementia? Dementia 5:133–136, 1994

Parkin ET, Watt NT, Hussain I, et al: Cellular prion protein regulates beta-secretase cleavage of the Alzheimer's amyloid precursor protein. Proc Natl Acad Sci U S A 104:11062–11067, 2007

Potter A, Corwin J, Lang J, et al: Acute effects of the selective cholinergic channel activator (nicotinic agonist) ABT-418 in Alzheimer's disease. Psychopharmacology (Berl) 142:334–342, 1999

Reisberg B, Doody R, Stoffler A, et al: Memantine in moderate-to-severe Alzheimer's disease. N Engl J Med 348:1333–1341, 2003

Rockwood K, Ebly E, Hachinski V, et al: Presence and treatment of vascular risk factors in patients with vascular cognitive impairment. Arch Neurol 54:33–39, 1997

Rose GM, Hopper A, De Vivo M, et al: Phosphodiesterase inhibitors for cognitive enhancement. Curr Pharm Des 11:3329–3334, 2005

Sarter M: Preclinical research into cognition enhancers. Trends Pharmacol Sci 27:602–608, 2006

Schwarz RD, Callahan MJ, Coughenour LL, et al: Milameline (CI-979/RU35926): a muscarinic receptor agonist with cognition-activating properties: biochemical and in vivo characterization. J Pharmacol Exp Ther 29:812–822, 1999

Selkoe DJ: Toward a comprehensive theory for Alzheimer's disease: hypothesis: Alzheimer's disease is caused by the cerebral accumulation and cytotoxicity of amyloid beta-protein. Ann N Y Acad Sci 924:17–25, 2000

Seltzer B: Cholinesterase inhibitors in the clinical management of Alzheimer's disease: importance of early and persistent treatment. J Int Med Res 34:339–347, 2006

Seltzer B: Donepezil: an update. Expert Opin Pharmacother 8:1011–1023, 2007

Siskou IC, Rekka EA, Kourounakis AP, et al: Design and study of some novel ibuprofen derivatives with potential nootropic and neuroprotective properties. Bioorg Med Chem 15:951–961, 2007

Solomon B: Alzheimer's disease immunotherapy: from in vitro amyloid immunomodulation to in vivo vaccination. J Alzheimers Dis 9:433–438, 2006

Solomon B: Clinical immunologic approaches for the treatment of Alzheimer's disease. Expert Opin Investig Drugs 16:819–828, 2007

Sunderland T, Tariot PN, Newhouse PA: Differential responsivity of mood, behavior, and cognition to cholinergic agents in elderly neuropsychiatric populations. Brain Res 472:371–389, 1988

Sunderland T, Molchan S, Lawlor B, et al: A strategy of "combination chemotherapy" in Alzheimer's disease: rationale and preliminary results with physostigmine plus deprenyl. Int Psychogeriatr 4:291–309, 1992

Tariot PN, Farlow MR, Grossberg GT, et al: Memantine treatment in patients with moderate to severe Alzheimer's disease already receiving donepezil: a randomized controlled trial. JAMA 291:317–324, 2004

Tasker A, Perry EK, Ballard CG: Butyrylcholinesterase: impact on symptoms and progression of cognitive impairment. Expert Rev Neurother 5:101–106, 2005

Terry AV, Buccafusco JJ: The cholinergic hypothesis of age and Alzheimer's disease-related cognitive deficits: recent challenges and their implications for novel drug development. J Pharmacol Exp Ther 306:821–827, 2003

Thompson S, Lanctot KL, Herrmann N: The benefits and risks associated with cholinesterase inhibitor therapy in Alzheimer's disease. Expert Opin Drug Saf 3:425–440, 2004

Ved HS, Koenig ML, Dave JR, et al: Huperzine A, a potential therapeutic agent for dementia, reduces neuronal cell death caused by glutamate. Neuroreport 8:963–968, 1997

Wallin AK, Andreasen N, Eriksson S, et al: Donepezil in Alzheimer's disease: what to expect after 3 years of treatment in a routine clinical setting. Dement Geriatr Cogn Disord 23:150–160, 2007

Whitehouse PJ, Price DL, Struble RG, et al: Alzheimer's disease and senile dementia: loss of neurons in the basal forebrain. Science 215:1237–1239, 1982

Wolozin B, Kellman W, Ruosseau P, et al: Decreased prevalence of Alzheimer disease associated with 3-hydroxy-3-methyglutaryl coenzyme A reductase inhibitors. Arch Neurol 57:1439–1443, 2000

Zhang W, Edvinsson L, Lee TJ: Mechanism of nicotine-induced relaxation in the porcine basilar artery. J Pharmacol Exp Ther 284:790–797, 1998

CHAPTER 33

Sedative-Hypnotics

Seiji Nishino, M.D., Ph.D.
Noriaki Sakai, D.V.M., Ph.D.
Kazuo Mishima, M.D., Ph.D.
Emmanuel Mignot, M.D., Ph.D.
William C. Dement, M.D., Ph.D.

In this chapter, we examine some of the pharmacological properties of benzodiazepines, barbiturates, and other sedative-hypnotic compounds. Sedative drugs moderate excitement, decrease activity, and induce calmness, whereas hypnotic drugs produce drowsiness and facilitate the onset and maintenance of a state that resembles normal sleep in its electroencephalographic characteristics. Although these agents are central nervous system (CNS) depressants, they usually produce therapeutic effects at doses that are far lower than those that cause coma and generalized depression of the CNS.

Some sedative-hypnotic drugs retain other therapeutic uses as muscle relaxants (especially benzodiazepines), antiepileptics, or preanesthetic medications. Although benzodiazepines are used widely as antianxiety drugs, whether their effect on anxiety is truly distinct from their effect on sleepiness remains unconfirmed.

Sedative-hypnotics are also important drugs to neuroscientists. These substances modulate basic behaviors such as arousal and response to stress. With increasing understanding of the molecular structure of the γ-aminobutyric acid type A ($GABA_A$) receptor, the cellular mechanisms of these compounds' mode of action have become elucidated. Further understanding of their mode of action could thus help to elucidate neurochemical and neurophysiological control of these behaviors.

Benzodiazepines

History and Discovery

Benzodiazepines were first synthesized in the 1930s. The introduction of chlorpromazine and meprobamate in the early 1950s led to the decade of development of sophisticated in vivo pharmacological screening methods that were used to identify the sedative properties of benzodiazepines. More than 3,000 benzodiazepines have been synthesized since chlordiazepoxide, which was synthesized by Sterbach in 1957, was introduced into clinical medicine. About 40 of them are in clinical use.

Several drugs chemically unrelated to the benzodiazepines have been shown to have sedative-hypnotic effects with a benzodiazepine-like profile, and these drugs have been determined to act via the benzodiazepine binding site on $GABA_A$ receptor.

Most of the benzodiazepines currently on the market were selected for their high anxiolytic potential relative to CNS depression. Nevertheless, all benzodiazepines have sedative-hypnotic properties to various degrees, and some compounds that facilitate sleep have been used as hypnotics.

Mainly because of their remarkably low capacity to produce fatal CNS depression, benzodiazepines have displaced barbiturates as sedative-hypnotic agents.

Structure-Activity Relations

The term *benzodiazepine* refers to the portion of the structure composed of benzene rings (A in Figure 33–1) fused to a seven-membered diazepine ring (*B*). However, most of the older benzodiazepines contain a 5-aryl substituent (C) and a 1,4-diazepine ring, and the term has come to mean 1,4-benzodiazepines.

A substituent (most often chloride) at position 7 is essential for biological activity. A carbonyl at position 2 enhances activity and is generally present. Most of the newest products also substitute the 2 position, as with flurazepam. These general features are important for the metabolic fate of the compounds. Because the 7 and 2 positions of the molecule are resistant to all major degradative pathways, many of the metabolites retain substantial pharmacological activity.

Pharmacological Profile

Benzodiazepines share anticonvulsant and sedative-hypnotic effects with the barbiturates. In addition, they have a remarkable ability to reduce anxiety and aggression (Cook and Sepinwall 1975). In the mammalian CNS, two subtypes of benzodiazepine omega (ω) receptors have been pharmacologically recognized. Benzodiazepine ω_1 (or BZ1) receptors are sensitive to β-carbolines, imidazopyridines (e.g., zolpidem), and triazolopyridazines. Benzodiazepine ω_2 (or BZ2) receptors have low affinity for these ligands but relatively high affinity for benzodiazepines. Benzodiazepine ω_1 sites are enriched in the cerebellum, whereas ω_2 sites are mostly present in the spinal cord, and both receptor subtypes are found in the cerebral cortex and hippocampus. Benzodiazepine ω_1 and ω_2 receptor subtypes are also located peripherally in adrenal chromaffin cells.

Another subtype, ω_3, was identified and is commonly labeled as the *peripheral benzodiazepine receptor subtype* because of its distribution on glial cell membranes in nonnervous tissues such as adrenal, testis, liver, heart, and kidney. The subtype was later detected in the CNS, especially on the mitochondrial membrane and not in association with $GABA_A$ receptors (Gavish et al. 1992). The ω_3 receptor subtype has high affinity for benzodiazepines and isoquinoline carboxamides (Awad and Gavish 1987). The functional role of this receptor subtype is unknown, but it may be involved in the biosynthesis and mediation of the sedative-hypnotic effects of some neuroactive steroids (e.g., pregnenolone, dehydroepiandrosterone [DHEA], allopregnanolone, tetrahydrodeoxycorticosterone) (Edgar et al. 1997; Friess et al. 1996; Rupprecht et al. 1996). Neurosteroids modulate $GABA_A$-mediated transmission through an allosteric mechanism that is distinct from that of benzodiazepines and barbiturates. By stimulation of ω_3 receptors with agonists, cholesterol is transferred from intracellular stores in mitochondria and becomes available to the mitochondrial P450 cholesterol side-chain cleav-

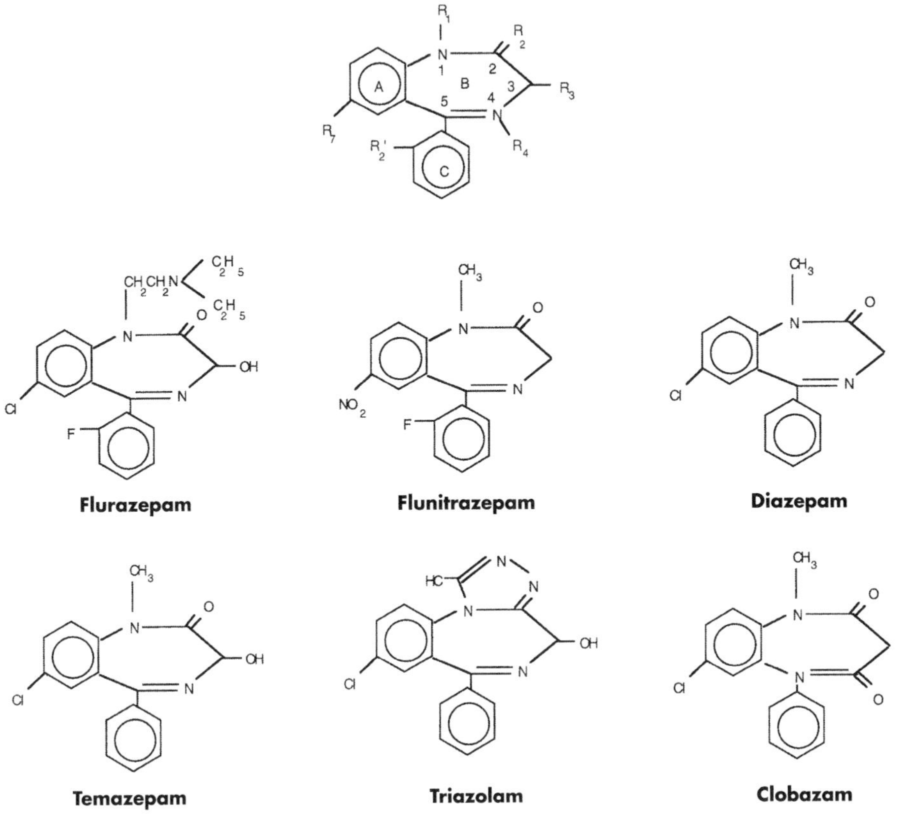

Flurazepam

Flunitrazepam

Diazepam

Temazepam

Triazolam

Clobazam

FIGURE 33–1. Chemical structures of some commonly used benzodiazepines.

age enzyme (P450scc), and neurosteroid biosynthesis begins (Papadopoulos et al. 2001). Benzodiazepine ω_3 receptor subtypes also may serve as mitochondrial membrane stabilizers and protect against pathologically induced mitochondrial and cell toxicity (Papadopoulos et al. 2001).

The $GABA_A$ receptor is a ligand-gated ion channel that mediates fast synaptic neurotransmission in the CNS. When the $GABA_A$ receptor is occupied by GABA or GABA agonists such as muscimol, the chloride channels open and chloride ions diffuse into the cell. Early research established that diazepam (and related benzodiazepines) does not act directly through GABA but modulates inhibitory transmission through the $GABA_A$ receptor in some other way. It was subsequently reported that benzodiazepines bind specifically to neural elements in the mammalian brain with high affinity and that an excellent correlation exists between drug affinities for these specific binding sites and in vivo pharmacological potencies (Möhler and Okada 1977; Squires and Braestrup 1977).

The binding of a benzodiazepine to this receptor site is enhanced in the presence of GABA or a GABA agonist, thereby suggesting that a functional (but independent) relationship exists between the $GABA_A$ receptor and the benzodiazepine binding sites (Tallman et al. 1978). Barbiturates (and to some extent alcohol) also seem to produce anxiolytic and sedative effects at least partly by facilitating GABAergic transmission (see section "Barbiturates" in this chapter). This common action for chemically unrelated compounds can be explained by the ability of these compounds to stimulate specific sites on the $GABA_A$ receptor.

The benzodiazepines bind with high affinity to their binding sites so that the action of GABA on its receptor is allosterically enhanced. GABA can produce stronger postsynaptic inhibition in the presence of a benzodiazepine. Benzodiazepine agonists are assumed to potentiate only ongoing physiologically initiated actions of GABA (at $GABA_A$ receptors), whereas barbiturates are thought to cause inhibition at all GABAergic synapses regardless of their physiological activity. In addition, barbiturates appear to increase the duration of the open state of the chloride channel, whereas benzodiazepines increase the frequency of channel openings with little effect on duration (Twyman et al. 1989). These fundamental differences between the allosteric effects of benzodiazepines within the $GABA_A$ receptor and the conducive effects of barbiturates on the chloride ion channel may explain why low doses of barbiturates have a pharmacological profile similar to that of benzodiazepines, whereas high doses of barbiturates cause a profound and sometimes fatal suppression of brain synaptic transmission. Note that selective $GABA_A$ agonists, such as muscimol, have no sedative or anxiolytic properties; thus, the whole $GABA_A$–benzodiazepine receptor complex must be involved to possess sedative-hypnotic properties.

Molecular Mechanism of $GABA_A$–Benzodiazepine Receptor Interaction

The structure of the $GABA_A$–benzodiazepine receptor complex has been elucidated by the cloning of all the implicated subunit genes and the study of the corresponding encoded proteins. The $GABA_A$ receptor is a pentameric protein consisting of five subunits that form a rosette surrounding a transmembrane ion channel pore for Cl^- (Figure 33–2). The $GABA_A$ receptor in humans includes the following known subunits: α_1–α_6, β_1–β_4, γ_1–γ_4, δ, ε, π, and τ (7 kinds of subunits, 18 isoforms total) (Mehta and Ticku 1999). Two alternatively spliced versions of the γ_2 subunit, γ_{2S} and γ_{2L}, are also known to exist (Kofuji et al. 1991).

Despite many studies, the physiological and neuroanatomical processes mediating benzodiazepine action on the $GABA_A$ receptor complex remain poorly understood. One reason is that the GABAergic system is the most widespread of all inhibitory neurotransmitters and could be involved in many circuits responsive to various effects of benzodiazepine agonists. In addition, the various subtypes of $GABA_A$ receptor have different ligand affinity and channel functions in response to benzodiazepine agonists. These subtypes of $GABA_A$ are broadly distributed in various brain areas to form a mosaic of receptor subtypes (Wisden and Stephens 1999), making it difficult to understand the functional mechanisms of interaction of benzodiazepine agonists on the $GABA_A$-ergic system from the physiological point of view (Rudolph et al. 1999). However, recent site-directed mutagenesis and gene knock-in techniques have identified several important findings about the benzodiazepine action sites on $GABA_A$ receptors and their physiological functions (Ueno et al. 2001).

It is postulated that the binding of GABA to *N*-terminal extracellular domains of α and β subunits causes conformational changes within the subunits. Ion channel pores subsequently open, and Cl^- flows across the neuronal membrane, resulting in neuronal inhibition (Amin and Weiss 1993; Boileau et al. 1999; Sigel et al. 1992; Smith and Olsen 1994) (see Figure 33–2). The extracellular domains of the α and γ subunits, which consist of about 220 amino acids in the *N*-terminal region, also have been shown to bind GABA and benzodiazepines. "Pharmacologically classified" ω_1 and ω_2 receptors are now thought to correspond to $GABA_A$

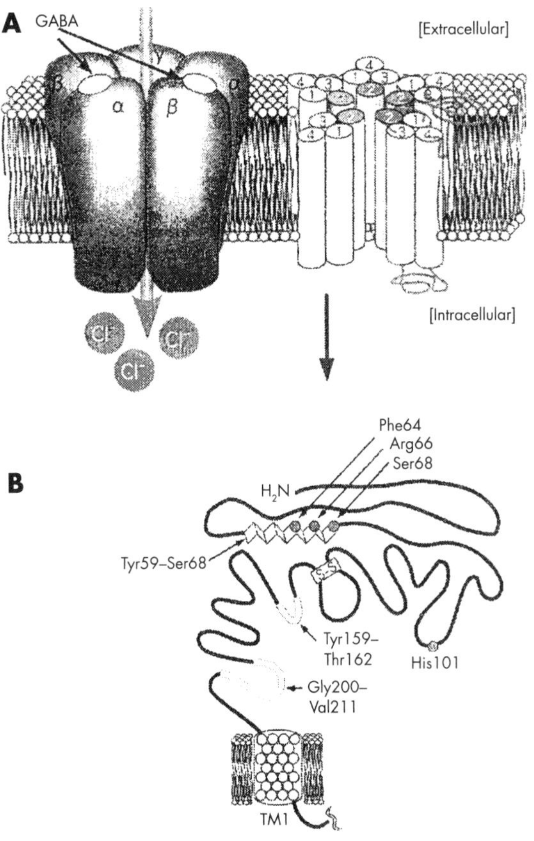

FIGURE 33–2. GABA$_A$–benzodiazepine receptor complex.

(A) Schematic model of the mammalian γ-aminobutyric acid type A (GABA$_A$) receptor embedded in the cell membrane, representatively possessing the α, β, and γ subunits (2:2:1). The binding of two molecules of GABA to the action site composed of α and β subunits causes the opening of the chloride channel pore, and the chloride ions diffuse into the cell. Each subunit comprises four transmembrane domains (TM1–TM4). The ion channel pore consists of TM2 of five subunits with a rosette formation. **(B)** Structure of the α_1 subunit, with amino acid sequence, indicating amino acid residues implicated in GABA and benzodiazepine binding domains.

Source. Modified from Ueno et al. 2001.

receptors possessing the α_1 and α_2 subunits and the α_3 and α_5 subunits, respectively.

Extracellular benzodiazepine binding sites on these subunits consist of several divided portions; His101, Tyr159–Thr162, and Gly200–Val211 on α_1 subunits, as well as Lys41–Trp82 and Arg114–Asp161 on γ_2 subunits, are essential to the formation of the binding pockets (Boileau et al. 1998). Most strikingly, His101 is a critical residue for diazepam to exhibit its sedative effect (Crestani et al. 2001; Low et al. 2000; McKernan et al. 2000; Rudolph et al. 1999). Knock-in mice with displacement of His101Arg are insensitive to benzodiazepine-induced allosteric modulation of the complex but have preserved physiological regulation by GABA (Rudolph et al. 1999). These knock-in mice failed to be sedated by diazepam but retained other effects of diazepam, such as anxiolytic-like, myorelaxant, motor-impairing, and ethanol-potentiating effects. This suggests the possibility that the sedative action of the benzodiazepine is mediated through $GABA_A$ receptors possessing the α_1 subunit. It is also noteworthy that His101Arg knock-in mice responded to diazepam and showed similar sleep changes as wild-type mice do, despite the lack of its sedative response in these animals (Tobler et al. 2001). Thus, hypnotic and sedative effects by benzodiazepines may be mediated via different subtypes, with hypnotic effects involving $GABA_A$ receptors possessing subunits other than α_1 (i.e., α_2, α_3, or α_5) (Tobler et al. 2001).

Nonbenzodiazepine Hypnotics (Acting on the Benzodiazepine Receptor)

Until about 1980, it was widely accepted that the benzodiazepine structure was a prerequisite for the anxiolytic profile and for benzodiazepine receptor recognition and binding. However, more recently, three chemically unrelated drugs—the imidazopyridine zolpidem, the cyclopyrrolone zopiclone (and its S[+]-enantiomer, eszopiclone), and the pyrazolopyrimidine zaleplon—have been shown to be useful sedative-hypnotics with benzodiazepine-like profiles (Figure 33–3). Other chemical classes of drugs that are structurally dissimilar to the benzodiazepines (e.g., triazolopyridazines) but act through the benzodiazepine receptor also have been developed and have anxiolytic activity in humans.

Nonbenzodiazepine hypnotics have a pharmacological profile slightly different from that of classic benzodiazepines. For example, zolpidem binds selectively to ω_1 (the 50% inhibitory concentration [IC_{50}] ratio for ω_1/ω_2 is nearly 1:10) and has sedative-hypnotic properties relative to other properties such as anxiolytic activity or muscle relaxation. Zolpidem and zopiclone have short half-lives (3 hours and 6 hours, respectively). These drugs were originally thought not to appreciably affect the rapid eye movement (REM) sleep pattern, whereas the quality of slow-wave sleep (SWS) may be slightly increased (Jovanovic and Dreyfus 1983; Shlarf 1992). Rebound effects (insomnia, anxiety), which are commonly seen following withdrawal of short-acting benzodiazepines, are minimal for zolpidem and zopiclone. These compounds also induce little respiratory depression and have less abuse potential than common clinical benzodiazepine hypnotics. However, much longer clinical trials are needed to demonstrate whether the imidazopyridines or cyclopyrrolones have any significant advantages over the short- to medium-half-life benzodiazepines in the treatment of insomnia. Eszopiclone, the active stereoisomer of zopiclone with a longer half-life, was recently approved by the U.S. Food and Drug Administration (FDA). It is claimed that the drug is helpful for sleep maintenance as well as for sleep induction. Because the compound induces little tolerance, it is suitable for long-term use.

Zaleplon, a pyrazolopyrimidine, also has been developed as a novel nonbenzodiazepine hypnotic (see Figure 33–3). Clinical trials have shown that zaleplon is a well-tolerated, safe, rapidly acting, and effective sedative with advantages over lorazepam with respect to unwanted cognitive and psychomotor impairments (Allen et al. 1993; Beer et al. 1994).

Benzodiazepine Antagonists, Partial Agonists, and Inverse Agonists

As knowledge of the relation between the structure of benzodiazepine receptor ligands and their pharmacological properties has increased, potent receptor agonists that stimulate the receptor and produce pharmacological effects qualitatively similar to those of classic benzodiazepines have been developed. *Antagonists*, which block the effects of the agonists without having any effects themselves, and *partial agonists*, which have a mixture of agonistic and antagonistic properties, also have been introduced (Haefley 1988). Partial agonists may be particularly important to develop in the future as sedative-hypnotics that lack common side effects such as ataxia and amnesia.

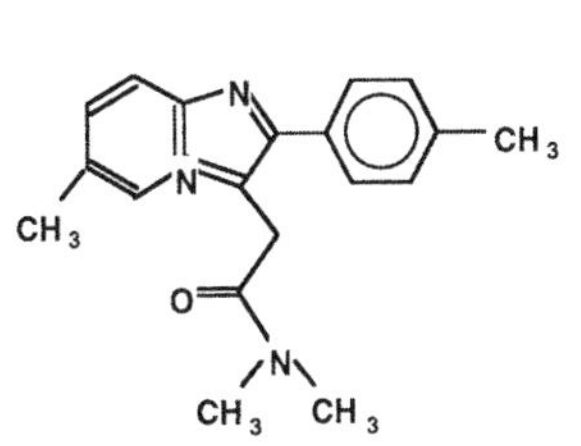

Zolpidem

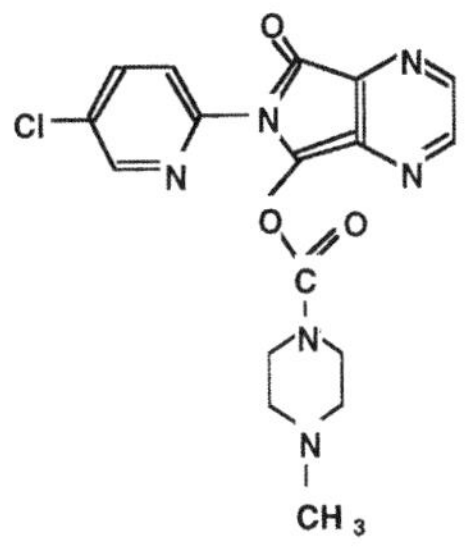

Zopiclone

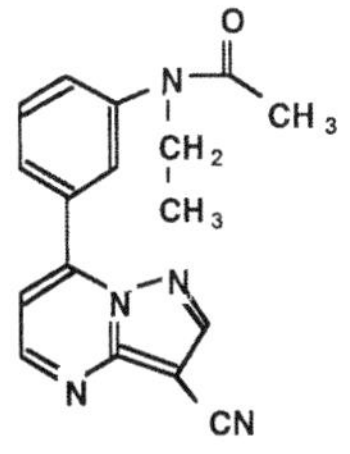

Zaleplon

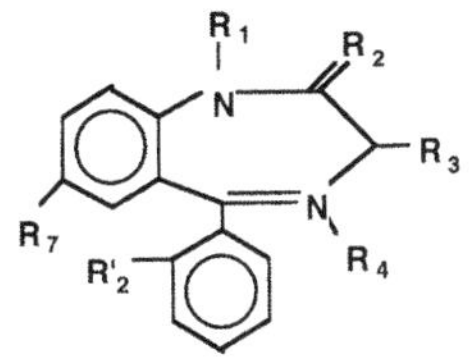

Benzodiazepines

FIGURE 33–3. Three nonbenzodiazepine hypnotics—zolpidem (an imidazopyridine), zopiclone (a cyclopyrrolone), and zaleplon (a pyrazolopyrimidine)—shown to be useful sedative-hypnotics with benzodiazepine-like profiles.

Braestrup and Nielsen (1986) found that a group of nonbenzodiazepine compounds, the β-carbolines, not only antagonized the action of the full agonists but also had intrinsic activity themselves. These compounds are called *benzodiazepine inverse agonists* because they have biological effects exactly opposite those of the pure agonists while also having intrinsic activity like that of agonists. Their effects are blocked by antagonists; thus, the benzodiazepine receptor is unique in that it has a bidirectional function (Figure 33–4).

Natural Ligands for Benzodiazepine Receptors in the Brain

The presence of benzodiazepine receptors in the brain suggests that natural ligands modulate GABAergic transmission through these sites. Small amounts of benzodiazepines, such as diazepam and desmethyldiazepam, can be detected in human and animal tissues. These benzodiazepines most likely originate from plants, such as wheat, corn, potatoes, or rice, and the levels that are detected are too low to be pharmacologically active (e.g., diazepam, <1 ng/g; desmethyldiazepam, 0.5 ng/g).

Other endogenous benzodiazepine-like substances with neuromodulatory effects probably exist in mammals. Endogenous ligands named *diazepam binding inhibitors*, or *endozepines*, that bind to the benzodiazepine site on the $GABA_A$-ergic receptor complex have been identified and are being isolated (Costa and Guidotti 1991; Marquardt et al. 1986; Rothstein et al. 1992). Their intrinsic action, like that of diazepam, is to potentiate $GABA_A$ receptor–mediated neurotransmission by acting as positive allosteric modulators of this receptor. Endozepines are present in the brain at pharmacologically active concentrations and may play a role both physio-

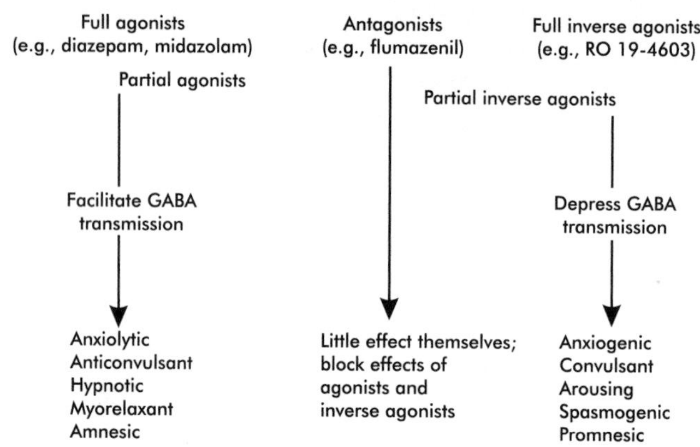

FIGURE 33–4. Properties of the various types of benzodiazepine receptor ligands.
GABA = γ-aminobutyric acid.

logically (e.g., regulation of memory, sleep, and learning) and pathologically (e.g., in panic attacks or hepatic encephalopathy) (Mullen et al. 1990; Nutt et al. 1990). Finally, endozepines have been involved in a newly described neurological condition, *idiopathic recurring stupor*, which is characterized by recurrent episodes of stupor or coma in the absence of any known toxic, metabolic, or structural brain damage. In this condition, the concentrations of endozepines are greatly increased in the plasma of affected individuals, and stupor can be interrupted by injections of flumazenil, a benzodiazepine antagonist. Thus, further knowledge of the roles of endozepines in physiological and pathological processes should be forthcoming once these endogenous ligands have been isolated and characterized (Rothstein et al. 1992).

Pharmacokinetics and Disposition

Benzodiazepines are generally absorbed rapidly and completely. Plasma binding is high (e.g., about 98% for diazepam). Benzodiazepines are very lipophilic (except for oxazepam), and penetration into the brain is rapid. For rapid onset of action, diazepam is available as an emulsion that is administered intravenously for rapid control of epilepsy; midazolam is a water-soluble benzodiazepine suitable for intravenous injection.

The major metabolic pathways for the 1,4-benzodiazepines are shown in Figure 33–5. Medazepam is metabolized to diazepam, which is *N*-desmethylated to desmethyldiazepam. Chlordiazepoxide is also partly converted to desmethyldiazepam. Clorazepate is transformed to desmethyldiazepam.

Desmethyldiazepam is a critical metabolite for biological activity because of its long half-life (>72 hours). Because diazepam's half-life is about 36 hours, the concentration of its desmethyl derivative soon exceeds that of diazepam during chronic administration. Desmethyldiazepam undergoes oxidation to oxazepam, which (like its 3-hydroxy analog temazepam) is rapidly conjugated with glucuronic acid and excreted.

Among the various benzodiazepines, triazolam has a particularly short half-life (<4 hours), and flurazepam and nitrazepam both have long half-lives. A major active metabolite of flurazepam, *N*-desalkylflurazepam, has a very long half-life of about 100 hours.

Because benzodiazepines are often prescribed for long periods, their long-term pharmacokinetics are particularly important. Concentrations of diazepam and desmethyldiazepam reach a plateau after a few weeks.

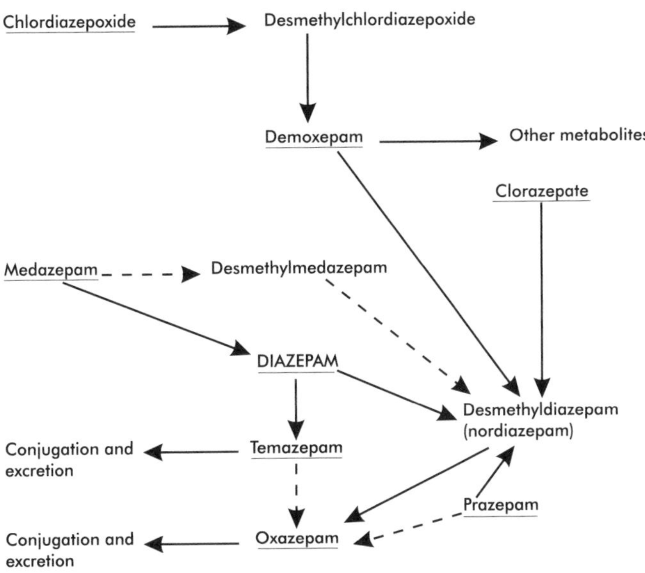

FIGURE 33–5. Metabolic pathways for the principal 1,4-benzodiazepines.
Solid arrows and *broken arrows* denote major and minor pathways, respectively; commercially available drugs are underscored. Flurazepam, flunitrazepam, nitrazepam, and triazolam have separate metabolic pathways.

Diazepam concentrations may then decline somewhat without much change in the concentration of the desmethyl metabolite.

Although benzodiazepines can stimulate liver metabolism in some animals, induction is of little clinical significance in humans.

Regarding the pharmacokinetics of nonbenzodiazepine hypnotics, no (or only weak) active metabolites exist for the compounds currently available.

Effects on Stages of Sleep

The hypnotic effects of benzodiazepines (and nonbenzodiazepine hypnotics) have been suggested to result from the inhibitory effects of the GABAergic system on the raphe and locus coeruleus monoaminergic ascending arousal systems, but this hypothesis may only partially explain their action. Magnocellular regions of the basal forebrain and the preoptic areas have been recognized as important sites for SWS regulation (Szymusiak 1995). Neurons that are selectively active during SWS have been described in these structures, most typically in the ventrolateral preoptic areas (Saper et al. 2001; Sherin et al. 1996). These neurons contain GABA and galanin, an inhibitory peptide, and project to the main components of the ascending arousal system, such as the raphe and locus coeruleus and brain stem cholinergic nuclei (Saper et al. 2001). The ventrolateral preoptic nucleus also sends a dense inhibitory projection to the tuberomammillary histaminergic nucleus, another important wake-promoting system (see Saper et al. 2001; Sherin et al. 1996). Benzodiazepines may thus indirectly modulate these wake-active monoaminergic neurons to promote their hypnotic effects.

Another important site of action for benzodiazepines might be the suprachiasmatic nucleus (SCN). In SCN-lesioned animals, benzodiazepine treatment does not induce sleep (Edgar et al. 1993), but the hypnotic effect is restored if the SCN-lesioned animal is sleep deprived before drug administration. Benzodiazepines thus may facilitate the release of a sleep debt accumulated during wakefulness rather than produce de novo sleep (Mignot et al. 1992).

The effects of benzodiazepines on sleep architecture are well known. Most benzodiazepines decrease sleep latency, especially when first used, and diminish the number of awakenings (Table 33–1). All benzodiazepines increase the time spent in stage 2 sleep. Benzodiazepines also affect the quality of the SWS pattern. Thus, stages 3 and 4 sleep are suppressed and remain so during the period of drug administration. The decrease in stage 4 sleep is accompanied by a reduction in nightmares.

Most benzodiazepines increase REM latency. The time spent in REM sleep is usually shortened; however, the reduction in percentage of REM sleep is minimal because the number of cycles of REM sleep usually increases late in the sleep time. Despite the shortening of SWS and REM sleep, the net effect of administration of benzodiazepines is usually an increase in total sleep time, so that the individual feels that the quality of sleep has improved. Furthermore, the hypnotic effect is greatest in subjects with the shortest baseline total sleep time.

If the benzodiazepine is discontinued after 3–4 weeks of nightly use, a considerable rebound in the amount and density of REM sleep and SWS may occur. However, this is not a consistent finding.

Because long-acting benzodiazepine hypnotics impair daytime performance and increase the risk of falls in geriatric patients, several shorter-acting compounds have been introduced and are the preferred choice for elderly patients (see section "General Considerations in the Pharmacological Treatment of Insomnia" later in this chapter). However, it has since been found that short-acting benzodiazepines induce rebound insomnia (a worsening of sleep difficulty beyond baseline levels on discontinuation of a hypnotic) (Kales et al. 1979), rebound anxiety, anterograde amnesia, and even paradoxical rage (Figure 33–6). Many other factors, such as the subtype of insomnia being treated and the dosage and duration of treatment, are also important in explaining the occurrence of these specific side effects that may also be observed with other benzodiazepines. Nevertheless, enthusiasm for shorter-acting compounds has been tempered.

Indications and Efficacy

Benzodiazepines are the drug treatment of choice in the management of anxiety, insomnia, and stress-related conditions. Although none of the currently available compounds has any significant advantage over the others, some drugs can be selected to match the patient's symptom patterns to the pharmacokinetics of the various drugs. If a patient has a persistently high level of anxiety, one of the precursors of desmethyldiazepam such as diazepam or clorazepate is most appropriate. Patients with fluctuating anxiety may prefer to take shorter-acting compounds, such as oxazepam or lorazepam, when stressful circumstances occur or are expected. The indications of nonbenzodiazepine hypnotics are equivalent to those of benzodiazepine hypnotics but may be more specific depending on the pharmacological property of each compound.

An ideal hypnotic should induce sleep rapidly without producing sedation the next day. Both flurazepam and nitrazepam have inappropriately long half-lives as hypnotics unless a persistent anxiolytic effect is desired the next day (see Figure 33–6). Even in such situations, diazepam given as one dose at night may be preferable. Oxazepam penetrates too slowly for a dependable hypnotic effect (slow onset of action). Both lorazepam and temazepam are appropriate treatments for insomnia, but the dosages available are quite high (Table 33–2). Triazolam is the shortest-acting hypnotic available. When very small doses of benzodiazepines (which were assumed to have no significant hypnotic action) are administered to patients with insomnia, sleep quality often improves greatly, and usually it is not necessary to use a

TABLE 33–1. Comparative effects of benzodiazepines and barbiturates on sleep parameters

	Benzodiazepines	**Barbiturates**
Total sleep time	↑ tolerance with short-acting agents	↑ rapid tolerance
Stage 2, %	↑	↑
Slow-wave sleep (stages 3 and 4), %	↓	↓ (slight)
REM latency	↑	↑
REM, %	↓ (slight)	↓
Withdrawal	Rebound insomnia with short-acting agents Carryover effectiveness with long-acting agents REM rebound (slight)	REM rebound Rebound decrease in stage 2 and total sleep time

Note. REM = rapid eye movement sleep; ↑ = increased; ↓ = decreased.

benzodiazepine at a hypnotic dose as a first-choice treatment.

Benzodiazepines can increase the frequency of apnea and exacerbate oxygen desaturation both in healthy subjects and in subjects with chronic bronchitis (Geddes et al. 1976). Although many reports suggest that benzodiazepines are safe in patients with obstructive sleep apnea, other authors disagree, and it seems wise to avoid hypnotics in patients with severe sleep apnea. One of the only other contraindications is myasthenia gravis, a condition in which muscle relaxation with benzodiazepines can exacerbate muscle atonia.

Side Effects and Toxicology

When a benzodiazepine is taken at high doses, tiredness, drowsiness, and profound feelings of detachment are common but can be minimized by a careful dose adjustment. Headache, dizziness, ataxia, confusion, and disorientation are less common except in the elderly. A marked potentiation of the depressant effect of alcohol occurs. Other less common side effects include weight gain, skin rash, menstrual irregularities, impairment of sexual function, and, very rarely, agranulocytosis.

Although otherwise asymptomatic subjects clearly show mental impairment with benzodiazepines, the situation with anxious patients is more complex. Because anxiety itself interferes with mental performance, alleviation of anxiety may result in improved functioning, which more than compensates for the direct drug-related decrement. The effects in some patients may be complicated and unpredictable, even at low dosages.

Because the safety of benzodiazepines in early pregnancy is not established, they should be avoided unless absolutely necessary. Diazepam is secreted in breast milk and may make the infant sleepy, unresponsive, and slow to feed.

Overdose

The benzodiazepines are extremely widely prescribed, so it is not surprising that they are used in many suicide attempts. For adults, overdoses of benzodiazepines reportedly are not fatal unless alcohol or other psychotropic drugs are taken simultaneously. Typically, the patient falls asleep but is arousable and wakes after 24–48 hours. Treatment is supportive. A stomach pump is usually more punitive than therapeutic, and dialysis is usually useless because of high plasma binding.

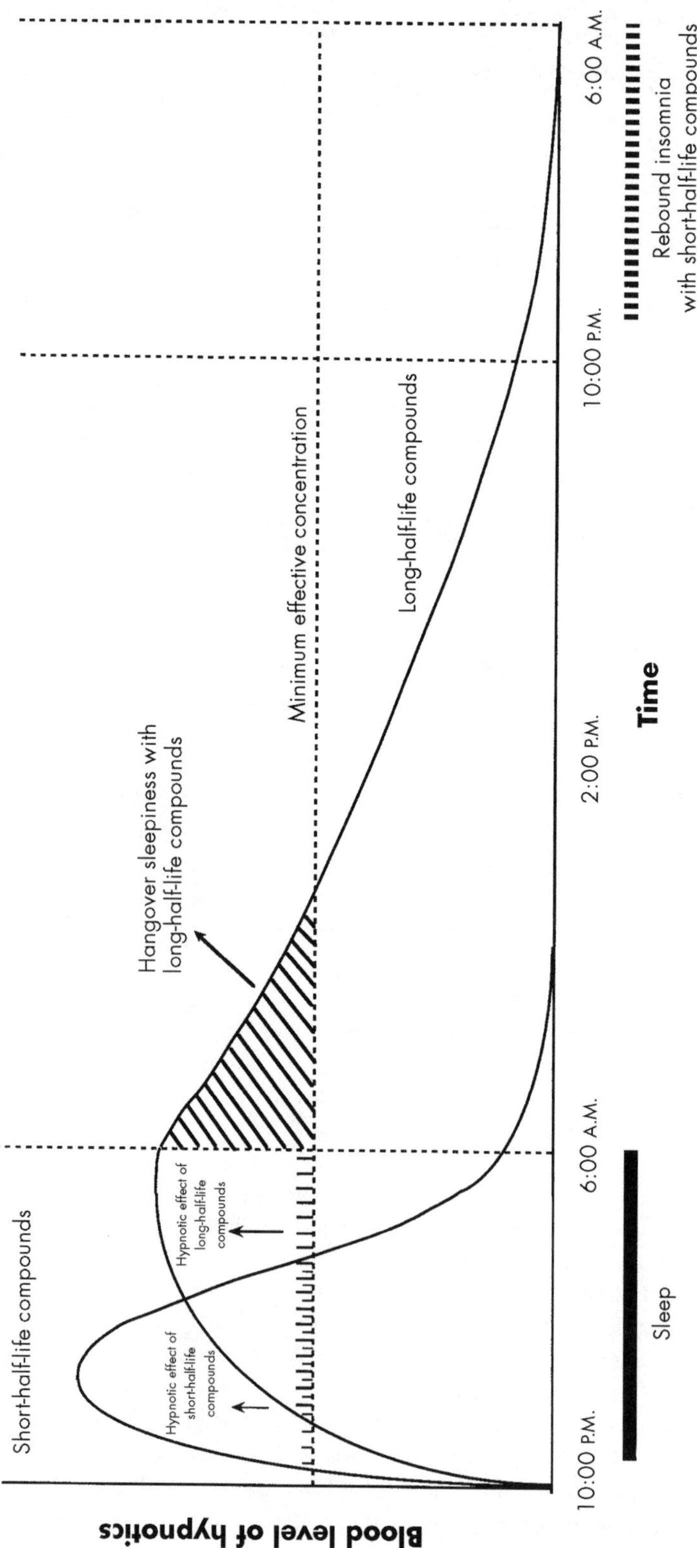

FIGURE 33–6. Duration of action of hypnotics and hangover and rebound insomnia.

Hypnotics with long half-lives may impair daytime performance the day after drug administration, whereas short-acting compounds may induce rebound insomnia on discontinuation.

TABLE 33–2. Pharmacokinetic properties of hypnotic compounds most commonly used in the United States

Hypnotic compounds	Usual dose (mg)	T_{MAX} (hours)[a]	Half-life (hours)[b]	Active metabolites
Benzodiazepines				
Flurazepam (Dalmane)	15–30	0.5–1.0	48–150	N-Desalkylflurazepam
Quazepam (Doral)	7.5–15	2	48–120	2-Oxoquazepam, N-dealkyl-2-oxoquazepam
Estazolam (ProSom)	1–2	4.9	18–30	1-Oxoestazolam
Temazepam (Restoril)	15–30	1.5	8–20	None
Triazolam (Halcion)	0.125–0.25	1.3	2–6	None
Nonbenzodiazepines				
Zolpidem (Ambien)	5–10	0.8	1.5–2.4	None
Zopiclone (Imovane in Canada)	3.75–7.5	1.5	5–6	N-Oxide zopiclone (weak agonist)
Eszopiclone (Lunesta)	1–3	1	6–9	S-Desmethylzopiclone (weak agonist)
Zaleplon (Sonata)	5–20	1.0	1.0–2.5	None

[a]T_{max} is the time required to reach the maximal plasma concentration.
[b]Half-life is the time required by the body to metabolize or inactivate half the amount of a substrate taken.

Tolerance and Dependence

The fact that some patients gradually increase the dose suggests tolerance, but increases in dose are sometimes related to particularly stressful crises.

Dependence, both psychological and physical, occurs with benzodiazepines as with other sedative-hypnotics. Abrupt discontinuation results in withdrawal phenomena such as anxiety, agitation, restlessness, and tension, which are usually delayed for several days because of the long half-life of the major metabolite, desmethyldiazepam. Even with the normal dose, some patients have withdrawal effects. Psychological dependence is also common, based on the high incidence of repeated prescriptions, but it is mild, and the drug-seeking behavior is much less persistent than with barbiturates.

Barbiturates

History and Discovery

Barbital, one of the derivatives of barbituric acid, was introduced in 1903 and soon became extremely popular in clinical medicine because of its sleep-inducing and anxiolytic effects (Maynert 1965). In 1912, phenobarbital was introduced as a sedative-hypnotic. Since then, more than 2,500 barbiturate analogs have been synthesized, about 50 of which have been made commercially available and only 20 of which remain on the market.

The success of the partial separation of anticonvulsant from sedative-hypnotic properties led to the development of nonsedative anticonvulsants such as phenytoin in the late 1930s and trimethadione in the early 1940s. The success of barbiturates as sedative-hypnotics was largely overshadowed by the discovery of benzodiazepines in the late 1960s. With pharmacological properties very similar to those of barbiturates, these compounds have a much safer pharmacological profile. Thus, benzodiazepines have replaced barbiturates in many incidents, especially for psychiatric conditions in which suicide is a possibility.

Structure-Activity Relations

Derivatives of barbituric acid, the parent compound of all barbiturates, do not dissolve readily in water but are quite soluble in nonpolar solvents. In general, structural changes that increase liposolubility also decrease these compounds' duration of action, decrease latency to onset of activity, accelerate metabolic degradation, and often increase hypnotic potency.

Derivatives with large aliphatic groups at position 5 have greater activity than do those with methyl groups but shorter duration of action. However, groups with more than seven carbons lose their hypnotic activity and tend to exhibit convulsant activity. Methylation of the 1-*N* atom increases liposolubility and shortens duration of action, and desmethylation may increase the duration of action (Rall 1990).

Pharmacological Profile and Mechanism of Action

The main effects of barbiturates are sedation, sleep induction, and anesthesia. Some of the barbiturates, such as phenobarbital, also have selective anticonvulsant properties. The mechanisms of action of barbiturates are complex and still not fully understood. Nonanesthetic doses of barbiturates preferentially suppress polysynaptic responses. Pertinent to their sedative-hypnotic effects is the fact that the mesencephalic reticular activating system is extremely sensitive to these drugs (Killam 1962). The synaptic site of inhibition is either postsynaptic (e.g., at the level of cortical and cerebellar pyramidal cells and in the cuneate nucleus, substantia nigra, and thalamus relay neurons) or presynaptic (e.g., in the spinal cord). This inhibition occurs only at synapses where physiological inhibition is GABAergic but not glycinergic or monoaminergic. Thus, barbiturates, like benzodiazepines, specifically potentiate GABA-mediated inhibitory processes in the brain. However, it remains unclear whether all of the effects of barbiturates are entirely mediated by GABAergic mechanisms.

Barbiturates do not displace benzodiazepines from their binding sites; instead, barbiturates enhance benzodiazepine binding by increasing the affinity of the receptor for benzodiazepines (Leeb-Lundberg et al. 1980). They also enhance the binding of GABA and its agonists to specific binding sites (Asano and Ogasawara 1981). These effects are almost completely dependent on the presence of chloride or other anions that are known to permeate the chloride channels associated with the GABA receptor complex, and they are competitively antagonized by picrotoxin (a convulsant) (Olsen et al. 1978).

The molecular correlations of the barbiturate-acting sites on the $GABA_A$ receptor have also been studied. However, neither the sequences important for the binding of

GABA and other direct receptor agonists nor the sequence important for the action of benzodiazepines is of vital importance to barbiturate function (Amin and Weiss 1993). Some reports suggest that the β subunit alone may form a site for barbiturates (Sanna et al. 1995). Although there is still much to be learned, new molecular experimental approaches hold great promise for resolving the most important pharmacological questions regarding which molecular species are important for the anticonvulsant, sedative, anesthetic, and toxic actions of the barbiturates.

Pharmacokinetics and Disposition

For hypnotic use, barbiturates usually are administered orally. Barbiturates are rapidly absorbed in the stomach, and their absorption decreases when the stomach is full.

Barbiturates are metabolized mainly in the liver. Oxidation of the larger of the two side chains at position 5 is a major catabolic pathway. It generally produces inactive polar metabolites that are rapidly excreted in the urine (Rall 1990). Changes in liver function can markedly alter the metabolic rate. Chronic administration leads to pharmacokinetic tolerance, even when low or infrequent doses of barbiturates are used (see section "Drug–Drug Interactions" later in this chapter).

In general, liposolubility decreases latency to onset of action and duration of action. Thiopental, for example, enters the CNS rapidly and is used to rapidly induce anesthesia; barbitone crosses into the brain so slowly that it is inappropriate as a hypnotic drug.

Effects on Stages of Sleep

Barbiturates decrease sleep latency; however, they also slightly increase fast electroencephalogram (EEG) activity during sleep. Barbiturates decrease body movement during sleep. Stage 2 sleep increases, whereas stage 3 and stage 4 SWS generally decreases, except in some patients who have anxiety and in patients who are addicted to barbiturates (see Table 33–1). REM sleep latency is prolonged, and both the total time spent in REM sleep and the number of REM cycles are diminished. With repeated nighttime administration of barbiturates, drug tolerance to the effects on sleep occurs in a few days. Discontinuation of barbiturates may lead to insomnia and disrupted sleep patterns (with a decrease in stage 2 sleep) and increases in REM sleep (Kay et al. 1976).

Indications and Efficacy

Although clinical trials have shown that the barbiturates have sedative and hypnotic properties, barbiturates generally compare poorly with benzodiazepines. The patient feels "drugged" the next day, and there is always the risk of fatal overdose because of the depressant effect on respiration. The therapeutic dose of barbiturates may cause fatal respiratory depression in patients with sleep apnea. Patients with sleep apnea should therefore avoid taking barbiturates. Because of these risks, many clinicians have stopped using barbiturates as hypnotics and sedatives (one exception is in the treatment of severe psychomotor excitation) and prescribe them only as anticonvulsants.

Barbiturates also have been administered intravenously to facilitate patient interviews (i.e., amobarbital interview).

Because they enhance porphyrin synthesis, barbiturates are contraindicated in patients with porphyria. Liver function should be checked before and during drug administration. Liver dysfunction can significantly prolong the sedative effects of these drugs and may lead to fatal overdose.

Side Effects and Toxicology

In treating many patients who are prescribed barbiturates, it is difficult to control symptoms without causing oversedation. Patients typically oscillate between anxiety and torpor. Mental performance is often impaired, and patients should not drive or operate dangerous machinery.

Patients whose conditions have been stabilized for years with barbiturates must be considered drug dependent. Withdrawal leads to anxiety, agitation, trembling, and, frequently, convulsions. Substitution with a benzodiazepine that can be withdrawn more easily later is often successful.

Overdose

An overdose of barbiturates leads to fatal respiratory and cardiovascular depression. Suicide attempts frequently involve overdoses of barbiturates, taken either alone or in combination with alcohol or other psychotropic drugs, particularly tricyclic antidepressants. These suicide attempts, unfortunately, are often successful. Depending on local factors such as proximity to a hospital and expertise of staff for intensive emergency care, death occurs in 0.5%–10% of these cases. Severe poisoning results at 10 times the hypnotic dose, and twice that amount may be fatal.

Tolerance and Dependence

Tolerance to barbiturates occurs rapidly and is a result of both pharmacokinetic factors (e.g., liver enzyme induction) and pharmacodynamic factors (e.g., neuronal adaptation to chronic drug administration). Cross-tolerance develops to alcohol, gas anesthetics, and other sedatives, including benzodiazepines.

Psychological dependence (i.e., drug-seeking behavior) is common. Patients typically visit several physicians to obtain more barbiturates. Physical dependence may be induced by dosages of 500 mg/day. Intoxication may occur, as evidenced by impaired mental functioning, emotional instability, and neurological signs. Abrupt discontinuation after high doses is likely to induce convulsions and delirium. After normal doses, withdrawal phenomena include anxiety, insomnia, restlessness, agitation, tremor, muscle twitching, nausea and vomiting, orthostatic hypotension, and weight loss.

Drug-Drug Interactions

Barbiturates used with other CNS depressants can cause severe depression. Ethanol is the drug most frequently used, and interactions with antihistaminic compounds are also common. Monoamine oxidase inhibitors and methylphenidate also increase the CNS depressant effect of barbiturates.

Barbiturates may increase the activity of hepatic microsomal enzymes two- to threefold. Clinically, this change is particularly important for patients who are also receiving metabolic competitors such as warfarin or digitoxin, for which careful control of plasma concentrations is vital (Rall 1990).

Other Sedative-Hypnotic Compounds

Alcohol-Type Hypnotics and Gamma-Hydroxybutyrate

The alcohol-type hypnotics include the chloral derivatives, of which chloral hydrate, clomethiazole, and ethchlorvynol are still used occasionally in the elderly. Chloral hydrate is metabolized to another active sedative-hypnotic—trichloroethanol. These drugs have short half-lives (about 4–6 hours) and decrease sleep latency and number of awakenings; SWS is slightly depressed, but overall REM sleep time is largely unaffected. Chloral hydrate and its metabolite have an unpleasant taste and frequently cause epigastric distress and nausea. Undesirable side effects include light-headedness, ataxia, and nightmares. Chronic use of these drugs can lead to tolerance and occasionally to physical dependence. As with barbiturates, overdosage can lead to respiratory and cardiovascular depression, and therapeutic use of these drugs has largely been superseded by the use of benzodiazepines.

γ-Hydroxybutyrate (GHB) is a hypnotic agent that has been used mostly in the treatment of insomnia in narcoleptic patients (Scrima et al. 1990). It is rarely used in other indications and is frequently abused. GHB was classified as a Schedule I controlled substance in March 2000 in the United States, but in July 2002, its sodium salt form, sodium oxybate (Xynem), was approved for the treatment of narcolepsy. Nighttime administration of GHB reduces excessive daytime sleepiness associated with narcolepsy. The mode of action involves specific non-GABAergic binding sites and a potent inhibitory effect on dopaminergic transmission (Vayer et al. 1987). The compound promotes SWS and REM sleep (Lapierre et al. 1990), but its effects on sleep architecture are short-lasting, and repeated administration usually is necessary during the night. GHB is also used for the treatment of cataplexy of narcolepsy, but the mechanisms of GHB's effect on cataplexy remain unknown.

Antihistamines

Antihistamines, such as promethazine, diphenhydramine, and doxylamine, are sometimes prescribed as sleep inducers. They decrease sleep latency but do not increase total sleep time (see Reite et al. 1997). These compounds are especially useful for patients who cannot sleep well because of acute allergic reactions or itching. Because sedative antihistamines lack abuse potential, they also may be prescribed for those persons who tend to abuse psychoactive drugs. Rapid tolerance is a problem.

In April 2008, the FDA approved the filing of a new drug application for doxepin hydrochloride, a tricyclic antidepressant with histaminergic$_1$ (H_1) antagonism, for the treatment of insomnia (marketed under the trade name Silenor). Doxepin (as Sinequan) reduces wake after sleep onset (WASO) and prolongs sleep time. Several other selective H_1 blockers and H_1 reverse agonists are also under development for hypnotic uses.

Melatonin

Melatonin is a neurohormone produced by the pineal gland during the dark phase of the day-night cycle. In animals, melatonin has been implicated in the circadian regulation of sleep and in the seasonal control of reproduction. Studies suggest that melatonin administration may have some therapeutic effects in various disturbances of circadian rhythmicity, such as jet lag (Arendt et al. 1987), shift work (Folkard et al. 1993), non-24-hour sleep-wake cycle in blind subjects (Arendt et al. 1988), and delayed-sleep-phase insomnia (Dahlitz et al. 1991), with few side effects (e.g., headaches or nausea). High doses of melatonin (3–100 mg), which increase serum melatonin levels far beyond the normal nocturnal range, have been suggested to produce hypnotic effects in humans. Lower and more physiological doses of melatonin (e.g., 0.3 mg) also might be active, but the data available to date are less convincing.

In humans, the production of melatonin during the dark period declines with age; this effect parallels declines in sleep quantity and quality (Van Coevorden et al. 1991), especially in elderly persons with insomnia (Haimov et al. 1994; Mishima et al. 2001). These results seemingly suggest that deficiency in nocturnal melatonin secretion might contribute to disrupted sleep in the elderly; thus, in this population, insomnia is a particularly attractive indication for melatonin. Indeed, some studies reported favorable effects with supplementary administration of melatonin in elderly persons with sleep maintenance disturbances (Garfinkel et al. 1995; Haimov et al. 1995). However, several studies reported contradictory findings indicating no significant relation between physiological melatonin secretion levels and sleep maintenance parameters (Hughes et al. 1998; Lushington et al. 1998; Youngstedt et al. 1998; Zeitzer et al. 1999) as well as no significant therapeutic effect of melatonin replacement on sleep maintenance in elderly persons with insomnia (Hughes et al. 1998).

One of the difficulties in establishing therapeutic efficacy of melatonin is its short half-life (20–30 minutes). Bedtime melatonin administration reduces sleep latency but has few objective effects on sleep architecture. It is also unclear whether the hypnotic effect of a physiological or pharmacological dose is a direct effect on sleep, an indirect effect on circadian timing that subsequently gates the release of sleep, or both. Finally, very few double-blind, placebo-controlled studies have been done, and most current reports are confounded by strong placebo effects in the context of a melatonin fad. Melatonin might be an effective hypnotic in some indications, but better-controlled studies are needed to establish efficacy in specific indications. The purity of the products sold in health food stores is also a problem, and the long-term effects of melatonin administration in humans are unknown.

There are at least three subtypes of melatonin receptors with high (MT_1) and low (MT_2 and MT_3) affinities for this ligand (Dubocovich 1995; Morgan et al. 1994). The MT_1 receptor is further divided into two subclasses, MT_{1a} and MT_{1b} (Reppert et al. 1994, 1995). The localization of the MT_{1a} receptor in the SCN and median eminence in humans and rodents suggests that this receptor is essential for circadian regulation and reproduction, whereas the MT_{1b} receptor is localized mainly in the retina.

Ramelteon, a melatonin receptor agonist with both high affinity for melatonin MT_1 and MT_2 receptors and selectivity over the MT_3 receptor and with a longer half-life than melatonin, has recently been approved by the FDA for long-term treatment of insomnia, particularly for delayed sleep onset. Ramelteon does not show any appreciable binding to $GABA_A$ receptors, which are associated with anxiolytic, myorelaxant, and amnesic effects. Ramelteon has not been demonstrated to produce dependence and has shown no potential for abuse, and the withdrawal and rebound insomnia typically seen with other GABA modulators are not present.

Animal studies demonstrated that sleep-enhancing effects of ramelteon are not associated with reduction in REM sleep (Miyamoto et al. 2004). It is currently the only nonscheduled prescription drug for the treatment of insomnia available in the United States. Ramelteon has no appreciable affinity for receptors that bind neuropeptides, cytokines, serotonin, dopamine, norepinephrine, acetylcholine, and opiates. It also does not interfere with the activity of a number of selected enzymes in a standard panel. The activity of ramelteon at the MT_1 and MT_2 receptors, especially on the SCN, is believed to contribute to its sleep-promoting properties, as these receptors, acted upon by endogenous melatonin, are thought to be involved in the maintenance of the circadian rhythm underlying the normal sleep-wake cycle.

The biological action of melatonin is similar to that of ramelteon. No published studies have indicated whether ramelteon is more or less safe or effective than melatonin, a much less expensive drug widely available in the United States without a prescription. Several other MT_1/MT_2 receptor agonists are under development.

A prolonged-release formulation of melatonin (marketed under the trade name Circadin) was approved by the European Commission in June 2007 as monotherapy for the short-term treatment of primary insomnia characterized by poor-quality sleep in patients 55 years and older (Lemoine et al. 2007).

General Considerations in the Pharmacological Treatment of Insomnia

Insomnia is a subjective complaint of insufficient, inadequate, or nonrestorative sleep (Buysse and Reynolds 1990). Disturbances in daytime functioning, such as fatigue, mood disturbances, and impaired performance, result from inadequate sleep. Insomnia is a common symptom. In 1983, a survey indicated that 35% of the general population reported having trouble sleeping in the past year, and 17% considered their problem serious (Mellinger et al. 1985). In the same survey, 7.1% of the population had used a hypnotic in the past year.

Insomnia is a symptom that must be explored clinically before treatment is initiated. Sleep disturbances often indicate a larger psychiatric problem, such as depression. As mentioned above, a complaint of insomnia is also common with old age, especially in an institutional setting. In other cases, environmental factors (e.g., noise) and associated sleep disorders (periodic leg movements, sleep apneas, parasomnias) may be involved.

A useful initial approach to the patient with insomnia is to consider the duration of the complaint. The duration of insomnia not only suggests its cause (Table 33–3) but also provides some guidance on how to use hypnotics.

Transient insomnias (1–2 days) are typically caused by an environmental acute stressor, jet lag, or shift work. In this indication, pharmacotherapy with benzodiazepine hypnotics or other hypnotics has no risks because dependence on the treatment is unlikely to develop when the therapy lasts less than 7–10 days.

Short-term (a few days to a few months) insomnias are particularly important to recognize because they may evolve into chronic psychophysiological insomnia if untreated or inadequately treated. Typically, patients develop insomnia during a stressful period of their lives. The condition frequently worsens if untreated, and the patient worries excessively about his or her sleep, which evolves into a behaviorally learned, chronic insomnia that does not resolve once the stressful period is over. In this indication, the daily use of benzodiazepine hypnotics is also dangerous because it may lead to tolerance and dependence. Reassurance regarding the favorable resolution of the stressful event is important, and the patient should be instructed to use hypnotic medications intermittently to avoid the development of tolerance. An education in sleep hygiene is also important to reduce the possibility of evolution into a chronic problem.

Chronic insomnia (several months or even years) should first be evaluated with a sleep log of a 2-week period. Most commonly, some degree of sleep-state misperception is present, and patients with insomnia greatly exaggerate the complaint. In rare cases, insomnia began in childhood and has persisted into adulthood (idiopathic insomnia). In chronic insomnia, improved sleep hygiene and various behavioral techniques that aim to reduce negative conditioning (stimulus control therapy), sleep restriction, and phototherapy are often helpful on a long-term basis, but these methods are successful only if the patient is motivated and if specialized clinical supervision is available. Drug use is most appropriate in patients whose sleep disturbance is clearly causing some daytime dysfunction. If the clinician decides to use pharmacotherapy, it is always helpful to start with the lowest dose of hypnotic possible to reduce the risk of tolerance and dependence and to try to avoid daily use.

Insomnia also can be classified on the basis of individual clinical features—that is, as sleep initiation, sleep maintenance, or termination (early-morning awakening). In this context, the most important pharmacological properties to consider when selecting a hypnotic for treatment are how quickly it acts and how long the effects last (see Table 33–2 for commonly used compounds). The rate of absorption is the most critical factor determining onset of action. The time required to reach the maximal plasma concentration (T_{max}) is the pharmacological parameter that best predicts onset of action. After absorption, hypnotics are distributed to various organs; distribution and drug elimination influence the duration of action. The elimination half-life (see Table 33–2) usually provides a good first estimate of the duration of action for drugs that have comparable absorption and distribution profiles. Hypnotics with long duration of action are helpful for pa-

TABLE 33–3. Nosological classification of insomnia (International Classification of Sleep Disorders diagnostic criteria)

CATEGORY AND PREVALENCE	DESCRIPTION
Adjustment insomnia (acute insomnia) (15%–20%)	Sleep disturbance of relatively short duration (typically a few days to a few weeks) associated with an identifiable stressor
Psychophysiological insomnia (1%–2%)	Persistent insomnia that develops as a result of physiological arousal and learned sleep-preventing associations marked by overconcern with the inability to sleep
Paradoxical insomnia (<5% of patients with insomnia)	Subjective insomnia that occurs without evidence of objective sleep disturbance and without the level of daytime impairment commensurate with the degree of sleep deficits reported
Idiopathic insomnia (0.7%–1.0%)	Lifelong insomnia with insidious onset occurring during infancy or early childhood
Insomnia due to mental disorder (~3%)	Psychiatric insomnia that is caused by underling mental disorders (including mood, anxiety, psychotic, and personality disorders)
Inadequate sleep hygiene (1%–2% [5%–10% of patients with insomnia])	Insomnia associated with daily living activities that are inconsistent with the maintenance of good quality sleep and full daytime alertness
Behavioral insomnia of childhood (10%–30% in childhood)	Difficulty falling asleep, staying asleep, or both that is related to an identified behavioral etiology
Insomnia due to drug or substance (~0.2%)	Insomnia caused by consumption of a prescription medication, recreational drug, caffeine, alcohol, or food item or by exposure to an environmental toxin
Insomnia due to medical condition (~0.5%)	Insomnia that is caused by a coexisting medical disorder or other physiologic factor
Insomnia not due to substance or known physiological condition, unspecified (nonorganic insomnia, NOS)	Insomnia that cannot be classified elsewhere but are suspected to be related to an underlying mental disorder, psychological factors, or sleep-disruptive practices
Physiological (organic) insomnia, unspecified	Insomnia that cannot be classified elsewhere but are suspected to be related to an underlying medical disorder, physiological state, or substance use or exposure

Note. NOS = not otherwise specified.

Source. Adapted from American Academy of Sleep Medicine: *The International Classification of Sleep Disorders: Diagnostic and Coding Manual*, 2nd Edition. Westchester, IL, American Academy of Sleep Medicine, 2005.

tients who have difficulty both initiating and maintaining sleep. One advantage of these long-acting compounds is that rebound insomnia is often delayed and milder if the drugs have to be withdrawn (see Figure 33–6). Patients who have difficulty initiating sleep might prefer short-acting compounds; however, for these compounds, it may be necessary, paradoxically, to switch to longer-acting hypnotics before withdrawal of all hypnotic treatment.

The importance of determining whether insomnia is the symptom of an underlying neuropsychiatric condition must be emphasized (see Table 33–3). For depression, trazodone (25–50 mg), amitriptyline (10 mg), trimipramine (25–50 mg), or doxepin (25–50 mg) can be used as a hypnotic or in combination with another hypnotic. Most individuals with schizophrenia also have persistent insomnia (affecting both initiation and maintenance of sleep), and phenothiazines, such as chlorpromazine, thioridazine, and levomepromazine, are effective therapies. When psychotic symptoms are associated with insomnia, butyrophenones, such as haloperidol, also can be used. For insomnia associated with anxiety disorders, hypnotics supplemented with anxiolytics can be used, and this treatment may prevent rebound insomnia and its related anxiety.

Sleep disturbances are very frequent complaints in old age, and treatment must be initiated carefully in this population. About 12% of the U.S. population is older than 60 years, and this segment of the population receives 35%–40% of all sedative-hypnotic prescriptions (Gottlieb 1990).

Before starting pharmacological therapy, all possible causes of insomnia should be examined (e.g., psychophysiological; associated with drugs and alcohol; due to disturbance of the sleep-wake cycle; associated with periodic leg movements, sleep apnea, or other physical or psychiatric conditions). Before selecting a specific hypnotic, the clinician should consider its pharmacological properties and side-effect profile, the patient's medical health and medical history, and the patient's history of sedative-hypnotic use. The special case of melatonin was discussed earlier in this chapter (see section "Other Sedative-Hypnotic Compounds"). Hypnotics or their active metabolites often accumulate during chronic use in elderly patients, and this accumulation may cause cognition problems, disorientation, confusion, and, occasionally, falls. Hypnotics with short or intermediate half-lives are thus recommended, and the lowest dose possible should be used. Compounds with a short half-life, such as triazolam or zolpidem, may be effective for problems with sleep initiation and sleep fragmentation. Zolpidem has little muscle relaxant effect and may be preferable. Compounds with an intermediate hypnotic profile, such as estazolam and temazepam, are also reported to be effective in elderly patients. Hypnotics with intermediate half-lives may alter daytime performance and memory to a lesser extent and are not as likely to induce rebound insomnia after withdrawal as are regular hypnotics.

Conclusion

The mechanism of action of most currently available hypnotics (benzodiazepines, barbiturates, alcohol, and recent nonbenzodiazepine hypnotics) involves a modulatory effect of GABAergic activity. These compounds stimulate GABAergic transmission by acting on the $GABA_A$–benzodiazepine–Cl^- macromolecular complex, known to contain multiple modulatory binding sites and many receptor subtypes. This recently discovered molecular diversity within the macromolecular complex suggests that new GABAergic hypnotic compounds with subtype selectivity may have better side-effect profiles.

Other non-GABAergic hypnotics, including mostly sedative antidepressants, antihistamines, and melatonin and melatonin receptor agonists, are viable strategies in the treatment of insomnia, especially because these hypnotics may lack some of the hampering side effects often seen with classical GABAergic hypnotics, such as abuse potential and amnesic effects. Their prescription, as with the prescription of other regular benzodiazepine-like hypnotic compounds, should be guided by the knowledge that insomnia is a heterogeneous condition that should be explored clinically before any pharmacological treatment is initiated.

References

Allen D, Curran HV, Lader M: The effects of single doses of CL284,846, lorazepam, and placebo on psychomotor and memory function in normal male volunteers. Eur J Clin Pharmacol 45:313–320, 1993

Amin J, Weiss DS: GABAA receptor needs two homologous domains of the beta-subunit for activation by GABA but not by pentobarbital. Nature 366:565–569, 1993

Arendt J, Aldhous M, Marks V, et al: Some effects of jet-lag and their alleviation by melatonin. Ergonomics 30:1379–1393, 1987

Arendt J, Aldhous M, Wright J: Synchronisation of a disturbed sleep-wake cycle in a blind man by melatonin treatment. Lancet 1(8588):772–773, 1988

Asano T, Ogasawara N: Chloride-dependent stimulation of GABA and benzodiazepine receptor binding by pentobarbital. Brain Res 225:212–216, 1981

Awad M, Gavish M: Binding of [3H]Ro 5–4864 and [3H]PK 11195 to cerebral cortex and peripheral tissues of various species: species differences and heterogeneity in peripheral benzodiazepine binding sites. J Neurochem 49:1407–1414, 1987

Beer B, Ieni JR, Wu WH, et al: A placebo-controlled evaluation of single, escalating doses of CL 284,846, a non-benzodiazepine hypnotic. J Clin Pharmacol 34:335–344, 1994

Boileau AJ, Kucken AM, Evers AR, et al: Molecular dissection of benzodiazepine binding and allosteric coupling using chimeric gamma-aminobutyric acid A receptor subunits. Mol Pharmacol 53:295–303, 1998

Boileau AJ, Evers AR, Davis AF, et al: Mapping the agonist binding site of the GABAA receptor: evidence for a beta-strand. J Neurosci 19:4847–4854, 1999

Braestrup C, Nielsen M: Benzodiazepine binding in vivo and efficacy, in Benzodiazepine/GABA Receptors and Chloride Channels: Structural and Functional Properties. Edited by Olsen RW, Venter JC. New York, Alan R Liss, 1986, pp 167–184

Buysse DJ, Reynolds CF III: Insomnia, in Handbook of Sleep Disorders. Edited by Thorpy MJ. New York, Marcel Dekker, 1990, pp 375–433

Cook L, Sepinwall J: Behavioral analysis of the effects and mechanisms of action of benzodiazepines. Adv Biochem Psychopharmacol 14:1–28, 1975

Costa E, Guidotti A: Diazepam binding inhibitor (DBI): a peptide with multiple biological actions. Life Sci 49:325–344, 1991

Crestani F, Low K, Keist R, et al: Molecular targets for the myorelaxant action of diazepam. Mol Pharmacol 59:442–445, 2001

Dahlitz M, Alvarez B, Vignan J, et al: Delayed sleep phase syndrome response to melatonin. Lancet 337:1121–1124, 1991

Dubocovich ML: Melatonin receptors: are there multiple subtypes? Trends Pharmacol Sci 16:50–56, 1995

Edgar DM, Dement WC, Fuller CA: Effect of SCN-lesions on sleep in squirrel monkeys: evidence for opponent processes in sleep-wake regulation. J Neurosci 13:1065–1079, 1993

Edgar DM, Seidel WF, Gee KW, et al: CCD-3693: an orally bioavailable analog of the endogenous neuroactive steroid, pregnanolone, demonstrates potent sedative hypnotic action in the rat. J Pharmacol Exp Ther 282:420–429, 1997

Folkard S, Arendt J, Clark M: Can melatonin improve shift workers' tolerance of the night shift? Some preliminary findings. Chronobiol Int 10: 315–320, 1993

Friess E, Lance M, Holster F: The effects of "neuroactive" steroids upon sleep in human and rats (abstract). J Sleep Res 5:S69, 1996

Garfinkel D, Laudon M, Nof D, et al: Improvement of sleep quality in elderly people by controlled-release melatonin. Lancet 346:541–544, 1995

Gavish M, Katz Y, Bar-Ami S, et al: Biochemical, physiological, and pathological aspects of the peripheral benzodiazepine receptor. J Neurochem 58:1589–1601, 1992

Geddes DM, Rudorf M, Saunders KB: Effect of nitrazepam and flurazepam on the ventilatory response to carbon dioxide. Thorax 31:548–551, 1976

Gottlieb GL: Sleep disorders and their management: special considerations in the elderly. Am J Med 88:29S–33S, 1990

Haefley W: Partial agonists of the benzodiazepine receptor: from animal data to results in patients, in Chloride Channels and Their Modulation by Neurotransmission and Drugs. Edited by Biggio G, Costa E. New York, Raven, 1988, pp 275–292

Haimov I, Laudon M, Zisapel N, et al: Sleep disorders and melatonin rhythms in elderly people. BMJ 309:167, 1994

Haimov I, Lavie P, Lauden M, et al: Melatonin treatment of sleep onset insomnia in the elderly. Sleep 18:598–603, 1995

Hughes RJ, Sack RL, Lewy AJ: The role of melatonin and circadian phase in age-related sleep-maintenance insomnia: assessment in a clinical trial of melatonin replacement. Sleep 21:52–68, 1998

Jovanovic UJ, Dreyfus JF: Polygraphical sleep recording in insomniac patients under zopiclone or nitrazepam. Pharmacology 27 (suppl 2): 136–145, 1983

Kales A, Shlarf MB, Kales JD, et al: Rebound insomnia: a potential hazard following withdrawal of certain benzodiazepines. JAMA 241:1691–1695, 1979

Kay DC, Blackburn AB, Buckingham JA, et al: Human pharmacology of sleep, in Pharmacology of Sleep. Edited by Williams RL, Karakan I. New York, Wiley, 1976, pp 83–210

Killam K: Drug action on the brainstem reticular formation. Pharmacol Rev 14:175–224, 1962

Kofuji P, Wang JB, Moss SJ, et al: Generation of two forms of the gamma-aminobutyric acidA receptor gamma 2-subunit in mice by alternative splicing. J Neurochem 56:713–715, 1991

Lapierre O, Montplaisir J, Lamarre M, et al: The effect of gamma-hydroxybutyrate on nocturnal and diurnal sleep of normal subjects: further consideration on REM sleep-triggering mechanisms. Sleep 13:24–30, 1990

Leeb-Lundberg F, Snowman A, Olsen RW: Barbiturate receptor sites are coupled to benzodiazepine receptors. Proc Natl Acad Sci U S A 77:7467–7472, 1980

Lemoine P, Nir T, Laudon M, et al: Prolonged-release melatonin improves sleep quality and morning alertness in insomnia patients aged 55 years and older and has no withdrawal effects. J Sleep Res 16:372–380, 2007

Low K, Crestani F, Keist R, et al: Molecular and neuronal substrate for the selective attenuation of anxiety. Science 290:131–134, 2000

Lushington K, Lack L, Kennaway DJ, et al: 6-Sulfatoxymelatonin excretion and self-reported sleep in good sleeping controls and 55–80-year-old insomniacs. J Sleep Res 7:75–83, 1998

Marquardt H, Todaro GJ, Shoyab M: Complete amino acid sequences of bovine and human endozepines: homology with rat diazepam binding inhibitor. J Biol Chem 261:9727–9731, 1986

Maynert EW: Sedative and hypnotics, II: barbiturates, in Drill's Pharmacology in Medicine. Edited by DiPalma IR. New York, McGraw-Hill, 1965, pp 188–209

McKernan RM, Rosahl TW, Reynolds DS, et al: Sedative but not anxiolytic properties of benzodiazepines are mediated by the GABAA receptor alpha1 subtype. Nature Neuroscience 3:587–592, 2000

Mehta AK, Ticku MK: An update on GABAA receptors. Brain Res Brain Res Rev 29:196–217, 1999

Mellinger GD, Balter MB, Uhlenhuth EH: Insomnia and its treatment: prevalence and correlates. Arch Gen Psychiatry 42:225–232, 1985

Mignot E, Edgar DM, Miller JD, et al: Strategies for the development of new treatments in sleep disorders medicine, in Target Receptors for Anxiolytics and Hypnotics: From Molecular Pharmacology to Therapeutics. Edited by Mendelwicz J, Racagni G, Karger AG. Basel, Switzerland, Karger, 1992, pp 129–150

Mishima K, Okawa M, Shimizu T, et al: Diminished melatonin secretion in the elderly caused by insufficient environmental illumination. J Clin Endocrinol Metab 86:129–134, 2001

Miyamoto M, Nishikawa H, Doken Y, et al: The sleep-promoting action of ramelteon (TAK-375) in freely moving cats. Sleep 27:1319–1325, 2004

Möhler H, Okada T: Benzodiazepine receptor: demonstration in the central nervous system. Science 198:849–851, 1977

Morgan PJ, Barrett P, Howell HE, et al: Melatonin receptors: localization, molecular pharmacology and physiological significance. Neurochem Int 24:101–146, 1994

Mullen KD, Szauter KM, Kaminsky-Russ K: "Endogenous" benzodiazepine activity in physiological fluids of patients with hepatic encephalopathy. Lancet 336:81–83, 1990

Nutt DJ, Glue P, Lawson C, et al: Flumazenil provocation of panic attacks. Arch Gen Psychiatry 47:917–925, 1990

Olsen RW, Tick MK, Miller T: Dihydropicotoxine binding to crayfish muscle sites possibly related to gamma-aminobutyric acid receptor-ionophores. Mol Pharmacol 14:381–390, 1978

Papadopoulos V, Amri H, Li H, et al: Structure, function and regulation of the mitochondrial peripheral-type benzodiazepine receptor. Therapie 56:549–556, 2001

Rall TR: Hypnotics and sedatives: ethanol, in The Pharmacological Basis of Therapeutics, 8th Edition. Edited by Gilman AG, Rall TW, Niles AS, et al. New York, Pergamon, 1990, pp 345–382

Reite M, Ruddy J, Nagel K: Concise Guide to Evaluation and Management of Sleep Disorders, 2nd Edition. Washington, DC, American Psychiatric Press, 1997

Reppert SM, Weaver DR, Ebisawa T: Cloning and characterization of a mammalian melatonin receptor that mediates reproductive and circadian responses. Neuron 13:1177–1185, 1994

Reppert SM, Godson C, Mahle CD, et al: Molecular characterization of a second melatonin receptor expressed in human retina and brain: the Mel1b melatonin receptor. Proc Natl Acad Sci U S A 92:8734–8738, 1995

Rothstein JD, Guidotti A, Tinuper P, et al: Endogenous benzodiazepine receptor ligands in idiopathic recurring stupor. Lancet 340:1002–1004, 1992

Rudolph U, Crestani F, Benke D, et al: Benzodiazepine actions mediated by specific gamma-aminobutyric acidA receptor subtypes. Nature 401:796–800, 1999

Rupprecht R, Hauser CAE, Trapp T, et al: Neurosteroids: molecular mechanisms of action and psychopharmacological significance. J Steroid Biochem Mol Biol 56:163–168, 1996

Sanna E, Garau F, Harris RA: Novel properties of homomeric b1 g-aminobutyric acid type A receptors: actions of the anesthetics propofol and pentobarbital. Mol Pharmacol 47:213–217, 1995

Saper CB, Chou TC, Scammell TE: The sleep switch: hypothalamic control of sleep and wakefulness. Trends Neurosci 24:726–731, 2001

Scrima L, Hartman PG, Johnson FH, et al: The effects of gamma-hydroxybutyrate on the sleep of narcolepsy patients: a double-blind study. Sleep 13:479–490, 1990

Sherin JE, Shiromani PJ, McCarley RW, et al: Activation of ventrolateral preoptic neurons during sleep. Science 271:216–219, 1996

Shlarf MB: Pharmacology of classic and novel hypnotic drugs, in Target Receptors for Anxiolytics and Hypnotics: From Molecular Pharmacology to Therapeutics. Edited by Mendelwicz J, Racagni G. Basel, Switzerland, Karger, 1992, pp 109–116

Sigel E, Baur R, Kellenberger S, et al: Point mutations affecting antagonist affinity and agonist dependent gating of GABAA receptor channels. EMBO J 11:2017–2023, 1992

Smith GB, Olsen RW: Identification of a [3H]muscimol photoaffinity substrate in the bovine gamma-aminobutyric acidA receptor alpha subunit. J Biol Chem 269:20380–20387, 1994

Squires RF, Braestrup C: Benzodiazepine receptors in rat brain. Nature 266:732–734, 1977

Szymusiak R: Magnocellular nuclei of the basal forebrain: substrates of sleep and arousal regulation. Sleep 18:478–500, 1995

Tallman JF, Thomas JW, Gllager DW: GABAergic modulation of benzodiazepine binding site sensitivity. Nature 274:383–385, 1978

Tobler I, Kopp C, Deboer T, et al: Diazepam-induced changes in sleep: role of the alpha 1 GABA(A) receptor subtype. Proc Natl Acad Sci U S A 98:6464–6469, 2001

Twyman RE, Rogers CJ, Macdonald RL: Differential regulation of gamma-aminobutyric acid receptor channels by diazepam and phenobarbital. Ann Neurol 25:213–220, 1989

Ueno S, Minami K, Yanagihara N: [Structure and function of GABAA receptors: recent studies by site-directed mutagenesis] (in Japanese). Protein, Nucleic Acid, and Enzyme 46:2042–2051, 2001

Van Coevorden A, Mockel J, Laurent E, et al: Neuroendocrine rhythms and sleep in aging men. Am J Physiol 260:651–661, 1991

Vayer P, Mandel P, Maitre M: Gamma-hydroxybutyrate, a possible neurotransmitter. Life Sci 41: 1547–1557, 1987

Wisden W, Stephens DN: Towards better benzodiazepines. Nature 401:751–752, 1999

Youngstedt SD, Kripke DF, Elliott JA: Melatonin excretion is not related to sleep in the elderly. J Pineal Res 24:142–145, 1998

Zeitzer JM, Daniels JE, Duffy JF, et al: Do plasma melatonin concentrations decline with age? Am J Med 107:432–436, 1999

CHAPTER 34

Psychostimulants and Wakefulness-Promoting Agents

Charles DeBattista, D.M.H., M.D.

Amphetamine, first discovered in 1887, and the subsequently developed stimulants have been used in clinical psychiatry with varying results. Beyond their use for attention-deficit/hyperactivity disorder (ADHD), stimulants have been used for symptomatic relief based on their effects on mood and hedonic drive. Research into the use of stimulants as adjunctive agents in the treatment of specific symptoms and syndromes has been increasing. Various common adjunctive psychotherapeutic uses for stimulants, such as depression, have not been well researched, whereas other indications, such as narcolepsy, are backed by considerable clinical data. In this chapter, I review the pharmacology of these medications and their indications (Tables 34–1 and 34–2).

Amphetamines

Structure-Activity Relations

Structurally, amphetamine is phenylisopropylamine. Ultimate pharmacological action is determined by alterations to any of the three basic parts of the amphetamine molecule.

Amine Changes

In terms of affecting clinical utility, substitution at the amine group is the most common alteration. Methamphetamine (both L and D

This chapter is an update and revision of Ballas CA, Evans DL, Dinges DF: "Psychostimulants and Wakefulness-Promoting Agents," in *The American Psychiatric Publishing Textbook of Psychopharmacology*, 4th Edition. Edited by Schatzberg AF, Nemeroff CB. Washington, DC, American Psychiatric Publishing, 2009, pp. 843–860.

TABLE 34–1. FDA classifications of psychostimulants and wakefulness-promoting agents

Agent	Schedule	Approved for	Medication type	Abuse potential
Amphetamine	II	ADHD, narcolepsy	Anorexiant/stimulant	Black box warning
Lisdexamfetamine	II	ADHD	Stimulant	Black box warning
Methylphenidate	II	ADHD, narcolepsy	Anorexiant/stimulant ("Mild stimulant")	Black box warning
Modafinil	IV	Excessive daytime sleepiness associated with narcolepsy, OSAHS, and SWSD	Wakefulness-promoting agent	Reinforcing
Armodafinil	IV	Excessive daytime sleepiness associated with narcolepsy, OSAHS, and SWSD	Wakefulness-promoting agent	Reinforcing

Note. ADHD=attention-deficit/hyperactivity disorder; FDA=U.S. Food and Drug Administration; OSAHS=obstructive sleep apnea/hypopnea syndrome; SWSD=shift-work sleep disorder.

Source. Adapted from *Physicians' Desk Reference*, 60th Edition. Montvale, NJ, Medical Economics Company, 2006.

isomers), which is characterized by an additional methyl group attached to the amine, making it a secondary substituted amine, is more potent than amphetamine. Usefully, one may think of the amine group as enhancing stimulant-like properties.

Isopropyl Changes

An intact isopropyl side chain appears to be needed in order to maintain the potency of amphetamine. For example, changing the propyl to an ethyl chain creates phenylethylamine, an endogenous neuroamine (and metabolite of the monoamine oxidase inhibitor [MAOI] phenelzine), which has mood- and energy-enhancing properties but less potency and a much shorter half-life than amphetamine (Janssen et al. 1999).

Aromatic Changes

Substitutions on the phenyl group are associated with a decrease in amphetamine-like properties. Interestingly, reduction of the phenyl to a cyclohexyl ring reduces the potency, but not the efficacy, of amphetamine properties. Unlike changes at the amine or isopropyl level, additions to the aromatic ring substantially alter the effects of the compound. The most common changes at the aromatic ring are of the methoxy type and are associated with hallucinogenic properties.

Stereospecificity

In recent years there has been renewed interest in drugs that are pure stereoisomers, as opposed to racemic mixtures, especially with the release of dexmethylphenidate (the dex-

TABLE 34–2. Amphetamine and methylphenidate preparations

STIMULANT	TIME TO EFFECT	PEAK (HOURS)	DURATION (HOURS)	DOSING
Amphetamine preparations				
Adderall[a]	~1 hour	3	6–9	bid
Adderall XR	1–2 hours	7	6–10	qd (or bid)
Dexedrine	1 hour	3	4–6	bid or tid
Dexedrine Spansules	1 hour	4	6–10	qd or bid
Desoxyn (methamphetamine)	40 minutes	1–3	4–24	qd, bid, or tid
Vyvanse (lisdexamfetamine)	~1 hour	2	9	qd
Methylphenidate preparations				
Methylphenidate	15–30 minutes	1–2	4–5	bid or tid
Focalin (dexmethylphenidate)	15–30 minutes	1–2	4–5	bid or tid
Ritalin SR (tablet)	1–2 hours	5	8	qd or bid
Concerta[b]	1–2 hours	6–8	12	qd or bid
Metadate-CD[c]	1 hour	Biphasic: 1–2 and 4–5	6–8	qd or bid

Note. bid = twice daily; qd = once daily; tid = three times daily.
[a]Amphetamine/dextroamphetamine, 1:3 ratio.
[b]Laser hole in capsule allows passage of drug; osmotically active push layer expels drug.
[c]Rapid-release and continuous-release beads give biphasic response.

tro isomer of methylphenidate) and escitalopram (the levo isomer of citalopram). In amphetamine isomers, it is true that the dextro form (i.e., dextro isomer, or dextroamphetamine) is almost twice as potent as the levo form (i.e., levo isomer, or levoamphetamine) in promoting wakefulness, but they are of equal potency in reducing cataplexy and rapid eye movement (REM) sleep (Nishino and Mignot 1997). The effect on dopamine reuptake is stereospecific; inhibition in rat brain, striatum, and hypothalamus has been found to be markedly different between the two isomers (Ferris and Tang 1979).

The clinical utility of stereospecificity is unclear. Urine levels of the levo isomer have been used to measure compliance in amphetamine-addicted patients prescribed dextroamphetamine for maintenance or detoxification; the logic is that the more levo isomer present in urine, the less compliance (George and Braithwaite 2000).

Perhaps the most clinically useful difference between amphetamine isomers involves their differential effects on reinforcement. Studies in rats have shown that the dextro isomer is four times more potent than the levo isomer in promoting lever pressing for intracranial stimulation (Hunt and Atrens 1992). However, that pure dextroamphetamine is better for the treatment of ADHD than, for example, the mixed salts of dextroamphetamine/amphetamine is neither obvious nor conclusively shown. In addition, the overall greater potency of the dextro form for central actions suggests that this form may have a higher potential for abuse.

Pharmacological Profile

Amphetamines are noncatecholamine, sympathomimetic amines with central nervous system (CNS) stimulant activity that causes catecholamine efflux and inhibits the reuptake of these neurotransmitters (see subsection "Mechanism of Action" later in this section).

Pharmacokinetics and Disposition

Amphetamine is highly lipid soluble and reaches peak levels in approximately 2 hours. Because of this lipid solubility, amphetamine has rapid distribution into tissues and transit across the blood-brain barrier. The protein binding is highly variable, but the average volume of distribution (V_d) is 5 L/kg.

The half-life of amphetamine is approximately 16–30 hours. On average, 30% of amphetamine is excreted unchanged.

Mechanism of Action

The classic mechanism of action of amphetamine involves rapid diffusion directly into neuron terminals; through dopamine and norepinephrine transporters, amphetamine enters vesicles, causing release of dopamine and norepinephrine. The release of these neurotransmitters into the synapse mediates some of the psychological and motoric effects of amphetamine, including euphoria, increased energy, and locomotor activation.

Side Effects and Toxicology

The side effects of amphetamines are predictable relative to their sympathomimetic pharmacology. The most common effects are nervousness, agitation, and decreased sleep. Serious adverse consequences have been observed with amphetamines and include arrhythmias, hyperpyrexia, rhabdomyolysis, and convulsions. Death, although uncommon, generally occurs only after the manifestation of one of these symptoms. Hallucinosis and psychosis are frequent complications of injected or inhaled amphetamines but are uncommon with oral intoxication.

Methamphetamine is more frequently associated with complications; because of its higher toxicity, it is not clear whether severe complications are dose dependent. For example, in a retrospective study of methamphetamine-related deaths in a large city, methamphetamine use was significantly associated with a higher risk of coronary artery disease, as well as a higher rate of subarachnoid hemorrhage, although it was of course impossible to determine whether the subjects were first-time users or chronic abusers (Karch et al. 1999). Of particular note in this study, however, was that blood levels of methamphetamine did not differ between the group in which methamphetamine was judged to be the cause of death and the group in which methamphetamine was detected but judged not to be related to the cause of death, suggesting that these toxicities are not necessarily dose dependent. Similarly, in one 5-year study, methamphetamine accounted for 43% of rhabdomyolysis cases in an emergency department setting.

Methamphetamine is more neurotoxic than amphetamine; it can cause destruction of dopaminergic neurons in the basal ganglia and thus is widely thought to increase the likelihood of future parkinsonism (Guilarte 2001). Although it is commonly believed that MDMA (3,4-methylenedioxy-N-methylamphetamine; "Ecstasy") is toxic primarily to serotonergic neurons (Sprague et al. 1998), evidence shows that it is also toxic to dopaminergic neurons (Ricaurte et al. 2002).

Seizures are fairly common in amphetamine abuse scenarios, especially with the more potent methamphetamine and hallucinogenic analogs.

Stimulant psychosis—often referred to as *paranoid psychosis*—is also common in amphetamine abuse scenarios because of the overwhelming presentation of the eponymous symptom. Visual hallucinations are also disproportionately common with amphetamine psychosis. Psychosis is often seen together with stereotypy. In humans, stereotypy can take many forms but usually is expressed as pacing, searching, or examining minute details.

The U.S. Food and Drug Administration (FDA) has added a black box warning to all stimulant medications, describing the risks of heart-related problems, especially sudden death in those with prior cardiac disease; stroke; and increased blood pressure and heart rate. Additionally, the warning describes the risk of new mental problems, especially bipolar disorder, hostility, or psychosis.

Drug-Drug Interactions

A comprehensive review found that drug interactions with amphetamine were mostly pharmacodynamic in nature (Markowitz and Patrick 2001); however, because a small portion of amphetamine metabolism occurs via the cytochrome P450 (CYP) 2D6 isoenzyme, those drugs that inhibit 2D6 metabolism can, theoretically, have the effect of increasing the plasma level of amphetamine.

Lisdexamfetamine

Lisdexamfetamine dimesylate, a prodrug that on absorption is metabolized to dextroamphetamine and L-lysine, was approved in 2007 for the treatment of ADHD. Food does not affect absorption of lisdexamfetamine, but acidification of the urine results in more rapid clearance.

Two small studies in children found good efficacy and tolerability for lisdexamfetamine in the treatment of ADHD. A 4-week randomized, double-blind, forced-dose, parallel-group study compared lisdexamfetamine 30, 50, or 70 mg with placebo in children (ages 6–12 years) with ADHD (Biederman et al. 2007b). Efficacy, as measured by the ADHD Rating Scale–Version IV (ADHD-RS-IV), the Conners Parent Rating Scale (CPR), and the Clinical Global Impression of Improvement scale, was statistically superior to that of placebo for all doses tested. A randomized, double-blind, placebo-controlled crossover study compared lisdexamfetamine with placebo and extended-release mixed amphetamine salts (Adderall XR) in 52 children (ages 6–12 years) with ADHD in an analog classroom setting (Biederman et al. 2007a). The study found comparable efficacy and safety for the active medications and superiority over placebo as measured by CGI and Swanson, Kotkin, Agler, M-Flynn, and Pelham (SKAMP)–Deportment scores.

In 420 adults, a 4-week forced-dose (30, 50, and 70 mg) study found lisdexamfetamine to have significantly greater efficacy over placebo as measured by ADHD-RS scores. Human liability studies have also found lower abuse-related drug-liking scores compared with immediate-release D-amphetamine at equivalent doses (Najib 2009).

Methylphenidate

Structure-Activity Relations

Although methylphenidate has two chiral centers, only one contributes to its clinical effect. The D- and L-threo enantiomers are in a racemic mixture, although a single-isomer form of methylphenidate, dexmethylphenidate [(R,R)-(+)], is currently being marketed under the brand name Focalin. There are some differences in the pharmacological parameters of the two isomers, as described in the following subsection.

Pharmacokinetics and Disposition

Methylphenidate is almost totally absorbed on oral administration (as is the single isomer dexmethylphenidate), although it is absorbed at a faster rate in the presence of food (Chan et al. 1983). Methylphenidate has low protein binding (15%) and is fairly short acting; the effects last approximately 4 hours, with a half-life of 3 hours. The primary means of clearance is through the urine, in which 90% is excreted.

Mechanism of Action

Although it is both a norepinephrine and a dopamine reuptake inhibitor, methylphenidate appears to exert its effects primarily through its action on dopamine neurobiology. It blocks the dopamine transporter (DAT) and increases extracellular dopamine. The amount of extracellular dopamine increase varies greatly among individuals depending on the extent of both DAT blockade and baseline dopamine release.

Side Effects and Toxicology

The common side effects of methylphenidate are similar to those of amphetamine and include nervousness, insomnia, and anorexia, as well as dose-related systemic effects such as increased heart rate and blood pressure. Overdose may lead to seizures, dysrhythmias, or hyperthermia (Klein-Schwartz 2002). At therapeutic doses, discontinuation symptoms tend to be slight, but with chronic abuse, symptoms similar to those in amphetamine withdrawal, including lethargy, depression, and paranoia, can occur (Klein-Schwartz 2002).

The FDA has added a black box warning to all stimulant medications, describing the risks of heart-related problems, especially sudden death in those with prior cardiac disease; stroke; and increased blood pressure and heart rate. Additionally, the warning describes the risk of new mental problems, especially bipolar disorder, hostility, or psychosis.

Drug-Drug Interactions

Although theoretically a substrate of CYP2D6, methylphenidate was found not to have any significant metabolism in humans via this enzyme (DeVane et al. 2000). The prescribing information (Novartis 2007) does cite methylphenidate's potential ability to inhibit the metabolism of warfarin, some antiepileptics, and tricyclic antidepressants (TCAs), and thus caution should be observed. However, a review found that methylphenidate is relatively safe and has minimal drug-drug interactions, with the exception of concomitant MAOI use (Markowitz and Patrick 2001).

Modafinil

Modafinil is the first FDA-designated "wakefulness-promoting agent." Modafinil is approved by the FDA for the treatment of excessive sleepiness associated with narcolepsy, sleep apnea, and residual sleepiness after standard treatment for shift-work sleep disorder (Cephalon Inc. 2008). As described below, modafinil does little to prevent or alter sleep when one is trying to do so; however, it appears to permit more stable wakefulness (i.e., reduced sleep propensity) when one is attempting to stay awake in the presence of elevated sleep pressure.

Structure-Activity Relations

Modafinil (2-[(diphenylmethyl)sulfinyl]acetamide) exists in racemic form. Both stereoisomers appear to have the same activity in animals.

Pharmacokinetics and Disposition

Modafinil, the primary metabolite of adrafinil, lacks many of the side effects found in adrafinil, such as increased liver enzymes, anxiety, and stomach pain. Modafinil is rapidly absorbed but slowly cleared. It has fairly high protein binding (60%) and a V_d of 0.8 L/kg. Its half-life is 11–14 hours.

The metabolism of modafinil is complex. In contrast to excretion of amphetamines, less than 10% of modafinil is excreted unchanged.

Metabolism is primarily via CYP3A4/5. It has been reported that modafinil also has in vitro capacity to induce CYP3A4 (Robertson et al. 2000), especially gastrointestinal 3A4. A clinically significant reduction of triazolam has been reported (Robertson et al. 2002).

Mechanism of Action

The precise mechanism by which modafinil exerts its wakefulness-promoting effect in patients with excessive sleepiness due to narcolepsy is not yet known. Modafinil, given its efficacy in narcolepsy, is not surprisingly observed to increase c-fos activity of hypocretin cells, as well as in the tuberomammillary nucleus (which is primarily histaminergic), striatum, and cingulate cortex at higher doses (Scammell et al. 2000). Additionally, in rats, an increase in histamine release in the anterior hypothalamus is seen (Ishizuka et al. 2003). However, modafinil's wakefulness-promoting effects were not decreased in histamine knockout mice (Bonaventure et al. 2007).

What may be an important aspect of the pharmacology of modafinil is its lack of effect on the neuroendocrine system. A comparison of healthy volunteers who were sleep deprived for 36 hours with those who received modafinil during sleep deprivation found no difference in cortisol, melatonin, or growth hormone levels (Brun et al. 1998).

Side Effects and Toxicology

Modafinil appears to be well tolerated, with the most frequent side effects being headache and nausea. Side effects have been found to increase with doses from 100 to 600 mg, and very high doses (800 mg) have been found to be associated with higher rates of tachycardia and hypertension (Wong et al. 1999). Overall, only 5% of the patients in Phase III trials discontinued modafinil because of side effects (Cephalon Inc. 2008).

Modafinil appears to be fairly safe in high doses. Reports indicate that 32 patients have safely taken 1,000 mg/day for more than 50 days; one individual safely took 1,200 mg/day for 21 consecutive days. Two patients took 4,000 mg and 4,500 mg, respectively, at once and experienced only transient (<24 hours) agitation and insomnia with mild elevations in heart rate and blood pressure (Cephalon Inc. 2008). There have been no reports of seizures with modafinil.

During the attempts to have modafinil approved for ADHD, concern arose over the possibility that modafinil may carry a risk of Stevens-Johnson syndrome. Three cases of drug-induced rash were reported during clinical trials (U.S. Food and Drug Administration 2007).

The package insert describes a risk of "serious rash, including Stevens-Johnson syndrome," in adults and children and cautions that modafinil is not indicated for children. The insert cites a rash incidence of 0.8% in pediatric patients, with one case of possible Stevens-Johnson syndrome and one case of multiorgan hypersensitivity reported, and concludes with the statement that although there are no known predictive factors, benign rashes do occur, and modafinil should be discontinued if rash develops.

Drug-Drug Interactions

As described earlier in this section, modafinil induces CYP3A4/5 and thus conceivably could lower the plasma concentrations of medications with substantial 3A4/5 metabolism. However, it is not clear if this induction is substantial only on the gastrointestinal cytochrome and is thus relevant only for other drugs undergoing significant first-pass metabolism.

Modafinil inhibits CYP2C19 in vitro (Robertson et al. 2000). It is prudent to assume that the effect of modafinil on the cytochrome system is not well characterized and to be vigilant for these potential drug-drug interactions.

Armodafinil

Armodafinil, properly L-*(R)*-modafinil (or [–]-*[R]*-modafinil), is the longer-acting isomer of racemic modafinil. In 2007, it received FDA approval for the same indications as modafinil—specifically, excessive sleepiness associated with narcolepsy, obstructive sleep apnea/hypopnea syndrome (OSAHS) as an adjunct to standard treatment, and shift-work sleep disorder (SWSD).

Armodafinil and racemic modafinil produce comparable peak plasma concentrations, although the peak for armodafinil occurs later than that for modafinil and is maintained for 6–14 hours postdose (Dinges et al. 2006).

Published data on armodafinil are still limited. Two 12-week double-blind studies using armodafinil 150 mg as an adjunct to continuous positive airway pressure (CPAP), both in patients who were otherwise stable except for some residual sleepiness (Hirshkowitz et al. 2006) and in patients who were still symptomatic (Roth et al. 2006), found improvements in wakefulness measures. Armodafinil also significantly improved the quality of episodic secondary memory (i.e., the ability to recall unrehearsed information). Whether this effect was due directly to the medication, to improved wakefulness, or to decreased hypoxia (as a function of being more awake) is unclear. However, armodafinil did not adversely affect the CPAP or any other physiological parameters.

A 12-week double-blind study of armodafinil in narcolepsy found improvements similar to those seen with modafinil. These included improved wakefulness (as measured by the Maintenance of Wakefulness Test), improved Clinical Global Impression of Change (CGI-C) scores, and improvement in memory and attention. Armodafinil 150 mg and 250 mg were similarly effective (Harsh et al. 2006).

In SWSD, armodafinil 150 mg/day was tested versus placebo in a 12-week study, showing significant prolongation of time to sleep onset and an improvement in overall clinical condition by CGI-C. Armodafinil had no effect on daytime sleep polysomnography (Roth et al. 2005).

Clinical Uses of Stimulants and Wakefulness-Promoting Agents

Although stimulants have been used for many years in a number of clinical scenarios, double-blind, randomized controlled trials examining their safety, efficacy, and effectiveness in neurobehavioral disorders other than ADHD are relatively rare. Most of the support for their use comes from open-label studies and case series. Randomized trials of modafinil for neurobehavioral disorders with symptoms of sleepiness and fatigue are beginning to be published.

Attention-Deficit/Hyperactivity Disorder

Multiple double-blind, placebo-controlled studies have shown the efficacy of stimulants for ADHD, and their use is well investigated in both adults and children (Greenhill et al. 2002; Wilens et al. 2002). Some studies are aimed at showing superiority of one preparation relative to another, although this approach is not always fruitful; for example, one study comparing various single-dose amphetamine preparations with one another and with placebo over 8 weeks found that they were all superior to placebo; however, immediate-release amphetamines had a faster onset but shorter duration of action; spansules, although much slower to take effect than the others, lasted several hours longer (James et al. 2001).

With respect to individual stimulants, all appear to be equally efficacious in the treatment of ADHD, but they have been reported to have different time courses. In a double-blind, double-control (placebo and methylphenidate) study, the mixed amphetamine salts of Adderall were found to exert their effects rapidly but to dissipate quickly over the course of the day, although Adderall lasted longer than methylphenidate (Swanson et al. 1998). Interestingly, higher doses of Adderall lasted longer than lower doses, indicating a dose-dependent effect in duration of action not found with methylphenidate. Thus, although stimulants may appear to be of equal efficacy overall, there is considerable variability in individual response to each stimulant.

The decision to choose amphetamines or methylphenidate for the treatment of ADHD is often based on the clinician's preference and degree of experience with the medication. At least one important blinded crossover study found that in performance tasks, both drugs were generally equally efficacious (Efron et al. 1997).

Modafinil is not FDA approved for the treatment of ADHD. A 4-week double-blind study with an 8-week open-label extension found modafinil to be efficacious across all ADHD rating subscales for the duration of the open-label extension (Boellner et al. 2006). Interestingly, 10% of the 220 children studied lost an average of 3 kg, while 4% gained the same amount. Another such double-blind study found significant efficacy with dosages of 300 mg/day, although heavier children (<30 kg) required 400 mg/day (Biederman et al. 2006). A pooled analysis of three trials (638 patients) found that modafinil produced similar and impressive improvements in ADHD rating scales between stimulant-naive and prior-stimulant subgroups, relative to placebo (Wigal et al. 2006). As in other studies, insomnia and headache were the most common, but infrequent, side effects. A 9-week trial (Biederman et al. 2005) found that almost half of patients (mean age 10 years, mean dose 368 mg) were much or very much improved, and efficacy was seen in both inattentive and hyperactive subgroups and both school and home ratings. Some small but controlled trials (Rugino and Samsock 2003; Turner et al. 2004) found efficacy with modafinil, and in one study (Taylor and Russo 2000) equivalence to dextroamphetamine. Modafinil is currently indicated only for the treatment of excessive sleepiness associated with narcolepsy, OSAHS, and SWSD.

Stroke and Traumatic Brain Injury

The results from studies on the effects of stimulants in patients who had strokes and traumatic brain injury are mixed. Although small early studies showed some superiority of amphetamine to placebo in improving motor function poststroke (Crisostomo et al. 1988; Walker-Batson et al. 1995), a double-blind study found that 10 mg/day of amphetamine combined with physiotherapy in geriatric stroke patients was not superior to placebo plus physiotherapy in improving activities of daily living or motor function 5 weeks later (Sonde et al. 2001). Neither was amphetamine found to be superior to placebo in improving somatosensory training outcomes (Knecht et al. 2001). Modafinil also has not been consistently effective in the treatment of fatigue associated with traumatic brain injury (Jha et al. 2008). In contrast, relative to placebo, dextroamphetamine 10 mg/day significantly improved language recovery in poststroke aphasic patients when immediately coupled with a session of speech therapy; this effect was seen as quickly as within 1 week (Walker-Batson et al. 2001). A review lamented the lack of good data in brain-injured patients but did note that available data suggest that the bulk of stimulant efficacy may lie with its improvements in mood and cognitive processing (Whyte et al. 2002).

Although there is a dearth of placebo-controlled studies, there are some interesting reports in which stimulants were compared with antidepressants in patients with poststroke depression. One such study, comparing methylphenidate with TCAs, found similar and significant response to both drugs, although the stimulant worked faster (Lazarus et al. 1994).

Modafinil has been reported to have some therapeutic efficacy in one type of brain injury. Two double-blind studies by the same group (Saletu et al. 1990, 1993) found modafinil effective in improving cognition and accelerating improvement in patients with alcoholic brain syndrome.

The very limited available evidence for

the efficacy of certain psychostimulants and modafinil in functional recovery from certain types of brain injury is promising, but much more work needs to be done in this area.

Cocaine and Stimulant Abuse Treatment

It may not be surprising that a double-blind study showed sustained-release dextroamphetamine to be superior to placebo in reducing cocaine use (Grabowski et al. 2001). However, similarly designed studies by the same authors did not find this effect with methylphenidate (Grabowski et al. 1997) or with risperidone (Grabowski et al. 2000). A double-blind, placebo-controlled study found that modafinil did not increase the euphoria or craving for cocaine; it may, in fact, have blunted the euphoria (Dackis et al. 2003). A double-blind, placebo-controlled study of 62 patients found that modafinil-treated patients had a longer duration of cocaine abstinence (>3 weeks), with no dropouts due to adverse events (Dackis et al. 2005). Likewise, a 48-day double-blind trial found that under controlled laboratory conditions, modafinil significantly attenuated self-administration and effects of cocaine (Hart et al. 2008). However, a large randomized controlled study of modafinil in the treatment of 210 subjects with cocaine dependence did not find modafinil generally efficacious in improving abstinence from cocaine use (Dackis et al. 2012), although there was a trend for male patients receiving a modafinil dosage of 400 mg/day to be less likely to use cocaine. More study is needed to determine which, if any, patients with cocaine dependence might benefit from modafinil treatment.

Alcohol Dependence

Basic research suggests that amphetamine appears to have an unexpected effect in alcohol abuse disorders. In rats, amphetamines reduced alcohol consumption during choice trials; this reduction was specific to alcohol intake, because amphetamine administration had no effect on rodents' intake of water (Yu et al. 1997). This effect of amphetamine on alcohol consumption may involve the neurobiology of reward systems. Much more research is needed to identify the mechanisms by which stimulants affect alcohol intake.

Narcolepsy

Stimulants have traditionally been used for the treatment of excessive sleepiness associated with narcolepsy. Narcolepsy is characterized by excessive sleepiness that is typically associated with cataplexy and other REM sleep phenomena such as sleep paralysis and hypnagogic hallucinations. Modafinil's approval for treatment of excessive sleepiness in narcolepsy was based on substantial evidence from large multicenter clinical trials (Broughton et al. 1997; U.S. Modafinil in Narcolepsy Multicenter Study Group 1998, 2000). Modafinil is less disruptive of sleep than amphetamines and is rated as having a lower abuse potential (Shelton et al. 1995) (see Table 34–1). One study found that taking an extra dose (200 mg) at midday improved wakefulness in patients with narcolepsy without causing insomnia at night (Schwartz et al. 2004). Importantly, cataplexy—the sudden occurrence of muscle weakness in association with experiencing laughter, anger, or surprise—is responsive to amphetamines but not to modafinil (Shelton et al. 1995).

Fatigue

The use of stimulants for the treatment of fatigue syndromes may seem intuitive, but evidence from large-scale controlled clinical trials to warrant this use is scant. In one of the only double-blind, placebo-controlled studies, men with HIV, depression, and fatigue had significantly less fatigue with dextroamphetamine (73% response) (Wagner and Rabkin 2000). Tolerance, dependence, and abuse were not observed, even across a 6-month open phase. A double-blind study of methylphenidate and pemoline in a similar group of 144 patients with HIV who had severe fatigue found both stimulants effective in improving fatigue and quality of life (Breitbart et al. 2001). Rabkin et al. (2011) found that a significant majority of HIV patients—including those with comorbid hepatitis C—reported an improvement in fatigue with armodafinil. Likewise, in a Phase III trial of modafinil treatment in 631 patients with cancer-related fatigue, Jean-Pierre et al. (2010) found that modafinil was more effective than placebo in helping patients with severe fatigue. However, modafinil did not separate from placebo in cancer patients with mild or moderate fatigue at baseline.

Two controlled trials (Adler et al. 2003; Hogl et al. 2002) found modafinil effective in reducing excessive sleepiness in Parkinson's disease. Open-label studies of modafinil for fatigue in multiple sclerosis (Rammohan et al. 2002) and myotonic dystrophy (Damian et al. 2001) are suggestive of modafinil's utility in management of fatigue. A small double-blind crossover study in myotonic dystrophy found reduction in fatigue but no improvement in activity measures (Wintzen et al. 2007). This would be consistent with modafinil's rather selective effect on wakefulness and minimal impact on motor or autonomic parameters. In the same vein, a study of 98 patients with fibromyalgia found that low doses of modafinil (mean 160 mg) substantially reduced fatigue (Schwartz et al. 2007).

Obstructive Sleep Apnea

There are two placebo-controlled studies of modafinil in the treatment of residual sleepiness in patients with OSA (Kingshott et al. 2001; Pack et al. 2001). The studies show modafinil's efficacy in treating the residual daytime sleepiness experienced by some OSA patients who were compliant in their use of CPAP treatment.

Importantly, modafinil's use was studied in—and should be limited to—the treatment of OSA only after CPAP has been instituted and maximized. OSA carries significant cardiovascular risks if the airway collapse during sleep is not treated appropriately with CPAP and related therapies. It is conceivable that lessened daytime sleepiness from use of modafinil might fool the patient into thinking that CPAP is unnecessary, thus posing a risk via the untreated underlying OSA disorder.

Obesity

That amphetamines are anorectic is well known; however, the extent of the effect may be overstated. Bray and Greenway (1999) summarized the studies of obesity treatments, wherein they cited a large review of more than 200 short-term (3 months) double-blind studies of various noradrenergic agents, including amphetamine and amphetamine derivatives. Patients taking stimulants were twice as likely as those taking placebo to lose 1 lb/week; however, the percentage of patients who lost 3 lb/week was quite small (10%). A small study found that high doses of amphetamine (30 mg) decreased overall caloric intake but did so primarily through a decrease in fat consumption; carbohydrate consumption actually increased (Foltin et al. 1995). This mild effect on appetite is important when considering the use of stimulants in elderly patients who lack both energy and motivation and have poor appetite.

Depression

No controlled trials have investigated the use of stimulants in depression to date. Most of the evidence for stimulant utility in depression derives from case series. The bulk of the current evidence derives from case series by Feighner et al. (1985) and Fawcett et al. (1991), which suggested the efficacy of stimulants combined with MAOIs and MAOI/TCA combinations as well as their safety in not causing hypertensive or hyperthermic crises, and case series by Stoll et al. (1996) and Metz and Shader (1991), in which a combination of stimulant and selective serotonin reuptake inhibitor (SSRI) was used. Another case series argued for amphetamine's ability to augment an antidepressant effect in patients with only partial response, although the effects were, not unexpectedly, primarily in improving fatigue and apathy (Masand et al. 1998).

In an open-label trial of depressed cancer patients, both amphetamine and methylphenidate were reported to improve depressive symptoms to the same extent, and effects were seen within 2 days. In this series, stimulants did not cause anorexia; in fact, they improved appetite in more than half of the patients studied (Olin and Masand 1996), suggesting that these agents are not contraindicated solely on the basis of concerns about anorexia.

In a review, Orr and Taylor (2007) noted the paucity of high-quality data and suggested a possible role for stimulants in depression, particularly as adjunctive agents, in specific patient subgroups.

The utility of modafinil in depressive states is still not well characterized, the majority of evidence being either anecdotal or retrospective. More work is likely forthcoming, but there are two studies that bear some examination. The mood-altering properties of modafinil were studied in 32 normal volunteers in a double-blind, crossover inpatient study (Taneja et al. 2007). Modafinil had positive results on general mood, especially on alertness and energy measures, but also had a negative effect on feeling calm (i.e., increased anxiety).

A double-blind, placebo-controlled trial (Dunlop et al. 2007) examining the effects of modafinil initiated at the outset of treatment with an SSRI in depressed patients with fatigue found no difference in the primary outcome measure of the Epworth Sleepiness Scale but found some improvement in the hypersomnia items of the 31-item Hamilton Rating Scale for Depression. Two other controlled trials (DeBattista et al. 2003; Fava et al. 2005) and two open-label trials (DeBattista et al. 2001; Menza et al. 2000) suggest that modafinil may have some utility as an augmentation agent to antidepressants in depressed patients with fatigue or excessive sleepiness.

Both modafinil and armodafinil have shown some preliminary benefit in the treatment of bipolar depression. Frye et al. (2007) found that the addition of modafinil at dosages of 100–200 mg/day for 6 weeks to a standard mood stabilizer was more effective than the addition of placebo in 85 patients with bipolar depression. In a larger randomized controlled multicenter study (Calabrese et al. 2010), 257 patients with bipolar depression on either lithium or valproate were randomly assigned to receive augmentation treatment with 150 mg/day armodafinil or placebo. Armodafinil appeared to help some—but not all—patients with bipolar depression, and the differences between groups did not reach statistical significance.

Negative Symptoms and Cognitive Deficits in Schizophrenia

While positive symptoms of schizophrenia are often responsive to antipsychotics, negative symptoms and cognitive deficits are often not (Tandon 2011). Because the negative symptoms and cognitive impairments of schizophrenia are frequently more disabling than the positive symptoms, there has been interest in developing effective treatments for these symptoms and deficits. A number of studies have explored the efficacy of modafinil and armodafinil in the treatment of negative symptoms and cognitive deficits in schizophrenia, with mixed results. For example, whereas some studies have found that modafinil or armodafinil improves negative symptoms (Arbabi et al. 2012; Kane et al. 2010) and working memory (Scoriels et al. 2012) in some schizophrenic patients, other studies have found no benefit (Bobo et al. 2011; Pierre et al. 2007; Sevy et al. 2005). Despite these mixed results, modafinil has been well tolerated in most studies in schizophrenia. By contrast, stimulants such as dextroamphetamine may worsen positive symptoms of schizophrenia and have been less commonly studied in the treatment of negative symptoms and cognitive impairments. Further study is required to determine the role of stimulants and wakefulness-promoting agents in schizophrenia.

Conclusion

The safety and efficacy of stimulants for the treatment of ADHD have been established. Modafinil and armodafinil are also firmly established as efficacious as wakefulness-promoting agents in narcolepsy, sleep apnea, and shift work sleep disorder. The utility of these drugs in other areas is being examined. Although there is intense interest in the potential use of stimulants and modafinil in other psychiatric and neurobehavioral conditions, controlled studies on their safety and efficacy are limited. It is unclear why stimulants have not been extensively investigated for clinical utility over the years, except for the treatment of ADHD. The approval of armodafinil, as the newest of the wakefulness-promoting compounds, may perhaps spur further research. Large-scale well-designed controlled trials are needed to define and characterize the role of stimulants and modafinil in various psychiatric illnesses. It is hoped that this will be an area of continued interest and development, from the elucidation of the molecular mechanisms of stimulants and modafinil to the demonstration through controlled trials of their potential clinical safety and benefits.

References

Adler CH, Caviness JN, Hentz JG, et al: Randomized trial of modafinil for treating subjective daytime sleepiness in patients with Parkinson's disease. Mov Disord 18:287–293, 2003

Arbabi M, Bagheri M, Rezaei F, et al: A placebo-controlled study of the modafinil added to risperidone in chronic schizophrenia. Psychopharmacology (Berl) 220:591–598, 2012

Biederman J, Swanson JM, Wigal SB, et al: Efficacy and safety of modafinil film-coated tablets in children and adolescents with attention-deficit/hyperactivity disorder: results of a randomized, double-blind, placebo-controlled, flexible-dose study. Pediatrics 116:e777–e784, 2005

Biederman J, Swanson JM, Wigal SB, et al: A comparison of once-daily and divided doses of modafinil in children with attention-deficit/hyperactivity disorder: a randomized, double-blind, and placebo-controlled study. Modafinil ADHD Study Group. J Clin Psychiatry 67:727–735, 2006

Biederman J, Boellner SW, Childress A, et al: Lisdexamfetamine dimesylate and mixed amphetamine salts extended-release in children with ADHD: a double-blind, placebo-controlled, crossover analog classroom study. Biol Psychiatry 62:970–976, 2007a

Biederman J, Krishnan S, Zhang Y, et al: Efficacy and tolerability of lisdexamfetamine dimesylate (NRP-104) in children with attention-deficit/hyperactivity disorder: a phase III multicenter, randomized, double-blind, forced-dose, parallel-group study. Clin Ther 29:450–463, 2007b

Bobo WV, Woodward ND, Sim MY, et al: The effect of adjunctive armodafinil on cognitive performance and psychopathology in antipsychotic-treated patients with schizophrenia/schizoaffective disorder: a randomized, double-blind, placebo-controlled trial. Schizophr Res 130:106–113, 2011

Boellner SW, Earl CQ, Arora S: Modafinil in children and adolescents with attention-deficit/hyperactivity disorder: a preliminary 8-week, open-label study. Curr Med Res Opin 22:2457–2465, 2006

Bonaventure P, Letavic M, Dugovic C, et al: Histamine H3 receptor antagonists: from target identification to drug leads. Biochem Pharmacol 73:1084–1096, 2007

Bray GA, Greenway FL: Current and potential drugs for treatment of obesity. Endocrinol Rev 20:805–875, 1999

Breitbart W, Rosenfeld B, Kaim M, et al: A randomized, double-blind, placebo-controlled trial of psychostimulants for the treatment of fatigue in ambulatory patients with human immunodeficiency virus disease. Arch Intern Med 161:411–420, 2001

Broughton RJ, Fleming JA, George CF, et al: Randomized, double-blind, placebo-controlled crossover trial of modafinil in the treatment of excessive daytime sleepiness in narcolepsy. Neurology 49:444–451, 1997

Brun J, Chamba G, Khalfallah Y, et al: Effect of modafinil on plasma melatonin, cortisol and growth hormone rhythms, rectal temperature and performance in healthy subjects during a 36 h sleep deprivation. J Sleep Res 7:105–114, 1998

Calabrese JR, Ketter TA, Youakim JM, et al: Adjunctive armodafinil for major depressive episodes associated with bipolar I disorder: a randomized, multicenter, double-blind, placebo-controlled, proof-of-concept study. J Clin Psychiatry 71:1363–1370, 2010

Cephalon Inc.: Provigil (modafinil) tablets: prescribing information. Frazer, PA, Cephalon, Inc., March 2008. Available at: http://www.provigil.com. Accessed December 2008.

Chan YP, Swanson JM, Soldin SS, et al: Methylphenidate hydrochloride given with or before breakfast, II: effects on plasma concentration of methylphenidate and ritalinic acid. Pediatrics 72:56–59, 1983

Crisostomo EA, Duncan PW, Propst M, et al: Evidence that amphetamine with physical therapy promotes recovery of motor function in stroke patients. Ann Neurol 23:94–97, 1988

Dackis CA, Lynch KG, Yu E, et al: Modafinil and cocaine: a double-blind, placebo-controlled drug interaction study. Drug Alcohol Depend 70:29–37, 2003

Dackis CA, Kampman KM, Lynch KG, et al: A double-blind, placebo-controlled trial of modafinil for cocaine dependence. Neuropsychopharmacology 30:205–211, 2005

Dackis CA, Kampman KM, Lynch KG, et al: A double-blind, placebo-controlled trial of modafinil for cocaine dependence. J Subst Abuse Treat Feb 27, 2012 [Epub ahead of print]

Damian MS, Gerlach A, Schmidt F, et al: Modafinil for excessive daytime sleepiness in myotonic dystrophy. Neurology 56:794–796, 2001

DeBattista C, Solvason HB, Kendrick E, et al: Modafinil as an adjunctive agent in the treatment of fatigue and hypersomnia associated with major depression, in New Research Program and Abstracts of the 154th Annual Meeting of the American Psychiatric Association, May 9, 2001, New Orleans, LA, USA Abstract NR532, 144, 2001

DeBattista C, Doghramji K, Menza MA, et al: Adjunct modafinil for the short-term treatment of fatigue and sleepiness in patients with major depressive disorder: a preliminary double-blind, placebo-controlled study. J Clin Psychiatry 64:1057–1064, 2003

DeVane CL, Markowitz JS, Carson SW, et al: Single-dose pharmacokinetics of methylphenidate in CYP2D6 extensive and poor metabolizers. J Clin Psychopharmacol 20:347–349, 2000

Dinges DF, Arora S, Darwish M, et al: Pharmacodynamic effects on alertness of single doses of armodafinil in healthy subjects during a nocturnal period of acute sleep loss. Curr Med Res Opin 22:159–167, 2006

Dunlop BW, Crits-Christoph P, Evans DL, et al: Coadministration of modafinil and a selective serotonin reuptake inhibitor from the initiation of treatment of major depressive disorder with fatigue and sleepiness: a double-blind, placebo-controlled study. J Clin Psychopharmacol 27:614–619, 2007

Efron D, Jarman F, Barker M: Methylphenidate versus dexamphetamine in children with attention deficit hyperactivity disorder: a double-blind, crossover trial. Pediatrics 100:E6, 1997

Fava M, Thase ME, DeBattista C: A multicenter, placebo-controlled study of modafinil augmentation in partial responders to selective serotonin reuptake inhibitors with persistent fatigue and sleepiness. J Clin Psychiatry 66:85–93, 2005

Fawcett J, Kravitz HM, Zajecka JM, et al: CNS stimulant potentiation of monoamine oxidase inhibitors in treatment-refractory depression. J Clin Psychopharmacol 11:127–132, 1991

Feighner JP, Herbstein J, Damlouji N: Combined MAOI, TCA, and direct stimulant therapy of treatment-resistant depression. J Clin Psychiatry 46:206–209, 1985

Ferris RM, Tang FL: Comparison of the effects of the isomers of amphetamine, methylphenidate and deoxypipradrol on the uptake of l-[3H]norepinephrine and [3H]dopamine by synaptic vesicles from rat whole brain, striatum and hypothalamus. J Pharmacol Exp Ther 210:422–428, 1979

Foltin RW, Kelly TH, Fischman MW: Effect of amphetamine on human macronutrient intake. Physiol Behav 58:899–907, 1995

Frye MA, Grunze H, Suppes T, et al: A placebo-controlled evaluation of adjunctive modafinil in the treatment of bipolar depression. Am J Psychiatry 164:1242–1249, 2007

George S, Braithwaite RA: Using amphetamine isomer ratios to determine the compliance of amphetamine abusers prescribed Dexedrine. J Anal Toxicol 24:223–227, 2000

Grabowski J, Roache JD, Schmitz JM, et al: Replacement medication for cocaine dependence: methylphenidate. J Clin Psychopharmacol 17:485–488, 1997

Grabowski J, Rhoades H, Silverman P, et al: Risperidone for the treatment of cocaine dependence: randomized, double-blind trial. J Clin Psychopharmacol 20:305–310, 2000

Grabowski J, Rhoades H, Schmitz J, et al: Dextroamphetamine for cocaine-dependence treatment: a double-blind randomized clinical trial. J Clin Psychopharmacol 21:522–526, 2001

Greenhill LL, Pliszka S, Dulcan MK, et al; American Academy of Child and Adolescent Psychiatry: Practice parameter for the use of stimulant medications in the treatment of children, adolescents, and adults. J Am Acad Child Adolesc Psychiatry 41 (2 suppl):26S–49S, 2002

Guilarte TR: Is methamphetamine abuse a risk factor in parkinsonism? Neurotoxicology 22:725–731, 2001

Harsh JR, Hayduk R, Rosenberg R, et al: The efficacy and safety of armodafinil as treatment for adults with excessive sleepiness associated with narcolepsy. Curr Med Res Opin 22:761–774, 2006

Hart CL, Haney M, Vosburg SK, et al: Smoked cocaine self-administration is decreased by modafinil. Neuropsychopharmacology 33:761–768, 2008

Hirshkowitz M, Black JE, Wesnes K, et al: Adjunct armodafinil improves wakefulness and memory in obstructive sleep apnea/hypopnea syndrome. Respir Med 101:616–627, 2006

Hogl B, Saletu M, Brandauer E, et al: Modafinil for the treatment of daytime sleepiness in Parkinson's disease: a double-blind, randomized, crossover, placebo-controlled polygraphic trial. Sleep 25:905–909, 2002

Hunt GE, Atrens DM: Reward summation and the effects of pimozide, clonidine, and amphetamine on fixed-interval responding for brain stimulation. Pharmacol Biochem Behav 42:563–577, 1992

Ishizuka T, Sakamoto Y, Sakurai T, et al: Modafinil increases histamine release in the anterior hypothalamus of rats. Neurosci Lett 339:143–146, 2003

James RS, Sharp WS, Bastain TM, et al: Double-blind, placebo-controlled study of single-dose amphetamine formulations in ADHD. J Am Acad Child Adolesc Psychiatry 40:1268–1276, 2001

Janssen PA, Leysen JE, Megens AA, et al: Does phenylethylamine act as an endogenous amphetamine in some patients? Int J Neuropsychopharmacol 2:229–240, 1999

Jean-Pierre P, Morrow GR, Roscoe JA, et al: A phase 3 randomized, placebo-controlled, double-blind, clinical trial of the effect of modafinil on cancer-related fatigue among 631 patients receiving chemotherapy: a University of Rochester Cancer Center Community Clinical Oncology Program Research base study. Cancer 116:3513–3520, 2010

Jha A, Weintraub A, Allshouse A, et al: A randomized trial of modafinil for the treatment of fatigue and excessive daytime sleepiness in individuals with chronic traumatic brain injury. J Head Trauma Rehabil 23:52–63, 2008

Kane JM, D'Souza DC, Patkar AA, et al: Armodafinil as adjunctive therapy in adults with cognitive deficits associated with schizophrenia: a 4-week, double-blind, placebo-controlled study. J Clin Psychiatry 71:1475–1481, 2010

Karch SB, Stephens BG, Ho CH: Methamphetamine-related deaths in San Francisco: demographic, pathologic, and toxicologic profiles. J Forens Sci 44:359–368, 1999

Kingshott RN, Vennelle M, Coleman EL, et al: Randomized, double-blind, placebo-controlled crossover trial of modafinil in the treatment of residual excessive daytime sleepiness in the sleep apnea/hypopnea syndrome. Am J Respir Crit Care Med 163:918–923, 2001

Klein-Schwartz W: Abuse and toxicity of methylphenidate. Curr Opin Pediatr 14:219–223, 2002

Knecht S, Imai T, Kamping S, et al: D-amphetamine does not improve outcome of somatosensory training. Neurology 57:2248–2252, 2001

Lazarus LW, Moberg PJ, Langsley PR, et al: Methylphenidate and nortriptyline in the treatment of poststroke depression: a retrospective comparison. Arch Phys Med Rehabil 75:403–406, 1994

Markowitz JS, Patrick KS: Pharmacokinetic and pharmacodynamic drug interactions in the treatment of attention-deficit hyperactivity disorder. Clin Pharmacokinet 40:753–772, 2001

Masand PS, Anand VS, Tanquary JF: Psychostimulant augmentation of second generation antidepressants: a case series. Depress Anxiety 7:89–91, 1998

Menza MA, Kaufman KR, Castellanos A: Modafinil augmentation of antidepressant treatment in depression. J Clin Psychiatry 61:378–381, 2000

Metz A, Shader RI: Combination of fluoxetine with pemoline in the treatment of major depressive disorder. Int Clin Psychopharmacol 6:93–96, 1991

Najib J: The efficacy and safety profile of lisdexamfetamine dimesylate, a prodrug of D-amphetamine, for the treatment of attention-deficit/hyperactivity disorder in children and adults. Clin Ther 31:142–176, 2009

Nishino S, Mignot E: Pharmacological aspects of human and canine narcolepsy. Prog Neurobiol 52:27–78, 1997

Novartis: Ritalin LA (methylphenidate hydrochloride) extended-release capsules: prescribing information. East Hanover, NJ, Novartis, April 2007. Available at: http://www.pharma.us.novartis.com/product/pi/pdf/ritalin_la.pdf. Accessed December 2008.

Olin J, Masand P: Psychostimulants for depression in hospitalized cancer patients. Psychosomatics 37:57–62, 1996

Orr K, Taylor D: Psychostimulants in the treatment of depression: a review of the evidence. CNS Drugs 21:239–257, 2007

Pack AI, Black JE, Schwartz JR, et al: Modafinil as adjunct therapy for daytime sleepiness in obstructive sleep apnea. Am J Respir Crit Care Med 164:1675–1681, 2001

Pierre JM, Peloian JH, Wirshing DA, et al: A randomized, double-blind, placebo-controlled trial of modafinil for negative symptoms in schizophrenia. J Clin Psychiatry 68:705–710, 2007

Rabkin JG, McElhiney MC, Rabkin R: Treatment of HIV-related fatigue with armodafinil: a placebo-controlled randomized trial. Psychosomatics 52:328–336, 2011

Rammohan KW, Rosenberg JH, Lynn DJ, et al: Efficacy and safety of modafinil (Provigil) for the treatment of fatigue in multiple sclerosis: a two centre phase 2 study. J Neurol Neurosurg Psychiatry 72:179–183, 2002

Ricaurte GA, Yuan J, Hatzidimitriou G, et al: Severe dopaminergic neurotoxicity in primates after a common recreational dose regimen of MDMA ("ecstasy"). Science 297:2260–2263, 2002

Robertson P, DeCory HH, Madan A, et al: In vitro inhibition and induction of human hepatic cytochrome P450 enzymes by modafinil. Drug Metab Dispos 28:664–671, 2000

Robertson P Jr, Hellriegel ET, Arora S, et al: Effect of modafinil on the pharmacokinetics of ethinyl estradiol and triazolam in healthy volunteers. Clin Pharmacol Ther 71:46–56, 2002

Roth T, Czeisler CA, Walsh JK, et al: Randomized, double-blind, placebo-controlled study of armodafinil for the treatment of excessive sleepiness associated with chronic shift work sleep disorder [abstract no. 161]. Neuropsychopharmacology 30:S140, 2005

Roth T, White D, Schmidt-Nowara W, et al: Effects of armodafinil in the treatment of residual excessive sleepiness associated with obstructive sleep apnea/hypopnea syndrome: a 12-week, multicenter, double-blind, randomized, placebo-controlled study in nCPAP-adherent adults. Clin Ther 28:689–706, 2006

Rugino TA, Samsock TC: Modafinil in children with attention-deficit hyperactivity disorder. Pediatr Neurol 29:136–142, 2003

Saletu B, Saletu M, Grunberger J, et al: On the treatment of the alcoholic organic brain syndrome with an alpha-adrenergic agonist modafinil: double-blind, placebo-controlled clinical, psychometric and neurophysiological studies. Prog Neuropsychopharmacol Biol Psychiatry 14:195–214, 1990

Saletu B, Saletu M, Grunberger J, et al: Treatment of the alcoholic organic brain syndrome: double-blind, placebo-controlled clinical, psychometric and electroencephalographic mapping studies with modafinil. Neuropsychobiology 27:26–39, 1993

Scammell TE, Estabrooke IV, McCarthy MT, et al: Hypothalamic arousal regions are activated during modafinil-induced wakefulness. J Neurosci 20:8620–8628, 2000

Scoriels L, Barnett JH, Soma PK, et al: Effects of modafinil on cognitive functions in first episode psychosis. Psychopharmacology (Berl) 220:249–258, 2012

Schwartz JR, Nelson MT, Schwartz ER, et al: Effects of modafinil on wakefulness and executive function in patients with narcolepsy experiencing late-day sleepiness. Clin Neuropharmacol 27:74–79, 2004

Schwartz TL, Rayancha S, Rashid A, et al: Modafinil treatment for fatigue associated with fibromyalgia. J Clin Rheumatol 13:52, 2007

Sevy S, Rosenthal MH, Alvir J, et al: Double-blind, placebo-controlled study of modafinil for fatigue and cognition in schizophrenia patients treated with psychotropic medications. J Clin Psychiatry 66:839–843, 2005

Shelton J, Nishino S, Vaught J, et al: Comparative effects of modafinil and amphetamine on daytime sleepiness and cataplexy of narcoleptic dogs. Sleep 18:817–826, 1995

Sonde L, Nordstrom M, Nilsson CG, et al: A double-blind placebo-controlled study of the effects of amphetamine and physiotherapy after stroke. Cerebrovasc Dis 12:253–257, 2001

Sprague JE, Everman SL, Nichols DE: An integrated hypothesis for the serotonergic axonal loss induced by 3,4-methylenedioxymethamphetamine. Neurotoxicology 19:427–441, 1998

Stoll AL, Pillay SS, Diamond L, et al: Methylphenidate augmentation of serotonin selective reuptake inhibitors: a case series. J Clin Psychiatry 57:72–76, 1996

Swanson JM, Wigal S, Greenhill LL, et al: Analog classroom assessment of Adderall in children with ADHD. J Am Acad Child Adolesc Psychiatry 37:519–526, 1998

Tandon R: Antipsychotics in the treatment of schizophrenia: an overview. J Clin Psychiatry 72 (suppl 1):4–8, 2011

Taneja I, Haman K, Shelton RC, et al: A randomized, double-blind, crossover trial of modafinil on mood. J Clin Psychopharmacol 27:76–79, 2007

Taylor FB, Russo J: Efficacy of modafinil compared to dextroamphetamine for the treatment of attention deficit hyperactivity disorder in adults. J Child Adolesc Psychopharmacol 10:311–320, 2000

Turner DC, Clark L, Dowson J, et al: Modafinil improves cognition and response inhibition in adult attention-deficit/hyperactivity disorder. Biol Psychiatry 55:1031–1040, 2004

U.S. Food and Drug Administration: Provigil (Modafinil): Follow-up to Hypersensitivity Reactions in the Pediatric Population. Pediatric Advisory Committee. November 28, 2007. Available at: http://www.fda.gov/ohrms/dockets/AC/07/slides/2007-4325s2_12_Modafinil,%20Villalba,%20MD%20(FDA).pdf. Accessed December 2008.

U.S. Modafinil in Narcolepsy Multicenter Study Group: Randomized trial of modafinil for the treatment of pathological somnolence in narcolepsy. Ann Neurol 43:88–97, 1998

U.S. Modafinil in Narcolepsy Multicenter Study Group: Randomized trial of modafinil as a treatment for the excessive daytime somnolence of narcolepsy. Neurology 54:1166–1175, 2000

Wagner GJ, Rabkin R: Effects of dextroamphetamine on depression and fatigue in men with HIV: a double-blind, placebo-controlled trial. J Clin Psychiatry 61:436–440, 2000

Walker-Batson D, Smith P, Curtis S, et al: Amphetamine paired with physical therapy accelerates motor recovery after stroke: further evidence. Stroke 26:2254–2259, 1995

Walker-Batson D, Curtis S, Natarajan R, et al: A double-blind, placebo-controlled study of the use of amphetamine in the treatment of aphasia. Stroke 32:2093–2098, 2001

Whyte J, Vaccaro M, Grieb-Neff P, et al: Psychostimulant use in the rehabilitation of individuals with traumatic brain injury. J Head Trauma Rehabil 17:284–299, 2002

Wigal SB, Biederman J, Swanson JM, et al: Efficacy and safety of modafinil film-coated tablets in children and adolescents with or without prior stimulant treatment for attention-deficit/hyperactivity disorder: pooled analysis of 3 randomized, double-blind, placebo-controlled studies. Prim Care Companion J Clin Psychiatry 8:352–360, 2006

Wilens TE, Spencer TJ, Biederman J: A review of the pharmacotherapy of adults with attention-deficit/hyperactivity disorder. J Atten Disord 5:189–202, 2002

Wintzen AR, Lammers GJ, van Dijk JG: Does modafinil enhance activity of patients with myotonic dystrophy? A double-blind placebo-controlled crossover study. J Neurol 254:26–28, 2007

Wong YN, Simcoe D, Hartman LN, et al: A double-blind, placebo-controlled, ascending-dose evaluation of the pharmacokinetics and tolerability of modafinil tablets in healthy male volunteers. J Clin Pharmacol 39:30–40, 1999

Yu YL, Fisher H, Sekowski A, et al: Amphetamine and fenfluramine suppress ethanol intake in ethanol-dependent rats. Alcohol 14:45–48, 1997

PART II

Psychopharmacological Treatment

CHAPTER 35

Treatment of Depression

Jonathan Shaywitz, M.D.

Mark Hyman Rapaport, M.D.

Major depressive disorder is a chronic syndrome with symptoms that fluctuate over a continuum of severity. Even the mildest form of depression is associated with both psychosocial morbidity and a risk for developing major depressive disorder (Beekman et al. 1997; Fergusson et al. 2005; Fogel et al. 2006; Hermens et al. 2004; Judd et al. 1994; Rieckmann et al. 2006). The goal of treatment of all forms of depression needs to be the return to an asymptomatic state of the patient's prior "normal" functioning. Thus, the treatment of patients with major depressive disorder requires aggressive and varied therapies that may need to continue for years, if not indefinitely.

Epidemiology

Prevalence of Depressive Disorders

Major depressive disorder is one of the most common medical disorders affecting adults in the world (Lopez and Murray 1998). In the United States, the lifetime prevalence of major depression is 9% for men and 17% for women (Hasin et al. 2005), whereas the lifetime prevalence of dysthymia is 4% for men and 8% for women (Kessler et al. 1994). The lifetime prevalence of minor depression is 10% for individuals between the ages of 15 and 54 years (Kessler et al. 1997). For persons 65 years and older, the 1-month point prevalence of minor depression is 13%, which is twice the prevalence of major depressive disorder for this age group (Judd and Akiskal 2002; McCusker et al. 2005). The lifetime prevalence for subsyndromal depression is 11.8% for the general population (Goldney et al. 2004; Judd et al. 1994).

Risk Factors for Depressive Disorders

Several factors seem to increase a person's vulnerability to developing a depressive disorder. Risk factors with the strongest body of evidence include female sex, age, a family history of a mood disorder, a history of trauma, and comorbid medical and psychiatric conditions.

A significant body of evidence indicates that the sex of an individual is an important risk factor for the development of depressive disorders. Prior to puberty, the prevalence of depression is equal in boys and girls. However, beginning with puberty, women demonstrate a twofold increase in the prevalence of major depressive disorder (Burt and Stein 2002; Weissman and Klerman 1977). This trend is seen across countries and ethnic groups (Weissman et al. 1996).

Age is another risk factor in the development of depressive disorders; the onset of major depressive disorder increases dramatically beginning in adolescence (12–16 years of age) and continuing through the age of about 44 years (Hasin et al. 2005). The mean age at onset has been reported to be 30 years, whereas the mean age at the start of treatment is 33.5 years of age, reflecting the amount of time depression often goes undiagnosed or untreated. In elderly populations, risk factors for depression are slightly different and include female sex, low socioeconomic status, bereavement, prior depression, medical comorbidity, disability, cognitive deterioration, and vascular disease (Helmer et al. 2004).

A family history of psychiatric illness is among the most profound risk factors for the development of an episode of major depressive disorder (Reinherz et al. 2003). No one gene has been clearly identified as a cause of major depression, and it may be concluded that depressive disorders are likely polygenetic in nature. This might further explain the heterogeneity of the disease and treatment response. Research has demonstrated that genetics coupled with environmental conditions may contribute to the development of depression.

Prolonged exposure to severe traumatic events in childhood has been linked to future depressive episodes. Trauma such as sexual abuse or the loss of a parent that occurs at a critical developmental period can result in permanent alteration of the hypothalamic-pituitary-adrenal (HPA) axis. It is recognized that individuals with depression, particularly those exposed to early trauma, have altered stress responses (Gillespie and Nemeroff 2005; Heim et al. 2000; Nemeroff and Vale 2005).

Other clinical and demographic variables have been linked to an increased risk of developing depressive disorders. These include stressful life events such as the death of a loved one, divorce, or job loss. Certain personality characteristics also may predispose an individual to develop a mood disorder. Individuals who score higher on measures of neuroticism, interpersonal dependency, or external locus of control may be vulnerable to stressful life events precipitating a major depressive episode (Hirschfeld et al. 1983; Paykel et al. 1996). Investigations suggesting that certain cultural groups may be at increased risk of a mood disorder (Native Americans) and that other cultural groups may have greater inherent resilience (Asian and Hispanic groups) are an area of renewed interest (Hasin et al. 2005).

Many medical illnesses are comorbid with major depressive disorder (Table 35–1). Cancer, AIDS, respiratory disease, cardiovascular disease, Parkinson's disease, and stroke are associated with an increased risk for depression. Depression is also associated with rehospitalization and mortality in patients with heart failure.

Major depressive disorder is highly comorbid with other psychiatric disorders. In primary care settings, more than 75% of patients with diagnosed depression also present with an anxiety disorder (Olfson et al. 1997). Patients with depression and anxiety have more chronic and severe illness, greater occupational and psychosocial impairment, and (when the comorbidity is unrecognized) a greater rate of psychiatric hospitalization and suicide attempts (Hirschfeld 2001). Fifty percent of schizophrenic patients have comorbid depression; depression is an additional risk factor for suicide and decreased social and performance status (Ginsberg et al. 2005). Substance abuse is also highly comorbid with depressive disorders. The prevalence of depressive disorders in patients with alcohol dependence is 15%–67%; for pa-

TABLE 35–1. Medical conditions often comorbid with major depressive disorder

INFECTIOUS	METABOLIC	NEUROLOGICAL	GENERAL MEDICAL
Encephalitis	Addison's disease	Brain tumor	Alcohol or sedative withdrawal
Hepatitis	Cushing's disease	Dementia, cortical	Arthritis
HIV/AIDS	Diabetes	Dementia, subcortical	Cancer
Influenza	Hyponatremia	Huntington's disease	Cardiovascular disease
Meningitis	Nutritional deficiencies	Migraine headaches	Chronic pain syndromes
Mononucleosis	Pituitary dysfunction	Multiple sclerosis	Cocaine or stimulant withdrawal
Pneumonia	Renal disease	Parkinson's disease	Connective tissue diseases
Postviral syndrome	Thyroid disease	Poststroke syndrome	Fibromyalgia
Syphilis		Seizure disorders	Heavy metal poisoning
Tuberculosis		Traumatic brain injury	Irritable bowel syndrome
Urinary tract infection			Liver failure
			Menopause
			Myocardial infarction
			Premenstrual syndrome
			Pulmonary disease
			Selenium toxicity
			Sleep disturbance

Note. AIDS=acquired immunodeficiency syndrome; HIV=human immunodeficiency virus.

tients with cocaine addiction, the prevalence is 33%–53%, and for patients with opiate dependence, the lifetime rate of affective disorders ranges from 16% to 75% (Nunes 2003; Rapaport et al. 1993).

In summary, it is clear that certain factors can increase the risk of developing a depressive disorder.

Disability and Costs Associated With Depressive Disorders

Major depressive disorder is associated with significant disease burden, exceeding that of cerebrovascular disease and cancer. It is the leading cause of years lived with disability worldwide for young adults (Lopez et al. 2006). It is estimated that depressive disorders cost employers in the United States $44 billion in productivity annually.

The greatest "cost" associated with depressive disorders is the increased likelihood that an individual suffering from a depressive disorder will commit suicide. According to the Centers for Disease Control and Prevention (Kochanek et al. 2011), suicide is the tenth leading cause of death in the United States: approximately 37,000 known suicides were identified in the 2009 census. In that year the overall suicide rate was more than double the homicide rate in the United States (12.0 per 100,000 vs. 5.5 per 100,000). Suicide is the second leading cause of death for individuals between the ages of 25 and 34 years and the third leading cause of death for young people between the ages of 15 and 24 years. Eighty percent of people who commit suicide are male. Suicide is more common in white than Hispanic or black individuals. Statistical risk factors for suicide include being male, being white, being single, having been hospitalized for a suicide attempt or having any history of a previous attempt, having a family history of suicide, and abusing substances. Women are more likely to attempt suicide, whereas men are more likely to complete it.

The elderly constitute a special at-risk group for successful completion of suicide. People older than 65 years constitute only 13% of the population and yet are responsible for 18% of all suicides: this is the highest suicide rate for any age group. Risk factors for suicide among older individuals include social isolation, physical illness, divorced or widowed status, and male sex. Older individuals who attempt suicide usually employ more lethal means (guns, drug overdoses) than younger individuals do (Clayton and Auster 2008). Despite recent guidance from the U.S. Food and Drug Administration (FDA) suggesting that suicidal thoughts and behavior among individuals younger than 25 years may increase during the first 10 days after starting an antidepressant, and despite a report based on the Sequenced Treatment Alternatives to Relieve Depression (STAR*D) study database that found an association between two ionotropic glutamate receptor genes (*GRIA3* and *GRIK2*) and an increased risk of selective serotonin reuptake inhibitor (SSRI)–induced suicidal thoughts, the vast majority of data suggest that antidepressant medication decreases suicidal thoughts and lowers rates of suicide completion (Gibbons et al. 2005; Henriksson and Isacsson 2006; Laje et al. 2007; Rich and Isacsson 1997; Søndergård et al. 2006). These observations are supported by the longitudinal work of Angst et al. (2005), who found that treatment with antidepressants, lithium, and clozapine reduced the number of suicides in their cohort. These data suggest that suicidal ideation with intent and a plan must be considered a medical emergency that merits the same type of care that a physician would give to other emergent conditions like a myocardial infarction.

Neurobiology of Depression

Depression has for many years been predominantly hypothesized to be marked by a depletion of monoamine neurotransmitters, specifically norepinephrine, serotonin, and dopamine. As our understanding of the mechanism of action of antidepressant therapies has grown, more attention has been given to the neurotransmitter systems involving glutamate and γ-aminobutyric acid (GABA). Evidence for the role of these neurotransmitter systems in depression comes from studies of therapies that have been shown to target the *N*-methyl-D-aspartate (NMDA) class of glutamate receptors, specifically lamotrigine, ketamine, and amantadine (Pittenger et al. 2007), and anticonvulsant therapies, which have a GABAergic route of action. Studies have demonstrated alterations of these systems in subjects with depression.

Depression is also marked by dysregulation of other important systems. External stressful stimuli are known to be a major risk factor for a depressive episode, and depressed individuals are often characterized by altered biological responses to stress. This is likely due to dysregulation and overstimulation of the HPA axis (Gertsik and Poland 2004; Holsboer 1995). Early studies (Brown and Shuey 1980; Carroll 1982; Coppen et al. 1983) found that in a large percentage of unmedicated individuals with depression, secretion of the stress hormone cortisol is not suppressed after dexamethasone administration, a condition known as *dexamethasone nonsuppression*. This impairment of HPA axis regulation has been traced upstream to dysregulation of corticotropin-releasing hormone (CRH), a hypothalamic hormone that controls the release of adrenocorticotropic hormone (ACTH) (Holsboer 2000). Depressed individuals have higher CRH neuronal activity (Raadsheer et al. 1994) and display a blunted ACTH and cortisol response to infusion of synthetic CRH (Gispen-de Wied et al. 1993; Gold et al. 1986). This global hyperactivity of the stress response in depressed individuals has been demonstrated to be a characteristic of the current depressed state, because the remission of clinical symptoms induces a normalization of responses to dexamethasone or CRH along with normalization of plasma cortisol levels (Amsterdam et al. 1988; Arana et al. 1985; Sachar et al. 1970). Dysregulation of the HPA axis activity and higher rates of depression are more prominent in individuals exposed to childhood trauma or abuse (Bremne and Vermetten 2001), suggesting that hyperactivity of the HPA axis during critical periods of brain development leads to higher rates of depression later in life.

This cascade of alterations in the HPA axis, and subsequent increase in glucocorticoids, is thought to be responsible for the structural and functional changes seen in the limbic structures of depressed individuals. Successful antidepressant therapy has been shown to increase cellular proliferation (Duman 2004; Warner-Schmidt and Duman 2006), and chronic stress induces the converse, giving further credence to the neurobiological component of depression.

Taken together, these observed alterations in monoamines and other neurotransmitters, in the HPA axis function, and in neuronal plasticity can be conceptualized as a state of depressive illnesses rather than a trait of such illnesses. Given that successful clinical therapies often reverse these trends, one has to ask what the underlying cause is. It is clear that a familial predisposition to depression is present, lending support to the idea of a genetic component to depression. Ongoing research has failed to pinpoint a specific genetic anomaly, a failure likely attributable to the heterogeneity of the disorder and the additive role that environmental factors play in triggering depressive episodes. Other studies have begun to examine the contribution of the immune system and cytokines in major depressive disorder, suggesting a new avenue for therapeutic alternatives. Cytokines are a heterogeneous group of signaling and regulatory molecules produced by immunocompetent cells and generally are categorized as proinflammatory or anti-inflammatory. The proinflammatory cytokines interferon alfa and interferon gamma have potent antiviral and immunomodulatory properties and are used to treat various forms of cancer and hepatitis C (Adams et al. 1984; Borgstrom et al. 1982; Meyers 1999). These cytokine therapies have been noted to be accompanied by depressive behavioral effects that can be significantly reduced by pretreatment with paroxetine (Capuron et al. 2002; Musselman et al. 2001), thus supporting the cytokine theory of depression. Furthermore, individuals with depressive disorders have higher plasma concentrations of the proinflammatory cytokines interleukin 1 (IL-1) and interleukin 6 (IL-6) than do nondepressed individuals, and concentrations correlate with the severity of depressive symptoms (Maes 1995, 1999).

It is clear that our understanding of the biological underpinnings of depressive disorders is rapidly increasing. In the future, the combined advances in molecular medicine, neuroimaging, and data analysis will begin to clarify the relationships among what currently appear to be disparate biological findings.

Treatment Options

Antidepressant Medications

Although the tricyclic antidepressants and the monoamine oxidase inhibitors have a long history of proven efficacy, these classes of agents have fallen out of favor because of their side-effect profiles. The majority of commonly used antidepressants work via one or more of the following mechanisms: 1) inhibition of serotonin reuptake, 2) inhibition of the reuptake of both serotonin and norepinephrine, 3) stimulation of noradrenergic and dopaminergic activity, or 4) α_2 antagonism of noradrenergic and serotonergic neurons. The pharmacokinetic profile of the agent can aid in the selection of an antidepressant medication. Antidepressants differ in protein binding, rate and mechanism of elimination, half-life, lipophilicity, and effects on metabolic pathways. Therefore, it is important to carefully determine what other medications the patient may be taking. Drug-drug interactions may increase blood levels of concomitant medications, and at times those interactions can be unpleasant or even life-threatening.

Somatic Therapies

Electroconvulsive therapy (ECT) is the best studied of the somatic interventions. It is clearly one of the treatments of choice for individuals with treatment-resistant depression. Although the mechanism of action of ECT is still not well understood, it is a safe and efficacious treatment. In repeated studies, ECT has been found to be more efficacious than placebo (sham ECT) and more efficacious than pharmacotherapy for treatment-resistant patients (UK ECT Review Group 2003).

Vagus nerve stimulation (VNS) was initially developed for the treatment of epilepsy. In 2005 it was approved by the FDA for use in treatment-resistant depression. One of the key findings to emerge from these studies of VNS is that its effect may be cumulative and one may not see the full benefit of VNS stimulation until 9–12 months after treatment is begun (Sackeim et al. 2007; Schlaepfer et al. 2008).

Repetitive transcranial magnetic stimulation (rTMS) was first identified as a treatment for depression by a group of National Institute of Mental Health (NIMH) researchers (George et al. 1995). Since that time, several smaller studies have supported the finding that rTMS may be an effective treatment for major depressive disorder. At present, rTMS is approved for individuals whose depressive episode has been unresponsive to one medication trial.

Deep brain stimulation (DBS) is an FDA-approved treatment for severe, intractable Parkinson's disease. In a large multisite study, DBS was performed in 20 individuals with treatment-refractory depression (Lozano et al. 2008). The initial 6-month response rate was 60%, and the remission rate was 30% (Lozano et al. 2008). Moreover, the long-term response rates were also promising (Kennedy et al. 2011).

Older literature suggested that phototherapy might be an effective augmentation therapy for individuals with certain forms of depressive disorders (Kripke 1981; Lewy and Sack 1986). Phototherapy has been best studied in patients with seasonal affective disorder. Light therapy for 90 minutes per day has been shown to effectively treat—and also to prevent the development of—depressive disorders (Even et al. 2007; Westrin and Lam 2007). Light therapy also was recently shown to improve depressive symptoms in pregnant women (Wirz-Justice et al. 2011).

In summary, at this time few somatic therapies have demonstrated efficacy for treatment-resistant depression. Two approaches are FDA approved, ECT and VNS, and at least three other somatic therapies show potential benefits. It is clear that more work needs to be done investigating somatic options for patients with treatment-resistant depression.

Psychotherapies

Cognitive-Behavioral Therapy

Cognitive-behavioral therapy (CBT) comprises a constellation of interventions that target, to varying degrees, maladaptive or self-disparaging thoughts and behavioral patterns that are destructive, such as inactivity, avoidance, and social withdrawal. Key to the CBT model is the observation that depressed individuals have negative mental self-representations of the world, themselves, and the future. An important aspect of the cognitive model of depression is the presence of negative self-schemata—that is, feelings of being worthless or helpless (Beck 1995; Feldman 2007; Jacobson et al. 1996; Kuyken et al. 2007).

The second component of most forms of CBT is the development of behaviorally oriented interventions to target specific symptoms and to enhance rewarding experiences. A number of modifications of classical CBT for depression are currently being investigated and are gaining significant attention. These include the use of behavioral activation as a stand-alone intervention for depression and the development of therapies that promote psychological well-being and that target cognitive reactivity (i.e., the tendency to respond to sad moods with more negative thinking) (Dimidjian et al. 2006). Well-being therapy is based on a theoretical model by Ryff (1989) that emphasizes the promotion of mental health and not merely the amelioration of mental illness. Another form of CBT that has become increasingly popular incorporates mindfulness-based interventions into CBT. Mindfulness-based cognitive therapy (MBCT) can be done either in individual settings or as part of group CBT treatment. This goal of this approach is to enable patients to become "decentered" with regard to depressogenic thoughts and to recognize such thoughts as mental events rather than accurate reflections of their reality or core aspects of themselves (Kabat-Zinn 1990; Segal et al. 2002). MBCT frequently employs alternative activities such as tai chi, yoga, or medication to facilitate "active disengaging." A third form of cognitively based psychotherapy that has gained acceptance in the research community and increasing acceptance in the clinical community is the cognitive-behavioral analysis system of psychotherapy (CBASP). This was initially designed as a treatment for chronic depression that targets problematic interpersonal patterns and uses situational analysis to challenge maladaptive thinking processes (McCullough 2000). One of the key differences between traditional CBT and CBASP is the integration of concepts of transference reactions into the therapy itself (Butler et al. 2006). This has been an exciting decade of development for CBT. Both the theoretical framework and the practice of cognitively based therapies continue to be refined and modified by researchers. This suggests that cognitive-behavioral psychotherapy will play an increasingly important role in the treatment of depression.

Efficacy of CBT. Findings from a meta-analysis and an NIMH-funded trial suggest that CBT and medication are equally effective in the acute treatment of major depressive disorder (DeRubeis et al. 1999, 2005). Behavioral activation therapy also has been found to be comparable to medication for the treatment of moderate to severe depression (Dimidjian et al. 2006). Several studies have evaluated the addition of CBT to maintenance antidepressant treatment, with mixed results. Findings from one continuation study suggested that after treatment discontinuation, CBT responders are more likely to maintain their remission status than are medication responders (Hollon et al. 2005a). Data from the NIMH-sponsored University of Pennsylvania–Vanderbilt University–Rush University treatment collaborative showed that 1-year relapse rates were equivalent for individuals treated with CBT with up to three optional booster sessions and those maintained on medication over 1 year of follow-up (Hollon et al. 2005a).

One large multisite study investigated the use of combined treatment—consisting of nefazodone plus CBASP (a therapy for chronic depression that also has elements of IPT)—versus CBASP alone or nefazodone alone. In this study, the effect sizes of combined treatment were significantly greater than the effect sizes of either treatment alone (Keller et al. 2000). These findings are consistent with reviews of the literature suggesting a slight advantage for combined treatment (medication plus CBT or IPT) over monotherapy (Hollon et al. 2005b).

Several studies have used some form of CBT either to augment antidepressants' effects or to attempt to treat residual symptoms (Fava et al. 1997; McPherson et al. 2005; Nemeroff et al. 2003). In the STAR*D study, augmentation of citalopram monotherapy with CBT and augmentation with pharmacological agents produced similar response rates; however, subjects receiving CBT augmentation tended to respond more slowly than those receiving pharmacological augmentation (Thase et al. 2007). CBT has also been used by investigators to treat residual symptoms of depressive disorders (Fava et al. 2004; Paykel et al. 1999); these studies suggest that adding CBT is more effective than continuing management with medication alone. Furthermore, follow-up evaluation of patients suggests that CBT augmentation may decrease the rate of relapse over time.

In summary, the data suggest that CBT is an effective first-line treatment for individuals with major depressive disorder. Furthermore, CBT may have an important role in facilitating remission for those who have residual symptoms of depression after adequate pharmacotherapy. Intriguing data suggest that CBT may play a powerful role in decreasing the risk of a relapse or recurrence of major depressive disorder.

Interpersonal Psychotherapy

Interpersonal psychotherapy (IPT) is a brief form of individual psychotherapy that focuses on one of four problem areas during acute treatment: grief, role transitions, role disputes, and interpersonal deficits. Acute therapy is tailored to the patient's specific presenting problems. IPT has been demonstrated to be an efficacious acute treatment both for outpatients and, more recently, for inpatients with major depressive disorder (Frank et al. 1990, 1991; Luty et al. 2007; Reynolds et al. 1999; Schramm et al. 2007). IPT has also been found to be an efficacious treatment for individuals with recurrent depressive disorder, older individuals with depression, and women with major depressive disorder (Frank et al. 1990, 1991; Luty et al. 2007; Reynolds et al. 1999). In a study designed to assess the treatment frequency necessary to prevent relapse into depression, Frank et al. (2007) reported that monthly booster sessions were as efficacious as twice-a-month booster sessions in preventing relapse for women who had been responsive to acute IPT as a monotherapy. However, maintenance IPT monotherapy was not efficacious as a relapse prevention technique for women who had initially required pharmacotherapy combined with IPT to achieve remission.

In conclusion, the data are clear that both CBT and IPT can be efficacious as monotherapies for the treatment of major depressive disorder. Growing data suggest that these psychotherapies may be effective not only in the acute treatment of depression but also in the maintenance treatment of depressive disorders. However, we are still not sure how to match the therapy to a specific patient.

Conclusion

Over the past decade, we have seen remarkable advances in our knowledge about the etiology, pathophysiology, and course of major depressive disorder and the prognosis for patients. The general consensus is that most people with major depressive disorder have a chronic lifelong syndrome that will wax and wane over time. An increasing body of evidence supports the postulate that some people with major depressive disorder have a syndrome that varies in presentation and symptom severity after the initial episode. Many people seem to traverse between having a full-blown episode of major depressive disorder and experiencing residual symptoms of depression, euthymia, minor depression, or new depressive symptoms. If the current evidence is correct, it suggests that our treatment approaches must be broadened to take into account both the chronic nature of the illness and its varied presentation. The implications for treatment are twofold: 1) we need to treat people until they achieve complete remission, and 2) we need to consider continuation and maintenance treatment for far more people than were previously considered.

Although the field has made significant progress with information from the STAR*D trial, there are many important unanswered questions. We have limited data about the persistence of remission even after vigorous acute treatment. Only a few studies have investigated the need for continuation augmentation therapy, and available reports suggest that it was not of significant value (Rapaport et al. 2006). No studies have addressed how patients whose condition worsens during continuation or maintenance therapy should be managed. However, advances in basic biological investigations of depression are greatly expanding our knowledge. Imaging data are beginning to define specific brain regions that seem to be altered in certain individuals with major depressive disorder. Preclinical studies are elucidating the roles played by a variety of neurotransmitter and neurohormonal systems—including the noradrenergic system, the serotonergic system, the HPA axis, the immune system, and the NMDA system—in the pathogenesis of depression. Advances in translational research will allow us to develop better and more personalized treatments for our patients.

References

Adams F, Quesada JR, Gutterman JU: Neuropsychiatric manifestations of human leukocyte interferon therapy in patients with cancer. JAMA 252:938–941, 1984

Amsterdam JD, Maislin G, Winokur A, et al: The oCRH stimulation test before and after clinical recovery from depression. J Affect Disord 14: 213–222, 1988

Angst J, Angst F, Gerber-Werder R, et al: Suicide in 406 mood-disorder patients with and without long-term medication: a 40 to 44 years' follow-up. Arch Suicide Res 9:279–300, 2005

Arana GW, Baldessarini RJ, Ornsteen M: The dexamethasone suppression test for diagnosis and prognosis in psychiatry: commentary and review. Arch Gen Psychiatry 42:1193–1204, 1985

Beck JS: Cognitive Therapy: Basics and Beyond. New York, Guilford, 1995

Beekman AT, Deeg DJ, Braam AW, et al: Consequences of major and minor depression in later life: a study of disability, well-being and service utilization. Psychol Med 27:1397–1409, 1997

Borgstrom S, von Eyben FE, Flodgren P, et al: Human leukocyte interferon and cimetidine for metastatic melanoma. N Engl J Med 307:1080–1081, 1982

Bremne JD, Vermetten E: Stress and development: behavioral and biological consequences. Dev Psychopathol 13:473–489, 2001

Brown WA, Shuey I: Response to dexamethasone and subtype of depression. Arch Gen Psychiatry 37:747–751, 1980

Burt VK, Stein K: Epidemiology of depression throughout the female life cycle. J Clin Psychiatry 63 (suppl 7):9–15, 2002

Butler AC, Chapman JE, Forman EM, et al: The empirical status of cognitive-behavioral therapy: a review of meta-analyses. Clin Psychol Rev 26:17–31, 2006

Capuron L, Gumnick JF, Musselman DL, et al: Neurobehavioral effects of interferon-alpha in cancer patients: phenomenology and paroxetine responsiveness of symptom dimensions. Neuropsychopharmacology 26:643–652, 2002

Carroll BJ: The dexamethasone suppression test for melancholia. Br J Psychiatry 140:292–304, 1982

Clayton P, Auster T: Strategies for the prevention and treatment of suicidal behavior. Focus 6:15–21, 2008

Coppen A, Abou-Saleh M, Milln P, et al: Dexamethasone suppression test in depression and other psychiatric illness. Br J Psychiatry 142: 498–504, 1983

DeRubeis RJ, Gelfand LA, Tang TZ, et al: Medications versus cognitive behavior therapy for severely depressed outpatients: mega-analysis of four randomized comparisons. Am J Psychiatry 156:1007–1013, 1999

DeRubeis RJ, Hollon SD, Amsterdam JD, et al: Cognitive therapy vs medications in the treatment of moderate to severe depression. Arch Gen Psychiatry 62:409–416, 2005

Dimidjian S, Hollon SD, Dobson KS, et al: Randomized trial of behavioral activation, cognitive therapy, and antidepressant medication in the acute treatment of adults with major depression. J Consult Clin Psychol 74:658–670, 2006

Duman RS: Depression: a case of neuronal life and death? Biol Psychiatry 56:140–145, 2004

Even C, Schröder CM, Friedman S, et al: Efficacy of light therapy in nonseasonal depression: a systematic review. J Affect Disord 108:11–23, 2007

Fava GA, Savron G, Grandi S, et al: Cognitive-behavioral management of drug-resistant major depressive disorder. J Clin Psychiatry 58:278–282; quiz 283–284, 1997

Fava GA, Ruini C, Rafanelli C, et al: Six-year outcome of cognitive behavior therapy for prevention of recurrent depression. Am J Psychiatry 161:1872–1876, 2004

Feldman G: Cognitive and behavioral therapies for depression: overview, new directions, and practical recommendations for dissemination. Psychiatr Clin North Am 30:39–50, 2007

Fergusson DM, Horwood LJ, Ridder EM, et al: Subthreshold depression in adolescence and mental health outcomes in adulthood. Arch Gen Psychiatry 62:66–72, 2005

Fogel J, Eaton WW, Ford DE: Minor depression as a predictor of the first onset of major depressive disorder over a 15-year follow-up. Acta Psychiatr Scand 113:36–43, 2006

Frank E, Kupfer DJ, Perel JM, et al: Three-year outcomes for maintenance therapies in recurrent depression. Arch Gen Psychiatry 47:1093–1099, 1990

Frank E, Kupfer DJ, Wagner EF, et al: Efficacy of interpersonal psychotherapy as a maintenance treatment of recurrent depression: contributing factors. Arch Gen Psychiatry 48:1053–1059, 1991

Frank E, Kupfer DJ, Buysse DJ, et al: Randomized trial of weekly, twice-monthly, and monthly interpersonal psychotherapy as maintenance treatment for women with recurrent depression. Am J Psychiatry 164:761–767, 2007

George MS, Wassermann EM, Williams WA, et al: Daily repetitive transcranial magnetic stimulation (rTMS) improves mood in depression. Neuroreport 6:1853–1856, 1995

Gertsik L, Poland RE: Psychoneuroendocrinology, in The American Psychiatric Publishing Textbook of Psychopharmacology, 3rd Edition. Edited by Schatzberg A, Nemeroff CB. Washington, DC, American Psychiatric Publishing, 2004, pp 115–129

Gibbons RD, Hur K, Bhaumik DK, et al: The relationship between antidepressant medication use and rate of suicide. Arch Gen Psychiatry 62:165–172, 2005

Gillespie CF, Nemeroff CB: Hypercortisolemia and depression. Psychosom Med 67 (suppl 1):S26–S28, 2005

Ginsberg DL, Schooler NR, Buckley PF, et al: Optimizing treatment of schizophrenia: enhancing affective/cognitive and depressive functioning. CNS Spectr 10:1–13; discussion 14–15, 2005

Gispen-de Wied CC, Kok FW, Koppeschaar HP, et al: Stimulation of the pituitary-adrenal system with graded doses of CRH and low dose vasopressin infusion in depressed patients and healthy subjects: a pilot study. Eur Neuropsychopharmacol 3:533–541, 1993

Gold PW, Loriaux DL, Roy A, et al: Responses to corticotropin-releasing hormone in the hypercortisolism of depression and Cushing's disease: pathophysiologic and diagnostic implications. N Engl J Med 314:1329–1335, 1986

Goldney RD, Fisher LJ, Dal Grande E, et al: Subsyndromal depression: prevalence, use of health services and quality of life in an Australian population. Soc Psychiatry Psychiatr Epidemiol 39:293–298, 2004

Hasin DS, Goodwin RD, Stinson FS, et al: Epidemiology of major depressive disorder: results from the National Epidemiologic Survey on Alcoholism and Related Conditions. Arch Gen Psychiatry 62:1097–1106, 2005

Heim C, Newport DJ, Heit S, et al: Pituitary-adrenal and autonomic responses to stress in women after sexual and physical abuse in childhood. JAMA 284:592–597, 2000

Helmer C, Montagnier D, Pérès K: Descriptive epidemiology and risk factors of depression in the elderly [in French]. Psychol Neuropsychiatr Vieil 2 (suppl 1):S7–S12, 2004

Henriksson S, Isacsson G: Increased antidepressant use and fewer suicides in Jämtland county, Sweden, after a primary care educational programme on the treatment of depression. Acta Psychiatr Scand 114:159–167, 2006

Hermens ML, van Hout HP, Terluin B, et al: The prognosis of minor depression in the general population: a systematic review. Gen Hosp Psychiatry 26:453–462, 2004

Hirschfeld RM: The comorbidity of major depression and anxiety disorders: recognition and management in primary care. Prim Care Companion J Clin Psychiatry 3:244–254, 2001

Hirschfeld RM, Klerman GL, Clayton PJ, et al: Personality and depression: empirical findings. Arch Gen Psychiatry 40:993–998, 1983

Hollon SD, DeRubeis RJ, Shelton RC, et al: Prevention of relapse following cognitive therapy vs medications in moderate to severe depression. Arch Gen Psychiatry 62:417–422, 2005a

Hollon SD, Jarrett RB, Nierenberg AA, et al: Psychotherapy and medication in the treatment of adult and geriatric depression: which monotherapy or combined treatment? J Clin Psychiatry 66:455–468, 2005b

Holsboer F: Neuroendocrinology of mood disorders, in Psychopharmacology: The Fourth Generation of Progress. Edited by Bloom FE, Kupfer DJ. New York, Raven, 1995, pp 957–971

Holsboer F: The corticosteroid receptor hypothesis of depression. Neuropsychopharmacology 23:477–501, 2000

Jacobson NS, Dobson KS, Truax PA, et al: A component analysis of cognitive-behavioral treatment for depression. J Consult Clin Psychol 64:295–304, 1996

Judd LL, Akiskal HS: The clinical and public health relevance of current research on subthreshold depressive symptoms to elderly patients. Am J Geriatr Psychiatry 10:233–238, 2002

Judd LL, Rapaport MH, Paulus MP, et al: Subsyndromal symptomatic depression: a new mood disorder? J Clin Psychiatry 55 (suppl):18–28, 1994

Kabat-Zinn J: Full Catastrophe Living: Using the Wisdom of Your Body and Mind to Face Stress, Pain, and Illness. New York, Delacorte Press, 1990

Keller MB, McCullough JP, Klein DN, et al: A comparison of nefazodone, the cognitive behavioral-analysis system of psychotherapy, and their combination for the treatment of chronic depression. N Engl J Med 342:1462–1470, 2000

Kennedy SH, Giacobbe P, Rizvi SJ, et al: Deep brain stimulation for treatment-resistant depression: follow-up after 3 to 6 years. Am J Psychiatry 168:502–510, 2011

Kessler RC, McGonagle KA, Zhao S, et al: Lifetime and 12-month prevalence of DSM-III-R psychiatric disorders in the United States: results from the National Comorbidity Survey. Arch Gen Psychiatry 51:8–19, 1994

Kessler RC, Zhao S, Blazer DG, et al: Prevalence, correlates, and course of minor depression and major depression in the National Comorbidity Survey. J Affect Disord 45:19–30, 1997

Kochanek KD, Xu J, Murphy SL, et al: Deaths: Final Data for 2009. National Vital Statistics Reports Vol 60 No 3. Hyattsville, MD, National Center for Health Statistics, 2012. Available at: http://www.cdc.gov/nchs/data/nvsr/nvsr60/nvsr60_03.pdf. Accessed October 2012.

Kripke DF: Photoperiodic mechanisms for depression and its treatment, in Biological Psychiatry. Edited by Perris C, Struwe G, Jansson B. Elsevier–North Holland Biomedical Press, 1981, pp 1249–1252

Kuyken W, Dalgleish T, Holden ER: Advances in cognitive-behavioural therapy for unipolar depression. Can J Psychiatry 52:5–13, 2007

Laje G, Paddock S, Manji H, et al: Genetic markers of suicidal ideation emerging during citalopram treatment of major depression. Am J Psychiatry 164:1530–1538, 2007

Lewy AJ, Sack RL: Light therapy and psychiatry. Proc Soc Exp Biol Med 183:11–18, 1986

Lopez AD, Murray CC: The global burden of disease, 1990–2020. Nat Med 4:1241–1243, 1998

Lopez AD, Mathers CD, Ezzati M, et al: Global and regional burden of disease and risk factors, 2001: systematic analysis of population health data. Lancet 367:1747–1757, 2006

Lozano AM, Mayberg HS, Giacobbe P, et al: Subcallosal cingulate gyrus deep brain stimulation for treatment-resistant depression. Biol Psychiatry 64:461–467, 2008

Luty SE, Carter JD, McKenzie JM, et al: Randomised controlled trial of interpersonal psychotherapy and cognitive-behavioural therapy for depression. Br J Psychiatry 190:496–502, 2007

Maes M: Evidence for an immune response in major depression: a review and hypothesis. Prog Neuropsychopharmacol Biol Psychiatry 19:11–38, 1995

Maes M: Major depression and activation of the inflammatory response system, in Cytokines, Stress, and Depression. Edited by Dantzer R, Wollman EE, Yirmiya R. New York, Kluwer Academic/Plenum, 1999, pp 25–46

McCullough JP: Treatment for Chronic Depression: Cognitive Behavioral Analysis System of Psychotherapy. New York, Guilford, 2000

McCusker J, Cole M, Dufouil C, et al: The prevalence and correlates of major and minor depression in older medical inpatients. J Am Geriatr Soc 53:1344–1353, 2005

McPherson S, Cairns P, Carlyle J, et al: The effectiveness of psychological treatments for treatment-resistant depression: a systematic review. Acta Psychiatr Scand 111:331–340, 2005

Meyers CA: Mood and cognitive disorders in cancer patients receiving cytokine therapy, in Cytokines, Stress, and Depression. Edited by Dantzer R, Wollman EE, Yirmiya R. New York, Kluwer Academic/Plenum, 1999, pp 75–81

Musselman DL, Lawson DH, Gumnick JF, et al: Paroxetine for the prevention of depression induced by high-dose interferon alfa. N Engl J Med 344:961–966, 2001

Nemeroff CB, Vale WW: The neurobiology of depression: inroads to treatment and new drug discovery. J Clin Psychiatry 66 (suppl 7):5–13, 2005

Nemeroff CB, Heim CM, Thase ME, et al: Differential responses to psychotherapy versus pharmacotherapy in patients with chronic forms of major depression and childhood trauma. Proc Natl Acad Sci U S A 100:14293–14296, 2003

Nunes EV: Substance abuse and depression. Paper presented at the annual meeting of the American Psychiatric Association, San Francisco, CA, May 2003

Olfson M, Fireman B, Weissman MM, et al: Mental disorders and disability among patients in a primary care group practice. Am J Psychiatry 154:1734–1740, 1997

Paykel ES, Cooper Z, Ramana R, et al: Life events, social support and marital relationships in the outcome of severe depression. Psychol Med 26: 121–133, 1996

Paykel ES, Scott J, Teasdale JD, et al: Prevention of relapse in residual depression by cognitive therapy: a controlled trial. Arch Gen Psychiatry 56:829–835, 1999

Pittenger C, Sanacora G, Krystal JH: The NMDA receptor as a therapeutic target in major depressive disorder. CNS Neurol Disord Drug Targets 6:101–115, 2007

Raadsheer FC, Hoogendijk WJ, Stam FC, et al: Increased numbers of corticotropin-releasing hormone expressing neurons in the hypothalamic paraventricular nucleus of depressed patients. Neuroendocrinology 60:436–444, 1994

Rapaport MH, Tipp JE, Schuckit MA: A comparison of ICD-10 and DSM-III-R criteria for substance abuse and dependence. Am J Drug Alcohol Abuse 19:143–151, 1993

Rapaport MH, Gharabawi GM, Canuso CM, et al: Effects of risperidone augmentation in patients with treatment-resistant depression: results of open-label treatment followed by double-blind continuation. Neuropsychopharmacology 31: 2505–2513, 2006

Reinherz HZ, Paradis AD, Giaconia RM, et al: Childhood and adolescent predictors of major depression in the transition to adulthood. Am J Psychiatry 160:2141–2147, 2003

Reynolds CF III, Frank E, Perel JM, et al: Nortriptyline and interpersonal psychotherapy as maintenance therapies for recurrent major depression: a randomized controlled trial in patients older than 59 years. JAMA 281:39–45, 1999

Rich CL, Isacsson G: Suicide and antidepressants in south Alabama: evidence for improved treatment of depression. J Affect Disord 45:135–142, 1997

Rieckmann N, Burg MM, Gerin W, et al: Depression vulnerabilities in patients with different levels of depressive symptoms after acute coronary syndromes. Psychother Psychosom 75:353–361, 2006

Ryff CD: Happiness is everything, or is it? Explorations on the meaning of psychological well-being. J Pers Soc Psychol 57:1069–1081, 1989

Sachar EJ, Hellman L, Fukushima DK, et al: Cortisol production in depressive illness: a clinical and biochemical clarification. Arch Gen Psychiatry 23:289–298, 1970

Sackeim HA, Brannan SK, Rush AJ, et al: Durability of antidepressant response to vagus nerve stimulation (VNS). Int J Neuropsychopharmacol 10:817–826, 2007

Schlaepfer TE, Frick C, Zobel A, et al: Vagus nerve stimulation for depression: efficacy and safety in a European study. Psychol Med 38:651–661, 2008

Schramm E, van Calker D, Dykierek P, et al: An intensive treatment program of interpersonal psychotherapy plus pharmacotherapy for depressed inpatients: acute and long-term results. Am J Psychiatry 164:768–777, 2007

Segal Z, Teasdale J, Williams M: Mindfulness-Based Cognitive Therapy for Depression. New York, Guilford, 2002

Søndergård L, Kvist K, Lopez AG, et al: Temporal changes in suicide rates for persons treated and not treated with antidepressants in Denmark during 1995–1999. Acta Psychiatr Scand 114: 168–176, 2006

Thase ME, Friedman ES, Biggs MM, et al: Cognitive therapy versus medication in augmentation and switch strategies as second-step treatments: a STAR*D report. Am J Psychiatry 164:739–752, 2007

UK ECT Review Group: Efficacy and safety of electroconvulsive therapy in depressive disorders: a systematic review and meta-analysis. Lancet 361:799–808, 2003

Warner-Schmidt JL, Duman RS: Hippocampal neurogenesis: opposing effects of stress and antidepressant treatment. Hippocampus 16:239–249, 2006

Weissman MM, Klerman GL: Sex differences and the epidemiology of depression. Arch Gen Psychiatry 34:98–111, 1977

Weissman MM, Bland RC, Canino GJ, et al: Cross-national epidemiology of major depression and bipolar disorder. JAMA 276:293–299, 1996

Westrin A, Lam RW: Long-term and preventative treatment for seasonal affective disorder. CNS Drugs 21:901–909, 2007

Wirz-Justice A, Bader A, Frisch U, et al: A randomized, double-blind, placebo-controlled study of light therapy for antepartum depression. J Clin Psychiatry 72:986–993, 2011

CHAPTER 36

Treatment of Bipolar Disorder

Paul E. Keck Jr., M.D.
Susan L. McElroy, M.D.

Bipolar disorder is a common, recurrent, often severe psychiatric illness that, without adequate treatment, is associated with high rates of morbidity and mortality (Goodwin and Jamison 2007). The goals of treatment of bipolar disorder are similar to those of management of many chronic illnesses: rapid, complete remission of acute episodes; prevention of further episodes; suppression of subsyndromal symptoms; and optimization of functional outcome and quality of life (Keck et al. 2001). However, the treatment of bipolar disorder is often complicated by the diversity of illness presentation, comorbidity, and course among individuals. Some medications have particular efficacy in one phase of illness but not in another, and some may actually increase the likelihood of precipitating a reciprocal mood episode.

In this chapter we review strategies for treating bipolar disorder, drawing primarily on data from randomized controlled trials. Where such data are lacking, strategies based on data from open trials, naturalistic studies, and expert consensus guidelines are included. The treatment of bipolar disorder in children and adolescents is covered elsewhere in this book (see Chapter 40 in this volume, "Treatment of Child and Adolescent Disorders," by Wagner and Pliszka).

Treatment of Acute Bipolar Manic and Mixed Episodes

Manic and mixed episodes are medical emergencies and frequently require treatment in a hospital to ensure safety of patients and those around them. The primary goal of treatment of manic and mixed episodes is rapid symptom reduction, followed by full remission of symptoms and restoration of psychosocial and vocational functioning (Hirschfeld et al. 2002).

Pharmacotherapy is the cornerstone of treatment of acute manic and mixed episodes and of bipolar disorder in general. A number of medications will be reviewed that have demonstrated efficacy in the treatment of acute manic and mixed episodes. Although these agents typically produce rates of response (defined as ≥50% reduction in manic symptoms from baseline to endpoint) of approximately 50% in short-term (3- to 4-week) trials, relatively few patients (<25%) actually achieve remission of symptoms within these time intervals while receiving monotherapy with any of these agents. Thus, use of combination therapy is common in clinical practice to improve response and remission rates (Suppes et al. 2005).

Lithium

Lithium has been a mainstay of treatment for acute mania for more than 50 years, with superior efficacy compared with placebo (reviewed in Goodwin and Jamison 2007) and comparable efficacy compared with divalproex (Bowden et al. 1994), carbamazepine (Lerer et al. 1987; Small et al. 1991), risperidone (Segal et al. 1998), olanzapine (Berk et al. 1999), quetiapine (Bowden et al. 2005), aripiprazole (Keck et al. 2003a), and typical antipsychotics (Garfinkel et al. 1980; Johnson et al. 1976; Platman 1970; Prien et al. 1972; Shopsin et al. 1975; Spring et al. 1970; Takahashi et al. 1975). Lithium resulted in improvement in psychotic as well as manic symptoms in these trials.

Lithium response for acute mania can be maximized by titrating to plasma concentrations at the upper end of the therapeutic range (1.0–1.4 mmol/L) as tolerated (Stokes et al. 1976). In randomized controlled trials, significant clinical improvement usually was reported within 7–14 days among responders (Keck and McElroy 2001). Common side effects associated with acute treatment with lithium include nausea, vomiting, tremor, somnolence, weight gain, and cognitive slowing. Lithium may also interfere with thyroid function and exacerbate renal disease; thus, monitoring of thyroid and renal function tests is an important part of lithium administration.

Antiepileptics

Divalproex

Divalproex and related formulations of valproic acid had superior efficacy compared with placebo (Bowden et al. 1994, 2006; Brennan et al. 1984; Emrich et al. 1981; Pope et al. 1991) and comparable efficacy compared with lithium (Bowden et al. 1994; Freeman et al. 1992), haloperidol (McElroy et al. 1996), and olanzapine (Zajecka et al. 2002) in randomized controlled acute treatment trials of bipolar manic or mixed episodes. Olanzapine was superior to divalproex in mean reduction of manic symptoms and in proportion of patients in remission at study completion in a second head-to-head comparison trial (Tohen et al. 2002a). Muller-Oerlinghausen et al. (2000) found that the combination of valproate and typical antipsychotics produced significantly lower mean antipsychotic doses and higher response rates compared with placebo added to typical antipsychotics in patients with acute mania.

Acute antimanic response is correlated with plasma concentrations between 50 and 125 mg/L, with some evidence of greater response at the upper end of the therapeutic range (Allen et al. 2006; Zajecka et al. 2002). Some patients may require plasma concentrations greater than 125 mg/L, but side effects become progressively more prevalent above this level. Divalproex can be administered at a therapeutic starting dosage of 20–30 mg/kg/day in inpatients with good tolerability, and some evidence indicates a more rapid response than with gradual titration from a lower (e.g., 750 mg/day) starting dosage (Hirschfeld et al. 1999; Keck et al. 1993).

Divalproex is generally well tolerated during treatment of acute manic or mixed episodes. Common side effects include somnolence, nausea, vomiting, tremor, weight gain, and cognitive slowing. Enteric-coated and extended-release formulations (the latter requiring a 20% dosage increase to yield plasma concentrations equivalent to those with immediate-release formulations) have improved tolerability compared with valproic acid formulations. Rare serious adverse events include pancreatitis, thrombocytopenia, significant hepatic transaminase elevation, hyperammonemic encephalopathy in patients with urea cycle disorders, and hepatic failure.

Carbamazepine and Oxcarbazepine

An extended-release formulation of carbamazepine was superior to placebo in two large randomized, placebo-controlled multicenter trials (Weisler et al. 2004b, 2005). These findings replicated earlier results from a placebo-controlled crossover trial (Ballenger and Post 1978). Common side effects of carbamazepine include diplopia, blurred vision, ataxia, somnolence, fatigue, and nausea. Less common side effects include rash, mild leukopenia and thrombocytopenia, and hyponatremia. Rare serious adverse events include agranulocytosis, aplastic anemia, thrombocytopenia, hepatic failure, pancreatitis, and exfoliative dermatitis.

In the only large randomized, placebo-controlled multicenter trial of oxcarbazepine in acute mania to date, a 7-week study in children and adolescents, oxcarbazepine was not superior to placebo in reduction of manic symptoms (Wagner et al. 2006). Thus, the use of oxcarbazepine in acute bipolar mania has not been substantiated based on evidence from clinical studies but rather is based on putative similarities in mechanism of action with carbamazepine and improved tolerability.

Antipsychotics

Typical (First-Generation) Antipsychotics

Chlorpromazine (Klein 1967) and haloperidol (McIntyre et al. 2005) were superior to placebo in randomized controlled trials. Typical antipsychotics bear the burden of neurological and neuroendocrinological side effects and may increase the risk of postmanic depressive episodes (Koukopoulos et al. 1980).

Atypical (Second-Generation) Antipsychotics

The atypical antipsychotics olanzapine, risperidone, quetiapine, ziprasidone, aripiprazole, and asenapine have all demonstrated efficacy in the treatment of acute bipolar mania in at least two randomized, placebo-controlled trials.

Olanzapine was found to be superior to placebo (Tohen et al. 1999, 2000), superior or equal in efficacy to divalproex (Tohen et al. 2002a; Zajecka et al. 2002), and comparable to lithium (Berk et al. 1999; Niufan et al. 2007), risperidone (Perlis et al. 2006), and haloperidol (Tohen et al. 2003a) in mean reduction of manic and mixed symptoms in 3- to 4-week monotherapy trials. Adjunctive treatment with olanzapine was superior to placebo in patients who were inadequately responsive to lithium or divalproex monotherapy (Tohen et al. 2002b). In short-term studies, the most common side effects associated with olanzapine were somnolence, constipation, dry mouth, increased appetite, weight gain, and orthostatic hypotension.

Risperidone was superior to placebo (Hirschfeld et al. 2004; Khanna et al. 2005) and comparable to olanzapine (Perlis et al. 2006), haloperidol (Smulevich et al. 2005), and lithium (Segal et al. 1998) in mean reduction of manic and mixed symptoms as monotherapy in 3- to 4-week trials. Risperidone was superior to placebo as adjunctive therapy with lithium or divalproex in one placebo-controlled trial (Sachs et al. 2002), but not in a second placebo-controlled trial in combination with lithium, divalproex, or carbamazepine (Yatham et al. 2003). The rate of extrapyramidal side effects associated with risperidone was low when the drug was administered at average dosages up to 4 mg/day (Hirschfeld et al. 2004; Sachs et al. 2002; Yatham et al. 2003) but not when administered at average dosages of 6 mg/day or greater (Khanna et al. 2005; Segal et al. 1998). In short-term trials, other commonly occurring side effects included prolactin elevation, akathisia, somnolence, dyspepsia, and nausea.

Quetiapine was superior to placebo as monotherapy in two 12-week studies in adult patients (Bowden et al. 2005; McIntyre et al. 2005) and was comparable to lithium in a 4-week study in adult patients (Li et al. 2008). Similarly, quetiapine was superior to placebo as adjunctive treatment with lithium or divalproex (Sachs et al. 2004; Yatham et al. 2004). The mean modal dosage of quetiapine associated with antimanic efficacy in most studies was approximately 600 mg/day (Vieta et al. 2005b). Quetiapine was also superior to placebo in the reduction of hypomanic or mild manic symptoms among outpatients in an 8-week trial (McElroy et al. 2010a). The most common side effects from quetiapine in monotherapy trials were headache, dry mouth, constipation, weight gain, somnolence, and dizziness.

Ziprasidone was superior to placebo (mean dosage 120–130 mg/day) in two 3-week monotherapy trials in adult patients (Keck et al. 2003b; Potkin et al. 2005) and comparable to haloperidol in a 12-week trial (Ramey et al. 2003). Ziprasidone was not superior to placebo as adjunctive treatment with lithium in a study designed to prove superior onset of action by 2 weeks of treatment (Weisler et al. 2004a). Ziprasidone-related side effects in monotherapy trials included headache, somnolence, extrapyramidal signs, akathisia, and dizziness.

Aripiprazole had significantly greater efficacy in the reduction of manic symptoms compared with placebo in three 3-week trials (Keck et al. 2003a, 2007; Sachs et al. 2006) and comparable efficacy with haloperidol (Vieta et al. 2005a) and lithium (Keck et al. 2009) in adequately powered 12-week comparison trials. Aripiprazole was initiated at 15 or 30 mg/day. Common side effects associated with aripiprazole in the placebo-controlled trials were headache, nausea, vomiting, constipation, insomnia, and akathisia.

Asenapine was superior to placebo in mean reduction of manic symptoms in two 3-week trials (McIntyre et al. 2009, 2010). Common side effects attributed to asenapine were extrapyramidal side effects (EPS) and mild weight gain.

In the studies of atypical antipsychotics reviewed above, there were no significant differences in response between patients with or without psychotic features or between patients with manic or mixed episodes among all agents, with the exception of trials of quetiapine, many of which excluded mixed patients. Lastly, the prototypical atypical agent clozapine has been reported to have substantial efficacy in a number of large case series of patients with treatment-refractory mania (Calabrese et al. 1996; Green et al. 2000) but has not been studied in placebo-controlled trials in mania.

Electroconvulsive Therapy

Electroconvulsive therapy (ECT) is an important treatment option for manic patients with severe, psychotic, or catatonic symptoms. ECT was superior in efficacy to lithium (Small et al. 1988) and the combination of lithium and haloperidol (Mukherjee et al. 1994) in prospective comparison studies. In addition, ECT in combination with chlorpromazine was superior to sham ECT and chlorpromazine (Sikdar et al. 1994). Although these were small studies, their findings are consistent with those of other naturalistic studies of ECT in the treatment of acute mania (Black et al. 1984; Thomas and Reddy 1982). There is a risk of neurotoxicity in patients receiving ECT while also receiving lithium; thus, lithium should be discontinued when ECT is administered (Hirschfeld et al. 2002).

Novel Treatments

In two short-term monotherapy pilot trials (Yildiz-Yesiloglu 2008; Zarate et al. 2007) and one adjunctive therapy trial (Amrollahi et al. 2011), the protein kinase C inhibitor tamoxifen was superior to placebo in reduction of manic symptoms. Placebo-controlled trials of the extended-release formulation of the atypical antipsychotic paliperidone in acute mania have thus far yielded mixed findings (Berwaerts et al. 2011, 2012; Vieta et al. 2010).

Treatment of Acute Bipolar Depressive Episodes

The goal of treatment of bipolar depression is full remission of symptoms (Hirschfeld et al. 2002). This straightforward goal is complicated by the limited efficacy of many mood stabilizers in bipolar depression (Zornberg and Pope 1993), often requiring the adjunctive use of unimodal antidepressants with the attendant risk of cycle acceleration or switching.

Lithium

Eight of nine placebo-controlled trials conducted in the 1960s and 1970s in patients with bipolar I and II disorders found lithium superior to placebo in acute bipolar depression (reviewed in Zornberg and Pope 1993). In an analysis of five studies in which it was possible to distinguish "unequivocal" lithium responders from patients who displayed partial but incomplete improvement in depression, Zornberg and Pope (1993) found that 36% had an unequivocal response, compared with 79% who had at least partial benefit.

Atypical Antipsychotics

Quetiapine

Quetiapine (300 mg/day and 600 mg/day) was superior to placebo in reduction of depressive symptoms in four large 8-week multicenter trials involving outpatients with bipolar I and II depression (Calabrese et al. 2005a; McElroy et al. 2010b; Thase et al. 2006; Young et al. 2010). There was no significant difference in efficacy between the two quetiapine dosage groups. However, the rate of side effects was lower in the 300 mg/day groups compared with the 600 mg/day groups. Switch rates were low across all treatment groups and were not significantly different among the quetiapine and placebo groups.

Olanzapine and Olanzapine-Fluoxetine Combination

Olanzapine and the combination of olanzapine and fluoxetine (OFC) were superior to placebo in reducing depressive symptoms in an 8-week trial of 833 patients with bipolar I depression (Tohen et al. 2003c). However, the OFC was superior not only to placebo throughout the trial but also to olanzapine for weeks 4–8. There were no significant differences in switch rates (6%–7%) among the three groups. Brown et al. (2006) compared OFC with lamotrigine (titrated to 200 mg/day) in a 7-week comparison trial in outpatients with bipolar I depression. Patients receiving OFC displayed greater reduction in depressive symptoms compared with patients receiving lamotrigine, although the lamotrigine group may have had a greater response with a longer trial, given the need for gradual lamotrigine titration. Switch rates were not significantly different between the two groups.

Antiepileptics

Lamotrigine

In an initial large 7-week randomized, placebo-controlled trial, lamotrigine (at 50 mg/day and 200 mg/day) was superior to placebo in patients with bipolar I depression (Calabrese et al. 1999). Switch rates (3%–8%) were not significantly different among the three groups. A second large placebo-controlled, parallel-group, flexible-dose trial involving patients with bipolar I and II depression did not find a significant advantage for lamotrigine over placebo (Bowden 2001). In a double-blind crossover trial, Frye et al. (2000) found lamotrigine superior to placebo in improving depression in patients with treatment-refractory rapid-cycling bipolar I and II disorders. Lamotrigine was superior to placebo when added to lithium treatment in an 8-week trial in patients with breakthrough depressive episodes (van der Loos et al. 2009). Common side effects of lamotrigine in these studies included headache, nausea, infection, and xerostomia. The risk of serious rash from lamotrigine can be reduced by carefully adhering to recommended titration schedules (GlaxoSmithKline 2012), but patients should be warned of the risk of rash and the need to report it immediately.

Carbamazepine

In two small controlled trials of patients with treatment-refractory bipolar depression, response to carbamazepine was superior to placebo (Post et al. 1986) and lithium (Small 1990). The results of these initial intriguing findings have not been followed up by large placebo-controlled, parallel-group trials.

Divalproex

Two small randomized, placebo-controlled trials of divalproex in the treatment of acute bipolar depression yielded opposite findings. Sachs and Collins (2001) did not find divalproex to be superior to placebo in one pilot trial, whereas Davis et al. (2005) found divalproex superior to placebo in reduction of depressive and anxiety symptoms in a later pilot study.

Antidepressants

Because of a thin evidence base, current recommendations regarding the use of antidepressants in conjunction with mood stabilizers for acute bipolar I depression tend toward the conservative (i.e., avoid antidepressants if possible). However, some general impressions can be gleaned from the available clinical trials. First, switch rates of newer antidepressants in short-term trials, in general, appear to be lower than those associated with tricyclic antidepressants (TCAs) in older studies (Thase and Sachs 2000). Second, among all of the antidepressants studied, the most substantial evidence for efficacy rests with the monoamine oxidase inhibitor (MAOI) tranylcypromine (Himmelhoch et al. 1991), but safety concerns often eliminate this agent from first-line therapy choices (Hirschfeld et al. 2002). Bupropion (Sachs et al. 1994) and selective serotonin reuptake inhibitors (SSRIs) (Nemeroff et al. 2001) are common first-line agents administered in conjunction with mood stabilizers.

Electroconvulsive Therapy

ECT had significantly greater efficacy than MAOIs, TCAs, or placebo in several randomized controlled trials in patients with bipolar depression (reviewed in Zornberg and Pope 1993). ECT may be particularly indicated for patients with severe, psychotic, or catatonic symptoms.

Psychotherapy

There are very few randomized controlled trials of any form of psychotherapy for patients with acute bipolar depression. Cognitive-behavioral and interpersonal therapy have demonstrated efficacy in the treatment of unipolar major depression, but these modalities have been examined only in very small preliminary studies in patients with bipolar depression, thus far without conclusive findings (Cole et al. 2002; Zaretsky et al. 1999).

Novel Treatments

Two preliminary placebo-controlled adjunctive trials found the dopamine D_2/D_3 receptor agonist pramipexole superior to placebo in patients with bipolar I and bipolar II depression (Goldberg et al. 2004; Zarate et al. 2004). Switch rates did not differ significantly from those with placebo.

Maintenance Treatment

Bipolar disorder is a recurrent lifelong illness in more than 90% of the patients who experience a manic episode (Goodwin and Jamison 2007). Because of the high risk of recurrence and morbidity associated with mood episodes and interepisode symptoms, maintenance treatment is usually recommended after a single manic episode (Hirschfeld et al. 2002). The goals of maintenance treatment include prevention of syndromal relapse and subsyndromal symptoms, optimization of functioning, and prevention of suicide.

Lithium

Lithium is the most extensively studied medication in the maintenance treatment of bipolar disorder. Data from randomized, placebo-controlled trials conducted in the 1960s and 1970s indicated that lithium protected against relapse, with a fourfold lower risk compared with placebo at 6-month and 1-year follow-up intervals (Keck et al. 2000). Lithium was superior to placebo in preventing relapse into mania in two randomized controlled parallel-group trials lasting 18 months (Bowden et al. 2003; Calabrese et al. 2003).

The optimal maintenance lithium serum concentration is an important consideration in successful maintenance treatment. Maintenance lithium serum concentrations usually are lower than those required to produce acute antimanic efficacy. Studies by Gelenberg et al. (1989) and Keller et al. (1992) found a serum level–response relationship, with levels of 0.4–0.6 mEq/L being associated with 2.6 times the relapse rate and a significantly greater likelihood of experiencing subsyndromal symptoms, compared with levels of 0.8 mEq/L or higher. There was also a serum level–side effect relationship, with patients at higher levels experiencing significantly higher rates of side effects, often leading to discontinuation. Perlis et al. (2002), in yet another reanalysis of the Gelenberg et al. (1989) data, reported that an abrupt drop in serum lithium levels, whether due to random reassignment or to nonadherence, was the most powerful predictor of relapse. The optimal lithium level for many patients will be the level that balances relapse prevention and suppression of subsyndromal symptoms against minimization of bothersome day-to-day side effects.

Antiepileptics

Two large 18-month placebo-controlled maintenance trials comparing lamotrigine (200–400 mg/day) with lithium (0.8–1.1 mEq/L) found lamotrigine, but not lithium, superior to placebo in preventing depressive episodes (Bowden et al. 2003; Calabrese et al. 2003). In contrast, lithium, but not lamotrigine, was superior to placebo in preventing manic episodes. Of the nearly 1,200 patients who received lamotrigine in these trials, 9% had benign rash (morbilliform or exanthematous eruptions), compared with 8% of the 1,056 patients receiving placebo. When patients who received lamotrigine during the open-label run-in phase of the studies were included in the analysis, the total incidence of rash was 13%, with two cases of serious rash requiring hospitalization (Calabrese 2002).

Calabrese et al. (2000) conducted a 6-month placebo-controlled relapse prevention study of lamotrigine (mean dosage, 288 mg/day) in 182 patients with rapid-cycling bipolar I and II disorders. There was no significant difference between the lamotrigine and placebo treatment groups in time to need for additional medications for recurrent mood symptoms.

In the only randomized, placebo-controlled maintenance trial that tested divalproex in bipolar I disorder, there was no significant difference in the time to development of any mood episode among patients receiving divalproex, lithium, or placebo (Bowden et al. 2000). A number of unforeseen methodological limitations in this trial complicated the interpretation of its results. In patients who received divalproex for treatment of the index manic episode in an open treatment period prior to randomization, divalproex was superior to placebo in early termination due to any mood episode (29% vs. 50%) during the subsequent year. Divalproex was also compared with olanzapine in a 47-week blinded maintenance trial (Tohen et al. 2003b) described earlier. Calabrese et al. (2005b) compared divalproex with lithium in a 20-month study of patients with rapid-cycling bipolar disorder and found comparable relapse rates in both treatment groups.

There are no data regarding the optimal maintenance valproic acid concentration in bipolar disorder. Current practice usually consists of titrating to therapeutic serum concentrations (50–125 μg/mL) and, as with lithium, balancing relapse and subsyndromal symptom prevention against minimization of side effects (Hirschfeld et al. 2002). Treatment with valproate appears to pose an increased risk of polycystic ovarian syndrome (PCOS), although the relationship between PCOS and weight gain as a possible mechanism is unclear (Hirschfeld et al. 2002).

Although a number of studies have examined the efficacy of carbamazepine in the maintenance treatment of bipolar disorder, most of these studies yielded results that were difficult to reliably interpret on methodological grounds (Dardennes et al. 1995).

Atypical Antipsychotics

Olanzapine was comparable to divalproex in a 47-week comparison trial (Tohen et al. 2003b) and to lithium in a 1-year comparison trial (Tohen et al. 2005). Olanzapine received an indication for maintenance treatment in bipolar disorder based on superiority over placebo in prevention of manic and depressive episodes over 48 weeks (Tohen et al. 2006). The combination of olanzapine and lithium or divalproex was superior to placebo and lithium or divalproex in relapse prevention over 18 months in patients who had initially responded to the active combination acutely (Tohen et al. 2002b) and then were re-randomized (Tohen et al. 2004). However, patients in the combination therapy group had twice the weight gain of patients in the monotherapy group.

Aripiprazole was superior to placebo in preventing manic relapse over a 6-month follow-up period in patients with bipolar disorder who were initially stabilized on aripiprazole monotherapy for an acute manic or mixed episode (Keck et al. 2006, 2007). There was no significant difference between treatment with aripiprazole and placebo in relapse into depressive episodes; however, the overall low relapse rate into depression of this trial may have been due to the inclusion of patients whose index episodes were manic or mixed, not depressed.

Two 104-week adjunctive placebo-controlled trials found quetiapine in combination with lithium or divalproex superior to placebo with lithium or divalproex in prolonging time to recurrence of a mood episode (Suppes et al. 2009; Vieta et al. 2008). The quetiapine combination groups also had lower proportions of patients experiencing a mood event.

In a 6-month maintenance trial, ziprasidone was superior to placebo in combination with lithium or divalproex in prolonging time to intervention for a mood episode and in proportion of patients requiring an intervention during the length of the trial (Bowden et al. 2010).

Electroconvulsive Therapy

The use of ECT in the maintenance treatment of bipolar disorder has never been studied systematically in a randomized controlled trial. However, a number of naturalistic studies suggest that maintenance ECT may be a useful treatment alternative for patients who are inadequately responsive to pharmacotherapy (Schwartz et al. 1995; Vanelle et al. 1994).

Psychotherapy

Most patients with bipolar disorder experience a common cluster of psychological problems stemming directly from the illness. A number of specific psychosocial interventions as adjuncts to mood stabilizer therapy have been shown to improve the long-term outcome of bipolar disorder (reviewed in Rizvi and Zaretsky 2007). The best-studied interventions include educational, interpersonal, family, and cognitive-behavioral therapies. Randomized controlled trials conducted over 1- to 2-year follow-up periods support the efficacy of cognitive-behavioral therapy (Lam et al. 2005), family-focused and related forms of therapy (Clarkin et al. 1990, 1998; Miklowitz et al. 2003; Rea et al. 2003), interpersonal and social rhythm therapies (Frank et al. 2005), and group psychoeducation (Colom et al. 2003) in reducing or delaying mood episode recurrence, increasing treatment adherence, and improving functioning. Family-focused, interpersonal, and social rhythm therapies were all associated with delaying time to depressive episode relapse compared with brief treatment (Miklowitz et al. 2007).

Conclusion

There have been substantial advances in the pharmacological treatment of bipolar disorder in the past decade. A number of medications have demonstrated efficacy in the treatment of acute mania in placebo-controlled trials, either as monotherapy or as an adjunct to mood stabilizers. In addition, data are available indicating that combination therapy with an antipsychotic and a mood stabilizer is more rapidly effective, with better overall response rates in acute mania, than either mood stabilizers or antipsychotics alone.

The treatment of bipolar depression remains one of the least-studied aspects of the illness. The "mood stabilizer first" strategy and combined use of mood stabilizers and antidepressants in moderate to severe bipolar depression are common approaches.

Most patients with bipolar disorder require treatment with more than one medication during the course of their illness. The efficacy of combination strategies is only now receiving close scrutiny. Recent studies suggest that the use of combinations of antidepressants and mood stabilizers as maintenance treatment for some patients to prevent depressive relapse may be important.

The role and efficacy of different types of psychotherapy at different phases of illness management in bipolar disorder are now becoming clearly established. These components of treatment are important in educating patients and families, improving insight and treatment adherence, enhancing coping skills, and dealing with the sequelae of mood symptoms and episodes—and, it is hoped, improving functioning and outcome. Treatment advances in bipolar disorder are finally occurring rapidly. Bringing these treatments to patients with bipolar disorder is both the challenge and the reward of helping people manage this illness.

References

Allen MH, Hirschfeld RM, Wozniak PJ, et al: Linear relationship of valproate serum concentration to response and optimal serum levels for acute mania. Am J Psychiatry 163:272–275, 2006

Amrollahi Z, Rezaei F, Salehi B, et al: Double-blind, randomized, placebo-controlled 6-week study on the efficacy and safety of tamoxifen adjunctive to lithium in acute bipolar mania. J Affect Disord 129:327–331, 2011

Ballenger JC, Post RM: Therapeutic effects of carbamazepine in affective illness: a preliminary report. Commun Psychopharmacol 2:159–175, 1978

Berk M, Ichim L, Brook S: Olanzapine compared to lithium in mania: a double-blind randomized controlled trial. Int Clin Psychopharmacol 14:339–343, 1999

Berwaerts J, Lane R, Nuamah IF, et al: Paliperidone extended-release as adjunctive therapy to lithium or valproate in the treatment of acute mania: a randomized, placebo-controlled study. J Affect Disord 129:252–260, 2011

Berwaerts J, Xu H, Nuamah I, et al: Evaluation of the efficacy and safety of paliperidone extended-release in the treatment of acute mania: a randomized, double-blind, dose-response study. J Affect Disord 136:e51–e60, 2012

Black DW, Winokur G, Nasrallah A: Treatment of mania: a naturalistic study of electroconvulsive therapy versus lithium in 438 patients. J Clin Psychiatry 48:132–139, 1984

Bowden CL: Novel treatments for bipolar disorder. Exp Opin Investig Drugs 10:661–671, 2001

Bowden CL, Brugger AM, Swann AC, et al: Efficacy of divalproex vs lithium and placebo in the treatment of mania. JAMA 271:918–924, 1994

Bowden CL, Calabrese JR, McElroy SL, et al: Efficacy of divalproex versus lithium and placebo in maintenance treatment of bipolar disorder. Arch Gen Psychiatry 57:481–489, 2000

Bowden CL, Calabrese JR, Sachs GS, et al: A placebo-controlled 18-month trial of lamotrigine and lithium maintenance treatment in recently manic or hypomanic patients with bipolar I disorder. Arch Gen Psychiatry 60:392–400, 2003

Bowden CL, Grunze H, Mullen J, et al: A randomized, double-blind, placebo-controlled efficacy and safety study of quetiapine or lithium as monotherapy for mania in bipolar disorder. J Clin Psychiatry 66:111–121, 2005

Bowden CL, Swann AD, Calabrese JR, et al: A randomized, placebo-controlled, multicenter study of divalproex sodium extended release in the treatment of acute mania. J Clin Psychiatry 67: 1501–1510, 2006

Bowden CL, Vieta E, Ice KS, et al: Ziprasidone plus a mood stabilizer in subjects with bipolar I disorder: a 6-month, randomized, placebo-controlled, double-blind trial. J Clin Psychiatry 71:130–137, 2010

Brennan MJ, Sandyk R, Borsook D: Use of sodium valproate in the management of affective disorders: basic and clinical aspects, in Anticonvulsants in Affective Disorders. Edited by Emrich HM, Okuma T, Muller AA. Amsterdam, Excerpta Medica, 1984, pp 56–65

Brown E, McElroy SL, Keck PE Jr, et al: A 7-week, randomized, double-blind trial of olanzapine/fluoxetine combination versus lamotrigine in the treatment of bipolar I depression. J Clin Psychiatry 67:1025–1033, 2006

Calabrese JR: Clinical Relevance and Management of Bipolar Disorders: Weighing Benefits Versus Risks (Presentations in Focus). New York, Medical Education Network, 2002

Calabrese JR, Kimmel SE, Woyshville MJ, et al: Clozapine for treatment-refractory mania. Am J Psychiatry 153:759–764, 1996

Calabrese JR, Bowden CL, Sachs GS, et al: A double-blind placebo-controlled study of lamotrigine monotherapy in outpatients with bipolar I depression. J Clin Psychiatry 60:79–88, 1999

Calabrese JR, Suppes T, Bowden CL, et al: A double-blind, placebo-controlled, prophylaxis study of lamotrigine in rapid-cycling bipolar disorder. J Clin Psychiatry 61:841–850, 2000

Calabrese JR, Bowden CL, Sachs GS, et al: A placebo-controlled 18-month trial of lamotrigine and lithium maintenance treatment in recently depressed patients with bipolar I disorder. J Clin Psychiatry 64:1013–1024, 2003

Calabrese JR, Keck PE Jr, Macfadden W, et al: A randomized, double-blind, placebo-controlled trial of quetiapine in the treatment of bipolar I or II depression. Am J Psychiatry 162:1351–1360, 2005a

Calabrese JR, Shelton MD, Rapport DJ, et al: A 20-month, double-blind, maintenance trial of lithium versus divalproex in rapid-cycling bipolar disorder. Am J Psychiatry 162:2152–2161, 2005b

Clarkin JF, Glick ID, Haas GL, et al: A randomized clinical trial of inpatient family intervention, V: results for affective disorders. J Affect Disord 18:17–28, 1990

Clarkin JF, Carpenter D, Hull J, et al: Effects of psychoeducational intervention for married patients with bipolar disorder and their spouses. Psychiatr Serv 49:531–533, 1998

Cole DP, Thase ME, Mallinger AG, et al: Slower treatment response in bipolar depression predicted by lower pretreatment thyroid function. Am J Psychiatry 159:116–121, 2002

Colom F, Vieta E, Martinez-Aran A, et al: A randomized trial on the efficacy of group psychoeducation in the prophylaxis of recurrences in bipolar patients whose disease is in remission. Arch Gen Psychiatry 60:402–407, 2003

Dardennes R, Even C, Bange F: Comparison of carbamazepine and lithium in the prophylaxis of bipolar disorders: a meta-analysis. Br J Psychiatry 166:375–381, 1995

Davis LL, Bartolucci A, Petty F: Divalproex in the treatment of bipolar depression: a placebo-controlled study. J Affect Disord 85:259–266, 2005

Emrich HM, von Zerssen D, Kissling W: On a possible role of GABA in mania: therapeutic efficacy of sodium valproate, in GABA and Benzodiazepine Receptors. Edited by Costa E, Dicharia G, Gessa GL. New York, Raven Press, 1981, pp 287–296

Frank E, Kupfer DJ, Thase ME, et al: Two-year outcomes for interpersonal and social rhythm therapy in individuals with bipolar I disorder. Arch Gen Psychiatry 62:996–1004, 2005

Freeman TW, Clothier JL, Pazzaglia P, et al: A double-blind comparison of valproate and lithium in the treatment of acute mania. Am J Psychiatry 149:108–111, 1992

Frye MA, Ketter TA, Kimbrell TA, et al: A placebo-controlled study of lamotrigine and gabapentin monotherapy in refractory mood disorders. J Clin Psychopharmacol 20:607–614, 2000

Garfinkel PE, Stancer HC, Persad E: A comparison of haloperidol, lithium and their combination in the treatment of mania. J Affect Disord 2:279–288, 1980

Gelenberg AJ, Kane JM, Keller MB, et al: Comparison of standard and low serum levels of lithium for maintenance treatment of bipolar disorder. N Engl J Med 321:1489–1493, 1989

GlaxoSmithKline: Lamictal (lamotrigine) full prescribing information. Research Triangle Park, NC, GlaxoSmithKline, September 2012. Available at: http://dailymed.nlm.nih.gov/dailymed/lookup.cfm?setid=d7e3572d-56fe-4727-2bb4-013ccca22678. Accessed October 2012.

Goldberg JF, Burdick KE, Endick CJ: Preliminary randomized, double-blind, placebo-controlled trial of pramipexole added to mood stabilizers for treatment-resistant bipolar depression. Am J Psychiatry 161:564–566, 2004

Goodwin FK, Jamison KR: Manic-Depressive Illness: Bipolar Disorders and Recurrent Depression. New York, Oxford University Press, 2007

Green AI, Tohen M, Patel JK, et al: Clozapine in the treatment of refractory psychotic mania. Am J Psychiatry 157:982–986, 2000

Himmelhoch JM, Thase ME, Mallinger AG, et al: Tranylcypromine versus imipramine in anergic bipolar depression. Am J Psychiatry 148:910–916, 1991

Hirschfeld RM, Allen MH, McEvoy JP, et al: Safety and tolerability of oral loading divalproex sodium in acutely manic bipolar patients. J Clin Psychiatry 60:815–818, 1999

Hirschfeld RM, Bowden CL, Gitlin MJ, et al: Practice guideline for the treatment of patients with bipolar disorder (revision). Am J Psychiatry 159 (suppl):1–50, 2002

Hirschfeld RM, Keck PE Jr, Kramer M, et al: Rapid antimanic effect of risperidone monotherapy: a 3-week multicenter, double-blind, placebo-controlled trial. Am J Psychiatry 161:1057–1065, 2004

Johnson G, Gershon S, Burdock EI, et al: Comparative effects of lithium and chlorpromazine in the treatment of acute manic states. Br J Psychiatry 119:267–276, 1976

Keck PE Jr, McElroy SL: Definition, evaluation, and management of treatment refractory mania. Psychopharmacol Bull 35:130–148, 2001

Keck PE Jr, McElroy SL, Tugrul KC, et al: Valproate oral loading in the treatment of acute mania. J Clin Psychiatry 54:305–308, 1993

Keck PE Jr, Welge JA, Strakowski SM, et al: Placebo effect in randomized, controlled maintenance studies of patients with bipolar disorder. Biol Psychiatry 47:756–765, 2000

Keck PE Jr, McElroy SL, Arnold LM: Bipolar disorder. Psychiatr Clin North Am 85:645–661, 2001

Keck PE Jr, Marcus R, Tourkodimitris S, et al: A placebo-controlled, double-blind study of the efficacy and safety of aripiprazole in patients with acute bipolar mania. Am J Psychiatry 160:1651–1658, 2003a

Keck PE Jr, Versiani M, Potkin S, et al: Ziprasidone in the treatment of acute bipolar mania: a three-week, placebo-controlled, double-blind, randomized trial. Am J Psychiatry 160:741–748, 2003b

Keck PE Jr, Calabrese JR, McQuade RD, et al: A randomized, double-blind, placebo-controlled 26-week trial of aripiprazole in recently manic patients with bipolar I disorder. J Clin Psychiatry 67:626–637, 2006

Keck PE Jr, Calabrese JR, McIntyre RS, et al: Aripiprazole monotherapy for maintenance therapy in bipolar I disorder: a 100-week, double-blind study versus placebo. J Clin Psychiatry 68:1480–1491, 2007

Keck PE Jr, Sanchez R, Torbeyns A, et al: Aripiprazole monotherapy in the treatment of acute bipolar I mania: a randomized, placebo- and lithium-controlled study. J Affect Disord 112:36–49, 2009

Keller MB, Lavori PW, Kane JM: Subsyndromal symptoms in bipolar disorder: a comparison of standard and low serum levels of lithium. Arch Gen Psychiatry 49:371–376, 1992

Khanna S, Vieta E, Lyons B, et al: Risperidone in the treatment of acute mania: double-blind, placebo-controlled study. Br J Psychiatry 187:229–234, 2005

Klein DF: Importance of psychiatric diagnosis in prediction of clinical drug effects. Arch Gen Psychiatry 16:118–126, 1967

Koukopoulos A, Reginaldi D, Laddomada P: Course of manic-depressive cycle and changes caused by treatments. Pharmakopsychiatrie Neuropsychopharmakologie 13:156–167, 1980

Lam DH, Hayward P, Watkins ER, et al: Relapse prevention in patients with bipolar disorder: cognitive therapy outcomes after 2 years. Am J Psychiatry 162:324–329, 2005

Lerer B, Moore N, Meyendorff E, et al: Carbamazepine versus lithium in mania: a double-blind study. J Clin Psychiatry 48:89–93, 1987

Li H, Ma C, Wang G, et al: Response and remission rates in Chinese patients with bipolar mania treated for 4 weeks with either quetiapine or lithium: a randomized and double-blind study. Curr Med Res Opin 24:1–10, 2008

McElroy SL, Keck PE Jr, Stanton SP, et al: A randomized comparison divalproex oral loading versus haloperidol in the initial treatment of acute psychotic mania. J Clin Psychiatry 57:142–146, 1996

McElroy SL, Martens BE, Winstanley EL, et al: Placebo-controlled study of quetiapine monotherapy in ambulatory bipolar spectrum patients with moderate-to-severe hypomania or mild mania. J Affect Disord 124:157–163, 2010a

McElroy SL, Weisler RH, Chang W, et al: A double-blind, placebo-controlled study of quetiapine and paroxetine as monotherapy in adults with bipolar depression (EMBOLDEN II). J Clin Psychiatry 7:163–174, 2010b

McIntyre RS, Brecher M, Paulsson B, et al: Quetiapine or haloperidol as monotherapy for bipolar mania—a 12-week, double-blind, randomized, parallel-group, placebo-controlled trial. Eur Neuropsychopharmacol 15:573–585, 2005

McIntyre RS, Cohen M, Zhao J, et al: A 3-week, randomized, placebo-controlled trial of asenapine in the treatment of acute mania in bipolar mania and mixed states. Bipolar Disord 11:673–686, 2009

McIntyre RS, Cohen M, Zhao J, et al: Asenapine in the treatment of acute mania in bipolar I disorder: a randomized, double-blind, placebo-controlled trial. J Affect Disord 122:27–38, 2010

Miklowitz DJ, George GL, Richards JA, et al: A randomized, controlled study of family focused psychoeducation and pharmacotherapy in outpatient management of bipolar disorder. Arch Gen Psychiatry 60:904–912, 2003

Miklowitz DJ, Otto MW, Frank E, et al: Psychosocial treatments for bipolar depression: a 1-year randomized trial from the Systematic Treatment Enhancement Program. Arch Gen Psychiatry 64:419–427, 2007

Mukherjee S, Sackeim HA, Schnur DB: Electroconvulsive therapy of acute manic episodes: a review of 50 years' experience. Am J Psychiatry 151:169–176, 1994

Muller-Oerlinghausen B, Retzow A, Henn FA, et al: Valproate as an adjunct to neuroleptic medication for the treatment of acute episodes of mania: a prospective, randomized, double-blind, placebo-controlled, multicenter study. European Valproate Mania Study Group. J Clin Psychopharmacol 20:195–203, 2000

Nemeroff CB, Evans DL, Gyulai L, et al: Double-blind, placebo-controlled comparison of imipramine and paroxetine in the treatment of bipolar depression. Am J Psychiatry 62:906–912, 2001

Niufan F, Tohen M, Qiuqing A, et al: Olanzapine versus lithium in the acute treatment of bipolar mania: a double-blind, randomized, controlled trial. J Affect Disord 23:117–122, 2007

Perlis RH, Sachs GS, Lafer B: Effect of abrupt change from standard to low serum levels of lithium: a re-analysis of double-blind lithium maintenance data. Am J Psychiatry 159:1155–1159, 2002

Perlis RH, Baker RW, Zarate CA Jr, et al: Olanzapine versus risperidone in the treatment of manic or mixed states in bipolar I disorder: a randomized, double-blind trial. J Clin Psychiatry 67:1747–1753, 2006

Platman SR: A comparison of lithium carbonate and chlorpromazine in mania. Am J Psychiatry 127:351–353, 1970

Pope HG Jr, McElroy SL, Keck PE Jr, et al: Valproate in the treatment of acute mania: a placebo-controlled study. Arch Gen Psychiatry 48:62–68, 1991

Post RM, Uhde TW, Roy-Byrne PP: Antidepressant effects of carbamazepine. Am J Psychiatry 43: 29–34, 1986

Potkin S, Keck PE Jr, Segal S, et al: Ziprasidone in acute bipolar mania: a 21-day randomized, double-blind, placebo-controlled replication trial. J Clin Psychopharmacol 25:301–310, 2005

Prien RF, Caffey EM Jr, Klett CJ: Comparison of lithium carbonate and chlorpromazine in the treatment of mania: report of the Veterans Administration and National Institute of Mental Health Collaborative Study Group. Arch Gen Psychiatry 26:146–153, 1972

Ramey TS, Giller EL, English EP: Ziprasidone efficacy and safety in acute bipolar mania: a 12-week study. Abstracts of the 6th International Conference on Bipolar Disorders, Pittsburgh, PA, June 16, 2003

Rea MM, Tompson M, Miklowitz DJ, et al: Family focused treatment vs. individual treatment for bipolar disorder: results from a randomized controlled trial. J Consult Clin Psychol 71:482–492, 2003

Rizvi S, Zaretsky AE: Psychotherapy through the phases of bipolar disorder: evidence for general efficacy and differential effects. J Clin Psychol 63:491–506, 2007

Sachs GS, Collins MC: A placebo-controlled trial of divalproex sodium in acute bipolar depression. Presented at the American College of Neuropsychopharmacology Annual Meeting, San Juan, PR, December 2001

Sachs GS, Lafer B, Stoll AL, et al: A double-blind trial of bupropion versus desipramine for bipolar depression. J Clin Psychiatry 55:391–393, 1994

Sachs GS, Grossman F, Ghaemi SN, et al: Combination mood stabilizer with risperidone or haloperidol for treatment of acute mania: a double-blind, placebo-controlled comparison of efficacy and safety. Am J Psychiatry 159:1146–1154, 2002

Sachs GS, Chengappa KN, Suppes T: Quetiapine with lithium or divalproex for the treatment of bipolar mania: a randomized, double-blind, placebo-controlled study. Bipolar Disord 6:213–223, 2004

Sachs GS, Sanchez R, Marcus R, et al: Aripiprazole in the treatment of acute manic or mixed episodes in patients with bipolar I disorder: a 3-week placebo controlled study. J Clin Psychopharmacol 20:536–546, 2006

Schwartz T, Loewenstein J, Isenberg KE: Maintenance ECT: indications and outcome. Convulsive Ther 11:14–23, 1995

Segal J, Berk M, Brook S: Risperidone compared with both lithium and haloperidol in mania: a double-blind randomized controlled trial. Clin Neuropharmacol 21:176–180, 1998

Shopsin B, Gershon S, Thompson H, et al: Psychoactive drugs in mania: a controlled comparison of lithium carbonate, chlorpromazine, and haloperidol. Arch Gen Psychiatry 32:34–42, 1975

Sikdar S, Kulhara P, Avasthi A: Combined chlorpromazine and electroconvulsive therapy in mania. Br J Psychiatry 164:806–810, 1994

Small JG: Anticonvulsants in affective disorders. Psychopharmacol Bull 26:25–36, 1990

Small JG, Klapper MH, Kellams JJ, et al: Electroconvulsive treatment compared with lithium in the management of manic states. Arch Gen Psychiatry 45:727–732, 1988

Small JG, Klapper MH, Milstein V, et al: Carbamazepine compared with lithium in the treatment of mania. Arch Gen Psychiatry 48:915–921, 1991

Smulevich AB, Khanna S, Eerdekens M, et al: Acute and continuation risperidone monotherapy in bipolar mania: a 3-week placebo-controlled trial followed by a 9-week double-blind trial of risperidone and haloperidol. Eur Neuropsychopharmacol 15:75–84, 2005

Spring G, Schweid D, Gray C, et al: A double-blind comparison of lithium and chlorpromazine in the treatment of manic states. Am J Psychiatry 126:1306–1310, 1970

Stokes PE, Kocsis JH, Orestes JA: Relationship of lithium chloride dose to treatment response in acute mania. Arch Gen Psychiatry 33:1080–1084, 1976

Suppes T, Dennehy EB, Hirschfeld RM, et al: The Texas Implementation of Medication Algorithms: update to the algorithms for the treatment of bipolar I disorder. J Clin Psychiatry 66:870–886, 2005

Suppes T, Vieta E, Liu S, et al: Maintenance treatment for patients with bipolar I disorder: results for a North American study of quetiapine in combination with lithium or divalproex (trial 127). Am J Psychiatry 166:476–488, 2009

Takahashi R, Sakuma A, Itoh K, et al: Comparison of efficacy of lithium carbonate and chlorpromazine in mania: report of collaborative study group on treatment of mania in Japan. Arch Gen Psychiatry 32:1310–1318, 1975

Thase ME, Sachs GS: Bipolar depression: pharmacotherapy and related therapeutic strategies. Biol Psychiatry 48:558–572, 2000

Thase ME, Macfadden W, Weisler RH, et al: Efficacy of quetiapine monotherapy in bipolar I and II depression: a double-blind, placebo-controlled study. J Clin Psychopharmacol 26:600–609, 2006

Thomas J, Reddy B: The treatment of mania: a retrospective evaluation of the effects of ECT, chlorpromazine, and lithium. J Affective Disorder 4:85–92, 1982

Tohen M, Sanger TM, McElroy SL, et al: Olanzapine versus placebo in the treatment of acute mania. Am J Psychiatry 156:702–709, 1999

Tohen M, Jacobs TG, Grundy SL, et al: Efficacy of olanzapine in acute bipolar mania: a double-blind, placebo-controlled study. Arch Gen Psychiatry 57:841–849, 2000

Tohen M, Baker RW, Altshuler LL, et al: Olanzapine versus divalproex in the treatment of acute mania. Am J Psychiatry 159:1011–1017, 2002a

Tohen M, Chengappa KNR, Suppes T, et al: Efficacy of olanzapine in combination with valproate or lithium in the treatment of mania in patients partially nonresponsive to valproate or lithium monotherapy. Arch Gen Psychiatry 59:62–69, 2002b

Tohen M, Goldberg JF, Gonzalez-Pinto A, et al: A 12-week, double-blind comparison of olanzapine vs haloperidol in the treatment of acute mania. Arch Gen Psychiatry 60:1218–1226, 2003a

Tohen M, Ketter TA, Zarate CA Jr, et al: Olanzapine versus divalproex sodium for the treatment of acute mania and maintenance of remission: a 47-week study. Am J Psychiatry 160:1263–1271, 2003b

Tohen M, Vieta E, Calabrese J, et al: Efficacy of olanzapine and olanzapine-fluoxetine combination in the treatment of bipolar I depression. Arch Gen Psychiatry 60:1079–1088, 2003c

Tohen M, Chengappa KN, Suppes T, et al: Relapse prevention in bipolar I disorder: 18-month comparison of olanzapine plus mood stabilizer vs mood stabilizer alone. Br J Psychiatry 184:337–345, 2004

Tohen M, Greil W, Calabrese JR, et al: Olanzapine versus lithium in the maintenance treatment of bipolar disorder: a 12-month, randomized, double-blind, controlled trial. Am J Psychiatry 162:1281–1290, 2005

Tohen M, Calabrese JR, Sachs GS, et al: Randomized, placebo-controlled trial of olanzapine as maintenance therapy in patients with bipolar I disorder. Am J Psychiatry 163:247–256, 2006

Van der Loos M, Mulder PG, Hartong EG, et al: Efficacy and safety of lamotrigine as add-on treatment to lithium in bipolar depression: a multicenter, double-blind, placebo-controlled trial. J Clin Psychiatry 70:223–231, 2009

Vanelle JM, Loo H, Galinowski A, et al: Maintenance ECT in intractable manic-depressive disorders. Convuls Ther 10:195–205, 1994

Vieta E, Bourin M, Sanchez R, et al: Effectiveness of aripiprazole vs haloperidol in acute bipolar mania: a double-blind, randomized, comparative 12-week trial. Br J Psychiatry 187:235–242, 2005a

Vieta E, Mullen J, Brecher M, et al: Quetiapine monotherapy for mania associated with bipolar disorder: combined analysis of two international, double-blind, randomized, placebo-controlled studies. Curr Med Res Opin 21:923–934, 2005b

Vieta E, Suppes T, Eggens I, et al: Efficacy and safety of quetiapine in combination with lithium or divalproex for maintenance of patients with bipolar disorder (international trial 126). J Affect Disord 109:251–263, 2008

Vieta E, Nuamah IF, Lim P, et al: A randomized, placebo- and active-controlled study of paliperidone extended release for the treatment of acute manic and mixed episodes of bipolar I disorder. Bipolar Disord 12:230–243, 2010

Wagner KD, Kowatch RA, Emslie GJ: A double-blind, randomized, placebo-controlled trial of oxcarbazepine in the treatment of bipolar disorder in children and adolescents. Am J Psychiatry 163:1179–1186, 2006

Weisler RH, Dunn J, English P: Ziprasidone adjunctive treatment of acute bipolar mania: a randomized, double-blind placebo-controlled trial. Abstracts of the 16th Annual Meeting of the European College of Neuropsychopharmacology, Prague, Czech Republic, September 24, 2004a

Weisler RH, Kalali AH, Ketter TA: A multicenter, randomized, double-blind, placebo-controlled trial of extended release carbamazepine capsules as monotherapy for bipolar patients with manic or mixed episodes. J Clin Psychiatry 65: 478–484, 2004b

Weisler RH, Keck PE Jr, Swann AC: Extended release carbamazepine capsules as monotherapy for acute mania in bipolar disorder: a multicenter, randomized, double-blind, placebo-controlled trial. J Clin Psychiatry 66:323–330, 2005

Yatham LN, Grossman F, Augustyns I, et al: Mood stabilizers plus risperidone or placebo in the treatment of acute mania. International, double-blind, randomized controlled trial. Br J Psychiatry 182:141–147, 2003

Yatham LN, Paulsson B, Mullen J, et al: Quetiapine versus placebo in combination with lithium or divalproex for the treatment of bipolar mania. J Clin Psychopharmacol 24:599–606, 2004

Yildiz-Yesiloglu A, Guleryuz S, Ankerst DP, et al. Protein kinase C inhibition in the treatment of mania: a double-blind, placebo-controlled trial of tamoxifen. Arch Gen Psychiatry 65:255–263, 2008

Young AH, McElroy SL, Bauer M, et al: A double-blind, placebo-controlled study of quetiapine and lithium monotherapy in adults in the acute phase of bipolar depression. J Clin Psychiatry 71:150–162, 2010

Zajecka JM, Weisler R, Swann AC, et al: A comparison of the efficacy, safety, and tolerability of divalproex sodium and olanzapine in the treatment of bipolar disorder. J Clin Psychiatry 63: 1148–1155, 2002

Zarate CA Jr, Payne LL, Quiroz J: Pramipexole for bipolar II depression: a placebo-controlled proof of concept study. Biol Psychiatry 56:54–60, 2004

Zarate CA Jr, Singh JB, Carlson PJ, et al: Efficacy of a protein kinase C inhibitor (tamoxifen) in the treatment of acute mania: a pilot study. Bipolar Disord 9:561–570, 2007

Zaretsky AE, Segal ZV, Gemar M: Cognitive therapy for bipolar depression: a pilot study. Can J Psychiatry 44:491–494, 1999

Zornberg GL, Pope HG Jr: Treatment of depression in bipolar disorder: new directions for research. J Clin Psychopharmacol 13:397–408, 1993

CHAPTER 37

Treatment of Schizophrenia

Tsung-Ung W. Woo, M.D., Ph.D.
Carla M. Canuso, M.D.
Joanne D. Wojcik, Ph.D., P.M.H.C.N.S.-B.C.
Mary F. Brunette, M.D.
Alan I. Green, M.D.

Schizophrenia is a debilitating brain disorder characterized by a chronic relapsing and remitting course of psychosis that is superimposed on persistent "deficit" features such as cognitive dysfunction and negative symptoms. It appears to be equally prevalent across geographical and cultural boundaries (see Jablensky et al. 1992), afflicting approximately 1% of the population (Perala et al. 2007).

Considerable progress has been made in the pharmacological treatment of schizophrenia since the serendipitous discovery in the early 1950s of chlorpromazine as the first effective antipsychotic medication (Lehmann and Hanrahan 1954). Many other antipsychotic agents, all sharing chlorpromazine's dopamine D_2 receptor–blocking ability, were subsequently developed. These "conventional," or first-generation, antipsychotics are all effective in the treatment of positive symptoms of psychosis, but they all have limited beneficial effects on negative symptoms and cognitive deficits. Since 1990, a second generation of antipsychotic drugs has become available in the United States. These second-generation agents are also commonly referred to as "atypical" or "novel" antipsychotics, largely because of the reduced propensity of many of these agents, compared with the conventional agents, to cause extrapyramidal side effects (EPS). It has been postulated that this unique property (i.e., the low risk of EPS) may reflect the potent serotonin$_{2A}$ (5-HT$_{2A}$) receptor antago-

The authors would like to acknowledge the contribution of Holly L. L. Pierce in the preparation of this chapter.

nistic effects or, more specifically, the high ratio of 5-HT_{2A} to D_2 receptor occupancy of these drugs (Meltzer 1989). More recently, it has been proposed that the rapid dissociation (high dissociation constant) of these drugs from D_2 receptors may be another very important pharmacological property that determines "atypicality" (Kapur and Remington 2001; Seeman 2002).

The focus of schizophrenia treatment has been gradually expanding beyond targeting psychotic or positive symptoms of the illness alone. Second-generation agents have been reported by some (but not all) investigators to improve some aspects of negative symptoms and cognitive impairment. Moreover, development of compounds that can improve cognition has become one of the main foci in schizophrenia research (Fenton et al. 2003; Hyman and Fenton 2003; Marder 2006).

In recent years, the field has developed a focused interest in early diagnosis and early intervention in patients who are just becoming psychotic. In the years to come, it is likely that this emphasis on early intervention will expand, with further research on the treatment of prodromal states, in an attempt to improve the overall course or perhaps even prevent the actual onset of overt illness in individuals who appear likely to develop schizophrenia.

Clinical Manifestations of Schizophrenia

There is a growing consensus, following the seminal work of several investigators (e.g., Andreasen 1985; Crow 1985), that schizophrenia can be conceptualized as a disorder with at least two more or less orthogonal dimensions of symptomatology: positive and negative symptoms.

Positive Symptoms

Positive symptoms are perceptual or cognitive features that "normal" individuals usually do not experience. They include hallucinations, delusions, and disorganized thinking, although disorganization also can be conceptualized as an independent symptom dimension (Liddle et al. 1989). As a general rule, positive symptoms tend to respond to treatment with antipsychotic medications. These symptoms do not appear to bear any significant association with or predict the long-term functional outcome of the illness (Green et al. 2000). It also should be emphasized that psychotic symptoms are not specific to schizophrenia; they can occur in a wide spectrum of other psychiatric, neurological, and medical disorders. Therefore, it is essential to rule out other possible causes of psychosis before a diagnosis of schizophrenia is made.

Negative Symptoms

Negative symptoms represent a "loss" of functions or abilities that people without schizophrenia normally possess. They include anhedonia, affective flattening, alogia, avolition, and asociality. Negative symptoms are somewhat associated with intellectual and neurocognitive impairment (Dickerson et al. 1996; Harvey et al. 1998), and they are better predictors of long-term functional outcome and psychosocial functioning of schizophrenia patients than are positive symptoms (Buchanan et al. 1994; Dickerson et al. 1996; Harvey and Keefe 1998). However, neurocognitive deficits in schizophrenia (see section with that title below) remain the strongest predictors of outcome (Green 1996). Importantly, EPS produced by antipsychotic medications can sometimes resemble negative symptoms of schizophrenia.

To clarify matters, the concept of primary versus secondary negative symptoms has been introduced (Carpenter et al. 1988). Thus, *primary* negative symptoms represent the core negative symptoms reflecting the schizophrenia disease process. *Secondary* negative symptoms, on the other hand, are caused by or are secondary to positive symptoms of psychosis or the antipsychotic medications themselves. A reduction in medication dosage may alleviate some secondary negative symptoms, but this strategy is unlikely to have a beneficial effect on primary negative symptoms.

Diagnosis of Schizophrenia

According to DSM-IV-TR (American Psychiatric Association 2000), to make the diagnosis of schizophrenia, there must be evidence of continuous symptomatic disturbance for at least 6 months accompanied by a decline from the premorbid level of functioning. Thus, in line with the Kraepelinian concept (Kraepelin 1919/1971), DSM-IV-TR emphasizes the longitudinal course of deterioration of the illness. This 6-month period can include functional deterioration occurring during the prodromal phase before the onset of overt psychosis. Within the 6-month period, the patient must have two or more of the following symptoms for at least 1 month: delusions, hallucinations, disorganized speech, grossly disorganized or catatonic behavior, and negative symptoms. If the duration of psychotic symptoms is less than 1 month because of successful treatment with antipsychotic medication, a diagnosis of schizophrenia still may be made. Of course, before the diagnosis of schizophrenia is made, other medical or psychiatric conditions need to be considered and ruled out.

Neurocognitive Deficits in Schizophrenia

Schizophrenia appears to be associated with a decline in general cognitive functions, including verbal declarative memory, working memory, executive function, and attention. Various studies have shown that this decline may either predate the onset of psychosis (Aylward et al. 1984; David et al. 1997; Nelson et al. 1990; Russell et al. 1997; Simon et al. 2007) or occur concurrently with or subsequent to the first psychotic episode (Nelson et al. 1990). It appears that after this initial decline, the level of cognitive impairment follows a relatively stable course for several decades without evidence of significant further deterioration (Elvevag and Goldberg 2000; Goldberg et al. 1993).

Course of Schizophrenia

Schizophrenia is a chronic illness with the onset of psychotic symptoms usually occurring around late adolescence and early adulthood (Lewis and Lieberman 2000). The age at onset is approximately 5 years later in women than in men (Angermeyer et al. 1990; Faraone et al. 1994; Hambrecht et al. 1992; Szymanski et al. 1995). Although there may be no clear sex differences in cross-sectional symptomatology of the illness (Hafner et al. 1993; Szymanski et al. 1995), women in general tend to have a more favorable outcome.

Accumulating evidence suggests that schizophrenia is a neurodevelopmental disorder (Lewis and Levitt 2002; Murray 1994; Pilowsky et al. 1993; Waddington 1993; Weinberger 1987, 1996). It has been postulated that disturbances in brain development during the first and second trimesters may contribute to the pathophysiology of the illness (Waddington 1993). Other factors such as obstetric complications may further alter the course of brain development (Cannon 1997; Geddes and Lawrie 1995).

For a period of 2–5 years before the onset of the first overt psychotic episode, up to three-quarters of the patients who eventually develop schizophrenia show a wide spectrum of "prodromal" symptoms and reduced functioning (Docherty et al. 1978; Freedman and Chapman 1973; Hafner et al. 1992, 1993, 1994; G. Huber et al. 1980; Lieberman 2006; Simon et al. 2007; Varsamis and Adamson 1971; Yung and McGorry 1996a, 1996b). Prodromal symptoms are usually affective or cognitive in nature (e.g., depressed mood, social withdrawal, decreased concentration and attention, decreased motivation, agitation, anxiety, and sleep disturbances). After the onset of the first episode of psychosis, the course of the illness is often characterized by a gradual deterioration, especially in the first 2–5 years (McGlashan 1998). Some evidence suggests that functional deterioration may be accompanied by a gradual loss of gray matter volume of the cerebral cortex (DeLisi et al. 1997; Kasai et al. 2003a, 2003b; Salisbury et al. 2007; van Haren et al. 2007; Zipursky et al. 1992). In addition, there has been speculation that these observations of functional and structural brain changes after the onset of psychosis may reflect a neurodegenerative process (DeLisi 1999; DeLisi et al. 1997; Lieberman 1999). However, the available evidence in support of the neurodegeneration hypothesis of schizophrenia remains weak (Carpenter 1998; Weinberger and McClure 2002).

After an initial period of functional deterioration, symptoms tend to become more or less stabilized. Positive symptoms usually respond to treatment, whereas negative symptoms are believed to be relatively treatment resistant and may tend to become increasingly prominent during the course of the illness (Breier et al. 1991). Many (but not all) studies (Ho et al. 2000) have implied that early intervention during the very first episode of psychosis could be associated with better overall prognosis; thus, a major goal in the treatment of schizophrenia is early recognition and timely treatment of the illness.

Management of Schizophrenia

Acute Psychosis

The acute phase of schizophrenia is characterized by psychotic symptoms and often by agitation. Affective symptoms such as depression and mania also may occur. Patients who are unable to care for themselves or who demonstrate a risk of harming themselves or others may require hospitalization. Acute psychosis requires treatment with antipsychotic medication.

Management of an acutely agitated and psychotic patient may require physical restraint and parenteral antipsychotic medication. Many physicians still use a high-potency first-generation antipsychotic either alone or in conjunction with a benzodiazepine (such as lorazepam) and/or an anticholinergic drug (such as benztropine).

If the patient has a history of treatment with antipsychotic medications, it needs to be ascertained whether the current psychosis is the result of noncompliance or of a "breakthrough" episode because of loss of therapeutic response to the medications. Noncompliance with antipsychotic medications is common and is one of the major causes of symptom exacerbation or full-blown relapse (Crow et al. 1986; Lieberman et al. 1993; Robinson et al. 1999). Causes of noncompliance vary, but the most common reasons are side effects, lack of insight into the illness, delusional interpretations about medication, substance abuse, and lack of a supportive environment (Kampman and Lehtinen 1999). With noncompliant patients, it is imperative to focus on improving adherence by providing psychoeducation to the patient (and family, if available), discussing with the patient the reasons for nonadherence, and developing a plan for improved adherence (which could include daily support and monitoring of medication doses). Depot or long-acting injectable medications also should be considered if noncompliance is a persistent or recurring problem. Of course, in the case of apparent breakthrough psychosis, change in the patient's medication regimen may be indicated. Other causes of exacerbation of psychosis may include comorbid substance abuse or dependence and comorbid depression, as well as psychosocial stressors including difficulties with housing, employment, benefits, insurance, disability, family, and friends. Therefore, although medications are undoubtedly the mainstay for initial treatment of psychosis, other treatment such as psychotherapy, group therapy, family therapy, dual-diagnosis treatment, social skills training, and case management are important adjuncts to pharmacological management.

First-Episode Psychosis

Emphasis on the early diagnosis and treatment of the first psychotic episode of schizophrenia arises from the recent evidence from some, but not all (Ho et al. 2000), studies suggesting that longer durations of untreated psychosis may be associated with poorer overall outcome (Birchwood 1992; Loebel et al. 1992; Wyatt 1991).

Because of their more favorable neurological side-effect profiles (mainly the reduced risks of adverse neurological events such as parkinsonism, akathisia, and tardive dyskinesia), the second-generation antipsychotics are often considered for the initial treatment of first-episode psychosis. However, as discussed below, many of these medications are associated with other medically important adverse effects, including weight gain, and because patients are likely to require long-term treatment, clinicians should pay close attention to all reported side effects and their potential morbidity. In general, a conservative titration schedule is appropriate for first-episode patients, in part to minimize side effects but also to take into account that these patients may require only low doses for the control and remission of symptoms (Remington et al. 1998; Robinson et al. 1999; Schooler et al. 2005; Wyatt 1995).

After remission of an initial episode of psychosis in a patient with a diagnosis of schizophrenia, potential discontinuation of medication, even if done very gradually, is controversial and often not attempted. Any decision about this should be made in light of studies showing that the relapse rate is very high after medication discontinuation in first-episode schizophrenia (Crow et al. 1986; Johnson 1985; Kane et al. 1982; Robinson et al. 1999). Gitlin et al. (2001), using a low threshold to define recurrence of symptoms, reported that the relapse rate in the first year after medication discontinuation was 78% and that this rate increased to 98% by the end of the second year.

Choice of Antipsychotics

Since the early 1990s, second-generation antipsychotics have been used widely. The National Institute of Mental Health (NIMH) sponsored the Clinical Antipsychotic Trials of Intervention Effectiveness (CATIE) study (Lieberman et al. 2005), which was designed to compare the effectiveness of four second-generation antipsychotics (olanzapine, quetiapine, risperidone, ziprasidone) and a representative first-generation antipsychotic (perphenazine) in "real world" schizophrenia patients. The primary outcome parameter was discontinuation of treatment. Of the 1,432 subjects who received at least one dose, 74% discontinued study medication before 18 months: 64% of subjects on olanzapine discontinued, compared with 74%–82% on perphenazine, quetiapine, risperidone, and ziprasidone. More subjects receiving olanzapine discontinued due to weight gain and metabolic effects, whereas more subjects assigned to perphenazine discontinued due to EPS (Lieberman et al. 2005). Interestingly, individuals assigned to olanzapine and risperidone who were continuing with their baseline medication had significantly longer times until discontinuation than did those assigned to switch antipsychotics (Essock et al. 2006). Phase II of the CATIE study included two treatment pathways (efficacy and tolerability) with randomized follow-up medication based on the reason for discontinuation of the previous antipsychotic drug (McEvoy et al. 2006; Stroup et al. 2006). For subjects who failed to improve with an atypical antipsychotic, clozapine was more effective than switching to another atypical antipsychotic (McEvoy et al. 2006), and in patients who failed to respond to perphenazine, olanzapine and quetiapine were more effective than risperidone (Stroup et al. 2006). Moreover, in subjects who discontinued an atypical agent for tolerability or efficacy reasons but who were unwilling to be randomly assigned to clozapine, risperidone and olanzapine were more effective than quetiapine or ziprasidone (Stroup et al. 2006).

(Note: Since the CATIE study was published, several new antipsychotics—asenapine, iloperidone, lurasidone, and paliperidone—have been approved by the U.S. Food and Drug Administration [FDA]. However, because they have not yet been directly compared against other first- or second-generation agents, little is known about the effectiveness of these newer antipsychotics relative to older agents.) Finally, although the CATIE cost-effectiveness analysis found perphenazine to be less costly than, and similar in effectiveness (based on quality-adjusted life-years) to, each of the atypical antipsychotics tested, the authors noted that their results could not be generalized to all patient populations; they therefore concluded that the study findings did not warrant policies that would unconditionally restrict access to a particular medication (Rosenheck et al. 2006).

Similar to the NIMH-sponsored CATIE study, the United Kingdom's National Health Service funded the Cost Utility of the Latest Antipsychotic Drugs in Schizophrenia Study (CUtLASS). This study of 227 schizophrenia-spectrum patients randomly assigned to first- and second-generation antipsychotics (other than clozapine) found no difference between the groups in quality of life, symptoms, or health care costs at 1 year (Jones et al. 2006).

Neither the CATIE nor the CUtLASS study addressed the comparative effects of oral and long-acting injectable antipsychotics. Older mirror-image studies in which patients served as their own controls provide evidence of substantial benefit for first-generation long-acting injectable (LAI) antipsychotics over first-generation oral medications (Schooler 2003). At present, risperidone, paliperidone, and olanzapine are the only second-generation antipsychotics available in LAI formulations.

Taken together, the CATIE and the CUtLASS studies indicate that antipsychotic medications are generally effective but have a variety of shortcomings. Physicians need to be well informed about the differential tolerability profiles among the antipsychotics. Several of the first-generation agents clearly have a high risk of EPS and tardive dyskinesia (Glazer 2000b; Jeste et al. 1998; Tollefson et al. 1997). Risperidone and paliperidone tend to elevate serum prolactin levels and may cause EPS at higher doses. Iloperidone may elevate serum prolactin to a lesser degree. Akathisia and other EPS may also be common with aripiprazole and lurasidone. Although weight gain and metabolic disturbances are associated with most of the second-generation agents, olanzapine and clozapine appear to have the highest likelihood of causing these side effects (Allison et al. 1999; American Diabetes Association et al. 2004). Sedation is most commonly observed in patients receiving asenapine, quetiapine, olanzapine, ziprasidone, or clozapine. Ziprasidone, paliperidone, and iloperidone carry product labeling for QTc prolongation and should be used with caution in patients at risk for QTc prolongation. Finally, clozapine, because of its side effects of agranulocytosis, seizures, and myocarditis, is generally reserved for patients with treatment-resistant illness or suicidality.

Maintenance Treatment

The major goals of maintenance treatment are prevention of relapse and improvement in psychosocial and vocational functioning. The primary methods used to achieve these goals are, as at all phases, an integration of optimal psychopharmacological and psychosocial treatments. Treatment and prevention of other psychiatric comorbidities, such as substance abuse and dependence, are important aspects of maintenance treatment. Also, prevention and treatment of medical comorbidities that may be associated with second-generation antipsychotics, as well as those that may result from the lifestyle of some patients with schizophrenia who are given these drugs, have become a very important part of long-term management.

Prevention of relapse improves long-term clinical outcomes (Wyatt et al. 1998) and reduces the associated economic burden of the illness (Bernardo et al. 2006). With each relapse, the time it takes to achieve clinical stability lengthens, with the possible consequence of ultimate unresponsiveness to treatment (Lieberman et al. 1993; Wyatt et al. 1998). Nonadherence to medication is a significant predictor of relapse (Schooler 2006). LAI antipsychotics may have the potential to improve medication adherence and thus improve long-term outcomes.

Treatment-Resistant Schizophrenia

At least 30% of patients have an incomplete to poor response to antipsychotics, with persistent psychotic symptoms (Kane et al. 1988, 2007; Tamminga 1999). However, failure to respond to one or two antipsychotic medications does not necessarily imply that a patient will not respond to a third agent. For research purposes, Kane et al. (1988) operationally defined *treatment resistance* as 1) lack of significant response to at least three adequate trials of neuroleptics from at least two different chemical classes in the past 5 years and 2) persistently poor social and occupational functioning.

Most of the available data suggest that clozapine is the most effective drug for treatment-resistant schizophrenia (Kane et al. 2001; S.W. Lewis et al. 2006; McEvoy et al. 2006). However, because of the serious side effects produced by clozapine and the requirement for frequent white blood cell count monitoring, some patients and some psychiatrists are reluctant to use it, and some patients are unable to tolerate it. However, whether the other second-generation agents even approach the effectiveness of clozapine for the treatment of these chronically ill patients is unclear. Evidence regarding whether either risperidone (Bondolfi et al. 1998; Breier et al. 1999; Volavka et al. 2002) or olanzapine (Buchanan et al. 2005; Tollefson et al. 2001; Volavka et al. 2002) is as effective as clozapine is mixed. Other preliminary data also suggest the possible utility of quetiapine, aripiprazole, and ziprasidone in treatment-resistant patients (Emsley et al. 2000; Kane et al. 2006, 2007).

Multiple controlled trials have assessed whether combining two antipsychotics is more effective than using antipsychotic monotherapy. Thus far, the evidence is mixed and inconclusive (Barbui 2008; Correll et al. 2009; Evins et al. 2005). In summary, clozapine remains the primary medication for treatment-resistant schizophrenia, although some studies suggest that other second-generation agents also may have a role in the management of this disorder. Clinically judicious addition of other agents, such as mood stabilizers, may be used. Clearly, more research is needed to guide treatment in such patients.

Neurocognitive Deficits

Neurocognitive deficits, especially disturbances in executive functioning, memory, and attention (Green 1996; Green et al. 2000), are closely associated with the long-term functional outcome of patients with schizophrenia. It appears that second-generation antipsychotics may improve some aspects of cognition in schizophrenia, as found in a meta-analysis of 15 studies on the cognition-enhancing effects of these drugs (Bilder et al. 2002). The therapeutic effects of the newer antipsychotics are most notable in measures of verbal fluency and executive functioning, whereas improvement in memory may be more limited. However, data obtained from the CATIE trial (Keefe et al. 2007) show that at 18 months of treatment, perphenazine was actually more effective than any of the second-generation drugs in improving all domains of neurocognitive deficits (Keefe et al. 2007). The authors postulate that a number of factors could potentially explain this unexpected finding, such as sample size, differences between midpotency drugs such as perphenazine and the high-potency drugs (e.g., haloperidol) that were commonly used in prior studies, the real-world features of the CATIE sample, and prior drug trials before entering the study (Keefe et al. 2007). Finally, it is not clear whether any of the apparent statistically significant improvements in neurocognitive deficits measured in the laboratory can actually be translated into improved functional outcomes, for example, in terms of employment, school performance, or social role (see Green 2002).

Psychosocial Treatment of Schizophrenia

Despite the proven efficacy of antipsychotics in the treatment of schizophrenia, most patients continue to have some degree of residual positive symptoms, negative symptoms, and cognitive deficits, and many have difficulty attaining or regaining their desired level of social and occupational functioning. To address functional goals, treatment is ideally offered by a multidisciplinary team that includes, at a minimum, a medication prescriber and a clinician who understands psychosocial rehabilitation but may also include employment and housing specialists. Programs that utilize clinical case managers to directly assist patients in accessing services and to provide the psychosocial interventions are ideal (Rapp and Goscha 2004). To date, several different types of psychosocial interventions have been empirically shown to reduce rates of relapse and rehospitalization, and a variety of treatments may assist patients in acquiring social and vocational skills and possibly in managing residual psychotic symptoms (Bustillo et al. 2001; Lauriello et al. 1999; Penn and Mueser 1996). Furthermore, the interaction between pharmacological and psychosocial treatments appears to be more than additive because each can enhance the effects of the other and affect different domains of outcome (Marder 2000).

Relapse Prevention

It has long been noted that patients with highly critical or overinvolved family members (so-called high-expressed-emotion [EE] families) have a higher risk of relapse (Brown and Rutter 1966). In a classic study, Goldstein et al. (1978) reported that a 6-week therapy focusing on teaching families more effective communication dispute-resolution skills reduced relapse rates for up to 6 months. Many other studies have since confirmed the efficacy of family psychoeducation interventions (involving education and training in problem-solving techniques and/or cognitive and behavioral management strategies) to prevent relapse and to improve other outcomes (Falloon et al. 1982; Pilling et al. 2002; Pitschel-Walz et al. 2001; Tarrier et al. 1988). In addition, the positive impact of family interventions seems to persist beyond the time of intervention (Sellwood et al. 2001) and is independent of either the specific form or the intensity of the intervention (Bustillo et al. 2001).

Another psychosocial intervention that has been shown to be effective in preventing relapse or rehospitalization in schizophrenia is assertive community treatment (ACT). This intervention, which involves intensive multidisciplinary team management and service delivery in both community and inpatient settings, is designed for individuals who experience intractable symptoms and high levels of functional impairment. At least 30 studies of ACT have shown advantages over standard community treatment in reducing symptoms, family burden, and hospitalization and in improving independent living, housing stability, and quality of life (Mueser et al. 1998; Phillips et al. 2001; Stein and Test 1980). However, it appears that the advantages of ACT do not persist after discontinuation of the program, even after prolonged delivery of services.

Improvement of Psychosocial Functioning

Most patients with schizophrenia have personal goals that involve social and occupational functioning in the community. Hence, psychosocial treatment of patients with schizophrenia targets impairments in these areas. In a 3-year study, Hogarty et al. (1997a) found that weekly individual personal therapy, in which an incremental psychoeducational approach based on the patient's phase of recovery was used, had a significant advantage over supportive therapy, family therapy, and combined treatment in improving social adjustment but not in preventing relapse (Hogarty et al. 1997b). Interestingly, cognitive-behavioral therapy (CBT) may have a role in the management of persistent psychotic symptoms (Chadwick et al. 1994; Granholm et al. 2005; Tarrier et al. 2000). CBT involves the use of techniques such as distraction, cognitive reframing of psychotic beliefs or experiences, and verbal challenge followed by reality testing (Penn and Mueser 1996). Reviews and meta-analyses of CBT for psychosis suggest a positive effect for reducing symptoms (Bellack 2004; Jones et al. 2004; Pilling et al. 2002).

Social skills training (SST) is one treatment strategy to help individuals acquire interpersonal disease management and independent living skills. Reviews of SST (Bellack and Mueser 1993; Kopelowicz et al. 2006) have described three models of SST: basic model, social problem-solving model, and cognitive remediation model. Within the *basic model*, complex social scenarios are broken down to simpler components, the therapist models correct behaviors, and the patient learns through repeated role-play. The combination of this form of SST with antipsychotic medication appears to be more effective than medication alone in reducing relapse (Hogarty et al. 1986).

The *social problem-solving model* focuses on impaired information processing, which is thought to cause social skills deficits. This model targets symptom and medication management, recreation, basic conversation, and self-care in educational modules, and it has been shown to be modestly effective in enhancing skills (Eckman et al. 1992; Liberman et al. 1998; Marder et al. 1996). Interventions that utilize cueing and support in everyday community interactions by friends or family seem to improve transfer of newly learned social skills to community functioning (e.g., Glynn et al. 2002).

Finally, the *cognitive remediation model* of SST targets more fundamental cognitive deficits, in areas such as attention, memory, and planning, with the aim of supporting more complex cognitive processes used in learning social skills. Small studies have reported mixed results for more complex cognitive and social skills (Hodel and Brenner 1994; Spencer et al. 1994; Wykes et al. 1999). An integrated approach to the concomitant training of neurocognitive and social cognitive abilities as well as social skills resulted in long-term improvement in social adjustment (Hogarty et al. 2006; McGurk et al. 2007).

Work to improve social functioning has focused on social cognition, the capacity to perceive the intentions and dispositions of others (Penn et al. 2006). A preliminary study of social cognition and interaction training during 18 weekly sessions consisting of emotion training, figuring out situations, and integrating skills into real life suggests that this may be a promising approach for improving interpersonal functioning and for directly managing symptoms of psychosis (Combs et al. 2007).

Illness management and recovery (IMR) is a manualized package of empirically supported approaches (psychoeducation, cognitive-behavioral approaches for medication adherence, relapse prevention planning, SST, and coping skills training) delivered in weekly group or individual sessions that are utilized with a recovery focus that targets each individual's personal life goals (Mueser et al. 2006). Preliminary research shows that this combination of approaches results in improved symptoms and better community functioning (Mueser et al. 2006).

Although family psychoeducation, CBT, SST, and IMR may improve symptoms and/or social functioning, they do not appear to affect employment status. However, more than 14 studies suggest that supported employment programs, which use rapid job searches, on-the-job training, continuous job support, and integration with mental health treatment, are more effective than traditional methods in helping patients obtain competitive employment (Bond 2004).

In addition to employment, the ability to maintain a residence in the community is an important marker of community functioning. Simple provision of access to affordable housing by Section 8 certificates improves housing stability (Hurlburt et al. 1996b). Supported housing, broadly defined as access to independent housing of the patient's choice (often supported with housing subsidies) that is coupled with access to community mental health and support services, improves residential stability and reduces hospitalization (Rog 2004). ACT for homeless individuals has also been shown to reduce homelessness (Coldwell and Bender 2007).

As multiple effective psychosocial interventions exist and are still being developed, the choice of which intervention to apply should depend not only on therapeutic efficacy but also on each individual's goals and preferences. Patients and their families need to be given information about treatment options and should be engaged in discussions with their treatment providers about how treatments can be useful in the context of an individual's symptoms, comorbidities, needs, and preferences.

Management of Medical Comorbidity

Obesity, Metabolic Syndrome, and Diabetes Mellitus

Medication side effects, as well as lifestyle and disease factors, place patients with schizophrenia at increased risk of developing obesity and metabolic side effects, including glucose intolerance, type 2 diabetes, diabetic ketoacidosis, and hyperlipidemia (Dixon et al. 2000; Meyer and Koro 2004; Wirshing et al. 2002, 2003). While clinically significant weight gain occurs in a substantial proportion of patients receiving an antipsychotic medication (Baptista 1999), a convincing body of evidence indicates that certain atypical antipsychotics cause more weight gain than other agents (Allison et al. 1999; Lieberman et al. 2005; Wirshing et al. 1999). A large meta-analytic study of atypical and typical antipsychotics (Wirshing et al. 1999) found a mean weight gain of 9.8 lbs with clozapine, 9.1 lbs with olanzapine, and 4.6 lbs with risperidone, compared with 2.4 lbs with haloperidol, whereas the atypical antipsychotic ziprasidone was associated with a less than 1-lb weight gain. Furthermore, the CATIE study demonstrated a greater than 7% weight gain from baseline in 30% of patients receiving olanzapine, 16% of those receiving quetiapine, 14% of those receiving risperidone, 12% of those receiving perphenazine, and 7% of those receiving ziprasidone (Lieberman et al. 2005). Compared with risperidone, the risk of weight gain may be higher for iloperidone (Weiden et al. 2008) and lower for asenapine (Potkin et al. 2007) and lurasidone (Citrome 2011a, 2011b). The propensity of an antipsychotic to cause weight gain and other cardiometabolic side effects may be substantially greater when it is given to children and young adults for the first time (Correll et al. 2009).

Diabetes mellitus is estimated to occur two to four times more frequently in patients with schizophrenia compared with the general population (Dixon et al. 2000; Goff et al. 2005; Henderson et al. 2000; Mukherjee et al. 1996; Wirshing et al. 1998). While the risk of diabetes in schizophrenia is likely multifactorial, accrued evidence clearly indicates that atypical antipsychotics are associated with glucose dysregulation (Jin et al. 2004). Numerous studies of hyperglycemia, new-onset diabetes mellitus, and diabetic ketoacidosis (Dixon et al. 2000; Gianfrancesco et al. 2002; Henderson et al. 2000; Wirshing et al. 2002) led to heightened concern, the issuance of warnings by regulatory authorities and class labeling (Jin et al. 2004), and published consensus guidelines on monitoring for cardiometabolic risk (American Diabetes Association et al. 2004). Some atypical antipsychotics appear to increase risk for diabetes beyond typical agents: clozapine and olanzapine are described as having the greatest risk for diabetes (Kessing et al. 2010; Leslie and Rosenheck 2004; Yood et al. 2009). The risk associated with other antipsychotics is not as clear, although the risk associated with aripiprazole, ziprasidone, and lurasidone is described as being low or not different from the risk associated with typical agents in adults with chronic schizophrenia.

Certain atypical antipsychotics (particularly clozapine, olanzapine, and quetiapine) and low-potency conventional agents have been shown to be associated with hyperlipidemia (Henderson et al. 2000; Meyer and Koro 2004; Osser et al. 1999), whereas ziprasidone and aripiprazole do not appear to carry this adverse effect (Kingsbury et al. 2001; Meyer and Koro 2004). The co-occurrence of atherogenic dyslipidemia along with abdominal adiposity, insulin resistance, impaired fasting glucose or overt diabetes mellitus, and hypertension constitutes the cluster of clinical features known as the metabolic syndrome. Baseline data from the CATIE study indicated that more than 40% of subjects had metabolic syndrome, with women carrying greater risk than men (McEvoy et al. 2005).

Centrally acting weight-loss drugs that have the potential to increase the activity of biogenic amines could theoretically exacerbate symptoms of psychosis in this population. However, controlled studies of metformin and nizatidine yielded mixed results (Ellinger et al. 2010; Praharaj et al. 2011), whereas controlled studies of topiramate, reboxetine, and modafinil showed beneficial effects on cardiometabolic risk factors, although topiramate treatment was associated with substantial side effects (Ellinger et al. 2010). Orlistat, the non–centrally acting weight-control drug, was not better than placebo in one controlled study (Joffe et al. 2008). A case series (Hamoui et al. 2004) suggested that bariatric surgery was as effective in promoting weight loss in patients with schizophrenia as it is in other obese patients.

The differential propensity of the various agents to cause weight gain, as well as glucose and lipid dysregulation, should be taken into consideration when selecting an antipsychotic medication. Clinicians should employ pre- and posttreatment monitoring such as that recommended by the American Diabetes Association–American Psychiatric Association consensus panel (American Diabetes Association et al. 2004). Patients who develop cardiometabolic abnormalities may require a medication switch, monitoring, and management of the new abnormalities with behavioral and pharmacological strategies in collaboration with an internist.

Cigarette Smoking

Reports indicate that up to 90% of patients with schizophrenia smoke cigarettes, a rate more than four times that seen in the general population (Brown et al. 2000; Dalack et al. 1998; Meyer and Nasrallah 2003). Treatment of nicotine addiction appears to be more difficult in the schizophrenia population compared with both the general and other psychiatric populations (Covey et al. 1994). Nonetheless, evidence suggests that a multimodality approach that integrates motivation-based treatment (Brunette et al. 2011; Steinberg et al. 2004), addiction treatment strategies, and tobacco dependence treatment into mental health settings may be beneficial (Ziedonis et al. 2003). FDA-approved cessation medications combined with group CBT lead to cessation in up to half of patients who initiate treatment (Evins et al. 2005; George et al. 2000; Nino-Gomez et al. 2010; Weiner et al. 2001; Williams et al. 2004).

Extrapyramidal Side Effects

Parkinsonism and acute dystonia are associated with the degree of dopamine D_2 receptor occupancy in the striatum (Kapur and Remington 1996). Thus, high-potency first-generation antipsychotics such as haloperidol have the greatest propensity (especially at high doses) to cause these side effects, but many second-generation agents also may cause EPS in a dose-dependent manner. The CATIE study found that the rate of drug discontinuation due to reported EPS was 8% in the patient group treated with the typical antipsychotic perphenazine, with rates of 4% for ziprasidone, 3% for risperidone and quetiapine, and 2% for olanzapine (Lieberman et al. 2005). Among the second-generation agents, iloperidone, asenapine, aripiprazole, olanzapine, quetiapine, and clozapine do not appear to produce clinically significant parkinsonism or dystonia (Citrome 2011a; Kane et al. 2008; Lieberman et al. 2005; Schoemaker et al. 2010; Stip and Tourjman 2010).

Akathisia, a disturbing sense of inner restlessness and the inability of the patient to stay still, is associated with seemingly purposeless movements (such as tapping or pacing) that may be noticeable to the examiner. Akathisia is less likely to occur with clozapine, olanzapine, quetiapine, iloperidone, and low-potency first-generation antipsychotic medications (Citrome 2011a; Kane et al. 2008; Lieberman et al. 2005; Schoemaker et al. 2010; Stip and Tourjman 2010). Although lowering the dose of the antipsychotic is an obvious treatment for akathisia, addition of a β-blocker (e.g., propranolol) is often effective. Anticholinergic drugs and benzodiazepines are generally not that effective but can be tried in patients who fail to respond to β-blockers, and anticholinergics also may be useful in patients with coexisting parkinsonism.

Parkinsonism (Osser 1999), characterized by tremor, rigidity, and bradykinesia, can occur early in treatment, usually within the initial weeks or months. Bradykinesia includes generalized slowing of movement and a mask-like face (with a loss of facial expression); it may be confused with depression or negative symptoms. One variant of parkinsonism, akinesia, can coexist with bradykinesia (but without tremor or rigidity) and may be associated with symptoms of apathy and fatigue. The "rabbit syndrome" (Casey 1999), occurring after months or years of antipsychotic drug treatment, is also a variant of parkinsonism and is characterized by a perioral and jaw tremor. Anticholinergic medications are the treatment of choice and usually are effective. Lower doses of antipsychotics and a switch to an agent less likely to produce EPS also may be helpful.

Acute dystonia occurs most commonly in young males during the week after initiation of antipsychotics or following an abrupt and rapid dose increase (Ayd 1961; Barnes and Spence 2000; Remington and Kapur 1996). The dystonia may appear as torticollis, trismus, tongue protrusion, pharyngeal constriction, laryngospasm, blepharospasm, oculogyric crisis, or abnormal contractions of any part of the body. Clinically, in addition to the dystonic muscular contractions that may be immediately noticeable, the patient may complain of tongue thickening, throat tightening, and difficulty speaking or swallowing. Acute treatment with either an anticholinergic agent or an antihistamine is usually highly effective but may need to be repeated at intervals. Should respiratory difficulty develop, medications may need to be given parenterally.

Tardive Dyskinesia and Tardive Dystonia

Tardive dyskinesia, which is a syndrome of potentially irreversible involuntary movements, and tardive dystonia, which is characterized by sustained muscle contractions, can gradually emerge after a prolonged period of treatment with antipsychotic medications. Accumulating evidence suggests that the second-generation antipsychotics are less likely to cause these tardive syndromes than the first-generation drugs (Jeste et al. 1998; Kane et al. 1993; Marder et al. 2002; Margolese et al. 2005; Shirzadi and Ghaemi 2006;

Tarsy and Baldessarini 2006; Tollefson et al. 1997). However, because many patients have had exposure to more than one second-generation agent, it is difficult to determine the risk associated with individual agents. It appears that in comparison with the first-generation agents, the second-generation drugs collectively carry one-third to one-twelfth the risk of causing tardive dyskinesia and tardive dystonia (Correll et al. 2004, 2009; Kane 2004; Leucht et al. 2003b; Margolese et al. 2005).

The most common form of tardive dyskinesia involves dyskinetic movements of the orofacial and buccolingual musculature, manifesting as grimacing, facial tics, lip smacking, chewing, and wormlike movements of the tongue. Involvement of the neck, axial, and extremity musculature also may occur in the form of choreoathetoid movements, which on rare occasions may involve laryngopharyngeal and respiratory muscles. Tardive dystonia may occur earlier in treatment than tardive dyskinesia and is characterized by slow, sustained twisting movements of the head, neck, trunk, and extremities; blepharospasm, torticollis, facial grimacing, back arching, and hyperextension and rotation of the limbs may also be seen (Simpson 2000).

Risk factors for tardive dyskinesia include older age and female sex (Kane 2004), whereas tardive dystonia is more common in younger patients and males. Other important risk factors for tardive dyskinesia include high doses of medication (Glazer 2000a, 2000c) and the presence of other extrapyramidal syndromes (Kane 2004).

Although no treatment has been proven to be effective for tardive dyskinesia, several management strategies may be clinically useful. Clinicians should screen patients taking antipsychotic medications on a regular basis. If tardive dyskinesia develops, switching from a first-generation to a second-generation drug may be helpful. For those patients who are taking a second-generation agent, a switch to another second-generation drug may be considered. Among the second-generation drugs, evidence suggests that clozapine may reduce symptoms of tardive dyskinesia (Glazer 2000a; Lieberman et al. 1991). Patients with tardive dyskinesia who are taking anticholinergic medications should discontinue these medications, because they can worsen tardive dyskinesia. Finally, the symptoms of tardive dystonia may be alleviated by reducing the dosages of the antipsychotics, by switching from first-generation to second-generation agents (including clozapine), by using anticholinergics, and/or by administering dopamine-depleting agents, such as reserpine or tetrabenazine (Simpson 2000).

Neuroleptic Malignant Syndrome

Neuroleptic malignant syndrome (NMS), which occurs in about 1%–2% of patients receiving typical antipsychotic medication and is potentially fatal in up to 20% of the cases (without treatment), has been reported to occur during treatment with both the typical (Caroff and Mann 1993) and the atypical (Ananth et al. 2004; Hasan and Buckley 1998; Wirshing et al. 2000) antipsychotics. Risk factors include intramuscular injections, rapid escalation to high doses, dehydration, restraint use, and high temperatures. Catatonia and severe disorganization are clinical symptoms that may be associated with a high risk for NMS (Berardi et al. 2002). Symptoms of NMS include hyperpyrexia, altered consciousness, muscle rigidity and dystonia, autonomic nervous system dysfunction, and laboratory tests indicating elevated creatine phosphokinase, liver enzymes, and white blood cell count. Early detection and rapid treatment of this medical emergency are crucial and include discontinuation of the antipsychotic, treatment in a medical setting that can support vital functioning, and in some cases the use of a dopamine agonist such as bromocriptine or dantrolene, a muscle relaxant (Koppel 1998; Susman 2001).

Hyperprolactinemia

Antipsychotic medications—particularly some of the typical agents, as well as risperidone, paliperidone, and lurasidone—can produce an increase in serum prolactin levels (Dickson and Glazer 1999; Marder et al. 2004). It is well known that hyperprolactinemia secondary to medical disorders (e.g., pituitary tumor) can produce galactorrhea, hypogonadism, and osteoporosis, all of which have also been reported in patients with schizophrenia (Abraham et al. 1996; Ghadirian et al. 1982; Riecher-Rossler et al. 1994; Windgassen et al. 1996; Yazigi et al. 1997). Yet the relationships between antipsychotic-induced hyperprolactinemia and these conditions, perhaps with the exception of galactorrhea (Windgassen et al. 1996), remain unclear, with conflicting reports in the literature (Canuso et al. 2002; Costa et al. 2007; Hummer et al. 2005; Kinon et al. 2006; Kleinberg et al. 1999; O'Keane and Meaney 2005).

Clinicians should inquire about possible adverse effects of hyperprolactinemia and aim to diminish them. If a patient is symptomatic, prolactin levels should be obtained and medical causes of hyperprolactinemia ruled out. Prolactin elevation associated with galactorrhea, or sexual and menstrual dysfunction, may be minimized by dosage reduction or by a medication change to an atypical antipsychotic with less prolactin-elevating potential (Canuso et al. 1998; Dickson and Glazer 1999).

Psychiatric Conditions Comorbid With Schizophrenia and Their Treatment

Substance-Related Disorders

Nearly one-half of the patients with schizophrenia are reported to have a lifetime history of an alcohol or a substance use disorder, compared with 16% of the general population (Regier et al. 1990). Alcohol is the most commonly abused substance in chronically ill patients, followed by cannabis and cocaine (Selzer and Lieberman 1993; Sevy et al. 1990). As in the general population, men with schizophrenia are more likely to abuse substances than are women (Mueser et al. 1995).

Comorbid substance use has a deleterious effect on the course of schizophrenia (Grech et al. 1999); use of even small amounts can produce negative effects (Drake et al. 2001; D'Souza et al. 2005). Patients with schizophrenia and substance abuse are at increased risk for infectious diseases such as HIV, hepatitis B, and hepatitis C (Rosenberg et al. 2001); in addition, alcohol and substance use is associated with clinical worsening, poor functioning, and an increased rate of hospitalizations and homelessness (Dixon et al. 1990; Drake and Mueser 1996; Hurlburt et al. 1996a; Negrete et al. 1986; Soni and Brownlee 1991). In some studies, more than 50% of the first-episode patients have been reported to have cannabis use disorder (Rolfe et al. 1999), often complicating the diagnosis of a psychotic disorder (Addington 1999).

Although obtaining information from patients about the use of substances of abuse should be a standard part of a medical history, alcohol or substance abuse is often underrecognized and undertreated in mental health settings (Ananth et al. 1989). Because patients often deny use of alcohol and drugs, clinicians also should pursue collateral reports from family members, case managers, and others involved in the delivery of services to patients. Patients with schizophrenia and a comorbid alcohol or substance use disorder require treatment for both disorders (Bellack and DiClemente 1999), optimally in programs that provide long-term comprehensive services along with integrated mental health and substance abuse treatment, including medication management (Drake and Mueser 2001; Minkoff 1989; Osher and Kofoed 1989).

Although there is no agreed-upon pharmacological treatment approach for patients with schizophrenia and comorbid alcohol or substance use disorders (Green et al. 2007, 2008; Wilkins 1997), some investigators have been interested in the potential role of atypical antipsychotics in these patients. The atypical antipsychotic that has been studied most in this population is clozapine. Preliminary studies of clozapine have reported promising results for reducing alcohol and drug use (Brunette et al. 2006; Buckley et al. 1999; Drake et al. 2000; Green et al. 2003; Lee et al. 1998; Zimmet et al. 2000). A recent small randomized trial provided some confirmation of these preliminary studies (Brunette et al. 2011).

Data concerning the potential effects of the other atypical antipsychotics on substance abuse and relapse prevention are even more preliminary. Reports are mixed for risperidone (Albanese 2000; Green et al. 2003; Petrakis et al. 2006; Rubio et al. 2006; Smelson et al. 2000), olanzapine (Littrell et al. 2001; Noordsy et al. 2001; Sayers et al. 2005; Smelson et al. 2006), quetiapine (Brown et al. 2003; Potvin et al. 2006), and aripiprazole (Beresford et al. 2005; Brown et al. 2005). No research has assessed the impact of ziprasidone, asenapine, iloperidone, and lurasidone.

Other possible pharmacological options with evidence for efficacy in the treatment of substance use disorders in schizophrenia include the following: 1) disulfiram for co-occurring alcohol dependence (note that use requires monitoring in patients with schizophrenia) (Kofoed et al. 1986; Mueser et al. 2003; Petrakis et al. 2005); 2) naltrexone for co-occurring alcohol disorders (Petrakis et al. 2004, 2005); 3) the tricyclic antidepressants desipramine and imipramine for comorbid cocaine disorders (Siris et al. 1993; Ziedonis et al. 1992); and 4) bupropion, nicotine replacement therapy, and varenicline for nicotine dependence (Evins et al. 2005; George et al. 2002; Nino-Gomez et al. 2010). Acamprosate, although shown to be effective for alcohol dependence in placebo-controlled trials, has yet to be studied in patients with schizophrenia.

Depression

Schizophrenia is often associated with depressive states, from dysphoria to major depression. The Epidemiologic Catchment Area study suggests that those with schizophrenia have a 14-fold greater risk of depression than the general population (Fenton 2001). At various times, depression has been viewed as an aspect of schizophrenia (McGlashan and Carpenter 1976; Sax et al. 1996), as a response to psychosis (McGlashan and Carpenter 1976; Sax et al. 1996), or as a state occurring after the cessation of frank psychotic symptoms (Birchwood et al. 2000).

Depression in patients with schizophrenia must be differentiated from negative symptoms and EPS; the presence of a core depressed mood and related neurovegetative symptoms should be distinguished from flatness of affect, parkinsonism, and anhedonia (McGlashan and Carpenter 1976). Depression occurring during an exacerbation of psychosis may remit with treatment of the psychosis (Birchwood et al. 2000; Koreen et al. 1993; Tollefson et al. 1999). However, postpsychotic depression classically develops after the resolution or improvement of psychotic symptoms (see Birchwood et al. 2000; Koreen et al. 1993). Dysphoria and demoralization (Iqbal et al. 2000; Siris 2000a) may occur as patients struggle with illness-related disability (Bartels and Drake 1988).

Treatment of depression in patients with schizophrenia may include both psychopharmacological and psychosocial components (Siris 2000b). Because depression may presage an increase in psychosis, the pharmacological treatment of psychotic symptoms should be optimized. Treatment of depression in acute psychosis may be accomplished through the use of antipsychotic medication alone, especially the atypical antipsychotics (Banov et al. 1994; Levinson et al. 1999; Marder et al. 1997; Tollefson et al. 1998).

However, major depression developing after the remission of psychosis often requires the addition of antidepressants (Hogarty et al. 1995; Kirli and Caliskan 1998; Levinson et al. 1999; Siris et al. 1987). Psychosocial interventions can help with demoralization and dysphoria (Siris 2000b).

Suicide

Suicide is one of the leading causes of premature death in patients with schizophrenia, who have a 10% lifetime risk of suicide. Nearly 50% of the patients with schizophrenia attempt suicide during their lifetime (Black et al. 1985; Tsuang et al. 1999). Risk factors include depression and the diagnosis of schizoaffective disorder (Harkavy-Friedman et al. 2004; Radomsky et al. 1999), social isolation (Drake et al. 1986; Goldstein et al. 2006; Potkin et al. 2003), and feelings of hopelessness and disappointment over failure to meet high self-expectations (Kim et al. 2003; Westermeyer et al. 1991). Patients with a higher level of insight and awareness of their illness may be at increased risk (Amador et al. 1996; Bourgeois et al. 2004; Crumlish et al. 2005), as may patients with a poor level of functioning (Kaplan and Harrow 1996).

A history of suicide attempts is one of the strongest predictors of suicide in patients with schizophrenia (Potkin et al. 2003; Rossau and Mortensen 1997; Roy 1982). Moreover, a meta-analysis of 29 case-control and cohort studies indicated that suicide risk factors included previous depressive disorders, drug abuse, agitation or motor restlessness, fear of mental disintegration, poor adherence to treatment, and recent loss (Hawton et al. 2005).

An increased risk of suicide is present in the early phase of the illness (Drake et al. 1985; Kuo et al. 2005; Ran et al. 2005). Suicide risk peaks immediately after admission and shortly after discharge (Qin and Nordentoft 2005; Rossau and Mortensen 1997). Patients in an active phase of the illness (Heila et al. 1997) or with positive symptoms (Kelly et al. 2004) may be at risk, especially if they have prominent symptoms of suspiciousness and delusions (Fenton et al. 1997).

The treating clinician should regularly evaluate the patient's condition, assess for suicide risk factors, and aim to enhance protective factors such as social support and positive coping skills (Montross et al. 2005). Patients who present with suicidal thoughts or behavior require close follow-up and intensive outreach (Drake et al. 1986; Harkavy-Friedman and Nelson 1997). Improved ward safety, effective substance abuse treatment, affective symptom control, and ensured medication adherence are all measures that may prevent suicide (Hawton et al. 2005; Hunt et al. 2006).

Psychopharmacological treatment plays a crucial role in the prevention of suicide. In one study, more than half of the patients who committed suicide were either medication noncompliant or prescribed inadequate doses of antipsychotics, and 23% of the sample were thought to be nonresponsive to treatment (Heila et al. 1999). Moreover, a landmark study of nearly 1,000 patients with schizophrenia and schizoaffective disorder who were at risk for suicide (but who were not necessarily classically treatment resistant) indicated that treatment with clozapine was more likely to decrease suicidality than was treatment with olanzapine (Meltzer et al. 2003).

Obsessive-Compulsive Symptoms

Obsessive-compulsive symptoms are seen in 8.8%–30% of patients with schizophrenia (Berman et al. 1995a; Byerly et al. 2005; Cassano et al. 1998; Ongur and Goff 2005). Although obsessive-compulsive symptoms may be difficult to distinguish from delusions (Eisen et al. 1997), they are important to identify because they may indicate a poor prognosis, yet they may be responsive to specialized treatment regimens (Byerly et al. 2005; Fenton and McGlashan 1986; Hwang et al. 2000; Ongur and Goff 2005). The obsessive-compulsive symptoms in schizophrenia are similar to those found in obsessive-compulsive disorder (Tibbo et al. 2000), although they may not be ego-dystonic in patients with schizophrenia.

Treatment of obsessive-compulsive schizophrenia may require the use of a tricyclic antidepressant or a serotonin reuptake inhibitor with a typical antipsychotic (Berman et al. 1995b; Chang and Berman 1999; Poyurovsky et al. 2000). Although the addition of a serotonin reuptake inhibitor to an atypical antipsychotic may decrease obsessive-compulsive symptoms in these patients (as the addition of a serotonin reuptake inhibitor to some typical agents does), the combined use of some of the serotonin reuptake inhibitors with clozapine, especially, may require care because of the possible increase in blood levels of clozapine.

Future Directions

Although all existing antipsychotic medications have effects on the dopamine system, modulation of other neurotransmitter systems, such as glutamatergic activity, could be a potential target for pharmacological treatment of schizophrenia. Another novel approach to the treatment of schizophrenia is the development of drugs that act as partial dopamine agonists. These drugs bind to dopamine receptors, including the presynaptic autoreceptors, with high affinity but with variable intrinsic activity, depending on the activity level of the target system. Because of this, they exert a wide range of modulatory effects on the dopaminergic system. The first FDA-approved drug with this mechanism was aripiprazole.

Given increasing evidence suggesting that neurocognitive deficits are pervasive in patients with schizophrenia and that they are important determinants of long-term functional outcome, there has been considerable interest in developing compounds that target such deficits. Drugs that may be effective, at least in theory, in the treatment of neurocognitive deficits include muscarinic agonists, $alpha_7$ nicotinic receptor agonists (Martin and Freedman 2007), ampakines (agonists of the AMPA [amino-3-hydroxy-5-methyl-4-isoxazole propionic acid] class of glutamate receptors) (Goff and Coyle 2001), class I metabotropic glutamate receptor agonists (Moghaddam 2004), dopamine D_1 receptor agonists (Williams and Castner 2006), and $alpha_2$ γ-aminobutyric acid type A ($GABA_A$) receptor agonists (Lewis and Gonzalez-Burgos 2006). Although clinical experience with these drugs is quite limited, ongoing clinical trials are under way to test the possible efficacy of at least some of these compounds.

References

Abraham G, Friedman RH, Verghese C: Osteoporosis demonstrated by dual energy x-ray absorptiometry in chronic schizophrenic patients. Biol Psychiatry 40:430–431, 1996

Addington J: Early intervention strategies for comorbid cannabis use and psychosis. Presented at the Inaugural International Cannabis and Psychosis Conference, Melbourne, Australia, February 16–19, 1999

Albanese MJ: Risperidone in substance abusers with bipolar disorder. Presented at the 39th Annual Meeting of the American College of Neuropsychopharmacology, San Juan, Puerto Rico, 2000

Allison DB, Mentore JL, Heo M, et al: Antipsychotic-induced weight gain: a comprehensive research synthesis. Am J Psychiatry 156:1686–1696, 1999

Amador XF, Friedman JH, Kasapis C, et al: Suicidal behavior in schizophrenia and its relationship to awareness of illness. Am J Psychiatry 153:1185–1188, 1996

American Diabetes Association, American Psychiatric Association, American Association of Clinical Endocrinologists, et al: Consensus development conference on antipsychotic drugs and obesity and diabetes. J Clin Psychiatry 65:267–272, 2004

American Psychiatric Association: Diagnostic and Statistical Manual of Mental Disorders, 4th Edition, Text Revision. Washington, DC, American Psychiatric Association, 2000

Ananth J, Vandewater S, Kamal M, et al: Missed diagnosis of substance abuse in psychiatric patients. Hosp Community Psychiatry 40:297–299, 1989

Ananth J, Parameswaran S, Gunatilake S, et al: Neuroleptic malignant syndrome and atypical antipsychotic drugs. J Clin Psychiatry 65:464–470, 2004

Andreasen NC: Positive vs. negative schizophrenia: a critical evaluation. Schizophr Bull 11:380–389, 1985

Angermeyer MC, Kuhn L, Goldstein JM: Gender and the course of schizophrenia: differences in treated outcomes. Schizophr Bull 16:293–307, 1990

Ayd FJ Jr: A survey of drug-induced extrapyramidal reactions. JAMA 175:1054–1060, 1961

Aylward E, Walker E, Bettes B: Intelligence in schizophrenia: meta-analysis of the research. Schizophr Bull 10:430–459, 1984

Banov MD, Zarate CA Jr, Tohen M, et al: Clozapine therapy in refractory affective disorders: polarity predicts response in long-term follow-up. J Clin Psychiatry 55:295–300, 1994

Baptista T: Body weight gain induced by antipsychotic drugs: mechanisms and management. Acta Psychiatr Scand 100:3–16, 1999

Barbui C: Intramuscular haloperidol plus promethazine is more effective and safer than haloperidol alone for rapid tranquillisation of agitated mentally ill patients. Evid Based Ment Health 11:86–87, 2008

Barnes TR, Spence SA: Movement disorders associated with antipsychotic drugs: clinical and biological implications, in Psychopharmacology of Schizophrenia. Edited by Reverly MA, Deakin JFW. New York, Oxford University Press, 2000, pp 178–210

Bartels SJ, Drake RE: Depressive symptoms in schizophrenia: comprehensive differential diagnosis. Compr Psychiatry 29:467–483, 1988

Bellack AS: Skills training for people with severe mental illness. Psychiatr Rehabil J 27:375–391, 2004

Bellack AS, DiClemente CC: Treating substance abuse among patients with schizophrenia. Psychiatr Serv 50:75–80, 1999

Bellack AS, Mueser KT: Psychosocial treatment for schizophrenia. Schizophr Bull 19:317–336, 1993

Berardi D, Dell'Atti M, Amore M, et al: Clinical risk factors for neuroleptic malignant syndrome. Hum Psychopharmacol 17:99–102, 2002

Beresford TP, Clapp L, Martin B, et al: Aripiprazole in schizophrenia with cocaine dependence: a pilot study. J Clin Psychopharmacol 25:363–366, 2005

Berman I, Kalinowski A, Berman SM, et al: Obsessive and compulsive symptoms in chronic schizophrenia. Compr Psychiatry 36:6–10, 1995a

Berman I, Sapers BL, Chang HH, et al: Treatment of obsessive-compulsive symptoms in schizophrenic patients with clomipramine. J Clin Psychopharmacol 15:206–210, 1995b

Bernardo M, Ramon Azanza J, Rubio-Terres C, et al: Cost-effectiveness analysis of schizophrenia relapse prevention: an economic evaluation of the ZEUS (Ziprasidone-Extended-Use-In-Schizophrenia) study in Spain. Clin Drug Investig 26:447–457, 2006

Bilder RM, Goldman RS, Volavka J, et al: Neurocognitive effects of clozapine, olanzapine, risperidone, and haloperidol in patients with chronic schizophrenia or schizoaffective disorder. Am J Psychiatry 159:1018–1028, 2002

Birchwood M: Early intervention in schizophrenia: theoretical background and clinical strategies. Br J Clin Psychol 31 (pt 3):257–278, 1992

Birchwood M, Iqbal Z, Chadwick P, et al: Cognitive approach to depression and suicidal thinking in psychosis, I: ontogeny of post-psychotic depression. Br J Psychiatry 177:516–521, 2000

Black DW, Warrack G, Winokur G: The Iowa record-linkage study, I: suicides and accidental deaths among psychiatric patients. Arch Gen Psychiatry 42:71–75, 1985

Bond GR: Supported employment: evidence for an evidence-based practice. Psychiatr Rehabil J 27:345–359, 2004

Bondolfi G, Dufour H, Patris M, et al: Risperidone versus clozapine in treatment-resistant chronic schizophrenia: a randomized double-blind study. The Risperidone Study Group. Am J Psychiatry 155:499–504, 1998

Bourgeois M, Swendsen J, Young F, et al: Awareness of disorder and suicide risk in the treatment of schizophrenia: results of the international suicide prevention trial. Am J Psychiatry 161:1494–1496, 2004

Breier A, Schreiber JL, Dyer J, et al: National Institute of Mental Health longitudinal study of chronic schizophrenia: prognosis and predictors of outcome. Arch Gen Psychiatry 48:239–246, 1991

Breier AF, Malhotra AK, Su TP, et al: Clozapine and risperidone in chronic schizophrenia: effects on symptoms, parkinsonian side effects, and neuroendocrine response. Am J Psychiatry 156:294–298, 1999

Brown ES, Nejtek VA, Perantie DC, et al: Cocaine and amphetamine use in patients with psychiatric illness: a randomized trial of typical antipsychotic continuation or discontinuation. J Clin Psychopharmacol 23:384–388, 2003

Brown ES, Jeffress J, Liggin JD, et al: Switching outpatients with bipolar or schizoaffective disorders and substance abuse from their current antipsychotic to aripiprazole. J Clin Psychiatry 66:756–760, 2005

Brown GW, Rutter M: The measurement of family activities and relationships: a methodological study. Human Relations 19:241–263, 1966

Brown S, Inskip H, Barraclough B: Causes of the excess mortality of schizophrenia. Br J Psychiatry 177:212–217, 2000

Brunette MF, Drake RE, Xie H, et al: Clozapine use and relapses of substance use disorder among patients with co-occurring schizophrenia and substance use disorders. Schizophr Bull 32:637–643, 2006

Brunette MF, Ferron JC, McHugo GJ, et al: An electronic decision support system to motivate people with severe mental illnesses to quit smoking. Psychiatr Serv 62:360–366, 2011

Buchanan RW, Strauss ME, Kirkpatrick B, et al: Neuropsychological impairments in deficit vs nondeficit forms of schizophrenia. Arch Gen Psychiatry 51:804–811, 1994

Buchanan RW, Ball MP, Weiner E, et al: Olanzapine treatment of residual positive and negative symptoms. Am J Psychiatry 162:124–129, 2005

Buckley P, McCarthy M, Chapman P, et al: Clozapine treatment of comorbid substance abuse in patients with schizophrenia. Schizophr Res 36:272, 1999

Bustillo J, Lauriello J, Horan W, et al: The psychosocial treatment of schizophrenia: an update. Am J Psychiatry 158:163–175, 2001

Byerly M, Goodman W, Acholonu W, et al: Obsessive compulsive symptoms in schizophrenia: frequency and clinical features. Schizophr Res 76:309–316, 2005

Cannon TD: On the nature and mechanisms of obstetric influences in schizophrenia: a review and synthesis of epidemiologic studies. Int Rev Psychiatry 9:387–397, 1997

Canuso CM, Hanau M, Jhamb KK, et al: Olanzapine use in women with antipsychotic-induced hyperprolactinemia. Am J Psychiatry 155:1458, 1998

Canuso CM, Goldstein JM, Wojcik J, et al: Antipsychotic medication, prolactin elevation, and ovarian function in women with schizophrenia and schizoaffective disorder. Psychiatry Res 111:11–20, 2002

Caroff SN, Mann SC: Neuroleptic malignant syndrome. Med Clin North Am 77:185–202, 1993

Carpenter WT Jr: New views on the course and treatment of schizophrenia. J Psychiatr Res 32:191–195, 1998

Carpenter WT Jr, Heinrichs DW, Wagman AM: Deficit and nondeficit forms of schizophrenia: the concept. Am J Psychiatry 145:578–583, 1988

Casey DE: Rabbit syndrome, in Movement Disorders in Neurology and Neuropsychiatry. Edited by Joseph AB, Young RR. Malden, MA, Blackwell Science, 1999, pp 119–122

Cassano GB, Pini S, Saettoni M, et al: Occurrence and clinical correlates of psychiatric comorbidity in patients with psychotic disorders. J Clin Psychiatry 59:60–68, 1998

Chadwick PD, Lowe CF, Horne PJ, et al: Modifying delusions: the role of empirical testing: innovations in cognitive-behavioral approaches to schizophrenia. Behav Ther 25:35–49, 1994

Chang HH, Berman I: Treatment issues for patients with schizophrenia who have obsessive-compulsive symptoms. Psychiatric Annals 29:529–532, 1999

Citrome L: Lurasidone for schizophrenia: a brief review of a new second-generation antipsychotic. Clin Schizophr Relat Psychoses 4:251–257, 2011a

Citrome L: Lurasidone for schizophrenia: a review of the efficacy and safety profile for this newly approved second-generation antipsychotic. Int J Clin Pract 65:189–210, 2011b

Coldwell CM, Bender WS: The effectiveness of assertive community treatment for homeless populations with severe mental illness: a meta-analysis. Am J Psychiatry 164:393–399, 2007

Combs DR, Adams SD, Penn DL, et al: Social Cognition and Interaction Training (SCIT) for inpatients with schizophrenia spectrum disorders: preliminary findings. Schizophr Res 91:112–116, 2007

Correll CU, Leucht S, Kane JM: Lower risk for tardive dyskinesia associated with second-generation antipsychotics: a systematic review of 1-year studies. Am J Psychiatry 161:414–425, 2004

Correll CU, Rummel-Kluge C, Corves C, et al: Antipsychotic combinations vs monotherapy in schizophrenia: a meta-analysis of randomized controlled trials. Schizophr Bull 35:443–457, 2009

Costa AM, de Lima MS, Faria M, et al: A naturalistic, 9-month follow-up, comparing olanzapine and conventional antipsychotics on sexual function and hormonal profile for males with schizophrenia. J Psychopharmacol 21:165–170, 2007

Covey L, Hughes DC, Glassman AH, et al: Ever-smoking, quitting, and psychiatric disorders: evidence from the Durham, North Carolina, Epidemiologic Catchment Area. Tobacco Control 3:222–227, 1994

Crow TJ: The two-syndrome concept: origins and current status. Schizophr Bull 11:471–486, 1985

Crow TJ, MacMillan JF, Johnson AL, et al: A randomised controlled trial of prophylactic neuroleptic treatment. Br J Psychiatry 148:120–127, 1986

Crumlish N, Whitty P, Kamali M, et al: Early insight predicts depression and attempted suicide after 4 years in first-episode schizophrenia and schizophreniform disorder. Acta Psychiatr Scand 112: 449–455, 2005

Dalack GW, Healy DJ, Meador-Woodruff JH: Nicotine dependence in schizophrenia: clinical phenomena and laboratory findings. Am J Psychiatry 155:1490–1501, 1998

David AS, Malmberg A, Brandt L, et al: IQ and risk for schizophrenia: a population-based cohort study. Psychol Med 27:1311–1323, 1997

DeLisi LE: Defining the course of brain structural change and plasticity in schizophrenia. Psychiatry Res 92:1–9, 1999

DeLisi LE, Sakuma M, Tew W, et al: Schizophrenia as a chronic active brain process: a study of progressive brain structural change subsequent to the onset of schizophrenia. Psychiatry Res 74:129–140, 1997

Dickerson F, Boronow JJ, Ringel N, et al: Neurocognitive deficits and social functioning in outpatients with schizophrenia. Schizophr Res 21:75–83, 1996

Dickson RA, Glazer WM: Neuroleptic-induced hyperprolactinemia. Schizophr Res 35 (suppl): S75–S86, 1999

Dixon L, Haas G, Weiden P, et al: Acute effects of drug abuse in schizophrenic patients: clinical observations and patients' self-reports. Schizophr Bull 16:69–79, 1990

Dixon L, Weiden P, Delahanty J, et al: Prevalence and correlates of diabetes in national schizophrenia samples. Schizophr Bull 26:903–912, 2000

Docherty JP, Van Kammen DP, Siris SG, et al: Stages of onset of schizophrenic psychosis. Am J Psychiatry 135:420–426, 1978

Drake RE, Mueser KT: Alcohol-use disorder and severe mental illness. Alcohol Health Res World 20:87–93, 1996

Drake RE, Mueser KT: Substance abuse comorbidity, in Comprehensive Care of Schizophrenia. Edited by Lieberman JA, Murray RM. London, Martin Dunitz, 2001, pp 243–254

Drake RE, Gates C, Whitaker A, et al: Suicide among schizophrenics: a review. Compr Psychiatry 26:90–100, 1985

Drake RE, Gates C, Cotton PG: Suicide among schizophrenics: a comparison of attempters and completed suicides. Br J Psychiatry 149:784–787, 1986

Drake RE, Xie H, McHugo GJ, et al: The effects of clozapine on alcohol and drug use disorders among patients with schizophrenia. Schizophr Bull 26:441–449, 2000

Drake RE, Essock SM, Shaner A, et al: Implementing dual diagnosis services for clients with severe mental illness. Psychiatr Serv 52:469–476, 2001

D'Souza DC, Abi-Saab WM, Madonick S, et al: Delta-9-tetrahydrocannabinol effects in schizophrenia: implications for cognition, psychosis, and addiction. Biol Psychiatry 57:594–608, 2005

Eckman TA, Wirshing WC, Marder SR, et al: Technique for training schizophrenic patients in illness self-management: a controlled trial. Am J Psychiatry 149:1549–1555, 1992

Eisen JL, Beer DA, Pato MT, et al: Obsessive-compulsive disorder in patients with schizophrenia or schizoaffective disorder. Am J Psychiatry 154: 271–273, 1997

Ellinger LK, Ipema HJ, Stachnik JM: Efficacy of metformin and topiramate in prevention and treatment of second-generation antipsychotic-induced weight gain. Ann Pharmacother 44: 668–679, 2010

Elvevag B, Goldberg TE: Cognitive impairment in schizophrenia is the core of the disorder. Crit Rev Neurobiol 14:1–21, 2000

Emsley RA, Raniwalla J, Bailey PJ, et al: A comparison of the effects of quetiapine ("Seroquel") and haloperidol in schizophrenic patients with a history of and a demonstrated, partial response to conventional antipsychotic treatment. PRIZE Study Group. Int Clin Psychopharmacol 15: 121–131, 2000

Essock SM, Covell NH, Davis SM, et al: Effectiveness of switching antipsychotic medications. Am J Psychiatry 163:2090–2095, 2006

Evins AE, Cather C, Deckersbach T, et al: A double-blind placebo-controlled trial of bupropion sustained-release for smoking cessation in schizophrenia. J Clin Psychopharmacol 25:218–225, 2005

Falloon IR, Boyd JL, McGill CW, et al: Family management in the prevention of exacerbations of schizophrenia: a controlled study. N Engl J Med 306:1437–1440, 1982

Faraone SV, Chen WJ, Goldstein JM, et al: Gender differences in age at onset of schizophrenia. Br J Psychiatry 164:625–629, 1994

Fenton WS: Comorbid conditions in schizophrenia. Curr Opin Psychiatry 14:17–23, 2001
Fenton WS, McGlashan TH: The prognostic significance of obsessive-compulsive symptoms in schizophrenia. Am J Psychiatry 143:437–441, 1986
Fenton WS, McGlashan TH, Victor BJ, et al: Symptoms, subtype, and suicidality in patients with schizophrenia spectrum disorders. Am J Psychiatry 154:199–204, 1997
Fenton WS, Stover EL, Insel TR: Breaking the logjam in treatment development for cognition in schizophrenia: NIMH perspective. Psychopharmacology (Berl) 169:365–366, 2003
Freedman B, Chapman LJ: Early subjective experience in schizophrenic episodes. J Abnorm Psychol 82:46–54, 1973
Geddes JR, Lawrie SM: Obstetric complications and schizophrenia: a meta-analysis. Br J Psychiatry 167:786–793, 1995
George TP, Ziedonis DM, Feingold A, et al: Nicotine transdermal patch and atypical antipsychotic medications for smoking cessation in schizophrenia. Am J Psychiatry 157:1835–1842, 2000
George TP, Vessicchio JC, Termine A, et al: A placebo controlled trial of bupropion for smoking cessation in schizophrenia. Biol Psychiatry 52:53–61, 2002
Ghadirian AM, Chouinard G, Annable L: Sexual dysfunction and plasma prolactin levels in neuroleptic-treated schizophrenic outpatients. J Nerv Ment Dis 170:463–467, 1982
Gianfrancesco FD, Grogg AL, Mahmoud RA, et al: Differential effects of risperidone, olanzapine, clozapine, and conventional antipsychotics on type 2 diabetes: findings from a large health plan database. J Clin Psychiatry 63:920–930, 2002
Gitlin M, Nuechterlein K, Subotnik KL, et al: Clinical outcome following neuroleptic discontinuation in patients with remitted recent-onset schizophrenia. Am J Psychiatry 158:1835–1842, 2001
Glazer WM: Expected incidence of tardive dyskinesia associated with atypical antipsychotics. J Clin Psychiatry 61 (suppl 4):21–26, 2000a
Glazer WM: Extrapyramidal side effects, tardive dyskinesia, and the concept of atypicality. J Clin Psychiatry 61 (suppl 3):16–21, 2000b
Glazer WM: Review of incidence studies of tardive dyskinesia associated with typical antipsychotics. J Clin Psychiatry 61 (suppl 4):15–20, 2000c
Glynn SM, Marder SR, Liberman RP, et al: Supplementing clinic-based skills training with manual-based community support sessions: effects on social adjustment of patients with schizophrenia. Am J Psychiatry 159:829–837, 2002
Goff DC, Coyle JT: The emerging role of glutamate in the pathophysiology and treatment of schizophrenia. Am J Psychiatry 158:1367–1377, 2001
Goff DC, Sullivan LM, McEvoy JP, et al: A comparison of ten-year cardiac risk estimates in schizophrenia patients from the CATIE study and matched controls. Schizophr Res 80:45–53, 2005
Goldberg TE, Hyde TM, Kleinman JE, et al: Course of schizophrenia: neuropsychological evidence for a static encephalopathy. Schizophr Bull 19:797–804, 1993
Goldstein G, Haas GL, Pakrashi M, et al: The cycle of schizoaffective disorder, cognitive ability, alcoholism, and suicidality. Suicide Life Threat Behav 36:35–43, 2006
Goldstein MJ, Rodnick EH, Evans JR, et al: Drug and family therapy in the aftercare of acute schizophrenics. Arch Gen Psychiatry 35:1169–1177, 1978
Granholm E, McQuaid JR, McClure FS, et al: A randomized, controlled trial of cognitive behavioral social skills training for middle-aged and older outpatients with chronic schizophrenia. Am J Psychiatry 162:520–529, 2005
Grech A, Van Os J, Murray RM: Influence of cannabis on the outcome of psychosis. Schizophr Res 36:41, 1999
Green AI, Burgess ES, Dawson R, et al: Alcohol and cannabis use in schizophrenia: effects of clozapine vs risperidone. Schizophr Res 60:81–85, 2003
Green AI, Drake RE, Brunette MF, et al: Schizophrenia and co-occurring substance use disorder. Am J Psychiatry 164:402–408, 2007
Green AI, Noordsy DL, Brunette MF, et al: Substance abuse and schizophrenia: pharmacotherapeutic intervention. J Subst Abuse Treat 34:61–71, 2008
Green MF: What are the functional consequences of neurocognitive deficits in schizophrenia? Am J Psychiatry 153:321–330, 1996
Green MF: Recent studies on the neurocognitive effects of second-generation antipsychotic medications. Curr Opin Psychiatry 15:25–29, 2002
Green MF, Kern RS, Braff DL, et al: Neurocognitive deficits and functional outcome in schizophrenia: are we measuring the "right stuff"? Schizophr Bull 26:119–136, 2000

Hafner H, Riecher-Rossler A, Maurer K, et al: First onset and early symptomatology of schizophrenia: a chapter of epidemiological and neurobiological research into age and sex differences. Eur Arch Psychiatry Clin Neurosci 242:109–118, 1992

Hafner H, Maurer K, Loffler W, et al: The influence of age and sex on the onset and early course of schizophrenia. Br J Psychiatry 162:80–86, 1993

Hafner H, Maurer K, Loffler W, et al: The epidemiology of early schizophrenia: influence of age and gender on onset and early course. Br J Psychiatry Suppl (23):29–38, 1994

Hambrecht M, Maurer K, Hafner H, et al: Transnational stability of gender differences in schizophrenia? An analysis based on the WHO study on determinants of outcome of severe mental disorders. Eur Arch Psychiatry Clin Neurosci 242:6–12, 1992

Hamoui N, Kingsbury S, Anthone GJ, et al: Surgical treatment of morbid obesity in schizophrenic patients. Obes Surg 14:349–352, 2004

Harkavy-Friedman JM, Nelson E: Management of the suicidal patient with schizophrenia. Psychiatr Clin North Am 20:625–640, 1997

Harkavy-Friedman JM, Nelson EA, Venarde DF, et al: Suicidal behavior in schizophrenia and schizoaffective disorder: examining the role of depression. Suicide Life Threat Behav 34:66–76, 2004

Harvey PD, Keefe RE: Cognition and the new antipsychotics. Journal of Advanced Schizophrenia Brain Research 1:2–8, 1998

Harvey PD, Howanitz E, Parrella M, et al: Symptoms, cognitive functioning, and adaptive skills in geriatric patients with lifelong schizophrenia: a comparison across treatment sites. Am J Psychiatry 155:1080–1086, 1998

Hasan S, Buckley P: Novel antipsychotics and the neuroleptic malignant syndrome: a review and critique. Am J Psychiatry 155:1113–1116, 1998

Hawton K, Sutton L, Haw C, et al: Schizophrenia and suicide: systematic review of risk factors. Br J Psychiatry 187:9–20, 2005

Heila H, Isometsa ET, Henriksson MM, et al: Suicide and schizophrenia: a nationwide psychological autopsy study on age- and sex-specific clinical characteristics of 92 suicide victims with schizophrenia. Am J Psychiatry 154:1235–1242, 1997

Heila H, Isometsa ET, Henriksson MM, et al: Suicide victims with schizophrenia in different treatment phases and adequacy of antipsychotic medication. J Clin Psychiatry 60:200–208, 1999

Henderson DC, Cagliero E, Gray C, et al: Clozapine, diabetes mellitus, weight gain, and lipid abnormalities: a five-year naturalistic study. Am J Psychiatry 157:975–981, 2000

Ho BC, Andreasen NC, Flaum M, et al: Untreated initial psychosis: its relation to quality of life and symptom remission in first-episode schizophrenia. Am J Psychiatry 157:808–815, 2000

Hodel B, Brenner HD: Cognitive therapy with schizophrenic patients: conceptual basis, present state, future directions. Acta Psychiatr Scand Suppl 384:108–115, 1994

Hogarty GE, Anderson CM, Reiss DJ, et al: Family psychoeducation, social skills training, and maintenance chemotherapy in the aftercare treatment of schizophrenia, I: one-year effects of a controlled study on relapse and expressed emotion. Arch Gen Psychiatry 43:633–642, 1986

Hogarty GE, McEvoy JP, Ulrich RF, et al: Pharmacotherapy of impaired affect in recovering schizophrenic patients. Arch Gen Psychiatry 52:29, 1995

Hogarty GE, Greenwald D, Ulrich RF, et al: Three-year trials of personal therapy among schizophrenic patients living with or independent of family, II: effects on adjustment of patients. Am J Psychiatry 154:1514–1524, 1997a

Hogarty GE, Kornblith SJ, Greenwald D, et al: Three-year trials of personal therapy among schizophrenic patients living with or independent of family, I: description of study and effects on relapse rates. Am J Psychiatry 154:1504–1513, 1997b

Hogarty GE, Greenwald DP, Eack SM: Durability and mechanism of effects of cognitive enhancement therapy. Psychiatr Serv 57:1751–1757, 2006

Huber G, Gross G, Schuttler R, et al: Longitudinal studies of schizophrenic patients. Schizophr Bull 6:592–605, 1980

Hummer M, Malik P, Gasser RW, et al: Osteoporosis in patients with schizophrenia. Am J Psychiatry 162:162–167, 2005

Hunt IM, Kapur N, Windfuhr K, et al: Suicide in schizophrenia: findings from a national clinical survey. J Psychiatr Pract 12:139–147, 2006

Hurlburt MS, Hough RL, Wood PA: Effects of substance abuse on housing stability of homeless mentally ill persons in supported housing. Psychiatr Serv 47:731–736, 1996a

Hurlburt MS, Wood PA, Hough RL: Providing independent housing for the homeless mentally ill: a novel approach to evaluating long-term longitudinal housing patterns. Journal of Community Psychology 24:291–310, 1996b

Hwang MY, Morgan JE, Losconzcy MF: Clinical and neuropsychological profiles of obsessive-compulsive schizophrenia: a pilot study. J Neuropsychiatry Clin Neurosci 12:91–94, 2000

Hyman SE, Fenton WS: Medicine. What are the right targets for psychopharmacology? Science 299:350–351, 2003

Iqbal Z, Birchwood M, Chadwick P, et al: Cognitive approach to depression and suicidal thinking in psychosis, II: testing the validity of a social ranking model. Br J Psychiatry 177:522–528, 2000

Jablensky A, Sartorius N, Ernberg G, et al: Schizophrenia: manifestations, incidence and course in different cultures. A World Health Organization ten-country study. Psychol Med Monogr Suppl 20:1–97, 1992

Jeste DV, Lacro JP, Bailey A: Lower incidence of tardive dyskinesia with risperidone compared with haloperidol in older patients. Presented at the 21st Congress of the Collegium Internationale Neuro-Psychopharmacologicum, Glasgow, Scotland, July 12–16, 1998

Jin H, Meyer JM, Jeste DV: Atypical antipsychotics and glucose dysregulation: a systematic review. Schizophr Res 71:195–212, 2004

Joffe G, Takala P, Tchoukhine E, et al: Orlistat in clozapine- or olanzapine-treated patients with overweight or obesity: a 16-week randomized, double-blind, placebo-controlled trial. J Clin Psychiatry 69:706–711, 2008

Johnson DA: Antipsychotic medication: clinical guidelines for maintenance therapy. J Clin Psychiatry 46:6–15, 1985

Jones C, Cormac I, Silveira da Mota Neto JI, et al: Cognitive behaviour therapy for schizophrenia. Cochrane Database Syst Rev (4):CD000524, 2004

Jones PB, Barnes TR, Davies L, et al: Randomized controlled trial of the effect on Quality of Life of second- vs first-generation antipsychotic drugs in schizophrenia: Cost Utility of the Latest Antipsychotic Drugs in Schizophrenia Study (CUtLASS 1). Arch Gen Psychiatry 63:1079–1087, 2006

Kampman O, Lehtinen K: Compliance in psychoses. Acta Psychiatr Scand 100:167–175, 1999

Kane JM: Tardive dyskinesia rates with atypical antipsychotics in adults: prevalence and incidence. J Clin Psychiatry 65 (suppl 9):16–20, 2004

Kane JM, Rifkin A, Quitkin F, et al: Fluphenazine vs placebo in patients with remitted, acute first-episode schizophrenia. Arch Gen Psychiatry 39: 70–73, 1982

Kane JM, Honigfeld G, Singer J, et al: Clozapine for the treatment-resistant schizophrenic: a double-blind comparison with chlorpromazine. Arch Gen Psychiatry 45:789–796, 1988

Kane JM, Woerner MG, Pollack S, et al: Does clozapine cause tardive dyskinesia? J Clin Psychiatry 54:327–330, 1993

Kane JM, Handan G, Malhotra AK: Clozapine, in Current Issues in the Psychopharmacology of Schizophrenia. Edited by Breier A, Tran PV, Herrea JM, et al. Philadelphia, PA, Lippincott Williams & Wilkins, 2001, pp 209–223

Kane JM, Khanna S, Rajadhyaksha S, et al: Efficacy and tolerability of ziprasidone in patients with treatment-resistant schizophrenia. Int Clin Psychopharmacol 21:21–28, 2006

Kane JM, Meltzer HY, Carson WH Jr, et al: Aripiprazole for treatment-resistant schizophrenia: results of a multicenter, randomized, double-blind, comparison study versus perphenazine. J Clin Psychiatry 68:213–223, 2007

Kane JM, Lauriello J, Laska E, et al: Long-term efficacy and safety of iloperidone: results from 3 clinical trials for the treatment of schizophrenia. J Clin Psychopharmacol 28:S29–S35, 2008

Kaplan KJ, Harrow M: Positive and negative symptoms as risk factors for later suicidal activity in schizophrenics versus depressives. Suicide Life Threat Behav 26:105–121, 1996

Kapur S, Remington G: Serotonin-dopamine interaction and its relevance to schizophrenia. Am J Psychiatry 153:466–476, 1996

Kapur S, Remington G: Dopamine D(2) receptors and their role in atypical antipsychotic action: still necessary and may even be sufficient. Biol Psychiatry 50:873–883, 2001

Kasai K, Shenton ME, Salisbury DF, et al: Progressive decrease of left Heschl gyrus and planum temporale gray matter volume in first-episode schizophrenia: a longitudinal magnetic resonance imaging study. Arch Gen Psychiatry 60:766–775, 2003a

Kasai K, Shenton ME, Salisbury DF, et al: Progressive decrease of left superior temporal gyrus gray matter volume in patients with first-episode schizophrenia. Am J Psychiatry 160:156–164, 2003b

Keefe RS, Bilder RM, Davis SM, et al: Neurocognitive effects of antipsychotic medications in patients with chronic schizophrenia in the CATIE Trial. Arch Gen Psychiatry 64:633–647, 2007

Kelly DL, Shim JC, Feldman SM, et al: Lifetime psychiatric symptoms in persons with schizophrenia who died by suicide compared to other means of death. J Psychiatr Res 38:531–536, 2004

Kessing LV, Thomsen AF, Mogensen UB, et al: Treatment with antipsychotics and the risk of diabetes in clinical practice. Br J Psychiatry 197:266–271, 2010

Kim CH, Jayathilake K, Meltzer HY: Hopelessness, neurocognitive function, and insight in schizophrenia: relationship to suicidal behavior. Schizophr Res 60:71–80, 2003

Kingsbury SJ, Fayek M, Trufasiu D, et al: The apparent effects of ziprasidone on plasma lipids and glucose. J Clin Psychiatry 62:347–349, 2001

Kinon BJ, Ahl J, Liu-Seifert H, et al: Improvement in hyperprolactinemia and reproductive comorbidities in patients with schizophrenia switched from conventional antipsychotics or risperidone to olanzapine. Psychoneuroendocrinology 31:577–588, 2006

Kirli S, Caliskan M: A comparative study of sertraline versus imipramine in postpsychotic depressive disorder of schizophrenia. Schizophr Res 33:103–111, 1998

Kleinberg DL, Davis JM, de Coster R, et al: Prolactin levels and adverse events in patients treated with risperidone. J Clin Psychopharmacol 19:57–61, 1999

Kofoed L, Kania J, Walsh T, et al: Outpatient treatment of patients with substance abuse and coexisting psychiatric disorders. Am J Psychiatry 143:867–872, 1986

Kopelowicz A, Liberman RP, Zarate R: Recent advances in social skills training for schizophrenia. Schizophr Bull 32 (suppl 1):S12–S23, 2006

Koppel BS: Neuroleptic malignant syndrome, in Principles and Practices of Emergency Medicine, 4th Edition. Edited by Schwartz GR, Hanke BK, Mayer TA. Baltimore, MD, Williams & Wilkins, 1998, pp 1155–1605

Koreen AR, Siris SG, Chakos M, et al: Depression in first-episode schizophrenia. Am J Psychiatry 150:1643–1648, 1993

Kraepelin E: Dementia Praecox and Paraphrenia (1919). New York, Robert E Krieger, 1971

Kuo CJ, Tsai SY, Lo CH, et al: Risk factors for completed suicide in schizophrenia. J Clin Psychiatry 66:579–585, 2005

Lauriello J, Bustillo J, Keith SJ: A critical review of research on psychosocial treatment of schizophrenia. Biol Psychiatry 46:1409–1417, 1999

Lee ML, Dickson RA, Campbell M, et al: Clozapine and substance abuse in patients with schizophrenia. Can J Psychiatry 43:855–856, 1998

Lehmann HE, Hanrahan GE: Chlorpromazine: new inhibiting agent for psychomotor excitement and manic states. AMA Arch Neurol Psychiatry 71:227–237, 1954

Leslie DL, Rosenheck RA: Incidence of newly diagnosed diabetes attributable to atypical antipsychotic medications. Am J Psychiatry 161:1709–1711, 2004

Leucht S, Wahlbeck K, Hamann J, et al: New generation antipsychotics versus low-potency conventional antipsychotics: a systematic review and meta-analysis. Lancet 361:1581–1589, 2003b

Levinson DF, Umapathy C, Musthaq M: Treatment of schizoaffective disorder and schizophrenia with mood symptoms. Am J Psychiatry 156:1138–1148, 1999

Lewis DA, Gonzalez-Burgos G: Pathophysiologically based treatment interventions in schizophrenia. Nat Med 12:1016–1022, 2006

Lewis DA, Levitt P: Schizophrenia as a disorder of neurodevelopment. Annu Rev Neurosci 25:409–432, 2002

Lewis DA, Lieberman JA: Catching up on schizophrenia: natural history and neurobiology. Neuron 28:325–334, 2000

Lewis SW, Davies L, Jones PB, et al: Randomised controlled trials of conventional antipsychotic versus new atypical drugs, and new atypical drugs versus clozapine, in people with schizophrenia responding poorly to, or intolerant of, current drug treatment. Health Technol Assess 10:iii–iv, ix–xi, 1–165, 2006

Liberman RP, Wallace CJ, Blackwell G, et al: Skills training versus psychosocial occupational therapy for persons with persistent schizophrenia. Am J Psychiatry 155:1087–1091, 1998

Liddle PF, Barnes TR, Morris D, et al: Three syndromes in chronic schizophrenia. Br J Psychiatry Suppl (7):119–122, 1989

Lieberman JA: Is schizophrenia a neurodegenerative disorder? A clinical and neurobiological perspective. Biol Psychiatry 46:729–739, 1999

Lieberman JA: Neurobiology and the natural history of schizophrenia. J Clin Psychiatry 67:e14, 2006

Lieberman JA, Saltz BL, Johns CA, et al: The effects of clozapine on tardive dyskinesia. Br J Psychiatry 158:503–510, 1991

Lieberman JA, Jody D, Geisler S, et al: Time course and biologic correlates of treatment response in first-episode schizophrenia. Arch Gen Psychiatry 50:369–376, 1993

Lieberman JA, Stroup TS, McEvoy JP, et al: Effectiveness of antipsychotic drugs in patients with chronic schizophrenia. N Engl J Med 353:1209–1223, 2005

Littrell KH, Petty RG, Hilligoss NM, et al: Olanzapine treatment for patients with schizophrenia and substance abuse. J Subst Abuse Treat 21: 217–221, 2001

Loebel AD, Lieberman JA, Alvir JM, et al: Duration of psychosis and outcome in first-episode schizophrenia. Am J Psychiatry 149:1183–1188, 1992

Marder SR: Integrating pharmacological and psychosocial treatments for schizophrenia. Acta Psychiatr Scand Suppl (407):87–90, 2000

Marder SR: Drug initiatives to improve cognitive function. J Clin Psychiatry 67 (suppl 9):31–35; discussion 36–42, 2006

Marder SR, Wirshing WC, Mintz J, et al: Two-year outcome of social skills training and group psychotherapy for outpatients with schizophrenia. Am J Psychiatry 153:1585–1592, 1996

Marder SR, Davis JM, Chouinard G: The effects of risperidone on the five dimensions of schizophrenia derived by factor analysis: combined results of the North American trials. J Clin Psychiatry 58:538–546, 1997

Marder SR, Essock SM, Miller AL, et al: The Mount Sinai conference on the pharmacotherapy of schizophrenia. Schizophr Bull 28:5–16, 2002

Marder SR, Essock SM, Miller AL, et al: Physical health monitoring of patients with schizophrenia. Am J Psychiatry 161:1334–1349, 2004

Margolese HC, Chouinard G, Kolivakis TT, et al: Tardive dyskinesia in the era of typical and atypical antipsychotics, part 2: incidence and management strategies in patients with schizophrenia. Can J Psychiatry 50:703–714, 2005

Martin LF, Freedman R: Schizophrenia and the alpha7 nicotinic acetylcholine receptor. Int Rev Neurobiol 78:225–246, 2007

McEvoy JP, Meyer JM, Goff DC, et al: Prevalence of the metabolic syndrome in patients with schizophrenia: baseline results from the Clinical Antipsychotic Trials of Intervention Effectiveness (CATIE) schizophrenia trial and comparison with national estimates from NHANES III. Schizophr Res 80:19–32, 2005

McEvoy JP, Lieberman JA, Stroup TS, et al: Effectiveness of clozapine versus olanzapine, quetiapine, and risperidone in patients with chronic schizophrenia who did not respond to prior atypical antipsychotic treatment. Am J Psychiatry 163:600–610, 2006

McGlashan TH: The profiles of clinical deterioration in schizophrenia. J Psychiatr Res 32:133–141, 1998

McGlashan TH, Carpenter WT Jr: Postpsychotic depression in schizophrenia. Arch Gen Psychiatry 33:231–239, 1976

McGurk SR, Twamley EW, Sitzer DI, et al: A meta-analysis of cognitive remediation in schizophrenia. Am J Psychiatry 164:1791–1802, 2007

Meltzer HY: Clinical studies on the mechanism of action of clozapine: the dopamine-serotonin hypothesis of schizophrenia. Psychopharmacology (Berl) 99 (suppl):S18–S27, 1989

Meltzer HY, Alphs L, Green AI, et al: Clozapine treatment for suicidality in schizophrenia: International Suicide Prevention Trial (InterSePT). Arch Gen Psychiatry 60:82–91, 2003

Meyer JM, Koro CE: The effects of antipsychotic therapy on serum lipids: a comprehensive review. Schizophr Res 70:1–17, 2004

Meyer J, Nasrallah H: Medical Illness and Schizophrenia. American Psychiatric Publishing, 2003

Minkoff K: An integrated treatment model for dual diagnosis of psychosis and addiction. Hosp Community Psychiatry 40:1031–1036, 1989

Moghaddam B: Targeting metabotropic glutamate receptors for treatment of the cognitive symptoms of schizophrenia. Psychopharmacology (Berl) 174:39–44, 2004

Montross LP, Zisook S, Kasckow J: Suicide among patients with schizophrenia: a consideration of risk and protective factors. Ann Clin Psychiatry 17:173–182, 2005

Mueser KT, Bennett M, Kushner MG: Epidemiology of substance use disorders among persons with chronic mental illnesses, in Double Jeopardy: Chronic Mental Illness and Substance Abuse. Edited by Lehman AF, Dixon L. New York, Harwood Academic Publishers, 1995, pp 9–25

Mueser KT, Bond GR, Drake RE, et al: Models of community care for severe mental illness: a review of research on case management. Schizophr Bull 24:37–74, 1998

Mueser KT, Noordsy DL, Fox L, et al: Disulfiram treatment for alcoholism in severe mental illness. Am J Addict 12:242–252, 2003

Mueser KT, Meyer PS, Penn DL, et al: The Illness Management and Recovery program: rationale, development, and preliminary findings. Schizophr Bull 32 (suppl 1):S32–S43, 2006

Mukherjee S, Decina P, Bocola V, et al: Diabetes mellitus in schizophrenic patients. Compr Psychiatry 37:68–73, 1996

Murray RM: Neurodevelopmental schizophrenia: the rediscovery of dementia praecox. Br J Psychiatry Suppl (25):6–12, 1994

Negrete JC, Knapp WP, Douglas DE, et al: Cannabis affects the severity of schizophrenic symptoms: results of a clinical survey. Psychol Med 16:515–520, 1986

Nelson HE, Pantelis C, Carruthers K, et al: Cognitive functioning and symptomatology in chronic schizophrenia. Psychol Med 20:357–365, 1990

Nino-Gomez J, Carlini S, Nemani K, et al: Safety and efficacy of varenicline in schizophrenia and schizoaffective disorder: preliminary data. Presented at Massachusetts General Hospital Clinical Research Day, Boston, MA, May 2010

Noordsy DL, O'Keefe C, Mueser KT, et al: Six-month outcomes for patients who switched to olanzapine treatment. Psychiatr Serv 52:501–507, 2001

O'Keane V, Meaney AM: Antipsychotic drugs: a new risk factor for osteoporosis in young women with schizophrenia? J Clin Psychopharmacol 25:26–31, 2005

Ongur D, Goff DC: Obsessive-compulsive symptoms in schizophrenia: associated clinical features, cognitive function and medication status. Schizophr Res 75:349–362, 2005

Osher FC, Kofoed LL: Treatment of patients with psychiatric and psychoactive substance abuse disorders. Hosp Community Psychiatry 40:1025–1030, 1989

Osser DN: Neuroleptic-induced pseudoparkinsonism, in Movement Disorders in Neurology and Neuropsychiatry. Edited by Joseph AB, Young RR. Malden, MA, Blackwell Science, 1999, pp 61–68

Osser DN, Najarian DM, Dufresne RL: Olanzapine increases weight and serum triglyceride levels. J Clin Psychiatry 60:767–770, 1999

Penn DL, Mueser KT: Research update on the psychosocial treatment of schizophrenia. Am J Psychiatry 153:607–617, 1996

Penn DL, Addington J, Pinkham A: Social cognitive impairments, in Textbook of Schizophrenia. Edited by Lieberman JA, Stroup TS, Perkins DO. Washington, DC, American Psychiatric Publishing, 2006, pp 261–274

Perala J, Suvisaari J, Saarni SI, et al: Lifetime prevalence of psychotic and bipolar I disorders in a general population. Arch Gen Psychiatry 64:19–28, 2007

Petrakis IL, O'Malley S, Rounsaville B, et al: Naltrexone augmentation of neuroleptic treatment in alcohol abusing patients with schizophrenia. Psychopharmacology (Berl) 172:291–297, 2004

Petrakis IL, Poling J, Levinson C, et al: Naltrexone and disulfiram in patients with alcohol dependence and comorbid psychiatric disorders. Biol Psychiatry 57:1128–1137, 2005

Petrakis IL, Leslie D, Finney JW, et al: Atypical antipsychotic medication and substance use-related outcomes in the treatment of schizophrenia. Am J Addict 15:44–49, 2006

Phillips SD, Burns BJ, Edgar ER, et al: Moving assertive community treatment into standard practice. Psychiatr Serv 52:771–779, 2001

Pilling S, Bebbington P, Kuipers E, et al: Psychological treatments in schizophrenia, II: meta-analyses of randomized controlled trials of social skills training and cognitive remediation. Psychol Med 32:783–791, 2002

Pilowsky LS, Kerwin RW, Murray RM: Schizophrenia: a neurodevelopmental perspective. Neuropsychopharmacology 9:83–91, 1993

Pitschel-Walz G, Leucht S, Bauml J, et al: The effect of family interventions on relapse and rehospitalization in schizophrenia—a meta-analysis. Schizophr Bull 27:73–92, 2001

Potkin SG, Alphs L, Hsu C, et al: Predicting suicidal risk in schizophrenic and schizoaffective patients in a prospective two-year trial. Biol Psychiatry 54:444–452, 2003

Potkin SG, Cohen M, Panagides J: Efficacy and tolerability of asenapine in acute schizophrenia: a placebo- and risperidone-controlled trial. J Clin Psychiatry 68:1492–1500, 2007

Potvin S, Stip E, Lipp O, et al: Quetiapine in patients with comorbid schizophrenia-spectrum and substance use disorders: an open-label trial. Curr Med Res Opin 22:1277–1285, 2006

Poyurovsky M, Dorfman-Etrog P, Hermesh H, et al: Beneficial effect of olanzapine in schizophrenic patients with obsessive-compulsive symptoms. Int Clin Psychopharmacol 15:169–173, 2000

Praharaj SK, Jana AK, Goyal N, et al: Metformin for olanzapine-induced weight gain: a systematic review and meta-analysis. Br J Clin Pharmacol 71:377–382, 2011

Qin P, Nordentoft M: Suicide risk in relation to psychiatric hospitalization: evidence based on longitudinal registers. Arch Gen Psychiatry 62:427–432, 2005

Ran MS, Xiang MZ, Mao WJ, et al: Characteristics of suicide attempters and nonattempters with schizophrenia in a rural community. Suicide Life Threat Behav 35:694–701, 2005

Rapp CA, Goscha RJ: The principles of effective case management of mental health services. Psychiatr Rehabil J 27:319–333, 2004

Regier DA, Farmer ME, Rae DS, et al: Comorbidity of mental disorders with alcohol and other drug abuse: results from the Epidemiologic Catchment Area (ECA) Study. JAMA 264:2511–2518, 1990

Remington G, Kapur S: Neuroleptic-induced extrapyramidal symptoms and the role of combined serotonin/dopamine antagonist. J Clin Psychiatry 14:14–24, 1996

Remington G, Kapur S, Zipursky R: APA Practice guideline for schizophrenia: risperidone equivalents. American Psychiatric Association. Am J Psychiatry 155:1301–1302, 1998

Riecher-Rossler A, Hafner H, Stumbaum M, et al: Can estradiol modulate schizophrenic symptomatology? Schizophr Bull 20:203–214, 1994

Robinson DG, Woerner MG, Alvir JM, et al: Predictors of treatment response from a first episode of schizophrenia or schizoaffective disorder. Am J Psychiatry 156:544–549, 1999

Rog DJ: The evidence on supported housing. Psychiatr Rehabil J 27:334–344, 2004

Rolfe TJ, McGory P, Cooks J, et al: Cannabis use in first episode psychosis: incidence and short-term outcome. Schizophr Res 36:313, 1999

Rosenberg SD, Goodman LA, Osher FC, et al: Prevalence of HIV, hepatitis B, and hepatitis C in people with severe mental illness. Am J Public Health 91:31–37, 2001

Rosenheck RA, Leslie DL, Sindelar J, et al: Cost-effectiveness of second-generation antipsychotics and perphenazine in a randomized trial of treatment for chronic schizophrenia. Am J Psychiatry 163:2080–2089, 2006

Rossau CD, Mortensen PB: Risk factors for suicide in patients with schizophrenia: nested case-control study. Br J Psychiatry 171:355–359, 1997

Roy A: Risk factors for suicide in psychiatric patients. Arch Gen Psychiatry 39:1089–1095, 1982

Rubio G, Martinez I, Ponce G, et al: Long-acting injectable risperidone compared with zuclopenthixol in the treatment of schizophrenia with substance abuse comorbidity. Can J Psychiatry 51:531–539, 2006

Russell AJ, Munro JC, Jones PB, et al: Schizophrenia and the myth of intellectual decline. Am J Psychiatry 154:635–639, 1997

Salisbury DF, Kuroki N, Kasai K, et al: Progressive and interrelated functional and structural evidence of post-onset brain reduction in schizophrenia. Arch Gen Psychiatry 64:521–529, 2007

Sax KW, Strakowski SM, Keck PE Jr, et al: Relationships among negative, positive, and depressive symptoms in schizophrenia and psychotic depression. Br J Psychiatry 168:68–71, 1996

Sayers SL, Campbell EC, Kondrich J, et al: Cocaine abuse in schizophrenic patients treated with olanzapine versus haloperidol. J Nerv Ment Dis 193:379–386, 2005

Schoemaker J, Naber D, Vrijland P, et al: Long-term assessment of asenapine vs. olanzapine in patients with schizophrenia or schizoaffective disorder. Pharmacopsychiatry 43:138–146, 2010

Schooler NR: Relapse and rehospitalization: comparing oral and depot antipsychotics. J Clin Psychiatry 64 (suppl 16):14–17, 2003

Schooler NR: Relapse prevention and recovery in the treatment of schizophrenia. J Clin Psychiatry 67 (suppl 5):19–23, 2006

Schooler NR, Rabinowitz J, Davidson M, et al: Risperidone and haloperidol in first-episode psychosis: a long-term randomized trial. Am J Psychiatry 162:947–953, 2005

Seeman P: Atypical antipsychotics: mechanism of action. Can J Psychiatry 47:27–38, 2002

Sellwood W, Barrowclough C, Tarrier N, et al: Needs-based cognitive-behavioural family intervention for carers of patients suffering from schizophrenia: 12-month follow-up. Acta Psychiatr Scand 104:346–355, 2001

Selzer JA, Lieberman JA: Schizophrenia and substance abuse. Psychiatr Clin North Am 16:401–412, 1993

Sevy S, Kay SR, Opler LA, et al: Significance of cocaine history in schizophrenia. J Nerv Ment Dis 178:642–648, 1990

Shirzadi AA, Ghaemi SN: Side effects of atypical antipsychotics: extrapyramidal symptoms and the metabolic syndrome. Harv Rev Psychiatry 14:152–164, 2006

Simon AE, Cattapan-Ludewig K, Zmilacher S, et al: Cognitive functioning in the schizophrenia prodrome. Schizophr Bull 33:761–771, 2007

Simpson GM: The treatment of tardive dyskinesia and tardive dystonia. J Clin Psychiatry 61 (suppl 4):39–44, 2000

Siris SG: Depression in schizophrenia: perspective in the era of "atypical" antipsychotic agents. Am J Psychiatry 157:1379–1389, 2000a

Siris SG: Management of depression in schizophrenia. Psychiatric Annals 30:13–19, 2000b

Siris SG, Morgan V, Fagerstrom R, et al: Adjunctive imipramine in the treatment of postpsychotic depression: a controlled trial. Arch Gen Psychiatry 44:533–539, 1987

Siris SG, Mason SE, Bermanzohn PC, et al: Adjunctive imipramine in substance-abusing dysphoric schizophrenic patients. Psychopharmacol Bull 29:127–133, 1993

Smelson DA, Williams J, Kaune M, et al: Reduced cue-elicited cocaine craving and relapses following treatment with risperidone. Presented at the 153rd Annual Meeting of the American Psychiatric Association, Chicago, IL, May 13–18, 2000

Smelson DA, Ziedonis D, Williams J, et al: The efficacy of olanzapine for decreasing cue-elicited craving in individuals with schizophrenia and cocaine dependence: a preliminary report. J Clin Psychopharmacol 26:9–12, 2006

Soni SD, Brownlee M: Alcohol abuse in chronic schizophrenics: implications for management in the community. Acta Psychiatr Scand 84:272–276, 1991

Spencer T, Biederman J, Wilens T, et al: Is attention-deficit hyperactivity disorder in adults a valid disorder? Harv Rev Psychiatry 1:326–335, 1994

Stein LI, Test MA: Alternative to mental hospital treatment, I: conceptual model, treatment program, and clinical evaluation. Arch Gen Psychiatry 37:392–397, 1980

Steinberg ML, Williams JM, Ziedonis DM: Financial implications of cigarette smoking among individuals with schizophrenia. Tob Control 13:206, 2004

Stip E, Tourjman V: Aripiprazole in schizophrenia and schizoaffective disorder: a review. Clin Ther 32 (suppl 1):S3–S20, 2010

Stroup TS, Lieberman JA, McEvoy JP, et al: Effectiveness of olanzapine, quetiapine, risperidone, and ziprasidone in patients with chronic schizophrenia following discontinuation of a previous atypical antipsychotic. Am J Psychiatry 163: 611–622, 2006

Susman VL: Clinical management of neuroleptic malignant syndrome. Psychiatr Q 72:325–336, 2001

Szymanski S, Lieberman JA, Alvir JM, et al: Gender differences in onset of illness, treatment response, course, and biologic indexes in first-episode schizophrenic patients. Am J Psychiatry 152:698–703, 1995

Tamminga CA: Principles of the pharmacotherapy of schizophrenia, in Neurobiology of Mental Illness. Edited by Charney DS, Nestler EJ, Bunney BS. New York, Oxford University Press, 1999, pp 272–290

Tarrier N, Barrowclough C, Vaughn C, et al: The community management of schizophrenia: a controlled trial of a behavioural intervention with families to reduce relapse. Br J Psychiatry 153:532–542, 1988

Tarrier N, Kinney C, McCarthy E, et al: Two-year follow-up of cognitive—behavioral therapy and supportive counseling in the treatment of persistent symptoms in chronic schizophrenia. J Consult Clin Psychol 68:917–922, 2000

Tarsy D, Baldessarini RJ: Epidemiology of tardive dyskinesia: is risk declining with modern antipsychotics? Mov Disord 21:589–598, 2006

Tibbo P, Kroetsch M, Chue P, et al: Obsessive-compulsive disorder in schizophrenia. J Psychiatr Res 34:139–146, 2000

Tollefson GD, Beasley CM Jr, Tamura RN, et al: Blind, controlled, long-term study of the comparative incidence of treatment-emergent tardive dyskinesia with olanzapine or haloperidol. Am J Psychiatry 154:1248–1254, 1997

Tollefson GD, Sanger TM, Lu Y, et al: Depressive signs and symptoms in schizophrenia: a prospective blinded trial of olanzapine and haloperidol. Arch Gen Psychiatry 55:250–258, 1998

Tollefson GD, Andersen SW, Tran PV: The course of depressive symptoms in predicting relapse in schizophrenia: a double-blind, randomized comparison of olanzapine and risperidone. Biol Psychiatry 46:365–373, 1999

Tollefson GD, Birkett MA, Kiesler GM, et al: Double-blind comparison of olanzapine versus clozapine in schizophrenic patients clinically eligible for treatment with clozapine. Biol Psychiatry 49:52–63, 2001

Tsuang MT, Fleming JA, Simpson JC: Suicide and schizophrenia, in The Harvard Medical School Guide to Suicide Assessment and Intervention. Edited by Jacobs DG. San Francisco, CA, Jossey-Bass, 1999, pp 287–299

van Haren NE, Pol HE, Schnack HG, et al: Progressive brain volume loss in schizophrenia over the course of the illness: evidence of maturational abnormalities in early adulthood. Biol Psychiatry 63:106–113, 2007

Varsamis J, Adamson JD: Early schizophrenia. Can Psychiatr Assoc J 16:487–497, 1971

Volavka J, Czobor P, Sheitman B, et al: Clozapine, olanzapine, risperidone, and haloperidol in the treatment of patients with chronic schizophrenia and schizoaffective disorder. Am J Psychiatry 159:255–262, 2002

Waddington JL: Schizophrenia: developmental neuroscience and pathobiology. Lancet 341:531–536, 1993

Weiden PJ, Cutler AJ, Polymeropoulos MH, et al: Safety profile of iloperidone: a pooled analysis of 6-week acute-phase pivotal trials. J Clin Psychopharmacol 28:S12–S19, 2008

Weinberger DR: Implications of normal brain development for the pathogenesis of schizophrenia. Arch Gen Psychiatry 44:660–669, 1987

Weinberger DR: On the plausibility of "the neurodevelopmental hypothesis" of schizophrenia. Neuropsychopharmacology 14:1S–11S, 1996

Weinberger DR, McClure RK: Neurotoxicity, neuroplasticity, and magnetic resonance imaging morphometry: what is happening in the schizophrenic brain? Arch Gen Psychiatry 59:553–558, 2002

Weiner E, Ball MP, Summerfelt A, et al: Effects of sustained-release bupropion and supportive group therapy on cigarette consumption in patients with schizophrenia. Am J Psychiatry 158:635–637, 2001

Westermeyer JF, Harrow M, Marengo JT: Risk for suicide in schizophrenia and other psychotic and nonpsychotic disorders. J Nerv Ment Dis 179:259–266, 1991

Wilkins JN: Pharmacotherapy of schizophrenia patients with comorbid substance abuse. Schizophr Bull 23:215–228, 1997

Williams GV, Castner SA: Under the curve: critical issues for elucidating D1 receptor function in working memory. Neuroscience 139:263–276, 2006

Williams JM, Ziedonis DM, Foulds J: A case series of nicotine nasal spray in the treatment of tobacco dependence among patients with schizophrenia. Psychiatr Serv 55:1064–1066, 2004

Windgassen K, Wesselmann U, Schulze Monking H: Galactorrhea and hyperprolactinemia in schizophrenic patients on neuroleptics: frequency and etiology. Neuropsychobiology 33:142–146, 1996

Wirshing DA, Spellberg BJ, Erhart SM, et al: Novel antipsychotics and new onset diabetes. Biol Psychiatry 44:778–783, 1998

Wirshing DA, Wirshing WC, Kysar L, et al: Novel antipsychotics: comparison of weight gain liabilities. J Clin Psychiatry 60:358–363, 1999

Wirshing DA, Erhart SM, Pierre JM: Nonextrapyramidal side effects of novel antipsychotics. Curr Opin Psychiatry 13:45–50, 2000

Wirshing DA, Boyd JA, Meng LR, et al: The effects of novel antipsychotics on glucose and lipid levels. J Clin Psychiatry 63:856–865, 2002

Wirshing DA, Pierre JM, Erhart SM, et al: Understanding the new and evolving profile of adverse drug effects in schizophrenia. Psychiatr Clin North Am 26:165–190, 2003

Wyatt RJ: Neuroleptics and the natural course of schizophrenia. Schizophr Bull 17:325–351, 1991

Wyatt RJ: Early intervention for schizophrenia: can the course of the illness be altered? Biol Psychiatry 38:1–3, 1995

Wyatt RJ, Damiani LM, Henter ID: First-episode schizophrenia: early intervention and medication discontinuation in the context of course and treatment. Br J Psychiatry Suppl 172:77–83, 1998

Wykes T, Reeder C, Corner J, et al: The effects of neurocognitive remediation on executive processing in patients with schizophrenia. Schizophr Bull 25:291–307, 1999

Yazigi RA, Quintero CH, Salameh WA: Prolactin disorders. Fertil Steril 67:215–225, 1997

Yood MU, DeLorenze G, Quesenberry CP Jr, et al: The incidence of diabetes in atypical antipsychotic users differs according to agent—results from a multisite epidemiologic study. Pharmacoepidemiol Drug Saf 18:791–799, 2009

Yung AR, McGorry PD: The initial prodrome in psychosis: descriptive and qualitative aspects. Aust N Z J Psychiatry 30:587–599, 1996a

Yung AR, McGorry PD: The prodromal phase of first-episode psychosis: past and current conceptualizations. Schizophr Bull 22:353–370, 1996b

Ziedonis D, Richardson T, Lee E, et al: Adjunctive desipramine in the treatment of cocaine abusing schizophrenics. Psychopharmacol Bull 28: 309–314, 1992

Ziedonis D, Williams JM, Smelson D: Serious mental illness and tobacco addiction: a model program to address this common but neglected issue. Am J Med Sci 326:223–230, 2003

Zimmet SV, Strous RD, Burgess ES, et al: Effects of clozapine on substance use in patients with schizophrenia and schizoaffective disorder: a retrospective survey. J Clin Psychopharmacol 20:94–98, 2000

Zipursky RB, Lim KO, Sullivan EV, et al: Widespread cerebral gray matter volume deficits in schizophrenia. Arch Gen Psychiatry 49:195–205, 1992

CHAPTER 38

Treatment of Anxiety Disorders

Daniella David, M.D.

Jonathan R. T. Davidson, M.D.

Over the past decade and a half, there has been substantial progress in the treatment of anxiety disorders. In this chapter, we review the main findings from double-blind and some open-label trials in each disorder.

Obsessive-Compulsive Disorder

According to the National Comorbidity Survey Replication (NCS-R), the lifetime and 12-month prevalence rates for obsessive-compulsive disorder (OCD) are 1.6% and 1.0%, respectively (Kessler et al. 2005a, 2005b). OCD has been recognized as the tenth leading cause of disability worldwide (Murray and Lopez 1996). Treatment can be grouped broadly into psychosocial and psychopharmacological approaches, the latter being our focus here. The chief rating scale for treatment studies of OCD remains the Yale-Brown Obsessive Compulsive Scale (Y-BOCS; Goodman et al. 1989), a 10-item observer-rated measure.

Monotherapy

A series of placebo-controlled studies completed in the late 1980s and the early 1990s led to the first approved treatment of OCD in the United States and other countries (Clomipramine Collaborative Study Group 1991). Clomipramine is a potent serotonin reuptake inhibitor (SRI) but is not selective for serotonin, because its demethylated metabolite is a norepinephrine reuptake inhibitor (NRI). The anti-OCD effect of clomipramine correlates with the plasma level of the SRI parent drug, suggesting that reuptake inhibition of serotonin is the critical factor underlying the drug's benefit. Moreover, selective NRIs, such as nortriptyline and desipramine, have been shown to lack efficacy in OCD (Leonard et al. 1988; Thoren et al. 1980).

In the Clomipramine Collaborative Study Group (1991) trial, the Y-BOCS score was reduced by about 40% in the active-drug group compared with 5% in the placebo group, consistent with findings by Huppert et al. (2004) that OCD has a remarkably low placebo response rate. Clomipramine and selective serotonin reuptake inhibitors (SSRIs) are equivalent in the treatment of OCD (Koran et al. 1996); however, because of its side effects, clomipramine is considered a second-line treatment.

Today, SSRIs are considered the first-line treatment for OCD, and fluvoxamine, fluoxetine, sertraline, and paroxetine have been approved by the U.S. Food and Drug Administration (FDA) for that indication (Greist et al. 1995a, 1995b; Tollefson et al. 1994). Clomipramine, fluvoxamine, fluoxetine, and sertraline are also effective and indicated for treating OCD in children (Flament et al. 1985; Liebowitz et al. 2002; March et al. 1998; Riddle et al. 2001). When an SSRI drug is to be used in the treatment of OCD, it may need to be given at higher doses, and it may take a longer time to work effectively (Ninan et al. 2006; Stein et al. 2007). Most clinicians believe that treatment should be long term to reduce the chance of relapse (Pato et al. 1990), although the dosage might be lowered without loss of benefit (Ravizza et al. 1996).

Long-Term Treatment and Relapse Prevention

Long-term pharmacological treatments of OCD have suggested sustained response beyond the acute treatment phase. In addition, clomipramine, paroxetine, sertraline, and (most recently) escitalopram all have been shown to be more effective than placebo in prevention of OCD relapse (Fineberg et al. 2005, 2007). SSRIs appear to be well tolerated in these studies.

Augmentation, Combination, and Other Strategies

Up to 60% of OCD patients show at least a partial response to SSRIs, although full remission is rare. Relapse can occur even during SSRI treatment, and comorbidity is common. The following augmentation, combination, and other novel strategies have been reported as offering benefit:

- The addition of fluvoxamine to clomipramine (Szegedi et al. 1996) may be helpful for partial responders, as fluvoxamine inhibits clomipramine's demethylation, thus increasing the amount of clomipramine and producing a potentiating effect. Monitoring of plasma levels and electrocardiograms is important with this combination to avoid toxicity and seizures.
- The use of intravenous clomipramine (Fallon et al. 1992) prevents first-pass metabolism, and side effects may be less severe. A double-blind trial of intravenous clomipramine suggested greater benefit with intravenous loading than with oral loading (Koran et al. 1997).
- In treatment-naive (i.e., nonrefractory) patients, the addition of quetiapine (moderate dose) to high-dose citalopram treatment was more effective than placebo augmentation (Vulink et al. 2009).
- The benzodiazepine clonazepam has been added to clomipramine treatment with mixed benefit (Pigott et al. 1992) and to sertraline treatment with no added benefit (Crockett et al. 1999).
- Patients with SRI-refractory OCD may benefit from antipsychotic augmentation. A meta-analysis demonstrated significant benefits for haloperidol and risperidone over placebo augmentation in OCD patients who failed to respond to an adequate SRI trial, whereas evidence for olanzapine and quetiapine was less robust (Bloch et al. 2006).
- The addition of lithium, buspirone, desipramine, or gabapentin to SRIs has produced very limited benefits in studies to date, although there may be occasional patients for whom such combinations are helpful.
- Topiramate augmentation of maximum-dose SSRI treatment in patients with treat-

ment-refractory OCD had a beneficial effect on compulsions, but not obsessions, and was poorly tolerated (Berlin et al. 2011).

- One report suggested that St. John's wort (*Hypericum perforatum*) produced some improvement after 12 weeks of treatment in 12 patients with OCD (Taylor and Kobak 2000). However, a subsequent and adequately powered placebo-controlled study was negative (Kobak et al. 2005).
- Inositol, a naturally occurring second-messenger precursor, led to greater OCD symptom improvement than placebo at a dosage of 18 g/day for 6 weeks (Fux et al. 1996).
- Neurosurgical approaches (cingulotomy or anterior capsulotomy) can be helpful for refractory OCD. Between 25% and 30% of subjects show marked improvement, and the side-effect burden of this procedure is small (Baer et al. 1995; Jenike et al. 1991).
- Small but promising studies also suggest benefits from deep brain stimulation for patients with treatment-refractory OCD (Denys et al. 2010; Greenberg et al. 2006).
- Repetitive transcranial magnetic stimulation (rTMS) studies to date have been limited in number of subjects and methodology and have yielded mixed results in patients with treatment-refractory OCD (Mantovani et al. 2010; Ruffini et al. 2009; Sachdev et al. 2007; Sarkhel et al. 2010).
- Cognitive-behavioral therapy (CBT) is well established in the treatment of OCD, and evidence for its efficacy is strong (Eddy et al. 2004; Foa et al. 2005). CBT employing exposure with response prevention is a first-choice option for OCD. One landmark study demonstrated that exposure with response prevention was superior to stress management training as an augmentation strategy in clomipramine partial responders (Simpson et al. 2008).

Panic Disorder

Treatment outcome in panic disorder can be measured with the Panic Disorder Severity Scale (PDSS), which can be administered both as a clinician-rated and as a self-rated scale (Shear et al. 1997). Other widely used measures include the Sheehan Panic and Anticipatory Anxiety Scale (PAAS; Sheehan 1986) and the self-rated Marks-Mathews Fear Questionnaire (FQ; Marks and Mathews 1979). Although not always attainable, the desired endpoint is full remission. Effective treatment results in reduced emergency department and laboratory resource utilization (Roy-Byrne et al. 2001).

First-Line Drug Treatments

Selective Serotonin Reuptake Inhibitors

In 1995, Boyer reported that SSRI drugs were more effective than imipramine and alprazolam in treating panic disorder, although a meta-analysis by Otto et al. (2001) failed to confirm these findings. Evidence is now available in support of citalopram (Wade et al. 1997), escitalopram (Stahl et al. 2003), fluoxetine (Michelson et al. 1998, 2001), fluvoxamine (Asnis et al. 2001; Black et al. 1993), paroxetine (Ballenger et al. 1998; Oehrberg et al. 1995; Sheehan et al. 2005), sertraline (Londborg et al. 1998), and also clomipramine (Lecrubier et al. 1997). Fluoxetine, paroxetine, and sertraline have been approved by the FDA for treatment of panic disorder.

Patients with panic disorder are often extremely sensitive to activating effects of antidepressants; have poor tolerance of symptoms such as palpitations, sweating, and tremor; and frequently discontinue treatment or drop out. This problem can almost always be prevented by coprescribing a benzodiazepine (Goddard et al. 2001; Pollack et al. 2003) or by starting with low doses of an SSRI and increasing them gradually as tolerated. Physician availability and thorough preparation and education of patients are crucial. Other common side effects of SSRIs include weight gain, sexual dysfunction, impairment of sleep, and potential drug-drug interactions.

Discontinuation of treatment can lead to relapse, which mimics panic symptoms and is quite distressing. Gradual dosage reduction is recommended, as are patient education, physician availability, and coping strategies, including behavior therapy (Otto et al. 1993). Switching to a long-acting SSRI such as fluoxetine may be considered. Serotonin$_2$ (5-HT$_2$) or serotonin$_3$ (5-HT$_3$) receptor antagonists, such as mirtazapine, nefazodone, and ondansetron, may be used to limit some of the symptoms that are mediated through these pathways (e.g., insomnia, agitation, gastrointestinal distress).

Benzodiazepines

The Cross-National Collaborative Panic Study (1992) showed that alprazolam, along with imipramine, was more effective than placebo in panic disorder; Lydiard et al. (1992) showed that alprazolam 2 mg/day was more effective than placebo. Efficacy for clonazepam was also demonstrated in panic disorder (Davidson and Moroz 1998; Rosenbaum et al. 1997; Tesar et al. 1991), and its use for this indication is now FDA approved.

Alprazolam is now regarded as a second-line treatment. Problems include sedation at higher doses, abuse liability, and discontinuation-related distress. Comparable efficacy and tolerability have been demonstrated for the sustained-release formulation of alprazolam (Pecknold et al. 1994; Schweizer et al. 1993), with decreased likelihood of adverse discontinuation effects.

Clonazepam has an advantage over alprazolam due to its longer half-life; however, it can also produce sedation, depression, and discontinuation symptoms. Bandelow et al. (1995) showed that overreliance on reduction of panic attacks as the principal outcome measure is an unsatisfactory marker of treatment benefits. Substantial improvement of quality of life and work productivity were demonstrated in the clonazepam trials compared to placebo (Jacobs et al. 1997).

A particular concern with benzodiazepines is their use in the elderly, who are more prone to sedation and falls that result in fractures and potential head injury and who are also more likely to experience discontinuation problems.

Other Pharmacological Approaches

Tricyclic Antidepressants

Although tricyclic antidepressants (TCAs) are effective (Andersch et al. 1991; Cross-National Collaborative Panic Study 1992; Fahy et al. 1992; Lecrubier et al. 1997; Lydiard et al. 1993; Mavissakalian and Perel 1989; Modigh et al. 1992), they are considered second-line treatments for panic disorder because of their side effects. Mavissakalian and Perel (1995) found that phobic symptoms responded best if the plasma level of imipramine and desmethylimipramine was in the range of 110–140 ng/mL, whereas control of panic attacks tended to occur at lower plasma levels. As with SSRIs, low starting dosages in the range of 10–25 mg/day are in order, with gradual titration thereafter as per patient tolerance.

Monoamine Oxidase Inhibitors

Sheehan et al. (1980) found that phenelzine, along with imipramine, was more effective than placebo in the treatment of panic disorder with agoraphobia, and Lydiard and Ballenger (1987) noted that monoamine oxidase inhibitors (MAOIs) may be superior to TCAs. Although MAOIs may still be the best treatment for some patients, the overall role of MAOIs in managing anxiety disorders is now fairly small because of their potential side effects and drug-drug interactions. The role of the safer reversible inhibitors of monoamine oxidase A (RIMAs) in panic disorder is unclear.

Other Drugs

The extended-release (XR) formulation of venlafaxine, a serotonin-norepinephrine reuptake inhibitor (SNRI), demonstrated greater efficacy than placebo in patients with panic disorder in a 10-week trial (Bradwejn et al. 2005), was as effective as paroxetine in a 12-week placebo-controlled trial (Pollack et al. 2007), and has received FDA approval for the treatment of panic disorder. The drug is well tolerated, with an adverse-effect profile comparable with that of the drug in depression and other anxiety disorders.

Mirtazapine, a noradrenergic and specific serotonergic antidepressant, demonstrated possible benefit in panic disorder in open trials (Boshuisen et al. 2001; Sarchiapone et al. 2003) and in a double-blind comparison with fluoxetine (Ribeiro et al. 2001); however, double-blind, placebo-controlled trials have yet to be conducted. It is noteworthy that mirtazapine has been associated with the induction of panic attacks in depressed patients undergoing dose escalation and discontinuation (Berigan 2003; Klesmer et al. 2000).

Reboxetine, a selective NRI, has been found to produce greater improvement than placebo in patients with panic disorder (Versiani et al. 2002) and in general to be well tolerated. In a more recent randomized, single-blind study comparing reboxetine with paroxetine, paroxetine was more effective on panic attacks, but no differences between the treatments were noted on anticipatory anxiety and avoidance (Bertani et al. 2004). These findings suggest perhaps different roles of norepinephrine and serotonin in the treatment of panic disorder. However, the selective NRI maprotiline appears to be ineffective in panic disorder (Den Boer and Westenberg 1988), whereas the data for bupropion are inconclusive (Sheehan et al. 1983; Simon et al. 2003).

Trazodone was less effective than imipramine and alprazolam in the treatment of panic disorder (Charney et al. 1986). The 5-HT_{1A} partial agonist buspirone and the anticonvulsant gabapentin were generally ineffective in panic disorder (Pande et al. 2000; Sheehan et al. 1990). Possible benefit has been reported in open-label trials for other anticonvulsant drugs, including levetiracetam, tiagabine, and valproic acid (Keck et al. 1993; Papp 2006; Zwanzger et al. 2001). A small double-blind, placebo-controlled trial with tiagabine did not show clinical benefits, although cholecystokinin-tetrapeptide (CCK-4)–induced sensitivity to panic attacks decreased (Zwanzger et al. 2009).

Preliminary data suggest improvement in refractory panic disorder when atypical antipsychotics are used as augmentation of SSRI treatment (olanzapine: Sepede et al. 2006; risperidone: Simon et al. 2006) or at higher doses as monotherapy (olanzapine: Hollifield et al. 2005). A single-blind comparison trial between paroxetine and low-dose risperidone found the low-dose risperidone to be as effective as paroxetine in the treatment of panic attacks (Prosser et al. 2009); however, double-blind, placebo-controlled trials are needed.

Metabotropic glutamate type 2 receptor agonists have shown promise in preclinical models of anxiety but have yet to demonstrate clinical efficacy in panic disorder (Bergink and Westenberg 2005). Similarly, the effect of a cholecystokinin-B receptor antagonist was no different from placebo in patients with panic disorder (Pande et al. 1999a).

Long-Term Management

Maintenance treatment is recommended for at least 12–24 months, if not longer. The long-term treatment of panic disorder has been reviewed elsewhere (Davidson 1998). In a controlled trial of paroxetine, clomipramine, and placebo, 84% of the paroxetine-treated patients eventually became panic free over the 9-month period (Lecrubier and Judge 1997). In a 4-year naturalistic follow-up study of 367 patients with panic disorder, greater improvements in panic attacks, phobic avoidance, and daily functioning were observed in those who received continuation treatment for 4 years, compared with 1 year (Katschnig et al. 1995), suggesting that recovery continues over several years.

Long-term randomized, controlled trials have reported efficacy for citalopram (Lepola et al. 1998), clomipramine (Fahy et al. 1992), fluoxetine (Michelson et al. 1999), paroxetine (Lecrubier and Judge 1997; Lydiard et al. 1998), and sertraline (Rapaport et al. 2001). In a relapse prevention trial following 3 months of successful open-label treatment, Ferguson et al. (2007) showed that over the course of 7 months, relapse on venlafaxine XR was 22%, compared with 50% on placebo.

Discontinuation

Even though there is some similarity between symptoms of relapse and symptoms of drug withdrawal, the existence of discontinuation symptoms is unarguable. A slow taper is recommended (for some benzodiazepines, it may be necessary to taper the drug over weeks or months). Timing of the taper may be important—it is best done when other variables in a patient's life are as stable as possible. Switching to a longer-acting benzodiazepine such as clonazepam, adding an anticonvulsant such as carbamazepine or valproate (Pages and Ries 1998), and utilizing behavior therapy (Otto et al. 1993) have all been used to ameliorate discontinuation symptoms.

Various elaborations of CBT have demonstrated consistent efficacy for panic disorder, with the common elements being education, cognitive strategies, and exposure to feared sensations and situations (Clum and Surls 1993; Royal Australian and New Zealand College of Psychiatrists Clinical Practice Guidelines Team for Panic Disorder and Agoraphobia 2003). CBT is a first-line choice, and even when pharmacotherapy is given as main treatment, principles of CBT should be incorporated into the management plan. It can be of benefit during the process of drug discontinuation and perhaps in lessening the chance of relapse afterwards.

Social Phobia

Social phobia (social anxiety disorder) has a lifetime prevalence of 12% (Kessler et al. 2005b). It can be grouped into generalized and nongeneralized types. Generalized social phobia is more common in clinical settings, is usually more disabling, and is associated with greater levels of comorbidity and genetic loading. Most of our knowledge about pharmacotherapy for social phobia derives from generalized social phobia, and the literature suggests that different medication approaches may be called for in treating the two subtypes.

Comprehensive treatment of social phobia requires that the symptoms of fear, avoidance, and physiological distress are brought under control; comorbidity is treated; disability and impairment are improved; and quality of life is enhanced. Furthermore, evidence from maintenance and relapse prevention studies has confirmed the value of long-term therapy in treatment responders.

Instruments commonly used to measure treatment change in social phobia include the clinician- and self-rated Liebowitz Social Anxiety Scale (LSAS; Liebowitz 1987), which assesses 24 performance or interpersonal situations for fear and avoidance. A score of 30 or less is considered to equate with remission. The Social Phobia Inventory (SPIN) is a 17-item self-rating instrument that assesses fear, avoidance, and physiological distress (Connor et al. 2000) and, like the LSAS, is able to detect treatment differences.

Pharmacotherapy

Most clinicians consider SSRIs as the first choice for generalized social phobia and β-blockers or benzodiazepines as the first choice for nongeneralized social phobia. Second-line drugs for generalized social phobia comprise the benzodiazepines, venlafaxine (an SNRI), and perhaps other antidepressants, including nefazodone, mirtazapine, and MAOIs. Bupropion and TCAs have been generally disappointing.

Serotonergic Drugs

Van Vliet et al. (1994) showed fluvoxamine's superiority over placebo, with response rates of 46% and 7%, respectively. Stein et al. (1999) confirmed the efficacy of fluvoxamine relative to placebo on all symptom domains (i.e., fear, avoidance, and physiological arousal). Controlled-released (CR) fluvoxamine was likewise found to be superior to placebo (Davidson et al. 2004c; Westenberg et al. 2004), and a study in Japan also found fluvoxamine to be effective versus placebo in reducing general social phobia symptoms and psychosocial disability (Asakura et al. 2007).

Sertraline also has been studied (Blomhoff et al. 2001; Katzelnick et al. 1995; Liebowitz et al. 2003; Van Ameringen et al. 2001; Walker et al. 2000). In the study by Van Ameringen et al. (2001), 53% responded to sertraline as compared with 29% to placebo, and sertraline-treated patients showed improvement on all three symptom domains of the Brief Social Phobia Scale. In a primary care setting, Haug et al. (2000) showed that cognitive therapy and sertraline could be effectively delivered, although the combination did not show any superiority over treatment with drug alone.

Paroxetine's superiority relative to placebo has been shown in both short-term efficacy and relapse prevention studies in social phobia. In the short-term studies by Stein et al. (1998), Allgulander (1999), and Baldwin et al. (1999), rates of response to paroxetine were 55%, 70%, and 66%, respectively, as compared with placebo response rates of 24%, 8%, and 32%. All subjects in the paroxetine trials fulfilled criteria for generalized social phobia and showed benefit on the LSAS within 2–4 weeks. Paroxetine CR was also shown to be effective (using LSAS as the primary outcome measure) and well tolerated in a 12-week double-blind, placebo-controlled trial (Lepola et al. 2004).

Fluoxetine, while superior to placebo on primary outcomes in one study (Davidson et al. 2004c), failed to separate from placebo in another study (Kobak et al. 2002), showing a relatively high placebo response rate (30%). Another study found cognitive therapy to be superior to either fluoxetine plus exposure exercises or placebo plus exposure exercises on measures of social phobia, with no difference between the latter two groups (Clark et al. 2003). Another serotonergic agent, nefazodone, also failed to separate from placebo on most outcome measures (Van Ameringen et al. 2007).

Trials with escitalopram have shown it to be superior to placebo in short-term, long-term, and relapse prevention studies of generalized social phobia (Kasper et al. 2005; Lader et al. 2004; Montgomery et al. 2005). Venlafaxine XR has also shown superiority over placebo in two double-blind trials of generalized social phobia (Allgulander et al. 2004; Liebowitz et al. 2005). A double-blind, placebo-controlled trial of mirtazapine in women showed statistically significant superiority for drug over placebo (Muehlbacher et al. 2005).

Paroxetine, paroxetine CR, sertraline, fluvoxamine CR, and venlafaxine XR are currently FDA approved for the treatment of social phobia.

Benzodiazepines

Three major placebo-controlled trials have shown efficacy for benzodiazepines in social phobia. Gelernter et al. (1991) showed a modest effect for alprazolam over placebo (38% vs. 20% response rate) at a mean daily dose of 4.2 mg, although it was generally inferior to phenelzine. Davidson et al. (1993) found a substantial 70% clonazepam response rate compared with a 20% placebo response rate in 75 subjects. Bromazepam was also found to be more effective than placebo (Versiani et al. 1997).

Benzodiazepines provide significant benefits yet are not considered first-line drugs because of their more limited spectrum of action and potential withdrawal difficulties. However, they work rapidly, are well tolerated, and may be particularly useful for individuals with periodic performance-related social anxiety.

Anticonvulsants

Gabapentin and pregabalin produce significant effects in social phobia. Pande et al. (1999b) found a superior effect for gabapentin over placebo in a flexible-dose trial (ranging from 900 mg/day to 3,600 mg/day, with 2,100 mg/day being the most common final dosage), with response rates of 39% and 17%, respectively. Baseline symptom scores were comparatively high and overall response rates relatively low, suggesting a degree of treatment resistance in the population. The newer anticonvulsant drug pregabalin has shown benefit in generalized social phobia (Feltner et al. 2003; Pande et al. 2003). Although 150 mg/day of pregabalin was no different from placebo, 600 mg/day produced greater effects than placebo, with response rates of 43% and 22%, respectively. At 600 mg/day, pregabalin produces a relatively high rate of side effects, and it is probably necessary to explore lower-dosage response. Levetiracetam failed to differentiate from placebo (Stein et al. 2010). Further work with anticonvulsants is needed, given that these agents are generally well tolerated, safe, and less likely to produce discontinuation symptoms compared with many SSRIs and benzodiazepines.

Reversible Inhibitors of Monoamine Oxidase

Moclobemide is safer than older MAOIs and was shown to be almost as effective as phenelzine and significantly better than placebo (Versiani et al. 1992). However, subsequent studies did not support these findings (Noyes et al. 1997; Schneier et al. 1998). The International Multicenter Clinical Trial Group on Moclobemide in Social Phobia (1997) found a modestly greater response rate (47%) for moclobemide at 600 mg/day than for placebo (34%). Moclobemide has received a license in some countries but is not available in the United States. Another RIMA, brofaromine, has shown promise in three trials, with response rates of 78%, 50%, and 73%, respectively, compared with placebo response rates of 23%, 19%, and 0% (Fahlen et al. 1995; Lott et al. 1997; van Vliet et al. 1992). Brofaromine is also not marketed in the United States.

Irreversible Inhibitors of Monoamine Oxidase

Phenelzine has been studied in four double-blind, placebo-controlled trials and showed positive benefit in all cases (Gelernter et al. 1991; Heimberg et al. 1998; Liebowitz et al. 1992; Versiani et al. 1992). Rates of response to phenelzine were 69%, 85%, 64%, and 65%, respectively, as compared with response rates of 20%, 15%, 23%, and 33%, respectively, to placebo. Even though phenelzine is so consistently effective, perhaps as a result of its combined noradrenergic, dopaminergic, and serotonergic effects, its poor tolerability, as well as greater risks, makes it an unsuitable choice for most patients. However, it should be considered for patients whose symptoms do not respond to other drugs and who are capable of being highly adherent to dietary and medication restrictions.

Other Drugs

Olanzapine yielded greater improvement than placebo in a small ($n=12$) double-blind, placebo-controlled monotherapy trial (Barnett et al. 2002), suggesting that atypical antipsychotics may deserve further investigation in social phobia, although their benefits will need to be weighed against their potential metabolic effects. Ondansetron, while producing a statistically significant effect relative to placebo, seems to be of limited clinical benefit (Bell and DeVeaugh-Geiss 1994; Davidson et al. 1997b), although it may be used adjunctively in some cases. Buspirone was ineffective in a double-blind trial, with a 7% response rate (van Vliet et al. 1997).

Despite their intuitive appeal, β-blockers have shown poor effect in treating generalized social phobia. For example, atenolol failed to separate from placebo in two trials (Liebowitz et al. 1992; Turner et al. 1994). β-Blockers do show some value in performance social anxiety, perhaps by virtue of their ability to reduce peripheral autonomic arousal and block negative feedback. A double-blind trial of mirtazapine failed to show benefit (Schutters et al. 2010). Nefazodone, bupropion, and selegiline have not shown impressive results in open-label reports (Emmanuel et al. 1991; Simpson et al. 1998; Van Ameringen et al. 1999).

A novel therapeutic approach is suggested by the findings of Hofmann et al. (2006), who administered a single dose of D-cycloserine or placebo to patients with social anxiety disorder treated with CBT. The drug was given prior to each CBT session and enhanced the benefit of CBT to a greater extent than did placebo. The postulated mechanism of action relates to drug-facilitated extinction of learned fear via glutamatergic pathways.

A study comparing the neurokinin-1 antagonist GR205171 against citalopram and placebo in 36 social phobia patients found response rates of 41.7%, 50%, and 8.3%, respectively, as well as a significant reduction in regional cerebral blood flow (rCBF) in the rhinal cortex, amygdala, and parahippocampal-hippocampal regions during a stressful public speaking task with the active agents (Furmark et al. 2005).

Treatment in Children and Adolescents

One placebo-controlled trial of fluvoxamine in children ages 6–17 years showed that it was superior to placebo in social phobia, generalized anxiety disorder (GAD), or the combination: 76% of the fluvoxamine group responded, as compared with 19% of the placebo group (Research Unit on Pediatric Psychopharmacology Anxiety Study Group 2001). Double-blind trials of immediate-release (IR) paroxetine (Wagner et al. 2004) and venlafaxine XR (March et al. 2007) have produced positive results in children and adolescents with generalized social anxiety disorder.

A multisite trial in 488 children (ages 7–17 years) with a primary diagnosis of separation anxiety disorder, GAD, or social phobia compared CBT alone, sertraline alone, combination CBT and sertraline, and placebo. CBT monotherapy and sertraline monotherapy were each superior to placebo in reducing anxiety symptoms in children (59.7% and 54.9% response rate, respectively); however, the combination treatment had the best response rate (80.7%) (Walkup et al. 2008).

Duration of Treatment

Social phobia is a chronic illness, and treatment is generally recommended for years. Sutherland et al. (1996) reported that at 2-year follow-up, subjects who had received an active drug rather than placebo were doing better. Relatively few relapse prevention studies have been done. In a 12-month trial with clonazepam, Connor et al. (1998) showed a 20% relapse rate in those switched to placebo compared with 0% in those who continued taking clonazepam. Stein et al. (1996) reported that 62% of the subjects relapsed when switched double-blind from paroxetine to placebo after 12 weeks, compared with only 12% who relapsed during maintenance treatment with paroxetine.

Other Issues

CBT is efficacious in social anxiety disorder, being comparable to pharmacotherapy (Davidson et al. 2004b; Fedoroff and Taylor 2001), but little is known as to whether adding CBT to medication lowers the relapse rate, and so far the limited evidence does not suggest any potentiating effects when the treatments are combined (Davidson et al. 2004b), except in children (Walkup et al. 2008). In a comparative study of drug and psychotherapy, Heimberg et al. (1998) showed that phenelzine and CBT were approximately similar, although phenelzine had an edge in more severely symptomatic patients. On the other hand, when subjects who had discontinued treatment were followed up, rates of relapse tended to be lower in those who had received CBT than in those who had taken phenelzine.

Specific Phobia

Specific phobia is among the most common psychiatric disorders, with a lifetime prevalence of 8%–12.5% (Alonso et al. 2004; Kessler et al. 2005b) and 12-month prevalence of 3.5%–9% (Alonso et al. 2004; Kessler et al. 2005a). Although the disorder is characterized by an early age of onset (median age at onset is 7 years) (Kessler et al. 2005b), most individuals are unimpaired by their symptoms and rarely seek treatment (Magee et al. 1996; Stinson et al. 2007; Zimmerman and Mattia 2000). However, for a minority of individuals, specific phobia causes significant disability and requires treatment. The generally accepted treatment of choice is exposure therapy, which is uniformly and rapidly effective, with techniques including virtual reality as well as in vivo exposure and muscle tension exercises (for blood-injury phobia) (Swinson et al. 2006). Few studies have evaluated the efficacy of pharmacological approaches, and no drug has yet been approved by the FDA for treating specific phobia. No standard ratings exist for this disorder, although the Marks-Mathews FQ is quite suitable for blood-injury phobia and some other fears. A modification of this scale, the Marks-Sheehan Main Phobia Severity Scale (MSMPSS; Sheehan 1986), can be recommended.

Serotonergic drugs have shown efficacy in treating symptoms of fear and avoidance in a variety of anxiety disorders and thus would seem logical choices in specific phobias. In a small (n=11) 4-week double-blind, controlled trial, subjects receiving paroxetine (up to 20 mg/day) showed a 60% response rate compared with 17% for subjects receiving placebo (Benjamin et al. 2000). A more recent randomized, double-blind pilot trial compared escitalopram versus placebo over 12 weeks in 12 adults with specific phobia (Alamy et al. 2008). No difference was observed on the primary outcome; however, 60% of escitalopram-treated subjects showed response (based on a Clinical Global Impression Scale [CGI] Improvement score of 1 or 2), compared with 29% of subjects receiving placebo (effect size=1.13). The findings from these two small trials require validation in larger controlled trials. In contrast, in a controlled trial of the serotonergic and noradrenergic TCA imipramine in 218 phobic subjects (agoraphobic, mixed phobic, or simple phobic) receiving 26 weeks of behavior therapy, no difference was observed between imipramine and placebo (Zitrin et al. 1983).

In a long-term controlled study of clonazepam in social phobia, Davidson et al. (1994) observed that clonazepam was superior in reducing symptoms of anxiety related to blood-injury phobia as measured by changes in the blood-injury phobia subscale of the Marks-Mathews FQ. Intermittent use of benzodiazepines also may be helpful in the acute treatment of the somatic anxiety that accompanies specific phobia, although this usage has not been an area of active investigation.

Using a novel approach, Ressler et al. (2004) investigated the effect of a cognitive enhancer, D-cycloserine, as an adjunct to psychotherapy. D-Cycloserine is an *N*-methyl-D-aspartate (NMDA) receptor partial agonist that has demonstrated improvement in extinction in rodents. Subjects with acrophobia (n=28) were randomly assigned to receive a single dose of D-cycloserine or placebo prior to each of two virtual reality exposure therapy sessions. The combination of D-cycloserine and exposure therapy was associated with greater improvement in the virtual reality setting, as well as on a variety of anxiety domains. These changes were noted early in treatment and were maintained at 3-month follow-up.

Specific phobia tends to be a chronic condition. Although psychotherapeutic approaches can be beneficial in the short term, evidence suggests that the initial gains noted with treatment may not be sustained over the long term (Lipsitz et al. 1999). Pharmacological augmentation may help to extend the benefits of exposure therapy over time.

Generalized Anxiety Disorder

GAD is a common disorder, with a lifetime prevalence of 5%–6% (Wittchen and Hoyer 2001), and is the most prevalent anxiety disorder in primary care, with rates that exceed 8% (Goldberg and Lecrubier 1995). GAD tends to be a chronic and disabling condition with lifetime rates of comorbidity as high as 90% (Wittchen et al. 1994), particularly depression (prevalence rate greater than 60%), which can increase the severity and burden of the disorder.

Assessment of response in almost all GAD pharmacotherapy trials has been with the clinician-administered Hamilton Anxiety Scale (Ham-A; Hamilton 1959), which measures psychic and somatic symptoms of anxiety; remission is usually defined as a Ham-A score of 7 or less. The self-rated Hospital Anxiety and Depression Scale (HADS; Zigmond and Snaith 1983) is also widely used and is capable of detecting differences in treatment efficacy.

Anxiolytics

Benzodiazepines

Benzodiazepines have been widely used to treat acute and chronic anxiety since their introduction in the 1960s. Their activity is mediated through potentiation of the inhibitory neurotransmitter γ-aminobutyric acid (GABA) at the $GABA_A$ receptor. The efficacy and relative safety of benzodiazepines in short-term use (i.e., several weeks or months) are well established (Rickels et al. 1983; Shader and Greenblatt 1993). However, the longer-term use of these drugs is more controversial and can be associated with the development of tolerance, physiological dependence, and withdrawal (if abruptly discontinued), as well as troublesome side effects, including ataxia, sedation, motor dysfunction, and cognitive impairment. Furthermore, these drugs should be avoided in patients with a history of substance use disorders, and long-term use may infrequently lead to the development of major depression (Lydiard et al. 1987).

Benzodiazepines have been shown to be effective in GAD, as reported by Rickels et al. (1993). The appeal of these drugs lies in their rapid onset of action, ease of use, tolerability, and relative safety. Findings from several 6- to 8-month trials of maintenance treatment for chronic anxiety have indicated continued efficacy of benzodiazepines over time (Rickels et al. 1983, 1988a, 1988b; Schweizer et al. 1993). Because GAD tends to be a chronic disorder, many patients may need to continue pharmacotherapy with benzodiazepines (or other drugs) for many years, and long-term use of benzodiazepines may lead to the complications listed above.

Approximately 70% of patients with GAD will respond to an adequate trial of a benzodiazepine (Greenblatt et al. 1983), which corresponds to the equivalent of a 3- to 4-week treatment course of up to 40 mg/day of diazepam or 4 mg/day of alprazolam (Schweizer and Rickels 1996). Discontinuation should be managed by slow taper to minimize withdrawal symptoms, rebound anxiety, and relapse potential. Some evidence suggests that benzodiazepines may be more effective in treating the autonomic arousal and somatic symptoms of GAD but less effective for the psychic symptoms of worry and irritability (Rickels et al. 1982; Rosenbaum et al. 1984).

As our understanding of the phenomenology of GAD has grown and as the diagnostic criteria have evolved from DSM-III (American Psychiatric Association 1980) to DSM-IV (American Psychiatric Association 1994), there has been a greater emphasis on the psychic component of the disorder. Given these changes, along with the high rates of comorbid depression in GAD and the anxiolytic activity of many of the newer classes of antidepressants, the use of benzodiazepines as a primary treatment for GAD is less recommended.

Azapirones

The azapirones are believed to exert their anxiolytic effect through partial agonism of 5-HT_{1A} receptors. Several trials have indicated that buspirone is superior to placebo and comparable to benzodiazepines in treating GAD, with fewer side effects and without concerns for abuse, dependence, and withdrawal (Cohn et al. 1986; Enkelmann 1991; Petracca et al. 1990; Rickels et al. 1988b; Strand et al. 1990), although other studies have reported conflicting results (Fontaine et al. 1987; Olajide and Lader 1987; Ross and Matas 1987). Buspirone appears more effective in treating the psychic component of anxiety (Rickels et al. 1982) and possibly anxiety with mixed depressive symptoms (Rickels et al. 1991) than the somatic and autonomic symptoms of anxiety (Schweizer and Rickels 1988; Sheehan et al. 1990). An adequate trial of buspirone in GAD would be 3–4 weeks of treatment at a dosage of up to 60 mg/day, in divided doses. Treatment-limiting effects of the drug include greater potential for side effects at higher dosages, slower onset of action, more variable antidepressant effects, and possibly reduced effectiveness in patients with a prior favorable response to benzodiazepines (Schweizer et al. 1986).

Tricyclic Antidepressants

In a 6-week trial comparing imipramine and alprazolam, similar improvement was observed with both treatments by week 2; however, imipramine appeared to be more effective in treating the psychic anxiety component, whereas alprazolam was more effective in attenuating somatic symptoms (Hoehn-Saric et al. 1988). In an 8-week double-blind, placebo-controlled trial of imipramine, trazodone, and diazepam (Rickels et al. 1993), diazepam showed an early-onset effect by week 2, primarily on somatic symptoms. Over the next 6 weeks, however, psychic anxiety symptoms were more responsive to the antidepressants. Overall, imipramine was more efficacious than diazepam, trazodone was comparable to diazepam, and all treatments were superior to placebo. In a controlled trial comparing imipramine, paroxetine, and 2′-chlordesmethyldiazepam, early onset of action was again noted with the benzodiazepine by week 2, but overall greater improvement was noted with the antidepressants by week 4, especially in psychic symptoms (Rocca et al. 1997).

Selective Serotonin Reuptake Inhibitors and Serotonin-Norepinephrine Reuptake Inhibitors

A number of SSRIs are effective in GAD. Paroxetine IR at 20–50 mg/day has been shown to be as effective as imipramine and more effective than 2′-chlordesmethyldiazepam (Rocca et al. 1997). Compared with placebo, a similar dosage range of paroxetine IR was associated with significant reduction in anxiety after 8 weeks of treatment (Bellew et al. 2000; Pollack et al. 2001; Rickels et al. 2003), with an improvement in Ham-A-rated psychic anxiety observed as early as 1 week after initiating treatment (Pollack et al. 2001). Paroxetine IR also improves social functioning in patients with GAD (Bellew et al. 2000).

Escitalopram was found to be superior to placebo in improving anxiety symptoms, disability, or quality of life in three 8-week trials at a 10- to 20-mg dose range (Davidson et al.

2004a; Goodman et al. 2005), and it was found equivalent to paroxetine IR in a 6-month trial (Bielski et al. 2005). In a larger placebo-controlled trial, 10 mg escitalopram was superior to 20 mg paroxetine, and 10 and 20 mg escitalopram were superior to placebo (Baldwin et al. 2006). A relapse prevention study found that sustained treatment with escitalopram 20 mg/day up to 74 weeks reduced the relapse rate (19%) relative to placebo substitution (56%) (Allgulander et al. 2006).

Sertraline was demonstrated to be superior to placebo in GAD in a 12-week (Allgulander et al. 2004) and a 10-week (Brawman-Mintzer et al. 2006) double-blind, placebo-controlled trial; sertraline was well tolerated and showed beneficial effects on Ham-A-rated psychic and somatic anxiety symptoms compared with placebo (Dahl et al. 2005).

Several placebo-controlled trials have confirmed the short-term efficacy of venlafaxine XR in GAD over 8 weeks on both psychic and somatic symptoms. In a trial of 365 adult outpatients treated with venlafaxine XR (75 mg/day or 150 mg/day), buspirone (30 mg/day), or placebo, the Ham-A-adjusted mean scores of the anxiety and tension items were significantly improved at both active drug doses compared with placebo; venlafaxine XR was superior to buspirone on the HADS Anxiety subscale (Davidson et al. 1999). In a second trial of 541 outpatients on either venlafaxine XR (37.5 mg/day, 75 mg/day, or 150 mg/day) or placebo (Allgulander et al. 2001), the 75-mg and 150-mg doses of venlafaxine showed superior efficacy compared with placebo on all primary outcome measures (with improvement in psychic anxiety noted earlier than somatic symptoms), whereas the 37.5-mg dose was superior on only one measure (the Anxiety subscale of the HADS). In a third trial of fixed dosages (75 mg/day, 150 mg/day, and 225 mg/day) of venlafaxine XR (Rickels et al. 2000), venlafaxine XR was superior to placebo on all outcome measures, with the most robust effects observed at 225 mg/day. Venlafaxine XR significantly reduced psychic anxiety but not somatic symptoms.

Venlafaxine XR also has shown long-term efficacy in GAD. In two 6-month controlled trials of fixed (37.5 mg, 75 mg, 150 mg/day) (Allgulander et al. 2001) and flexible (75–225 mg/day) (Gelenberg et al. 2000) dosages of venlafaxine XR, significant improvement in anxiety was observed as early as 1 week, and efficacy was sustained over the 28-week treatment period. In the fixed-dosage study of venlafaxine XR, the greatest effect was observed with the 150-mg/day dosage. Significant improvement in social functioning was noted at the two higher dosages by week 8 and was sustained over the 6 months of the trial.

Venlafaxine XR is also effective in treating GAD with comorbid depression (Silverstone and Salinas 2001). After 12 weeks of treatment with venlafaxine XR (75–225 mg/day), fluoxetine, or placebo, significant reduction was observed in both Ham-A-rated anxiety and Hamilton Rating Scale for Depression (Ham-D; Hamilton 1960)–rated depression only in subjects receiving venlafaxine XR. The response was delayed somewhat in subjects with comorbid GAD and depression, as compared with those with depression alone, suggesting that individuals with comorbidity may benefit from a longer course of treatment.

The traditional treatment goal for GAD and many other psychiatric disorders has been attainment of response, defined as 50% improvement relative to baseline. There is a growing consensus in the field, however, that the goal of treatment should instead be remission, defined as 70% or greater improvement from baseline and/or minimal or absent symptoms (i.e., Ham-A score ≤7). Pooled analysis of data from the two long-term studies noted earlier (Allgulander et al. 2001; Gelenberg et al. 2000) has determined that remission is attainable in GAD (Meoni and Hackett 2000). By 2 months, approximately 40% of those receiving venlafaxine responded to treatment, and 42% attained remission. By 6 months, the proportion of those in remission increased to almost 60%, whereas responders declined to 20%, in contrast to a remission rate of less than 40% with placebo.

Venlafaxine XR has some advantages over the benzodiazepines—notably, antidepressant activity, lack of potential for abuse and dependence, and efficacy in treating symptoms of psychic anxiety. Nonetheless, venlafaxine can be associated with some adverse effects in the long term, including sexual dysfunction and blood pressure elevation in some patients. Abrupt discontinuation of treatment can be associated with unpleasant side effects, most commonly dizziness, lightheadedness, tinnitus, nausea, vomiting, and loss of appetite, and the discontinuation syndrome is worse if one abruptly stops at higher dosage levels (Allgulander et al. 2001).

Duloxetine, another SNRI antidepressant, has shown efficacy superior to placebo in GAD (Allgulander et al. 2007; Rynn et al. 2008) in the range of 60–120 mg/day and also appears to lessen the chance of relapse during maintenance therapy.

One interesting application of SSRIs in GAD is in combination with nonbenzodiazepine hypnotics such as eszopiclone (Pollack et al. 2008a) and zolpidem (Fava et al. 2009), which may be particularly suited where insomnia is a major problem.

Noradrenergic and Specific Serotonergic Antidepressants (Mirtazapine, Bupropion)

The antidepressant mirtazapine also has demonstrated anxiolytic properties (Ribeiro et al. 2001). However, published reports of its effect in GAD are limited to a small open-label study in major depression and comorbid GAD (Goodnick et al. 1999) and a small open-label GAD trial in 44 outpatients (Gambi et al. 2005). Although the results were encouraging, data from controlled trials are needed to adequately assess a possible role for mirtazapine in GAD.

A 12-week double-blind active comparison trial of bupropion XL at 150–300 mg/day versus escitalopram at 10–20 mg/day in 24 subjects found similar Ham-A-rated anxiolytic efficacy of bupropion XL and escitalopram (Bystritsky et al. 2008). Notwithstanding these intriguing findings, the current body of clinical evidence supports the use of SSRIs or SNRIs before agents that are primarily noradrenergic in action.

Hydroxyzine

Hydroxyzine, a drug that blocks both histamine$_1$ (H_1) and muscarinic receptors, has been studied in GAD. In one controlled study, hydroxyzine was superior to placebo following 1 week of treatment, and this difference was maintained over a 4-week trial (Ferreri and Hantouche 1998). In a larger controlled multicenter trial, hydroxyzine was compared with buspirone over 4 weeks (Lader and Scotto 1998). Changes in the Ham-A from baseline to day 28 indicated that hydroxyzine was superior to placebo, with no difference observed between buspirone and placebo, although both hydroxyzine and buspirone were more efficacious than placebo on the secondary outcomes. Llorca et al. (2002) found that hydroxyzine 50 mg/day was superior to placebo and comparable to bromazepam in a 12-week trial.

Anticonvulsants

The $\alpha_2\delta$ calcium channel antagonist pregabalin was superior to placebo in four studies of GAD (Feltner et al. 2003; Pande et al. 2003; Pohl et al. 2005; Rickels et al. 2005). Efficacy was noted early in treatment, but the ability of this drug to successfully treat some of the comorbid disorders associated with GAD is unknown. A recent review of six short-term double-blind, placebo-controlled pregabalin trials in GAD showed that pregabalin treatment significantly improved both psychic and somatic Ham-A-rated GAD symptoms, with a dose-response effect that plateaued at 300 mg/day (Lydiard et al.

2010). Pregabalin has shown efficacy and reasonably good tolerability in elderly patients with GAD (Montgomery 2006). In a long-term trial in 624 GAD patients, responders to 8 weeks of open-label pregabalin at 450 mg/day were randomly assigned to pregabalin or placebo for 24 weeks (Feltner et al. 2008). Relapse rates were significantly lower for pregabalin (42%) than for placebo (65%), although attrition rates for pregabalin were higher (21.4% vs. 15.3%).

The GABA reuptake inhibitor tiagabine failed to separate from placebo on key measures in three placebo-controlled multicenter trials (Pollack et al. 2008b).

Antipsychotics

Evidence for antipsychotic monotherapy in GAD is limited for some agents and more robust for others. An open-label trial suggested benefit for ziprasidone (Snyderman et al. 2005). Flupenthixol is approved for the treatment of depression in some countries and was shown in one controlled study to be superior to amitriptyline, clotiazepam, and placebo in subjects with refractory GAD (Wurthmann et al. 1995). Sulpiride is also used in similar situations (Bruscky et al. 1974; Chen et al. 1994).

The strongest evidence supporting atypical antipsychotic use in GAD at present is for quetiapine XR, which was shown to be effective and superior to placebo in a multicenter trial, and at 150 mg/day was effective for both psychic and somatic anxiety symptoms, with improvement being noted as early as 4 days (Bandelow et al. 2010). The active comparator in this trial, paroxetine 20 mg/day, showed lesser effect on somatic anxiety and a higher prevalence of sexual side effects. Remission rates were 42.6%, 38.8%, and 27.2% for quetiapine XR, paroxetine, and placebo, respectively. A longer-term double-blind, placebo-controlled multicenter maintenance trial with quetiapine XR at 50–300 mg/day in 432 patients found it to be effective in preventing recurrence of anxiety symptoms (Katzman et al. 2011).

Long-term use of atypical antipsychotics carries some concerns about tolerability and safety, especially in regard to weight gain and metabolic adverse effects, and these concerns need to be balanced against the long-term benefits in GAD in terms of reduction of disability and improved functionality.

Other Drugs

Riluzole, a presynaptic glutamate release inhibitor, showed promise in a small open-label study at a daily dose of 100 mg (Mathew et al. 2005). Agomelatine, a serotonin 5-HT_{2C} antagonist and $melatonin_{1/2}$ receptor agonist, is efficacious in GAD (Stein et al. 2008).

Complementary treatments have had mixed results in GAD. Homeopathy was found to be ineffective in one trial (Bonne et al. 2003). The herbal remedy kava did not separate from placebo in one trial (Connor and Davidson 2002), although Sarris et al. (2009) showed some evidence supporting the benefit of a water-soluble formulation of kava in subjects with short-term GAD-like symptoms. Liver damage remains a potentially devastating concern, however, and even the preferred aqueous extract cannot be regarded as entirely safe, particularly at kava dosages above 250 mg/day (Teschke and Schulze 2010). Two small, placebo-controlled trials suggest that chamomile and Ginkgo biloba may have modest anxiolytic effects in patients with mild to moderate GAD (Amsterdam et al. 2009; Woelk et al. 2007).

A meta-analysis of GAD studies by Hidalgo et al. (2007) showed that the effect sizes (in diminishing order from strongest to weakest) for each drug or drug group versus placebo were as follows: pregabalin, 0.50; hydroxyzine, 0.45; venlafaxine XR, 0.42; benzodiazepines, 0.38; SSRIs, 0.36; buspirone, 0.17; and homeopathy and herbal treatment, –0.31.

Drugs that have been approved in the United States for treating GAD or historical forerunners of the disorder include a large number of benzodiazepines, buspirone, paroxetine IR, escitalopram, venlafaxine XR, and duloxetine. Pregabalin is not approved in the United States but is approved for GAD in Europe.

There is also convincing evidence in favor of efficacy for CBT in GAD, with sustained benefit over 2 years of follow-up. These findings have been well reviewed by Swinson et al. (2006). There are no clinically informative studies to compare, or combine, CBT and pharmacotherapy in GAD, but on pragmatic grounds, one may consider their combination in patients who have shown only a partial response to a thorough course of either CBT or medication alone.

Posttraumatic Stress Disorder

Posttraumatic stress disorder (PTSD) is a chronic and disabling disorder, with a lifetime prevalence of about 7% (Kessler et al. 2005a). It can lead to significant functional impairment and inflict an enormous burden on society.

Treatment of PTSD must target the core symptoms of the disorder, focusing on improving resilience and quality of life and reducing comorbidity and disability. Widely used instruments include the DSM-IV criteria–linked Clinician-Administered PTSD Scale (CAPS; Weathers et al. 2001) and the more globally oriented Short PTSD Rating Instrument (SPRINT; Connor and Davidson 2001). Self-rating scales include the Davidson Trauma Scale (DTS; Davidson et al. 1997a), the PTSD Checklist (PCL; Weathers et al. 1991), and the SPRINT, which also has been validated as a self-rating.

Antidepressants

The TCAs and MAOIs were among the first pharmacological agents studied in controlled trials of PTSD. More recently, several controlled multicenter trials have shown efficacy for the SSRIs and SNRIs. With the documented antidepressant and anxiolytic effects of these agents and the high rates of comorbid depression in PTSD (Kessler et al. 1995), antidepressants would seem a logical choice for PTSD treatment.

Tricyclic Antidepressants

Two controlled trials of TCAs in male combat veterans with DSM-III-defined PTSD showed benefit for amitriptyline and imipramine (Davidson et al. 1990; Kosten et al. 1991).

Monoamine Oxidase Inhibitors

In a study of male combat veterans, Kosten et al. (1991) compared phenelzine (15–75 mg/day) with placebo and found a 45% decrease in Impact of Event Scale (IES) scores from baseline for phenelzine, compared with a 5% decrease for placebo, but no improvement was noted in depressive symptoms with either treatment. The RIMA brofaromine has been assessed in two controlled trials of PTSD: a U.S. sample composed predominantly of combat veterans (n=114) (Baker et al. 1995) and a civilian European sample with few veterans (n=68) (Katz et al. 1994). The U.S. study failed to show a difference between the treatments, and findings from the European study were mixed. Finally, the RIMA moclobemide was assessed in 20 subjects with PTSD meeting DSM-III-R (American Psychiatric Association 1987) criteria (Neal et al. 1997). Following 12 weeks of treatment, 11 subjects no longer met the full PTSD criteria, providing a signal that the drug might be effective in PTSD.

Selective Serotonin Reuptake Inhibitors and Serotonin-Norepinephrine Reuptake Inhibitors

Three controlled trials support the efficacy of fluoxetine in PTSD. In these studies, fluoxetine was administered at dosages of 20–80 mg/day for 5–12 weeks in samples including both civilians and combat veterans with PTSD meeting DSM-III-R (Connor et al. 1999; van der Kolk et al. 1994) or DSM-IV (Martenyi et al. 2002a) criteria. Significant improvement in clinician-rated structured interviews from baseline to end of treatment were noted, as were significant improvement in resilience and reductions in disability (Connor et al. 1999). Symptomatic improvement was noted as early as week 6 (Martenyi et al. 2002a).

Two studies of maintenance therapy with fluoxetine over a period of 1 year have shown reductions in the rate of relapse, as compared with placebo substitution (Davidson et al. 2005; Martenyi et al. 2002b).

Sertraline has been compared against placebo in 10 trials, and positive results have emerged in 3 (Brady et al. 2000; Davidson et al. 2001; Panahi et al. 2011), while 7 were either ambiguous or negative. A pooled analysis of the two positive trials showed an early effect on anger at 1 week (Davidson et al. 2002). This finding is of significance, given that angry temperament can be associated with violence and a greater risk for cardiac events (Williams et al. 2001), as well as increased heart rate and blood pressure, in PTSD (Beckham et al. 2002). A recent placebo-controlled trial of sertraline in Iranian veterans of the Iran-Iraq war showed that sertraline was superior to placebo and was well tolerated (Panahi et al. 2011). Other short-term studies of sertraline in PTSD have been negative (Brady et al. 2005; Davidson et al. 2006b; Friedman et al. 2007; Tucker et al. 2003) or inconclusive (Zohar et al. 2002). A trial in children by Robb et al. (2010) failed to show any difference between drug and placebo.

Continued sertraline treatment over 9 months was associated with sustained improvement in more than 90% of subjects, and more than 50% of initial nonresponders responded with continued treatment (Londborg et al. 2001). Improvement was sustained over 15 months, with a relapse rate of 5% for sertraline and 26% for placebo, suggesting that the drug provides prophylactic protection against relapse (Davidson et al. 2001). Sertraline was also effective in improving quality of life and reducing functional impairment, with more than 55% of patients functioning at levels within 10% of the general population. These gains were maintained with long-term treatment, whereas treatment discontinuation was more likely to lead to deteriorating function, although not to levels observed prior to treatment (Rapaport et al. 2002).

The efficacy of paroxetine in PTSD has been shown in two 12-week controlled multicenter trials, including flexible-dose (n=307; paroxetine 20–50 mg) (Tucker et al. 2001) and fixed-dose (n=451; paroxetine 20 or 40 mg) (Marshall et al. 2001) regimens. Compared with placebo, paroxetine produced significant improvement in overall PTSD symptomatology, individual symptom clusters, and functional impairment. Response rates ranged from 54% to 62% for paroxetine compared with 37% to 40% for placebo.

Findings from two open-label studies of fluvoxamine at dosages of 100–250 mg/day—an 8-week study in civilians (n=15; Davidson et al. 1998) and a 10-week study in combat veterans (n=10; Marmar et al. 1996)—showed that the drug was effective in treating PTSD symptoms. Treatment with fluvoxamine (mean=194 mg/day) also was associated with significant improvement in autonomic reactivity, with reductions in heart rate and blood pressure on exposure to trauma cues to levels that are indistinguishable from those of control subjects (Tucker et al. 2000). These findings are encouraging, although larger controlled trials are needed to determine the efficacy of the drug in PTSD.

In contrast, Shalev et al. (2012) found that escitalopram administered in the acute aftermath of trauma was no different from placebo in treating acute PTSD and did not prevent chronic PTSD.

Two large multicenter studies have established efficacy for venlafaxine XR up to 300 mg per day, in one case for as long as 6 months. Rates of remission exceeded 50% in the longer-term trial, and resilience was significantly improved in one of the two studies (Davidson et al. 2006a, 2006b).

In summary, the SSRIs are efficacious in the treatment of PTSD, and paroxetine IR and sertraline are approved for PTSD treatment. SSRIs and SNRIs show a broad spectrum of activity, with significant reduction in some symptoms as early as 1–2 weeks after treatment initiation, sustained and continued improvement, and in some cases remission, with long-term treatment up to 15 months. These drugs are generally well tolerated, although some adverse effects (e.g., sexual dysfunction, sleep disturbances, and weight gain) may lead to treatment discontinuation.

Other Antidepressants

An 8-week controlled trial of mirtazapine in 29 outpatients with PTSD showed a 65% response rate on clinician-rated global assessment with mirtazapine compared with a rate of 20% with placebo, with significant improvement on several measures of PTSD as well as general anxiety (Davidson et al. 2003).

Six open-label studies of nefazodone in civilians and combat veterans with PTSD have been reported (Hidalgo et al. 1999). Treatment with nefazodone (50–600 mg/day) over 6–12 weeks was associated with significant reduction in severity of overall PTSD, as well as in each of the symptom clusters. Of particular note was improvement in sleep, which is often disrupted in PTSD and sometimes worsened by treatment with SSRIs. Davis et al. (2004) have demonstrated superior efficacy for the drug, relative to placebo, in combat veterans.

Anxiolytics

Benzodiazepines are often prescribed to treat acute anxiety in the aftermath of a trauma; however, findings have been disappointing. An open-label study of alprazolam and clonazepam in 13 outpatients with PTSD found reduced hyperarousal symptoms but no change in intrusion or avoidance/numbing (Gelpin et al. 1996). In a crossover design, subjects received 5 weeks of treatment with either alprazolam or placebo followed by 5 weeks of the alternative therapy (Braun et al. 1990). Minimal improvement was observed in anxiety symptoms overall, with no improvement in core PTSD symptoms. Clonazepam 2 mg was not different from placebo in controlling nightmares in a 2-week single-blind crossover study, where the test drug was added to preexisting treatment (Cates et al. 2004). Thus, the evidence does not support the use of benzodiazepines in the management of core PTSD symptoms, even though they appear to be widely used for that purpose (Mellman et al. 2003).

Anticonvulsants

Lipper et al. (1986) proposed that the pathophysiology of PTSD may involve sensitization and kindling processes and, to this end, that anticonvulsants might be of therapeutic benefit. In testing this hypothesis, Lipper and colleagues found that 7 of 10 Vietnam War veterans who received open-label carbamazepine (600–1,000 mg/day) for 5 weeks reported improvement, particularly in intrusion and hyperarousal symptoms. Three subsequent open-label studies, two with sodium valproate in combat veterans (Clark et al. 1999; Fesler 1991) and one with adjunctive topiramate in a civilian PTSD sample (Berlant and van Kammen 2002) also reported positive effects. However, two more recent double-blind, placebo-controlled trials of divalproex monotherapy in combat veterans with PTSD were negative (Davis et al. 2008a, $n=85$; Hamner et al. 2009, $n=29$). Topiramate has also been shown to have no effect in PTSD (Tucker et al. 2007).

The largest placebo-controlled trial of an anticonvulsant to date found no difference between tiagabine, dosed up to 16 mg/day, and placebo in a 12-week multicenter trial in 232 patients (Davidson et al. 2007). In a small placebo-controlled trial of lamotrigine (200–500 mg/day) in 15 outpatients (Hertzberg et al. 1999), a response rate of 50% was noted with lamotrigine, compared with a placebo response rate of 25%.

Other Treatments

Antipsychotics

In a monotherapy trial of olanzapine (Butterfield et al. 2001), 15 subjects were randomly assigned 2:1 to treatment with olanzapine (up to 20 mg/day) or placebo. No differences were observed between the treatments; however, it is difficult to interpret the findings in this small sample, especially given the high placebo response rate (60%). In a recent small randomized, placebo-controlled trial of flexible-dose olanzapine monotherapy in a noncombat-related chronic PTSD population, olanzapine was found to be superior to placebo, though approximately half of the patient sample experienced significant weight gain (Carey et al. 2012). Other reports of antipsychotics are based on augmentation therapy in SSRI partial responders. Several placebo-controlled studies, mainly as augmentation, have found superior efficacy for low-dose risperidone in both civilian and veteran populations (Bartzokis et al. 2005; Hamner et al. 2003; Monnelly et al. 2003; Reich et al. 2004; Rothbaum et al. 2008) and olanzapine (Stein et al. 2002). In the Monnelly et al. (2003) study, particular benefit was noted for irritability, and in the Hamner et al. (2003) study, psychotic symptoms were relieved. However, a recent large double-blind, placebo-controlled trial of adjunctive risperidone treatment in a patient population with military-related PTSD and SRI-resistant symptoms found no major benefit for risperidone, although statistically significant changes occurred on some measures (Krystal et al. 2011).

In a recently completed double-blind, placebo-controlled monotherapy trial of quetiapine in 80 patients with chronic PTSD, a significant improvement in CAPS scores, as well as in reexperiencing and hyperarousal subscores, was seen by the end of the 12-week trial (Canive et al. 2009).

Prazosin and Guanfacine

Raskind et al. (2003) reported encouraging results for intractable PTSD-related nightmares in a placebo-controlled crossover study of prazosin, an α_1-adrenergic antagonist, at dosages of up to 10 mg/day. The initial findings were confirmed in a second and larger placebo-controlled, double-blind augmentation trial in combat veterans, using dosages of up to 15 mg daily; benefits were most apparent on nightmares and sleep quality, but the drug also produced greater global improvement (Raskind et al. 2007). In a randomized, placebo-controlled crossover study of prazosin in 13 patients with civilian trauma–related PTSD, Taylor et al. (2008) found that prazosin significantly increased total and rapid eye movement (REM) sleep time, reduced trauma-related nightmares and awakenings, and improved PCL and CGI scores. A recent study comparing prazosin with quetiapine for nighttime PTSD symptoms found similar short-term effectiveness for the two drugs but a greater likelihood of treatment discontinuation due to adverse effects for quetiapine (Byers et al. 2010).

In contrast, two placebo-controlled studies of the α_2-adrenergic agonist guanfacine in veterans with PTSD found no benefit (Davis et al. 2008b; Neylan et al. 2006).

Additional Approaches

Given the prevalence of comorbid depression with PTSD and the effectiveness of triiodothyronine (T_3) augmentation in some individuals with treatment-refractory depression, it is possible that T_3 augmentation also may be of benefit in PTSD. Five subjects with PTSD currently taking an SSRI were treated with open-label T_3 (25 μg/day) for 8 weeks (Agid et al. 2001). Improvement was noted as early as 2 weeks, and by the end of treatment, four of the five subjects showed at least partial improvement in depressive symptoms and hyperarousal. The mechanism for these effects is unknown, and further controlled studies of this augmentation strategy are needed. Cyproheptadine, an antihistaminic drug, was no more effective than placebo for nightmares over 2 weeks in a series of 69 combat veterans with PTSD (Jacobs-Rebhun et al. 2000). The naturally occurring compound inositol was ineffective in a small placebo-controlled trial (Kaplan et al. 1996). Innovative treatments with some promise include the NMDA agonist D-serine (Heresco-Levy et al. 2009; de Kleine et al. 2012) and the neurokinin-1 receptor antagonist GR205171(Mathew et al. 2011).

Low-intensity rTMS—in particular, right-sided rTMS applied to the dorsolateral prefrontal cortex (Boggio et al. 2010)—has shown some promise in PTSD, as has acupuncture (Hollifield et al. 2007). A recent electroconvulsive therapy (ECT) open trial in 20 patients with chronic, treatment-refractory PTSD showed improvement in CAPS-rated PTSD symptoms, independent of depressive symptoms (Margoob et al. 2010). Larger double-blind studies are needed before these somatic treatments can be recommended for PTSD.

CBT has been extensively studied in PTSD and shows overall efficacy (Bisson and Andrew 2005). In one large well-designed multicenter trial (Schnurr et al. 2007), the effect size and number-needed-to-treat results for CBT were of the same order of magnitude as those found in comparable trials of antidepressant drugs for PTSD, but there have been no head-to-head trials of CBT and medication. Exposure is regarded as the key therapeutic principle in the numerous variants of CBT and is recommended as a first-line treatment for PTSD. Modest preservation of gains is found at long-term follow-up (Bradley et al. 2005), but much pathology remains.

Acute Stress Disorder and the Immediate Aftermath of Trauma

Acute stress disorder (ASD) develops shortly after a traumatic event; symptoms include dissociation and intrusive recollections, avoidance, and hyperarousal that persist for 2–28 days following the trauma and cause significant distress and/or impairment. ASD was first included in DSM-IV, and it has been suggested that early intervention might help to alter the course of PTSD, which would imply early identification and treatment of those with or at risk for ASD.

The effects of open-label treatment with risperidone have been reported in four inpatient survivors of physical trauma with ASD; this drug showed possible benefit in flashback symptoms (Eidelman et al. 2000).

A controlled pilot study assessed the effects of low-dose imipramine compared with chloral hydrate in 25 pediatric burn patients with ASD (Robert et al. 1999a). After 1 week of treatment, 38% of the subjects responded to treatment with placebo, compared with 83% to imipramine, with an earlier report noting reduction in intrusion and hyperarousal symptoms (Robert et al. 1999b). Unfortunately, a subsequent placebo-controlled trial failed to replicate these promising initial findings (Robert et al. 2008).

The effects of β-adrenergic blockade in reducing subsequent PTSD following acute trauma were also evaluated (Pitman et al. 2002). Within 6 hours of the trauma, subjects were treated with either propranolol (n=18; 40 mg four times per day) or placebo (n=23) for 10 days, followed by a 9-day taper period. PTSD was noted in 30% of the placebo group compared with 10% of the propranolol group 1 month after the trauma, and at 3-month follow-up, physiological arousal rate to trauma cues was 43% in the placebo group compared with 0% of the propranolol group. However, a more recent double-blind, randomized controlled 14-day trial of propranolol and gabapentin versus placebo, administered within 48 hours of admission to a surgical trauma unit, did not demonstrate any benefits of the two active drugs over placebo on depressive or PTSD symptoms (Stein et al. 2007).

A short-term trial with temazepam versus placebo in the acute aftermath of trauma showed no long-term benefits and possibly worse PTSD outcomes at 6-week follow-up (Mellman et al. 2002).

Three promising studies have found greater long-term benefit for short-term hydrocortisone versus placebo in high-risk subjects recovering from septic shock, cardiac surgery, or acute respiratory distress syndrome (Hauer et al. 2009; Schelling et al. 2006). In subpopulations with critical illness–related corticosteroid insufficiency, this might be an attractive treatment approach for preventing PTSD. One limitation of the authors' work, however, has been the absence of baseline PTSD ratings before administration of hydrocortisone.

Shortened forms of CBT appear to be effective for acute PTSD-like states, with persistence of gain at 4-year follow-up (Bryant et al. 1998, 2003).

Conclusion

Twenty years ago, few would have thought that one class of drugs, the SSRIs, which were all introduced initially for depression, would have established primacy in five of the six major anxiety disorder categories. Their position is based on numerous placebo-controlled trials, and they are considered first-line drugs for treatment of these disorders, followed closely by the SNRIs. There is evidence that these drugs also offer some protection against relapse. However, they are not 100% successful, they carry some limiting side effects, and they may require supplementation with, or substitution by, drugs from other categories. We have reviewed what is known about these other drugs and expect further progress in the pharmacotherapy of anxiety, with both established drugs and novel categories. Among many unexplored areas, we need to know more about the treatment of resistant and comorbid anxiety disorders, combined psychotherapy and pharmacotherapy interventions, and the comparative efficacy of pharmacotherapy and psychosocial treatment in anxiety.

References

Agid O, Shalev AY, Lerer B, et al: Triiodothyronine augmentation of selective serotonin reuptake inhibitors in posttraumatic stress disorder. J Clin Psychiatry 62:169–173, 2001

Alamy S, Zhang W, Varia I, et al: Escitalopram in specific phobia: results of a placebo-controlled pilot trial. J Psychopharmacol 22:157–161, 2008

Allgulander C: Paroxetine in social anxiety disorder: a randomized placebo-controlled study. Acta Psychiatr Scand 100:193–198, 1999

Allgulander C, Hackett D, Salinas E: Venlafaxine extended release (ER) in the treatment of generalised anxiety disorder: twenty-four-week placebo-controlled dose-ranging study. Br J Psychiatry 179:15–22, 2001

Allgulander C, Dahl AA, Austin C, et al: Efficacy of sertraline in a 12-week trial for generalized anxiety disorder. Am J Psychiatry 161:1642–1649, 2004

Allgulander C, Florea I, Huusom AK: Prevention of relapse in generalized anxiety disorder by escitalopram treatment. Int J Neuropsychopharmacol 9:495–505, 2006

Allgulander C, Hartford J, Russell J, et al: Pharmacotherapy of generalized anxiety disorder: results of duloxetine treatment from a pooled analysis of three clinical trials. Curr Med Res Opin 23:1245–1252, 2007

Alonso J, Angermeyer MC, Bernert S, et al: Sampling and methods of the European Study of the Epidemiology of Mental Disorders (ESEMeD) project. Acta Psychiatr Scand Suppl (420):8–20, 2004

American Psychiatric Association: Diagnostic and Statistical Manual of Mental Disorders, 3rd Edition. Washington, DC, American Psychiatric Association, 1980

American Psychiatric Association: Diagnostic and Statistical Manual of Mental Disorders, 3rd Edition, Revised. Washington, DC, American Psychiatric Association, 1987

American Psychiatric Association: Diagnostic and Statistical Manual of Mental Disorders, 4th Edition. Washington, DC, American Psychiatric Association, 1994

Amsterdam JD, Li Y, Soeller I, et al: A randomized, double-blind, placebo-controlled trial of oral *Matricaria recutita* (chamomile) extract therapy for generalized anxiety disorder. J Clin Psychopharmacol 29:378–382, 2009

Andersch S, Rosenberg NK, Kullingsjo H, et al: Efficacy and safety of alprazolam, imipramine and placebo in treating panic disorder. A Scandinavian multicenter study. Acta Psychiatr Scand Suppl 365:18–27, 1991

Asakura S, Tajima O, Koyama T: Fluvoxamine treatment of generalized social anxiety disorder in Japan: a randomized double-blind, placebo-controlled study. Int J Neuropsychopharmacol 10:263–274, 2007

Asnis GM, Hameedi FA, Goddard AW, et al: Fluvoxamine in the treatment of panic disorder: a multi-center, double-blind, placebo-controlled study in outpatients. Psychiatry Res 103:1–14, 2001

Baer L, Rauch SL, Ballantine HT Jr, et al: Cingulotomy for intractable obsessive-compulsive disorder. Prospective long-term follow-up of 18 patients. Arch Gen Psychiatry 52:384–392, 1995

Baker DG, Diamond BI, Gillette G, et al: A double-blind, randomized, placebo-controlled, multicenter study of brofaromine in the treatment of post-traumatic stress disorder. Psychopharmacology (Berl) 122:386–389, 1995

Baldwin D, Bobes J, Stein DJ, et al: Paroxetine in social phobia/social anxiety disorder. Randomised, double-blind, placebo-controlled study. Paroxetine Study Group. Br J Psychiatry 175:120–126, 1999

Baldwin DS, Huusom AK, Maehlum E: Escitalopram and paroxetine in the treatment of generalised anxiety disorder: randomised, placebo-controlled, double-blind study. Br J Psychiatry 189:264–272, 2006

Ballenger JC, Wheadon DE, Steiner M, et al: Double-blind, fixed-dose, placebo-controlled study of paroxetine in the treatment of panic disorder. Am J Psychiatry 155:36–42, 1998

Bandelow B, Hajak G, Holzrichter S, et al: Assessing the efficacy of treatments for panic disorder and agoraphobia, I: methodological problems. Int Clin Psychopharmacol 10:83–93, 1995

Bandelow B, Chouinard G, Bobes J et al: Extended-release quetiapine fumarate (quetiapine XR): a once-daily monotherapy effective in generalized anxiety disorder. Data from a randomized, double-blind, placebo- and active-controlled study. Int J Neuropsychopharmacol 13:305–320, 2010

Barnett SD, Kramer ML, Casat CD, et al: Efficacy of olanzapine in social anxiety disorder: a pilot study. J Psychopharmacol (Oxf) 16:365–368, 2002

Bartzokis G, Lu PH, Turner J, et al: Adjunctive risperidone in the treatment of chronic combat-related posttraumatic stress disorder. Biol Psychiatry 57:474–479, 2005

Beckham JC, Vrana SR, Barefoot JC, et al: Magnitude and duration of cardiovascular responses to anger in Vietnam veterans with and without posttraumatic stress disorder. J Consult Clin Psychol 70:228–234, 2002

Bell J, DeVeaugh-Geiss J: Multicenter trial of a 5-HT antagonist, ondansetron, in social phobia. Paper presented at the 33rd Annual Meeting of the American College of Neuropsychopharmacology, San Juan, Puerto Rico, December 12–16, 1994

Bellew KM, McCafferty JP, Iyengar M: Short-term efficacy of paroxetine in generalized anxiety disorder: a double-blind placebo-controlled trial (NR253). Paper presented at the 153rd Annual Meeting of the American Psychiatric Association, Chicago, IL, May 13–18, 2000

Benjamin J, Ben-Zion IZ, Karbofsky E, et al: Double-blind placebo-controlled pilot study of paroxetine for specific phobia. Psychopharmacology 149:194–196, 2000

Bergink V, Westenberg HG: Metabotropic glutamate II receptor agonists in panic disorder: a double blind clinical trial with LY354740. Int Clin Psychopharmacol 20:291–293, 2005

Berigan TR: Panic attacks during escalation of mirtazapine (abstract). Prim Care Companion J Clin Psychiatry 5:93, 2003

Berlant J, van Kammen DP: Open-label topiramate as primary or adjunctive therapy in chronic civilian posttraumatic stress disorder: a preliminary report. J Clin Psychiatry 63:15–20, 2002

Berlin HA, Koran LM, Jenike MA, et al: Double-blind, placebo-controlled trial of topiramate augmentation in treatment-resistant obsessive-compulsive disorder. J Clin Psychiatry 72:716–721, 2011

Bertani A, Perna G, Migliarese G, et al: Comparison of the treatment with paroxetine and reboxetine in panic disorder: a randomized, single-blind study. Pharmacopsychiatry 37:206–210, 2004

Bielski RJ, Bose A, Chang CC: A double-blind comparison of escitalopram and paroxetine in the long-term treatment of generalized anxiety disorder. Ann Clin Psychiatry 17:65–69, 2005

Bisson J, Andrew M: Psychological treatment of post-traumatic stress disorder (PTSD). Cochrane Database Syst Rev (2):CD003388, 2005

Black DW, Wesner R, Bowers W, et al: A comparison of fluvoxamine, cognitive therapy, and placebo in the treatment of panic disorder. Arch Gen Psychiatry 50:44–50, 1993

Bloch MH, Landeros-Weisenberger A, Kelmendi B, et al: A systematic review: antipsychotic augmentation with treatment refractory obsessive-compulsive disorder. Mol Psychiatry 11:622–632, 2006

Blomhoff S, Haug TT, Hellstrom K, et al: Randomised controlled general practice trial of sertraline, exposure therapy and combined treatment in generalised social phobia. Br J Psychiatry 179:23–30, 2001

Boggio PS, Rocha M, Oliveira MO, et al: Noninvasive brain stimulation with high-frequency and low-intensity repetitive transcranial magnetic stimulation treatment for posttraumatic stress disorder. J Clin Psychiatry 71:992–999, 2010

Bonne O, Shemer Y, Gorali Y, et al: A randomized, double-blind, placebo-controlled study of classical homeopathy in generalized anxiety disorder. J Clin Psychiatry 64:282–287, 2003

Boshuisen ML, Slaap BR, Vester-Blokland ED, et al: The effect of mirtazapine in panic disorder: an open label pilot study with a single-blind placebo run-in period. Int Clin Psychopharmacol 16:363–368, 2001

Boyer W: Serotonin uptake inhibitors are superior to imipramine and alprazolam in alleviating panic attacks: a meta-analysis. Int Clin Psychopharmacol 10:45–49, 1995

Bradley R, Greene J, Russ E, et al: A multidimensional meta-analysis of psychotherapy for PTSD. Am J Psychiatry 162:214–227, 2005

Bradwejn J, Ahokas A, Stein DJ, et al: Venlafaxine extended-release capsules in panic disorder: flexible-dose, double-blind, placebo-controlled study. Br J Psychiatry 187:352–359, 2005

Brady K, Pearlstein T, Asnis GM, et al: Efficacy and safety of sertraline treatment of posttraumatic stress disorder: a randomized controlled trial. JAMA 283:1837–1844, 2000

Brady KT, Sonne S, Anton RF, et al: Sertraline in the treatment of co-occurring alcohol dependence and posttraumatic stress disorder. Alcohol Clin Exp Res 29:395–401, 2005

Braun P, Greenberg D, Dasberg H, et al: Core symptoms of posttraumatic stress disorder unimproved by alprazolam treatment. J Clin Psychiatry 51:236–238, 1990

Brawman-Mintzer O, Knapp RG, Rynn M, et al: Sertraline treatment for generalized anxiety disorder: a randomized, double-blind, placebo-controlled study. J Clin Psychiatry 67:874–881, 2006

Bruscky SB, Caldeira MV, Bueno JR: Clinical trials of sulpiride. Arq Neuropsiquiatr 32:234–239, 1974

Bryant RA, Harvey AG, Dang ST, et al: Treatment of acute stress disorder: a comparison of cognitive-behavioral therapy and supportive counseling. J Clin Psychol 66:862–866, 1998

Bryant RA, Moulds ML, Nixon RV, et al: Cognitive behaviour therapy of acute stress disorder: a four-year follow-up. Behav Res Ther 41:489–494, 2003

Butterfield MI, Becker ME, Connor KM, et al: Olanzapine in the treatment of post-traumatic stress disorder: a pilot study. Int Clin Psychopharmacol 16:197–203, 2001

Byers MG, Allison KM, Wendell CS, et al: Prazosin versus quetiapine for nighttime posttraumatic stress disorder symptoms in veterans: an assessment of long-term comparative effectiveness and safety. J Clin Psychopharmacol 30:225–229, 2010

Bystritsky A, Kerwin L, Feusner JD, et al: A pilot controlled trial of bupropion XL versus escitalopram in generalized anxiety disorder. Psychopharmacol Bull 41:46–51, 2008

Canive J, Hamner MB, Calais LA, et al: Quetiapine monotherapy in chronic PTSD: a randomized, double-blind, placebo-controlled trial. Paper presented at Collegium International Neuro-psychopharmacologicum Thematic Meeting, Edinburgh, Scotland, April 24–27, 2009

Carey P, Suliman S, Ganesan K, et al: Olanzapine monotherapy in posttraumatic stress disorder: efficacy in a randomized, double-blind, placebo-controlled study. Hum Psychopharmacol 27:386–391, 2012

Cates ME, Bishop MH, Davis LL, et al: Clonazepam for treatment of sleep disturbances associated with combat-related posttraumatic stress disorder. Ann Pharmacother 38:1395–1399, 2004

Charney DS, Woods SW, Goodman WK, et al: Drug treatment of panic disorder: the comparative efficacy of imipramine, alprazolam, and trazodone. J Clin Psychiatry 47:580–586, 1986

Chen A, Zhao Y, Yu X: The clinical study of anti-anxiety and antidepressive effect of sulpiride. Chin J Neurol Psychiatry 27:220–222, 1994

Clark DM, Ehlers A, McManus F, et al: Cognitive therapy versus fluoxetine in generalized social phobia: a randomized placebo-controlled trial. J Consult Clin Psychol 71:1058–1067, 2003

Clark RD, Canive JM, Calais LA, et al: Divalproex in posttraumatic stress disorder: an open-label clinical trial. J Trauma Stress 12:395–401, 1999

Clomipramine Collaborative Study Group: Clomipramine in the treatment of patients with obsessive-compulsive disorder. Arch Gen Psychiatry 48:730–738, 1991

Clum GA, Surls R: A meta-analysis of treatments for panic disorder. J Consult Clin Psychol 61:317–326, 1993

Cohn JB, Bowden CL, Fisher JG, et al: Double-blind comparison of buspirone and clorazepate in anxious outpatients. Am J Med 80:10–16, 1986

Connor KM, Davidson JRT: SPRINT: a brief global assessment of post-traumatic stress disorder. Int Clin Psychopharmacol 16:279–284, 2001

Connor KM, Davidson JRT: A placebo-controlled study of kava kava in generalized anxiety disorder. Int Clin Psychopharmacol 17:185–188, 2002

Connor KM, Davidson JRT, Potts NL, et al: Discontinuation of clonazepam in the treatment of social phobia. J Clin Psychopharmacol 18:373–378, 1998

Connor KM, Sutherland SM, Tupler LA, et al: Fluoxetine in post-traumatic stress disorder. Randomised, double-blind study. Br J Psychiatry 175:17–22, 1999

Connor KM, Davidson JRT, Churchill EL, et al: Psychometric properties of the Social Phobia Inventory (SPIN). A new self-rating scale. Br J Psychiatry 176:379–386, 2000

Crockett BA, Davidson JRT, Churchill LE: Treatment of obsessive-compulsive disorder with clonazepam and sertraline versus placebo and sertraline. Paper presented at the 39th Annual Meeting of the New Clinical Drug Evaluation Unit, Boca Raton, FL, June 1, 1999

Cross-National Collaborative Panic Study: Drug treatment of panic disorder. Comparative efficacy of alprazolam, imipramine, and placebo. Br J Psychiatry 160:191–202, 1992

Dahl AA, Ravindran A, Allgulander C, et al: Sertraline in generalized anxiety disorder: efficacy in treating the psychic and somatic anxiety factors. Acta Psychiatr Scand 111:429–435, 2005

Davidson JRT: The long-term treatment of panic disorder. J Clin Psychiatry 59 (suppl 8):17–21, 1998

Davidson JRT, Moroz G: Pivotal studies of clonazepam in panic disorder. Psychopharmacol Bull 34:169–174, 1998

Davidson JRT, Kudler H, Smith R, et al: Treatment of posttraumatic stress disorder with amitriptyline and placebo. Arch Gen Psychiatry 47:259–266, 1990

Davidson JRT, Hughes DL, George LK, et al: The epidemiology of social phobia: findings from the Duke Epidemiological Catchment Area Study. Psychol Med 23:709–718, 1993

Davidson JRT, Tupler LA, Potts NL: Treatment of social phobia with benzodiazepines. J Clin Psychiatry 55 (suppl):28–32, 1994

Davidson JRT, Book SW, Colket JT, et al: Assessment of a new self-rating scale for post-traumatic stress disorder. Psychol Med 27:153–160, 1997a

Davidson JRT, Miner CM, DeVeaugh-Geiss J, et al: The Brief Social Phobia Scale: a psychometric evaluation. Psychol Med 27:161–166, 1997b

Davidson JRT, Weisler RH, Malik M, et al: Fluvoxamine in civilians with posttraumatic stress disorder. J Clin Psychopharmacol 18:93–95, 1998

Davidson JRT, DuPont RL, Hedges D, et al: Efficacy, safety, and tolerability of venlafaxine extended release and buspirone in outpatients with generalized anxiety disorder. J Clin Psychiatry 60:528–535, 1999

Davidson JRT, Pearlstein T, Londborg P, et al: Efficacy of sertraline in preventing relapse of posttraumatic stress disorder: results of a 28-week double-blind, placebo-controlled study. Am J Psychiatry 158:1974–1981, 2001

Davidson JRT, Landerman LR, Farfel GM, et al: Characterizing the effects of sertraline in posttraumatic stress disorder. Psychol Med 32:661–670, 2002

Davidson JRT, Weisler RH, Butterfield MI, et al: Mirtazapine vs. placebo in posttraumatic stress disorder: a pilot trial. Biol Psychiatry 53:188–191, 2003

Davidson JRT, Bose A, Korotzer A, et al: Escitalopram in the treatment of generalized anxiety disorder: double-blind, placebo controlled, flexible-dose study. Depress Anxiety 19:234–240, 2004a

Davidson JRT, Foa EB, Huppert JD, et al: Fluoxetine, comprehensive cognitive behavioral therapy (CCBT) and placebo in generalized social phobia. Arch Gen Psychiatry 61:1005–1013, 2004b

Davidson JRT, Yaryura-Tobias J, DuPont R, et al: Fluvoxamine-controlled release formulation for the treatment of generalized social anxiety disorder. J Clin Psychopharmacol 24:118–225, 2004c

Davidson JRT, Connor KM, Hertzberg MA, et al: Maintenance therapy with fluoxetine in posttraumatic stress disorder: a placebo-controlled discontinuation study. J Clin Psychopharmacol 25:166–169, 2005

Davidson JRT, Baldwin D, Stein DJ, et al: Treatment of posttraumatic stress disorder with venlafaxine extended release: a 6-month randomized controlled trial. Arch Gen Psychiatry 63:1158–1165, 2006a

Davidson JRT, Rothbaum BO, Tucker P, et al: Venlafaxine extended release in posttraumatic stress disorder: a sertraline- and placebo-controlled study. J Clin Psychopharmacol 26:259–267, 2006b

Davidson JRT, Brady K, Mellman TA, et al: The efficacy and tolerability of tiagabine in adult patients with post-traumatic stress disorder. J Clin Psychopharmacol 27:85–88, 2007

Davis LL, Jewell ME, Ambrose S, et al: A placebo-controlled study of nefazodone for the treatment of chronic posttraumatic stress disorder: a preliminary study. J Clin Psychopharmacol 24:291–297, 2004

Davis LL, Davidson JR, Ward LC, et al: Divalproex in the treatment of posttraumatic stress disorder: a randomized, double-blind, placebo-controlled trial in a veteran population. J Clin Psychopharmacol 28:84–88, 2008a

Davis LL, Ward C, Rasmusson A, et al: A placebo-controlled trial of guanfacine for the treatment of posttraumatic stress disorder in veterans. Psychopharmacol Bull 41:8–18, 2008b

de Kleine RA, Hendriks GJ, Kusters WJ, et al: A randomized placebo-controlled trial of D-cycloserine to enhance exposure therapy for posttraumatic stress disorder. Biol Psychiatry 71:962–968, 2012

Den Boer JA, Westenberg HG: Effect of a serotonin and noradrenaline uptake inhibitor in panic disorder: a double-blind comparative study with fluvoxamine and maprotiline. Int Clin Psychopharmacol 3:59–74, 1988

Denys D, Mantione M, Figee M, et al: Deep brain stimulation of the nucleus accumbens for treatment-refractory obsessive-compulsive disorder. Arch Gen Psychiatry 67:1061–1068, 2010

Eddy K, Dutra L, Bradley R, et al: A multidimensional meta-analysis of psychotherapy and pharmacotherapy for obsessive-compulsive disorder. Clin Psychol Rev 24:1–30, 2004

Eidelman I, Seedat S, Stein DJ: Risperidone in the treatment of acute stress disorder in physically traumatized in-patients. Depress Anxiety 11: 187–188, 2000

Emmanuel NP, Lydiard RB, Ballenger JC: Treatment of social phobia with bupropion. J Clin Psychopharmacol 11:276–277, 1991

Enkelmann R: Alprazolam versus buspirone in the treatment of outpatients with generalized anxiety disorder. Psychopharmacology (Berl) 105: 428–432, 1991

Fahlen T, Nilsson HL, Borg K, et al: Social phobia: the clinical efficacy and tolerability of the monoamine oxidase-A and serotonin uptake inhibitor brofaromine. A double-blind placebo-controlled study. Acta Psychiatr Scand 92:351–358, 1995

Fahy TJ, O'Rourke D, Brophy J, et al: The Galway Study of Panic Disorder, I: clomipramine and lofepramine in DSM-III-R panic disorder. A placebo controlled trial. J Affect Disord 25:63–75, 1992

Fallon BA, Campeas R, Schneier FR, et al: Open trial of intravenous clomipramine in five treatment-refractory patients with obsessive-compulsive disorder. J Neuropsychiatry Clin Neurosci 4:70–75, 1992

Fava M, Asnis GM, Shrivastava R, et al: Zolpidem extended-release improves sleep and next-day symptoms in comorbid insomnia and generalized anxiety disorder. J Clin Psychopharmacol 29:222–230, 2009

Fedoroff I, Taylor S: Psychological and pharmacological treatments of social phobia: a meta-analysis. J Clin Psychopharmacol 21:311–324, 2001

Feltner DE, Crockatt JG, Dubovsky SJ, et al: A randomized, double-blind, placebo-controlled, fixed-dose, multicenter study of pregabalin in patients with generalized anxiety disorder. J Clin Psychopharmacol 23:240–249, 2003

Feltner D, Wittchen HU, Kavoussi R, et al: Long-term efficacy of pregabalin in generalized anxiety disorder. Int Clin Psychopharmacol 23:18–28, 2008

Ferguson JM, Khan A, Mangano R, et al: Relapse prevention of panic disorder in adult outpatient responders to treatment with venlafaxine extended release. J Clin Psychiatry 68:58–68, 2007

Ferreri M, Hantouche EG: Recent clinical trials of hydroxyzine in generalized anxiety disorder. Acta Psychiatr Scand Suppl 393:102–108, 1998

Fesler FA: Valproate in combat-related posttraumatic stress disorder. J Clin Psychiatry 52:361–364, 1991

Fineberg NA, Sivakumaran T, Roberts A, et al: Adding quetiapine to SRI in treatment-resistant obsessive-compulsive disorder: a randomized controlled treatment study. Int Clin Psychopharmacol 20:223–226, 2005

Fineberg NA, Tonnoir B, Lemming O, et al: Escitalopram prevents relapse of obsessive-compulsive disorder. Eur Neuropsychopharmacol 17:430–439, 2007

Flament MF, Rapoport JL, Berg CJ, et al: Clomipramine treatment of childhood obsessive-compulsive disorder. A double-blind controlled study. Arch Gen Psychiatry 42:977–983, 1985

Foa EB, Liebowitz MR, Kozak MJ, et al: Randomized, placebo-controlled trial of exposure and ritual prevention, clomipramine, and their combination in the treatment of obsessive-compulsive disorder. Am J Psychiatry 162:151–161, 2005

Fontaine R, Beaudry P, Beauclair L, et al: Comparison of withdrawal of buspirone and diazepam: a placebo controlled study. Prog Neuropsychopharmacol Biol Psychiatry 11:189–197, 1987

Friedman MJ, Marmar CR, Baker DG, et al: Randomized double-blind comparison of sertraline and placebo for posttraumatic stress disorder in a Department of Veterans Affairs setting. J Clin Psychiatry 68:711–720, 2007

Furmark T, Appel L, Micelgard A, et al: Cerebral blood flow changes after treatment of social phobia with the neurokinin-1 antagonist GR205171, citalopram, or placebo. Biol Psychiatry 58:132–142, 2005

Fux M, Levine J, Aviv A, et al: Inositol treatment of obsessive-compulsive disorder. Am J Psychiatry 153:1219–1221, 1996

Gambi F, De Berardis D, Campanella D, et al: Mirtazapine treatment of generalized anxiety disorder: a fixed dose, open label study. J Psychopharmacol 19:483–487, 2005

Gelenberg AJ, Lydiard RB, Rudolph RL, et al: Efficacy of venlafaxine extended-release capsules in nondepressed outpatients with generalized anxiety disorder: a 6-month randomized controlled trial. JAMA 283:3082–3088, 2000

Gelernter CS, Uhde TW, Cimbolic P, et al: Cognitive-behavioral and pharmacological treatments of social phobia. A controlled study. Arch Gen Psychiatry 48:938–945, 1991

Gelpin E, Bonne O, Peri T, et al: Treatment of recent trauma survivors with benzodiazepines: a prospective study. J Clin Psychiatry 57:390–394, 1996

Goddard AW, Brouette T, Almai A, et al: Early coadministration of clonazepam with sertraline for panic disorder. Arch Gen Psychiatry 58:681–686, 2001

Goldberg DP, Lecrubier Y: Form and frequency of mental disorders across centers, in Mental Illness in General Health Care: An International Study. Edited by Üstürn TB, Sartorius N. New York, Wiley, 1995, pp 323–334

Goodman WK, Price LH, Rasmussen SA, et al: The Yale-Brown Obsessive Compulsive Scale, II: validity. Arch Gen Psychiatry 46:1012–1016, 1989

Goodman WK, Bose A, Wang Q: Treatment of generalized anxiety disorder with escitalopram: pooled results from double-blind, placebo-controlled trials. J Affect Disord 87:161–167, 2005

Goodnick PJ, Puig A, DeVane CL, et al: Mirtazapine in major depression with comorbid generalized anxiety disorder. J Clin Psychiatry 60:446–448, 1999

Greenberg BD, Malone DA, Friehs GM, et al: Three-year outcomes in deep brain stimulation for highly resistant obsessive-compulsive disorder. Neuropsychopharmacology 31:2384–2393, 2006

Greenblatt DJ, Shader RI, Abernethy DR: Drug therapy. Current status of benzodiazepines. N Engl J Med 309:410–416, 1983

Greist JH, Chouinard G, DuBoff E, et al: Double-blind parallel comparison of three dosages of sertraline and placebo in outpatients with obsessive-compulsive disorder. Arch Gen Psychiatry 52:289–295, 1995a

Greist JH, Jefferson JW, Kobak KA, et al: Efficacy and tolerability of serotonin transport inhibitors in obsessive-compulsive disorder. A meta-analysis. Arch Gen Psychiatry 52:53–60, 1995b

Hamilton M: The assessment of anxiety states by rating. Br J Med Psychol 32:50–55, 1959

Hamilton M: A rating scale for depression. J Neurol Neurosurg Psychiatry 23:56–62, 1960

Hamner MB, Faldowski RA, Ulmer HG, et al: Adjunctive risperidone treatment in post-traumatic stress disorder: a preliminary controlled trial of effects on comorbid psychotic symptoms. Int Clin Psychopharmacol 18:1–8, 2003

Hamner MB, Faldowski RA, Robert S, et al: A preliminary controlled trial of divalproex in post-traumatic stress disorder. Ann Clin Psychiatry 21:89–94, 2009

Hauer D, Weis F, Krauseneck T, et al: Traumatic memories, post-traumatic stress disorder and serum cortisol levels in long-term survivors of the acute respiratory distress syndrome. Brain Res 1293:114–120, 2009

Haug TT, Hellstrom K, Blomhoff S, et al: The treatment of social phobia in general practice: is exposure therapy feasible? Fam Pract 17:114–118, 2000

Heimberg RG, Liebowitz MR, Hope DA, et al: Cognitive behavioral group therapy vs phenelzine therapy for social phobia: 12-week outcome. Arch Gen Psychiatry 55:1133–1141, 1998

Heresco-Levy U, Vass A, Bloch B, et al: Pilot controlled trial of D-serine for the treatment of post-traumatic stress disorder. Int J Neuropsychopharmacol 12:1275–1282, 2009

Hertzberg MA, Butterfield MI, Feldman ME, et al: A preliminary study of lamotrigine for the treatment of posttraumatic stress disorder. Biol Psychiatry 45:1226–1229, 1999

Hidalgo R, Hertzberg MA, Mellman T, et al: Nefazodone in post-traumatic stress disorder: results from six open-label trials. Int Clin Psychopharmacol 14:61–68, 1999

Hidalgo RB, Tupler LA, Davidson JRT: An effect-size analysis of pharmacological treatments for generalized anxiety disorder. J Psychopharmacol 21:864–872, 2007

Hoehn-Saric R, McLeod DR, Zimmerli WD: Differential effects of alprazolam and imipramine in generalized anxiety disorder: somatic versus psychic symptoms. J Clin Psychiatry 49:293–301, 1988

Hofmann SG, Meuret AE, Smits JA, et al: Augmentation of exposure therapy with D-cycloserine for social anxiety disorder. Arch Gen Psychiatry 63:298–304, 2006

Hollifield M, Thompson PM, Ruiz JE, et al: Potential effectiveness and safety of olanzapine in refractory panic disorder. Depress Anxiety 21:33–40, 2005

Hollifield M, Sinclair-Lian N, Warner TD, et al: Acupuncture for posttraumatic stress disorder: a randomized controlled pilot trial. J Nerv Ment Dis 195:504–513, 2007

Huppert JD, Schultz LT, Foa EB, et al: Differential response to placebo among patients with social phobia, panic disorder, and obsessive-compulsive disorder. Am J Psychiatry 161:1485–1487, 2004

International Multicenter Clinical Trial Group on Moclobemide in Social Phobia: Moclobemide in social phobia. A double-blind, placebo-controlled clinical study. Eur Arch Psychiatry Clin Neurosci 247:71–80, 1997

Jacobs RJ, Davidson JRT, Gupta S, et al: The effects of clonazepam on quality of life and work productivity in panic disorder. Am J Manag Care 3:1187–1196, 1997

Jacobs-Rebhun S, Schnurr PP, Friedman MJ, et al: Posttraumatic stress disorder and sleep difficulty. Am J Psychiatry 157:1525–1526, 2000

Jenike MA, Baer L, Ballantine T, et al: Cingulotomy for refractory obsessive-compulsive disorder. A long-term follow-up of 33 patients. Arch Gen Psychiatry 48:548–555, 1991

Kaplan Z, Amir M, Swartz M, et al: Inositol treatment of post-traumatic stress disorder. Anxiety 2:51–52, 1996

Kasper S, Stein DJ, Loft H, et al: Escitalopram in the treatment of social anxiety disorder: randomised, placebo-controlled, flexible-dosage study. Br J Psychiatry 186:222–226, 2005

Katschnig H, Amering M, Stolk JM, et al: Long-term follow-up after a drug trial for panic disorder. Br J Psychiatry 167:487–494, 1995

Katz RJ, Lott MH, Arbus P, et al: Pharmacotherapy of post-traumatic stress disorder with a novel psychotropic. Anxiety 1:169–174, 1994

Katzelnick DJ, Kobak KA, Greist JH, et al: Sertraline for social phobia: a double-blind, placebo-controlled crossover study. Am J Psychiatry 152:1368–1371, 1995

Katzman MA, Brawman-Mintzer O, Reyes EB, et al: Extended release quetiapine fumarate (quetiapine XR) monotherapy as maintenance treatment for generalized anxiety disorder: a long-term, randomized, placebo-controlled trial. Int Clin Psychopharmacol 26:11–24, 2011

Keck PE Jr, McElroy SL, Tugrul KC, et al: Antiepileptic drugs for the treatment of panic disorder. Neuropsychobiology 27:150–153, 1993

Kessler RC, Sonnega A, Bromet E, et al: Posttraumatic stress disorder in the National Comorbidity Survey. Arch Gen Psychiatry 52:1048–1060, 1995

Kessler RC, Berglund P, Demler O, et al: Lifetime prevalence and age-of-onset distributions of DSM-IV disorders in the National Comorbidity Survey Replication. Arch Gen Psychiatry 62:593–602, 2005a

Kessler RC, Chiu WT, Demler O, et al: Prevalence, severity, and comorbidity of 12-month DSM-IV disorders in the National Comorbidity Survey Replication [see comment]. Arch Gen Psychiatry 62:617–627, 2005b

Klesmer J, Sarcevic A, Fomari V: Panic attacks during discontinuation of mirtazapine. Can J Psychiatry 45:570–571, 2000

Kobak KA, Greist JH, Jefferson JW, et al: Fluoxetine in social phobia: a double-blind, placebo-controlled pilot study. J Clin Psychopharmacol 22:257–262, 2002

Kobak KA, Taylor LV, Bystritsky A, et al: St. John's wort versus placebo in obsessive-compulsive disorder: results from a double-blind study. Int Clin Psychopharmacol 20:299–304, 2005

Koran LM, McElroy SL, Davidson JR, et al: Fluvoxamine versus clomipramine for obsessive-compulsive disorder: a double-blind comparison. J Clin Psychopharmacol 16:121–129, 1996

Koran LM, Sallee FR, Pallanti S: Rapid benefit of intravenous pulse loading of clomipramine in obsessive-compulsive disorder. Am J Psychiatry 154:396–401, 1997

Kosten TR, Frank JB, Dan E, et al: Pharmacotherapy for posttraumatic stress disorder using phenelzine or imipramine. J Nerv Ment Dis 179:366–370, 1991

Krystal JH, Rosenheck RA, Cramer JA, et al; Veterans Affairs Cooperative Study No. 504 Group: Adjunctive risperidone treatment for antidepressant-resistant symptoms of chronic military service-related PTSD: a randomized trial. JAMA 306:493–502, 2011

Lader M, Scotto JC: A multicentre double-blind comparison of hydroxyzine, buspirone and placebo in patients with generalized anxiety disorder. Psychopharmacology (Berl) 139:402–406, 1998

Lader M, Stender K, Burger V, et al: Efficacy and tolerability of escitalopram in 12- and 24-week treatment of social anxiety disorder: randomised, double-blind, placebo-controlled, fixed-dose study. Depress Anxiety 19:241–248, 2004

Lecrubier Y, Judge R: Long-term evaluation of paroxetine, clomipramine and placebo in panic disorder. Collaborative Paroxetine Panic Study Investigators. Acta Psychiatr Scand 95:153–160, 1997

Lecrubier Y, Bakker A, Dunbar G, et al: A comparison of paroxetine, clomipramine and placebo in the treatment of panic disorder. Collaborative Paroxetine Panic Study Investigators. Acta Psychiatr Scand 95:145–152, 1997

Leonard H, Swedo S, Rapoport JL, et al: Treatment of childhood obsessive compulsive disorder with clomipramine and desmethylimipramine: a double-blind crossover comparison. Psychopharmacol Bull 24:93–95, 1988

Lepola UM, Wade AG, Leinonen EV, et al: A controlled, prospective, 1-year trial of citalopram in the treatment of panic disorder. J Clin Psychiatry 59:528–534, 1998

Lepola U, Bergtholdt B, St Lambert J, et al: Controlled-release paroxetine in the treatment of patients with social anxiety disorder. J Clin Psychiatry 65:222–229, 2004

Liebowitz MR: Social phobia. Mod Probl Pharmacopsychiatry 22:141–173, 1987

Liebowitz MR, Schneier F, Campeas R, et al: Phenelzine vs atenolol in social phobia. A placebo-controlled comparison. Arch Gen Psychiatry 49:290–300, 1992

Liebowitz MR, Turner SM, Piacentini J, et al: Fluoxetine in children and adolescents with OCD: a placebo-controlled trial. J Am Acad Child Adolesc Psychiatry 41:1431–1438, 2002

Liebowitz MR, DeMartinis NA, Weihs K, et al: Efficacy of sertraline in severe generalized social anxiety disorder: results of a double-blind, placebo-controlled study. J Clin Psychiatry 64:785–792, 2003

Liebowitz MR, Mangano RM, Bradwejn J, et al: A randomized controlled trial of venlafaxine extended release in generalized social anxiety disorder. J Clin Psychiatry 66:238–247, 2005

Lipper S, Davidson JR, Grady TA, et al: Preliminary study of carbamazepine in post-traumatic stress disorder. Psychosomatics 27:849–854, 1986

Lipsitz JD, Mannuzza S, Klein DF, et al: Specific phobia 10–16 years after treatment. Depress Anxiety 10:105–111, 1999

Llorca PM, Spadone C, Sol O, et al: Efficacy and safety of hydroxyzine in the treatment of generalized anxiety disorder: a 3-month double-blind study [see comment]. J Clin Psychiatry 63:1020–1027, 2002

Londborg PD, Wolkow R, Smith WT, et al: Sertraline in the treatment of panic disorder. A multisite, double-blind, placebo-controlled, fixed-dose investigation. Br J Psychiatry 173:54–60, 1998

Londborg PD, Hegel MT, Goldstein S, et al: Sertraline treatment of posttraumatic stress disorder: results of 24 weeks of open-label continuation treatment. J Clin Psychiatry 62:325–331, 2001

Lott M, Greist JH, Jefferson JW, et al: Brofaromine for social phobia: a multicenter, placebo-controlled, double-blind study. J Clin Psychopharmacol 17:255–260, 1997

Lydiard RB, Ballenger JC: Antidepressants in panic disorder and agoraphobia. J Affect Disord 13:153–168, 1987

Lydiard RB, Laraia MT, Ballenger JC, et al: Emergence of depressive symptoms in patients receiving alprazolam for panic disorder. Am J Psychiatry 144:664–665, 1987

Lydiard RB, Lesser IM, Ballenger JC, et al: A fixed-dose study of alprazolam 2 mg, alprazolam 6 mg, and placebo in panic disorder. J Clin Psychopharmacol 12:96–103, 1992

Lydiard RB, Morton WA, Emmanuel NP, et al: Preliminary report: placebo-controlled, double-blind study of the clinical and metabolic effects of desipramine in panic disorder. Psychopharmacol Bull 29:183–188, 1993

Lydiard RB, Steiner M, Burnham D, et al: Efficacy studies of paroxetine in panic disorder. Psychopharmacol Bull 34:175–182, 1998

Lydiard RB, Rickels K, Herman B, et al: Comparative efficacy of pregabalin and benzodiazepines in treating the psychic and somatic symptoms of generalized anxiety disorder. Int J Neuropsychopharmacol 13:229–241, 2010

Magee WJ, Eaton WW, Wittchen HU, et al: Agoraphobia, simple phobia, and social phobia in the National Comorbidity Survey. Arch Gen Psychiatry 53:159–168, 1996

Mantovani A, Simpson HB, Fallon BA, et al: Randomized sham-controlled trial of repetitive transcranial magnetic stimulation in treatment-resistant obsessive-compulsive disorder. Int J Neuropsychopharmacol 13:217–227, 2010

March JS, Biederman J, Wolkow R, et al: Sertraline in children and adolescents with obsessive-compulsive disorder: a multicenter randomized controlled trial. JAMA 280:1752–1756, 1998

March JS, Entsuah AR, Rynn M, et al: A randomized controlled trial of venlafaxine ER versus placebo in pediatric social anxiety disorder. Biol Psychiatry 62:1149–1154, 2007

Margoob MA, Ali Z, Andrade C: Efficacy of ECT in chronic, severe, antidepressant- and CBT-refractory PTSD: an open, prospective study. Brain Stimul 3:28–35, 2010

Marks IM, Mathews AM: Brief standard self-rating for phobic patients. Behav Res Ther 17:263–267, 1979

Marmar CR, Schoenfeld F, Weiss DS, et al: Open trial of fluvoxamine treatment for combat-related posttraumatic stress disorder. J Clin Psychiatry 57 (suppl 8):66–70, 1996

Marshall RD, Beebe KL, Oldham M, et al: Efficacy and safety of paroxetine treatment for chronic PTSD: a fixed-dose, placebo-controlled study. Am J Psychiatry 158:1982–1988, 2001

Martenyi F, Brown EB, Zhang H, et al: Fluoxetine versus placebo in posttraumatic stress disorder. J Clin Psychiatry 63:199–206, 2002a

Martenyi F, Brown EB, Zhang H, et al: Fluoxetine vs placebo in prevention of relapse in post-traumatic stress disorder. Br J Psychiatry 181:315–320, 2002b

Mathew SJ, Amiel JM, Coplan JD, et al: Open-label trial of riluzole in generalized anxiety disorder. Am J Psychiatry 162:2379–2381, 2005

Mathew SJ, Vythilingham M, Murrough JW, et al: A selective neurokinin-1 receptor antagonist in chronic PTSD: a randomized, double-blind, placebo-controlled, proof-of-concept trial. Eur Neuropsychopharmacol 21:221–229, 2011

Mavissakalian MR, Perel JM: Imipramine dose-response relationship in panic disorder with agoraphobia. Preliminary findings. Arch Gen Psychiatry 46:127–131, 1989

Mavissakalian MR, Perel JM: Imipramine treatment of panic disorder with agoraphobia: dose ranging and plasma level-response relationships. Am J Psychiatry 152:673–682, 1995

Mellman TA, Bustamante V, David D, et al: Hypnotic medication in the aftermath of trauma. J Clin Psychiatry 63:1183–1184, 2002

Mellman TA, Clark RE, Peacock WJ: Prescribing patterns for patients with posttraumatic stress disorder. Psychiatr Serv 54:1618–1621, 2003

Meoni P, Hackett D: Characterization of the longitudinal course of long-term venlafaxine-ER treatment of GAD. Paper presented at the 13th Annual Meeting of the European College of Neuropsychopharmacology, Munich, Germany, September 11, 2000

Michelson D, Lydiard RB, Pollack MH, et al: Outcome assessment and clinical improvement in panic disorder: evidence from a randomized controlled trial of fluoxetine and placebo. The Fluoxetine Panic Disorder Study Group. Am J Psychiatry 155:1570–1577, 1998

Michelson D, Pollack M, Lydiard RB, et al: Continuing treatment of panic disorder after acute response: randomised, placebo-controlled trial with fluoxetine. The Fluoxetine Panic Disorder Study Group. Br J Psychiatry 174:213–218, 1999

Michelson D, Allgulander C, Dantendorfer K, et al: Efficacy of usual antidepressant dosing regimens of fluoxetine in panic disorder: randomised, placebo-controlled trial. Br J Psychiatry 179:514–518, 2001

Modigh K, Westberg P, Eriksson E: Superiority of clomipramine over imipramine in the treatment of panic disorder: a placebo-controlled trial. J Clin Psychopharmacol 12:251–261, 1992

Monnelly EP, Ciraulo DA, Knapp C, et al: Low-dose risperidone as adjunctive therapy for irritable aggression in posttraumatic stress disorder. J Clin Psychopharmacol 23:193–196, 2003

Montgomery SA: Pregabalin for the treatment of generalized anxiety disorder. Exp Opin Pharmacother 7:2139–2154, 2006

Montgomery SA, Nil R, Durr-Pal N, et al: A 24-week randomized, double-blind, placebo-controlled study of escitalopram for the prevention of generalized social anxiety disorder. J Clin Psychiatry 66:1270–1278, 2005

Muehlbacher M, Nickel MK, Nickel C, et al: Mirtazapine treatment of social phobia in women: a randomized, double-blind, placebo controlled trial. J Clin Psychopharmacol 25:580–583, 2005

Murray CJL, Lopez AD: The Global Burden of Disease. Cambridge, MA, Harvard School of Public Health, 1996

Neal LA, Shapland W, Fox C: An open trial of moclobemide in the treatment of post-traumatic stress disorder. Int Clin Psychopharmacol 12:231–237, 1997

Neylan TC, Lenoci M, Samuelson KW, et al: No improvement of posttraumatic stress disorder symptoms with guanfacine treatment. Am J Psychiatry 163:2186–2188, 2006

Ninan PT, Koran LM, Kiev A, et al: High-dose sertraline strategy for nonresponders to acute treatment for obsessive-compulsive disorder: a multicenter double-blind trial. J Clin Psychiatry 67:15–22, 2006

Noyes R Jr, Moroz G, Davidson JR, et al: Moclobemide in social phobia: a controlled dose-response trial. J Clin Psychopharmacol 17:247–254, 1997

Oehrberg S, Christiansen PE, Behnke K, et al: Paroxetine in the treatment of panic disorder. A randomised, double-blind, placebo-controlled study. Br J Psychiatry 167:374–379, 1995

Olajide D, Lader M: A comparison of buspirone, diazepam, and placebo in patients with chronic anxiety states. J Clin Psychopharmacol 7:148–152, 1987

Otto MW, Pollack MH, Sachs GS, et al: Discontinuation of benzodiazepine treatment: efficacy of cognitive-behavioral therapy for patients with panic disorder. Am J Psychiatry 150:1485–1490, 1993

Otto MW, Tuby KS, Gould RA, et al: An effect-size analysis of the relative efficacy and tolerability of serotonin selective reuptake inhibitors for panic disorder. Am J Psychiatry 158:1989–1992, 2001

Pages KP, Ries RK: Use of anticonvulsants in benzodiazepine withdrawal. Am J Addict 7:198–204, 1998

Panahi Y, Moghaddam BR, Sahebkar A, et al: A randomized, double-blind, placebo-controlled trial on the efficacy and tolerability of sertraline in Iranian veterans with post-traumatic stress disorder. Psychol Med 41:2159–2166, 2011

Pande AC, Davidson JR, Jefferson JW, et al: Treatment of social phobia with gabapentin: a placebo-controlled study. J Clin Psychopharmacol 19:341–348, 1999a

Pande AC, Greiner M, Adams JB, et al: Placebo-controlled trial of the CCK-B antagonist, CI-988, in panic disorder. Biol Psychiatry 46:860–862, 1999b

Pande AC, Pollack MH, Crockatt J, et al: Placebo-controlled study of gabapentin treatment of panic disorder. J Clin Psychopharmacol 20:467–471, 2000

Pande AC, Crockatt JG, Feltner DE, et al: Pregabalin in generalized anxiety disorder: a placebo-controlled trial. Am J Psychiatry 160:533–540, 2003

Papp LA: Safety and efficacy of levetiracetam for patients with panic disorder: results of an open-label, fixed-flexible dose study. J Clin Psychiatry 67:1573–1576, 2006

Pato MT, Hill JL, Murphy DL: A clomipramine dosage reduction study in the course of long-term treatment of obsessive-compulsive disorder patients. Psychopharmacol Bull 26:211–214, 1990

Pecknold J, Luthe L, Munjack D, et al: A double-blind, placebo-controlled, multicenter study with alprazolam and extended-release alprazolam in the treatment of panic disorder. J Clin Psychopharmacol 14:314–321, 1994

Petracca A, Nisita C, McNair D, et al: Treatment of generalized anxiety disorder: preliminary clinical experience with buspirone. J Clin Psychiatry 51 (suppl):31–39, 1990

Pigott T, L'Hereux F, Rubinstein CS: A controlled trial of clonazepam augmentation in OCD patients treated with clomipramine or fluoxetine (NR82). Paper presented at the 145th Annual Meeting of the American Psychiatric Association, Washington, DC, May 2–7, 1992

Pitman RK, Sanders KM, Zusman RM, et al: Pilot study of secondary prevention of posttraumatic stress disorder with propranolol. Biol Psychiatry 51:189–192, 2002

Pohl RB, Feltner DE, Fieve RR, et al: Efficacy of pregabalin in the treatment of generalized anxiety disorder: double-blind, placebo-controlled comparison of BID versus TID dosing. J Clin Psychopharmacol 25:151–158, 2005

Pollack MH, Zaninelli R, Goddard A, et al: Paroxetine in the treatment of generalized anxiety disorder: results of a placebo-controlled, flexible-dosage trial. J Clin Psychiatry 62:350–357, 2001

Pollack MH, Simon NM, Worthington JJ, et al: Combined paroxetine and clonazepam treatment strategies compared to paroxetine monotherapy for panic disorder. J Psychopharmacol (Oxf) 17:276–282, 2003

Pollack MH, Mangano R, Entsuah R, et al: A randomized controlled trial of venlafaxine ER and paroxetine in the treatment of outpatients with panic disorder. Psychopharmacology (Berl) 194: 233–242, 2007

Pollack MH, Kinrys G, Krystal A, et al: Eszopiclone coadminstered with escitalopram in patients with insomnia and comorbid generalized anxiety disorder. Arch Gen Psychiatry 65:551–562, 2008a

Pollack MH, Tiller J, Xie F, et al: Tiagabine in adult patients with generalized anxiety disorder: results from three randomized, double-blind, placebo-controlled, parallel-group studies. J Clin Psychopharmacol 28:308–316, 2008b

Prosser JM, Yard S, Steele A, et al: A comparison of low-dose risperidone to paroxetine in the treatment of panic attacks: a randomized, single-blind study. BMC Psychiatry 9:25, 2009

Rapaport MH, Wolkow R, Rubin A, et al: Sertraline treatment of panic disorder: results of a long-term study. Acta Psychiatr Scand 104:289–298, 2001

Rapaport MH, Endicott J, Clary CM: Posttraumatic stress disorder and quality of life: results across 64 weeks of sertraline treatment. J Clin Psychiatry 63:59–65, 2002

Raskind MA, Peskind ER, Kanter ED, et al: Reduction of nightmares and other PTSD symptoms in combat veterans by prazosin: a placebo-controlled study. Am J Psychiatry 160:371–373, 2003

Raskind MA, Peskind ER, Hoff DJ, et al: A parallel group placebo controlled study of prazosin for trauma nightmares and sleep disturbance in combat veterans with post-traumatic stress disorder. Biol Psychiatry 61:928–934, 2007

Ravizza L, Barzega G, Bellino S, et al: Drug treatment of obsessive-compulsive disorder (OCD): long-term trial with clomipramine and selective serotonin reuptake inhibitors (SSRIs). Psychopharmacol Bull 32:167–173, 1996

Reich DB, Winternitz S, Hennen J, et al: A preliminary study of risperidone in the treatment of posttraumatic stress disorder related to childhood abuse in women. J Clin Psychiatry 65: 1601–1606, 2004

Research Unit on Pediatric Psychopharmacology Anxiety Study Group: Fluvoxamine for the treatment of anxiety disorders in children and adolescents. N Engl J Med 344:1279–1285, 2001

Ressler KJ, Rothbaum BO, Tannenbaum L, et al: Cognitive enhancers as adjuncts to psychotherapy: use of D-cycloserine in phobic individuals to facilitate extinction of fear. Arch Gen Psychiatry 61:1136–1144, 2004

Ribeiro L, Busnello JV, Kauer-Sant'Anna M, et al: Mirtazapine versus fluoxetine in the treatment of panic disorder. Braz J Med Biol Res 34:1303–1307, 2001

Rickels K, Weisman K, Norstad N, et al: Buspirone and diazepam in anxiety: a controlled study. J Clin Psychiatry 43:81–86, 1982

Rickels K, Case WG, Downing RW, et al: Long-term diazepam therapy and clinical outcome. JAMA 250:767–771, 1983

Rickels K, Fox IL, Greenblatt DJ, et al: Clorazepate and lorazepam: clinical improvement and rebound anxiety. Am J Psychiatry 145:312–317, 1988a

Rickels K, Schweizer E, Csanalosi I, et al: Long-term treatment of anxiety and risk of withdrawal. Prospective comparison of clorazepate and buspirone. Arch Gen Psychiatry 45:444–450, 1988b

Rickels K, Amsterdam JD, Clary C, et al: Buspirone in major depression: a controlled study. J Clin Psychiatry 52:34–38, 1991

Rickels K, Downing R, Schweizer E, et al: Antidepressants for the treatment of generalized anxiety disorder. A placebo-controlled comparison of imipramine, trazodone, and diazepam. Arch Gen Psychiatry 50:884–895, 1993

Rickels K, Pollack MH, Sheehan DV, et al: Efficacy of extended-release venlafaxine in nondepressed outpatients with generalized anxiety disorder. Am J Psychiatry 157:968–974, 2000

Rickels K, Zaninelli R, McCafferty J, et al: Paroxetine treatment of generalized anxiety disorder: a double-blind, placebo-controlled study. Am J Psychiatry 160:749–756, 2003

Rickels K, Pollack MH, Feltner DE, et al: Pregabalin for treatment of generalized anxiety disorder: a 4-week, multicenter, double-blind, placebo-controlled trial of pregabalin and alprazolam. Arch Gen Psychiatry 62:1022–1030, 2005

Riddle MA, Reeve EA, Yaryura-Tobias JA, et al: Fluvoxamine for children and adolescents with obsessive-compulsive disorder: a randomized, controlled, multicenter trial. J Am Acad Child Adolesc Psychiatry 40:222–229, 2001

Robb AS, Cueva JE, Sporn J, et al: Sertraline treatment of children and adolescents with posttraumatic stress disorder: a double-blind, placebo-controlled trial. J Child Adolesc Psychopharmacol 20:463–471, 2010

Robert R, Blakeney PE, Villarreal C, et al: Imipramine treatment in pediatric burn patients with symptoms of acute stress disorder: a pilot study. J Am Acad Child Adolesc Psychiatry 38:873–882, 1999a

Robert R, Meyer WJ III, Villarreal C, et al: An approach to the timely treatment of acute stress disorder. J Burn Care Rehabil 20:250–258, 1999b

Robert R, Tcheung WJ, Rosenberg L, et al: Treating thermally injured children suffering symptoms of acute stress with imipramine and fluoxetine: a randomized, double-blind study. Burns 34:919–928, 2008

Rocca P, Fonzo V, Scotta M, et al: Paroxetine efficacy in the treatment of generalized anxiety disorder. Acta Psychiatr Scand 95:444–450, 1997

Rosenbaum JF, Woods SW, Groves JE, et al: Emergence of hostility during alprazolam treatment. Am J Psychiatry 141:792–793, 1984

Rosenbaum JF, Moroz G, Bowden CL: Clonazepam in the treatment of panic disorder with or without agoraphobia: a dose-response study of efficacy, safety, and discontinuance. Clonazepam Panic Disorder Dose-Response Study Group. J Clin Psychopharmacol 17:390–400, 1997

Ross CA, Matas M: A clinical trial of buspirone and diazepam in the treatment of generalized anxiety disorder. Can J Psychiatry 32:351–355, 1987

Rothbaum BO, Killeen TK, Davidson JR, et al: Placebo-controlled trial of risperidone augmentation for selective serotonin reuptake inhibitor-resistant civilian posttraumatic stress disorder. J Clin Psychiatry 69:520–525, 2008

Royal Australian and New Zealand College of Psychiatrists Clinical Practice Guidelines Team for Panic Disorder and Agoraphobia: Australian and New Zealand clinical practice guidelines for the treatment of panic disorder and agoraphobia. Aust N Z J Psychiatry 37:641–656, 2003

Roy-Byrne PP, Clary CM, Miceli RJ, et al: The effect of selective serotonin reuptake inhibitor treatment of panic disorder on emergency room and laboratory resource utilization. J Clin Psychiatry 62:678–682, 2001

Ruffini C, Locatelli M, Lucca A, et al: Augmentation effect of repetitive transcranial magnetic stimulation over the orbitofrontal cortex in drug-resistant obsessive-compulsive disorder patients: a controlled investigation. Prim Care Companion J Clin Psychiatry 11:226–230, 2009

Rynn M, Russell JM, Erickson J, et al: Efficacy and safety of duloxetine in the treatment of generalized anxiety disorder: a flexible-dose, progressive-titration, placebo-controlled trial. Depress Anxiety 25:182–189, 2008

Sachdev PS, Loo CK, Mitchell PB, et al: Repetitive transcranial magnetic stimulation for the treatment of obsessive compulsive disorder: a double-blind controlled investigation. Psychol Med 37:1645–1649, 2007

Sarkhel S, Sinha VK, Praharaj SK: Adjunctive high-frequency right prefrontal repetitive transcranial magnetic stimulation (rTMS) was not effective in obsessive-compulsive disorder but improved secondary depression. J Anxiety Disord 24:535–539, 2010

Sarchiapone M, Amore M, De Risio S, et al: Mirtazapine in the treatment of panic disorder: an open-label trial. Int Clin Psychopharmacol 18:35–38, 2003

Sarris J, Kavanaugh DJ, Byrne G, et al: The kava anxiety depression spectrum study (KADSS): a randomized, placebo-controlled crossover trial using an aqueous extract of Piper methysticum. Psychopharmacology (Berl) 205:399–407, 2009

Schelling G, Roozendaal B, Krauseneck T, et al: Efficacy of hydrocortisone in preventing posttraumatic stress disorder following critical illness and major surgery. Ann N Y Acad Sci 1071:46–53, 2006

Schneier FR, Goetz D, Campeas R, et al: Placebo-controlled trial of moclobemide in social phobia. Br J Psychiatry 172:70–77, 1998

Schnurr PP, Friedman MJ, Engel CC, et al: Cognitive behavioral therapy for PTSD in women: a randomized controlled trial. JAMA 297:820–830, 2007

Schutters SI, Van Megen HJ, Van Veen JF, et al: Mirtazapine in generalized social anxiety disorder: a randomized, double-blind, placebo-controlled study. Int Clin Psychopharmacol 25:302–304, 2010

Schweizer E, Rickels K: Buspirone in the treatment of panic disorder: a controlled pilot comparison with clorazepate (abstract). J Clin Psychopharmacol 8:303, 1988

Schweizer E, Rickels K: Pharmacological treatment for generalized anxiety disorder, in Long-term Treatments of Anxiety Disorders. Edited by Mavissakalian M, Prien RF. Washington, DC, American Psychiatric Press, 1996, pp 201–220

Schweizer E, Rickels K, Lucki I: Resistance to the anti-anxiety effect of buspirone in patients with a history of benzodiazepine use. N Engl J Med 314:719–720, 1986

Schweizer E, Patterson W, Rickels K, et al: Double-blind, placebo-controlled study of a once-a-day, sustained-release preparation of alprazolam for the treatment of panic disorder. Am J Psychiatry 150:1210–1215, 1993

Sepede G, De Berardis D, Gambi F, et al: Olanzapine augmentation in treatment-resistant panic disorder: a 12-week, fixed-dose, open-label trial. J Clin Psychopharmacol 26:45–49, 2006

Shader RI, Greenblatt DJ: Use of benzodiazepines in anxiety disorders. N Engl J Med 328:1398–1405, 1993

Shalev AY, Ankri Y, Israeli-Shalev Y, et al: Prevention of posttraumatic stress disorder by early treatment: results from the Jerusalem Trauma Outreach and Prevention study. Arch Gen Psychiatry 69:166–176, 2012

Shear MK, Brown TA, Barlow DH, et al: Multicenter collaborative Panic Disorder Severity Scale. Am J Psychiatry 154:1571–1575, 1997

Sheehan DV: The Anxiety Disease. Bantam Books, New York, 1986

Sheehan DV, Ballenger J, Jacobsen G: Treatment of endogenous anxiety with phobic, hysterical, and hypochondriacal symptoms. Arch Gen Psychiatry 37:51–59, 1980

Sheehan DV, Davidson J, Manschreck T, et al: Lack of efficacy of a new antidepressant (bupropion) in the treatment of panic disorder with phobias. J Clin Psychopharmacol 3:28–31, 1983

Sheehan DV, Raj AB, Sheehan KH, et al: Is buspirone effective for panic disorder? J Clin Psychopharmacol 10:3–11, 1990

Sheehan DV, Burnham DB, Iyengar MK, et al: Efficacy and tolerability of controlled-release paroxetine in the treatment of panic disorder. J Clin Psychiatry 66:34–40, 2005

Silverstone PH, Salinas E: Efficacy of venlafaxine extended release in patients with major depressive disorder and comorbid generalized anxiety disorder. J Clin Psychiatry 62:523–529, 2001

Simon NM, Emmanuel N, Ballenger J, et al: Bupropion sustained release for panic disorder. Psychopharmacol Bull 37:66–72, 2003

Simon NM, Hoge EA, Fischmann D, et al: An open-label trial of risperidone augmentation for refractory anxiety disorders. J Clin Psychiatry 67:381–385, 2006

Simpson HB, Schneier FR, Marshall RD, et al: Low dose selegiline (L-deprenyl) in social phobia. Depress Anxiety 7:126–129, 1998

Simpson HB, Foa EB, Liebowitz MR, et al: A randomized, controlled trial of cognitive-behavioral therapy for augmenting pharmacotherapy in obsessive-compulsive disorder. Am J Psychiatry 165:621–630, 2008

Snyderman SH, Rynn MA, Rickels K: Open-label pilot study of ziprasidone for refractory generalized anxiety disorder. J Clin Psychopharmacol 25:497–499, 2005

Stahl SM, Gergel I, Li D: Escitalopram in the treatment of panic disorder: a randomized, double-blind, placebo-controlled trial. J Clin Psychiatry 64:1322–1327, 2003

Stein DJ, Andersen EW, Tonnoir B, et al: Escitalopram in obsessive-compulsive disorder: a randomized, placebo-controlled, paroxetine-referenced, fixed-dose, 24-week study. Curr Med Res Opin 23:701–711, 2007

Stein DJ, Ahokas AA, de Bodinat C: Efficacy of agomelatine in generalized anxiety disorder: a randomized, double-blind, placebo-controlled trial. J Clin Psychopharmacol 28:561–566, 2008

Stein MB, Chartier MJ, Hazen AL, et al: Paroxetine in the treatment of generalized social phobia: open-label treatment and double-blind placebo-controlled discontinuation. J Clin Psychopharmacol 16:218–222, 1996

Stein MB, Liebowitz MR, Lydiard RB, et al: Paroxetine treatment of generalized social phobia (social anxiety disorder): a randomized controlled trial. JAMA 280:708–713, 1998

Stein MB, Fyer AJ, Davidson JR, et al: Fluvoxamine treatment of social phobia (social anxiety disorder): a double-blind, placebo-controlled study. Am J Psychiatry 156:756–760, 1999

Stein MB, Kline NA, Matloff JL: Adjunctive olanzapine for SSRI-resistant combat-related PTSD: a double-blind, placebo-controlled study. Am J Psychiatry 159:1777–1779, 2002

Stein MB, Ravindran LN, Simon NM, et al: Levetiracetam in generalized social anxiety disorder: a double-blind, randomized controlled trial. J Clin Psychiatry 71:627–631, 2010

Stinson FS, Dawson DA, Patricia Chou S, et al: The epidemiology of DSM-IV specific phobia in the USA: results from the National Epidemiologic Survey on Alcohol and Related Conditions. Psychol Med 37:1047–1059, 2007

Strand M, Hetta J, Rosen A, et al: A double-blind, controlled trial in primary care patients with generalized anxiety: a comparison between buspirone and oxazepam. J Clin Psychiatry 51 (suppl):40–45, 1990

Sutherland SM, Tupler LA, Colket JT, et al: A 2-year follow-up of social phobia. Status after a brief medication trial. J Nerv Ment Dis 184:731–738, 1996

Swinson RP, Antony MM, Bleau P, et al: Clinical practice guidelines. Management of anxiety disorders. Can J Psychiatry 51 (suppl 2):1–92, 2006

Szegedi A, Wetzel H, Leal M, et al: Combination treatment with clomipramine and fluvoxamine: drug monitoring, safety, and tolerability data. J Clin Psychiatry 57:257–264, 1996

Taylor LH, Kobak KA: An open-label trial of St John's wort (Hypericum perforatum) in obsessive-compulsive disorder. J Clin Psychiatry 61:575–578, 2000

Taylor FB, Martin P, Thompson C, et al: Prazosin effects on objective sleep measures and clinical symptoms in civilian trauma posttraumatic stress disorder: a placebo-controlled study. Biol Psychiatry 63:629–632, 2008

Tesar GE, Rosenbaum JF, Pollack MH, et al: Double-blind, placebo-controlled comparison of clonazepam and alprazolam for panic disorder. J Clin Psychiatry 52:69–76, 1991

Teschke R, Schulze J: Role of kava hepatotoxicity and the FDA consumer advisory. JAMA 304:2174–2175, 2010

Thoren P, Asberg M, Cronholm B, et al: Clomipramine treatment of obsessive-compulsive disorder, I: a controlled clinical trial. Arch Gen Psychiatry 37:1281–1285, 1980

Tollefson GD, Rampey AH Jr, Potvin JH, et al: A multicenter investigation of fixed-dose fluoxetine in the treatment of obsessive-compulsive disorder. Arch Gen Psychiatry 51:559–567, 1994

Tucker P, Smith KL, Marx B, et al: Fluvoxamine reduces physiologic reactivity to trauma scripts in posttraumatic stress disorder. J Clin Psychopharmacol 20:367–372, 2000

Tucker P, Zaninelli R, Yehuda R, et al: Paroxetine in the treatment of chronic posttraumatic stress disorder: results of a placebo-controlled, flexible-dosage trial. J Clin Psychiatry 62:860–868, 2001

Tucker P, Potter-Kimball R, Wyatt DB, et al: Can physiologic assessment and side effects tease out differences in PTSD trials? A double-blind comparison of citalopram, sertraline, and placebo. Psychopharmacol Bull 37:135–149, 2003

Tucker P, Trautman RP, Wyatt DB, et al: Efficacy and safety of topiramate monotherapy in civilian posttraumatic stress disorder: a randomized, double-blind, placebo-controlled study. J Clin Psychiatry 68:201–206, 2007

Turner SM, Beidel DC, Jacob RG: Social phobia: a comparison of behavior therapy and atenolol. J Consult Clin Psychol 62:350–358, 1994

Van Ameringen M, Mancini C, Oakman JM: Nefazodone in social phobia. J Clin Psychiatry 60:96–100, 1999

Van Ameringen MA, Lane RM, Walker JR, et al: Sertraline treatment of generalized social phobia: a 20-week, double-blind, placebo-controlled study. Am J Psychiatry 158:275–281, 2001

Van Ameringen M, Mancini C, Oakman J, et al: Nefazodone in the treatment of generalized social phobia: a randomized, placebo-controlled trial. J Clin Psychiatry 68:288–295, 2007

van der Kolk BA, Dreyfuss D, Michaels M, et al: Fluoxetine in posttraumatic stress disorder [see comment]. J Clin Psychiatry 55:517–522, 1994

van Vliet IM, den Boer JA, Westenberg HG: Psychopharmacological treatment of social phobia: clinical and biochemical effects of brofaromine, a selective MAO-A inhibitor. Eur Neuropsychopharmacol 2:21–29, 1992

van Vliet IM, den Boer JA, Westenberg HG: Psychopharmacological treatment of social phobia: a double blind placebo controlled study with fluvoxamine. Psychopharmacology (Berl) 115:128–134, 1994

van Vliet IM, den Boer JA, Westenberg HG, et al: Clinical effects of buspirone in social phobia: a double-blind placebo-controlled study. J Clin Psychiatry 58:164–168, 1997

Versiani M, Nardi AE, Mundim FD, et al: Pharmacotherapy of social phobia. A controlled study with moclobemide and phenelzine. Br J Psychiatry 161:353–360, 1992

Versiani M, Nardi AE, Figueria J: Double-blind placebo-controlled trial with bromazepam in social phobia. J Bras Psiquiatr 46:167–171, 1997

Versiani M, Cassano G, Perugi G, et al: Reboxetine, a selective norepinephrine reuptake inhibitor, is an effective and well-tolerated treatment for panic disorder. J Clin Psychiatry 63:31–37, 2002

Vulink NC, Denys D, Fluitman SB, et al: Quetiapine augments the effect of citalopram in non-refractory obsessive-compulsive disorder: a randomized, double-blind, placebo-controlled study of 76 patients. J Clin Psychiatry 70:1001–1008, 2009

Wade AG, Lepola U, Koponen HJ, et al: The effect of citalopram in panic disorder. Br J Psychiatry 170:549–553, 1997

Wagner KD, Berard R, Stein MB, et al: A multicenter, randomized, double-blind, placebo-controlled trial of paroxetine in children and adolescents with social anxiety disorder. Arch Gen Psychiatry 61:1153–1162, 2004

Walker JR, Van Ameringen MA, Swinson R, et al: Prevention of relapse in generalized social phobia: results of a 24-week study in responders to 20 weeks of sertraline treatment. J Clin Psychopharmacol 20:636–644, 2000

Walkup JT, Albano AM, Piacentini J, et al: Cognitive behavioral therapy, sertraline, or a combination in childhood anxiety. N Engl J Med 359:2753–2766, 2008

Weathers FW, Huska JA, Keane TM: PCL-C for DSM-IV. Boston, MA, National Center for PTSD—Behavioral Science Division, 1991

Weathers FW, Keane TM, Davidson JRT: Clinician-Administered PTSD Scale: a review of the first ten years of research. Depress Anxiety 13:132–156, 2001

Westenberg HG, Stein DJ, Yang H, et al: A double-blind placebo-controlled study of controlled release fluvoxamine for the treatment of generalized social anxiety disorder. J Clin Psychopharmacol 24:49–55, 2004

Williams JE, Nieto FJ, Sanford CP, et al: Effects of an angry temperament on coronary heart disease risk: the Atherosclerosis Risk in Communities Study. Am J Epidemiol 154:230–235, 2001

Wittchen HU, Hoyer J: Generalized anxiety disorder: nature and course. J Clin Psychiatry 62 (suppl 11):15–19, 2001

Wittchen HU, Zhao S, Kessler RC, et al: DSM-III-R generalized anxiety disorder in the National Comorbidity Survey. Arch Gen Psychiatry 51:355–364, 1994

Woelk H, Arnoldt KH, Kieser M, et al: Ginkgo biloba special extract EGb 761 in generalized anxiety disorder and adjustment disorder with anxious mood: a randomized, double-blind, placebo-controlled trial. J Psychiatr Res 41:472–480, 2007

Wurthmann C, Klieser E, Lehmann E: [Differential pharmacologic therapy of generalized anxiety disorders—results of a study with 30 individual case experiments]. Fortschritte der Neurologie-Psychiatrie 63:303–309, 1995

Zigmond AS, Snaith RP: The Hospital Anxiety and Depression Scale. Acta Psychiatr Scand 67:361–370, 1983

Zimmerman M, Mattia JI: Principal and additional DSM-IV disorders for which outpatients seek treatment. Psychiatr Serv 51:1299–1304, 2000

Zitrin CM, Klein DF, Woerner MG, et al: Treatment of phobias, I: comparison of imipramine hydrochloride and placebo. Arch Gen Psychiatry 40:125–138, 1983

Zohar J, Amital D, Miodownik C, et al: Double-blind placebo-controlled pilot study of sertraline in military veterans with posttraumatic stress disorder. J Clin Psychopharmacol 22:190–195, 2002

Zwanzger P, Baghai TC, Schule C, et al: Tiagabine improves panic and agoraphobia in panic disorder patients. J Clin Psychiatry 62:656–657, 2001

Zwanzger P, Eser D, Nothdurfter C, et al: Effects of the GABA-reuptake inhibitor tiagabine on panic and anxiety in patients with panic disorder. Pharmacopsychiatry 42:266–269, 2009

CHAPTER 39

Treatment of Substance-Related Disorders

James W. Cornish, M.D.

Laura F. McNicholas, M.D., Ph.D.

Charles P. O'Brien, M.D., Ph.D.

Alcohol

Experimentation with alcohol is very common, and a large proportion of users find the experience pleasant. More than 90% of American adults have consumed alcohol at least once, and approximately 70% report some level of current use (Hasin et al. 2007). In a national survey in 2009 (Substance Abuse and Mental Health Services Administration 2010), a little more than half (51.9%) of Americans 12 years and older reported having at least one alcoholic drink in the past 30 days. With respect to heavier drinking in the population 12 years and older, 23.7% reported binge drinking (5 or more drinks on one occasion for males, 4 or more for women) and 6.8% reported heavy drinking (5 or more drinks on one occasion on 5 or more days).

Alcoholism is the most prevalent substance use disorder in the United States (excluding nicotine), affecting approximately 7.3% of the population at some point in their lifetime (Substance Abuse and Mental Health Services Administration 2010). The natural history of excessive alcohol consumption is known. The amount and pattern of alcohol consumption and the harmful effects of drinking are associated in a predictable manner (Kranzler et al. 1990). The aim of long-term treatment of alcoholism is complete abstinence from drinking, although reduction in heavy drinking has been found in clinical trials to have beneficial effects.

Psychosocial Treatment

The principal forms of treatment for alcoholism have been self-help/support groups, such as Alcoholics Anonymous, or psychosocial treatments in inpatient or outpatient rehabilitation programs or sheltered living situations. Many 28-day treatment programs provide group and individual therapy for alcoholic rehabilitation.

Cognitive-behavioral therapy and 12-step facilitation have shown significant efficacy in the treatment of alcohol dependence in several controlled clinical trials (McCaul and Petry 2003). Cognitive-behavioral therapy is based on teaching patients new, alternative adaptive skills to deal with situations that lead to drinking.

Unfortunately, a large percentage of persons relapse to drinking following psychosocial treatment alone. For over two decades, this has been a prime motivation to find effective pharmacotherapies for alcohol dependence to complement existing psychosocial treatments.

Cognitive-behavioral therapy has been successfully combined with various pharmacotherapies to treat alcohol dependence. However, in their review of this area, Weiss and Kueppenbender (2006) stated, "There is no evidence that any single form of psychosocial treatment is the criterion standard for alcohol-dependent patients receiving pharmacotherapy."

Pharmacotherapy

Pharmacotherapy has been directed at specific indications that often occur during the course of treatment for alcoholism. Studies have been conducted involving alcohol detoxification treatments, alcohol sensitization agents, anticraving agents, and agents that diminish drinking by modifying neurotransmitter systems associated with the reinforcement of alcohol.

Frequently, the first step in management of an alcoholic patient is treatment of alcohol withdrawal symptoms. This initial step is followed by long-term treatment that aims for complete abstinence from alcohol consumption. *Detoxification* refers to the clearing of alcohol from the body and the readjustment of all systems to functioning in the absence of alcohol. The alcohol withdrawal syndrome at the mild end may include only headache and irritability, but about 5% of alcoholic patients have severe withdrawal symptoms (Schuckit 1991) manifested by tremulousness, tachycardia, perspiration, and even seizures (rum fits). The presence of malnutrition, electrolyte imbalance, or infection increases the possibility of cardiovascular collapse.

Alcohol Withdrawal Management: Benzodiazepines and Other Agents

Significant progress has been made in establishing safe and effective medications for alcohol withdrawal. Pharmacotherapy with a benzodiazepine is the treatment of choice for the prevention and treatment of the signs and symptoms of alcohol withdrawal (Ntais et al. 2005). Many patients detoxify from alcohol dependence without specific treatment or medications; however, it is difficult to determine accurately which patients will require medication for alcohol withdrawal. Patients in good physical condition with uncomplicated mild to moderate alcohol withdrawal symptoms can usually be treated as outpatients. Patients with medical complications, significant psychosocial problems, and severe alcohol dependence do better with inpatient treatment (Ait-Daoud et al. 2006).

A typical detoxification regimen requires frequent clinical evaluations, multiple vitamins, and benzodiazepine pharmacotherapy. A typical dosing regimen involves giving enough benzodiazepine on the first day of treatment to relieve withdrawal symptoms; the dose should be adjusted if withdrawal symptoms increase or if the patient complains of excessive sedation. Over the next 5–7 days, the dose of benzodiazepine is tapered to zero. Most clinicians use longer-acting benzodiazepines such as clonazepam, chlordiazepoxide, or diazepam. In outpatient settings, oxazepam may be particularly useful because it is associated with less abuse and does not require hepatic biotransformation. Carbamazepine and other anticonvulsants have been shown to effectively treat alcohol withdrawal symptoms. These agents are less effective than benzodiazepines in relieving subjective symptoms of withdrawal.

The diagnosis of delirium tremens is given to patients who have marked confusion and severe agitation in addition to the usual alcohol withdrawal symptoms. It is important to remember that the risk of mortality is 5% for patients with severe alcohol withdrawal symptoms (Eyer et al. 2011). Patients who have medically complicated or severe alcoholic withdrawal must be treated in a hospital. Benzodiazepines will usually be sufficient to calm agitated patients; however, some patients may require intravenous barbiturates to control extreme agitation.

Alcohol-Sensitizing Agent: Disulfiram

In 1951, disulfiram was the first medication to be approved by the U.S. Food and Drug Administration (FDA) for the treatment of alcohol dependence other than detoxification. Disulfiram inhibits a key enzyme, aldehyde dehydrogenase, involved in breakdown of ethyl alcohol. After drinking, the alcohol-disulfiram reaction produces excess blood levels of acetaldehyde, which is toxic in that it produces facial flushing, tachycardia, hypotension, nausea and vomiting, and physical discomfort. The usual maintenance dosage of disulfiram is 250 mg/day.

There have been only a few randomized controlled trials of disulfiram, and these trials have had mixed results for drug efficacy (Peachy and Naranjo 1984). The most comprehensive trial was the Veterans Administration (VA) Cooperative Study of disulfiram treatment of alcoholism. This study was conducted with male veterans and found no differences between disulfiram, 250 mg/day and 1 mg/day (an ineffective dose), and placebo groups in total abstinence, time to first drink, employment, or social stability. Among patients who drank, those in the 250-mg disulfiram group reported significantly fewer drinking days (Fuller et al. 1986).

Disulfiram is most effective when it is used in a clinical setting that emphasizes abstinence and offers a mechanism to ensure that the medication is taken. Drug compliance may be successfully ensured either by giving the medication at 3- to 4-day intervals in the physician's office or at the treatment center or by having a spouse or family member administer it.

Opioid Receptor Antagonists

Naltrexone and naloxone. It has been shown in animal and human studies that endogenous opioids are involved in the reinforcing properties of alcohol (Gianoulakis et al. 1996; Volpicelli et al. 1986). Alcohol increases the release of endogenous opioids. The opioid receptor antagonists naloxone and naltrexone block this effect and reduce alcohol consumption in several animal models.

Naltrexone is an FDA-approved medication used as an adjunct in the treatment of alcoholism. This opioid receptor antagonist has been shown to block some of the reinforcing properties of alcohol and has resulted in a decreased rate of relapse to alcohol drinking in the majority of published double-blind clinical trails (Pettinati et al. 2006). In clinical trials on alcoholism, naltrexone-treated subjects, compared with placebo-treated subjects, have significantly better results in delaying the time to relapse to drinking, reducing relapse to heavy drinking, and reducing the amount of alcohol consumed when they sample alcohol.

Naltrexone has a better treatment response in alcoholic patients who have a family history of alcoholism, a strong craving for alcohol, and good compliance with taking the medication.

A significant development in identifying a potential endophenotype of alcoholism has grown out of the clinical experience with naltrexone. Animal studies have demonstrated that alcohol causes the release of endogenous opioids in brain reward systems and the disinhibition or activation of dopamine neurons, a condition common to all drugs of abuse. Blocking opioid receptors prevents this dopaminergic effect and results in less stimulation or reward from alcohol (Ray and Hutchison 2007). A functional allele of the gene for the μ opioid receptor has been associated with alcohol stimulation that is blocked by the opioid antagonist naltrexone, and this allele has also been associated with good response to naltrexone treatment among alcoholic individuals (Anton et al. 2008).

For several years, research was conducted to develop a long-acting naltrexone. In 2006, the FDA approved naltrexone in an injectable sustained-release formulation under the trade name Vivitrol. An intramuscular injection of 380 mg of depot naltrexone provides effective plasma concentrations of the medication for at least 30 days. This formulation maximizes drug-taking compliance by replacing daily pills with a monthly injection.

The pivotal efficacy data for depot naltrexone was derived from a large randomized multicenter clinical trial with a 24-week medication phase (Garbutt et al. 2006). The results showed that compared with placebo-injected subjects, those who received 380 mg depot naltrexone injections had significantly fewer heavy-drinking days. Interestingly, a secondary data analysis revealed that the beneficial effect from naltrexone was mainly seen in male subjects. There is no explanation for this finding. Further specific research is needed to confirm the existence of gender differences in patient response to depot naltrexone treatment.

Nalmefene. The efficacy of naltrexone in reducing alcohol drinking led to the testing of another opioid receptor antagonist. Nalmefene, like naltrexone, is an antagonist at μ, δ, and κ receptors and was found to be effective in one clinical trial in the United States (Mason et al. 1999). However, a second 12-week double-blind, placebo-controlled multisite study reported no difference between the nalmefene group and the placebo group on measures of efficacy (Anton et al. 2004).

Recently completed European trials tested a different protocol in which nalmefene was to be taken whenever the patient experienced alcohol craving. The goal was to reduce relapse to heavy drinking. Positive results for "as-needed" nalmefene from three unpublished clinical trials involving 1,997 subjects were reported at the 2012 European Congress of Psychiatry. All three trials were double-blind, placebo-controlled multisite studies in which a standard nalmefene dosage of 18 mg/day was tested. Two of the trials had 6-month treatment phases; results of one of these 6-month trials (Mann et al. 2012) was presented as a poster at the Congress. The third trial had a 52-week treatment phase with an aim to study long-term safety and efficacy. The data presented showed that after 6 months of treatment, nalmefene-treated subjects reduced their total alcohol consumption by 65% on average. It is anticipated that these clinical studies will soon be published.

Anticraving Agents

Acamprosate. Acamprosate was developed in Europe, where placebo-controlled trials found it to be effective in treating alcoholism. Although trials conducted in the United States did not show efficacy, acamprosate nevertheless received FDA approval because of the positive European trials. It has been found to be effective when used to decrease craving and relapse in patients who have already undergone detoxification. Acamprosate requires dosing 2–3 times per day, but side effects are minimal, and some patients report a remarkable reduction in alcohol craving.

Topiramate. Developed for the treatment of epilepsy, topiramate has been used off-label to treat alcoholism and cocaine addiction. Although there are placebo-controlled studies that show topiramate's efficacy in addiction (Johnson et al. 2004; Kampman et al. 2004), at present there appears to be no plan to obtain FDA approval for this indication.

Ondansetron. Ondansetron, an antagonist of the ionotropic serotonin$_3$ (5-HT$_3$) receptor, was reported to reduce heavy drinking in individuals with early-onset alcoholism, a clinical subtype characterized by onset of alcohol dependence before the age of 25 years, frequently by the teenage years. Ondansetron is not yet available to clinicians, but clinical trials continue.

Sedatives

Sedative abuse at present consists mainly in the overuse of benzodiazepine tranquilizers and sleeping pills. Dependence and drug seeking can occur, but many users of unprescribed sedative-hypnotics use them to self-medicate withdrawal from other drugs, such as alcohol. Benzodiazepines are useful in the detoxification of patients dependent on alcohol, but they are not indicated in the long-term treatment of alcoholism because alcoholic individuals are at risk of developing dependence on these medications.

Nicotine

According to the 2009 National Survey on Drug Use and Health (NSDUH), an estimated 69.7 million Americans, or 27.7% of the population, reported current use of tobacco. Most tobacco users, 58.7 million, smoked cigarettes, whereas the remainder smoked cigars and pipes or used smokeless tobacco (Substance Abuse and Mental Health Services Administration 2010). Tobacco accounts for about 400,000 deaths per year. Since the mid-1960s, the incidence of smoking in the United States has progressively decreased by about 1% per year. This remarkable change in tobacco use is a consequence of the realization by society that tobacco-related mortality and morbidity are entirely preventable. Most smokers have symptoms that meet the DSM-IV-TR (American Psychiatric Association 2000) criteria for the substance use disorder nicotine dependence. The behavioral aspects of nicotine dependence are similar to those of alcohol and opiate dependence and include the production of tolerance and physical dependence. In about 80% of smokers (Gross and Stitzer 1989), nicotine abstinence leads to well-described withdrawal signs and symptoms (Hughes and Hatsukami 1986).

Nicotine replacement therapy and the nonnicotine medications bupropion and varenicline have emerged as very effective pharmacotherapies for nicotine dependence. These treatments have the key elements of reducing withdrawal symptoms, aiding smoking cessation, and decreasing the reinforcement effects of smoking.

Nicotine Replacement Therapy

Nicotine replacement medications deliver nicotine to a person without the use of tobacco products. The aim with each medication is to relieve withdrawal symptoms in abstaining smokers by replacing nicotine that is usually derived from tobacco products.

The nicotine replacement products available in the United States include chewing gum, an inhaler, a nasal spray, sublingual tablets, lozenges, and skin patches. With the exception of skin patches, all of these products provide nicotine that is absorbed through the oral mucosa. Skin patches are formulated to allow nicotine to be absorbed through the skin. Nicotine gum, skin patches, and lozenges are available as over-the-counter (OTC) medications. The nicotine inhaler and nasal spray are by prescription.

An analysis of several clinical trials found that compared with placebo, nicotine replacement therapies increase the likelihood of long-term abstinence from smoking by 50%–70% (Stead et al. 2008). Based on a wealth of empirical data over the past 20 years, these medications have emerged as effective, well-recognized, and accepted first-line treatments for persons desiring to stop smoking cigarettes (Fiore et al. 2008).

Nicotine polacrilex gum, 2 mg and 4 mg, is typically prescribed so that patients have free access to it for periods up to 4 months. Clinical studies indicate that strongly dependent smokers (25 or more cigarettes per day) have more success with the 4-mg dose (Glover et al. 1996; Sachs 1995). Abstaining smokers are to chew the gum to relieve acute cravings to smoke. Chewing the gum releases nicotine that then is absorbed through the oral mucosa. Peak nicotine plasma levels are reached at 20 minutes. The correct chewing technique is needed to get the full dose of nicotine. This requires that the patient chew the piece of gum a few times and then "park" the gum in his or her cheek to allow the nicotine to be absorbed; the patient repeats this for up to 30 minutes. Individuals with poor teeth, dentures, or temporomandibular joint disease may have difficulty using nicotine gum.

Nicotine nasal spray is the most rapidly delivered form of nicotine replacement therapy. The spray delivers nicotine to the nasal mucosa where it is quickly absorbed. Following administration, peak nicotine plasma levels are reached in 10 minutes. The major and limiting side effect of nasal irritation reportedly occurs in more than 80% of patients after 3 weeks of use.

The nicotine lozenge is very similar to the gum but does not require chewing. Patients are instructed to let the lozenge dissolve in the mouth for 30 minutes. Consequently, even patients who have poor teeth or dentures may use it successfully. It is available as OTC medication in 2-mg and 4-mg dosages.

The nicotine inhaler is a device with the appearance of a cigarette that has a mouthpiece and a cartridge containing nicotine. It is available only by prescription. To use it, the person inhales through the mouthpiece, which releases nicotine vapor that is then absorbed through the oral mucosa. In addition to providing nicotine, the inhaler has the unique benefit of providing oral and sensory stimulation similar to that of the physical act of cigarette smoking but without harmful smoke. The initial dose range is 6–16 cartridges daily for up to 12 weeks, followed by a gradual taper of dose over the next 12 weeks.

The transdermal nicotine patch is an OTC medication that is available as a 24-hour patch system (7, 14, or 21 mg of nicotine) or a 16-hour patch that provides 15 mg of nicotine. It is a first-line treatment. Among nicotine replacement therapies, the patch provides the most continuous nicotine plasma level over the longest period of time. It is the simplest to use, since it requires only that each morning the user apply the patch to a bare area of skin. The 24-hour patch allows for three levels of dose adjustment but no same-day dose changes. Research has shown that the 16-hour (waking hours) patch is equal in efficacy to the 24-hour patch (Stead et al. 2008).

The recommendation from clinical practice guidelines (Fiore et al. 2008) is to use nicotine patches for a minimum of 8 weeks. Patients are usually initiated on the high-dose patches, maintained on these for 4–6 weeks, and then tapered over the next 6 weeks. Although it seems intuitive that longer treatment with the nicotine patch would improve the sustained abstinence rate, this has not been scientifically supported. A double-blind, placebo-controlled smoking cessation trial of nicotine patch therapy in 3,575 smokers enrolled in a pulmonary clinic showed no difference in abstinence rates between subjects who received 8 weeks of pharmacotherapy versus those who received 22 weeks (Tønnesen et al. 1999).

Nonnicotine Pharmacotherapies

Bupropion

Bupropion, a monocyclic antidepressant with noradrenergic and dopaminergic effects, has been in use for more than 25 years as an antidepressant. In 1997, a sustained-release (SR) formulation of bupropion, marketed under the trade name Zyban, was approved by the FDA for use as a smoking cessation aid. Bupropion reduces craving for nicotine, but the mechanism by which this occurs is not well understood. The results from several studies indicate that bupropion's anticraving effect is related to its action on central nervous system dopamine (Covey et al. 2000). The results from a meta-analysis of 31 controlled trials found that compared with placebo, bupropion SR doubled long-term abstinence rates (Hughes et al. 2004).

The target dosage of bupropion SR is 150 mg twice a day. Because approximately 7 days are required to reach steady-state blood levels with bupropion, patients are instructed to start the medication 1 week before their target quit date. An initial treatment trial is for 7–12 weeks; if successful, treatment may be extended for relapse prevention for up to 6 months. Bupropion was recommended as a first-line treatment for smoking cessation in the two most recent clinical practice guidelines from the Tobacco Use and Dependence Guideline Panel (2000, 2008).

The common side effects for Zyban are the same as for bupropion that is used as an antidepressant medication. These include dry mouth, headache, insomnia, and anxiety. Bupropion may induce seizures because it reduces the seizure threshold, but this serious adverse reaction is infrequent and estimated to occur in about 1:1,000 treated patients (Aubin 2002).

Varenicline

Approved by the FDA in 2006, varenicline is the newest medication available for smoking cessation. Varenicline is an $\alpha_4\beta_2$ nicotinic receptor partial agonist that relieves symptoms of nicotine withdrawal. It also has antagonist effects, because it binds very tightly to the nicotinic receptor and blocks administered nicotine from attaching (Hays et al. 2001; Henningfield et al. 2005).

Several controlled trials support the efficacy of varenicline as a medication for smoking cessation. The largest of these were two studies that included more than 2,000 subjects (Gonzales et al. 2006; Jorenby et al. 2006). Both studies were 12-week trials that compared varenicline, bupropion, and placebo. Rates of continuous abstinence for the last 4 weeks of the treatment phase were 44%, 30%, and 18% for varenicline, bupropion, and placebo, respectively. In one of these studies (Jorenby et al. 2006), continuous abstinence rates for 1 year for varenicline, bupropion, and placebo were 23%, 14.6%, and 10.3%, respectively. Overall, the clinical trails show that compared with bupropion, varenicline is better for both quitting smoking and preventing relapse.

The target dosage of varenicline is 1 mg twice a day. Because it takes approximately 7 days to reach steady-state blood levels with varenicline, patients are instructed to start the medication 1 week before their target quit date. An initial treatment trial is for 12 weeks; if successful, treatment may be extended for another 12 weeks.

Black Box Warnings

In 2009, following a review of postmarketing data for bupropion and varenicline, the FDA concluded that both of these medications may increase suicidal behavior in treated individuals. As a consequence, the FDA mandated that labeling for bupropion and varenicline include the same black box warnings about the risk of serious neuropsychiatric symptoms and suicidality (U.S. Food and Drug Administration 2009). These warnings call for close monitoring of treated patients for symptoms of changes in behavior.

Combination Pharmacotherapy

Although nicotine patch plus bupropion is the only FDA-approved combination pharmacotherapy for smoking cessation, other medication combinations have been shown to be effective.

A meta-analysis of combination therapy for smoking cessation (Shah et al. 2008) found that nicotine patch plus bupropion, nicotine patch plus nicotine inhaler, and long-term patch plus ad lib nicotine replacement therapy were each significantly more effective than the respective placebo combinations.

In a clinical trial evaluating five smoking-cessation pharmacotherapies (Piper et al. 2009), 1,504 subjects were randomly assigned to treatment with nicotine lozenge, nicotine patch, bupropion, nicotine patch plus nicotine lozenge, bupropion plus nicotine lozenge, or placebo. At the end of the treatment phase (12 weeks for lozenge and lozenge placebo; 8 weeks for all other treatments), all active-medication groups had higher quit rates than the placebo group. At 6-month follow-up, only the nicotine patch plus nicotine lozenge group significantly outperformed the placebo group (abstinence rates of 40% and 22%, respectively).

Psychological Interventions

It is well recognized that smoking is maintained by both behavioral and pharmacological aspects (Jaffe and Kranzler 1979; Leventhal and Cleary 1980). It is not surprising that the combination of nicotine gum replacement and behavioral modification therapy is superior to either treatment alone (Hall et al. 1985; Killen et al. 1984). Hall and Killen (1985) conducted a controlled combined treatment trial for smoking cessation. They found that the abstinence rates from these studies, 44% at 12 months and 50% at 10.5 months, were "some of the highest abstinence rates ever reported" (Hall and Killen 1985, p. 139). To determine the minimum behavioral treatment necessary to optimize abstinence, we need more controlled trials involving combined therapy.

Smoking and Psychiatric Disorders

There is a high incidence of smoking among persons who have psychiatric illnesses and persons who abuse alcohol. Several investigators have reported data showing markedly increased smoking rates associated with schizophrenia and depression (Dani and Harris 2005; Glassman et al. 1988; Goff et al. 1992).

There is no known reason for the high rate of nicotine use by persons with schizophrenia. Some have speculated that the dopamine-augmenting effect of nicotine may counterbalance a relative dopamine deficiency that exists in schizophrenia patients (Dalack et al. 1998; Glassman 1993). Reports from two small trials in smokers with schizophrenia indicate that smoking-cessation pharmacotherapy is effective in this population (Evins et al. 2005; George et al. 2002). In each study, subjects were randomly assigned to receive treatment with either bupropion or placebo. The results of these studies showed an increased quit rate for the bupropion-treated subjects compared with those who received placebo. There is also some evidence that the atypical antipsychotic medication olanzapine reduces smoking in schizophrenia patients (Rohsenow et al. 2008).

Glassman et al. (1988) conducted pioneering research establishing a link between major depression and cigarette smoking. Based on data from the Epidemiologic Catchment Area (ECA) survey (Regier et al. 1984), they found that 76% of persons with a lifetime history of major depression "had ever smoked" compared with 52% of persons without a depression history. Similarly, the incidence of depression was 6.6% in smokers compared with 2.9% in nonsmokers, and smokers with a history of depression had a low rate of cessation. These findings have been replicated by several investigators, and the association between depression and smoking is well supported.

Another observation is that depressive symptoms appear during smoking cessation in persons with a history of depression (Covey et al. 1990). Hughes (2007) conducted a literature review of clinical trials that investigated smoking cessation among smokers with a history of depression. He found that these smokers developed depressive symptoms more frequently than smokers who had no history of depression (Hughes 2007). It is advisable to closely follow patients with a history of depression who are undergoing smoking-cessation treatment. Should patients develop depressed mood, it is important to determine whether the symptoms are the typical self-limited low mood seen in recently abstinent smokers or the beginning of clinical depression.

Summary of Smoking Cessation Treatments

Nicotine replacement combined with behavioral modification therapy is very effective in relieving nicotine withdrawal symptoms and in initiating smoking cessation. The two nonnicotine medications bupropion and varenicline have been shown to be effective pharmacotherapies for smoking cessation. Findings from one study (Piper et al. 2009) suggest that the combination nicotine patch plus nicotine lozenge is the most effective pharmacological treatment for smoking cessation.

Opioids

Pharmacotherapy for opioid dependence has a long history, in part because "heroinism" was one of the first recognized drug problems in the United States and because therapeutically used congeners of the drug of abuse, heroin, were readily available. More recently, the abuse of prescription opioids has far outpaced the abuse of heroin. Later studies have shown only limited success with nonpharmacological treatment.

Detoxification From Opioid Dependence

The classical method of opioid detoxification was, and remains, short-term substitution therapy. The medication traditionally used has been methadone, at a sufficient dose to suppress signs and symptoms of opioid withdrawal (opioid abstinence syndrome); the methadone is then tapered over a period ranging from 1 week to 6 months. More recently, a partial agonist, buprenorphine, has been studied for efficacy in suppressing the signs and symptoms of opioid withdrawal/abstinence (Bickel et al. 1988; Kosten and Kleber 1988). The point of a detoxification regimen is to achieve total opioid abstinence so that treatment can be continued in a drug-free setting. This approach continues to be employed despite evidence showing the superiority of agonist maintenance over drug-free treatment or placebo maintenance of opioid-addicted persons. Maddux and Desmond (1992) reported on six long-term (3 years or longer) follow-up studies of drug-free treatment of opiate abuse and dependence. Methadone was used for initial withdrawal, and one study used naltrexone to increase the chances of compliance with a drug-free program. Abstinence rates at follow-up in these studies ranged from 10% to 19%; the percentage of patients with unknown status at follow-up ranged from 10% to 32%. Kakko et al. (2003) compared detoxification versus maintenance treatment using buprenorphine and found that no subjects remained in treatment on placebo after 60 days. Furthermore, all regimens, regardless of the detoxification agent involved, must be individualized; this eliminates the possibility of standard protocols for opioid detoxification.

There has always been concern about substitution detoxification on the grounds that the physician is prolonging the problem by prescribing an addictive medication, even with a tapering regimen. Many of the symptoms of opioid withdrawal/abstinence (e.g., diaphoresis, hyperactivity, irritability) appear to be mediated by overactivity in the sympathetic nervous system. This led Gold et al. (1978, 1980) to attempt to depress this overactivity and thereby ameliorate the abstinence syndrome by using adrenergic agents that have no abuse potential. Clonidine, an α-adrenergic agonist with inhibitory action primarily at an autoreceptor in the locus coeruleus, was effective in inpatient populations in decreasing the signs and symptoms of opioid withdrawal. However, outpatient detoxification with clonidine has not been as successful as inpatient treatment. Inpatient studies reported an 80%–90% success rate, whereas outpatient studies reported success rates as low as 31% for methadone detoxification and 36% for heroin detoxification. Because the side effects of clonidine are unacceptable to many patients, other α-adrenergic agonists have been investigated for use in detoxification treatment of opioid-dependent patients. Lofexidine, guanabenz, and guanfacine have all been investigated, to varying degrees, as detoxification agents. The data thus far indicate that all of these agents have fewer cardiovascular side effects than clonidine. Because clonidine was much less successful in the outpatient setting than in the inpatient setting, various approaches, including the previously mentioned alternative α-adrenergic agonists, were studied in efforts to improve on the efficacy of clonidine. One of the major reasons clonidine was less successful in the outpatient setting was that heroin and other opioids were available to the patient. Naltrexone, a competitive opioid antagonist, was added to the clonidine regimen both to speed up the time course of withdrawal and to block the effect of any opioid used illicitly by the patient. As reported by Stine and Kosten (1992), 82% of the patients successfully completed detoxification as outpatients in 4–5 days with a single daily dosage of clonidine and 12.5 mg of naltrexone. This represented a significant reduction in the time required for detoxification. Furthermore, the patients reported few signs or symptoms of withdrawal except restlessness, insomnia, and muscle aches. This protocol allowed the patients not only to detoxify from opioids but also to simultaneously begin naltrexone maintenance treatment (see section "Relapse Prevention: Naltrexone" later in this chapter).

Loimer and colleagues have studied very rapid opioid detoxification. These methods have involved anesthetizing patients with either methohexital (Loimer et al. 1990) or midazolam (Loimer et al. 1991) and then using naltrexone to precipitate abstinence. These protocols successfully detoxified patients in 48 hours but required major medical intervention (intubation, mechanical ventilation, and intravenous fluids) and exposed patients to the risks of general anesthesia. This very rapid detoxification procedure has gained acceptance in some areas in treating opioid dependence. However, follow-up studies of patients undergoing rapid detoxification versus other detoxification methods found no superiority of the anesthesia-assisted arm and serious medical complications in the anesthesia-assisted arm (Collins et al. 2005).

Because drug-free treatment of opioid users has such high relapse rates, other modalities of treatment have been developed.

Maintenance Treatment of Opioid Dependence

Methadone maintenance has been the mainstay of the pharmacotherapy for opioid dependence since its introduction by Dole and Nyswander (1965). Buprenorphine received FDA approval in 2002 and can be prescribed by physicians for the treatment of opioid dependence.

Methadone

As discussed earlier in this chapter (see section "Detoxification From Opioid Dependence"), methadone has been used for both short- and long-term detoxification from opioids. Methadone maintenance, however, is designed to support a patient with opioid dependence for months or years while the patient engages in counseling and other therapy to change his or her lifestyle. Experience with methadone encompassing approximately 1.5 million person-years strongly demonstrated methadone to be safe and effective (Gerstein 1992). Furthermore, this experience has shown that although patients on methadone maintenance show physiological signs of opioid tolerance, there are minimal side effects, and patients' general health and nutritional status improve.

This approach to the treatment of opioid dependence has been controversial since its beginning. Physicians and other treatment professionals who regard opioid dependence according to a disease model have little or no problem treating patients with an active drug for long periods of time, especially in light of repeated treatment failures in the absence of active medication therapy. However, many people view methadone maintenance as simply substituting a legal drug for an illegal one and refuse to accept any outcome other than total abstinence from all drugs. These people point to long-term follow-up studies of methadone maintenance patients (see Maddux and Desmond 1992) that show that only 10%–20% of the patients are completely abstinent (defined as not being enrolled in methadone maintenance and not using illicit opioids) 5 years after discharge from the maintenance program. However, long-term follow-up studies of patients discharged from drug-free treatment programs show that only 10%–19% of opioid-dependent patients are abstinent at 3- or 5-year time points (see Maddux and Desmond 1992) when the same definition is used.

Despite these results of patients discharged from programs, studies of outcome measures other than total abstinence for patients in maintenance treatment consistently show that these patients have marked improvement in various measures. Investigators have shown up to an 85% decrease in criminal behavior, as measured by self-report or arrest records, among patients in treatment, whereas employment among maintenance patients ranges from 40% to 80%. Gerstein (1992) quoted a Swedish study published in 1984 showing the results over 5 years in 34 patients who applied for treatment to the only methadone clinic in Sweden at the time. These patients were randomly assigned to either methadone maintenance or outpatient drug-free therapy; the patients in drug-free treatment could not apply for methadone for a minimum of 24 months after being accepted into the study. After 2 years, 71% of the methadone patients were doing well, compared with 6% of the patients admitted to drug-free treatment. After 5 years, 13 of 17 (76%) patients remained on methadone and were free of illicit drugs, whereas 4 of 17 (24%) patients had been discharged from treatment for continued drug use. Of the 17 drug-free treatment patients, 9 (53%) had subsequently been switched to methadone treatment, were free of illicit drug use, and were "socially productive." Of the remaining 8 patients, 5 (63%) were dead (allegedly from overdose), 2 (25%) were in prison, and 1 (13%) was drug free.

Methadone maintenance programs in the United States are accredited by various federal agencies. A program must be accredited and its physicians licensed for a methadone maintenance program in order to prescribe or dispense more than a 2-week supply of any opioid to a patient known or suspected to be dependent on opioids. Most clinics treat ambulatory outpatients and are open 6–7 days per week, requiring patients to come into the clinic daily to receive medication unless and until a patient has "earned" privileges (take-home medication) by compliance with the clinic rules and abstinence from illicit substances. For a person to be eligible for methadone maintenance, he or she must be at least 18 years old (or have consent of the legal guardian) and must be physiologically dependent on heroin or other opioids for at least 1 year. The treatment regulations define a 1-year history of addiction to mean that the patient was addicted to an opioid narcotic at some time at least 1 year before admission and was addicted, either continuously or episodically, for most of the year immediately before admission to the methadone maintenance program. A physician must document evidence of current physiological dependence on opioids before a patient can be admitted to the program; such evidence may be a precipitated abstinence syndrome in response to a naloxone challenge or, more commonly, signs and symptoms of opioid withdrawal, evidence of intravenous injections, or evidence of medical complications of intravenous injections. Exceptions to these requirements include patients recently in penal or chronic care, previously treated patients, and pregnant patients; in these cases, patients need not show evidence of current physiological dependence, but the physician must justify their enrollment in methadone maintenance. An individual younger than 18 years must have documented evidence of at least two attempts at short-term detoxification or drug-free treatment (the episodes must be separated by at least 1 week) and have the consent of his or her parent or legal guardian.

Each clinic sets its own rules within the guidelines established by state and federal agencies. Many clinics are open only 6 days per week, thus giving all patients at least one dose of take-home medication weekly; others are open 7 days a week. All clinics must obtain urine drug screens on patients; Center for Substance Abuse Treatment regulations mandate a minimum of eight drug tests yearly. All methadone maintenance clinics are required to provide counseling for patients, but the amount provided is up to the individual clinic.

Clinic practice varies widely and is sometimes mandated by state regulators. The importance of psychosocial services in substance abuse treatment was eloquently demonstrated by McLellan et al. (1993) in a comparison of three levels of treatment services in which all patients received at least 60 mg/day of methadone. "Enhanced methadone services" patients (methadone plus counseling and on-site medical/psychiatric, employment, and family counseling) had fewer positive urine test results for illicit substances than did patients in the "standard services" (methadone plus counseling) group or the "minimum services" (methadone alone) group. The standard services group did significantly better in treatment than the minimum services group, and in fact, 69% of the minimum services group required transfer to a standard program 12 weeks into the study because of unremitting use of opioids or other illicit drugs.

More recently, an issue has emerged regarding a connection between methadone use and prolonged QTc interval with the potential for torsades de pointes. The clinical significance of this prolongation has engendered much discussion, particularly because the subjects in the various studies that reported methadone-induced QTc prolongation had predisposing factors for prolonged QTc in addition to the use of methadone (Ehret et al. 2006; Krantz et al. 2002). However, in 2006 the FDA issued a black box warning for methadone cautioning clinicians about the potential for prolonged QTc. The Substance Abuse and Mental Health Services Administration currently recommends that clinicians inform patients about the risk of cardiac complications; screen patients for a history of cardiac conditions; and, if indicated, obtain a pretreatment and 1-month electrocardiogram for patients at heightened risk (Center for Substance Abuse Treatment 2009).

Another issue that has engendered a great deal of controversy is the treatment of opioid dependence in pregnant women. Because many women with substance abuse problems fear all organizations, including medical ones, they frequently have little or no prenatal care, exposing themselves and their children to the complications of unsupervised pregnancy in addition to the severe stressor of maternal addiction. The complications and treatment of maternal opioid addiction and the effects on the fetus and neonate have been discussed by Finnegan (1991) and Finnegan and Kandall (1992). For the purposes of this chapter, it should be noted that current evidence shows that pregnant women who wish to be detoxified from opioids (either heroin or methadone) should not be detoxified before gestational week 14 because of the potential risk of inducing abortion or after gestational week 32 because of possible withdrawal-induced fetal stress (see Finnegan 1991). Most clinicians dealing with pregnant opioid-dependent patients advocate methadone maintenance at a dose of methadone that maintains homeostasis and eliminates opioid craving; this dose must be individualized for each patient and managed in concert with the obstetrician.

Buprenorphine

Buprenorphine is a partial agonist of the μ opioid receptor and is a clinically effective analgesic agent with an estimated potency of 25–40 times that of morphine (Cowan et al. 1977). A sublingual formulation of buprenorphine, as a monoproduct and as a buprenorphine/naloxone combination, was approved for treatment of opioid dependence in 2002. Human pharmacology studies have shown buprenorphine to be 25–30 times as potent as morphine in producing pupillary constriction, but buprenorphine was less effective in producing morphine-like subjective effects (Jasinski et al. 1978). Furthermore, these studies demonstrated that the physiological and subjective effects of morphine (15–120 mg) were significantly attenuated when morphine was administered 3 hours after buprenorphine in patients maintained on 8 mg/day of buprenorphine; the physiological and subjective effects of 30 mg of morphine also were tested at 29.5 hours after the last dose of chronically administered buprenorphine and were again significantly attenuated.

Studies in opiate-abusing patients have shown that buprenorphine is effective when administered sublingually. Early clinical trials with opioid-dependent patients found that patients would tolerate the sublingual route, that the dose of buprenorphine could be rapidly escalated to effective doses without significant side effects or toxicity (Johnson et al. 1989), and that detoxification from heroin dependence using buprenorphine was as effective as using methadone (Bickel et al. 1988) or clonidine (Kosten and Kleber 1988). Johnson et al. (1992) compared buprenorphine (8 mg/day sublingually) and methadone (20 mg/day or 60 mg/day) in a 25-week maintenance study and found that buprenorphine was as effective as 60 mg/day of methadone in reducing illicit opioid use and keeping patients in treatment. Both buprenorphine and methadone 60 mg/day were superior to methadone 20 mg/day in this study. A multicenter study compared sublingual doses of 1 mg of buprenorphine with 8 mg of buprenorphine in more than 700 patients. The 8-mg dose was significantly better than the 1-mg dose on outcome measures of opiate-free urine tests and retention in treatment (Ling et al. 1998).

Several other clinical trials have established the effectiveness of buprenorphine in treating heroin addiction. These have included studies comparing buprenorphine with placebo (Johnson et al. 1995; Ling et al. 1998) as well as with methadone (Johnson et al. 1992; Ling et al. 1996; Schottenfeld et al. 1997; Strain et al. 1994a, 1994b). Results from the latter studies suggest that buprenorphine is just as effective as moderate dosages of methadone (e.g., 60 mg/day), although it is not clear whether it can be as effective as higher dosages of methadone (80–100 mg/day) in patients who require such dosages for maintenance therapy.

Johnson et al. (2000) compared buprenorphine (16–32 mg/day), levo-α-acetylmethadol (LAAM; 75–115 mg), and methadone (low [20 mg/day] and high [60–100 mg/day] dosages) in patients with opioid dependence. Buprenorphine, LAAM, and the high-dose methadone arm were all effective in reducing the use of illicit opioids; the low-dose methadone condition was much less effective. The high-dose methadone arm had the best treatment retention rate of all conditions.

Both detoxification and maintenance studies have shown that the abrupt discontinuation of buprenorphine in a blind fashion causes only very minor elevations in withdrawal scores on any withdrawal scale (Bickel et al. 1988; Fudala et al. 1990; Jasinski et al. 1978; Johnson et al. 1989; Kosten and Kleber 1988).

Because the issue of take-home medication is likely to arise in any opiate maintenance program and because methadone take-home medication is likely to be diverted, the option of alternate-day buprenorphine dosing has been explored. After 19 heroin-dependent patients were stabilized on buprenorphine 8 mg/day for 2 weeks, 9 patients continued to receive buprenorphine daily while the other 10 patients, in a blind fashion, received alternate-day buprenorphine doses (8 mg/dose) for 4 weeks. Patients reported some dysphoria on days on which they received placebos, and it was also noted that pupils were less constricted on placebo days in the patients on alternate-day therapy, but patients tolerated the 48-hour dosing interval without significant signs or symptoms of opiate withdrawal abstinence (Fudala et al. 1990). This leaves open the possibility of alternate-day medication in the treatment setting, much like dosing regimens with LAAM, eliminating the need for take-home medication; however, unlike LAAM, buprenorphine can be administered on a daily basis until the patient "earns" days away from the clinic. The main concern with buprenorphine take-home medication is the potential for diversion of the sublingual tablets, particularly diversion to the injection route.

In order to decrease the abuse liability of sublingual buprenorphine products by the injection route, adding naloxone to the sublingual formulation of buprenorphine was proposed. Mendelson et al. (1999) showed that buprenorphine-to-naloxone combination ratios of 2:1 and 4:1 might be useful in treating opiate dependence by causing significant opiate withdrawal symptoms when administered by the intravenous route. A multicenter clinical trial compared the efficacy of a sublingual tablet of combination buprenorphine-naloxone (in a 4:1 ratio) with that of placebo and a buprenorphine monotherapy sublingual tablet. Preliminary results showed that both the buprenorphine-naloxone combination and the buprenorphine monotherapy tablets were significantly more effective than placebo in reducing illicit opioid use, reducing opioid craving, and improving global functioning. No difference was noted between the efficacy of the combination and the monotherapy products, and subjects found the combination product to be as acceptable as the monotherapy product (Fudala et al. 1999). Since 2002, the most common formulation of buprenorphine for the treatment of opioid dependence has been the combination product.

Drug Addiction Treatment Act of 2000

The Drug Addiction Treatment Act of 2000 (DATA 2000) allowed for the use of opioid medications in the office-based treatment of opioid dependence, provided that both the medication and the physician meet the criteria set forth by the law. The medication must be approved by the FDA for the treatment of opioid dependence and be scheduled in C-III, C-IV, or C-V; medications in Schedule C-II are not included in the act. The physician must be a "qualified" physician and have a "unique identifier" added to his or her U.S. Drug Enforcement Administration license to prescribe medications under DATA 2000. Qualifying physicians under this law, however, will be able to more effectively treat opioid dependence in their offices, without referring patients to opioid treatment clinics. The only medications approved by the FDA that may meet the requirements of DATA 2000 are sublingual buprenorphine and buprenorphine-naloxone combinations.

Relapse Prevention: Naltrexone

As was noted earlier in this chapter, various methods of detoxifying patients from opioids have been developed, from substitution and rapidly tapering the dose of opioid to long-term methadone maintenance and a very gradual methadone taper. These methodologies are, by and large, unsuccessful in achieving permanent opioid abstinence in patients. It has long been thought that both conditioned reactivity to drug-associated cues (Wikler 1973) and protracted withdrawal symptoms (Martin and Jasinski 1969) contribute to the high rate of opioid relapse. The use of a blocking dose of a pure opioid antagonist would allow the patient to extinguish the conditioned responses to opioids by blocking the positive reinforcing effects of the illicit drugs. Naltrexone was shown to be orally effective in blocking the subjective effects of morphine for up to 24 hours (Martin et al. 1973). Patients using naltrexone maintenance for relapse prevention need to be carefully screened because they must be opioid free at the start of naltrexone administration. Many practitioners administer a naloxone challenge, which must be negative, before starting naltrexone. Naltrexone usually is administered either daily (50 mg) or three times weekly (100 mg, 100 mg, and 150 mg). Although naltrexone is pharmacologically able to block the reinforcing effects of opioids, the patient must take the medication in order for it to be effective. Many opioid-addicted patients have very little motivation to remain abstinent. Fram et al. (1989) reported that of 300 inner-city patients offered naltrexone, only 15 (5%) agreed to take the medication, and 2 months later, only 3 patients were still taking naltrexone. However, patients with better-identified motivation—among them groups of recovering professionals (e.g., physicians, attorneys) and federal probationers, who face loss of license to practice a profession or legal consequences—have significantly better success with naltrexone.

A major advance occurred in 2010 with the approval of a slow-release depot formulation of naltrexone for the prevention of relapse to opioid addiction. One injection provides coverage for 30–40 days against the effects of usual doses of heroin or other opioids. Very high doses of opioids can eventually override this competitive blockade, but usual doses produce no effect. Thus, the patient is able to function in the community without opioid effects, often the first such experience in years. Early reports suggest that this treatment option represents a major improvement over oral naltrexone and is a realistic alternative to agonist maintenance for patients motivated to become drug free.

Summary of Treatments for Opioid Dependence

A variety of well-developed and well-studied treatments for opiate-dependent patients are available; these include detoxification from opioids; maintenance therapy; and effective, if not well-accepted, relapse prevention pharmacotherapies. However, even though opioid dependence is probably the most widely studied area of drug abuse, we can "cure" only a small percentage of patients seeking help. We must be content with assisting the rest of this patient population to improve their lives and the lives of their families while they continue to deal with the effects of ongoing opioid dependence.

References

Ait-Daoud N, Malcolm RJ, Johnson BA: An overview of medications for the treatment of alcohol withdrawal and alcohol dependence with an emphasis on the use of older and newer anticonvulsants. Addict Behav 31:1628–1649, 2006

American Psychiatric Association: Diagnostic and Statistical Manual of Mental Disorders, 4th Edition, Text Revision. Washington, DC, American Psychiatric Association, 2000

Anton RF, Pettinati H, Zweben A, et al: A multisite dose ranging study of nalmefene in the treatment of alcohol dependence. J Clin Psychopharmacol 24:421–428, 2004

Anton RF, Oroszi G, O'Malley S, et al: An evaluation of mu-opioid receptor (OPRM1) as a predictor of naltrexone response in the treatment of alcohol dependence: results from the Combined Pharmacotherapies and Behavioral Interventions for Alcohol Dependence (COMBINE) study. Arch Gen Psychiatry 65:135–144, 2008

Aubin HJ: Tolerability and safety of sustained-release bupropion in the management of smoking cessation. Drugs 62 (suppl 2):45–52, 2002

Bickel WE, Stitzer ML, Bigelow GE, et al: A clinical trial of buprenorphine: comparison with methadone in the detoxification of heroin addicts. Clin Pharmacol Ther 43:72–78, 1988

Center for Substance Abuse Treatment: Emerging issues in the use of methadone (HHS Publ No. SMA 09-4368). Substance Abuse Treatment Advisory 8(1), 2009. Available at: http://kap.samhsa.gov/products/manuals/advisory/pdfs/Methadone-Advisory.pdf. Accessed September 2012.

Collins ED, Kleber HD, Whittington RA, et al: Anesthesia-assisted vs buprenorphine- or clonidine-assisted heroin detoxification and naltrexone induction: a randomized trial. JAMA 294:903–913, 2005

Covey LS, Glassman AH, Stetner F: Depression and depressive symptoms in smoking cessation. Compr Psychiatry 31:350–354, 1990

Covey LS, Sullivan MA, Johnston J, et al: Advances in non-nicotine pharmacotherapy for smoking cessation. Drugs 59:17–31, 2000

Cowan A, Lewis JW, Macfarlane IR: Agonist and antagonist properties of buprenorphine, a new antinociceptive agent. Br J Pharmacol 60:537–545, 1977

Dalack GW, Healy DJ, Meador-Woodruff JH: Nicotine dependence in schizophrenia: clinical phenomena and laboratory findings. Am J Psychiatry 155:1490–1501, 1998

Dani JA, Harris RA: Nicotine addiction and comorbidity with alcohol abuse and mental illness. Nat Neurosci 8:1465–1470, 2005

Dole VP, Nyswander M: A medical treatment for diacetylmorphine (heroin) addiction: a clinical trial with methadone hydrochloride. JAMA 193:646–650, 1965

Ehret GB, Voide C, Gex-Fabry M, et al: Drug-induced long QT syndrome in injection drug users receiving methadone: high frequency in hospitalized patients and risk factors. Arch Intern Med 166:1280–1287, 2006

Evins AE, Cather C, Deckersbach T, et al: A double-blind placebo-controlled trial of bupropion sustained-release for smoking cessation in schizophrenia. J Clin Psychopharmacol 25:218–225, 2005

Eyer F, Schuster T, Felgenhauer N, et al: Risk assessment of moderate to severe alcohol withdrawal: predictors for seizures and delirium tremens in the course of withdrawal. Alcohol Alcohol 46:427–433, 2011

Finnegan LP: Treatment issues for opioid-dependent women during the perinatal period. J Psychoactive Drugs 23:191–201, 1991

Finnegan LP, Kandall SR: Maternal and neonatal effects of alcohol and drugs, in Substance Abuse: A Comprehensive Textbook. Edited by Lowinson JH, Ruiz P, Millman RB, et al. Baltimore, MD, Williams & Wilkins, 1992, pp 628–656

Fiore MC, Jaen CR, Baker TB: Treating Tobacco Use and Dependence: 2008 Update. Clinical Practice Guideline. In: Services USDoHaH, editor. Rockville, MD, U.S. Public Health Service, 2008, pp 106–116

Fram DH, Marmo J, Holden R: Naltrexone treatment—the problem of patient acceptance. J Subst Abuse Treat 6:119–122, 1989

Fudala PJ, Jaffe JH, Dax EM, et al: Use of buprenorphine in the treatment of opiate addiction, II: physiologic and behavioral effects of daily and alternate-day administration and abrupt withdrawal. Clin Pharmacol Ther 47:525–534, 1990

Fudala PJ, Bridge TP, Herbert S, et al: A multi-site efficacy evaluation of a buprenorphine/naloxone product for opiate dependence treatment. NIDA Res Monogr 179:105, 1999

Fuller RK, Branchey L, Brightwell DR, et al: Disulfiram treatment of alcoholism: a Veterans Administration cooperative study. JAMA 256:1449–1455, 1986

Garbutt JC, Kranzler HR, O'Malley SS, et al: Efficacy and tolerability of long-acting injectable naltrexone for alcohol dependence: a randomized controlled trial. JAMA 293:1617–1625, 2005

George TP, Vessicchio JC, Termine A, et al: A placebo controlled trial of bupropion for smoking cessation in schizophrenia. Biol Psychiatry 52:53–61, 2002

Gerstein DR: The effectiveness of drug treatment, in Addictive States, Vol 70. Edited by O'Brien CP, Jaffe JH. New York, Raven, 1992, pp 253–282

Gianoulakis C, de Waele JP, Thavundayil J: Implication of the endogenous opioid system in excessive ethanol consumption. Alcohol 13:19–23, 1996

Glassman AH: Cigarette smoking: implications for psychiatric illness. Am J Psychiatry 150:546–553, 1993

Glassman AH, Stetner F, Walsh Raizman PS, et al: Heavy smokers, smoking cessation, and clonidine: results of a double-blind, randomized trial. JAMA 259:2863–2866, 1988

Glover ED, Sachs DPL, Stitzer ML: Smoking cessation in highly dependent smokers with 4 mg nicotine polacrilex. American Journal of Health and Behavior 20:319–332, 1996

Goff DC, Henderson DC, Amico E: Cigarette smoking in schizophrenia: relationship to psychopathology and medication side effects. Am J Psychiatry 149:1189–1194, 1992

Gold MS, Redmond DE, Kleber HD: Clonidine blocks acute opiate withdrawal symptoms. Lancet 2(8090):599–602, 1978

Gold MS, Pottach AC, Sweeney DR, et al: Opiate withdrawal using clonidine. JAMA 243:343–346, 1980

Gonzales D, Rennard SI, Nides M, et al: Varenicline, an alpha4beta2 nicotinic acetylcholine receptor partial agonist, vs sustained-release bupropion and placebo for smoking cessation: a randomized controlled trial. JAMA 296:47–55, 2006

Gross J, Stitzer ML: Nicotine replacement: ten-week effects on tobacco withdrawal symptoms. Psychopharmacology 93:334–341, 1989

Hall SM, Killen JD: Psychological and pharmacological approaches to smoking relapse prevention. NIDA Research Monograph 53:131–143, 1985

Hall SM, Tunstall C, Rugg D, et al: Nicotine gum and behavioral treatment in smoking cessation. J Consult Clin Psychol 53:256–258, 1985

Hasin DS, Stinson FS, Ogburn E, et al: Prevalence, correlates, disability, and comorbidity of DSM-IV alcohol abuse and dependence in the United States: results from the National Epidemiologic Survey on Alcohol and Related Conditions. Arch Gen Psychiatry 64:830–842, 2007

Hays JT, Hurt RD, Rigotti NA, et al: Sustained-release bupropion for pharmacologic relapse prevention after smoking cessation. a randomized, controlled trial. Ann Intern Med 135:423–433, 2001

Henningfield JE, Fant RV, Buchhalter AR, et al: Pharmacotherapy for nicotine dependence. CA Cancer J Clin 55:281–299, 2005

Hughes JR: Depression during tobacco abstinence. Nicotine Tob Res 9:443–446, 2007

Hughes JR, Hatsukami D: Signs and symptoms of tobacco withdrawal. Arch Gen Psychiatry 43:289–294, 1986

Hughes J, Stead L, Lancaster T: Antidepressants for smoking cessation. Cochrane Database Syst Rev (4):CD000031, 2004

Jaffe JH, Kranzler M: Smoking as a addictive disorder. NIDA Research Monograph 23:4–43, 1979

Jasinski DR, Pevnick JS, Griffith JD: Human pharmacology and abuse potential of the analgesic buprenorphine. Arch Gen Psychiatry 35:501–516, 1978

Jasinski DR, Fudala PJ, Johnson RE: Sublingual versus subcutaneous buprenorphine in opiate abusers. Clin Pharmacol Ther 45:513–519, 1989

Johnson BA, Ait-Daoud N, Akhtar FZ, et al: Oral topiramate reduces the consequences of drinking and improves the quality of life of alcohol-dependent individuals: a randomized controlled trial. Arch Gen Psychiatry 61:905–912, 2004

Johnson RE, Cone EJ, Henningfield JE, et al: Use of buprenorphine in the treatment of opiate addiction, I: physiologic and behavioral effects during a rapid dose induction. Clin Pharmacol Ther 46:335–343, 1989

Johnson RE, Jaffe JH, Fudala PJ: A controlled trial of buprenorphine treatment for opioid dependence. JAMA 267:2750–2755, 1992

Johnson RE, Eissenberg T, Stitzer ML, et al: A placebo controlled clinical trial of buprenorphine as a treatment for opioid dependence. Drug Alcohol Depend 40:17–25, 1995

Johnson RE, Chutuape MA, Strain EC, et al: A comparison of levomethadyl acetate, buprenorphine, and methadone for opioid dependence. N Engl J Med 343:1290–1297, 2000

Jorenby DE, Hays JT, Rigotti NA, et al: Efficacy of varenicline, an alpha4beta2 nicotinic acetylcholine receptor partial agonist, vs placebo or sustained-release bupropion for smoking cessation: a randomized controlled trial. JAMA 296:56–63, 2006

Kakko J, Svanborg KD, Kreek MJ, et al: 1-year retention and social function after buprenorphine-assisted relapse prevention treatment for heroin dependence in Sweden: a randomised, placebo-controlled trial. Lancet 361:662–668, 2003

Kampman KM, Pettinati H, Lynch KG, et al: A pilot trial of topiramate for the treatment of cocaine dependence. Drug Alcohol Depend 75:233–240, 2004

Killen JD, Maccoby N, Taylor CB: Nicotine gum and self-regulation training in smoking relapse prevention. Behav Res Ther 15:234–248, 1984

Kosten TR, Kleber HD: Buprenorphine detoxification from opioid dependence: a pilot study. Life Sci 42:635–641, 1988

Krantz MJ, Lewkowiez L, Hays H, et al: Torsade de pointes associated with very-high-dose methadone. Ann Intern Med 137:501–504, 2002

Kranzler HR, Babor TF, Lauerman RJ: Problems associated with average alcohol consumption and frequency of intoxication in a medical population. Alcohol Clin Exp Res 14:119–126, 1990

Leventhal H, Cleary P: The smoking problem: a review of the research and theory in behavioral risk modification. Psychol Bull 88:370–405, 1980

Ling W, Wesson D, Charuvastra C, et al: A controlled trial comparing buprenorphine and methadone maintenance in opioid dependence. Arch Gen Psychiatry 53:401–407, 1996

Ling W, Charuvastra C, Collins JF, et al: Buprenorphine maintenance treatment of opiate dependence: a multicenter, randomized clinical trial. Addiction 93:475–486, 1998

Loimer N, Schmid R, Lenz K, et al: Acute blocking of naloxone-precipitated opiate withdrawal symptoms by methohexitone. Br J Psychiatry 157:748–752, 1990

Loimer N, Lenz K, Schmid R, et al: Technique for greatly shortening the transition from methadone to naltrexone maintenance of patients addicted to opiates. Am J Psychiatry 148:933–935, 1991

Maddux JF, Desmond DP: Methadone maintenance and recovery from opioid dependence. Am J Drug Alcohol Abuse 18:63–74, 1992

Mann K, Bladstrom A, Torup L, et al: Shifting the paradigm: reduction of alcohol consumption in alcoholic dependent patients. A randomized, double-blind placebo-controlled study of nalmefene as-needed use. Poster presentation (no. 710) at the 20th European Congress of Psychiatry, Prague, Czech Republic, March 3–6, 2012

Martin WR, Jasinski DR: Physical parameters of morphine dependence in man: tolerance, early abstinence, protracted abstinence. J Psychiatry Res 7:9–17, 1969

Martin WR, Jasinski D, Mansky P: Naltrexone, an antagonist for the treatment of heroin dependence. Arch Gen Psychiatry 28:784–791, 1973

Mason BJ, Salvato FR, Williams LD, et al: A double-blind, placebo-controlled study of oral nalmefene for alcohol dependence. Arch Gen Psychiatry 56:719–724, 1999

McCaul ME, Petry NM: The role of psychosocial treatments in pharmacotherapy for alcoholism. Am J Addict 12 (suppl 1):S41–S52, 2003

McLellan AT, Arndt IO, Metzger DS, et al: The effects of psychosocial services on substance abuse treatment. JAMA 269:1953–1959, 1993

Mendelson J, Jones RT, Welm S, et al: Buprenorphine and naloxone combinations: the effects of three dose ratios in morphine-stabilized, opiate-dependent volunteers. Psychopharmacology 141:37–46, 1999

Ntais C, Pakos E, Kyzas P, et al: Benzodiazepines for alcohol withdrawal. Cochrane Database Syst Rev (3):CD005063, 2005

Peachy JE, Naranjo CA: The role of drugs in the treatment of alcoholism. Drugs 27:171–182, 1984

Pettinati HM, O'Brien CP, Rabinowitz AR, et al: The status of naltrexone in the treatment of alcohol dependence: specific effects on heavy drinking. J Clin Psychopharmacol 26:610–625, 2006

Piper ME, Smith SS, Schlam TR, et al: A randomized placebo-controlled clinical trial of 5 smoking cessation pharmacotherapies. Arch Gen Psychiatry 66:1253–1262, 2009

Ray LA, Hutchison KE: Effects of naltrexone on alcohol sensitivity and genetic moderators of medication response: a double-blind placebo-controlled study. Arch Gen Psychiatry 64:1069–1077, 2007

Regier DA, Myers JK, Kramer M, et al: The NIMH Epidemiologic Catchment Area Program: historical context, major objectives, and study population characteristics. Arch Gen Psychiatry 41:934–941, 1984

Rohsenow DJ, Tidey JW, Miranda R, et al: Olanzapine reduces urge to smoke and nicotine withdrawal symptoms in community smokers. Exp Clin Psychopharmacol 16:215–222, 2008

Sachs DP: Effectiveness of the 4-mg dose of nicotine polacrilex for the initial treatment of high-dependent smokers. Arch Intern Med 155:1973–1980, 1995

Schottenfeld RS, Pakes JR, Oliveto A, et al: Buprenorphine versus methadone maintenance for concurrent opioid dependence and cocaine abuse. Arch Gen Psychiatry 54:713–720, 1997

Schuckit MA: Alcohol and alcoholism, in Harrison's Principles of Internal Medicine. Edited by Wilson JD, Braunwald E, Isselbacher KJ, et al. New York, McGraw-Hill, 1991, pp 2149–2151

Shah SD, Wilken LA, Winkler SR, et al: Systematic review and meta-analysis of combination therapy for smoking cessation. J Am Pharm Assoc (2003) 48:659–665, 2008

Stead LF, Bergson G, Lancaster T: Physician advice for smoking cessation. Cochrane Database Syst Rev (2):CD000165, 2008

Stine SM, Kosten TR: Use of drug combinations in treatment of opioid withdrawal. J Clin Psychopharmacol 12:203–209, 1992

Strain EC, Stitzer ML, Liebson IA, et al: Buprenorphine versus methadone in the treatment of opioid-dependent cocaine users. Psychopharmacology 116:401–406, 1994a

Strain EC, Stitzer ML, Liebson IA, et al: Comparison of buprenorphine versus methadone in the treatment of opioid dependence. Am J Psychiatry 151:1025–1030, 1994b

Substance Abuse and Mental Health Services Administration: Results From the 2009 National Survey on Drug Use and Health, Vol I: Summary of National Findings (Office of Applied Studies, NSDUH Series H-38A, HHS Publication No. SMA 10-4586). Rockville, MD, Substance Abuse and Mental Health Services Administration, 2010

Tobacco Use and Dependence Practice Guideline Panel: A clinical practice guideline for treating tobacco use and dependence: a US Public Health Service report. JAMA 283:3244–3254, 2000

Tobacco Use and Dependence Guideline Panel: Treating Tobacco Use and Dependence: 2008 Update. Guideline Update Development and Use. Rockville, MD, U.S. Department of Health and Human Services, May 2008. Available at: http://www.ncbi.nlm.nih.gov/books/NBK63947. Accessed September 2012.

Tønnesen P, Paoletti P, Gustavsson G, et al: Higher dosage nicotine patches increase one-year smoking cessation rates: results from the European CEASE trial. Collaborative European Anti-Smoking Evaluation. European Respiratory Society. Eur Respir J 13:238–246, 1999

U.S. Food and Drug Administration: The smoking cessation aids varenicline (marketed as Chantix) and bupropion (marketed as Zyban and generics): suicidal ideation and behavior. FDA Drug Safety Newsletter 2(1):1–4, 2009. Available at: http://www.fda.gov/downloads/Drugs/DrugSafety/DrugSafetyNewsletter/UCM107318.pdf. Accessed September 2012.

Volpicelli JR, Davis MA, Olgin JE: Naltrexone blocks the post-shock increase of ethanol consumption. Life Sci 38:841–847, 1986

Weiss RD, Kueppenbender KD: Combining psychosocial treatment with pharmacotherapy for alcohol dependence. J Clin Psychopharmacol 26 (suppl 1):S37–S42, 2006

Wikler A: Dynamics of drug dependence. Arch Gen Psychiatry 28:611–616, 1973

CHAPTER 40

Treatment of Child and Adolescent Disorders

Karen Dineen Wagner, M.D., Ph.D.

Steven R. Pliszka, M.D.

This chapter focuses on the psychopharmacology of psychiatric disorders in children and adolescents. However, nonpharmacological treatment interventions are also an important component of a child's psychiatric care. Individual psychotherapy, group therapy, and family therapy may improve clinical outcome. Working closely with school personnel is another ingredient in the treatment of a child with a psychiatric disorder. Case management for the child and support for the family are other facets of treatment for children.

It is important for clinicians to be aware of the evidence base for the use of psychotropic medications for children and adolescents. In this chapter, data from the literature, with a focus on controlled studies, are presented. On the basis of these findings, clinical recommendations regarding pharmacotherapy for childhood psychiatric disorders are offered. The Appendix and tables contain specific information about dosages, monitoring, and adverse effects of psychotropics in children.

Psychotropic Medication for Children and Adolescents

Evaluation

Prior to the initiation of psychotropic medication for children and adolescents, it is essential to conduct a comprehensive evaluation to ensure the accuracy of the diagnosis. A thorough history and careful attention to the clinical presentation are central components

---

Portions of the Attention-Deficit/Hyperactivity Disorder section of this chapter were adapted from Wagner KD: "Management of Treatment Refractory Attention-Deficit/Hyperactivity Disorder in Children and Adolescents." *Psychopharmacology Bulletin* 36:130–142, 2002. Used with permission.

of the evaluation. The clinician should interview the child and parents separately so that both may have the opportunity to freely express their concerns. Extended family members, school personnel, and school records are other potential sources of information.

Clinicians must be skilled at differential diagnosis of childhood disorders, given that there is a significant overlap of symptoms among these disorders. Knowledge of commonly occurring comorbid disorders is also necessary. Medical conditions should be considered within the differential diagnosis and adequately assessed.

Disorder-specific rating scales at baseline and during the course of treatment may be useful in assisting with the measurement of clinical outcome.

Clinical Issues Affecting Response to Pharmacotherapy

Whenever a child fails to respond to initial pharmacotherapy, several clinical issues should be addressed before initiating alternative or adjunctive medication.

Diagnostic Accuracy

The diagnosis should be reassessed. Often there is symptomatic overlap among disorders that may lead to misdiagnosis. For example, symptoms of excessive energy and distractibility are common features of both attention-deficit/hyperactivity disorder (ADHD) and bipolar disorder.

Comorbid Disorders

Unrecognized comorbid disorders may adversely affect treatment outcome. As an example, comorbid ADHD may lower response rates in the treatment of bipolar disorder (Pavuluri et al. 2006).

Psychosocial Factors

Child abuse, domestic violence, family conflict, parental psychopathology, and bullying by peers may lead to symptoms that mimic or exacerbate a preexisting psychiatric disorder.

Medication Compliance

Some children and adolescents are reluctant to take medication because of such reasons as denial of illness, perceived stigma, and side effects. To increase medication compliance, it is essential that the child or adolescent, as well as the parents, understand the youth's disorder, course of illness, and goals of treatment. It is important for parents to participate in monitoring their child's medication compliance.

Nonpharmacological Treatment

Psychotherapy may be a component of treatment, either alone or in conjunction with medication. Specific psychotherapies have been found to be effective in the treatment of some childhood disorders. For example, cognitive-behavioral therapy (CBT) (Brent et al. 1997) and interpersonal therapy (Mufson and Sills 2006) have demonstrated efficacy in the treatment of adolescents with depression. Similarly, CBT is commonly used for the treatment of childhood anxiety disorders (Roblek and Piacentini 2005). Behavior therapy has led to improvement in symptoms of ADHD for children (Pelham et al. 1998). Adjunctive psychoeducation to medication treatment has shown benefit in the treatment of children with bipolar disorder (Fristad et al. 2003). Social skills training can be a useful component of treatment in autism spectrum disorders (Krasny et al. 2003).

Informed Consent

Informed consent is necessary prior to prescribing psychotropic medication to any patient, but it is particularly important in pediatric psychopharmacology because there are few U.S. Food and Drug Administration (FDA)–approved medications. There are five recommended components of informed consent for prescribing psychotropic medications to children and adolescents (Popper 1987). The child's parent(s) and the child/adolescent should be provided with the following information:

1. The purpose (benefits) of the treatment
2. A description of the treatment process
3. An explanation of the risks of the treatment, including risks that would ordinarily be described by the psychiatrist and risks that would be relevant to making the decision
4. A statement of the alternative treatments, including nontreatment
5. A statement that there may be unknown risks of these medications (This is particularly essential for children, because there is a paucity of information on the potential long-term effects of psychotropic medications.)

Evidence Base

It is important for clinicians to be aware of the evidence base for medication treatment of each childhood psychiatric disorder. Clinical treatment guidelines generally rely on the strength of the available data in determining first-line agents (Hughes et al. 2007; Kowatch et al. 2005). In most cases, clinicians should select a medication within the group of first-line agents when initiating medication treatment with a child. Additional factors that will dictate medication choice are prior medication history, medical history, side-effect profile of the drug, and adolescent and parent preferences.

Major Depressive Disorder

The prevalence of major depression in children and adolescents is estimated to range from 1.8% to 4.6% (Kashani and Sherman 1988; Kroes et al. 2001). DSM-IV-TR (American Psychiatric Association 2000) criteria are used to establish a diagnosis of major depression in children and adolescents. The mean length of an episode of major depression in youth ranges from 8 to 13 months, and relapse rates range from 30% to 70% (Birmaher et al. 2002). There is increasing evidence for the continuity of depression from youth into adulthood (Dunn and Goodyer 2006).

Selective Serotonin Reuptake Inhibitors

Two selective serotonin reuptake inhibitor (SSRI) medications have FDA approval for the acute and maintenance treatment of major depression in children and adolescents: fluoxetine (≥8 years old) and escitalopram (≥12 years old).

Fluoxetine

There have been three positive controlled medication trials of fluoxetine in the treatment of major depression in children and adolescents.

In the first study of fluoxetine, 96 child and adolescent outpatients (ages 8–17 years) with major depression were randomly assigned to fluoxetine (20 mg/day) or placebo for an 8-week trial (Emslie et al. 1997). The fluoxetine group, with 27 youths (56%) much or very much improved, showed statistically significant greater improvement in Clinical Global Impression (CGI) Scale scores than did the placebo group, with 16 youths (33%) much or very much improved. Medication side effects leading to discontinuation in the study were manic symptoms in 3 patients and severe rash in 1 patient.

In a double-blind, placebo-controlled multicenter study of fluoxetine, 219 child and adolescent outpatients (ages 8–17 years) with major depression were randomly assigned to fluoxetine (20 mg/day) or placebo for an 8-week trial (Emslie et al. 2002). The fluoxetine group showed statistically significant greater improvement in depression, as assessed by Children's Depression Rating Scale—Revised (CDRS-R) scores, than did the placebo group. Fifty-two percent of patients treated with fluoxetine were rated as much or very much improved, compared with 37% of patients treated with placebo. Headache was the only side effect that was reported more frequently in the group treated with fluoxetine than in the group treated with placebo.

Fluoxetine alone, fluoxetine with CBT, CBT alone, and placebo were compared in a multicenter trial of 439 adolescent outpatients with a diagnosis of major depression (Treatment for Adolescents with Depression Study [TADS] Team 2004). Patients were randomly assigned to 12 weeks of fluoxetine (10–40 mg/day), fluoxetine (10–40 mg/day) with CBT, CBT alone, or placebo. Compared with placebo, the combination of fluoxetine with CBT was significantly superior on CDRS-R scores. Combination treatment with fluoxetine and CBT was significantly superior to fluoxetine alone and CBT alone. Fluoxetine monotherapy was superior to CBT. Based on CGI scores of much or very much improved, the response rates were 71% for fluoxetine-CBT combination therapy, 61% for fluoxetine, 43% for CBT, and 35% for placebo.

Citalopram

There have been two controlled trials of citalopram in the treatment of depression in youth, one with positive and one with negative results.

The efficacy of citalopram was demonstrated in a double-blind, placebo-controlled multicenter trial of 174 outpatient children and adolescents (ages 7–17 years) with major depression (Wagner et al. 2004b). Patients were randomly assigned to citalopram (dosage range = 20–40 mg/day; mean daily dose = 23 mg for children, 24 mg for adolescents) or placebo for an 8-week trial. The group treated with citalopram showed statistically significant greater improvement in depression (CDRS-R scores) than did the placebo group. The most frequent adverse events were headache, nausea, rhinitis, abdominal pain, and influenza-like symptoms. A European double-blind, placebo-controlled multicenter study (Knorring et al. 2006) of citalopram in 224 adolescents with major depression failed to show superiority of citalopram to placebo on the primary efficacy measures of Schedule for Affective Disorders and Schizophrenia for School-Aged Children—Present Episode Version (Kiddie-SADS-P; Chambers et al. 1985) and the Montgomery-Åsberg Depression Rating Scale (MADRS; Montgomery and Åsberg 1979). The most commonly reported adverse events were headache, nausea, and vomiting.

Paroxetine

There have been three double-blind, placebo-controlled trials of paroxetine for treatment of depression in children and adolescents, all of which had negative findings on the primary outcome measure.

In a study of 275 adolescent outpatients (ages 12–18 years) with major depression, patients were randomly assigned to paroxetine (dosage range = 20–40 mg/day; mean daily dose = 28 mg), imipramine (dosage range = 200–300 mg; mean daily dose = 205 mg/day), or placebo for an 8-week trial (Keller et al. 2001). There was no statistically significant difference among the treatment groups on the primary efficacy measure of reduction in the Hamilton Rating Scale for Depression (Ham-D; Hamilton 1960) total score. The most common side effects reported for paroxetine were headache, nausea, dizziness, dry mouth, and somnolence.

Two hundred six children and adolescents (ages 7–17 years) with major depression were included in an 8-week double-blind, placebo-controlled, randomized multicenter study of paroxetine treatment (Emslie et al. 2006). There was no statistically significant difference between paroxetine-treated patients and placebo-treated patients on change from baseline in CDRS-R total score at endpoint. Adverse events reported for paroxetine with an incidence of >5% and at least twice that of placebo were dizziness, cough, dyspepsia, and vomiting.

A 12-week international placebo-controlled multicenter trial of paroxetine in 286 adolescents with major depression failed to show superiority for paroxetine compared with placebo on change from baseline in MADRS or Schedule for Affective Disorders and Schizophrenia for School-Aged Children—Lifetime Version (Kiddie-SADS-L; Kaufman et al. 1997) total scores (Berard et al. 2006).

Sertraline

The efficacy of sertraline was assessed in two identical double-blind, placebo-controlled multicenter studies in 376 outpatient children and adolescents with major depression (Wagner et al. 2003a). Patients were randomly assigned to sertraline (dosage range = 50–200 mg/day; mean daily dose = 131 mg) or placebo for a 10-week trial. The group receiving sertraline showed a statistically significant greater improvement in depression (CDRS-R scores) than did the placebo group. Response rates (decrease >40% in baseline CDRS-R scores) were 69% in the group treated with sertraline and 59% in the group treated with placebo. The most common side effects in the group treated with sertraline were headache, nausea, insomnia, upper respiratory tract infection, abdominal pain, and diarrhea.

Sertraline, CBT, and combined CBT plus medication were compared for the treatment of 73 adolescents with depressive disorders (Melvin et al. 2006). All treatments showed statistically significant improvement on all outcome measures; there were no significant advantages of combined treatment.

In the Adolescent Depression and Psychotherapy Trial (ADAPT; Goodyer et al. 2008), 208 adolescents with major depression were randomly assigned to receive an SSRI alone or an SSRI plus CBT for 12 weeks. No significant differences were found between the groups; 44% of the SSRI-alone group and 42% of the SSRI-plus-CBT group were much or very much improved on the CGI-I.

Escitalopram

There have been two controlled trials of escitalopram in the treatment of youth with depression, one positive and one negative.

The efficacy of escitalopram in adolescents was demonstrated in a double-blind, placebo-controlled multicenter trial of 157 adolescents with major depression (Emslie et al. 2009). Patients were randomly assigned to escitalopram (dosage range 10–20 mg/day) or placebo for an 8-week trial. The group treated with escitalopram showed statistically significant greater improvement in depression (CDRS-R scores) than did the placebo group. Sixty-four percent of escitalopram-treated patients were much or very much improved, compared with 53% of placebo-treated patients. In a study that included 264 children and adolescents with major depression (Wagner et al. 2006a), there was no significant improvement on CDRS-R scores at endpoint between escitalopram and placebo. The most common adverse events with escitalopram were headache, abdominal pain, nausea, insomnia, and menstrual cramps.

Other Antidepressants

Venlafaxine

Two double-blind, placebo-controlled multicenter studies have evaluated the efficacy of venlafaxine extended-release in the treatment of major depression in 165 and 169 child and adolescent outpatients, respectively (Emslie et al. 2007a, 2007b). Patients were randomly assigned to venlafaxine extended-release (37.5–225 mg/day) for 8-week trials. Both studies were negative on the primary outcome measure of change from baseline to endpoint in the CDRS-R scores. The most common adverse events were anorexia and abdominal pain (Emslie et al. 2007a).

Nefazodone

There have been two double-blind, placebo-controlled multicenter trials of nefazodone in the treatment of major depression in youth (Rynn et al. 2002; U.S. Food and Drug Administration 2004b). These studies failed to find statistically significant improvement in baseline-to-endpoint CDRS-R scores between the nefazodone-treated group and the placebo-treated group. The most common adverse events with nefazodone were headache, abdominal pain, nausea, vomiting, somnolence, and dizziness.

Bupropion

There are no controlled trials of bupropion for the treatment of pediatric depression.

In an 8-week study of bupropion sustained release (dosage range=100–400 mg/day; mean daily dose=362 mg) for treating 11 adolescents with major depression, 8 adolescents (79%) showed a 50% reduction in depression scores from baseline (Glod et al. 2000). Bupropion sustained release was assessed in an 8-week open study for the treatment of comorbid depression and ADHD in 24 adolescents (Daviss et al. 2001). Global improvement was reported in 14 subjects (58%) for both depression and ADHD and in 7 subjects (29%) for depression only. Common side effects were headache, nausea, rash, and irritability.

Mirtazapine

There have been two double-blind, placebo-controlled multicenter trials of mirtazapine in the treatment of child and adolescent outpatients with major depression. In these studies, mirtazapine was not superior to placebo on the primary efficacy measure of change from baseline to endpoint in CDRS-R scores (U.S. Food and Drug Administration 2004b).

Duloxetine

There are no controlled trials of duloxetine in the treatment of children and adolescents with major depression. In an open-label study of 72 pediatric patients with major depression, 76% of patients needed dosages of 60–120 mg/day for efficacy (Prakash et al. 2012).

Suicidality and Black Box Warning

In a combined analysis of 24 short-term placebo-controlled trials of antidepressant medications in child and adolescent major depressive disorder, obsessive-compulsive disorder (OCD), or other psychiatric disorders, the risk of suicidality (suicidal thinking and behavior) was 4%, twice the placebo rate (2%). There were no suicides in any of the clinical trials. The FDA directed manufacturers to add a black box warning to the health professional label of antidepressant medications to describe the increased risk of suicidal thoughts and behavior in children and adolescents being treated with antidepressant medications and to emphasize the need for close monitoring of patients on the medications (U.S. Food and Drug Administration 2004a). Parents and patients should be advised of the black box warning for an-tidepressant medication.

In a subsequent meta-analysis of 27 trials of antidepressants in pediatric major depression, the rates of suicidal ideation and attempts were 3% in the youth treated with antidepressants and 2% in the youth who received placebo (Bridge et al. 2007). These investigators reported that the number needed to treat was 10, whereas the number needed to harm was 112, and therefore the benefits of antidepressants outweigh the potential risk from suicidal ideation or attempt.

A number of studies, in both the United States and Europe, have failed to demonstrate an association between antidepressant use and youth suicide (Gibbons et al. 2006; Markowitz and Cuellar 2007; Simon et al. 2006; Søndergård et al. 2006). It is noteworthy that there was an increase in the suicide rate in youth following the addition of the black box warning on antidepressants (Hamilton et al. 2007). The FDA advisory has been associated with significant decreases in the rates of diagnosis and treatment in pediatric depression (Libby et al. 2007).

Treatment-Resistant Depression

In the National Institute of Mental Health (NIMH)–funded multisite Treatment of SSRI-Resistant Depression in Adolescents (TORDIA) trial (Brent et al. 2008), 334 adolescents with SSRI-resistant depression were randomly assigned to one of four treatments for 12 weeks: 1) switch to an alternate SSRI, 2) switch to an alternate SSRI plus CBT, 3) switch to venlafaxine, or 4) switch to venlafaxine plus CBT. CBT plus a switch to either medication produced the highest rate of response (54.8%). Response rates (CGI-I score ≤2 and CDRS-R ≥50% reduction) were similar for switching to an alternate SSRI and switching to venlafaxine (47% and 48.2%, respectively). Adverse events of increase in diastolic blood pressure and pulse and skin problems were more frequent in venlafaxine-treated patients than in SSRI-treated patients.

Clinical Recommendations for Major Depressive Disorder

An evidence-based consensus medication algorithm for the treatment of childhood major depression is available (Texas Children's Medication Algorithm Project [TMAP]; Hughes et al. 2007). Based on research evidence and panel discussion, four stages of medication treatment are identified:

- Stage 1: SSRI
- Stage 2: Alternate SSRI
- Stage 2A (if partial response to SSRI): SSRI + lithium, bupropion, or mirtazapine
- Stage 3: Different class of antidepressant medication (venlafaxine, bupropion, mirtazapine, duloxetine)
- Stage 4: Reassessment, treatment guidance

It was further recommended that antidepressants be continued for 6–12 months after symptom remission. At the time of discontinuation of an antidepressant, the dose should be tapered slowly (i.e., no more than 25% per week). The typical tapering and discontinuation period is 2–3 months.

Bipolar Disorder

The prevalence of bipolar disorder in a community sample of adolescents was found to be 1% (Lewinsohn et al. 1995). Although DSM-IV-TR criteria are used to diagnose bipolar disorder in youth, the clinical features in children may differ from those in adolescents and adults. Children with bipolar disorder frequently exhibit mixed mania and rapid cycling (B. Geller et al. 2000). One-year recovery rates of 87% and relapse rates of 64% have been reported in children with bipolar disorder (B. Geller et al. 2004).

Five medications have FDA approval for the acute treatment of bipolar I disorder, mixed or manic episode, in youth: aripiprazole (≥10 years old), risperidone (≥10 years old), quetiapine (≥10 years old), lithium (≥12 years old), and olanzapine (≥13 years old).

Lithium

In an NIMH-funded study, 153 children and adolescents with bipolar I disorder, mixed or manic episode, were randomly assigned to treatment with lithium, divalproex, or placebo in an 8-week trial (Kowatch et al. 2007). Target lithium serum levels were 0.8–1.2 mEq/L. Lithium was not significantly superior to placebo.

There is one small double-blind, placebo-controlled study of lithium treatment for adolescent bipolar disorder and substance dependence (B. Geller et al. 1998). Twenty-five adolescent outpatients were randomly assigned to either lithium (mean serum level = 0.97 mEq/L) or placebo for a 6-week trial. There was significantly greater improvement in global functioning with lithium than with placebo. Side effects in the group treated with lithium were polyuria, thirst, nausea, vomiting, and dizziness.

There have been six controlled studies of lithium in the treatment of bipolar disorder in youths. In four of these double-blind crossover studies, significant improvement was found with lithium, compared with placebo (DeLong and Nieman 1983; Gram and Rafaelsen 1972; Lena 1979; McKnew et al. 1981). However, small sample size, diagnostic issues, and short treatment duration limit these findings.

Anticonvulsants

Divalproex

A 4-week double-blind, placebo-controlled multicenter trial of 150 youths (ages 10–17 years) with bipolar I disorder, mixed or manic episode, failed to show a significant difference in scores on the Young Mania Rating Scale (YMRS) from baseline to endpoint between extended-release divalproex and placebo (Wagner et al. 2009). The mean modal dose of divalproex extended release was 1,286 mg. There were no statistically significant differences in adverse-event incidents between the divalproex extended release and placebo groups. Gastrointestinal symptoms were more commonly reported in divalproex extended release than in placebo groups.

In an NIMH-funded trial comparing divalproex, lithium, and placebo (Kowatch et al. 2007), response rates (≥50% reduction in YMRS) were significantly greater for divalproex (56%) compared with placebo (30%). The target serum level for divalproex was 85–110 μg/L.

Carbamazepine

In a 6-week active-comparator study of lithium, divalproex, and carbamazepine (Kowatch et al. 2000b), carbamazepine had a response rate (defined as ≥50% reduction in YMRS from baseline to endpoint) of 38% (vs. 38% for lithium and 53% for divalproex) and an effect size of 1.00 (vs. 1.6 for lithium and 1.63 for divalproex). The most common side effects of carbamazepine were sedation, nausea, dizziness, and rash.

Oxcarbazepine

There is one double-blind, placebo-controlled multicenter trial of oxcarbazepine for the treatment of children and adolescents with bipolar I disorder, current episode mixed or manic, that failed to show superiority of oxcarbazepine to placebo. One hundred sixteen youths (ages 7–18 years) were randomly assigned to oxcarbazepine (mean dosage = 1,515 mg/day) or placebo for a 7-week trial (Wagner et al. 2006b). There was no significant difference in YMRS scores at endpoint between the oxcarbazepine and placebo groups. The most common side effects in the oxcarbazepine-treated patients were dizziness, nausea, somnolence, diplopia, fatigue, and rash.

Topiramate

A double-blind, randomized, placebo-controlled multicenter study assessing the efficacy of topiramate treatment in children and adolescents with acute mania was designed as a 200-patient study but was terminated after randomization of 56 patients (ages 6–17 years) when adult mania trials failed to show efficacy (DelBello et al. 2005). Dosages were titrated to 400 mg/day (mean dosage = 278 mg/day). Over a 4-week period, no significant difference was found between the topiramate and placebo groups. The most common adverse events in the topiramate group included decreased appetite, nausea, diarrhea, paresthesias, and somnolence.

Lamotrigine

In a 12-week open-label trial, the efficacy of lamotrigine was assessed in 30 children and adolescents with bipolar spectrum disorders (Biederman et al. 2010). The mean endpoint lamotrigine dosage was 160.7 mg/day. Significant improvement in mean YMRS scores was reported; however, only about half of the participants completed the trial, and 7 participants discontinued lamotrigine because of rash.

Atypical Antipsychotics

Olanzapine

There is one reported double-blind, placebo-controlled multicenter study of olanzapine (2.5–20 mg/day) in the treatment of adolescent outpatients with bipolar I disorder, mixed or manic episode (Tohen et al. 2007).

Adolescents were randomly assigned to receive olanzapine (n=107) or placebo (n=54) for 3 weeks. Response rates (defined as ≥50% decrease in YMRS and a CGI-BP mania score ≤3) were significantly greater for the olanzapine group (44.8%) than for the placebo group (18.5%). Remission rates (defined as YMRS <12 and CGI-BP mania score ≤3) were significantly greater for the olanzapine (35.2%) than for the placebo (11.1%) group. Adverse effects in the olanzapine group were hyperprolactinemia, weight gain (mean=3.7 kg), somnolence, and sedation.

Risperidone

In a 3-week double-blind, placebo-controlled trial, the efficacy of risperidone was assessed in 169 children and adolescents with bipolar I disorder, manic or mixed episode (Haas et al. 2009). Both low-dose risperidone (0.5–2.5 mg/day) and high-dose risperidone (3.0–6 mg/day) were significantly superior to placebo in reduction of YMRS scores. The response rate (≥50% reduction in baseline YMRS) was 59% for low-dose risperidone and 63% for high-dose risperidone, compared with a placebo response rate of 26%. The most common adverse events with risperidone were somnolence, headache, and fatigue. Extrapyramidal symptoms were more frequent in the high-dose risperidone group than in the low-dose group.

Quetiapine

In a 3-week double-blind, placebo-controlled trial, the efficacy of quetiapine was assessed in 277 youths with bipolar I disorder, manic or mixed episode (DelBello et al. 2007). Both low-dose quetiapine (400 mg/day) and high-dose quetiapine (600 mg/day) were significantly superior to placebo in reduction of YMRS scores. The response rate (≥50% reduction in baseline YMRS) was 64% for low-dose quetiapine, 58% for high-dose quetiapine, and 37% for placebo. The most common adverse events with quetiapine were somnolence, sedation, dizziness, and headache.

Aripiprazole

The efficacy of aripiprazole was assessed in a 4-week double-blind, placebo-controlled trial that included 296 youths with bipolar I disorder, mixed or manic episode (Findling et al. 2009). Both low-dose aripiprazole (10 mg/day) and high-dose aripiprazole (30 mg/day) were significantly superior to placebo in reduction of YMRS scores. The response rate (≥50% reduction in YMRS) was 44.8% for low-dose aripiprazole, 63.6% for high-dose aripiprazole, and 26.1% for placebo. The most common adverse events with ziprasidone were somnolence, extrapyramidal symptoms, and tremor, which were more frequent in the high-dose aripiprazole group.

Ziprasidone

The efficacy of ziprasidone was assessed in a 4-week double-blind, placebo-controlled trial that included 150 youths with bipolar I disorder, manic or mixed episode (DelBello et al. 2008). Ziprasidone dosages ranged from 80 to 160 mg/day. Ziprasidone was significantly superior to placebo in reduction of YMRS scores. The response rate (≥50% reduction in YMRS) was 62% for ziprasidone and 35% for placebo. The most common side effects were sedation, somnolence, nausea, fatigue, and dizziness.

Comparator Studies

A comparator analysis of the efficacy of antipsychotics and mood stabilizers for the treatment of pediatric bipolar disorder showed significantly greater improvement in YMRS scores for antipsychotics compared with mood stabilizers (Correll et al. 2010). Effect sizes were 0.65 for antipsychotics and 0.24 for mood stabilizers.

The efficacy of lithium, divalproex, and carbamazepine was compared in a 6-week randomized open-label trial in 42 children and adolescents with bipolar disorder (Kowatch et al. 2000b). There were no significant differences in response rates (≥50% reduction in YMRS) among the lithium

(38%), divalproex (53%), and carbamazepine (38%) groups.

The efficacy of risperidone and divalproex was compared in an 8-week double-blind, randomized trial in 66 children and adolescents with bipolar disorder (Pavuluri et al. 2010). Significantly higher response rates (≥50% reduction in YMRS) were found for risperidone (78.1%) compared with divalproex (45.5%), and improvement was more rapid in risperidone-treated patients than in divalproex-treated patients.

The efficacy of quetiapine and divalproex was compared in a 4-week double-blind, placebo-controlled trial involving 50 adolescents with bipolar I disorder, manic or mixed episode (DelBello et al. 2006). No significant group differences were found in YMRS scores during the trial.

In an 8-week open-label trial, the efficacy of olanzapine and risperidone was compared in preschool-age children with bipolar disorder (Biederman et al. 2005). There were no significant differences in response rates between risperidone (69%) and olanzapine (53%).

Combination Treatment

Some children may not respond to initial monotherapy treatment or may need combination treatment over the course of the illness. For example, following acute 6-week treatment with one mood stabilizer, Kowatch et al. (2000a) reported that 20 of 35 youths (58%) required additional psychotropic medication over the next 16 weeks. The response rate to combination treatment with two mood stabilizers was high (80%) for those youths who did not respond to monotherapy.

Quetiapine and aripiprazole are FDA approved for use as an adjunct to lithium or valproate treatment in children ages 10 years and older with bipolar I disorder, mixed or manic episode.

The effectiveness of combination treatment with lithium and divalproex sodium was assessed in an open trial (Findling et al. 2003). Ninety youths (ages 5–17 years) with bipolar I or II disorder were treated for up to 20 weeks with divalproex sodium (mean blood level = 79.8 μg/mL) and lithium (mean blood level = 0.9 mmol/L). The clinical remission rate (defined as contiguous weekly ratings of YMRS ≤12.5, CDRS-R ≤40, Children's Global Assessment Scale [CGAS] ≥51, clinical stability, and no mood cycling) was 42%.

The efficacy of risperidone in combination with lithium or divalproex sodium was assessed in a 6-month open-label trial (Pavuluri et al. 2004). Thirty-seven youths (ages 5–18 years) with bipolar I disorder (manic or mixed episode) received risperidone (mean dosage = 0.75 mg) plus divalproex sodium (mean serum level = 106 μg/mL) or risperidone (mean dosage = 0.70 mg) plus lithium (mean serum level = 0.9 mEq/L). Response rates (≥50% reduction in baseline YMRS scores) were similar for both combinations: 80% for divalproex sodium plus risperidone, and 82.4% for lithium plus risperidone. There were no significant differences between the groups in safety and tolerability.

Risperidone augmentation of lithium nonresponders was assessed in a 1-year open-label study (Pavuluri et al. 2006). Twenty-one of 38 youths (ages 4–17 years) who failed to respond to lithium monotherapy or relapsed after initial response were given risperidone (mean dosage = 0.99 mg) for 11 months. Response rates in the lithium plus risperidone group were 85.7%.

In a double-blind, placebo-controlled study of quetiapine, 30 adolescents with bipolar disorder received divalproex (20 mg/kg) and were randomly assigned to adjunctive quetiapine (mean daily dose = 432 mg) or placebo for 6 weeks (DelBello et al. 2002). Response rates (YMRS reduction from baseline ≥50%) were significantly higher in the group receiving divalproex and quetiapine (87%) than in the group receiving divalproex and placebo (53%).

Maintenance Treatment

Sixty youths who had responded to a combination of lithium and divalproex in a 20-week trial were randomly assigned in a double-blind trial to either lithium or divalproex for 18 months (Findling et al. 2005). There was no significant difference in the time to relapse between the groups (median days: divalproex 112, lithium 114).

Clinical Recommendations for Bipolar Disorder

Treatment guidelines were developed by expert consensus and review of the available treatment literature for children and adolescents (ages 6–17 years) with bipolar I disorder, manic or mixed episode (Kowatch et al. 2005). Six stages were identified:

- Stage 1: Monotherapy with mood stabilizer or atypical antipsychotic
- Stage 2: Switch monotherapy agent (drug class not tried in stage 1)
- Stage 3: Switch monotherapy agent (drug class not tried in stage 1 or 2) OR combination treatment (2 agents)
- Stage 4: Combination treatment (2 agents) OR combination treatment (3 agents)
- Stage 5: Alternative monotherapy (drugs not tried in stages 1, 2, 3)
- Stage 6: Electroconvulsive therapy (adolescents) or clozapine

If a child fails to respond to treatment in one stage, the clinician should move to the next stage of treatment. For treatment of bipolar I disorder, manic or mixed episode with psychosis, it was recommended that initial treatment be a mood stabilizer plus an atypical antipsychotic. A minimum of 4–6 weeks at therapeutic blood levels and/or adequate doses for each medication was recommended. Following sustained remission of at least 12–24 months, medication taper should be considered.

Anxiety Disorders

Obsessive-Compulsive Disorder

OCD has a prevalence rate of 2%–4% in youth (Douglass et al. 1995; Zohar 1999). The DSM-IV-TR criteria for OCD are the same in children and adults, with the exception that children may not recognize that their obsessions or compulsions are unreasonable (American Psychiatric Association 2000). The course of OCD in youth is chronic.

Serotonin Reuptake Inhibitors

Four medications have received FDA approval for the treatment of OCD in children and adolescents: sertraline (≥6 years old), fluoxetine (≥7 years old), fluvoxamine (≥7 years old), and clomipramine (≥10 years old).

Fluvoxamine. The safety and efficacy of fluvoxamine were evaluated in a double-blind, placebo-controlled multicenter study (Riddle et al. 2001). One hundred twenty outpatient children and adolescents (ages 8–17 years) with OCD were randomly assigned to fluvoxamine (dosage range = 50–200 mg/day; mean daily dose = 165 mg) or placebo for a 10-week trial. Patients who did not respond after 6 weeks could discontinue the double-blind phase and enter an open-label trial of fluvoxamine. Mean Children's Yale-Brown Obsessive Compulsive Scale (CY-BOCS; Goodman et al. 1991) scores were significantly different between the group treated with fluvoxamine and the group treated with placebo at weeks 1, 2, 3, 4, 6, and 10. Response rates (>25% reduction in CY-BOCS scores) were 42% in the group being treated with placebo. Adverse events occurring at a placebo-adjusted frequency of >10% were insomnia and asthenia.

To assess the safety and effectiveness of fluvoxamine in the long-term treatment of pediatric OCD, 99 patients who completed the acute double-blind, placebo-controlled fluvoxamine study (Riddle et al. 2001) participated in a 1-year open-label extension study (Walkup et al. 1998). Fluvoxamine dosages were titrated to 200 mg/day over the first 4 weeks. Patients experienced a 42% reduction in CY-BOCS scores by the end of long-term treatment. Clinical improvement plateaued at about 6 months of treatment. The most common side effects were insomnia, asthenia, nausea, hyperkinesias, and nervousness.

Sertraline. In a double-blind, placebo-controlled multicenter study, 187 children and adolescents (ages 6–17 years) with OCD were randomly assigned to sertraline or placebo (March et al. 1998). Sertraline dosages were titrated to a maximum of 200 mg/day during the first 4 weeks of the trial, and these dosages were maintained for an additional 8 weeks. The mean dosage of sertraline was 167 mg/day at endpoint. Compared with patients receiving placebo, patients receiving sertraline showed significantly greater improvement on the CY-BOCS, the NIMH Global Obsessive Compulsive Rating Scale (NIMH GOCS), and the CGI Severity of Illness (CGI-S) and Improvement (CGI-I) rating scales. Forty-two percent of patients in the sertraline group and 26% of patients in the placebo group were rated as very much or much improved. Side effects of insomnia, nausea, agitation, and tremor occurred significantly more often in the group receiving sertraline than in the group receiving placebo.

To assess the long-term safety and effectiveness of sertraline for pediatric OCD, 137 patients who completed the 12-week double-blind, placebo-controlled sertraline study (March et al. 1998) were given open-label sertraline (mean dosage = 120 mg/day) in a 52-week extension study. Significant improvement was found on CY-BOCS, NIMH GOCS, and CGI scores. Rates of response (defined as >25% decrease in CY-BOCS and a CGI-I score of 1 or 2) were 72% for children and 61% for adolescents (Cook et al. 2001). Full remission (defined as a CY-BOCS score >8) was achieved in 47% of patients, and an additional 25% achieved partial remission (CY-BOCS score <15 but >8) (Wagner et al. 2003b). The most common side effects were headache, nausea, diarrhea, somnolence, abdominal pain, hyperkinesias, nervousness, dyspepsia, and vomiting.

The relative and combined efficacy of sertraline and CBT was assessed in a 12-week trial for 112 children and adolescents (ages 7–17 years) with OCD (Pediatric OCD Treatment Study [POTS] Team 2004). Patients were randomly assigned to sertraline, CBT, combined sertraline and CBT, or placebo. Combined treatment was significantly superior to CBT alone and sertraline alone, which did not differ from each other.

Paroxetine. The efficacy and safety of paroxetine were assessed in a double-blind, placebo-controlled multicenter study of 203 outpatient children and adolescents (ages 7–17 years) with OCD (D.A. Geller et al. 2004). Patients were randomly assigned to paroxetine (dosage range = 10–50 mg/day; mean daily dose = 23 mg) or placebo for a 10-week trial. There was a statistically significant greater reduction in CY-BOCS scores from baseline to endpoint in patients treated with paroxetine than in patients treated with placebo. Response rates (>25% reduction in CY-BOCS scores) were 64.9% in the paroxetine-treated patients and 41.2% in the placebo-treated patients. The most common adverse effects in the paroxetine group were headache, abdominal pain, nausea, respiratory disorder, somnolence, hyperkinesias, and trauma.

The efficacy of paroxetine in 335 outpatients (ages 7–17 years) with OCD was assessed in a 16-week open-label multicenter study of paroxetine (10–60 mg/day), followed by double-blind randomization of responders to paroxetine or placebo for an additional 16 weeks (Emslie et al. 2000). No significant differences in response rates were found between the group receiving paroxetine and the group receiving placebo in the randomization phase.

Fluoxetine. The safety and efficacy of fluoxetine were assessed in a 13-week double-blind, placebo-controlled multicenter trial (D.A. Geller et al. 2001). One hundred three children and adolescents (ages 7–17 years) with OCD were randomly assigned in a 2:1 ratio to either fluoxetine (dosage range = 10–60 mg/day; mean daily dose = 24.6 mg) or placebo. The group treated with fluoxetine showed a statistically significant reduction in OCD severity compared with the group treated with placebo, as assessed by CY-BOCS scores. Rates of response (defined as >40% reduction in CY-BOCS score) were 49% in the fluoxetine group and 25% in the placebo group. There were no significant differences in treatment-emergent adverse events between the fluoxetine and placebo groups.

Fluoxetine was compared with placebo in a controlled trial in 43 children and adolescents with OCD (Liebowitz et al. 2002). It was found that after 16 (but not 8) weeks of treatment, the fluoxetine group had significantly lower CY-BOCS scores than the placebo group.

Citalopram. Twenty-three child and adolescent outpatients (ages 9–18 years) with OCD were administered open-label citalopram (dosage range = 10–40 mg/day; mean daily dose = 37 mg) in a 10-week trial (Thomsen 1997). There was a statistically significant improvement in CY-BOCS scores from baseline to endpoint. Adverse effects were minimal and transient.

In an 8-week open-label citalopram study of 15 youths (ages 6–17 years) with OCD, 14 patients showed significant improvement in CY-BOCS scores from baseline to endpoint (Mukaddes and Abali 2003).

In a long-term open study of 30 adolescents with OCD, citalopram (dosage range = 20–70 mg/day; mean daily dose = 46.5 mg) was administered for 1–2 years (Thomsen et al. 2001). There was a significant reduction in CY-BOCS scores from baseline to assessment at 2 years. No serious adverse events were reported, and the most common side effects were sedation, sexual dysfunction, and weight gain.

Clomipramine

Clomipramine has been shown to be efficacious in the treatment of pediatric OCD in two double-blind, placebo-controlled trials. In the first study (Flament et al. 1985), 19 children (ages 10–18 years) with OCD were randomly assigned to clomipramine (dosage range = 100–200 mg/day; mean daily dose = 141 mg) or placebo for 5 weeks. Significant improvement in observed and self-reported obsessions and compulsions was found for patients who received clomipramine. The most common side effects were tremor, dry mouth, dizziness, and constipation. One patient had a grand mal seizure.

In an 8-week double-blind, placebo-controlled multicenter study of 60 children and adolescents (ages 10–17 years) with OCD, it was found that patients who received clomipramine (up to 200 mg/day) had significantly greater reductions in scores on the CY-BOCS compared with the placebo group (37% and 8%, respectively). Forty-seven patients continued in a 1-year open-label extension trial, and effectiveness was maintained with long-term treatment. The most frequent side effects were dry mouth, somnolence, dizziness, fatigue, tremor, headache, constipation, and anorexia (DeVeaugh-Geiss et al. 1992).

Atypical Antipsychotic Augmentation

Adjunctive risperidone (≤2 mg daily) was investigated in an open trial for 17 adolescents with OCD who failed to respond to two serotonin reuptake inhibitor monotherapy trials. A significant reduction in CY-BOCS scores was reported (Thomsen 2004).

Aripiprazole augmentation of CBT was found to be effective in the case of an adolescent who had a partial response to combined CBT and sertraline (Storch et al. 2008).

In a naturalistic sample of 220 children and adolescents with OCD, 43 children were treated with an atypical antipsychotic as an augmenting agent (Masi et al. 2009). Twenty-five (58.1%) of these youths responded to treatment.

The efficacy of aripiprazole augmentation of an SSRI was assessed in 39 youths with OCD who had not responded to two trials with SSRI monotherapy (Masi et al. 2010). Fifty-nine percent of the youths responded to treatment.

Generalized Anxiety Disorder

The prevalence of generalized anxiety disorder (GAD) in children and adolescents is estimated to range from 2.9% to 7.3% (Anderson et al. 1987; Kashani and Orvaschel 1988). Children with GAD have excessive anxiety and worry about several events or activities (e.g., school performance), have difficulty controlling the worry, and have at least one associated symptom, such as restlessness, fatigue, concentration difficulties, irritability, muscle tension, and sleep disturbance (American Psychiatric Association 2000). The course of GAD in youth tends to be chronic (Keller et al. 1992).

Venlafaxine

The efficacy of extended-release venlafaxine in children and adolescents with GAD (N= 320) was evaluated in two double-blind, placebo-controlled trials (Rynn et al. 2007). Venlafaxine was dosed up to 225 mg/day. In one study, venlafaxine extended release was superior to placebo on primary and secondary measures; however, in the other study, the results were negative.

Sertraline

Twenty-two children and adolescents (ages 5–17 years) with GAD were randomly assigned to sertraline or placebo in a 9-week double-blind trial (Rynn et al. 2001). The maximum dosage of sertraline was 50 mg/day. Significant differences in favor of sertraline over placebo were observed on Hamilton Anxiety Scale (Ham-A; Hamilton 1959) scores and on CGI-S and CGI-I ratings. Side effects found to be more common (but not statistically significant so) with sertraline than with placebo were dry mouth, drowsiness, leg spasm, and restlessness.

Buspirone

In an open study of adolescents with GAD, a significant decrease in anxiety clinical ratings after 6 weeks of treatment with buspirone (mean dosage range = 15–30 mg/day) was reported (Kutcher et al. 1992). Simeon (1993) reported the results of an open trial of buspirone for 13 children with anxiety disorders; 9 of these children had DSM-III-R (American Psychiatric Association 1987) overanxious disorder as a primary or secondary diagnosis. Participants received buspirone (maximum dosage = 30 mg/day) over 4 weeks. Significant improvement in anxiety was found on clinical ratings and parent, teacher, and participant reports. Mild and transient side effects were reported and included sleep difficulties, tiredness, nausea, stomachaches, and headaches.

Social Anxiety Disorder

The prevalence of social anxiety disorder (social phobia) is estimated to range from 0.9% to 7% of children and adolescents (Anderson et al. 1987; Stein et al. 2001). The diagnostic criteria for social anxiety disorder in children and adolescents are the same as the diagnostic criteria used in adults (American Psychiatric Association 2000). Social anxiety disorder in youth is a chronic condition, and it increases the risk of depression (Stein et al. 2001).

Selective Serotonin Reuptake Inhibitors

Paroxetine. The efficacy and safety of paroxetine were evaluated in a 16-week double-blind, placebo-controlled multicenter trial in 322 outpatient children and adolescents (ages 8–17 years) with social anxiety disorder

(Wagner et al. 2004a). Paroxetine was significantly superior to placebo, with rates of response (defined as CGI-I score = 1 or 2) of 77.6% and 38.3%, respectively. Side effects more common with paroxetine than with placebo were insomnia, decreased appetite, and vomiting.

Sertraline. Fourteen outpatient children and adolescents (ages 10–17 years) with a diagnosis of social anxiety disorder received sertraline (dosage range = 100–200 mg/day; mean daily dose = 123 mg) in an 8-week open trial (Compton et al. 2001). Five of the patients (36%) were much or very much improved, and four of the patients (29%) had a partial response by the end of the 8-week trial. Sertraline was well tolerated, and no patient developed significant behavioral disinhibition or mania (Compton et al. 2001).

Escitalopram. Twenty children with social anxiety disorder participated in a 12-week open-label study of escitalopram (Isolan et al. 2007). Sixty-five percent of participants were much or very much improved.

Citalopram. Chavira and Stein (2002) investigated the effectiveness of a combined psychoeducational and pharmacological treatment program for youth with social anxiety disorder. Twelve children and adolescents (ages 8–17 years) with social anxiety disorder received citalopram (mean daily dose = 35 mg) and eight 15-minute counseling sessions over a 12-week period. On the basis of clinical global ratings of change, 41.7% of youth (n=5) were very much improved, and 41.7% of youth (n=5) were much improved.

Venlafaxine

In a 16-week double-blind, placebo-controlled trial, 293 children and adolescents with social anxiety disorder were randomly assigned to extended-release venlafaxine (dosage range 37.5 mg–225 mg) or placebo (March et al. 2007). Venlafaxine extended release was significantly superior to placebo in reducing ratings of social anxiety. Response rates (CGI-I score ≤2) were 56% for the venlafaxine extended release group and 37% for the placebo group.

Posttraumatic Stress Disorder

The prevalence of posttraumatic stress disorder (PTSD) in adolescents is reported to be 6.3% (Giaconia et al. 1995). The criteria for diagnosing PTSD in youth are the same as those used for adults (American Psychiatric Association 2000). PTSD symptoms in children tend to vary over time, and although the disorder is chronic, the course is prolonged with greater severity of the stressor (Clarke et al. 1993).

Sertraline

The efficacy of sertraline was evaluated in a 10-week double-blind, placebo-controlled trial in 131 children and adolescents with PTSD (Robb et al. 2010). Sertraline dosages ranged from 50 to 200 mg/day. There was no difference between sertraline-treated patients and placebo-treated patients on the primary outcome measure, the UCLA PTSD-I score.

The benefit of adding sertraline versus placebo to trauma-focused CBT was assessed in a controlled 12-week trial (Cohen et al. 2007). Although both groups showed significant improvement in symptoms of PTSD, there was no significant advantage from the addition of sertraline to CBT.

Citalopram

Eight adolescents with PTSD received citalopram in a fixed daily dose of 20 mg in a 12-week open-label study (Seedat et al. 2001). Core PTSD symptoms of reexperiencing, avoidance, and hyperarousal showed statistically significant improvement at week 12, with a 38% reduction in total score on the Clinician-Administered PTSD Scale—Child and Adolescent Version (CAPS-CA; Nader et al. 1996). Citalopram was well tolerated, and the most common side effects were increased sweating, nausea, headache, and tiredness.

In a larger 8-week open trial, Seedat et al. (2002) treated 24 children and adolescents with citalopram (dosage range = 20–40 mg/day; mean daily dose 20 mg). Both the children and the adolescents had a significant reduction in CAPS-CA scores at endpoint. Common side effects of citalopram were drowsiness, headache, nausea, and increased sweating.

Clonidine

Seven preschool children (ages 3–6 years) with a diagnosis of PTSD received open treatment with clonidine at a dosage range of 0.05–0.15 mg/day (Harmon and Riggs 1996). To decrease sedation, oral clonidine was subsequently converted to a clonidine patch. The majority of children showed at least moderate improvements in hyperarousal, hypervigilance, insomnia, nightmares, and mood lability.

Carbamazepine

Twenty-eight children and adolescents (ages 8–17 years) with a diagnosis of PTSD received carbamazepine (dosage range = 300–1,200 mg/day) for an average of 35 days. Twenty-two patients (78%) became asymptomatic, and the remaining six patients were significantly improved during the course of treatment (Looff et al. 1995).

Propranolol

Eleven children (ages 6–12 years) with a diagnosis of PTSD participated in an off-on-off medication design of 4 weeks of propranolol treatment (Famularo et al. 1988). Propranolol was initiated at 0.8 mg/kg/day and titrated to a maximum of 2.5 mg/kg/day. A significant improvement in PTSD symptoms was found during the treatment period. Side effects included sedation and mildly lowered blood pressure and pulse.

Panic Disorder

The prevalence of panic disorder in children and adolescents ranges from 0.6% to 5.0% in the community and from 0.2% to 9.6% in clinical settings (Masi et al. 2001). The diagnostic criteria for panic disorder in children and adolescents are the same as those for adults (American Psychiatric Association 2000). Panic disorder in youth is a chronic condition, and there is continuity between pediatric and adult panic disorder (Biederman et al. 1997).

Selective Serotonin Reuptake Inhibitors

In an open-label trial, 12 children and adolescents (ages 7–17 years) with panic disorder were treated with an SSRI for 6–8 weeks (Renaud et al. 1999). Mean daily doses of SSRIs were fluoxetine 34 mg, paroxetine 20 mg, and sertraline 125 mg. Adjunctive benzodiazepines were used for 8 patients. Seventy-five percent of patients showed much to very much clinical improvement while receiving treatment with SSRIs. At the end of the trial, 8 patients (67%) no longer fulfilled panic disorder criteria.

Paroxetine. A chart review was conducted of 18 child and adolescent outpatients (ages 7–16 years) with a diagnosis of panic disorder who received monotherapy with paroxetine (dosage range = 10–40 mg/day; mean daily dose = 23 mg) (Masi et al. 2001). The mean paroxetine treatment duration was 11.7 months. Fifteen patients (83%) had a CGI score of much or very much improved. The most common side effects were nausea, tension-agitation, sedation, insomnia, palpitations, and headache.

Citalopram. Three youths (ages 9, 13, and 16 years) with panic disorder and school phobia were treated with citalopram (up to 20 mg/day) over an 8- to 15-month period.

All patients experienced resolution of panic attacks during the course of citalopram treatment (Lepola et al. 1996).

Benzodiazepines

In a 2-week open trial, four adolescents with panic disorder were treated with clonazepam (0.5 mg twice daily). A significant reduction in panic attacks (from 3 attacks per week to 0.25 per week) was reported (Kutcher and MacKenzie 1988).

Mixed Anxiety Disorders

Selective Serotonin Reuptake Inhibitors

Fluvoxamine. One hundred twenty-eight outpatient children and adolescents (ages 6–17 years) with GAD, social anxiety disorder, or separation anxiety disorder (who had received 3 weeks of open treatment with supportive psychoeducational therapy without improvement) were randomly assigned to fluvoxamine (up to 300 mg) or placebo for an 8-week trial (Research Units on Pediatric Psychopharmacology Anxiety Study Group 2001). The group treated with fluvoxamine had a significantly greater reduction in scores on the Pediatric Anxiety Rating Scale (Research Units on Pediatric Psychopharmacology Anxiety Study Group 2002a) than did the group treated with placebo. On the CGI-I scale, the response rate was 76% in the group being treated with fluvoxamine and 29% in the group receiving placebo. After completion of the 8-week placebo-controlled study, the 128 patients entered a 6-month open-label treatment phase (Research Units on Pediatric Psychopharmacology Anxiety Study Group 2002b). Anxiety symptoms remained low in 33 of 35 (94%) subjects who initially responded to fluvoxamine. Of 14 fluvoxamine nonresponders switched to fluoxetine, anxiety symptoms significantly improved in 10 (71%) patients. Among 48 placebo nonresponders, 27 (56%) showed significant improvement in anxiety on fluvoxamine.

Fluoxetine. Seventy-four youths (ages 7–17 years) with GAD, separation anxiety disorder, and/or social phobia were randomly assigned to fluoxetine (20 mg/day) or to placebo for 12 weeks (Birmaher et al. 2003). Sixty-one percent of fluoxetine-treated patients and 35% of placebo-treated patients were much or very much improved.

Fluoxetine's efficacy in long-term treatment of children with GAD, separation anxiety disorder, and/or social phobia was assessed in a 1-year open treatment (Clark et al. 2005) following the acute-phase study (Birmaher et al. 2003). Compared with youth taking no medication, those taking fluoxetine ($n=42$) showed significantly superior outcome in anxiety measures.

Sertraline. The comparative efficacy of sertraline, CBT, sertraline plus CBT, and placebo was evaluated in a 12-week randomized controlled trial (the Child Anxiety Multimodal Study [CAMS]) involving 488 children and adolescents with a diagnosis of GAD, separation anxiety disorder, or social phobia (Walkup et al. 2008). Combination treatment was significantly superior to sertraline alone or CBT alone. Rates of response (CGI-I ≤ 2) were 80.7% for combined treatment, 59.7% for CBT, and 54.9% for sertraline. All treatments were significantly superior to placebo (23.7%).

Clinical Recommendations for Anxiety Disorders

SSRIs are the medication treatment of choice for OCD in children and adolescents (Riddle 1998). Clomipramine is also effective in the treatment of this disorder; however, anticholinergic side effects often make this a less tolerable agent than SSRIs. A 10- to 12-week trial at adequate dosages is required to determine whether a child with OCD will respond to an SSRI (Greist et al. 1995). If a child fails to respond to one SSRI, switching to another SSRI is a reasonable strategy. Clomipramine may be a third treatment option, either as monotherapy or as augmentation of an SSRI. Other possible SSRI augmentation strategies are clonazepam, antipsychotics, lithium, and buspirone; however, these agents have not received systematic study in children (American Academy of Child and Adolescent Psychiatry 1998). Some children may require long-term medication maintenance; however, it is reasonable to attempt medication discontinuation 1 year after symptom resolution. Medication should be tapered gradually to assess for relapse and to avoid discontinuation symptoms (Grados et al. 1999). SSRIs are also the first-line treatment for non-OCD anxiety disorders.

In regard to other childhood anxiety disorders, SSRIs are first-line treatment (Reinblatt and Walkup 2005). Venlafaxine has also demonstrated efficacy for the treatment of childhood GAD. Other treatment options include buspirone, tricyclic antidepressants, and benzodiazepines (Bernstein et al. 1996). However, benzodiazepines should be used only on a short-term basis (i.e., weeks) because of the potential for abuse and dependence in youth (Riddle et al. 1999).

Attention-Deficit/Hyperactivity Disorder

The prevalence of ADHD in children and adolescents is estimated to range from 5% to 12%. In addition to the core behavioral features of inattention, hyperactivity, and impulsivity, children with ADHD often have significant impairment in social and academic functioning (Barkley 2005). About 4% of adults in the general population meet criteria for ADHD (Kessler et al. 2006). Of all of the childhood psychiatric disorders, ADHD has the greatest number of pharmacological treatment studies.

Psychostimulants

The classes of psychostimulants include methylphenidate, dexmethylphenidate, dextroamphetamine, mixed amphetamine salts, and L-lysine-D-amphetamine (lisdexamfetamine). By the 1980s, there were already hundreds of randomized controlled trials showing the efficacy of stimulants in the treatment of ADHD in school-age children (Greenhill et al. 1999). Arnold (2000) reviewed studies in which subjects underwent a trial of both amphetamine and methylphenidate. This review suggested that approximately 41% of subjects with ADHD responded equally to methylphenidate and amphetamine, whereas 44% responded preferentially to one of the classes of stimulants. This suggests that the initial response rate to stimulants may be as high as 85% if both stimulants are tried (in contrast to the finding of 65%–75% response when only one stimulant is tried). In contrast, placebo response rates in stimulant trials are rarely above 20%–30%, making the effect size of the stimulants (0.8–1.0) one of the largest among all the psychotropics. At present, however, no method is available to predict which stimulant will produce the best response in a given patient. The past decade has seen the emergence of the long-acting stimulants; studies of these agents have been the focus of major reviews (Biederman and Spencer 2008; Pliszka 2007).

Initial research with stimulants was carried out in school-age children, but more recent controlled trials of stimulants have focused on adolescents (Spencer et al. 2006b; Wilens et al. 2006a) and adults (Biederman et al. 2006a; Weisler et al. 2006). These studies in older individuals show response rates to stimulants similar to those of children, with adequate response for most subjects being obtained with 70–100 mg of methylphenidate or 40–60 mg of amphetamine a day.

Preschoolers with ADHD have also been the focus of investigation. In the NIMH Preschool ADHD Treatment Study (PATS), 183 children (ages 3–5 years) underwent an open-label trial of methylphenidate, with 165 of these subjects subsequently randomly assigned to a double-blind, placebo-controlled crossover trial of methylphenidate lasting 6 weeks (Greenhill et al. 2006; Wigal et al. 2006). The mean optimal dosage of methylphenidate was found to be 0.7+0.4 mg/kg/day, which is lower than the mean of 1.0 mg/kg/day found to be optimal in school-age children. Eleven percent of subjects discontinued methylphenidate because of adverse events. Compared with the school-age children, the preschool group showed a higher rate of emotional adverse events, including crabbiness, irritability, and proneness to crying. The conclusion was that the dose of methylphenidate (or any stimulant) should be titrated more conservatively in preschoolers than in school-age patients, and lower mean doses may be effective.

The Appendix shows the recommended dosage ranges for these agents. The Appendix also discusses adverse events with stimulants, particularity growth suppression.

Atomoxetine

Atomoxetine is a noradrenergic reuptake inhibitor that has indirect effects on dopamine reuptake in cortex but not in the striatum (Bymaster et al. 2002). Numerous double-blind, placebo-controlled trials have demonstrated its efficacy in the treatment of ADHD in children, adolescents, and adults (Michelson et al. 2001, 2002, 2003). Given its pharmacokinetic half-life of 5 hours, it is generally dosed twice a day. While open trials comparing methylphenidate with atomoxetine showed the two agents to have similar efficacy (Kratochvil et al. 2002), double-blind, placebo-controlled trials comparing atomoxetine with amphetamine (Biederman et al. 2006b; Wigal et al. 2005) and methylphenidate (Newcorn et al. 2008) have shown the stimulants to be more efficacious.

Atomoxetine is effective in treating ADHD in those with comorbid tics and may also reduce tics (Allen et al. 2005). It is also useful in children with ADHD who have comorbid anxiety, showing effectiveness in treating anxiety and inattention (Sumner et al. 2005). Atomoxetine is well tolerated in long-term use. In a global multicenter study, 416 children and adolescents who responded to an initial 12-week open-label period of treatment with atomoxetine were randomly assigned to continued atomoxetine treatment or placebo for 9 months under double-blind conditions. Atomoxetine was significantly superior to placebo in preventing relapse (defined as a return to 90% of baseline symptom severity), 22.3% and 37.9%, respectively (Michelson et al. 2001). Data from 13 atomoxetine studies (6 double-blind, 7 open-label) were pooled for subjects ages 12–18 years with ADHD (Wilens et al. 2006b). Of the 601 atomoxetine-treated subjects in this meta-analysis, 537 (89.4%) completed 3 months of acute treatment. At the time of publication, a total of 259 subjects (48.4%) were continuing atomoxetine treatment; 219 of these subjects had completed at least 2 years of treatment. Symptoms remained improved up to 24 months without dosage escalation. During the 2-year treatment period, 99 (16.5%) subjects discontinued treatment due to lack of effectiveness, and 31 (5.2%) subjects discontinued treatment due to adverse events. No clinically significant abnormalities in height, weight, blood pressure, pulse, mean laboratory values, or electrocardiography parameters were found.

Clonidine

A review of the literature from 1980 to 1999 found 39 studies regarding the use of clonidine for symptoms of childhood ADHD, and 11 of these studies (n=150) had sufficient data to be included in a meta-analysis (Connor et al. 1999). Of these 150 subjects, 42 received clonidine for ADHD, and the others received clonidine for ADHD comorbid with tic disorders (n=67), developmental disorders (n=15), or conduct disorders (n=26). The mean daily dose of clonidine was 0.18 mg, and the average length of treatment was 10.9 weeks. Clonidine showed a moderate effect size of 0.58 on symptoms of ADHD, which is smaller than the effect size (0.82) reported for stimulant treatment of ADHD (Swanson et al. 1995b). An extended-release form of clonidine was recently developed, and this formulation was evaluated in a double-blind, placebo-controlled trial (Jain et al. 2011) in which patients (n=236) were randomly assigned to receive clonidine extended release 0.2 mg/day, clonidine extended release 0.4 mg/day, or placebo. Improvement in ADHD symptoms was significantly greater in the clonidine extended release groups relative to the placebo group, with this difference apparent at week 2 and greatest at week 5. Somnolence was the most common side effect, and the rate of withdrawal due to adverse events was higher in the clonidine extended release 0.4 mg/day group than in the other groups. There were no serious adverse events, and bradycardia was the most common cardiovascular side effect.

Guanfacine

In a study by Hunt et al. (1995), 13 children and adolescents with ADHD received guanfacine (mean daily dose=3.2 mg) for 1 month. Significant improvements in hyperactivity and inattention were found. In an 8-week double-blind, placebo-controlled trial, 34 children and adolescents (ages 7–14 years) with ADHD and tic disorder were randomly assigned to guanfacine (dosage range=1.5–3.0 mg/day) or placebo (Scahill et al. 2001). There was a 37% improvement in ADHD symptoms for children treated with guanfacine, compared with an 8% improvement in ADHD symptoms for children receiving placebo. The most common side effects of guanfacine were sedation and dry mouth. There were no significant changes in pulse or blood pressure with guanfacine.

An extended-release formulation of guanfacine was recently approved for the treatment of ADHD (Biederman et al. 2008; Sallee et al. 2009). In a double-blind, placebo-controlled Phase III multicenter trial (Melmed et al. 2006), children and adolescents ages 6–17 years were randomly assigned to placebo or 2, 3, or 4 mg/day of extended-release guanfacine. All three dosages of guanfacine were superior to placebo in reducing symptoms of ADHD. The most commonly reported side effects were headache, somnolence, and fatigue. No serious adverse events were reported. In healthy young adults (ages 19–24 years), abrupt discontinuation of 4 mg/day of extended-release guanfacine did not lead to increases in blood pressure or electrocardiogram (ECG) abnormalities (Kisicki et al. 2006).

Clinical Recommendations for Attention-Deficit/Hyperactivity Disorder

Based on the strength of clinical trial data, stimulants should be regarded as the first line for treatment of ADHD, and generally a different stimulant class should be used if the first stimulant prescribed has failed. Either atomoxetine or guanfacine is an appropriate second-line agent. Stimulants have been combined with atomoxetine in an open trial, with results suggesting that the two agents are superior to atomoxetine alone (Wilens et al. 2009). Placebo-controlled studies have shown that the addition of either guanfacine (Wilens et al. 2012) or clonidine (Kollins et al. 2011) can further reduce symptoms of ADHD after a partial response to psychostimulants. Thus, alpha-2 agonists are increasingly used in this adjunctive role.

The stages of pharmacological treatment of ADHD can be summarized as follows:

- Stage 1: Psychostimulant
- Stage 2: Alternative psychostimulant
- Stage 3: Atomoxetine or alpha-2 agonist
- Stage 4: Combination of alpha-2 agonist or atomoxetine with stimulant

Disruptive Behavior Disorders and Aggression

Oppositional defiant disorder (ODD) and conduct disorder (CD) are highly comorbid with ADHD, particularly in younger children (Pliszka et al. 1999). While ODD and CD are *syndromes*, aggression is a *symptom*. Although many children and adolescents with CD are aggressive, a child can meet criteria for CD without being aggressive; aggression may present as a problematic symptom in children with depression, psychosis, or bipolar disorder without the child meeting criteria for CD. Thus, the clinician must be clear whether ODD/CD or aggression is the target of treatment, as studies have addressed the problems separately. Treatments for ADHD have been used to target ODD/CD, whereas mood stabilizers and antipsychotics have been used in patients with severe aggressive outbursts, regardless of diagnosis (Pappadopulos et al. 2006).

Oppositional Defiant Disorder and Conduct Disorder

Psychostimulants

In a 5-week double-blind, placebo-controlled trial of methylphenidate in 84 youths (ages 6–15 years) with CD (with and without ADHD), ratings of antisocial behaviors specific to CD were significantly reduced by methylphenidate treatment (up to 60 mg/day) (Klein et al. 1997). The severity of the ADHD did not affect the response of CD symptoms to the stimulant studies. Since this study, multiple double-blind, placebo-controlled trials have shown that ODD responds to stimulant medication, yielding an effect size similar to that for the ADHD symptoms (Spencer et al. 2006a).

Atomoxetine

Children and adolescents (ages 8–18 years) with ADHD were treated for approximately 8 weeks with placebo or atomoxetine under randomized, double-blind conditions. Of the 293 subjects, 39% were diagnosed with comorbid ODD and 61% were not (Newcorn et al. 2005). Treatment group differences and differences between patients with and without comorbid ODD were examined post hoc for changes on numerous clinical measures. Treatment response was similar in youth with and without ODD, although the comorbid group may require higher doses to achieve response than those with ADHD alone.

In general, a child with ODD or CD should be treated with a stimulant or atomoxetine before proceeding to the use of other psychotropic agents. The use of more potent agents (mood stabilizers, antipsychotics) is generally reserved for those with severe aggression, and then only after a behavioral treatment has failed.

Aggression

Psychostimulants

In a meta-analysis of the literature from 1970 to 2001 that utilized 28 studies to determine the effect size for stimulants on overt and covert aggression-related behaviors in children with ADHD, it was found that the mean effect size for aggressive behaviors was similar to that for core behaviors of ADHD (Connor et al. 2002).

Risperidone

A significant body of research has accumulated showing the effectiveness of risperidone in the treatment of aggression, although most of these studies involve patients with subaverage intelligence (Snyder et al. 2002). Eighty percent of subjects had comorbid ADHD. Risperidone dosages ranged from 0.02 to 0.06 mg/kg/day. The risperidone-treated subjects showed a significant ($P<0.001$) reduction (47.3%) in conduct problems compared with placebo-treated subjects (20.9%). The effect of risperidone was unaffected by diagnosis, presence/absence of ADHD, psychostimulant use, and IQ status. Risperidone produced no changes on the cognitive variables, and the most common side effects were somnolence, headache, appetite increase, and dyspepsia. Somnolence did not predict response of aggressive symptoms. Side effects related to extrapyramidal symptoms were reported in 7 (13.2%) and 3 (5.3%) of the subjects in the risperidone and placebo groups, respectively ($P=0.245$).

Other double-blind, placebo-controlled trials of risperidone in children and adolescents with disruptive behavior disorders (and subaverage IQ) have yielded similar results, with no negative trials reported (Aman et al. 2002; Buitelaar et al. 2001; LeBlanc et al. 2005). Weight gain was a significant side effect in these studies, but there has not been evidence of adverse neuropsychological effects (Gunther et al. 2006). Addition of risperidone to a stimulant does not appear to increase rates of side effects and enhances treatment of hyperactivity (Aman et al. 2004). Indeed, adding risperidone to a stimulant to control aggression has become a common practice, although a controlled study showed that aggression was equally reduced when either placebo or risperidone was added to psychostimulant medication (Armenteros et al. 2007). The sample in this study was small ($N=25$), but the study should caution clinicians that aggression can respond to psychosocial events, like the expectations of a study.

A full review of all studies of risperidone in the treatment of childhood aggression has been published (Pandina et al. 2006). This review pooled adverse-event data from these studies ($n=688$), showing the most common side effects of risperidone to be somnolence (33%), weight gain (20%), hyperprolactinemia (10.2%), and fatigue (10%). In the pooled studies, there was an excess mean weight gain (over normal growth) of 6.0+7 kg after 35–43 weeks of treatment. Of the 688 patients, 651 were free of dyskinetic movements at baseline, and only 1 patient developed new dyskinetic movements during the follow-up period (these symptoms resolved even though risperidone was continued). There was no worsening of dyskinetic movements in those with such preexisting symptoms. Rates of extrapyramidal side effects were low throughout the long-term follow-up period. It should be noted that the dosages of risperidone used in these studies were quite low (1–2 mg/day); thus, these results may not apply to dosages in the 6 mg/day range.

Quetiapine

Quetiapine has been studied in an open trial with aggressive children with CD (Findling et al. 2006) The 8-week trial enrolled 17 children ages 6–12 years. Outcome measures included the Rating of Aggression Against People and/or Property Scale (RAAPPS) and the Conners Parent Rating Scale (CPRS-48). The mean dose of quetiapine at week 8 was 4.4±1.1 mg/kg. Significant decreases in baseline scores of the RAAPPS, and in several subscales of the CPRS, were found by the end of the study. No patients discontinued because of an adverse event or experienced extrapyramidal side effects. These preliminary data suggest that aggressive children with CD may benefit from quetiapine. Nine of the subjects in this study were subsequently enrolled in a 26-week open-label trial; they were treated with dosages of quetiapine ranging from 75 to 300 mg/day. Aggression remained well controlled, no subject developed extrapyramidal side effects, and 1 subject had a significant weight gain but remained in the study.

Other Atypical Antipsychotics

There have only been small open trials and case reports of the use of aripiprazole, olanzapine, and ziprasidone in the treatment of aggression (Hazaray et al. 2004; Khan et al. 2006; Rugino and Janvier 2005; Staller and Staller 2004; Stephens et al. 2004; Valicenti-McDermott and Demb 2006). In most of these studies, children had primary psychiatric diagnoses other than ODD or CD, such as mood disorders or developmental disorders.

Rugino and Janvier (2005) reported on the use of aripiprazole in a mixed sample ($n=17$) of children with bipolar disorder and developmental disorders. Only 4 of the subjects responded, but coadministration of alpha-2 agonists in a large proportion of the sample may have confounded the results. A retrospective chart review of 32 children (ages 5–19 years) with developmental disabilities treated with aripiprazole was conducted (Valicenti-McDermott and Demb 2006). Twenty-four had diagnoses within the autistic spectrum, and 18 had mental retardation. Other disorders included ADHD/disruptive behavior disorders (n=13), mood disorders (n=7), reactive attachment disorder (n=2), and sleep disorders (n=2). Target symptoms included aggression, hyperactivity, impulsivity, and self-injurious behaviors. The mean daily aripiprazole starting dose was 7.1±0.32 mg (0.17 mg/kg/day), and the mean daily maintenance dose was 10.55±6.9 mg (0.27 mg/kg/day). While improvement in target symptoms was found in 56% of the sample, side effects were reported in 16 (50%), with the most frequent being sleepiness (n=6). Mean body mass index (BMI) rose significantly, and weight gain was more pronounced in children younger than 12 years.

The effects of olanzapine on aggressive behavior and tic severity were examined in 10 subjects (ages 7–13 years) with a primary diagnosis of Tourette syndrome and a history of aggressive behavior (Stephens et al. 2004). They were treated in a 2-week single-blind placebo run-in followed by an 8-week treatment-phase trial. The starting dosage of olanzapine was 1.25–2.5 mg/day, with dosage was titrated upward at biweekly intervals, as tolerated. The mean dosage at the end of the trial was 14.5 mg/day. Olanzapine produced clinically and statistically significant reductions in aggression and tic severity from baseline to trial completion. Weight gain during the treatment period was the most common adverse effect.

Lithium

The efficacy of lithium in the treatment of CD in youth has been demonstrated in three of the four double-blind, placebo-controlled studies reported to date. Haloperidol, lithium, and placebo were compared in a double-blind, randomized trial for 61 hospitalized children with aggression (ages 5–12 years) and CD. The optimal dosages of haloperidol ranged from 1 to 6 mg/day; the optimal dosages of lithium ranged from 500 to 2,000 mg/day. Both haloperidol and lithium were found to be significantly superior to placebo in reducing aggression. However, there were more adverse effects associated with haloperidol than with lithium, including excessive sedation, acute dystonic reaction, and drooling. Stomachache, headache, and tremor were more common with lithium than with haloperidol (Campbell et al. 1984).

In a subsequent study, Campbell et al. (1995) conducted a 6-week double-blind, placebo-controlled trial of lithium treatment for 50 hospitalized children (ages 5–12 years) with aggression and CD. The mean optimal daily dose of lithium was 1,248 mg, and the mean serum level was 1.12 mEq/L. Lithium was significantly superior to placebo in reducing aggression. The most common lithium side effects were stomachache, nausea, vomiting, headache, tremor, and urinary frequency.

Eighty-six inpatients (ages 10–17 years) with CD were randomly assigned to treatment with lithium (mean daily dose= 1,425 mg; mean serum level=1.07 mmol/L) or placebo in a 4-week double-blind trial. Aggression ratings decreased significantly for the group treated with lithium, compared with the group treated with placebo. More than 50% of patients in the lithium group experienced nausea, vomiting, and urinary frequency (Malone et al. 2000).

Rifkin et al. (1997) found no significant differences between lithium and placebo in aggression ratings in a 2-week double-blind study of 33 inpatients with CD. The short duration of treatment may have accounted for the lack of efficacy, suggesting that a 4- to 6-week trial is necessary to show response.

Divalproex

Twenty outpatient children and adolescents (ages 10–18 years) with CD or ODD were randomly assigned to divalproex (dosage range=750–1,500 mg/day; mean blood level=82 μg/mL) or placebo in a 6-week double-blind, placebo-controlled crossover study. Of the 15 patients who completed both phases, 12 patients (80%) had a statistically significant superior response to divalproex. Increased appetite was the only significant side effect (Donovan et al. 2000). Steiner et al. (2003) randomly assigned 71 adolescents with CD in a residential facility for juvenile offenders to either therapeutic or low doses of divalproex for 7 weeks; both subjects and outcome raters were blind to treatment status. Reduction in aggression severity ($P = 0.02$), improvement in impulse control ($P < 0.05$), and global improvement ($P = 0.0008$) were greater in the group with therapeutic divalproex levels than in the low-dose condition. Serum level and "Immature defenses" (as assessed by the Weinberger Adjustment Inventory) predicted response to divalproex, but psychiatric comorbidity did not (Saxena et al. 2005).

Blader et al. (2009) treated children with ADHD and aggression ($n = 74$) with open stimulant treatment during a lead-in phase that averaged 5 weeks. Children whose aggressive behavior persisted at the conclusion of the lead-in phase ($n = 30$) were randomly assigned to receive double-blind, flexibly dosed divalproex or a placebo adjunctive to stimulant for 8 weeks. Families received weekly behavioral therapy throughout the trial. A significantly higher proportion of the children randomly assigned to divalproex met remission criteria (8 of 14; 57%) than of those randomly assigned to placebo (2 of 13; 15%).

Clonidine

Despite controversy over its safety (Swanson et al. 1995a; see Appendix), clonidine has often been combined with stimulants to treat comorbid aggression in children with ADHD. In a 2-month randomized comparison of clonidine, methylphenidate, and clonidine combined with methylphenidate in the treatment of 24 children and adolescents (ages 6–16 years) with ADHD and CD or ODD, it was found that all three treatment groups showed significant improvement in oppositional and CD symptoms (Connor et al. 2000). No significant ECG changes were noted.

Children ages 6–14 years with ADHD currently taking methylphenidate were randomly assigned to receive clonidine syrup 0.10–0.20 mg/day ($n = 37$) or placebo ($n = 29$) for 6 weeks (Hazell and Stuart 2003). Analysis showed that significantly more clonidine-treated children than control subjects were responders on the Conduct subscale (21 of 37 vs. 6 of 29; $P < 0.01$) of the parent-report Conners Behavior Checklist but not the Hyperactive Index subscale (13 of 37 vs. 5 of 29). Compared with placebo, clonidine was associated with a greater reduction in systolic blood pressure measured standing and with transient sedation and dizziness. Clonidine-treated individuals had a greater reduction in a number of unwanted effects associated with psychostimulant treatment compared with placebo. The findings supported the use of clonidine in combination with psychostimulant medication to reduce conduct symptoms associated with ADHD.

Clinical Recommendations for Disruptive Behavior Disorders and Aggression

The Center for the Advancement of Children's Mental Health at Columbia University joined with the New York State Office of Mental Health to develop guidelines for treatment of aggression, which led to the Treatment Recommendations for the Use of Antipsychotics for Aggressive Youth (TRAAY; Pappadopulos et al. 2003; Schur et al. 2003). These recommendations call first for a thorough psychiatric evaluation of the child with severe aggression. Next, a psychosocial intervention should be used first when the aggression is the primary problem (such as in ODD/CD or intermittent explosive disorder). The clinician should then treat any primary condition, such as ADHD, psychosis, or mood disorder, that may be causing or contributing to the aggression. If the aggression does not respond to these steps, then an atypical antipsychotic should be used. Different atypical antipsychotics should be tried as monotherapy before moving to polypharmacy (e.g., adding a classic mood stabilizer such as lithium or divalproex to the antipsychotic). Monitoring of weight and laboratory measures of glucose, cholesterol, and triglycerides is mandatory (Correll and Carlson 2006).

Alpha-2 agonists may be used in milder aggression or temper outbursts since their effect size on aggression is more modest (Hazell and Stuart 2003).

Tourette Syndrome

The prevalence of Tourette syndrome is estimated to be 0.7% in children (Comings et al. 1990). Tourette syndrome is characterized by multiple motor tics and by one or more vocal tics that occur frequently for longer than 1 year.

Alpha$_2$-Adrenergic Receptor Agonists

Clonidine

Two of three controlled studies support the efficacy of clonidine treatment for Tourette syndrome. In a 12-week double-blind, placebo-controlled trial, 39 children and adolescents with Tourette syndrome were randomly assigned to clonidine (dosage range = 3.2–5.7 μg/kg/day; mean daily dose = 4.4 μg/kg) or placebo. The group treated with clonidine had a statistically significant greater improvement on Tourette's Syndrome Global Scale (TSGS) scores than did the group receiving placebo. Clonidine was most effective for motor tics and tics that were noticeable to others. The most common side effects were sedation, fatigue, dry mouth, dizziness, and irritability (Leckman et al. 1991).

Thirteen children and adolescents (ages 9–16 years) with Tourette syndrome were randomly assigned to a 20-week single-blind, placebo-controlled trial of clonidine (mean daily dose = 5.5 μg/kg). Six patients (46%) had a positive response to clonidine, as determined by TSGS scores. The most common side effects of clonidine were sedation, headache, and early-morning awakening (Leckman et al. 1985).

Twenty-four children and adolescents with Tourette syndrome were randomized in a double-blind crossover design that included two 12-week treatment phases—one phase with clonidine (either 0.0075 mg/kg/day or 0.015 mg/kg/day) and the other phase with placebo. However, in this study, clonidine did not significantly reduce motor tics, vocalizations, or associated behaviors. The most common side effects were sedation, dry mouth, and restlessness. There were no clinically significant changes in blood pressure or pulse (Goetz et al. 1987).

A retrospective study of 53 children and adolescents (ages 5–18 years) with Tourette syndrome was conducted to determine predictors of response to clonidine treatment. Patients who had a longer duration of vocal tics had a good behavioral response to clonidine. Of 47 patients who received clonidine for tic control, 57% had a good tic response. The authors concluded that clonidine is a useful medication for 40%–60% of patients who have mild to moderate tics (Lichter and Jackson 1996).

Clonidine was compared with risperidone in the treatment of children and adolescents with Tourette syndrome (Gaffney et al. 2002). Following a single-blind placebo lead-in, 21 subjects (ages 7–17 years) were randomly assigned to 8 weeks of double-blind treatment with clonidine or risperidone. Risperidone (mean dosage = 1.5±0.9 mg/day) and clonidine (mean dosage = 0.175±0.075 mg/day) appeared equally effective in the treatment of tics in an intent-to-treat analysis, as rated by the Yale Global Tic Severity Scale (YGTSS). Risperidone produced a mean reduction in the YGTSS of 21%; clonidine produced a 26% reduction. There was a nonsignificant trend for subjects with comorbid obsessive-compulsive symptoms to respond better to risperidone (63%) than to clonidine (33%). Both treatments caused mild sedation that resolved with time; no clinically significant extrapyramidal symptoms were observed.

In a 16-week double-blind, placebo-controlled multicenter study, 136 youths with tic disorder and ADHD were randomly assigned to clonidine (mean daily dose = 0.25 mg), methylphenidate (mean daily dose = 26 mg), combination methylphenidate plus clonidine (mean daily dose = 0.28 mg), or placebo. Compared with the placebo group, the active treatment groups showed a significant reduction in tic severity, with combination treatment producing the greatest improvement in tics (Tourette's Syndrome Study Group 2002).

Guanfacine

Scahill et al. (2001) randomly assigned 34 children (mean age 10.4 years) with comorbid ADHD and tic disorders to receive either placebo or guanfacine for 8 weeks in a double-blind fashion. Tic severity declined by an average of 31% in the guanfacine group versus 0% in the placebo group. Globally, 9 of 17 subjects were rated as much or very much improved on the CGI compared with none so rated in the placebo group. One subject withdrew due to sedation; guanfacine was associated with insignificant decreases in blood pressure. In contrast, in a 4-week double-blind, placebo-controlled study of guanfacine in 24 children (ages 6–16 years) with Tourette syndrome, there was no significant improvement in tic severity for guanfacine-treated patients compared with placebo-treated patients (Cummings et al. 2002).

Atypical Antipsychotics

Risperidone

In a double-blind, placebo-controlled trial in 48 adolescent and adult outpatients (ages 14–49 years) with Tourette syndrome, patients were randomly assigned to risperidone (dosage range = 1–6 mg/day; median daily dose = 2.5 mg) or placebo for an 8-week trial. Risperidone was significantly superior to placebo on the global severity rating of the Tourette's Syndrome Severity Scale (TSSS; Shapiro et al. 1988). Adverse effects more common in the group treated with risperidone than in the group treated with placebo were hypokinesia, tremor, fatigue, and somnolence (Dion et al. 2002).

The efficacy of risperidone in Tourette syndrome was further assessed in an 8-week randomized, double-blind, placebo-controlled trial using the Total Tic score of the YGTSS as the primary outcome variable (Scahill et al. 2003). Thirty-four medication-free subjects (26 children and 8 adults) ranging in age from 6 to 62 years (mean = 19.7±17.0 years) participated. After 8 weeks of treatment, the 16 subjects receiving risperidone (mean daily dose = 2.5±0.85) demonstrated a 32% reduction in tic severity from baseline, compared with a 7% reduction for the 18 subjects receiving placebo (P = 0.004). The 12 children randomly assigned to risperidone showed a 36% reduction in tic symptoms, compared with an 11% decrease in the 14 children receiving placebo (P = 0.004). Two children on risperidone showed acute social phobia, which resolved with dose reduction in 1 subject but resulted in medication discontinuation in the other. A mean increase in body weight of 2.8 kg was observed in the risperidone group compared with no change in placebo (P = 0.0001). No extrapyramidal symptoms and no clinically significant alterations in cardiac conduction times or laboratory measures were observed.

Risperidone was compared with pimozide in the treatment of children and adolescents with tic disorders in a randomized, double-blind crossover study (Gilbert et al. 2004). Nineteen children (ages 7–17 years) with Tourette syndrome or chronic motor tic disorder were randomly assigned to 4 weeks of treatment with pimozide or risperidone, followed by the alternate treatment after a

2-week placebo washout. The primary efficacy outcome measure was change in tic severity assessed by the YGTSS. Compared with pimozide treatment, risperidone treatment was associated with significantly lower tic severity scores. Weight gain during the 4-week treatment periods was greater for risperidone (mean 1.9 kg) than pimozide (1.0 kg). No participant suffered a serious adverse event, but 6 of 19 subjects failed to complete the protocol. Neither medication was associated with ECG changes. Although risperidone appeared superior to pimozide for tic suppression, it was associated with greater weight gain.

More recently, a 6-week open-label study examined the effects of risperidone in the treatment of chronic tic disorder or Tourette's disorder in children and adolescents (Kim et al. 2005). The participants were 15 young children and adolescents (mean age 10±2.4 years). Ten of the 15 participants were administered risperidone for the first time, and 5 of the 15 participants had been previously treated with traditional drugs (haloperidol or pimozide). Comparisons between periods on the YGTSS showed significant differences for weeks 1 through 3. After 6 weeks, tic severity scale scores revealed a 36% reduction in overall tic symptoms, with 13 of the 15 participants showing significant improvement.

Olanzapine

An open-label trial was performed to explore efficacy and safety of olanzapine for treatment of Tourette's disorder (Budman et al. 2001). Ten adult patients (ages 20–44 years) with Tourette's disorder were treated using an open-label, flexible-dosing schedule for 8 weeks. The YGTSS was used to rate tic severity; weight, vital signs, and adverse effects were assessed weekly. Two of 10 patients prematurely discontinued olanzapine owing to excessive sedation. Of 8 patients who completed the 8-week trial, 4 (50%) demonstrated significant reductions in global tic severity scores. Sedation, weight gain, increased appetite, dry mouth, and transient asymptomatic hypoglycemia were the most common side effects. Improvements in tic severity were maintained in 3 patients reassessed 6 months later. Final olanzapine dosages ranged from 2.5 mg to 20 mg daily (mean = 10.9 mg/day).

Ziprasidone

In an 8-week double-blind, placebo-controlled trial, 28 children and adolescents (ages 7–17 years) with Tourette syndrome were randomly assigned to ziprasidone (dosage range = 10–40 mg/day; mean daily dose = 28 mg) or placebo. The group treated with ziprasidone showed a statistically significant reduction in scores on the YGTSS, compared with the group treated with placebo. The most common adverse event was somnolence. No clinically significant changes in vital signs or ECG parameters were reported (Sallee et al. 2000).

Nonetheless, concerns continue to be raised about possible cardiovascular effects of ziprasidone. A sudden death occurred in a child who participated in a clinical trial of ziprasidone for Tourette syndrome (Scahill et al. 2005). Despite the fact that a single dose of ziprasidone did not produce abnormal ECG changes (Sallee et al. 2006), ECG changes were observed in the children treated with ziprasidone for Tourette syndrome in a long-term open-label safety study (Blair et al. 2005). These findings, occurring at doses low by current treatment standards, suggest that electrocardiographic monitoring is warranted when prescribing ziprasidone to children.

Quetiapine

The short-term safety and effectiveness of quetiapine in the treatment of children and adolescents with Tourette's disorder were studied in an 8-week open-label trial that included 12 subjects with a mean age of 11.4± 2.4 years (Mukaddes and Abali 2003). Clinical responses, as measured by the Turkish version of the YGTSS, revealed a statistically significant reduction in tic scores ranging from 30% to 100%. The mean dosage of quetiapine at the end of the study was 72.9±22.5 mg/day. Three subjects complained of sedation in the first week of treatment.

In a retrospective study of clinic patients, 12 patients (ages 8–18 years) with Tourette syndrome received quetiapine therapy at a starting dosage of 25 mg/day, which was increased to a mean dosage of 175.0±116.6 mg/day by the eighth week of the study (Copur et al. 2007). The YGTSS score showed significant decreases at 4 and 8 weeks. Routine laboratory parameters and serum prolactin levels were all normal and did not change throughout treatment. Mild but significant increases in both body weight and BMI at 4 and 8 weeks compared with baseline were observed. No controlled trials of quetiapine in the treatment of tic disorders have been performed.

Aripiprazole

Murphy et al. (2005) reported six cases of children and adolescents (age range = 8–19 years; mean age = 12.1 years) who had comorbid tic disorder and OCD and were treated with aripiprazole (mean dosage = 11.7 mg/day; range = 5–20 mg/day) for 12 weeks. The subjects experienced a mean reduction of 56% in the severity of their tics as assessed by the YGTSS. Similarly, Yoo et al. (2006) treated 15 children and adolescents with tic disorder with aripiprazole (mean dosage = 10.89 mg/day; range = 12.5–15 mg/day) and reported a mean reduction of 40% in YGTSS scores; side effects were minimal. Two subjects experienced nausea, 1 experienced weight gain, and 1 experienced sedation that responded to dosage reduction.

A case series of 11 consecutive patients with Tourette syndrome (age range = 7–50 years; mean age = 7 years) were treated with aripiprazole; the majority of these cases had been refractory to previous treatments with other antipsychotics (Davies et al. 2006). Ten of the 11 patients who were treated with aripiprazole improved, although to variable degrees. In the majority of patients, response was sustained with aripiprazole doses ranging from 10 to 20 mg daily. Side effects were mild and transient.

Pimozide and Haloperidol

Sallee et al. (1997) conducted a 24-week double-blind, placebo-controlled, double-crossover study of pimozide (mean daily dose = 3.4 mg) and haloperidol (mean daily dose = 3.5 mg) in 22 children and adolescents (ages 7–16 years) with Tourette syndrome. Only pimozide was significantly superior to placebo on TSGS scores. There was a threefold higher frequency of serious side effects (depression, anxiety, and severe dyskinesias) with haloperidol (41%) than with pimozide (14%) in these youths. Extrapyramidal side effects were reported significantly more often with haloperidol than with pimozide.

Long-term (6–84 months) treatment with pimozide (0.5–9 mg/day) was reported to produce a good clinical response in 81% of 65 patients (ages 6–54 years) (Regeur et al. 1986). A 1- to 15-year follow-up of 33 patients (ages 9–50 years) with Tourette syndrome treated with pimozide (2–18 mg/day), haloperidol (2–15 mg/day), or no medications found that significantly more patients discontinued haloperidol than pimozide because of adverse side effects, especially dyskinesias and dystonias (Sandor et al. 1990). Thus, pimozide appears superior to haloperidol for treatment of tics. However, both drugs are rarely used today due to the risk of tardive dyskinesia.

Clinical Recommendations for Tourette Syndrome

If a tic is not severe or socially impairing, observation may be in order, as the natural history of tics is to wax and wane; in general, tics improve over time (Leckman 2002). Often, psychosocial treatment such as habit reversal training is highly effective at reducing tics (Piacentini and Chang 2006). If conservative treatment fails, use of an alpha-2 agonist would be desirable, owing to the risk of weight gain and dyslipidemia with atypical antipsychotics. Because of the lower efficacy and higher risk of tardive dyskinesia with typical antipsychotics, the atypical antipsychotics are preferred. Haloperidol and pimozide should be used only as a last resort when several atypical agents have failed.

In children with comorbid ADHD, a stimulant can be used, but a nonstimulant is indicated if the stimulant exacerbates tics (Pliszka et al. 2006a). Often stimulants must be combined with alpha-2 agonists or antipsychotics to control both the ADHD and the tics (Pliszka et al. 2006a; Tourette's Syndrome Study Group 2002).

Schizophrenia

Cases of schizophrenia in children younger than 13 years are very rare; however, the prevalence rises in adolescence, with peak onset from 15 to 30 years (McClellan and Werry 2001). The clinical features of the disorder are similar in youth and adults, and the same DSM-IV-TR criteria are used to establish a diagnosis (American Psychiatric Association 2000). The outcome of childhood-onset schizophrenia is reported to be poor (Eggers and Bunk 1997).

Atypical Antipsychotics

Four atypical antipsychotics have FDA approval for the treatment of schizophrenia in adolescents (≥age 13 years): olanzapine, risperidone, aripiprazole, and quetiapine.

Clozapine

A 6-week double-blind, placebo-controlled comparison of clozapine and haloperidol was conducted in 21 children and adolescents (ages 6–18 years) with schizophrenia (Kumra et al. 1996). Clozapine (mean dosage = 176 mg/day; range = 25–525 mg/day) was significantly superior to haloperidol (mean dosage = 16 mg/day; range = 7–27 mg/day) in reducing positive and negative symptoms of schizophrenia. Clozapine improved interpersonal functioning and enabled patients to live in a less restrictive setting. Side effects, however, were significant with clozapine. One patient had a seizure, and 3 patients were given anticonvulsants after they became more irritable and aggressive and experienced epileptiform changes on electroencephalogram (EEG). Mild to moderate neutropenia, weight gain, and sinus tachycardia were the other major side effects.

Olanzapine

In a double-blind, placebo-controlled multicenter study of olanzapine (mean dosage = 11.1 mg/day) for the treatment of adolescents with schizophrenia (Kryzhanovskaya et al. 2009), 107 adolescents were randomly assigned to receive olanzapine (n = 72) or placebo (n = 35) for a 6-week trial. Olanzapine-treated adolescents had significant improvements on the Brief Psychiatric Rating Scale for Children (BPRS-C; Overall and Pfefferbaum 1984) and CGI-S compared with the placebo group. There was no significant difference in response rate (≥30% decrease in BPRS-C and CGI severity ≤3) between the olanzapine (37.5%) and placebo (25.7%) groups. Significantly more olanzapine-treated adolescents had treatment-emergent high AST/SGOT, ALT/SGPT, and prolactin and low bilirubin and hematocrit during treatment. There was a significant increase in fasting triglycerides at endpoint in the olanzapine-treated adolescents.

Risperidone

Positive findings were reported in a double-blind, placebo-controlled multicenter trial of risperidone in the treatment of adolescents with schizophrenia (Haas et al. 2007). One hundred sixty adolescents were randomly assigned to risperidone 1–3 mg/day (n = 55), risperidone 4–6 mg/day (n = 51), or placebo (n = 54) for a 6-week trial. Both dosage ranges of risperidone were significantly superior to placebo on the primary efficacy measure, Positive and Negative Syndrome Scale (PANSS) total change score at endpoint. The most common adverse events were somnolence (24%), agitation (15%), and headache (13%) in the risperidone 1–3 mg/day group. Extrapyramidal disorder (16%), dizziness (14%), and hypertonia (14%) were the most common adverse events in the risperidone 4–6 mg/day group. The investigators concluded that the overall risk-benefit ratio favored the lower dosage range of risperidone.

Aripiprazole

In a large double-blind, placebo-controlled multicenter trial of aripiprazole for the treatment of schizophrenia in adolescents (Findling et al. 2008), 302 adolescents were randomly assigned to receive aripiprazole 10 mg, aripiprazole 30 mg (after 5- or 11-day titration), or placebo over a 6-week period. Both the 10-mg and 30-mg doses of aripiprazole showed statistically significant differences from placebo on the PANSS total score at week 6. The most common adverse events associated with aripiprazole were extrapyramidal disorder, somnolence, and tremor.

Quetiapine

The efficacy of quetiapine in the treatment of schizophrenia in adolescents was evaluated in a 6-week double-blind, placebo-controlled trial in which subjects (N = 222) were randomly assigned to quetiapine 400 mg/day, quetiapine 800 mg/day, or placebo. Both quetiapine dosages were significantly superior to placebo in reduction of total PANSS scores (AstraZeneca 2011).

Comparison of Atypical Antipsychotics

In a 12-week open-label trial, risperidone (mean dosage = 1.6 mg/day) was compared with olanzapine (mean dosage = 8.2 mg/day) in the treatment of 25 children with schizophrenia (Mozes et al. 2006). Both treatment groups showed similar significant improvement as measured by PANSS total and subscale scores.

In an 8-week double-blind study, 50 children and adolescents (ages 8–19 years) with psychotic disorders were randomly assigned to receive risperidone (mean dosage = 4 mg/day), olanzapine (mean dosage = 12.3 mg/day), or haloperidol (mean dosage = 5 mg/day) (Sikich et al. 2004). Eighty-eight percent of patients treated with olanzapine, 74% treated with risperidone, and 53% treated with haloperidol met response criteria (CGI-I scores of much or very much improved and at least a 20% reduction in BPRS-C total score).

Clozapine was compared with olanzapine in an 8-week double-blind, randomized trial (Shaw et al. 2006). Twenty-five youths (ages 7–16 years) with schizophrenia who were resistant to treatment with at least two antipsychotics participated in the trial. Clozapine (mean dosage = 327 mg/day) showed significant improvement in all outcome measures, compared with olanzapine (mean dosage = 19.1 mg/day), which showed improvement on some outcome measures. Improvement in negative symptoms was significantly greater for the clozapine group.

In an 8-week double-blind trial comparing olanzapine and risperidone against the typical antipsychotic molindone in 116 children and adolescents with early-onset schizophrenia or schizoaffective disorder (Sikich et al. 2008), no significant differences were observed in rates of response (CGI-I score ≤2 and ≥20% reduction in PANSS total score) among the treatment groups (risperidone 46%, olanzapine 34%, and molindone 50%). Significantly greater weight gain occurred with olanzapine and risperidone compared with molindone.

A double-blind maintenance study followed this acute controlled trial in children and adolescents with early-onset schizophrenia or schizoaffective disorder (Findling et al. 2010). Among the 54 youths eligible for the maintenance phase, 14 (26%) completed 44 weeks of treatment. No significant differences were found among olanzapine, risperidone, and molindone in reduction of symptoms or time to discontinuation.

Typical Antipsychotics

Haloperidol

Haloperidol has been compared with placebo and other typical antipsychotics in controlled trials in youth. In a 10-week double-blind, placebo-controlled crossover study, the safety and efficacy of haloperidol were assessed in 12 hospitalized children (ages 5–12 years) with schizophrenia. Haloperidol (optimal dosage range = 0.5–3.5 mg/day) was significantly superior to placebo in improving overall clinical functioning and reducing ideas of reference, delusions, and hallucinations. Common side effects were acute dystonic reaction, drowsiness, and dizziness (Spencer et al. 1992).

Haloperidol and loxapine were compared in a 4-week double-blind, placebo-controlled study of 75 adolescent inpatients with schizophrenia. Both haloperidol and loxapine were significantly superior to placebo, and there was no significant difference in efficacy between the two medications. Response rates (based on CGI improvement) were 87.5% for loxapine, 70% for haloperidol, and 36.4% for placebo. Common side effects were sedation, extrapyramidal symptoms, and somnolence (Pool et al. 1976).

Thiothixene

Thiothixene was compared with thioridazine in a 6-week single-blind study in 21 adolescent inpatients with schizophrenia. Thiothixene (optimal mean dosage = 16.2 mg/day) and thioridazine (optimal mean dosage = 178 mg/day) were equally effective in controlling symptoms, although most of the adolescents continued to be quite impaired. Thiothixene was less sedating than thioridazine (Realmuto et al. 1984). Thiothixene was also compared with trifluoperazine in an 8-week double-blind study of 16 children (ages 8–15 years) with schizophrenia (Wolpert et al. 1967). The effects of both medications were similar in terms of decreasing avoidance behavior, reducing stereotypic behavior, and increasing peer socialization.

Clinical Recommendations for Schizophrenia

Both typical and atypical antipsychotics have demonstrated some effectiveness in the treatment of schizophrenia in youth, although the sample sizes have been small in the trials of typical antipsychotics. Given fewer reported extrapyramidal side effects and tardive dyskinesia with atypical antipsychotics, it would be reasonable to initiate treatment with an atypical antipsychotic for a child with schizophrenia. Clozapine, however, should not be initiated unless at least two other antipsychotics have been tried without success. It is important to monitor weight and metabolic parameters for children who receive atypical antipsychotics.

Antipsychotics should be administered at adequate dosages for a period of no less than 4–6 weeks in order to determine efficacy. If there is no response or if there are intolerable side effects, a trial of a different antipsychotic should be initiated (American Academy of Child and Adolescent Psychiatry 2001).

There are no data to guide maintenance treatment. Because the majority of youth will have a second psychotic episode within 5–7 years of stabilization, there is a significant risk of relapse with medication withdrawal (Kumra 2000). It is recommended that first-episode patients receive maintenance pharmacological treatment for 1–2 years after the initial episode, given the risk of relapse (American Academy of Child and Adolescent Psychiatry 2001). If medication discontinuation is attempted, the dosage should be gradually reduced over several months.

Autistic Disorder and Other Pervasive Developmental Disorders

The prevalence of autistic disorder and other pervasive developmental disorders is estimated to be up to 18.7 per 10,000 population (Howlin 2000). Core features of these disorders are impairments in communication and social skills and the restriction of interests and activities (American Psychiatric Association 2000). Associated behavioral features include hyperactivity, stereotypies, attentional problems, self-injurious behavior, aggression, mood lability, anxiety, obsessions, and compulsions. The majority of children with autistic disorder will continue to have significant social and communication impairments throughout adulthood (Buitelaar and Willemsen-Swinkels 2000).

Atypical Antipsychotics

Risperidone (≥5 years old) and aripiprazole (≥6 years old) have FDA approval for the treatment of irritability associated with autistic disorder.

Risperidone

One hundred one children ranging in age from 5 to 17 years with autistic disorder participated in an 8-week double-blind, placebo-controlled trial of risperidone (dosage range = 0.5–3.5 mg/day; mean dosage = 1.8 mg/day). A significantly greater positive response (defined as a 25% decrease in the irritability subscale of the Aberrant Behavior Checklist and a rating of much or very much improved on the CGI-I scale) was found for the risperidone group (69%) compared with the placebo group (12%). Adverse events of increased appetite, fatigue, drowsiness, dizziness, and drooling were more common in the risperidone group than in the placebo group. Mean weight gain was 2.7 kg in the risperidone group and 0.8 kg in the placebo group. An 18-month follow-up showed that the majority of subjects who responded to risperidone during intermediate-length treatment continued to show improvement (McDougle et al. 2004).

In an 8-week double-blind, placebo-controlled trial, 79 children (ages 5–12 years) with autism and other pervasive developmental disorders were randomly assigned to either placebo or risperidone (mean dosage = 1.5 mg/day). Risperidone-treated patients exhibited a 64% improvement over baseline irritability, compared with a 30.7% improvement in placebo-treated subjects (Shea et al. 2004).

In a 6-month placebo-controlled study of 40 children (ages 2–9 years) with autism, risperidone (1 mg/day) decreased aggressiveness, hyperactivity, and irritability and improved social responsiveness and nonverbal communication. Appetite increase, weight gain, sedation, and transient dyskinesias in the risperidone-treated children were reported (Nagaraj et al. 2006).

The long-term effects of risperidone were assessed in youth (ages 5–17 years) with autism spectrum disorders (Troost et al. 2005). Twenty-four youths received risperidone for 6 months, followed by a double-blind discontinuation to placebo or continued risperidone. Risperidone was superior to placebo in preventing relapse, with relapse rates of 25% and 75%, respectively.

The efficacy of risperidone and haloperidol was compared in an 8-week double-blind trial that included 30 children and adolescents with autistic disorder (Miral et al. 2008). Risperidone produced significantly greater reductions in scores on the Aberrant Behavior Checklist as well as on other scales used to assess symptoms of autism. An open-label continuation study (Gencer et al. 2008) of this controlled trial showed that risperidone-treated patients had greater improvement than haloperidol-treated patients on CGI ratings and on the Aberrant Behavior Checklist.

Aripriprazole

The efficacy of aripiprazole in the treatment of irritability was evaluated in 218 children and adolescents with autistic disorder in an 8-week double-blind, placebo-controlled trial (Marcus et al. 2009). Aripiprazole dosages were 5, 10, or 15 mg/day. Compared with placebo, all aripiprazole dosages produced significantly greater improvement on mean Aberrant Behavior Checklist irritability subscale scores. The most common adverse events were sedation, tremor, and somnolence. The efficacy of aripiprazole was assessed in another 8-week double-blind, placebo-controlled trial that included 98 children and adolescents with autistic disorder (Owen et al. 2009). Aripiprazole dosages were 5, 10, or 15 mg/day. Significantly greater improvements in mean Aberrant Behavior Checklist irritability subscale scores were seen with aripiprazole versus placebo. Rates of extrapyramidal symptom–related adverse events were 14.9% with aripiprazole and 8% with placebo.

Olanzapine

The efficacy of olanzapine was evaluated in an 8-week double-blind, placebo-controlled trial that included 11 children and adolescents with pervasive developmental disorders (Hollander et al. 2006). Rates of response (CGI-I score ≤2) were 50% for olanzapine-treated patients and 20% for placebo-treated patients. Olanzapine-treated patients experienced significantly greater weight gain (mean 7.5 lbs for olanzapine vs. 1.5 lbs for placebo-treated patients).

In a 12-week open-label study of olanzapine (mean dosage = 7.8 mg/day) in eight patients (ages 5–42 years) with autistic disorder or pervasive developmental disorder not otherwise specified, the six patients who completed the trial showed much or very much global improvement (Potenza et al. 1999). Significant improvements were found in hyperactivity, social relatedness, affectual responses, sensory responses, language usage, self-injurious behavior, aggression, irritability, anxiety, and depression. The most significant adverse effects were increased appetite and weight gain in six patients and sedation in three patients.

In a 3-month open study of olanzapine (dosage range = 1.25–20 mg/day) in 25 subjects (ages 6–16 years) with pervasive developmental disorder, significant global improvement was reported. The most common side effect was weight gain (mean = 4.8 kg) (Kemner et al. 2002).

Olanzapine was compared with haloperidol in a 6-week open trial in 12 children (ages 4–11 years) with autistic disorder (Malone et al. 2001). Both the olanzapine treatment (mean dosage = 7.9 mg/day) and the haloperidol treatment (mean dosage = 1.4 mg/day) reduced symptoms of social withdrawal and stereotypies and improved speech and object relations.

Quetiapine

The effectiveness of quetiapine (dosage range = 100–350 mg/day) was assessed in a 16-week open-label trial in six children with autistic disorder (Martin et al. 1999). No significant behavioral improvements were found from baseline to endpoint.

In a 12-week open-label study of quetiapine of nine adolescents (mean age = 14.6 years) with autistic disorder, only two patients were much or very much improved at study endpoint (Findling et al. 2004).

Ziprasidone

The efficacy of ziprasidone was evaluated in a 6-week open-label study in 12 adolescents with autism (Malone et al. 2007). Ziprasidone dosages ranged from 20 mg/day to 160 mg/day (mean dosage = 98.3 mg/day). Of the 12 patients, 9 (75%) were considered treatment responders (based on CGI-I scores ≤2). The mean change in QTc from baseline to endpoint was 14.7, which was a statistically significant increase. There was no significant weight change.

The efficacy and safety of ziprasidone in autistic children, adolescents, and young adults were evaluated in an open-label study in which 12 patients (ages 8–20 years) were treated with ziprasidone (mean daily dose = 59.23 mg) for at least 6 weeks (McDougle et al. 2002). Fifty percent of patients were responders based on a CGI Scale rating of much improved or very much improved. Transient sedation was the most common side effect.

Typical Antipsychotics

Haloperidol

Haloperidol has been the most widely studied typical antipsychotic for the treatment of autism in children and adolescents. In double-blind, placebo-controlled studies, haloperidol has been shown to be significantly superior to placebo in reducing maladaptive behaviors and facilitating learning on discrimination tasks (Campbell et al. 1982); in increasing retention of discrimination learning and decreasing maladaptive behaviors in the classroom (Anderson et al. 1984); in decreasing occurrence of stereotypies and increasing orienting reactions of children (Cohen et al. 1980); and in decreasing hyperactivity, temper tantrums, withdrawal, and stereotypies and increasing relatedness (Anderson et al. 1989). Optimal dosages of haloperidol in these studies ranged from 0.25 to 4 mg/day. The most common side effects were sedation, increased irritability, and acute dystonic reactions. Weight gain was modest (0.2 kg) in autistic children who received haloperidol 0.25–3.5 mg/day for a 6-month period (Silva et al. 1993).

The long-term efficacy of haloperidol was assessed in 48 children (ages 2–8 years) with autism who received haloperidol for 6 months (Perry et al. 1989). Haloperidol remained effective throughout the 6-month treatment period, and it was equally effective whether it was given continuously or on a discontinuous schedule consisting of 5 days on haloperidol and 2 days on placebo. Children who had symptoms of irritability, angry and labile affect, and uncooperativeness were the best responders to haloperidol.

Serotonin Reuptake Inhibitors

Fluoxetine

The efficacy of liquid fluoxetine in treating repetitive behaviors in autism was assessed in 45 children and adolescents with autism spectrum disorders. Subjects were randomly assigned to two 8-week acute phases in a double-blind crossover study (Hollander et al. 2005). Low-dose liquid fluoxetine (mean dosage = 9.9 mg/day) was superior to placebo in reducing repetitive behaviors.

In an open study of fluoxetine (dosage range = 20 mg every other day to 80 mg/day) in 23 patients (ages 7–28 years) with autistic disorder, 15 patients (65%) experienced significant clinical global improvement (Cook et al. 1992). The most common side effects were restlessness, hyperactivity, agitation, decreased appetite, and insomnia.

Fluvoxamine

A double-blind, placebo-controlled study of fluvoxamine treatment (mean dosage = 106.9 mg/day) in 34 children and adolescents with autistic disorder did not find significant clinical improvement with fluvoxamine (McDougle et al. 2000).

Sertraline

Open-label sertraline (dosage range = 25–50 mg/day) was administered to nine children with autistic disorder (Steingard et al. 1997). Eight of the nine patients showed clinically significant improvement in ability to tolerate changes in their routine or environment without displaying symptoms of anxiety, irritability, or agitation.

Citalopram

The efficacy of citalopram was evaluated for treatment of repetitive behavior in children with autistic spectrum disorders (King et al. 2009). One hundred forty-nine children and adolescents with autistic spectrum disorders were randomly assigned to receive citalopram or placebo in a 12-week controlled trial. The mean dosage of citalopram at endpoint was 16.5 mg/day. There was no significant difference in rates of response (CGI-I score ≤2) between citalopram-treated patients (39.2%) and placebo-treated patients (34.2%). No difference was found in reduction in CY-BOCS scores between the citalopram group and the placebo group. Adverse events that were significantly more common in the citalopram group were increased energy level, impulsiveness, hyperactivity, stereotypy, decreased concentration, diarrhea, insomnia, and dry skin or pruritus.

Escitalopram

In a 10-week open-label study, 28 children and adolescents (ages 6–17 years) with pervasive developmental disorder received escitalopram. There was significant improvement in irritability and clinical global functioning. Twenty-five percent of youths responded at escitalopram daily doses less than 10 mg, and 36% of youths responded at doses greater than or equal to 10 mg (Owley et al. 2005).

Other Antidepressants

Clomipramine

The results of controlled trials with clomipramine in the treatment of autistic disorder have yielded mixed results. Clomipramine and haloperidol were compared in a placebo-controlled crossover study for 7 weeks with active treatment (Remington et al. 2001). Thirty-six patients (ages 10–36 years) with autistic disorder were randomly assigned to clomipramine (mean dosage = 128.4 mg/day; range = 100–150 mg/day), haloperidol (mean dosage = 1.3 mg/day; range = 1–1.5 mg), or placebo. A significant advantage for haloperidol was found on global measures of autistic symptom severity and on specific measures of irritability and hyperactivity. Clomipramine was comparable to haloperidol only among patients who were able to complete a full therapeutic trial. However, significantly fewer patients receiving clomipramine versus haloperidol were able to complete the trial (37.5% vs. 69.7%, respectively) for reasons related to inefficacy, side effects, or behavioral problems.

Mirtazapine

In an open-label study of mirtazapine (dosage range = 7.5–45 mg/day; mean = 30.3 mg/day) in 26 patients (ages 3–23 years) with pervasive developmental disorders, 9 patients (34.6%) were judged much or very much improved in symptoms of aggression, self-injury, irritability, hyperactivity, anxiety, depression, and insomnia (Posey et al. 2001). Mirtazapine did not improve symptoms of social or communication impairment. Common side effects included increased appetite, irritability, and transient sedation.

Venlafaxine

The effectiveness of venlafaxine was assessed in an open retrospective study of 10 patients (ages 3–21 years) with pervasive developmental disorders (Hollander et al. 2000). Six of 10 patients who received venlafaxine (mean dosage = 24.4 mg/day; range = 6.25–50 mg/day) over an average of 5 months were much or very much improved. Improvements were observed in repetitive behaviors, restricted interests, social deficits, communication and language function, inattention, and hyperactivity. Side effects of venlafaxine included behavioral activation, nausea, inattention, and polyuria.

Mood Stabilizers

Lamotrigine

Twenty-eight children (ages 3–11 years) with autistic disorder participated in a double-blind, placebo-controlled study of lamotrigine (mean maintenance dosage = 5 mg/kg/day) for a 12-week study period (Belsito et al. 2001). There were no significant differences between the lamotrigine and placebo groups on severity of behavioral symptoms. Insomnia and hyperactivity were the most frequently reported side effects. No children in the study were withdrawn because of rash.

Other Agents

Clonidine

A double-blind, placebo-controlled crossover study with transdermal clonidine (0.005 mg/kg/day or placebo by a weekly transdermal patch) in nine patients (ages 5–33 years) with autistic disorder was conducted for a total 8-week active period (Fankhauser et al. 1992). Significant improvement with clonidine, compared with placebo, was found on measures of social relationship, affectual responses, and sensory responses. In a double-blind, placebo-controlled crossover trial of clonidine in eight children with autistic disorder, clonidine was found to be modestly effective in reducing irritability and hyperactivity (Jaselskis et al. 1992).

Methylphenidate

There have been two small double-blind, placebo-controlled crossover studies of methylphenidate for the treatment of autistic disorder in children ranging in age from 5 to 11 years. In a study that included 10 children, a modest but statistically significant improvement in hyperactivity was found with methylphenidate treatment, compared with placebo (Quintana et al. 1995). No significant side effects, such as worsening of behavior or of stereotypic movements, were observed. In a study that included 13 children, 6 patients had a significant decrease in hyperactivity, stereotypies, and inappropriate speech (Handen et al. 2000). However, no changes were found on the Child Autism Rating Scale. Significant adverse side effects occurred in some children and included social withdrawal and irritability, particularly at a methylphenidate dosage of 0.6 mg/kg/day.

Clinical Recommendations for Autistic Disorder and Other Pervasive Developmental Disorders

There is no evidence that pharmacotherapy is effective in treating the core social and communication deficits in autistic disorder. However, medications have been shown to be useful in treating associated symptoms, such as hyperactivity, inattention, stereotypies, self-injurious behavior, tantrums, aggression, mood lability, and anxiety. Antipsychotics may decrease withdrawal, stereotypies, and aggression and may facilitate learning. To date, the most data available support the use of risperidone or aripiprazole for treating irritability, aggression, self-injurious behavior, temper tantrums, and mood lability associated with autistic disorder in children and adolescents. Serotonin reuptake inhibitors and other antidepressants have been shown to reduce compulsions, anxiety, and depression in children with autism.

There are limited data on the long-term use of pharmacotherapy in children with autism. After receiving an intermediate-length (4–6 months) course of treatment with risperidone, children withdrawn from the medication through placebo substitution had high relapse rates (Research Units on Pediatric Psychopharmacology Autism Network et al. 2005; Troost et al. 2005). Therefore, clinicians must weigh the risk-benefit ratio of maintenance medication treatment in this population and carefully monitor children for side effects.

References

Allen AJ, Kurlan RM, Gilbert DL, et al: Atomoxetine treatment in children and adolescents with ADHD and comorbid tic disorders. Neurology 65:1941–1949, 2005

Aman MG, De Smedt G, Derivan A, et al: Double-blind, placebo-controlled study of risperidone for the treatment of disruptive behaviors in children with subaverage intelligence. Am J Psychiatry 159:1337–1346, 2002

Aman MG, Binder C, Turgay A: Risperidone effects in the presence/absence of psychostimulant medicine in children with ADHD, other disruptive behavior disorders, and subaverage IQ. J Child Adolesc Psychopharmacol 14:243–254, 2004

American Academy of Child and Adolescent Psychiatry: Practice parameters for the assessment and treatment of children and adolescents with obsessive-compulsive disorder. J Am Acad Child Adolesc Psychiatry 37 (10 suppl):27S–45S, 1998

American Academy of Child and Adolescent Psychiatry: Practice parameters for the assessment and treatment of children and adolescents with schizophrenia. J Am Acad Child Adolesc Psychiatry 40 (7 suppl):4S–23S, 2001

American Academy of Child and Adolescent Psychiatry: Practice parameter for the assessment and treatment of children and adolescents with attention-deficit/hyperactivity disorder. J Am Acad Child Adolesc Psychiatry 46:894–921, 2007

American Diabetes Association, American Psychiatric Association, American Association of Clinical Endocrinologists, et al: Consensus development conference on antipsychotic drugs and obesity and diabetes. Diabetes Care 27:596–601, 2004

American Psychiatric Association: Diagnostic and Statistical Manual of Mental Disorders, 3rd Edition, Revised. Washington, DC, American Psychiatric Association, 1987

American Psychiatric Association: Diagnostic and Statistical Manual of Mental Disorders, 4th Edition, Text Revision. Washington, DC, American Psychiatric Association, 2000

Anderson JC, Williams S, McGee R, et al: DSM-III disorders in preadolescent children. Prevalence in a large sample from the general population. Arch Gen Psychiatry 44:69–76, 1987

Anderson LT, Campbell M, Grega DM, et al: Haloperidol in the treatment of infantile autism: effects on learning and behavioral symptoms. Am J Psychiatry 141:1195–1202, 1984

Anderson LT, Campbell M, Adams P, et al: The effects of haloperidol on discrimination learning and behavioral symptoms in autistic children. J Autism Dev Disord 19:227–239, 1989

Armenteros JL, Lewis JE, Davalos M: Risperidone augmentation for treatment-resistant aggression in attention-deficit/hyperactivity disorder: a placebo-controlled pilot study. J Am Acad Child Adolesc Psychiatry 46:558–565, 2007

Arnold LE: Methylphenidate vs amphetamine: comparative review. J Attention Disord 3:200–211, 2000

AstraZeneca Pharmaceuticals: Seroquel (quetiapine fumarate) tablets, full prescribing information. Revised December 2011. Available at: http://www1.astrazeneca-us.com/pi/Seroquel.pdf. Accessed August 2012.

Barbey JT, Roose SP: SSRI safety in overdose. J Clin Psychiatry 59 (suppl 15):42–48, 1998

Barkley RA: Attention Deficit Hyperactivity Disorder: A Clinical Handbook, 3rd Edition. New York, Guilford, 2005

Barrickman LL, Perry PJ, Allen AJ, et al: Bupropion versus methylphenidate in the treatment of attention-deficit hyperactivity disorder. J Am Acad Child Adolesc Psychiatry 34:649–657, 1995

Belsito KM, Law PA, Kirk KS, et al: Lamotrigine therapy for autistic disorder: a randomized, double-blind, placebo-controlled trial. J Autism Dev Disord 31:175–181, 2001

Berard R, Fond R, Carpenter DJ, et al: An international, multicenter, placebo-controlled trial of paroxetine in adolescents with major depressive disorder. J Child Adolesc Psychopharmacol 16:59–75, 2006

Bernstein GA, Borchardt CM, Perwien AR: Anxiety disorders in children and adolescents: a review of the past 10 years. J Am Acad Child Adolesc Psychiatry 35:1110–1119, 1996

Biederman J, Spencer TJ: Psychopharmacological interventions. Child Adolesc Psychiatr Clin N Am 17:439–458, xi, 2008

Biederman J, Faraone SV, Marrs A, et al: Panic disorder and agoraphobia in consecutively referred children and adolescents. J Am Acad Child Adolesc Psychiatry 36:214–223, 1997

Biederman J, Mick E, Hammerness P, et al: Open-label, 8-week trial of olanzapine and risperidone for the treatment of bipolar disorder in preschool-age children. Biol Psychiatry 58:589–594, 2005

Biederman J, Mick E, Surman C, et al: A randomized, placebo-controlled trial of OROS methylphenidate in adults with attention-deficit/hyperactivity disorder. Biol Psychiatry 59:829–835, 2006a

Biederman J, Wigal SB, Spencer TJ, et al: A post hoc subgroup analysis of an 18-day randomized controlled trial comparing the tolerability and efficacy of mixed amphetamine salts extended release and atomoxetine in school-age girls with attention-deficit/hyperactivity disorder. Clin Ther 28:280–293, 2006b

Biederman J, Melmed RD, Patel A, et al: A randomized, double-blind, placebo-controlled study of guanfacine extended release in children and adolescents with attention-deficit/hyperactivity disorder. Pediatrics 121:e73–e84, 2008

Biederman J, Joshi G, Mick E, et al: A prospective open-label trial of lamotrigine monotherapy in children and adolescents with bipolar disorder. CNS Neurosci Ther 16:91–102, 2010

Birmaher B, Arbelaez C, Brent D: Course and outcome of child and adolescent major depressive disorder. Child Adolesc Psychiatry Clin North Am 11:619–637, 2002

Birmaher B, Axelson DA, Monk K, et al. Fluoxetine for the treatment of childhood anxiety disorders. J Am Acad Child Adolesc Psychiatry 42:415–423, 2003

Blader JC, Schooler NR, Jensen PS, et al: Adjunctive divalproex versus placebo for children with ADHD and aggression refractory to stimulant monotherapy. Am J Psychiatry 166:1392–1401, 2009

Blair J, Scahill L, State M, et al: Electrocardiographic changes in children and adolescents treated with ziprasidone: a prospective study. J Am Acad Child Adolesc Psychiatry 44:73–79, 2005

Brent DA, Holder D, Kolko D, et al: A clinical psychotherapy trial for adolescent depression comparing cognitive, family, and supportive therapy. Arch Gen Psychiatry 54:877–885, 1997

Brent DA, Emslie G, Clarke G, et al: Switching to another SSRI or to venlafaxine with or without cognitive behavioral therapy for adolescents with SSRI-resistant depression: the TORDIA randomized controlled trial. JAMA 299:901–913, 2008

Bridge JA, Iyengar S, Salary CB, et al: Clinical response and risk for reported suicidal ideation and suicide attempts in pediatric antidepressant treatment: a meta-analysis of randomized controlled trials. JAMA 297:1683–1696, 2007

Budman CL, Gayer A, Lesser M, et al: An open-label study of the treatment efficacy of olanzapine for Tourette's disorder. J Clin Psychiatry 62:290–294, 2001

Buitelaar JK, Willemsen-Swinkels SH: Medication treatment in subjects with autistic spectrum disorders. Eur Child Adolesc Psychiatry 9 (suppl 1): I85–I97, 2000

Buitelaar JK, Van der Gaag RJ, Cohen-Kettenis P, et al: A randomized controlled trial of risperidone in the treatment of aggression in hospitalized adolescents with subaverage cognitive abilities [comment]. J Clin Psychiatry 62:239–248, 2001

Bymaster FP, Katner JS, Nelson DL, et al: Atomoxetine increases extracellular levels of norepinephrine and dopamine in prefrontal cortex of rat: a potential mechanism for efficacy in attention deficit/hyperactivity disorder. Neuropsychopharmacology 27:699–711, 2002

Campbell M, Anderson LT, Small AM, et al: The effects of haloperidol on learning and behavior in autistic children. J Autism Dev Disord 12:167–175, 1982

Campbell M, Small AM, Green WH, et al: Behavioral efficacy of haloperidol and lithium carbonate: a comparison in hospitalized aggressive children with conduct disorder. Arch Gen Psychiatry 41:650–656, 1984

Campbell M, Adams PB, Small AM, et al: Lithium in hospitalized aggressive children with conduct disorder: a double blind and placebo controlled study. J Am Acad Child Adolesc Psychiatry 34:445–453, 1995

Cantwell DP, Swanson J, Connor DF: Case study: adverse response to clonidine. J Am Acad Child Adolesc Psychiatry 36:539–544, 1997

Chambers WJ, Puig-Antich J, Hirsch M, et al: The assessment of affective disorders in children and adolescents by semistructured interview. Test-retest reliability of the Schedule for Affective Disorders and Schizophrenia for School-Age Children, Present Episode Version. Arch Gen Psychiatry 42:696–702, 1985

Chappell PB, Riddle MA, Scahill L, et al: Guanfacine treatment of comorbid attention-deficit hyperactivity disorder and Tourette's syndrome: preliminary clinical experience. J Am Acad Child Adolesc Psychiatry 34:1140–1146, 1995

Charach A, Figueroa M, Chen S, et al: Stimulant treatment over 5 years: effects on growth. J Am Acad Child Adolesc Psychiatry 45:415–421, 2006

Chavira DA, Stein MB: Combined psychoeducation and treatment with selective serotonin reuptake inhibitors for youth with generalized social anxiety disorder. J Child Adolesc Psychopharmacol 12:47–54, 2002

Clark DB, Birmaher B, Axelson D, et al: Fluoxetine for the treatment of childhood anxiety disorder: open-label, long-term extension to a controlled trial. J Am Acad Child Adolesc Psychiatry 44:1263–1270, 2005

Clarke GN, Sack WH, Ben R, et al: English language skills in a group of previously traumatized Khmer adolescent refugees. J Nerv Ment Dis 181:454–456, 1993

Cohen JA, Mannarino AP, Perel JM, et al: A pilot randomized controlled trial of combined trauma-focused CBT and sertraline for childhood PTSD symptoms. J Am Acad Child Adolesc Psychiatry 46:811–819, 2007

Cohen IL, Campbell M, Posner D, et al: Behavioral effects of haloperidol in young autistic children. An objective analysis using a within-subjects reversal design. J Am Acad Child Psychiatry 19:665–677, 1980

Comings DE, Himes JA, Comings BG: An epidemiologic study of Tourette's syndrome in a single school district. J Clin Psychiatry 51:463–469, 1990

Compton SN, Grant PJ, Chrisman AK, et al: Sertraline in children and adolescents with social anxiety disorder. J Am Acad Adolesc Psychiatry 40:564–571, 2001

Conners CK, Casat CD, Gualtieri CT, et al: Bupropion hydrochloride in attention deficit disorder with hyperactivity. J Am Acad Child Adolesc Psychiatry 35:1314–1321, 1996

Connor DF, Fletcher KE, Swanson JM: A meta-analysis of clonidine for symptoms of attention-deficit hyperactivity disorder. J Am Acad Child Adolesc Psychiatry 38:1551–1559, 1999

Connor DF, Barkley RA, Davis HT: A pilot study of methylphenidate, clonidine, or the combination in ADHD comorbid with aggressive oppositional defiant disorder or conduct disorder. Clin Pediatr 39:15–25, 2000

Connor DF, Glatt SJ, Lopez ID, et al: Psychopharmacology and aggression, I: a meta-analysis of stimulant effects on overt/covert aggression-related behaviors in ADHD. J Am Acad Child Adolesc Psychiatry 41:253–261, 2002

Cook EH, Rowlett R, Jaselskis C, et al: Fluoxetine treatment of children and adults with autistic disorder and mental retardation. J Am Acad Child Adolesc Psychiatry 31:739–745, 1992

Cook EH, Wagner KD, March JS, et al: Long-term sertraline treatment of children and adolescents with obsessive-compulsive disorder. J Am Acad Child Adolesc Psychiatry 40:1175–1181, 2001

Copur M, Arpaci B, Demir T, et al: Clinical effectiveness of quetiapine in children and adolescents with Tourette's syndrome: a retrospective case-note survey. Clin Drug Investig 27:123–130, 2007

Correll CU, Carlson HE: Endocrine and metabolic adverse effects of psychotropic medications in children and adolescents. J Am Acad Child Adolesc Psychiatry 45:771–791, 2006

Correll CU, Penzer JB, Parikh UH, et al: Recognising and monitoring adverse events of second-generation antipsychotics in children and adolescents. Child Adolesc Psychiatric Clin N Am 15:177–206, 2006

Correll CU, Sheridan EM, DelBello MP: Antipsychotic and mood stabilizer efficacy and tolerability in pediatric and adult patients with bipolar I mania: a comparative analysis of acute, randomized, placebo-controlled trials. Bipolar Disord 12:116–141, 2010

Cummings DD, Singer HS, Krieger M, et al: Neuropsychiatric effects of guanfacine in children with mild Tourette syndrome: a pilot study. Clin Neuropharmacol 25:325–332, 2002

Davanzo PA, McCracken JT: Mood stabilizers in the treatment of juvenile bipolar disorder: advances and controversies. Child Adolesc Psychiatr Clin N Am 9:159–182, 2000

Davies L, Stern JS, Agrawal N, et al: A case series of patients with Tourette's syndrome in the United Kingdom treated with aripiprazole. Hum Psychopharmacol. 21:447–453, 2006

Daviss WB, Bentivoglio P, Racusin R, et al: Bupropion sustained release in adolescents with comorbid attention-deficit/hyperactivity disorder and depression. J Am Acad Child Adolesc Psychiatry 40:307–314, 2001

DelBello MP, Kowatch RA: Pharmacological interventions for bipolar youth: developmental considerations. Dev Psychopathol 18:1231–1246, 2006

DelBello M, Schwiers ML, Rosenberg HL: A double-blind, randomized, placebo-controlled study of quetiapine as adjunctive treatment for adolescent mania. J Am Acad Child Adolesc Psychiatry 41:1216–1223, 2002

DelBello MP, Findling RL, Kushner S, et al: A pilot controlled trial of topiramate for mania in children and adolescents with bipolar disorder. J Am Acad Child Adolesc Psychiatry 44:539–547, 2005

DelBello MP, Kowatch RA, Adler CM, et al: A double-blind randomized pilot study comparing quetiapine and divalproex for adolescent mania. J Am Acad Child Adolesc Psychiatry 45:305–313, 2006

DelBello MP, Findling RL, Earley WR, et al: Efficacy of quetiapine in children and adolescents with bipolar mania: a 3-week, double-blind, randomized, placebo-controlled trial. Presented at the 46th Annual Meeting of the American College of Neuropsychopharmacology, Boca Raton, FL, December 9–13, 2007

DelBello MP, Findling R, Wang RP, et al: Safety and efficacy of ziprasidone in pediatric bipolar disorder. Presented at the 63rd Annual Meeting of the Society of Biological Psychiatry, Washington, DC, May 1–3, 2008

DeLong GR, Nieman GW: Lithium-induced behavior changes in children with symptoms suggesting manic-depressive illness. Psychopharmacol Bull 19:258–265, 1983

DeVeaugh-Geiss J, Moroz G, Biederman J, et al: Clomipramine hydrochloride in childhood and adolescent obsessive-compulsive disorder—a multicenter trial. J Am Acad Child Adolesc Psychiatry 31:45–49, 1992

Dion Y, Annable L, Sandor P, et al: Risperidone in the treatment of Tourette syndrome: a double blind, placebo controlled trial. J Clin Psychopharmacol 22:31–39, 2002

Donovan SJ, Stewart JW, Nunes EV, et al: Divalproex treatment for youth with explosive temper and mood lability: a double-blind, placebo-controlled crossover design. Am J Psychiatry 157:818–820, 2000

Douglass HM, Moffitt TE, Dar R, et al: Obsessive-compulsive disorder in a birth cohort of 18-year-olds: prevalence and predictors. J Am Acad Child Adolesc Psychiatry 34:1424–1431, 1995

Dunn V, Goodyer IM: Longitudinal investigation into childhood- and adolescence-onset depression: psychiatric outcome in early adulthood. Br J Psychiatry 188:216–222, 2006

Eggers C, Bunk D: The long-term course of childhood-onset schizophrenia: a 42-year follow-up. Schizophr Bull 23:105–117, 1997

Emslie GJ, Rush AJ, Weinberg WA, et al: A double-blind, randomized, placebo-controlled trial of fluoxetine in children and adolescents with depression. Arch Gen Psychiatry 54:1031–1037, 1997

Emslie GJ, Wagner KD, Riddle M, et al: Efficacy and safety of paroxetine in juvenile OCD. Poster presented at the 153rd annual meeting of the American Psychiatric Association, Chicago, IL, May 13–18, 2000

Emslie GJ, Heiligenstein JH, Wagner KD, et al: Fluoxetine for acute treatment of depression in children and adolescents: a placebo-controlled, randomized clinical trial. J Am Acad Child Adolesc Psychiatry 41:1205–1215, 2002

Emslie GJ, Wagner KD, Kutcher S, et al: Paroxetine treatment in children and adolescents with major depressive disorder: a randomized, multicenter, double-blind, placebo-controlled trial. J Am Acad Child Adolesc Psychiatry 45:709–719, 2006

Emslie GJ, Findling RL, Yeung PP, et al: Venlafaxine ER for the treatment of pediatric subjects with depression: results of two placebo-controlled trials. J Am Acad Child Adolesc Psychiatry 46:479–488, 2007a

Emslie GJ, Yeung PP, Kunz NR: Long-term, open-label venlafaxine extended-release treatment in children and adolescents with major depressive disorder. CNS Spectr 12:223–233, 2007b

Emslie GJ, Ventura D, Korotzer A, et al: Escitalopram in the treatment of adolescent depression: a randomized placebo-controlled multisite trial. J Am Acad Child Adolesc Psychiatry 48:721–729, 2009

Famularo R, Kinscherff R, Fenton T: Propranolol treatment for childhood posttraumatic stress disorder, acute type: a pilot study. Am J Dis Child 142:1244–1247, 1988

Fankhauser MP, Karumanchi VC, German ML, et al: A double blind, placebo-controlled study of the efficacy of transdermal clonidine in autism. J Clin Psychiatry 53:77–82, 1992

Fenichel R: Combining methylphenidate and clonidine: the role of post-marketing surveillance. J Child Adolesc Psychopharmacol 5:155–156, 1995

Findling RL, McNamara NK, Gracious BL, et al: Combination lithium and divalproex sodium in pediatric bipolarity. J Am Acad Child Adolesc Psychiatry 42:895–901, 2003

Findling RL, McNamara NK, Gracious BL: Quetiapine in nine youths with autistic disorder. J Child Adolesc Psychopharmacol 14:287–294, 2004

Findling RL, McNamara NK, Youngstrom EA, et al: Double-blind 18-month trial of lithium versus divalproex maintenance treatment in pediatric bipolar disorder. J Am Acad Child Adolesc Psychiatry 44:409–417, 2005

Findling RL, Reed MD, O'Riordan MA, et al: Effectiveness, safety, and pharmacokinetics of quetiapine in aggressive children with conduct disorder. J Am Acad Child Adolesc Psychiatry 45:792–800, 2006

Findling RL, Robb A, Nyilas M, et al: A multiple-center, randomized, double-blind, placebo-controlled study of oral aripiprazole for treatment of adolescents with schizophrenia. Am J Psychiatry 165:1432–1441, 2008

Findling RL, Nyilas M, Forbes RA, et al: Acute treatment of pediatric bipolar I disorder, manic or mixed episode, with aripiprazole: a randomized, double-blind, placebo-controlled study. J Clin Psychiatry 70:1441–1451, 2009

Findling RL, Johnson JL, McClellan J, et al: Double-blind maintenance safety and effectiveness findings from the treatment of early-onset schizophrenia spectrum (TEOSS) study. J Am Acad Child Adolesc Psychiatry 49:583–594, 2010

Flament MF, Rapoport JL, Berg CJ, et al: Clomipramine treatment of childhood obsessive-compulsive disorder. A double-blind controlled study. Arch Gen Psychiatry 42:977–983, 1985

Fristad MA, Goldberg-Arnold JS, Gavazzi SM, et al: Multifamily psychoeducation groups in the treatment of children with mood disorders. J Marital Fam Ther 29:491–504, 2003

Gaffney GR, Perry PJ, Lund BC, et al: Risperidone versus clonidine in the treatment of children and adolescents with Tourette's syndrome. J Am Acad Child Adolesc Psychiatry 41:330–336, 2002

Geller B, Cooper TB, Sun K, et al: Double blind and placebo controlled study of lithium for adolescent bipolar disorders with secondary substance dependency. J Am Acad Child Adolesc Psychiatry 37:171–178, 1998

Geller B, Zimerman B, Williams M, et al: Diagnostic characteristics of 93 cases of prepubertal and early adolescent bipolar disorder phenotype by gender, puberty and comorbid attention deficit hyperactivity disorder. J Child Adolesc Psychopharmacol 10:157–164, 2000

Geller B, Tillman MS, Craney JL, et al: Four-year prospective outcome and natural history of mania in children with a prepubertal and early adolescent bipolar disorder phenotype. Arch Gen Psychiatry 61:459–467, 2004

Geller DA, Hoog SL, Heiligenstein JH, et al: Fluoxetine treatment for obsessive-compulsive disorder in children and adolescents: a placebo-controlled clinical trial. J Am Acad Child Adolesc Psychiatry 40:773–779, 2001

Geller DA, Wagner KD, Emslie G, et al: Paroxetine treatment in children and adolescents with obsessive-compulsive disorder: a randomized, multicenter, double-blind, placebo-controlled trial. J Am Acad Child Adolesc Psychiatry 43:1387–1396, 2004

Gelperin K: Psychiatric adverse events associated with drug treatment of ADHD: review of postmarketing safety data. U.S. Food and Drug Administration Pediatric Advisory Committee, March 22, 2006. Available at: http://www.fda.gov/ohrms/dockets/ac/06/slides/2006-4210s_15_Gelperin_Review%20of%20Postmarking%20Safety.ppt. Accessed December 2008.

Gencer O, Emiroglu FN, Miral S, et al: Comparison of long-term efficacy and safety of risperidone and haloperidol in children and adolescents with autistic disorder. Eur Child Adolesc Psychiatry 17:217–225, 2008

Gibbons RD, Hur K, Bhaumik DK, et al: The relationship between antidepressant prescription rates and rate of early adolescent suicide. Am J Psychiatry 163:1898–1904, 2006

Gilbert DL, Batterson JR, Sethuraman G, et al: Tic reduction with risperidone versus pimozide in a randomized, double-blind, crossover trial. J Am Acad Child Adolesc Psychiatry 43:206–214, 2004

Gittelman-Klein R, Mannuzza S: Hyperactive boys almost grown up, III: methylphenidate effects on ultimate height. Arch Gen Psychiatry 45:1131–1134, 1988

Glod CA, Lynch A, Flynn E, et al: Bupropion SR in the treatment of adolescent depression. Poster presented at the 40th Annual Meeting of the New Clinical Drug Evaluation Unit, Boca Raton, FL, 2000

Goetz CG, Tanner CM, Wilson RS, et al: Clonidine and Gilles de la Tourette's syndrome: double-blind study using objective rating methods. Ann Neurol 21:307–310, 1987

Goodman WK, Price LH, Rasmusen SA, et al: Children's Yale-Brown Obsessive Compulsive Scale (CY-BOCS). New Haven, CT, Department of Psychiatry, Yale University School of Medicine, 1991

Goodyer IM, Dubicka B, Wilkinson P, et al: A randomised controlled trial of cognitive behaviour therapy in adolescents with major depression treated by selective serotonin reuptake inhibitors. The ADAPT trial. Health Technol Assess 12(14):iii–iv, ix–60, 2008

Grados M, Scahill L, Riddle MA: Pharmacotherapy in children and adolescents with obsessive-compulsive disorder. Child Adolesc Clin N Am 8:617–634, 1999

Gram LF, Rafaelsen OJ: Lithium treatment of psychotic children and adolescents. A controlled clinical trial. Acta Psychiatr Scand 48:253–260, 1972

Green WH: Child and Adolescent Clinical Psychopharmacology, 3rd Edition. Philadelphia, PA, Lippincott Williams & Wilkins, 2001

Greenhill LL, Halperin JM, Abikoff H: Stimulant medications. J Am Acad Child Adolesc Psychiatry 38:503–512, 1999

Greenhill LL, Kollins S, Abikoff H, et al: Efficacy and safety of immediate-release methylphenidate treatment for preschoolers with ADHD. J Am Acad Child Adolesc Psychiatry 45:1284–1293, 2006

Greist JH, Jefferson JW, Kobak KA, et al: Efficacy and tolerability of serotonin transport inhibitors in obsessive-compulsive disorder. Arch Gen Psychiatry 52:53–60, 1995

Gunther T, Herpertz-Dahlmann B, Jolles J, et al: The influence of risperidone on attentional functions in children and adolescents with attention-deficit/hyperactivity disorder and co-morbid disruptive behavior disorder. J Child Adolesc Psychopharmacol 16:725–735, 2006

Haas M, Unis AS, Copenhaver M, et al: Efficacy and safety of risperidone in adolescents with schizophrenia. Presented at the 160th Annual Meeting of the American Psychiatric Association, San Diego, CA, May 19–24, 2007

Haas M, DelBello MP, Pandina G, et al: Risperidone for the treatment of acute mania in children and adolescents with bipolar disorder: a randomized, double-blind, placebo-controlled study. Bipolar Disord 11:687–700, 2009

Hamilton BE, Minino AM, Martin JA, et al: Annual summary of vital statistics: 2005. Pediatrics 119:345–360, 2007

Hamilton M: The assessment of anxiety states by rating. Br J Med Psychol 32:50–55, 1959

Hamilton M: A rating scale for depression. J Neurol Neurosurg Psychiatry 23:56–62, 1960

Hammerness PG, Vivas FM, Geller DA: Selective serotonin reuptake inhibitors in pediatric psychopharmacology: a review of the evidence. J Pediatr 148:158–165, 2006

Handen BL, Johnson CR, Lubetsky M: Efficacy of methylphenidate among children with autism and symptoms of attention-deficit hyperactivity disorder. J Autism Dev Disord 30:245–255, 2000

Harmon RJ, Riggs PD: Clonidine for posttraumatic stress disorder in preschool children. J Am Acad Child Adolesc Psychiatry 35:1247–1249, 1996

Hazaray E, Ehret J, Posey DJ, et al: Intramuscular ziprasidone for acute agitation in adolescents. J Child Adolesc Psychopharmacol 14:464–470, 2004

Hazell PL, Stuart JE: A randomized controlled trial of clonidine added to psychostimulant medication for hyperactive and aggressive children. J Am Acad Child Adolesc Psychiatry 42:886–894, 2003

Hollander E, Kaplan A, Cartwright C, et al: Venlafaxine in children, adolescents, and young adults with autism spectrum disorders: an open retrospective clinical report. J Child Neurol 15:132–135, 2000

Hollander E, Phillips A, Chaplin W, et al: A placebo controlled crossover trial of liquid fluoxetine on repetitive behaviors in childhood and adolescent autism. Neuropsychopharmacology 30:582–589, 2005

Hollander E, Wasserman S, Swanson EN, et al: A double-blind placebo-controlled pilot study of olanzapine in childhood/adolescent pervasive developmental disorder. J Child Adolesc Psychopharmacol 16:541–548, 2006

Howlin P: Autism and intellectual disability: diagnostic and treatment issues. J R Soc Med 93:351–355, 2000

Hughes CW, Emslie GJ, Crismon MJ, et al: The Texas Children's Medication Algorithm Project: Update from Texas Consensus Conference Panel on Medication Treatment of Childhood Major Depressive Disorder. J Am Acad Child Adolesc Psychiatry 46:667–686, 2007

Hunt RD, Capper L, O'Connell P: Clonidine in child and adolescent psychiatry. J Child Adolesc Psychopharmacol 1:87–102, 1990

Hunt RD, Amsten AF, Asbell MD: An open trial of guanfacine in the treatment of attention-deficit hyperactivity disorder. J Am Acad Child Adolesc Psychiatry 34:50–54, 1995

Isolan L, Pheula G, Salum GA, et al: An open-label trial of escitalopram in children and adolescents with social anxiety disorder. J Child Adolesc Psychopharmacol 17:751–759, 2007

Jain R, Segal S, Kollins SH, et al: Clonidine extended-release tablets for pediatric patients with attention-deficit/hyperactivity disorder. J Am Acad Child Adolesc Psychiatry 50:171–179, 2011

Jaselskis CA, Cook EH, Fletcher KE, et al: Clonidine treatment of hyperactive and impulsive children with autistic disorder. J Clin Psychopharmacol 12:322–327, 1992

Kaufman J, Birmaher B, Brent D, et al: Schedule for Affective Disorders and Schizophrenia for School Age Children, Present and Lifetime Versions (K-SADS-PL): initial reliability and validity data. J Am Acad Child Adolesc Psychiatry 36:980–988, 1997

Kappagoda C, Schell DN, Hanson RM, et al: Clonidine overdose in childhood: implications of increased prescribing. J Paediatr Child Health 34:508–512, 1998

Kashani JH, Orvaschel H: Anxiety disorders in mid-adolescence: a community sample. Am J Psychiatry 145:960–964, 1988

Kashani JH, Sherman DD: Childhood depression: epidemiology, etiological models, and treatment implications. Integr Psychiatry 6:1–8, 1988

Keller MB, Lavori PW, Wunder J, et al: Chronic course of anxiety disorder in children and adolescents. J Am Acad Child Adolesc Psychiatry 31:595–599, 1992

Keller MB, Ryan ND, Strober M, et al: Efficacy of paroxetine in the treatment of adolescent major depression: a randomized, controlled trial. J Am Acad Child Adolesc Psychiatry 40:762–772, 2001

Kemner C, Willemsen-Swinkels SH, DeJonge M, et al: Open-label study of olanzapine in children with pervasive developmental disorder. J Clin Psychopharmacol 22:455–460, 2002

Kessler RC, Adler L, Barkley R, et al: The prevalence and correlates of adult ADHD in the United States: results from the National Comorbidity Survey Replication. Am J Psychiatry 163:716–723, 2006

Khan SS, Mican LM, Khan SS, et al: A naturalistic evaluation of intramuscular ziprasidone versus intramuscular olanzapine for the management of acute agitation and aggression in children and adolescents. J Child Adolesc Psychopharmacol 16:671–677, 2006

Kim BN, Lee CB, Hwang JW, et al: Effectiveness and safety of risperidone for children and adolescents with chronic tic or Tourette disorders in Korea. J Child Adolesc Psychopharmacol 15:318–324, 2005

King BH, Hollander E, Sikich L, et al: Lack of efficacy of citalopram in children with autism spectrum disorders and high levels of repetitive behavior. Arch Gen Psychiatry 66:583–590, 2009

Kisicki J, Fiske K, Scheckner B, et al: Abrupt cessation of guanfacine extended release in healthy young adults. Presented at the 53rd Annual Meeting of the American Academy of Child and Adolescent Psychiatry, San Diego, CA, October 24–29, 2006

Klein RG, Abikoff H, Klass E, et al: Clinical efficacy of methylphenidate in conduct disorder with and without attention deficit hyperactivity disorder. Arch Gen Psychiatry 54:1073–1080, 1997

Knorring A, Olsson GI, Thomsen PH, et al: A randomized, double-blind, placebo-controlled study of citalopram in adolescents with major depressive disorder. J Clin Psychopharmacol 26:311–315, 2006

Kofoed L, Tadepalli G, Oesterheld JR, et al: Case series: clonidine has no systematic effects on PR or QTc intervals in children. J Am Acad Child Adolesc Psychiatry 38:1193–1196, 1999

Kollins SH, Jain R, Brams M, et al: Clonidine extended-release tablets as add-on therapy to psychostimulants in children and adolescents with ADHD. Pediatrics 127:e1406–e1413, 2011

Kowatch RA, Carmody TJ, Suppes T, et al: Acute and continuation pharmacological treatment of children and adolescents with bipolar disorders: a summary of two previous studies. Acta Neuropsychiatrica 12:145–149, 2000a

Kowatch RA, Suppes T, Carmody TJ, et al: Effect size of lithium, divalproex sodium, and carbamazepine in children and adolescents with bipolar disorder. J Am Acad Child Adolesc Psychiatry 39:713–720, 2000b

Kowatch RA, Fristad M, Birmaher B, et al: Treatment guidelines for children and adolescents with bipolar disorder. J Am Acad Child Adolesc Psychiatry 44:213–235, 2005

Kowatch RA, Findling RL, Scheffer RE, et al: Pediatric bipolar collaborative mood stabilizer trial. Presented at the 54th Annual Meeting of the American Academy of Child and Adolescent Psychiatry, Boston, MA, October 23–28, 2007

Kramer JR, Loney J, Ponto LB, et al: Predictors of adult height and weight in boys treated with methylphenidate for childhood behavior problems. J Am Acad Child Adolesc Psychiatry 39:517–524, 2000

Krasny L, Williams BJ, Provencal S, et al: Social skills interventions for the autism spectrum: essential ingredients and a model curriculum. Child Adolesc Psychiatric Clin N Am 12:107–122, 2003

Kratochvil CJ, Heiligenstein JH, Dittmann R, et al: Atomoxetine and methylphenidate treatment in children with ADHD: a prospective, randomized, open-label trial. J Am Acad Child Adolesc Psychiatry 41:776–784, 2002

Kratochvil CJ, Vaughan BS, Harrington MJ, et al: Atomoxetine: a selective noradrenaline reuptake inhibitor for the treatment of attention-deficit/hyperactivity disorder. Expert Opin Pharmacother 4:1165–1174, 2003

Kroes M, Kalfe AC, Kessels AG, et al: Child psychiatric diagnoses in a population of Dutch schoolchildren aged 6 to 8 years. J Am Acad Child Adolesc Psychiatry 40:1401–1409, 2001

Kryzhanovskaya L, Schulz S, McDougle C, et al: Olanzapine versus placebo in adolescents with schizophrenia: a 6-week, randomized, double-blind, placebo-controlled trial. J Am Acad Child Adolesc Psychiatry 48:60–70, 2009

Kumra S: The diagnosis and treatment of children and adolescents with schizophrenia: "My mind is playing tricks on me." Child Adolesc Psychiatr Clin N Am 9:183–199, 2000

Kumra S, Frazier JA, Jacobsen LK, et al: Childhood-onset schizophrenia. A double-blind clozapine-haloperidol comparison. Arch Gen Psychiatry 53:1090–1097, 1996

Kutcher SP, MacKenzie S: Successful clonazepam treatment of adolescents with panic disorder. J Clin Psychopharmacol 8:299–301, 1988

Kutcher SP, Reiter S, Gardner DM, et al: The pharmacotherapy of anxiety disorders in children and adolescents. Psychiatr Clin North Am 15: 41–67, 1992

Law SF, Schachar RJ: Do typical clinical doses of methylphenidate cause tics in children treated for attention-deficit hyperactivity disorder? J Am Acad Child Adolesc Psychiatry 38:944–951, 1999

LeBlanc JC, Binder CE, Armenteros JL, et al: Risperidone reduces aggression in boys with a disruptive behaviour disorder and below average intelligence quotient: analysis of two placebo-controlled randomized trials. Int Clin Psychopharmacol 20:275–283, 2005

Leckman JF: Tourette's syndrome. Lancet 360:1577–1586, 2002

Leckman JF, Detlor J, Harcherik DF, et al: Short- and long-term treatment of Tourette's syndrome with clonidine: a clinical perspective. Neurology 35:343–351, 1985

Leckman JF, Hardin MT, Riddle MA, et al: Clonidine treatment of Gilles De La Tourette's syndrome. Arch Gen Psychiatry 48:324–328, 1991

Lena B: Lithium in child and adolescent psychiatry. Arch Gen Psychiatry 36:854–855, 1979

Lepola U, Leinonen E, Koponen H: Citalopram in the treatment of early onset panic disorder and school phobia. Pharmacopsychiatry 29:30–32, 1996

Lewinsohn PM, Klein DN, Seeley JR: Bipolar disorders in a community sample of older adolescents: prevalence, phenomenology, comorbidity, and course. J Am Acad Child Adolesc Psychiatry 34:454–463, 1995

Libby AM, Brent DA, Morrato EH, et al: Decline in treatment of pediatric depression after FDA advisory on risk suicidality with SSRIs. Am J Psychiatry 164:884–891, 2007

Liberthson RR: Sudden death from cardiac causes in children and young adults. N Engl J Med 334:1039–1044, 1996

Lichter DG, Jackson LA: Predictors of clonidine response in Tourette's syndrome: implications and inferences. J Child Neurol 11:93–97, 1996

Liebowitz MR, Turner SM, Piacentini J, et al: Fluoxetine in children and adolescents with OCD: a placebo-controlled trial. J Am Acad Child Adolesc Psychiatry 41:1431–1438, 2002

Looff D, Grimley P, Kuller F, et al: Carbamazepine for PTSD. J Am Acad Child Adolesc Psychiatry 34:703–704, 1995

Malone RP, Delaney MA, Luebbert JF, et al: A double-blind placebo-controlled study of lithium in hospitalized aggressive children and adolescents with conduct disorder. Arch Gen Psychiatry 57:649–654, 2000

Malone RP, Cater J, Sheikh RM, et al: Olanzapine versus haloperidol in children with autistic disorder: an open pilot study. J Am Acad Child Adolesc Psychiatry 40:887–894, 2001

Malone RP, Delaney MA, Hyman SB, et al: Ziprasidone in adolescents with autism: an open-label pilot study. J Child Adolesc Psychopharmacol 17:779–790, 2007

March JS, Biederman J, Wolkow R, et al: Sertraline in children and adolescents with obsessive-compulsive disorder: a multicenter randomized controlled trial. JAMA 280:1752–1756, 1998

March JS, Entusah R, Rynn M, et al: A randomized controlled trial of venlafaxine ER versus placebo in pediatric social anxiety disorder. Biol Psychiatry 62:1149–1154, 2007

Marcus RN, Owen, R, Kamen, L, et al: A placebo-controlled, fixed-dose study of aripiprazole in children and adolescents with irritability associated with autistic disorder. J Am Acad Child Adolesc Psychiatry 48:1110–1119, 2009

Markowitz S, Cuellar A: Antidepressants and youth: healing or harmful? Soc Sci Med 64:2138–2151, 2007

Martin A, Koenig K, Scahill L, et al: Open-label quetiapine in the treatment of children and adolescents with autistic disorder. J Child Adolesc Psychopharmacol 9:99–107, 1999

Masi G, Toni C, Mucci M, et al: Paroxetine in child and adolescent outpatients with panic disorder. J Child Adolesc Psychopharmacol 11:151–157, 2001

Masi G, Millepiedi S, Perugi G, et al: Pharmacotherapy in paediatric obsessive-compulsive disorder: a naturalistic, retrospective study. CNS Drugs 23:241–252, 2009

Masi G, Pfanner C, Millepiedi S, et al: Aripiprazole augmentation in 39 adolescents with medication-resistant obsessive-compulsive disorder. J Clin Psychopharmacol 30:688–693, 2010

McClellan J, Werry J: Practice parameter for the assessment and treatment of children and adolescents with schizophrenia. American Academy of Child and Adolescent Psychiatry. J Am Acad Child Adolesc Psychiatry 40 (7 suppl):4S–23S, 2001

McClellan J, Kowatch R, Findling RL: Practice parameter for the assessment and treatment of children and adolescents with bipolar disorder. J Am Acad Child Adolesc Psychiatry 46:107–125, 2007

McDougle CJ, Kresch LE, Posey DJ: Repetitive thoughts and behavior in pervasive developmental disorders: treatment with serotonin reuptake inhibitors. J Autism Dev Disord 30:427–435, 2000

McDougle CJ, Kem DL, Posey DJ: Case series: use of ziprasidone for maladaptive symptoms in youths with autism. J Am Acad Child Adolesc Psychiatry 41:921–927, 2002

McDougle CJ, Martin A, Aman M, et al: New findings from the RUPP autism network study of risperidone. Presented at the 51st Annual Meeting of the American Academy of Child and Adolescent Psychiatry, Washington, DC, October 19–24, 2004

McKnew DH, Cytryn L, Buchsbaum MS, et al: Lithium in children of lithium-responding parents. Psychiatry Res 4:171–180, 1981

Mei Z, Grummer-Strawn LM, Thompson D, et al: Shifts in percentiles of growth during early childhood: analysis of longitudinal data from the California Child Health and Development Study. Pediatrics 113:e617–e627, 2004

Melmed RD, Patel A, Konow J, et al: Efficacy and safety of guanfacine extended release for ADHD treatment. Presented at the 53rd Annual Meeting of the American Academy of Child and Adolescent Psychiatry, San Diego, CA, October 24–29, 2006

Melvin GA, Tonge BJ, King NJ, et al: A comparison of cognitive-behavioral therapy, sertraline, and their combination for adolescent depression. J Am Acad Child Adolescent Psychiatry 45: 1151–1161, 2006

Messenheimer JA: Rash in adult and pediatric patients treated with lamotrigine. Can J Neurol Sci 25:S14–S18, 1998

Michelson D, Faries D, Wernicke J, et al: Atomoxetine in the treatment of children and adolescents with attention-deficit/hyperactivity disorder: a randomized, placebo-controlled, dose-response study. Pediatrics 108:1–9, 2001

Michelson D, Allen AJ, Busner J, et al: Once-daily atomoxetine treatment for children and adolescents with attention deficit hyperactivity disorder: a randomized, placebo-controlled study. Am J Psychiatry 159:1896–1901, 2002

Michelson D, Adler L, Spencer T, et al: Atomoxetine in adults with ADHD: two randomized, placebo-controlled studies. Biol Psychiatry 53:112–120, 2003

Miral S, Gencer O, Inal-Emiroglu FN, et al: Risperidone versus haloperidol in children and adolescents with AD. A randomized, controlled, double-blind trial. Eur Child Adolesc Psychiatry 17:1–8, 2008

Molina BS, Hinshaw SP, Swanson JM, et al: MTA at 8 years: prospective follow-up of children treated for combined-type ADHD in a multisite study. J Am Acad Child Adolesc Psychiatry 48:484–500, 2009

Montgomery SA, Asberg M: A new depression scale designed to be sensitive to change. Br J Psychiatry 134:382–389, 1979

Mosholder A: Psychiatric adverse events in clinical trials of drugs for attention deficit hyperactivity disorder (ADHD). FDA Report PID D060163. U.S. Food and Drug Administration, March 3, 2006. Available at: http://www.fda.gov/ohrms/dockets/ac/06/briefing/2006-4210b_10_01_Mosholder.pdf. Accessed September 2012.

Mozes T, Ebert T, Michal SE, et al: An open-label randomized comparison of olanzapine versus risperidone in the treatment of childhood-onset schizophrenia. J Child Adolesc Psychopharmacol 16:393–403, 2006

MTA Cooperative Group: National Institute of Mental Health Multimodal Treatment Study of ADHD follow-up: changes in effectiveness and growth after the end of treatment. Pediatrics 113:762–769, 2004

MTA Cooperative Group: Effects of stimulant medication on growth rates across 3 years in the MTA follow-up. J Am Acad Child Adolesc Psychiatry 46:1015–1027, 2007

Mufson L, Sills R: Interpersonal Psychotherapy for depressed adolescents (IPT-A): an overview. Nord J Psychiatry 60:431–437, 2006

Mukaddes NM, Abali O: Quetiapine treatment of children and adolescents with Tourette's disorder. J Child Adolesc Psychopharmacol 13:295–299, 2003

Murphy TK, Bengtson MA, Soto O, et al: Case series on the use of aripiprazole for Tourette syndrome. Int J Neuropsychopharmacol 8:489–490, 2005

Nader KO, Kriegler JA, Blake DD, et al: Clinician Administered PTSD Scale for Children and Adolescents for (DSM-IV) (CAPS-CA). Current and Lifetime Diagnostic Version, and Instruction Manual. A National Center for PTSD/UCLA Trauma Psychiatry Program. Los Angeles, CA, National Center for PTSD and UCLA Trauma Psychiatry Program, 1996

Nagaraj R, Singhi P, Malhi P: Risperidone in children with autism: randomized, placebo-controlled, double-blind study. J Child Neurol 21:450–455, 2006

Newcorn JH, Spencer TJ, Biederman J, et al: Atomoxetine treatment in children and adolescents with attention-deficit/hyperactivity disorder and comorbid oppositional defiant disorder. J Am Acad Child Adolesc Psychiatry 44:240–248, 2005

Newcorn JH, Kratochvil CJ, Allen AJ, et al: Atomoxetine and osmotically released methylphenidate for the treatment of attention deficit hyperactivity disorder: acute comparison and differential response. Am J Psychiatry 165:721–730, 2008

Overall J, Pfefferbaum B: A Brief Psychiatric Rating Scale for Children. Innovations 3:264, 1984

Owen R, Sikich L, Marcus RN, et al: Aripiprazole in the treatment of irritability in children and adolescents with autistic disorder. Pediatrics 124:1533–1540, 2009

Owley T, Walton L, Salt J, et al: An open-label trial of escitalopram in pervasive developmental disorders. J Am Acad Child Adolesc Psychiatry 44:343–348, 2005

Pandina GJ, Aman MG, Findling RL, et al: Risperidone in the management of disruptive behavior disorders. J Child Adolesc Psychopharmacol 16:379–392, 2006

Pappadopulos E, Macintyre Ii JC, Crismon ML, et al: Treatment Recommendations for the Use of Antipsychotics for Aggressive Youth (TRAAY), Part II. J Am Acad Child Adolesc Psychiatry 42:145–161, 2003

Pappadopulos E, Woolston BA, Chait A, et al: Pharmacotherapy of aggression in children and adolescents: efficacy and effect size. J Am Acad Child Adolesc Psychiatry 15:27–39, 2006

Pavuluri MN, Henry DB, Carbray JA, et al: Open-label prospective trial of risperidone in combination with lithium or divalproex sodium in pediatric mania. J Affect Disord 82 (suppl 1): S103–S111, 2004

Pavuluri MN, Henry DB, Carbray JA, et al: A one-year open-label trial of risperidone augmentation in lithium nonresponder youth with preschool-onset bipolar disorder. J Child Adolesc Psychopharmacol 16:336–350, 2006

Pavuluri MN, Henry DB, Findling RL, et al: Double-blind randomized trial of risperidone versus divalproex in pediatric bipolar disorder. Bipolar Disord 12:593–605, 2010

Pediatric OCD Treatment Study (POTS) Team: Cognitive-behavior therapy, sertraline, and their combination for children and adolescents with obsessive-compulsive disorder. JAMA 292:1969–1976, 2004

Pelham WE, Wheeler T, Chronis A: Empirically supported psychosocial treatments for attention deficit hyperactivity disorder. J Clin Child Psychol 27:190–205, 1998

Perry R, Campbell M, Adams P, et al: Long-term efficacy of haloperidol in autistic children: continuous versus discontinuous drug administration. J Am Acad Child Adolesc Psychiatry 28:87–92, 1989

Piacentini JC, Chang SW: Behavioral treatments for tic suppression: habit reversal training. Adv Neurol 99:227–233, 2006

Pliszka S: Practice parameter for the assessment and treatment of children and adolescents with attention-deficit/hyperactivity disorder. J Am Acad Child Adolesc Psychiatry 46:894–921, 2007

Pliszka SR, Carlson CL, Swanson JM: ADHD With Comorbid Disorders: Clinical Assessment and Management. New York, Guilford, 1999

Pliszka SR, Crismon ML, Hughes CW, et al: The Texas Children's Medication Algorithm Project: revision of the algorithm for pharmacotherapy of attention-deficit/hyperactivity disorder. J Am Acad Child Adolesc Psychiatry 45:642–657, 2006a

Pliszka SR, Matthews TL, Braslow KJ, et al: Comparative effects of methylphenidate and mixed salts amphetamine on height and weight in children with attention-deficit/hyperactivity disorder (ADHD). J Am Acad Child Adolesc Psychiatry 45:520–526, 2006b

Pool D, Bloom W, Mielke DH, et al: A controlled evaluation of loxitane in seventy-five adolescent schizophrenic patients. Curr Ther Res Clin Exp 19:99–104, 1976

Popper CW: Medical unknowns and ethical consent: prescribing psychotropic medications for children in the face of uncertainty, in Psychiatric Pharmacosciences of Children and Adolescents. Edited by Popper CW. Washington, DC, American Psychiatric Press, 1987, pp 127–161

Popper CW: Pharmacologic alternatives to psychostimulants for the treatment of attention-deficit/hyperactivity disorder. Child Adolesc Psychiatr Clin N Am 9:605–646, 2000

Posey DJ, Guenin KD, Kohn AE, et al: A naturalistic open-label study of mirtazapine in autistic and other pervasive developmental disorders. J Child Adolesc Psychiatry 11:267–277, 2001

Potenza MN, Holmes JP, Kanes SJ, et al: Olanzapine treatment of children, adolescents, and adults with pervasive developmental disorders: an open-label pilot study. J Clin Psychopharmacol 19:37–44, 1999

Poulton A: Growth on stimulant medication: clarifying the confusion: a review. Arch Dis Child 90:801–806, 2005

Prakash A, Lobo E, Kratochvil CJ, et al: An open-label safety and pharmacokinetics study of duloxetine in pediatric patients with major depression. J Child Adolesc Psychopharmacol 22:48–55, 2012

Quintana H, Birmaher B, Stedge D, et al: Use of methylphenidate in the treatment of children with autistic disorder. J Autism Dev Disord 25:283–294, 1995

Rasgon NL: The relationship between polycystic ovary syndrome and antiepileptic drugs: a review of the evidence. J Clin Psychopharmacol 24:322–334, 2004

Realmuto GM, Erickson WD, Yellin AM, et al: Clinical comparison of thiothixene and thioridazine in schizophrenic adolescents. Am J Psychiatry 141:440–442, 1984

Regeur L, Pakkenberg B, Fog R, et al: Clinical features and long-term treatment with pimozide in 65 patients with Gilles de la Tourette's syndrome. J Neurol Neurosurg Psychiatry 49:791–795, 1986

Reinblatt SP, Walkup JT: Psychopharmacologic treatment of pediatric anxiety disorders. Child Adolesc Psychiatric Clin N Am 14:877–908, 2005

Remington G, Sloman L, Konstantareas M, et al: Clomipramine versus haloperidol in the treatment of autistic disorder: a double-blind, placebo-controlled, crossover study. J Clin Psychopharmacol 21:440–444, 2001

Renaud J, Birmaher B, Wassick SC, et al: Use of selective serotonin reuptake inhibitors for the treatment of childhood panic disorder: a pilot study. J Child Adolescent Psychopharmacology 9:73–83, 1999

Research Units on Pediatric Psychopharmacology Anxiety Study Group: Fluvoxamine for the treatment of anxiety disorders in children and adolescents. N Engl J Med 344:1279–1285, 2001

Research Units on Pediatric Psychopharmacology Anxiety Study Group: The Pediatric Anxiety Rating Scale (PARS): development and psychometric properties. J Am Acad Child Adolesc Psychiatry 41:1061–1069, 2002a

Research Units on Pediatric Psychopharmacology Anxiety Study Group: Treatment of pediatric anxiety disorders: an open-label extension of the Research Units on Pediatric Psychopharmacology anxiety study. J Am Acad Child Adolesc Psychiatry 12:175–188, 2002b

Research Units on Pediatric Psychopharmacology Autism Network: Risperidone treatment of autistic disorder: longer-term benefits and blinded discontinuation after 6 months. Am J Psychiatry 162:1361–1369, 2005

Riddle M: Obsessive-compulsive disorder in children and adolescents. Br J Psychiatry 173 (35 suppl): 91–96, 1998

Riddle MA, Bernstein GA, Cook EH, et al: Anxiolytics, adrenergic agents, and naltrexone. J Am Acad Child Adolesc Psychiatry 38:546–556, 1999

Riddle MA, Reeve EA, Yaryura-Tobias JA, et al: Fluvoxamine for children and adolescents with obsessive-compulsive disorder: a randomized, controlled, multicenter trial. J Am Acad Child Adolesc Psychiatry 40:222–229, 2001

Rifkin A, Karajgi B, Dicker R, et al: Lithium treatment of conduct disorders in adolescents. Am J Psychiatry 154:554–555, 1997

Robb AS, Cueva JE, Sporn J, et al: Sertraline treatment of children and adolescents with posttraumatic stress disorder: a double-blind, placebo-controlled trial. J Child Adolesc Psychopharmacol 20:463–471, 2010

Roblek T, Piacentini J: Cognitive-behavior therapy for childhood anxiety disorders. Child Adolesc Psychiatric Clin N Am 14:863–876, 2005

Rugino TA, Janvier YM: Aripiprazole in children and adolescents: clinical experience. J Child Neurol 20:603–610, 2005

Rynn MA, Siqueland L, Rickels K: Placebo-controlled trial of sertraline in the treatment of children with generalized anxiety disorder. Am J Psychiatry 158:2008–2014, 2001

Rynn MA, Findling RL, Emslie GJ, et al: Efficacy and safety of nefazodone in adolescents with MDD. Poster presented at the 155th Annual Meeting of the American Psychiatric Association, Philadelphia, PA, May 18–23, 2002

Rynn MA, Riddle M, Yeung PP, et al: Efficacy and safety of extended-release venlafaxine in the treatment of generalized anxiety disorder in children and adolescents: two placebo-controlled trials. Am J Psychiatry 164:290–300, 2007

Sallee FR, Nesbitt L, Jackson C, et al: Relative efficacy of haloperidol and pimozide in children and adolescents with Tourette's disorder. Am J Psychiatry 154:1057–1062, 1997

Sallee FR, Kurlan R, Goetz CG, et al: Ziprasidone treatment of children and adolescents with Tourette's syndrome: a pilot study. J Am Acad Child Adolesc Psychiatry 39:292–299, 2000

Sallee FR, Miceli JJ, Tensfeldt T, et al: Single-dose pharmacokinetics and safety of ziprasidone in children and adolescents. J Am Acad Child Adolesc Psychiatry 45:720–728, 2006

Sallee FR, Lyne A, Wigal T, et al: Long-term safety and efficacy of guanfacine extended release in children and adolescents with attention-deficit/hyperactivity disorder. J Child Adolesc Psychopharmacol 19:215–226, 2009

Sandor P, Musisi S, Moldofsky H, et al: Tourette syndrome: a follow-up study. J Clin Psychopharmacol 10:197–199, 1990

Saxena K, Silverman MA, Chang K, et al: Baseline predictors of response to divalproex in conduct disorder. J Clin Psychiatry 66:1541–1548, 2005

Scahill L, Chappell PB, Kim YS, et al: A placebo-controlled study of guanfacine in the treatment of children with tic disorders and attention deficit hyperactivity disorder. Am J Psychiatry 158:1067–1074, 2001

Scahill L, Leckman JF, Schultz RT, et al: A placebo-controlled trial of risperidone in Tourette syndrome. Neurology 60:1130–1135, 2003

Scahill L, Blair J, Leckman JF, et al: Sudden death in a patient with Tourette syndrome during a clinical trial of ziprasidone. J Psychopharmacol 19:205–206, 2005

Schur SB, Sikich L, Findling RL, et al: Treatment recommendations for the use of antipsychotics for aggressive youth (TRAAY), part I: a review. J Am Acad Child Adolesc Psychiatry 42:132–144, 2003

Seedat S, Lockhat R, Kaminer D, et al: An open trial of citalopram in adolescents with posttraumatic stress disorder. Int Clin Psychopharmacol 16:21–25, 2001

Seedat S, Stein DJ, Ziervogel C, et al: Comparison of response to a selective serotonin reuptake inhibitor in children, adolescents, and adults with posttraumatic stress disorder. J Child Adolesc Psychopharmacology 12:37–46, 2002

Shapiro A, Shapiro E, Young J, et al: Gilles de la Tourette Syndrome, 2nd Edition. New York, Raven, 1988

Shaw P, Sporn A, Gogtay N, et al: Childhood-onset schizophrenia: a double-blind, randomized clozapine-olanzapine comparison. Arch Gen Psychiatry 63:721–730, 2006

Shea S, Turgay A, Carroll A, et al: Risperidone in the treatment of disruptive behavioral symptoms in children with autistic and other pervasive developmental disorders. Pediatrics 114:634–641, 2004

Sikich L, Hamer RM, Bashford RA, et al: A pilot study of risperidone, olanzapine, and haloperidol in psychotic youth: a double-blind, randomized, 8-week trial. Neuropsychopharmacology 29:133–145, 2004

Sikich L, Frazier JA, McClellan J, et al: Double-blind comparison of first- and second-generation antipsychotics in early-onset schizophrenia and schizoaffective disorder: findings from the treatment of early-onset schizophrenia spectrum disorders (TEOSS) study. Am J Psychiatry 165:1420–1431, 2008

Silva RR, Malone RP, Anderson LT, et al: Haloperidol withdrawal and weight changes in autistic children. Psychopharmacol Bull 29:287–291, 1993

Simeon JG: Use of anxiolytics in children. Encephale 19:71–74, 1993

Simon GE, Savarino J, Operskalski B, et al: Suicide risk during antidepressant treatment. Am J Psychiatry 163:41–47, 2006

Snyder R, Turgay A, Aman M, et al: Effects of risperidone on conduct and disruptive behavior disorders in children with subaverage IQs. J Am Acad Child Adolesc Psychiatry 41:1026–1036, 2002

Søndergård L, Kvist K, Andersen PK, et al: Do antidepressants precipitate youth suicide? A nationwide pharmacoepidemiological study. Eur Child Adolesc Psychiatry 15:232–240, 2006

Spencer EK, Kafantaris V, Padron-Gayol MV, et al: Haloperidol in schizophrenic children: early findings from a study in progress. Psychopharmacol Bull 28:183–186, 1992

Spencer TJ, Abikoff HB, Connor DF, et al: Efficacy and safety of mixed amphetamine salts extended release (Adderall XR) in the management of oppositional defiant disorder with or without comorbid attention-deficit/hyperactivity disorder in school-aged children and adolescents: a 4-week, multicenter, randomized, double-blind, parallel-group, placebo-controlled, forced-dose-escalation study. Clin Ther 28:402–418, 2006a

Spencer TJ, Wilens TE, Biederman J, et al: Efficacy and safety of mixed amphetamine salts extended release (Adderall XR) in the management of attention-deficit/hyperactivity disorder in adolescent patients: a 4-week, randomized, double-blind, placebo-controlled, parallel-group study. Clin Ther 28:266–279, 2006b

Staller JA, Staller JA: Intramuscular ziprasidone in youth: a retrospective chart review. J Child Adolesc Psychopharmacol 14:590–592, 2004

Stein MB, Fuetsch M, Muller N, et al: Social anxiety disorder and the risk of depression: a prospective community study of adolescents and young adults. Arch Gen Psychiatry 58:251–256, 2001

Steiner H, Petersen ML, Saxena K, et al: Divalproex sodium for the treatment of conduct disorder: a randomized controlled clinical trial. J Clin Psychiatry 64:1183–1191, 2003

Steingard RJ, Zimnitzky B, DeMaso RD, et al: Sertraline treatment of transition-associated anxiety and agitation in children with autistic disorder. J Child Adolesc Psychopharmacol 7:9–15, 1997

Stephens RJ, Bassel C, Sandor P, et al: Olanzapine in the treatment of aggression and tics in children with Tourette's syndrome—a pilot study. J Child Adolesc Psychopharmacol 14:255–266, 2004

Storch EA, Lehmkuhl H, Geffken GR, et al: Aripiprazole augmentation of incomplete treatment response in an adolescent male with obsessive-compulsive disorder. Depress Anxiety 25:172–174, 2008

Sumner CS, Donnelly C, Lopez FA, et al: Atomoxetine treatment for pediatric patients with ADHD and comorbid anxiety. Presented at the annual meeting of the American Psychiatric Association, Atlanta, GA, May 2005

Swanson JM, Flockhart D, Udrea D, et al: Clonidine in the treatment of ADHD: questions about safety and efficacy. J Child Adolesc Psychopharmacol 5:301–304, 1995a

Swanson JM, McBurnett K, Christian DL, et al: Stimulant medications and the treatment of children with ADHD. Adv Clin Child Psychol 17:232–265, 1995b

Swanson JM, Greenhill LL, Wigal T, et al: Stimulant-related reduction of growth rates in the Preschool ADHD Treatment Study (PATS). J Am Acad Child Adolesc Psychiatry 45:1304–1313, 2006

Thomsen PH: Child and adolescent obsessive-compulsive disorder treated with citalopram: findings from an open trial of 23 cases. J Child Adolesc Psychopharmacol 7:157–166, 1997

Thomsen PH: Risperidone augmentation in the treatment of severe adolescent OCD in SSRI-refractory cases: a case-series. Ann Clin Psychiatry 16:201–207, 2004

Thomsen PH, Ebbesen C, Persson C: Long-term experience with citalopram in the treatment of adolescent OCD. J Am Acad Child Adolesc Psychiatry 40:895–902, 2001

Tohen M, Kryzhanovskaya L, Carlson G, et al: Olanzapine versus placebo in the treatment of adolescents with bipolar mania. Am J Psychiatry 164:1547–1556, 2007

Tourette's Syndrome Study Group: Treatment of ADHD in children with tics: a randomized controlled trial. Neurology 58:527–536, 2002

Treatment for Adolescents with Depression Study (TADS) Team: Fluoxetine, cognitive-behavioral therapy, and their combination for adolescents with depression. TADS randomized controlled trial. JAMA 292:807–820, 2004

Troost PW, Lahuis BE, Steenhuis MP, et al: Long-term effects of risperidone in children with autism spectrum disorders: a placebo discontinuation study. J Am Acad Child Adolesc Psychiatry 44:1137–1144, 2005

U.S. Food and Drug Administration: FDA News: FDA launches a multi-pronged strategy to strengthen safeguards for children treated with antidepressant medication. October 15, 2004a. Available at: http://www.fda.gov/NewsEvents/Newsroom/PressAnnouncements/2004/ucm108363.htm. Accessed September 2012.

U.S. Food and Drug Administration: Joint Meeting of the Psychopharmacologic Drugs Advisory Committee and Pediatric Advisory Committee. September 13–14, 2004b. Available at: http://www.fda.gov/ohrms/dockets/ac/04/briefing/2004-4065b1.htm. Accessed September 2012.

U.S. Food And Drug Administration: New warning for strattera. ScienceDaily. December 22, 2004c. Available at: http://www.sciencedaily.com/releases/2004/12/041219133156.htm. Accessed September 2012.

U.S. Food and Drug Administration: FDA Alert [09/05]: Suicidal thinking in children and adolescents. September 2005. Available at: http://www.fda.gov/Drugs/DrugSafety/PostmarketDrugSafetyInformationforPatientsandProviders/ucm124391.htm. Accessed September 2012.

U.S. Food and Drug Administration: Pediatric Advisory Committee briefing information. March 22, 2006. Available at: http://www.fda.gov/ohrms/dockets/ac/06/briefing/2006-4210B-Index.htm. Accessed September 2012.

U.S. Food and Drug Administration: FDA News: FDA Proposes New Warnings About Suicidal Thinking, Behavior in Young Adults Who Take Antidepressant Medications. May 2, 2007. Available at: http://www.fda.gov/NewsEvents/Newsroom/PressAnnouncements/2007/ucm108905.htm. Accessed September 2012.

Valicenti-McDermott MR, Demb H: Clinical effects and adverse reactions of off-label use of aripiprazole in children and adolescents with developmental disabilities. J Child Adolesc Psychopharmacol 16:549–560, 2006

Villalaba L: Follow-up review of AERS search identifying cases of sudden death occurring with drugs used for the treatment of attention deficit hyperactivity disorder (ADHD). February 28, 2006. Available at: http://www.fda.gov/ohrms/dockets/ac/06/briefing/2006-4210b_07_01_safetyreview.pdf. Accessed September 2012.

Wagner KD, Ambrosini P, Rynn M, et al: Efficacy of sertraline in the treatment of children and adolescents with major depressive disorder: two randomized controlled trials. JAMA 290:1033–1041, 2003a

Wagner KD, Cook EH, Chung H, et al: Remission status after long-term sertraline treatment of pediatric obsessive-compulsive disorder. J Child Adolesc Psychopharmacol 13 (suppl 1):S53–S60, 2003b

Wagner KD, Berard R, Stein MB, et al: A multicenter, randomized, double-blind, placebo-controlled trial of paroxetine in children and adolescents with social anxiety disorder. Arch Gen Psychiatry 61:1153–1162, 2004a

Wagner, KD, Robb AS, Findling RL, et al: A randomized, placebo-controlled trial of citalopram for the treatment of major depression in children and adolescents: Am J Psychiatry 161:1079–1083, 2004b

Wagner KD, Jonas J, Findling RL, et al: A double-blind, randomized, placebo-controlled trial of escitalopram in the treatment of pediatric depression. J Am Acad Child Adolesc Psychiatry 45:280–288, 2006a

Wagner KD, Kowatch RA, Emslie GJ, et al: A double-blind, randomized, placebo-controlled trial of oxcarbazepine in the treatment of bipolar disorder in children and adolescents. Am J Psychiatry 163:1179–1186, 2006b

Wagner KD, Redden L, Kowatch R, et al: A double-blind, randomized, placebo-controlled trial of divalproex extended-release in the treatment of bipolar disorder in children and adolescents. J Am Acad Child Adolesc Psychiatry 48:519–532, 2009

Walkup JT, Reeve E, Yaryura-Tobias J, et al: Fluvoxamine for childhood OCD: long-term treatment. Poster presented at the 45th Annual Meeting of the American Academy of Child and Adolescent Psychiatry, Anaheim, CA, October 27–November 1, 1998

Walkup JT, Albano AM, Piacentini J, et al: Cognitive behavioral therapy, sertraline, or a combination in childhood anxiety. N Engl J Med 359:2753–2766, 2008

Weisler RH, Biederman J, Spencer TJ, et al: Mixed amphetamine salts extended-release in the treatment of adult ADHD: a randomized, controlled trial. CNS Spectr 11:625–639, 2006

Weiss G, Hechtman L: Hyperactive Children Grown Up, 2nd Edition. New York, Guilford, 2003

Wigal SB, McGough JJ, McCracken JT, et al: A laboratory school comparison of mixed amphetamine salts extended release (Adderall XR) and atomoxetine (Strattera) in school-aged children with attention deficit/hyperactivity disorder. J Atten Disord 9:275–289, 2005

Wigal T, Greenhill LL, Chuang S, et al: Safety and tolerability of methylphenidate in preschool children with ADHD. J Am Acad Child Adolesc Psychiatry 45:1294–1303, 2006

Wilens TE, McBurnett K, Bukstein O, et al: Multisite controlled study of OROS methylphenidate in the treatment of adolescents with attention-deficit/hyperactivity disorder. Arch Pediatr Adolesc Med 160:82–90, 2006a

Wilens TE, Newcorn JH, Kratochvil CJ, et al: Long-term atomoxetine treatment in adolescents with attention-deficit/hyperactivity disorder. J Pediatr 149:112–119, 2006b

Wilens TE, Hammerness P, Utzinger L, et al: An open study of adjunct OROS-methylphenidate in children and adolescents who are atomoxetine partial responders, I: effectiveness. J Child Adolesc Psychopharmacol 19:485–492, 2009

Wilens TE, Bukstein O, Brams M, et al: A controlled trial of extended-release guanfacine and psychostimulants for attention-deficit/hyperactivity disorder. J Am Acad Child Adolesc Psychiatry 51:74–85, 2012

Wolpert A, Hagamen MB, Merlis S: A comparative study of thiothixene and trifluoperazine in childhood schizophrenia. Curr Ther Res Clin Exp 9:482–485, 1967

Yoo HK, Kim JY, Kim CY: A pilot study of aripiprazole in children and adolescents with Tourette's disorder. J Child Adolesc Psychopharmacol 16:505–506, 2006

Zohar AH: The epidemiology of obsessive-compulsive disorder in children and adolescents. Child Adolesc Psychiatr Clin N Am 8:445–460, 1999

Appendix

Psychotropic Medications Commonly Prescribed for Children and Adolescents

This Appendix describes common classes of psychotropic medications used to treat children and adolescents. Dosages, monitoring schedules, and common side effects are presented for each medication class.

Antidepressants

Dosage and monitoring. The starting and target doses of antidepressants for children and adolescents are listed in Table 40–1.

Premedication laboratory testing should include complete blood count, blood chemistries, and liver function tests. Blood pressure should be monitored during dosage titration with venlafaxine.

The U.S. Food and Drug Administration (2007) has issued the following black box warning, which applies to all antidepressants:

> Antidepressants increased the risk compared to placebo of suicidal thinking and behavior (suicidality) in children, adolescents, and young adults in short-term studies of major depressive disorder (MDD) and other psychiatric disorders. Anyone considering the use of [*Name of Antidepressant*] or any other antidepressant in a child, adolescent, or young adult must balance this risk with the clinical need. Short-term studies did not show an increase in the risk of suicidality with antidepressants compared with placebo in adults beyond age 24 years; there was a reduction in risk with antidepressants compared with placebo in adults ages 65 years and older. Depression and certain other psychiatric disorders are themselves associated with increases in the risk of suicide. Patients of all ages who are started on antidepressant therapy should be monitored appropriately and observed closely for clinical worsening, suicidality, or unusual changes in behavior. Families and caregivers should be advised of the need for close observation and communication with the prescriber.

Side effects. Common side effects of selective serotonin reuptake inhibitors (SSRIs) are headache, nausea, abdominal pain, dry mouth, insomnia, and somnolence (Emslie et al. 2002; Keller et al. 2001; Wagner et al. 2003a, 2004b, 2006a). Potential serious adverse events include serotonin syndrome, extrapyramidal symptoms (tics, myoclonus), amotivational syndrome, and increased bleeding (Hammerness et al. 2006). A major advantage of SSRIs is their safety in overdose (Barbey and Roose 1998).

Common side effects of mirtazapine are somnolence, increased appetite, weight gain, dizziness, dry mouth, and constipation (Green 2001).

Common side effects of venlafaxine include anorexia, abdominal pain, insomnia, somnolence, dizziness, dry mouth, increased sweating and nervousness, and elevated blood pressure with dose increase (Emslie et al. 2007a; Green 2001).

Common side effects of bupropion are headache, nausea, rash, irritability, drowsiness, fatigue, and anorexia (Barrickman et al. 1995; Conners et al. 1996; Daviss et al. 2001). Bupropion is contraindicated in children with seizure disorders, because it may lower the seizure threshold.

Atomoxetine

Dosage and monitoring. Atomoxetine can be given in the late afternoon or evening, whereas stimulants generally cannot; atomoxetine may have less pronounced effects on appetite and sleep than stimulants, though it may produce relatively more nausea or sedation. Gastrointestinal distress can be minimized by taking the medication after a meal. In children and young adolescents, atomoxetine is initiated at a dosage of 0.3 mg/kg/day and titrated over 1–3 weeks to a maximum dosage of 1.2–1.8 mg/kg/day (Kratochvil et

TABLE 40–1. Clinical use of antidepressants in children and adolescents

Medication	Typical starting dose (mg)		Target dosage (mg/day)
	Child	Adolescent	
Citalopram	5–10	10	20–40
Escitalopram	5	10	10–20
Fluoxetine	5–10	10	20–40
Paroxetine	5–10	10	20–40
Sertraline	25	50	100–200
Mirtazapine	15	15	30–45
Venlafaxine	37.5	37.5	150–225
Bupropion	50 twice daily	50 twice daily	100–200

al. 2003). Adults or adult-sized adolescents should be started on atomoxetine 40 mg daily and titrated to atomoxetine 80–100 mg/day over 1–3 weeks, if needed (Kratochvil et al. 2003). Atomoxetine's labeling recommends both once-daily and twice-daily dosing, although its elimination half-life of 5 hours (as well as clinical experience) suggests that twice-daily dosing (early A.M. and early P.M.) is more effective and less prone to cause side effects. Michelson et al. (2002) showed that while atomoxetine was superior to placebo at week 1 of the trial, its greatest effects were observed at week 6, suggesting that patients should be maintained at the full therapeutic dose for at least several weeks in order to observe the drug's full effects.

Side effects. Side effects of atomoxetine that occurred more often than placebo in clinical trials included gastrointestinal distress, sedation, and decreased appetite. These can generally be managed by dosage adjustment and often attenuate with time. In December 2004, the FDA announced a new warning for atomoxetine due to reports of two patients (an adult and a child) who developed severe liver disease (U.S. Food and Drug Administration 2004c). Both patients recovered. The FDA has also issued an alert regarding suicidal thinking with atomoxetine in children and adolescents (U.S. Food and Drug Administration 2005). A black box warning is included in the package insert. In 12 controlled trials involving 1,357 patients on atomoxetine and 851 on placebo, the average risk of suicidal thinking was 4 per 1,000 patients in the atomoxetine-treated group versus none in the placebo group.

Atypical Antipsychotics

Dosage and monitoring. Usual starting and target dosages of atypical antipsychotics are listed in Table 40–2.

Premedication laboratory testing should include complete blood count, blood chemistries, and liver function tests. In addition, the American Diabetes Association et al. (2004) recommendations should be followed. These include baseline body mass index (BMI), waist circumference, blood pressure, and fasting glucose and lipid panels. BMI should be followed monthly for 3 months and then measured quarterly. Blood pressure, fasting glucose, and lipid panels should be followed up at 3 months and then yearly. Monitoring should also be done for extrapyramidal side effects.

Side effects. Side effects of atypical antipsychotics include weight gain, dyslipidemia, insulin resistance and diabetes, hyperprolactin-

TABLE 40–2. Clinical use of atypical antipsychotics in children and adolescents

MEDICATION	TYPICAL STARTING DOSE (MG)	TARGET DOSAGE (MG/DAY)
Clozapine	25 twice daily	200–400
Olanzapine	2.5 twice daily	10–20
Quetiapine	50 twice daily	400–600
Risperidone	0.25 twice daily	1–2
Ziprasidone	20 twice daily	80–120
Aripiprazole	2.5–5.0 at bedtime	10–25

Source. DelBello and Kowatch 2006.

emia, extrapyramidal side effects and akathisia, QTc prolongation, sedation, liver toxicity, neutropenia, and neuroleptic malignant syndrome. Clozapine has also been associated with seizures, agranulocytosis, and myocarditis (Correll et al. 2006).

Clonidine

Dosage and monitoring. Clonidine is initiated at 0.05 mg/day, with dose increases of 0.05 mg every 3 days. Typical dosages for attention-deficit/hyperactivity disorder (ADHD) are in the range of total 0.15–0.3 mg/day (on a three-times-per-day schedule). Transdermal clonidine delivers doses of 0.1, 0.2, or 0.3 mg/day. During initial treatment, a temporary worsening of motor and phonic tics in Tourette syndrome may occur, which usually resolves within 2–4 weeks. Clonidine should be tapered by 0.05 mg/day upon discontinuation (Hunt et al. 1990).

Given the reports of adverse cardiovascular side effects in children taking clonidine, recommendations have been made regarding cardiovascular monitoring (Cantwell et al. 1997). Pulse and blood pressure should be measured at baseline, weekly during titration of dose, and every 4–6 weeks during maintenance treatment. Electrocardiograms (ECGs) should be obtained at baseline and after the maximal dosage of clonidine is achieved. Abrupt discontinuation of clonidine is not recommended, because it increases the risk of adverse cardiovascular side effects, particularly hypertension.

Side effects. Common side effects of clonidine in children are sedation, depression, irritability, hypotension, sleep disturbance, dry mouth, and dizziness. Skin irritation and erythema are common with the clonidine patch (Connor et al. 1999; Hunt et al. 1990). Rebound tachycardia and hypertension may occur if clonidine is abruptly discontinued, particularly after chronic use (Popper 2000).

Safety concerns have been raised about the combination of clonidine and methylphenidate, following the report of 4 cases of sudden death in children on this medication combination (Cantwell et al. 1997; Fenichel 1995). Swanson et al. (1995a) described two types of clonidine-related cardiovascular side effects. In one type, fatigue and sedation were associated with a decrease in pulse and blood pressure and changes in ECG. In the other, tachycardia and tachypnea occurred, which led to anxiety, fever, and changes in mental status. Adverse cardiovascular side effects, including bradycardia and depressed level of consciousness, have been reported with clonidine overdose in children (Kappagoda et al. 1998). However, in a retrospective study of 42 children treated with clonidine alone or clonidine plus stimulants, no systematic effects were found on ECG parameters of pulse rate or QTc intervals (Kofoed et al. 1999).

Guanfacine

Dosage and monitoring. Guanfacine is initiated at a daily dose of 0.5 mg, with an upward titration of 0.5 mg every 3 days, based on clinical response and tolerability, to a maximum daily dose of 4 mg (Hunt et al. 1995).

Pulse and blood pressure should be monitored during guanfacine treatment. Guanfacine should be tapered over a 4-day period upon discontinuation.

Side effects. Common side effects of guanfacine in children are sedation, fatigue, headache, dizziness, stomachache, and decreased appetite (Chappell et al. 1995; Hunt et al. 1995; Melmed et al. 2006; Scahill et al. 2001). Rebound hypertension, nervousness, and anxiety may occur if guanfacine is abruptly discontinued (Green 2001).

Mood Stabilizers

Dosage and monitoring. The starting dose and target doses and therapeutic serum levels of mood stabilizers are listed in Table 40–3.

Premedication laboratory testing in general should include complete blood count, liver function tests, and a pregnancy test (for females).

For lithium, baseline thyroid function tests, electrolytes, urinalysis, blood urea nitrogen, creatinine, and serum calcium should also be obtained. Lithium levels, renal function, thyroid function, and urinalysis should be monitored every 3–6 months.

For divalproex, drug serum levels, complete blood count, and liver function tests should be monitored every 3–6 months. Given concerns about a possible relationship between divalproex and polycystic ovarian syndrome (PCOS; Rasgon 2004), female adolescents taking divalproex should be monitored for signs of PCOS, including menstrual abnormalities, weight gain, acne, and hirsutism (DelBello and Kowatch 2006; McClellan et al. 2007). Parents and their female adolescents should be apprised about this possible association prior to initiating medication.

For oxcarbazepine, children should be monitored for hyponatremia.

Side effects. Common side effects of lithium in children and adolescents include hypothyroidism, nausea, polyuria, polydypsia, acne, tremor, and weight gain (DelBello and Kowatch 2006).

Common side effects of divalproex in children and adolescents include weight gain, nausea, sedation, and tremor (DelBello and Kowatch 2006). Concerns have been raised about a possible association between divalproex and PCOS (Rasgon 2004). Other potential adverse effects of concern are hepatic failure, pancreatitis, thrombocytopenia, behavioral deterioration, and hair loss (Davanzo and McCracken 2000; Green 2001).

Side effects of topiramate include decreased appetite, weight loss, nausea, diarrhea, paresthesias, somnolence, and word-finding difficulties (DelBello and Kowatch 2006; DelBello et al. 2005).

Side effects of oxcarbazepine in children include dizziness, nausea, somnolence, diplopia, fatigue, and rash (Wagner et al. 2006b). Hyponatremia is also a side effect of oxcarbazepine.

Common side effects of lamotrigine in children include ataxia, nausea, vomiting, and constipation. Of particular concern, the incidence of serious rash, including Stevens-Johnson syndrome, in pediatric populations is reported to be 1%. This high incidence of serious rash may be attributable to the prior use of high doses of lamotrigine with concomitant divalproex (Messenheimer et al. 1998). The current dosing guidelines may reduce this rash incidence in pediatric patients.

Psychostimulants

Dosage and monitoring. The American Academy of Child and Adolescent Psychiatry (2007) has developed practice parameters for the diagnosis and treatment of

TABLE 40–3. Clinical use of mood stabilizers in children and adolescents

Medication	**Typical starting dose (mg)**	**Target dosage**	**Therapeutic serum level**
Carbamazepine	7 mg/kg/day	Based on response and serum level	8–11 μg/L
Lamotrigine	12.5 mg once daily	Based on response	NA
Lithium	25 mg/kg/g (2–3 daily doses)	30 mg/kg/day (2–3 daily doses)	0.8–1.2 mEq/L
Oxcarbazepine	150 mg twice daily	20–29 kg (900 mg/day) 30–39 kg (1,200 mg/day) >39 kg (1,800 mg/day)	NA
Topiramate	25 mg once daily	100–400 mg/day	NA
Valproic acid, divalproex sodium	20 mg/kg/day (2 daily doses)	20 mg/kg/day (2–3 daily doses)	90–120 μg/mL

Source. DelBello and Kowatch 2006.

ADHD. A wide variety of stimulant preparations are available; Table 40–4 describes their use in clinical practice. Each stimulant has a maximum dose suggested by the FDA-approved package insert, but higher off-label doses are commonly used with careful monitoring. In terms of safety monitoring, pulse, blood pressure, weight, and height should be obtained at baseline and at least annually. No laboratory measures or ECG monitoring is required.

Side effects. Common side effects of psychostimulants are insomnia, diminished appetite, weight loss, irritability, abdominal pain, and headaches (American Academy of Child and Adolescent Psychiatry 2007). Rebound symptoms of worsening behavior may occur when the effects of the short-acting psychostimulants dissipate. Switching to sustained-release or longer-acting psychostimulants may ameliorate rebound symptoms.

Although earlier reports of a protective effect from psychostimulants were not borne out (Molina et al. 2009), there is no evidence that psychostimulants increase substance abuse in youth with ADHD. Motor tics may develop during treatment with stimulants, but one study reported no increase in tics for children with or without preexisting tics who received typical clinical doses of methylphenidate compared with placebo (Law and Schachar 1999).

The FDA and its Pediatric Advisory Committee have reviewed data regarding psychiatric adverse events related to stimulant medication (U.S. Food and Drug Administration 2006). Data from both controlled trials and postmarketing safety data from sponsors and the FDA Adverse Events Reporting System (AERS), also referred to as MedWatch, were reviewed. For most of the agents, these events were slightly more common in the active-drug group relative to placebo in the controlled trials, but these differences did not reach statistical significance (Mosholder 2006). Postmarketing safety data were also reviewed for reports of mania/psychotic symptoms, aggression, and suicidality (Gelperin 2006). Rare events of suicidal thoughts, manic-like activation, or psychosis were reported. At the time, the Pediatric Advisory Committee did not recommend a black box warning regarding psychiatric adverse events but did suggest clarifying labeling regarding these phenomena. No changes to the

TABLE 40–4. Clinical use of psychostimulants in children and adolescents

MEDICATION	DOSAGE FORM	TYPICAL STARTING DOSAGE	FDA MAX/DAY	OFF-LABEL MAX/DAY
Amphetamine preparations				
Adderall	5, 7.5, 10, 12.5, 15, 20, 30 mg	3–5 yr: 2.5 mg qd ≥6 yr: 5 mg qd–bid	40 mg	≥50 kg: 60 mg
Dexedrine	5 mg	3–5 yr: 2.5 mg qd ≥6 yr: 5 mg qd–bid	40 mg	≥50 kg: 60 mg
DextroStat	5, 10 mg	3–5 yr: 2.5 mg qd ≥6 yr: 5 mg qd–bid	40 mg	≥50 kg: 60 mg
Dexedrine Spansule	5, 10, 15 mg	≥6 yr: 5–10 mg qd–bid	40 mg	≥50 kg: 60 mg
Adderall XR	5, 10, 15, 20, 25, 30 mg	≥6 yr: 10 mg qd	30 mg	≥50 kg: 60 mg
Vyvanse	30, 50, 70 mg	30 mg qd	70 mg	Not determined
Methylphenidate preparations				
Focalin	2.5, 5, 10 mg	2.5 mg bid	20 mg	50 mg
Focalin XR	5, 10, 15, 20 mg	5 mg q A.M.	30 mg	50 mg
Methylin	5, 10, 20 mg	5 mg bid	60 mg	≥50 kg: 100 mg
Metadate ER	10, 20 mg	10 mg q A.M.	60 mg	≥50 kg: 100 mg
Methylin ER	10, 20 mg	10 mg q A.M.	60 mg	≥50 kg: 100 mg
Ritalin SR	20 mg	10 mg q A.M.	60 mg	≥50 kg: 100 mg
Metadate CD	10, 20, 30, 40, 50, 60 mg	20 mg q A.M.	60 mg	≥50 kg: 100 mg
Ritalin LA	20, 30, 40 mg	20 mg q A.M.	60 mg	Not yet known
Concerta	18, 27, 36, 54 mg	18 mg q A.M.	72 mg	108 mg
Daytrana patch	10-, 15-, 20-, 30-mg patches	Begin with 10-mg patch qd; then titrate up by patch strength	30 mg	Not yet known

Note. bid = twice daily; q A.M. = every morning; qd = once daily.

stimulant medication labeling were suggested regarding suicide or suicidal ideation.

There have been rare reports of sudden death in patients taking stimulant medication The FDA has record of 20 cases of sudden death with amphetamine or dextroamphetamine (14 children, 6 adults), while there were 14 pediatric and 4 adult cases of sudden death with methylphenidate (Villalaba 2006). It is important to note that the rate of sudden death in the general pediatric population has been estimated at 1.3–8.5 per 100,000 patient-years (Liberthson 1996). The rate of sudden death among those with a history of congenital heart disease can be as high as 6% by age 20 years (Liberthson 1996). Villalaba (2006) estimated the rate of sudden death in treated ADHD children for the exposure period January 1, 1992, to December 31, 2004, to be 0.2 per 100,000 patient-years for methylphenidate, 0.3 per 100,000 patient-years for amphetamine, and 0.5 per 100,000 patient-years for atomoxetine (the differences between the agents are not clinically meaningful). Thus, the rate of sudden death of children on ADHD medications does not appear to exceed the base rate of sudden death in the general population; therefore, cardiac monitoring of healthy children during treatment with stimulants is not required. Children with preexisting heart disease (or significant symptoms suggesting the condition) should obtain a cardiology consultation prior to starting a stimulant.

Poulton (2005) reviewed growth data and concluded that stimulant treatment may be associated with a reduction in expected height gain, at least in the first 1–3 years of treatment. The National Institute of Mental Health (NIMH) Multimodal Treatment of ADHD (MTA) study showed reduced growth rates in ADHD patients after 2 years of stimulant treatment compared with patients who received no medication (MTA Cooperative Group 2004), and these deficits persisted at 36 months (MTA Cooperative Group 2007). The Preschool ADHD Treatment Study (PATS) followed a group of 140 preschoolers who received methylphenidate for up to a year for ADHD (Swanson et al. 2006). The subjects had less than expected mean gains in height (−1.38 cm) and weight (−1.3 kg). Charach et al. (2006) found that higher doses of stimulant correlated with reduced gains in height and weight and that the effect did not become significant until the dosage in methylphenidate equivalents was >2.5 mg/kg/day for 4 years. Pliszka et al. (2006b) did not find that children with ADHD treated with monotherapy with either amphetamine or methylphenidate showed any failure to achieve expected height; furthermore, the two stimulant classes did not have any differential effect on height, but amphetamine had somewhat greater effects on weight than methylphenidate. The subjects in this study had drug holidays averaging 31% of time during their treatment course, which may have contributed to the lack of effect of the stimulant on height.

In assessing for clinically significant growth reduction, it is recommended to use serial plotting of height and weight on growth charts labeled with lines showing the major percentiles (5th, 10th, 25th, 50th, 75th, 90th, and 95th) (Mei et al. 2004). This should occur one to two times per year and more frequently if practical. If the patient has a change in height or weight that crosses 2 percentile lines, this suggests an aberrant growth trajectory. In these cases, a drug holiday should be considered, if return of symptoms during weekends or summers does not lead to marked impairment of functioning. The clinician should also consider switching the patient to another ADHD medication. It is important for the clinician to carefully balance the benefits of medication treatment with the risks of small reductions in height gain, which as of yet have not been shown to be related to reductions in adult height (Gittelman-Klein and Mannuzza 1988; Kramer et al. 2000; Weiss and Hechtman 2003).

CHAPTER 41

Psychopharmacology During Pregnancy and Lactation

D. Jeffrey Newport, M.D.
Zachary N. Stowe, M.D.

The management of mental illness during pregnancy and lactation is a complex task encompassing two concomitant medical conditions (i.e., pregnancy and a psychiatric disorder) and the welfare of at least two patients (i.e., mother and child). Unfortunately, definitive treatment guidelines for perinatal psychotropic therapy remain unavailable. In this chapter, we posit that minimizing infant exposure to the risks of both maternal mental illness and maternal psychotropic therapy is the preeminent clinical objective. We review the available data regarding pharmacokinetic alterations during pregnancy and lactation and describe the clinical relevance of these data for psychotropic dose management. We then review the reproductive safety data available for specific psychotropic agents. We conclude the chapter with a review of the future directions for perinatal psychiatric research and a discussion of potential modifications of previously suggested treatment guidelines.

Minimizing Exposure of Offspring: The Primary Therapeutic Objective

The clinical management of any medical condition during pregnancy and lactation is one of relative safety that must consider the reproductive safety of available therapies, the likelihood of illness recurrence without continued treatment, and the potential impact of untreated maternal illness. Minor ailments, including headaches, nausea, and insomnia, are routinely treated during pregnancy with medications that often have limited reproductive safety data. Conversely, women with mental illness are frequently encouraged to discontinue psychotropic medication during pregnancy and lactation. The underlying desire to avoid offspring psychotropic exposure is laudable; however, such recommendations are often made with limited knowledge of the potential adverse obstetrical effects of maternal mental illness.

An assessment of the risks of offspring exposure to maternal psychiatric illness must consider both the likelihood that an episode of illness will occur and the evidence that the illness may be harmful to the child. The clinician can estimate a patient's likelihood of peripartum recurrence or exacerbation by carefully synthesizing prevalence data from epidemiological studies with evidence from the patient's own history. Patients with frequent episodes of psychiatric illness, a declining course, or a history of prior perinatal illness are more likely to become ill in the current puerperium.

Research data also aid in estimating recurrence risk. Despite the common notion that pregnancy is a time of emotional well-being, prenatal depression rates rival those of nonpuerperal depression (Buesching et al. 1988; Cutrona 1986; Kumar and Robson 1984; Manly et al. 1982; O'Hara et al. 1982; Watson et al. 1984). Two large studies, collectively comprising 122,400 women, found a 14%–20% incidence of prenatal major depressive disorder (MDD) (Marcus et al. 2003; Oberlander et al. 2006). In fact, 11% of women presenting for evaluation of postpartum depression report symptom onset before delivery (Stowe et al. 2005). Pregnant women with histories of MDD or bipolar disorder are especially vulnerable if treatment is discontinued (Cohen et al. 2006; Newport et al. 2008c; Viguera et al. 2007b). Psychotic disorders may also worsen during pregnancy (Glaze et al. 1991; McNeil et al. 1984a, 1984b). The course of obsessive-compulsive disorder (OCD) appears to be variable during pregnancy, with 14% of patients experiencing exacerbation and 14% improvement (Jenike et al. 1990; Williams and Koran 1997). Panic disorder during gestation is also variable, with 19% of patients experiencing more frequent panic attacks and 30% less frequent attacks (Hertzberg and Wahlbeck 1999; Wisner et al. 1996a). Finally, obstetrical trauma and pregnancy loss can precipitate posttraumatic stress disorder (PTSD) (Allen 1998; Engelhard et al. 2001; Fones 1996), with PTSD symptoms following stillbirth persisting into the next pregnancy (Turton et al. 2001).

Postpartum mental illness has been documented for millennia and is substantiated by modern research. For example, psychiatric hospitalization rates rise dramatically in the first postpartum month (Kendler et al. 1993). Up to 12.5% of all psychiatric admissions for women occur during the first postpartum year (Duffy 1983). Postpartum depression affects 10%–22% of adult women and up to 26% of adolescent mothers (Stowe and Nemeroff 1995; Troutman and Cutrona 1990). Women with bipolar disorder also face considerable postpartum risk (Kendell et al. 1987; Targum et al. 1979). Postpartum OCD, often manifested by violence and contamination obsessions, may affect 9% of new mothers (Zambaldi et al. 2009). Thankfully, postpartum psychosis, the most severe postpartum syndrome, is a rare condition, but its prevalence is at least 100-fold higher among women with bipolar disorder (Brockington et al. 1982; Kendell et al. 1987).

Effect of Maternal Psychiatric Disorders

Not only the likelihood but also the potential impact of maternal mental illness on child well-being must be considered. Obstetrical and developmental outcomes have been best studied in offspring of women experiencing perinatal depression. Maternal depression during pregnancy may slow fetal growth (Hedegaard et al. 1996; Schell 1981), increase the risk of preterm delivery and other obstetrical complications (Korebrits et al. 1998; Oberlander et al. 2006; Orr and Miller 1995; Perkin et al. 1993; Steer et al. 1992), and precipitate long-standing cognitive, behavioral, and emotional changes in the offspring (Luoma et al. 2001, 2004; Meijer 1985; Nulman et al. 2002; O'Connor et al. 2003; Sondergaard et al. 2003; Stott 1973). Depressed pregnant women are less compliant with prenatal vitamins and obstetrical care, receive poorer nutrition, and have greater use of prescription opiates, hypnotics, alcohol, tobacco, and illicit substances (Newport et al. 2012; Zuckerman et al. 1989). Finally, depressed pregnant women, and those with PTSD, often experience suicidal thoughts (Newport et al. 2007b; Smith et al. 2006) and may engage in suicidal behavior.

Postnatal maternal depression also carries deleterious consequences for infant development. As early as 3 months, infants of depressed mothers exhibit less facial expression, less head orientation, less crying, and more fussiness than do infants of nondepressed mothers (Martinez et al. 1996). As they age, the children of depressed mothers show ineffective emotional regulation (Downey and Coyne 1990), delayed motor development (Galler et al. 2000), poor interpersonal interactions (Jameson et al. 1997), lower self-esteem (Downey and Coyne 1990), more fear and anxiety (Lyons-Ruth et al. 2000), more aggression (Jameson et al. 1997), and more insecure and disorganized attachment behaviors (Martins and Gaffan 2000). Children of depressed mothers are ultimately more likely to experience emotional instability, to have behavioral problems, to exhibit suicidal behavior, and to require psychiatric treatment (Lyons-Ruth et al. 2000; Weissman et al. 1984).

Perinatal exacerbation of schizophrenia and other psychotic illnesses also warrants concern. Women with schizophrenia have a higher prevalence of substance abuse during pregnancy (Miller and Finnerty 1996) and may exhibit bizarre ideas regarding contraception, pregnancy, and child rearing that complicate their perinatal course (McEvoy et al. 1983; Riordan et al. 1999). Maternal schizophrenia has been associated with elevated rates of obstetrical complications (Bennedsen et al. 2001; Miller and Finnerty 1996), including a higher rate of perinatal death (Rieder et al. 1975).

The effect of other maternal psychiatric disorders is less well investigated. Formal studies on the impact of maternal bipolar disorder are lacking. The impact of anxiety disorders also remains obscure; however, our group recently reported that prenatal anxiety is associated with noncompliance with prenatal vitamins and increased use of tobacco, benzodiazepines, and hypnotics (Newport et al. 2012). Another study indicated that prenatal maternal anxiety is related to subsequent anxiety and attention-deficit/hyperactivity symptoms in school-age offspring (Van den Bergh et al. 2004).

The clinical data regarding the obstetrical and developmental consequences of maternal mental illness are supported by an extensive line of laboratory animal research. Preclinical studies across a variety of species indicate that stress during pregnancy and the early postpartum period adversely affects offspring growth, learning ability, and postnatal development, producing a range of biobehavioral aberrations that may persist into adulthood (for a review, see Newport et al. 2002).

Risks of Perinatal Psychotropic Medication Exposure

Clinical decisions during pregnancy and the postpartum period must consider the risks attributable to fetal and neonatal medication exposure. These risks may be classified as either acute or developmental adverse effects (Table 41–1). *Acute effects* are typically immediately evident and are not dependent on the developmental window of exposure. Examples of acute effects include drug toxicity, drug withdrawal, and drug-drug interactions. *Developmental effects* are, by definition, dependent on the developmental win-

TABLE 41–1. Risks of perinatal medication exposure

	Acute	Developmental
Pregnancy	Neonatal toxicity Neonatal withdrawal Drug-drug interactions	Somatic teratogenesis Neurobehavioral teratogenesis
Lactation	Infant toxicity Drug-drug interactions	Neurobehavioral teratogenesis

dow of exposure and are often not evident until later. These effects include somatic teratogenesis (i.e., major and minor malformations) and so-called neurobehavioral teratogenesis (i.e., alterations in brain development that affect the child's subsequent behavior, cognitive abilities, and emotional regulation). The window of vulnerability to somatic teratogenesis is limited to the embryonic phase of development, but because central nervous system (CNS) development continues long after delivery, the fetus and breast-feeding infant are vulnerable to the theoretical risk of neurobehavioral teratogenesis.

The decision to use psychotropic medication during pregnancy and/or lactation has complicated clinical, ethical, and potentially legal consequences. Although a rapidly expanding base of reproductive safety data has begun to address many of these concerns, review of the current literature reveals numerous methodological problems. The most glaring deficiencies are a frequent lack of appropriate control groups and an overreliance on retrospective data collection—deficiencies demonstrated to introduce systematic biases that potentially lead to overestimation of the impact of psychotropic exposure (Newport et al. 2008a). Despite these limitations, ethical considerations preclude the use of randomized clinical trials to evaluate psychotropic efficacy and safety during pregnancy and lactation. As a result, the reproductive safety database for psychotropic medications is composed of a diverse conglomeration of case reports, case series by pharmaceutical companies and academic centers, birth registries, retrospective surveys, reports from teratology or poison control centers, clinical and preclinical pharmacokinetic investigations, review articles summarizing data from these primary sources, and medication safety rating systems (Table 41–2).

Published reproductive safety data are not the only resource available to inform treatment selection. A meticulous review of the patient's clinical history is also important. Obtaining comprehensive medical and obstetrical histories, particularly screening for a history of placental insufficiency, preeclampsia, and urinary or gastrointestinal disorders, is imperative. Early identification of probable perinatal comorbidities may guide the selection of psychotropic agents. For example, psychotropics with potent antihistaminic properties may complicate the course of gestational diabetes. Obtaining the patient's personal and family psychiatric histories is pivotal, not only for clarifying the psychiatric diagnosis but also for documenting responses to previous therapeutic trials of psychotropic medications. Regardless of the favorability of its reproductive safety profile, a medication that has previously been ineffective for or poorly tolerated by a particular patient is of little value in the perinatal period.

Dosage Management: Perinatal Pharmacokinetics

Prescribing the *minimal effective dose* is especially important during pregnancy and lactation. Upon learning that a patient is pregnant, clinicians and patients often instinc-

TABLE 41–2. U.S. Food and Drug Administration (FDA) use-in-pregnancy ratings

CATEGORY	INTERPRETATION
A	**Controlled studies show no risk:** Adequate, well-controlled studies in pregnant women have failed to demonstrate risk to the fetus.
B	**No evidence of risk in humans:** Either animal findings show risk, but human findings do not; or, if no adequate human studies have been done, animal findings are negative.
C	**Risk cannot be ruled out:** Human studies are lacking, and animal studies are either positive for fetal risk or lacking as well. However, potential benefits may justify the potential risk.
D	**Positive evidence of risk:** Investigational or postmarketing data show risk to the fetus. Nevertheless, potential benefits may outweigh risks.
X	**Contraindicated in pregnancy:** Studies in animals or humans, or investigational or postmarketing reports, have shown fetal risk that clearly outweighs any possible benefit to the patient.

tively lower psychotropic dosages in an effort to reduce fetal exposure, but indiscriminate dosage reduction may increase the vulnerability to relapse. If the therapeutic objective is to eliminate the child's exposure to maternal illness while minimizing the child's psychotropic exposure, then perinatal dose management must be informed by an understanding of the factors governing the alterations in drug disposition across gestation, the placental passage, and excretion into breast milk.

Dosage adjustments may be required to maintain medication efficacy during pregnancy. For example, it may be necessary to increase the dose of tricyclic antidepressants (TCAs) to approximately 1.6 times the preconception dose to maintain therapeutic concentrations in late pregnancy (Altshuler et al. 1996; Wisner et al. 1993). Similar increases may be required with selective serotonin reuptake inhibitors (SSRIs) during the third trimester (Hostetter et al. 2000). However, the pattern of dose adjustment during gestation is not uniform for all medications. For example, among anticonvulsant/mood-stabilizing medications, serum concentrations of lamotrigine (Ohman et al. 2000; Pennell et al. 2004; Tran et al. 2002) and valproate (Otani 1985; Philbert et al. 1985) decline steadily across gestation, whereas carbamazepine concentrations (Bardy et al. 1982b; Battino et al. 1982; Bologa et al. 1991; Dam et al. 1979; Lander et al. 1980; Omtzigt et al. 1993; Otani 1985; Tomson et al. 1994; Yerby et al. 1985) exhibit smaller changes that are primarily evident only in late pregnancy. These alterations in drug concentrations and dosing requirements are likely a consequence of the impact of the physiological changes of pregnancy on the pharmacokinetics (Boobis and Lewis 1983; Frederiksen 2001; Little 1999; Wyska and Jusko 2001) and possibly the pharmacodynamics (Wyska and Jusko 2001) of psychotropic medications. Ultimately, an improved understanding of the factors governing perinatal pharmacokinetic and pharmacodynamic alterations may enable the construction of personalized dosing strategies during gestation.

The level of fetal psychotropic exposure is another key consideration. All psychotropics presumably cross the placenta, yet there are significant differences in placental passage rates. Bidirectional placental transfer is mediated primarily by simple diffusion, and determinants of the transplacental diffusion rate include molecular weight, lipid solubility, degree of ionization, and protein-binding affinity (Audus 1999; Moore et al. 1966; Pacifici and Nottoli 1995). In addition, placental P-glycoprotein (P-gp), which actively transports substrates from the fetal to the maternal circulation, is likely a key determinant of fetal psychotropic exposure. Consequently, medications with greater affinity for P-gp should be associated with lower fetal-to-maternal medication ratios, as in fact has been demonstrated in an investigation of antipsychotic placental passage (Newport et al. 2007a). Further clarification of the factors governing placental passage may ultimately contribute to the development of psychotropic agents with minimal rates of placental transfer (Wang et al. 2007).

Fetal plasma concentrations are not, however, the ultimate measure of functional psychotropic exposure and may even underestimate the more critical measure, fetal brain concentration. Certain physiological attributes of the human fetus, including high cardiac output, increased blood-brain barrier permeability, low plasma protein concentrations and plasma protein binding affinity, and low hepatic enzyme activity (Bertossi et al. 1999; Morgan 1997; Oesterheld 1998), may produce higher-than-anticipated fetal CNS concentrations of psychotropic medications than might be anticipated from circulating levels. Preclinical investigations from our group have demonstrated that transplacental passage results in high levels in fetal CNS tissues and significant binding at neurotransmitter receptor and transporter sites (Capello et al. 2011).

Similar considerations apply when endeavoring to minimize the psychotropic exposure of nursing infants. Because the neonate exhibits relatively low hepatic enzyme activity (Warner 1986) and glomerular filtration and tubular secretion rates (Welch and Findlay 1981), psychotropic exposure may be higher than anticipated for breast-fed infants. A model to predict rates of breast milk excretion from characteristics of the molecular structure of candidate medications has been proposed (Agatonovic-Kustrin et al. 2002). Such models may allow clinicians to estimate a nursing infant's exposure without subjecting the infant to invasive procedures.

Antidepressants

Selective Serotonin Reuptake Inhibitors

Reproductive safety data on the SSRIs have rapidly accrued over the past two decades. Prospective reports of first-trimester SSRI use consist of 4,679 fluoxetine exposures resulting in 126 (2.7%) children with major malformations (Briggs et al. 2005; Chambers et al. 1996; GlaxoSmithKline 2005; Goldstein et al. 1997; Hallberg and Sjöblom 2005; McElhatton et al. 1996; Pastuszak et al. 1993; Wilton et al. 1998), 3,393 sertraline exposures with 66 (1.9%) major malformations (GlaxoSmithKline 2005; Hallberg and Sjöblom 2005; Kulin et al. 1998; Wilton et al. 1998), 2,688 citalopram exposures with 73 (2.7%) major malformations (Ericson et al. 1999; GlaxoSmithKline 2005; Hallberg and Sjöblom 2005; Heikkinen et al. 2002; Sivojelezova et al. 2005), 2,687 paroxetine exposures with 94 (3.5%) major malformations (GlaxoSmithKline 2005; Hallberg and Sjöblom 2005; Kulin et al. 1998; McElhatton et al. 1996; Wilton et al. 1998), 235 escitalopram exposures with 8 (3.4%) major malformations (GlaxoSmithKline 2005), 147 fluvoxamine exposures with 1 (0.7%) major malformation (GlaxoSmithKline 2005; Kulin et al. 1998; McElhatton et al. 1996; Wilton et al. 1998), and 395 exposures to unspecified SSRIs with 6 (1.5%) major malformations (Einarson et al. 2001; Ericson et al. 1999; Hendrick et al. 2003a; Simon et al. 2002; Sivojelezova et al. 2005). The 2.6% ($n = 374$) overall malformation rate among these 14,224 pregnancies is consistent with rates reported in the general population (New York State Department of Health 2005; Rimm et al. 2004; Swedish Centre for Epidemiology 2004).

Despite these reassuring data, some concerns have emerged. Analysis of a managed care database revealed a higher odds ratio (OR) for cardiovascular malformations with exposure to paroxetine compared with other antidepressants (GlaxoSmithKline 2005). Similarly, three large case-control studies (Alwan et al. 2007; Berard et al. 2007; Louik et al. 2007) have produced largely reassuring results, though with some concerns. The first (Alwan et al. 2007) reported small increases in the risk for three uncommon malformations—anencephaly (OR=2.4), craniosynostosis (OR=2.5), and omphalocele (OR= 2.8). The second study (Louik et al. 2007) reported an increased risk for omphalocele (OR=5.7) and septal defects (OR=2.0) with sertraline exposure and for right ventricular outflow tract obstruction defects (OR=3.3) with paroxetine exposure. The third study (Berard et al. 2007) found no evidence of increased risk for cardiovascular or other malformations with SSRI or paroxetine use, unless women were taking ≥25 mg of paroxetine per day, in which case an increased risk for cardiovascular (OR=3.1) and overall malformations (OR=2.2) was observed.

A handful of studies have systematically assessed child development after prenatal exposure to antidepressants. Two studies (Nulman et al. 1997a, 2002) assessed children (ages 15–86 months) who had been prenatally exposed to fluoxetine (n=90) or TCAs (n= 126), collectively comparing them with nonexposed children (n=120). No differences were observed with respect to global cognitive, psychomotor, or language development. A similar study that compared children (ages 6–40 months) with prenatal SSRI exposure (n=31) and without antidepressant exposure (n=13) observed no differences in global cognition but reported lower psychomotor scores for the SSRI-exposed children (Casper et al. 2003). Unfortunately, limitations of these studies render their implications speculative at best. First, children were not age-matched in any of these studies. Although the researchers reported age-adjusted index scores, the predictive validity of these indices across child developmental stages has not been established (Black and Matula 2000). Consequently, groupwise differences in the ages of the children might confound the results. Second, the Casper et al. (2003) study is further confounded by the fact that 29% of the participants were enrolled after delivery. This inclusion of a retrospective (postnatally enrolled) sampling could result in an overrepresentation of children with developmental abnormalities. A study of 69 (46 SSRI exposed; 23 nonexposed) children that eliminated the age confound by examining the children at two fixed time points—2 months and 8 months of age—reported no differences between the exposed and nonexposed children in cognitive or motor development (Oberlander et al. 2004). Finally, an assessment of 4-year-old children found no evidence that prenatal SSRI exposure affected externalizing or attentional behaviors (Oberlander et al. 2007). It is noteworthy that several of these developmental studies involved a significant overlap in the cohort of children, thereby limiting further the cumulative sample size of extant follow-up studies.

Data regarding the impact of prenatal antidepressant exposure on rates of miscarriage, preterm delivery, and low birth weight are decidedly mixed. Some investigators have reported an association with such outcomes (Chambers et al. 1996; Chun-Fai-Chan et al. 2005; Oberlander et al. 2006; Pastuszak et al. 1993; Simon et al. 2002), whereas others have not (Einarson et al. 2001, 2003; Kulin et al. 1998; Sivojelezova et al. 2005). Interpretation is complicated by other reports that prematurity and low birth weight are associated with prenatal maternal stress and/or depression (Orr et al. 2002; Steer et al. 1992). As a result, no definitive conclusions can be drawn as to whether antidepressant use during gestation conveys an adverse impact on fetal growth or the timing of parturition.

Finally, concerns have been expressed regarding neonatal SSRI syndromes, typically manifested by transient symptoms including respiratory difficulty and tremulousness (Moses-Kolko et al. 2005). Most controlled prospective studies suggest that SSRI exposure is associated with poor neonatal adaptation (Chambers et al. 1996; Costei et al. 2002; Källén 2004; Laine et al. 2003; Oberlander et al. 2004, 2006; Sivojelezova et al. 2005; Zeskind and Stephens 2004), although one study found no such association (Maschi et al. 2008). Closer scrutiny of these reports reveals a cadre of methodological shortcomings. Limited effort was made to mask those evaluating the neonates as to exposure status, only one study (Oberlander et al. 2006) controlled for the impact of maternal mental illness, and key confounding factors such as gestational age at delivery and maternal use of other medications and/or habit-forming substances were either ignored altogether or controlled in a rudimentary manner. A case-control study comparing the exposures of neonates who "required observation" with those of "healthy" neonates (Misri et al. 2004) underscores the importance of controlling for confounding factors. In this study of antidepressant-exposed neonates ($n = 46$) born to mothers with MDD, the mothers of infants who required observation had more severe symptoms of depression and anxiety, were more likely to have a comorbid anxiety disorder, and were exposed to higher doses of clonazepam.

Debate has also focused on a more serious neonatal concern—a possible connection between late-pregnancy SSRI exposure and persistent pulmonary hypertension of the neonate (PPHN). The first evaluation of this potential association, a case-control study (Chambers et al. 2006) of 1,213 neonates (377 with PPHN), reported data supporting an association between SSRI exposure and PPHN (OR = 6.1). However, a similar study of 1,104 SSRI-exposed neonates and 1,104 matched control subjects found no association between SSRI exposure and PPHN (Andrade et al. 2009). By far the largest study conducted to date, a case-control study (Källén and Olausson 2008) of more than 831,000 neonates (of whom 506 were diagnosed with PPHN) from the Swedish Medical Birth Register, observed a more modest association (OR = 2.9). The overall rate of PPHN in this population-wide study was approximately 1 in 2,000, and the rate of PPHN with SSRI exposure was approximately 1 in 600. Finally, a recent study concluded that PPHN was associated not with SSRI exposure but rather with cesarean delivery prior to onset of labor (Wilson et al. 2011), underscoring the importance of controlling for potential confounding factors. Overall, the SSRI-PPHN data are mixed, although the absolute rate of PPHN is very low.

Pharmacokinetic data regarding the placental passage of SSRI antidepressants remain limited. However, existing studies have demonstrated that mean fetal-maternal ratios for numerous SSRIs and their active metabolites are uniformly less than 1.0, although considerable differences exist between agents (Hendrick et al. 2003b; Rampono et al. 2009).

Published reports pertaining to SSRIs and lactation now encompass data on 173 mother-infant pairs, including 121 exposures to sertraline (Altshuler et al. 1995; Birnbaum et al. 1999; Dodd et al. 2000; Epperson et al. 1997, 2001; Hendrick et al. 2001a; Kristensen et al. 1998; Mammen et al. 1997; Stowe et al. 1997, 2003; Wisner et al. 1998), 86 to fluoxetine (Birnbaum et al. 1999; Burch and Wells 1992; Hendrick et al. 2001b; Kristensen et al. 1999; Lester et al. 1993; Suri et al. 2002; Taddio et al. 1996; Yoshida et al. 1998a), 52 to paroxetine (Birnbaum et al. 1999; Hendrick et al. 2001a; Ohman et al. 1999; Spigset et al. 1996; Stowe et al. 2000), 8 to escitalopram (Rampono et al. 2006), 7 to fluvoxamine (Hendrick et al. 2001a; Piontek et al. 2001;

Wright et al. 1991), and 5 to citalopram (Jensen et al. 1997; Schmidt et al. 2000; Spigset et al. 1997). Although infant follow-up data are limited, only a few isolated cases of adverse effects have been reported. Long-term neurobehavioral studies of infants exposed to SSRI antidepressants during lactation have not been conducted. The pharmacokinetic profiles of breast milk excretion, including delineation of distribution gradients and time gradients, are best defined for sertraline (Stowe et al. 1997, 2003), paroxetine (Stowe et al. 2000), and fluoxetine (Suri et al. 2002). These studies indicate that quantitative infant SSRI exposure during lactation is considerably lower than transplacental exposure.

Atypical Antidepressants

Reproductive safety data are more limited for the assortment of so-called atypical antidepressants, including bupropion, desvenlafaxine, duloxetine, mirtazapine, nefazodone, trazodone, venlafaxine, and vilazodone.

Prospective reports of first-trimester use of these agents consist of 2,550 bupropion exposures producing 56 (2.2%) children with major malformations (Boshier et al. 2003; Briggs et al. 2005; Chun-Fai-Chan et al. 2005; Cole et al. 2007; GlaxoSmithKline 2005), 771 venlafaxine exposures with 14 (1.4%) major malformations (Einarson et al. 2001; GlaxoSmithKline 2005), 404 trazodone exposures with 10 (2.5%) major malformations (Briggs et al. 2005; GlaxoSmithKline 2005; McElhatton et al. 1996), 140 nefazodone exposures with 2 (1.4%) major malformations (GlaxoSmithKline 2005), 125 mirtazapine exposures with 2 (1.6%) major malformations (Djulus et al. 2006; GlaxoSmithKline 2005), and a combined report of 121 nefazodone or trazodone exposures with 2 (1.7%) major malformations (Einarson et al. 2003). There are no published data on first-trimester duloxetine or vilazodone exposure.

There have been no reports regarding neonatal or developmental outcomes following prenatal exposure to atypical antidepressants. However, in lieu of formal investigation, it should be assumed that concerns regarding neonatal exposure to SSRIs are equally applicable to exposure to atypical antidepressants that work via serotonergic mechanisms.

Prenatal pharmacokinetic data are limited. High rates of placental transfer (umbilical cord concentrations in excess of maternal concentrations) have been reported both for venlafaxine (Hendrick et al. 2003b) and for its active metabolite, desvenlafaxine (Hendrick et al. 2003b; Rampono et al. 2009). This higher rate of placental passage may be a consequence of certain physicochemical properties of the compound, including its relatively low molecular weight and low binding to plasma proteins.

Lactation data also remain limited. Best studied are venlafaxine/desvenlafaxine, for which three studies (Ilett et al. 1998; Newport et al. 2009; Rampono et al. 2011) encompassing 26 mother-infant nursing dyads have reported relative infant doses of 6.8%–8.1%, which is within the notional 10% presumed safety level and 10 times lower than the placental passage rate (Hendrick et al. 2003b; Rampono et al. 2009). A small series of 6 women receiving duloxetine therapy during lactation reported relative infant doses of less than 1% (Lobo et al. 2008). The sole report of bupropion in lactation noted that the drug could not be detected in the plasma of a nursing infant (Briggs et al. 1993). There are no published lactation data for mirtazapine or vilazodone.

Tricyclic Antidepressants

Before the introduction of the SSRIs, TCAs were widely used during pregnancy and lactation. No clear association has been demonstrated between TCA exposure and congenital malformations. Early studies raised concerns regarding limb anomalies (Barson 1972; Elia et al. 1987; McBride 1972), but a meta-analysis by Altshuler et al. (1996)

identified a congenital malformation incidence of only 3.14% ($n = 13$) among 414 infants exposed to a TCA during the first trimester. A review of data from the European Network of Teratology Information Services revealed similar rates of malformation after TCA exposure (McElhatton et al. 1996). Moreover, no adverse neurodevelopmental effects were reported in two studies involving 126 children with prenatal TCA exposure (Nulman et al. 1997a, 2002).

Few data exist regarding the acute effects of TCA exposure on fetal and neonatal well-being. There are case reports of fetal tachycardia and neonatal symptoms including tachypnea, tachycardia, cyanosis, irritability, hypertonia, clonus, and spasm (Eggermont 1973). A small ($n = 18$) prospective study identified no evidence of increased complications during labor and delivery but did report transient withdrawal symptoms among TCA-exposed neonates (Misri and Sivertz 1991).

TCAs have been widely used during lactation. The only adverse event reported to date is respiratory depression in a nursing infant exposed to doxepin, leading the authors to conclude that doxepin should be avoided but that most TCAs are safe for use during breast-feeding (Matheson et al. 1985). This clinical finding is paralleled by the pharmacokinetic data indicating that whereas all TCAs are evident in breast milk, infant plasma concentrations are considerably higher for doxepin than for other TCAs (for a review, see Wisner et al. 1996b).

Monoamine Oxidase Inhibitors

Although the monoamine oxidase inhibitors (MAOIs) were introduced almost 50 years ago, reproductive safety data are sparse. The utility of MAOIs during pregnancy and lactation is severely limited by the potential for hypertensive crisis, which necessitates dietary constraints and avoidance of numerous medications that are commonly used during pregnancy (e.g., pseudoephedrine) or labor and delivery (e.g., meperidine).

Mood Stabilizers

Lithium

Early retrospective data suggested that lithium exposure was associated with a 400-fold increase in cardiac malformations, with particular susceptibility to a defect of the tricuspid valve known as Ebstein's anomaly (Nora et al. 1974; Weinstein and Goldfield 1975). However, a subsequent meta-analysis calculated the risk ratio for cardiac malformations as 1.2–7.7 and the risk ratio for overall congenital malformations as 1.5–3.0 (Cohen et al. 1994). Altshuler et al. (1996) estimated that the risk for Ebstein's anomaly after prenatal lithium exposure rises from 1 in 20,000 to 1 in 1,000. Additional studies (albeit small ones) also failed to confirm the early estimates regarding lithium's teratogenic potential (Friedman and Polifka 2000; Jacobsen et al. 1992; Källén and Tandberg 1983). Laboratory animal studies had indicated that neurobehavioral alterations also might be a concern for prenatal lithium exposure, but a study of 60 school-age children exposed to lithium during gestation found no evidence of adverse neurobehavioral sequelae (Schou 1976).

Prenatal assessment for fetal anomalies, including a fetal echocardiogram between weeks 18–20 of gestation, should be performed for women treated with lithium during the first trimester. In the event of unplanned conception during lithium therapy, the decision to continue or discontinue lithium should also be informed by the severity and course of the patient's illness as well as the time point in gestation when the exposure comes to attention. Discontinuing lithium therapy after cardiogenesis is complete at approximately 9–11 weeks' gestation may be ill-advised.

Lithium's low therapeutic index raises concerns regarding acute perinatal toxicities. Lithium exposure later in gestation can produce fetal and neonatal cardiac arrhythmias (Wilson et al. 1983), hypoglycemia and nephrogenic diabetes insipidus (Mizrahi et al. 1979), thyroid dysfunction (Karlsson et al. 1975), polyhydramnios, premature delivery, and floppy infant syndrome (Llewellyn et al. 1998). Neonatal symptoms of lithium toxicity, including flaccidity, lethargy, and poor suck reflexes, may persist for more than 7 days (Woody et al. 1971).

In a pooled analysis of lithium placental passage and neonatal outcomes (Newport et al. 2005), we determined that 1) higher neonatal lithium concentrations were associated with significantly lower Apgar scores, longer hospital stays, and higher rates of CNS and neuromuscular complications; 2) umbilical cord (i.e., fetal) plasma concentrations were uniformly equivalent to maternal concentrations, suggesting that lithium rapidly equilibrates across the placenta; and 3) withholding lithium therapy for 24–48 hours prior to delivery resulted in a 0.28 mEq/L reduction in maternal (and presumably fetal) lithium concentrations, thereby likely improving neonatal outcomes. Consequently, scheduled deliveries, which afford opportunity for temporary suspension of lithium therapy for 24–48 hours, are advised for women taking lithium during late gestation.

The physiological alterations of pregnancy are of particular importance in the perinatal management of lithium. Changes in renal clearance across pregnancy and the potential for abrupt volume changes during delivery due to copious diaphoresis and the loss of blood and amniotic fluid mandate careful monitoring of lithium levels during pregnancy and especially at delivery. Furthermore, nonsteroidal anti-inflammatory drugs, which inhibit renal clearance of lithium, should be avoided in mother and infant alike during the early postpartum period.

The existing database regarding lithium and lactation encompasses 21 maternal-infant nursing dyads (Fries 1970; Schou and Amdisen 1973; Skausig and Schou 1977; Sykes et al. 1976; Tunnessen and Hertz 1972; Viguera et al. 2007a; Weinstein and Goldfield 1969; Woody et al. 1971). Adverse events, including lethargy, hypotonia, hypothermia, cyanosis, electrocardiogram changes, and elevated thyroid-stimulating hormone level, were reported in 4 (19%) of these children (Skausig and Schou 1977; Tunnessen and Hertz 1972; Viguera et al. 2007a; Woody et al. 1971), including 1 infant who developed frank lithium toxicity with a serum concentration of 1.4 mEq/L, which was double the maternal level (Skausig and Schou 1977). The American Academy of Pediatrics (2001) discourages the use of lithium during lactation. The largest pharmacokinetic study of lithium in lactation demonstrated a milk-to-plasma ratio of 0.53 and an infant-to-maternal plasma ratio of 0.24 (Viguera et al. 2007a). In other studies, nursing infants have exhibited lithium concentrations generally ranging from 5% to 65% of maternal levels (Fries 1970; Kirksey and Groziak 1984; Schou and Amdisen 1973; Sykes et al. 1976; Tunnessen and Hertz 1972; Weinstein and Goldfield 1969), excluding the lone infant whose serum concentration was 200% of the maternal concentration (Skausig and Schou 1977). Because dehydration can increase the vulnerability to lithium toxicity, the hydration status of nursing infants of mothers taking lithium should be carefully monitored (Llewellyn et al. 1998). There are no available reports regarding the long-term neurobehavioral sequelae of lithium exposure during lactation.

Valproate (Valproic Acid)

Prenatal exposure to valproate has been associated with numerous congenital malformations, including neural tube defects (Bjerkedal et al. 1982; Centers for Disease Control 1992; Jager-Roman et al. 1986; Lindhout and Schmidt 1986), craniofacial anomalies (Assencio-Ferreira et al. 2001; Lajeunie et al. 1998, 2001; Paulson and Paulson 1981), limb abnormalities (Rodriguez-Pinilla et al. 2000), and cardiovascular anomalies (Dalens et al. 1980; Koch et al. 1983; Sodhi et al. 2001). Valproate exposure prior to neural tube closure, during the fourth week of gestation, confers a 1%–2% risk for spina bifida, which is 10–20 times greater than the prevalence in the general population (Bjerkedal et al. 1982; Centers for Disease Control 1992; Rosa 1991). One meta-analysis placed the risk for neural tube defects even higher, at 3.8%, with particular vulnerability for the infants of women whose daily dose exceeds 1,000 mg (Samrén et al. 1997). Other studies support this dose-response relationship (Canger et al. 1999; Kaneko et al. 1999; Omtzigt et al. 1992; Samrén et al. 1999), leading one group to recommend that daily dosages not exceed a maximum of 1,000 mg and that maternal serum concentrations not exceed a maximum of 70 μg/mL to reduce the risk for malformations (Kaneko et al. 1999). In a case-control study examining the incidence of limb malformations in a cohort of more than 44,000 children, 67 of whom were exposed to valproate in the first trimester, Rodriguez-Pinilla et al. (2000) reported an odds ratio of 6.17 for limb abnormalities among children exposed to valproate and estimated the risk of limb abnormalities from valproate exposure at 0.42%.

A *fetal valproate syndrome* was initially reported by Di Liberti et al. (1984) and subsequently confirmed by other investigators (Ardinger et al. 1988; Martinez-Frias 1990; Winter et al. 1987). The phenotypic attributes of fetal valproate syndrome include stereotypical facial features such as bifrontal narrowing, midface hypoplasia, a broad nasal bridge, a short nose with anteverted nares, epicanthal folds, micrognathia, a shallow philtrum, a thin upper lip, and a thick lower lip (McMahon and Braddock 2001; Moore et al. 2000). Many of the congenital malformations previously associated with valproate exposure have been recognized as attributes of fetal valproate syndrome (McMahon and Braddock 2001). Valproate's antagonism of folate activity may underlie the risk for both spina bifida and fetal valproate syndrome. A case-control study comparing 57 children with fetal anticonvulsant syndromes, 46 of whose mothers were treated with valproate, with 152 control children found a significantly higher rate of homozygosity for a mutation in the gene for methylenetetrahydrofolate reductase (MTHFR), a key enzyme in folate metabolism (Dean et al. 1999).

Neurodevelopmental outcomes associated with prenatal valproate exposure are equally of concern. A review indicated that developmental delay is evident in 20% and mental retardation in 10% of children exposed to valproate monotherapy prenatally (Kozma 2001). An interim report from a prospective multicenter investigation of the neurodevelopmental effects of prenatal antiepileptic drug exposure indicated that 24% of 2-year-olds with prenatal valproate exposure had mental developmental indexes of less than 70, more than doubling the rate of other antiepileptic drugs (Meador et al. 2006). More recent studies have consistently shown deleterious neurodevelopmental effects from prenatal valproate exposure (Meador et al. 2009; Shallcross et al. 2011), with particular consequences for verbal cognition (McVearry et al. 2009; Meador et al. 2011; Nadebaum et al. 2011a, 2011b). Retrospective reports indicate that varying degrees of cognitive impairment may be present in children manifesting the physical sequelae of fetal valproate syndrome (Adab et al. 2001; Gaily et al. 1990; Moore et al. 2000). Fetal valproate syndrome has also been associated with autism spectrum disorders (Bescoby-Chambers et al. 2001; Moore et al. 2000; Williams et al. 2001; Williams and Hersh 1997).

Valproate exposure during gestation is also associated with risks for numerous fetal and neonatal toxicities, including hepatotoxicity (Kennedy and Koren 1998), coagulopathies (Mountain et al. 1970), and neonatal hypoglycemia (Ebbesen et al. 2000; Thisted and Ebbesen 1993). Ten of 13 infants who demonstrated neonatal hypoglycemia after prenatal valproate exposure developed withdrawal symptoms—including irritability, jitteriness, hypertonia, seizures, and vomiting—that began 12–24 hours after delivery and lasted up to 1 week (Ebbesen et al. 2000).

Pharmacokinetic studies in women with epilepsy indicate that maternal valproate concentrations steadily decline across pregnancy, reaching levels up to 50% lower than preconception concentrations (Yerby et al. 1990, 1992). Consistent findings from other studies demonstrate that valproate is more rapidly cleared during gestation, and especially during the final month of pregnancy (Nau et al. 1982b; Otani 1985; Philbert et al. 1985). Dosage increases during pregnancy may therefore be required to maintain therapeutic efficacy. Valproate readily crosses the human placenta, with umbilical cord concentrations at delivery equal to or slightly higher than maternal concentrations (Froescher et al. 1984b; Philbert et al. 1985; Yerby et al. 1990, 1992).

The literature regarding valproate and lactation includes 41 mother-infant nursing dyads (Alexander 1979; Bardy et al. 1982a; Dickinson et al. 1979; Froescher et al. 1981; Nau et al. 1981; Piontek et al. 2000; Stahl et al. 1997; Tsuru et al. 1988; von Unruh et al. 1984; Wisner and Perel 1998). From these cases, only one adverse event, thrombocytopenia and anemia in an infant, has been reported (Stahl et al. 1997). The pharmacokinetic data indicate that valproate milk-to-plasma ratios are uniformly low and that serum concentrations of nursing infants are 2%–40% of maternal concentrations (Alexander 1979; Bardy et al. 1982a; Piontek et al. 2000; Stahl et al. 1997; von Unruh et al. 1984; Wisner et al. 1996b). Studies of the neurobehavioral effects of valproate exposure during lactation have not been conducted.

In summary, prenatal valproate raises grave safety concerns. In women of childbearing age, valproate should never be used except as a treatment of last resort. If valproate must be used during pregnancy, its risk may be reduced by being careful not to exceed 1,000 mg/day or a serum concentration of 70 μg/mL. Folate supplementation (4–5 mg/day) is also recommended, although there is no definitive evidence that it reduces the risk of valproate-associated anomalies. All women of childbearing potential who are treated with valproate should receive concomitant folate supplementation, regardless of whether they plan to conceive. The preliminary evidence that aspects of fetal valproate syndrome other than neural tube defects may be associated with valproate's antagonism of folate metabolism suggests that folate supplementation should be administered not only in the first trimester but also throughout gestation. Because of the potential for valproate-associated neonatal coagulopathies, oral vitamin K supplementation (10–20 mg/day) may be considered during the final month of gestation. Prenatal surveillance for congenital abnormalities should include maternal serum α-fetoprotein, fetal echocardiography, and a level 2 ultrasound at approximately 16–18 weeks' gestation. Finally, genetic screening of women taking valproate for mutations in the MTHFR gene warrants future consideration. In contrast to the marked risks of its use during pregnancy, valproate therapy during lactation appears to be well tolerated by nursing infants. Nevertheless, periodic assays of platelet count and serum liver enzymes of nursing infants are recommended because the neurodevelopmental impact of nursing exposure to valproate is unclear.

Carbamazepine

Carbamazepine is associated with many of the same risks as valproate during gestation, although in many cases with less frequency or severity. For example, first-trimester carbamazepine exposure is associated with a risk for neural tube defects, although the 0.5%–1.0% risk in carbamazepine-exposed infants (Rosa 1991) is approximately half that seen with valproate exposure (Lindhout and Schmidt 1986; Rosa 1991). A meta-analysis of five prospective studies encompassing 1,255 prenatal exposures indicated that carbamazepine exposure in utero is associated with an increased risk of neural tube defects, cleft palate, cardiovascular abnormalities, and urinary tract anomalies (Matalon et al. 2002). The European Surveillance of Congenital Anomalies (EUROCAT) study (Jentink et al. 2010), a large case-control investigation, reported that carbamazepine exposure was associated with an increased risk for spina bifida (OR = 2.6) but no other major malformations. An epidemiological study indicated that periconceptional folate supplementation was associated with a lower rate of neural tube defects among the children of women taking carbamazepine during pregnancy (Hernandez-Diaz et al. 2001).

A *fetal carbamazepine syndrome*—manifested by a short nose, long philtrum, epicanthal folds, hypertelorism, upslanting palpebral fissures, and fingernail hypoplasia—has been described (Jones et al. 1989), and in one study, the phenotypic characteristics of this syndrome were observed in 6 of 47 children prenatally exposed to carbamazepine (Ornoy and Cohen 1996). Other studies have confirmed the association with facial anomalies (Moore et al. 2000; Nulman et al. 1997b; Scolnick et al. 1994; Wide et al. 2000), but one of these studies demonstrated similar facial abnormalities among children born to women with epilepsy who were untreated during pregnancy (Nulman et al. 1997b).

Data regarding the neurodevelopmental sequelae of prenatal carbamazepine exposure have been mixed. Some early studies reported developmental delay in up to 20% of children exhibiting the physical characteristics of fetal carbamazepine syndrome (Jones et al. 1989; Moore et al. 2000; Ornoy and Cohen 1996), but others failed to demonstrate that association (Gaily et al. 1990; Scolnick et al. 1994; van der Pol 1991; Wide et al. 2000). Recent systematic studies have generally found no evidence of developmental delay in children exposed to carbamazepine during gestation (McVearry et al. 2009; Meador et al. 2006, 2009, 2011; Nadebaum et al. 2011b). However, one recent study reported that carbamazepine exposure was associated with poorer verbal performance in school-age children (Meador et al. 2011).

Potential fetal/neonatal toxicities associated with carbamazepine exposure include blood dyscrasias, coagulopathies, skin reactions, and hepatotoxicity. Most of these risks remain theoretical, although neonatal hepatotoxicity has been reported in a carbamazepine-exposed infant (Frey et al. 2002).

Pharmacokinetic studies of carbamazepine clearance during gestation have yielded mixed results. Some investigators have reported statistically significant increases in carbamazepine clearance during the third trimester (Battino et al. 1982; Dam et al. 1979; Lander et al. 1980), but others have found no changes in carbamazepine clearance (Bardy et al. 1982b; Otani 1985; Yerby et al. 1985). Placental pharmacokinetic studies indicate that the placental transfer of carbamazepine is lower than that of other anticonvulsants (Nau et al. 1982a; Yerby et al. 1990, 1992), with umbilical cord–to–maternal plasma ratios equaling 0.5–0.8 (Nau et al. 1982a).

The literature on carbamazepine and lactation encompasses 12 published reports and 144 mother-infant nursing pairs (Brent and Wisner 1998; Frey et al. 1990, 2002; Froescher et al. 1984a; Kaneko et al. 1982; Kok et al. 1982; Kuhnz et al. 1983; Merlob et al. 1992; Niebyl et al. 1979; Pynnonen and Sillanpaa 1975; Pynnonen et al. 1977; Wisner and Perel 1998), representing the most extensive data set for any mood stabilizer in lactation. Included are 8 reports of adverse events: 1 drowsy, irritable infant with an undetectable serum concentration of carbamazepine (Kok et al. 1982); 2 "hyperexcitable" infants in whom carbamazepine levels were not reported (Kuhnz et al. 1983); 2 infants with cholestatic hepatitis in whom carbamazepine levels were not reported (Frey et al. 1990, 2002); 1 infant with poor nursing effort (Froescher et al. 1984a); 1 infant with an increased serum concentration of γ-glutamyl transpeptidase (GGT) but no overt clinical sequelae whose serum concentration was 33% of the maternal concentration (Merlob et al. 1992); and 1 infant with a "seizurelike" phenomenon whose carbamazepine level was 8% of the maternal level (Brent and Wisner 1998). Serum carbamazepine concentrations in the 8 nursing infants in whom these levels were assessed ranged from undetectable to 65% of the maternal level (Brent and Wisner 1998; Kok et al. 1982; Merlob et al. 1992; Pynnonen and Sillanpaa 1975; Pynnonen et al. 1977; Wisner and Perel 1998).

Although the risks associated with prenatal carbamazepine exposure are marginally better than those for valproate exposure, the clinical recommendations are quite similar. Carbamazepine should be avoided in pregnancy, especially during the first trimester. Folate supplementation (4–5 mg/day) is also recommended not only during gestation but also throughout the reproductive years because of the high prevalence of inadvertent conception in the United States. Women taking carbamazepine during gestation should receive prenatal surveillance for congenital abnormalities, including maternal serum α-fetoprotein, fetal echocardiography, and a level 2 ultrasound at approximately 16–18 weeks' gestation. Carbamazepine has by far the most extensive database for mood stabilizers in lactation, but reports of hepatic dysfunction in nursing infants certainly raise concern. Periodic assays of blood counts and serum liver enzymes of nursing infants are recommended in light of the risks for blood dyscrasias and hepatotoxicity associated with carbamazepine therapy.

Lamotrigine

Reproductive safety data regarding lamotrigine have rapidly accrued during the past decade and compare favorably with safety data for other mood stabilizers. The overall risk of major fetal malformations following first-trimester prenatal exposure to lamotrigine is 2.9% (121 per 4,195 exposures, including 0.32% [8 per 2,537 exposures] for midline cleft formations) (Dominguez-Salgado et al. 2004; GlaxoSmithKline 2007; Holmes et al. 2006; Meador et al. 2006; Molgaard-Nielsen and Hviid 2011; Morrow et al. 2006; Sabers et al. 2004; Vajda et al. 2003), rates that are within the range of births not involving drug exposures. A report by the North American Pregnancy Registry (Holmes et al. 2006) noted a relatively high rate of midline facial clefts (0.89% of 564 exposures); however, the collective rate of orofacial clefts in the other registries was only 0.10% (3 per 2,956 exposures) (Dominguez-Salgado et al. 2004; GlaxoSmithKline 2007; Meador et al. 2006; Molgaard-Nielsen and Hviid 2011; Morrow et al. 2006; Sabers et al. 2004; Vajda et al. 2003). Furthermore, the EUROCAT case-control study, encompassing 5,511 children with orofacial clefts and 80,052 children without clefts, reports an adjusted odds ratio of 0.67 for clefts with lamotrigine exposure (Dolk et al. 2008). The UK Epilepsy and Pregnancy Register reported a higher risk of malformations at maternal dosages exceeding 200 mg/day (Morrow et al. 2006), although this was not confirmed in subsequent analyses (GlaxoSmithKline 2007; Molgaard-Nielsen and Hviid 2011). Despite these reassuring findings, folate supplementation is recommended for all women of childbearing age taking any antiepileptic drug, including lamotrigine.

Prospective neurodevelopmental data have been consistently favorable among children with prenatal lamotrigine exposure (McVearry et al. 2009; Meador et al. 2006, 2009, 2011; Nadebaum et al. 2011b).

Numerous pharmacokinetic studies have reported that lamotrigine clearance steadily increases across gestation (De Haan et al. 2004; Fotopoulou et al. 2009; Franco et al.

2008; Pennell et al. 2004, 2008; Petrenaite et al. 2005; Tran et al. 2002). These studies are limited by the cotherapy of lamotrigine with other anticonvulsants, which are known to alter the metabolism of lamotrigine. It is unclear whether similar dose changes would be necessary to maintain mood stability in patients with bipolar disorder and whether the common adjunctive agents used to treat bipolar disorder would have similar effects on lamotrigine metabolism. Studies in epilepsy patients taking lamotrigine also reveal that its rate of clearance abruptly declines after delivery (Ohman et al. 2000; Pennell et al. 2004; Tran et al. 2002). Therefore, dosage reductions may be necessary after delivery to avoid maternal symptoms of lamotrigine toxicity, such as dizziness, nausea and vomiting, and diplopia (Tran et al. 2002). Published reports regarding the placental passage of lamotrigine indicate that lamotrigine concentrations in fetal circulation at delivery are equal to maternal concentrations (Myllynen et al. 2003; Ohman et al. 2000; Sathanandar et al. 2000; Tomson et al. 1997). There have been no reports of acute adverse events observed in neonates exposed to lamotrigine.

Reports regarding lamotrigine and lactation (GlaxoSmithKline 2007; Liporace et al. 2004; Newport et al. 2008c; Nordmo et al. 2009; Ohman et al. 2000; Page-Sharp et al. 2006; Rambeck et al. 1997; Tomson et al. 1997) collectively encompass 56 maternal-infant nursing dyads. The only reported adverse event was an apneic episode in a nursing infant whose mother was being treated with lamotrigine 850 mg/day (Nordmo et al. 2009). Seven other infants were observed to have a benign thrombocytosis (Newport et al. 2008b). In the largest ($n = 30$) of these studies (Newport et al. 2008b), the mean milk-to-plasma ratio was 41.3%, the relative infant dose equaled 9.2%, and the infant-to-maternal plasma ratio equaled 18.3%. Long-term neurobehavioral outcomes have not been studied in nursing infants exposed to lamotrigine.

Antipsychotics

Second-Generation Antipsychotics

Commonly prescribed antipsychotic medications, as well as agents used to treat the side effects of first-generation antipsychotics (FGAs), are covered in Chapters 15–25 of this volume. The second-generation antipsychotics (SGAs) currently available in the United States are aripiprazole, clozapine, lurasidone, olanzapine, paliperidone, quetiapine, risperidone, and ziprasidone. The SGAs have supplanted the FGAs as first-line medications for psychotic disorders and are also used for other psychiatric indications, including bipolar disorder, anxiety disorders, and treatment-resistant depression. Despite these agents' rapidly expanding use, the reproductive safety database regarding SGAs remains limited.

Clozapine

Reproductive safety data for clozapine, the oldest of the SGAs, are limited to case reports (Barnas et al. 1994; Di Michele et al. 1996; Kornhuber and Weller 1991; Waldman and Safferman 1993), case series (McKenna et al. 2005; Stoner et al. 1997; Tenyi and Tixler 1998), and a retrospective review (Dev and Krupp 1995), collectively encompassing 79 children exposed to clozapine during pregnancy and/or lactation. Adverse sequelae associated with perinatal clozapine therapy include maternal gestational diabetes (Dickson and Hogg 1998); several minor anomalies, including cephalohematoma, hyperpigmentation folds, and a coccygeal dimple, in an infant (Stoner et al. 1997); transient low-grade fever in an infant also exposed to lithium (Stoner et al. 1997); and floppy infant syndrome in a newborn also exposed to lorazepam (Di Michele et al. 1996). In a review of 61 children exposed to clozapine perinatally, Dev and Krupp (1995) reported 5 cases of congenital malformations and 5 cases of neonatal syndromes, although many of these mothers were taking other psychotropic medications during pregnancy. The lone case report of clozapine use during lactation reported no adverse impact on the nursing infant (Kornhuber and Weller 1991).

The only investigation of the perinatal pharmacokinetics of clozapine demonstrated similar medication concentrations in maternal serum and amniotic fluid but markedly higher concentrations in fetal serum and breast milk (Barnas et al. 1994), leading the authors to conclude that clozapine accumulates in the fetal circulation and breast milk. Although no cases of agranulocytosis have been reported in clozapine-exposed infants, this potential risk and the requisite laboratory monitoring limit the utility of clozapine during the peripartum.

Olanzapine

A published birth registry of 23 prospectively ascertained olanzapine-exposed pregnancies from the Lilly Worldwide Pharmacovigilance Safety Database reported no major malformations, 13% spontaneous abortions, 5% preterm deliveries, and 5% fetal deaths (Goldstein et al. 2000). A prospective study comparing outcomes among 151 pregnant women with SGA exposure (olanzapine, $n=60$; risperidone, $n=49$; quetiapine, $n=36$; clozapine, $n=6$) to 151 pregnant control subjects reported no differences in rates of spontaneous abortion, stillbirth, major malformations, prematurity, or low birth weight (McKenna et al. 2005). In this study, only one SGA-exposed child (olanzapine) was observed to have any major malformations (a series of midline defects including an oral cleft, encephalocele, and aqueductal stenosis). There are no available data regarding the neurodevelopmental effects of olanzapine exposure during pregnancy or lactation.

In a study of antipsychotic placental passage rates and neonatal outcomes (Newport et al. 2007a), umbilical cord concentrations in olanzapine-exposed neonates ($n=14$) were 72.1% of maternal concentrations (higher than rates for haloperidol, risperidone, and quetiapine). In this study, there were trends toward higher rates of low birth weight (30.8%; $P<0.06$) and neonatal intensive care unit admission (30.8%; $P<0.09$) among neonates exposed to olanzapine than those exposed to the other antipsychotics.

Case reports of 17 infants exposed to olanzapine during lactation with no evidence of infant toxicity currently appear in the literature (Croke et al. 2002; Friedman and Rosenthal 2003; Gardiner et al. 2003; Goldstein et al. 2000; Kirchheiner et al. 2000; Whitworth et al. 2010). Pharmacokinetic studies of olanzapine exposure during lactation have reported that plasma concentrations were undetectable in infants during nursing (Gardiner et al. 2003; Kirchheiner et al. 2000) and that the median infant daily dose via breast-feeding was approximately 1.0%–1.6% of the maternal dose (Ambresin et al. 2004; Croke et al. 2002; Gardiner et al. 2003).

Risperidone

There are two prospective reports of pregnancy outcomes for women with first-trimester risperidone exposure. The first, which reported collective outcomes for several SGAs (McKenna et al. 2005), found no major malformations among 49 risperidone-exposed infants. The second study, including 68 women with first-trimester exposure and known outcomes, reported 9 (13.2%) spontaneous abortions, 1 (1.5%) stillbirth, and 2 (2.9%) children with major malformations (Coppola et al. 2007). There are no available data regarding the neurodevelopmental effects of risperidone exposure during pregnancy or lactation.

Pharmacokinetic studies have reported placental passage concentrations among neonates ($n=6$) of 49.2% (Newport et al. 2007a), milk-to-plasma ratios of less than 0.5 for both risperidone and 9-hydroxyrisperidone (Hill et al. 2000; Ilett et al. 2004), and infant doses ranging from 2.3% to 4.7% of the maternal dose (Ilett et al. 2004).

Quetiapine

The reproductive safety literature for first-trimester quetiapine exposure is limited to the McKenna et al. (2005) study, which reported no major malformations among 36 infants exposed to quetiapine. In the Newport et al. (2007a) study of antipsychotic placental passage, quetiapine concentrations among neonates (n=21) were 23% of maternal concentrations. To our knowledge, this is the lowest placental passage rate ever reported for a psychotropic agent. There are no available data regarding the neurodevelopmental effects of quetiapine exposure during pregnancy or lactation.

A single case of quetiapine use during lactation following use during pregnancy estimated the nursing infant dose at 0.09% of the maternal daily dose (Lee et al. 2004).

Aripiprazole

There are currently no reports regarding the use of aripiprazole during pregnancy. There are two case reports of aripiprazole in lactation, but milk excretion profiles in these two reports are questionable (Lutz et al. 2010; Schlotterbeck et al. 2007).

Paliperidone

There are currently no reports regarding the use of paliperidone during pregnancy or lactation.

Ziprasidone

There are currently no reports regarding the use of ziprasidone during pregnancy. A single case report of ziprasidone in lactation reported a milk-to-plasma ratio of 0.06 (Schlotterbeck et al. 2009).

Lurasidone

There are currently no reports regarding the use of lurasidone during pregnancy or lactation.

First-Generation Antipsychotics

In contrast to the SGAs, the FGAs have an extensive reproductive safety database addressing both somatic and neurobehavioral teratogenicity. Furthermore, the historical use of phenothiazine antipsychotics to treat pregnancy-associated emesis aids in separating the effects of psychiatric illness and antipsychotic drugs on pregnancy outcome. Chlorpromazine, haloperidol, and perphenazine have received the greatest scrutiny, with no significant associations between these compounds and major malformations (Goldberg and DiMascio 1978; Hill and Stern 1979; Nurnberg and Prudic 1984). In a study of 100 women treated with haloperidol (mean dosage = 1.2 mg/day) for hyperemesis gravidarum, no differences in gestational duration, fetal viability, or birth weight were noted (Van Waes and Van de Velde 1969). In a prospective study encompassing nearly 20,000 women treated primarily with phenothiazines for emesis, Milkovich and Van den Berg (1976) found no significant association with neonatal survival rates or severe anomalies after controlling for maternal age, medication, and gestational age at exposure. Similar results have been obtained in several retrospective studies of women treated with trifluoperazine for repeated abortions and emesis (Moriarty and Nance 1963; Rawlings et al. 1963). In contrast, Rumeau-Rouquette et al. (1977) reported a significant association of major anomalies with prenatal exposure to aliphatic phenothiazines but not piperazine- or piperidine-class agents. Reanalysis of the data obtained by Milkovich and Van den Berg (1976) did find a significant risk of malformations associated with phenothiazine exposure in weeks 4 through 10 of gestation (Edlund and Craig 1976).

Neurobehavioral outcome studies encompassing 203 children exposed to FGAs during gestation detected no significant differences in IQ scores at 4 years of age (Kris 1965; Slone et al. 1977), although relatively low antipsychotic doses were used by many women in these studies. Conversely, several laboratory animal studies (Hoffeld et al. 1968; Ordy et al. 1966; Robertson et al. 1980), although not all (Dallemagne and Weiss 1982), have demonstrated persistent deficits in learning and memory among offspring prenatally exposed to FGA medications.

Beyond the teratogenic potential of the FGAs lies the possibility of fetal and infant toxicities such as neuroleptic malignant syndrome (James 1988) and extrapyramidal side effects (EPS) manifested by heightened muscle tone and increased rooting and tendon reflexes persisting for several months (Cleary 1977; Hill et al. 1966; O'Connor et al. 1981). Furthermore, prenatal exposure to FGAs has been associated with neonatal jaundice (Scokel and Jones 1962) and postnatal intestinal obstruction (Falterman and Richardson 1980).

In our study of antipsychotic placental passage, neonatal haloperidol ($n = 13$) concentrations were 66% of maternal concentrations (Newport et al. 2007a).

In lactation, chlorpromazine is the most widely studied typical antipsychotic, with 7 infants exposed to chlorpromazine during nursing exhibiting no developmental deficits at 16-month and 5-year follow-up evaluations (Kris and Carmichael 1957). However, 3 infants in another study whose mothers were prescribed both chlorpromazine and haloperidol exhibited evidence of developmental delay at 12–18 months (Yoshida et al. 1998b). Pharmacokinetic investigations of FGAs during lactation, including haloperidol (Stewart et al. 1980; Whalley et al. 1981; Yoshida et al. 1998b), trifluoperazine (Wilson et al. 1980; Yoshida et al. 1998b), perphenazine (Wilson et al. 1980), thioxanthenes (Matheson and Skjaeraasen 1988), and chlorpromazine (Yoshida et al. 1998b), have uniformly reported milk-to-plasma ratios of less than 1, although adequate control for distribution and time gradients is lacking in these studies. One group postulated that the physicochemical properties of perphenazine could lead it to become "trapped" in breast milk (Wilson et al. 1980); however, this speculation is unconfirmed.

Fetal and infant exposure to any of the various agents available for the management of EPS (e.g., diphenhydramine, benztropine, amantadine) also raises concern. Results of the Collaborative Perinatal Project indicate that first-trimester exposure to diphenhydramine, the best studied of these medications, is associated with major and minor congenital anomalies (Miller 1991; Wisner and Perel 1988). A case-control study demonstrated a significantly higher rate of prenatal diphenhydramine exposure among 599 infants with oral clefts than among 590 control infants (Saxén 1974). Despite these data, diphenhydramine has maintained a relatively favorable FDA Category B rating and is routinely utilized during pregnancy, underscoring the potential discordance between category systems, clinical experience, and formal investigation. Clinical studies of the teratogenic potential of benztropine and amantadine are lacking, although laboratory animal studies indicate that amantadine is associated with an elevated risk of congenital malformations (Hirsch and Swartz 1980). Perinatal toxicities, including neonatal intestinal obstruction after gestational exposure to benztropine (Falterman and Richardson 1980) and a possible neonatal diphenhydramine withdrawal syndrome manifested by tremulousness and diarrhea (Parkin 1974), also warrant concern.

In summary, FGAs have been widely used for more than 40 years, and the paucity of data linking these agents to either teratogenic or toxic effects suggests that their risks are minimal. In particular, piperazine phenothiazines (e.g., trifluoperazine, perphenazine) may have especially limited teratogenic potential (Rumeau-Rouquette et al. 1977). Given the greater perinatal risks associated with anticholinergic medications (e.g., diphenhydramine), their use should be avoided if possible. Consequently, FGAs used during the peripartum should be kept at the lowest effective dose to minimize the need for adjunctive medications to manage EPS. Early data regarding the teratogenic potential of the SGAs have been reassuring; however, the limited volume of SGA data to date precludes definitive conclusions regarding their reproductive safety. Therefore, the routine use of SGAs during pregnancy and lactation cannot yet be recommended. Nonetheless, if a woman who is taking an SGA inadvertently conceives, a comprehensive risk-benefit assessment may indicate that continuing the SGA (to which the fetus has already been exposed) during gestation is preferable to switching to an FGA (to which the fetus has not yet been exposed).

Anxiolytics

Pharmacotherapy for anxiety disorders includes antidepressants, benzodiazepines, buspirone, and certain atypical antipsychotics.

Benzodiazepines

A retrospective analysis including more than 100,000 women found that at least 2% were prescribed a benzodiazepine during gestation (Bergman et al. 1992). The earliest benzodiazepine teratogenicity studies reported an increased risk of oral clefts after diazepam exposure (Aarskog 1975; Saxén 1975; Saxén and Saxén 1974), but later studies failed to confirm this association (Entman and Vaughn 1984; Rosenberg et al. 1984; Shiono and Mills 1984). Prospective studies of first-trimester alprazolam exposure encompassing approximately 1,300 pregnancies demonstrated no excess of oral clefts or other birth defects (Barry and St. Clair 1987; Schick-Boschetto and Zuber 1992; St. Clair and Schirmer 1992). A subsequent meta-analysis demonstrated that prenatal benzodiazepine exposure does confer an increased risk of oral cleft, although the absolute risk increased by only 0.01% (Altshuler et al. 1996). This conclusion is consistent with that of a later case-control study that found no difference in the rate of prenatal benzodiazepine exposure between more than 38,000 infants with congenital anomalies and nearly 23,000 control children without congenital defects (Eros et al. 2002).

Studies to evaluate the neurobehavioral effects of prenatal benzodiazepine exposure are urgently needed. A benzodiazepine exposure syndrome—consisting of growth retardation, dysmorphism, and mental and psychomotor retardation in infants exposed prenatally to benzodiazepines (Laegreid et al. 1987)—has been reported, although other investigators have disputed this finding (Gerhardsson and Alfredsson 1987; Winter 1987). One group found no differences in the incidence of behavioral abnormalities at age 8 months or in IQ scores at age 4 years among children exposed to chlordiazepoxide during gestation (Hartz et al. 1975). Nevertheless, a series of laboratory animal studies raised concerns that prenatal benzodiazepine exposure may produce deficits in memory and learning ability (Frieder et al. 1984; Hassmannova and Myslivecek 1994; Jaiswal and Bhattacharya 1993; Myslivecek et al. 1991).

Although benzodiazepine teratogenicity data are somewhat mixed, benzodiazepine neonatal syndromes are well documented. Numerous groups have described a floppy infant syndrome characterized by hypothermia, lethargy, poor respiratory effort, and feeding difficulties following benzodiazepine exposure in late pregnancy (Erkkola et al. 1983; Fisher et al. 1985; Haram 1977; Kriel and Cloyd 1982; McAuley et al. 1982; Sanchis et al. 1991; Speight 1977; Woods and Malan 1978). In a study of 53 infants with late-pregnancy lorazepam exposure, term infants whose mothers had taken oral lorazepam (up to 2.5 mg three times daily) showed no evidence of toxicity other than a brief delay in establishing feeding, whereas preterm infants and term infants whose mothers had received larger intravenous doses of lorazepam exhibited symptoms consistent with floppy infant syndrome

(Whitelaw et al. 1981). Neonatal withdrawal syndromes characterized by restlessness, hypertonia, hyperreflexia, tremulousness, apnea, diarrhea, and vomiting have been described in infants whose mothers were taking alprazolam (Barry and St. Clair 1987), chlordiazepoxide (Athinarayanan et al. 1976; Bitnum 1969; Stirrat et al. 1974), or diazepam (Backes and Cordero 1980; Mazzi 1977). Benzodiazepine neonatal syndromes have been reported to persist for as long as 3 months after delivery (for a review, see Miller 1991).

Pharmacokinetic studies during pregnancy indicate that benzodiazepines readily traverse the placenta and with prolonged administration may accumulate in the fetus (Mandelli et al. 1975; Shannon et al. 1972). For example, fetal concentrations of diazepam at delivery are typically higher than maternal concentrations (Erkkola et al. 1974). Because benzodiazepine metabolism in the fetus is slower than that in the adult, it is understandable that an agent like diazepam (which has multiple active metabolites) might accumulate in the fetus. In addition, high concentrations of diazepam are sequestered in lipophilic fetal tissues, including the brain, lungs, and heart (Mandelli et al. 1975). In contrast, fetal-maternal ratios of lorazepam (which has no active metabolites) are typically less than 1 (Whitelaw et al. 1981). Yet neonatal clearance of lorazepam is slow, with detectable levels evident 8 days after delivery (Whitelaw et al. 1981), and the clearance of chlordiazepoxide appears to be even slower (Athinarayanan et al. 1976).

Buist et al. (1990) concluded that benzodiazepines at relatively low doses present no contraindication to nursing. However, infants with impaired metabolic capacity may exhibit sedation and poor feeding even with low maternal doses (Wesson et al. 1985). Overall, benzodiazepines exhibit lower milk-to-plasma ratios than other classes of psychotropics. For example, Wreitland (1987) found a milk-to-plasma ratio of 0.1–0.3 for oxazepam and calculated that the infant daily dose via lactation is 1/1,000th of the maternal dose. The percentage of the maternal dose of lorazepam to which a nursing infant is exposed has been estimated to be 2.2% (Summerfield and Nielsen 1985).

In summary, benzodiazepines do not appear to carry a significant risk of somatic teratogenesis, but neurobehavioral sequelae remain obscure. Because benzodiazepines are associated with neonatal risks, they should be used judiciously and tapered before delivery if possible. Benzodiazepines should not, however, be abruptly withdrawn during pregnancy. Clonazepam (FDA Category C) appears to have minimal teratogenic risks (Sullivan and McElhatton 1977). Because lorazepam and oxazepam are less dependent on hepatic metabolism, they theoretically have less potential for fetal accumulation during pregnancy. Finally, when judicious doses are utilized, benzodiazepines can be safely administered during lactation. However, breastfeeding should be discontinued if an infant exhibits sedation or other signs of benzodiazepine toxicity, regardless of maternal dose.

Buspirone

Buspirone has garnered a unique, and arguably illogical, position within the psychotropic armamentarium. It is the only psychotropic agent that still carries an FDA Category B designation for pregnancy. While this would seem to imply that buspirone is the safest psychotropic agent to administer during gestation, published data are in fact extremely limited. The only report of prenatal administration of buspirone identified 1 infant born with a major malformation among 14 infants with first-trimester buspirone exposure (Wilton et al. 1998). There are no published reports regarding buspirone's safety during lactation.

Future Directions and General Recommendations

The development of perinatal treatment guidelines is hampered by the haphazard accrual of clinical research data with inconsistent methodologies. Whereas clinical data have confirmed the teratogenic potential for only a few psychotropic agents, animal studies, which commonly use maternal concentrations exponentially higher than those seen in clinical care, demonstrate clear somatic and neurobehavioral teratogenicity (Elia et al. 1987). Such inconsistencies between clinical and preclinical data further confound efforts to construct reliable treatment recommendations. Because pregnant and nursing women are generally excluded from clinical trials of pharmacological agents, definitive clarification is unlikely to be forthcoming in the near future. Consequently, treatment decisions must be made using incomplete or uncertain information.

Reproductive Safety Ratings

The current FDA pregnancy rating system has numerous shortcomings. For example, medications that have been available longer have had more time to accrue adverse reports than newer, less studied medications, and as a result, they often have less favorable safety classifications. Furthermore, it is often difficult to ascertain the process that contributed to a specific medication's rating, leading to rating inconsistencies and controversies. As currently formulated, the FDA pregnancy rating system arguably possesses greater medicolegal than clinical relevance. In 2008, the FDA proposed the introduction of new pregnancy and lactation labeling requirements (U.S. Food and Drug Administration 2008). As proposed, the new labeling requirements will constitute an exponential advance over existing rating systems, providing a standard format for presenting clinical and preclinical safety data and risk summaries derived from those data.

Informed Consent

The importance of a thorough informed consent process cannot be overemphasized. Informed consent should include the following:

1. Agreement on the primary treatment objective, which typically is to minimize potential harm to the fetus (Acceptance of and adherence to this objective help reduce the potential for subsequent maternal self-recrimination.)
2. Discussion of the availability, affordability, and potential efficacy of nonpharmacological treatments
3. Consideration of the likelihood and severity of illness without continued pharmacotherapy
4. Review of the potential risks of untreated mental illness to the fetus and mother.
5. Review of the potential risks of fetal psychotropic exposure
6. Acknowledgment that there is no risk-free alternative other than deciding not to conceive
7. Acknowledgment that our understanding of risks remains incomplete (Ultimately, it is impossible to provide an exhaustive list of all risks for any given psychotropic agent, but the evidence—or lack of evidence—for adverse effects should be reviewed.)

Nonpsychotropic Treatment Strategies

Nonpsychotropic treatment includes measures to maximize maternal health during pregnancy, such as prenatal vitamins, adequate hydration, daily exercise, and avoidance of alcohol, tobacco, caffeine, and illicit substances. It also includes psychotherapy alternatives appropriate for administration during pregnancy and the postpartum period.

Medication Selection

Psychotropic therapy is administered only when the clinician and patient agree that the risks to the fetus of untreated mental illness likely exceed the risks of fetal psychotropic exposure. Consequently, both the safety and the efficacy of the psychotropic regimen are important considerations. A psychotropic agent is preferred if 1) it has previously been effective for the patient; 2) it has previously been well tolerated by the patient; 3) the fetus has already been exposed to it (i.e., the patient was taking the agent at knowledge of conception); and 4) it has a favorable reproductive safety profile. Switching agents during pregnancy or lactation should generally be avoided (unless there are well-defined risks associated with the current regimen), as it increases the number of medications to which the baby has been exposed and may heighten the mother's vulnerability to illness.

Dosage Management

Maintaining maternal emotional well-being is the goal of perinatal psychotropic treatment. Partial or subtherapeutic treatment enhances risk by continuing to expose the mother and infant to both illness and medications. The minimum effective dose should be maintained throughout treatment, and the clinician should remain mindful that dosage requirements may change during pregnancy. Similarly, clinicians and patients should be aware that dosage adjustment may not significantly alter exposure during pregnancy (i.e., the fetus is exposed to the maternal plasma concentration, not the maternal dose). To minimize the potential for neonatal withdrawal and maternal toxicity after delivery, careful monitoring of side effects and serum concentrations may be indicated. Adjusting the feeding and dose schedule and discarding breast milk at peak concentrations can minimize the exposure of nursing infants.

Monitoring of Nursing Infants

Because clinical laboratory assays typically lack the sensitivity necessary to detect the serum concentrations of nursing infants, infant plasma monitoring for psychotropic medications is not routinely indicated. If there is an index of suspicion that a child is experiencing an adverse effect from nursing exposure to a psychotropic medication, then breastfeeding should be discontinued. However, routine laboratory monitoring (e.g., blood counts, electrolytes, hepatic profiles) is required when nursing mothers are taking medications (e.g., valproate, carbamazepine) with low therapeutic indices or known systemic toxicities.

References

Aarskog D: Letter: Association between maternal intake of diazepam and oral clefts. Lancet 2(7941):921, 1975

Adab N, Jacoby A, Smith D, et al: Additional educational needs in children born to mothers with epilepsy. J Neurol Neurosurg Psychiatry 70:15–21, 2001

Agatonovic-Kustrin S, Ling LH, Tham SY, et al: Molecular descriptors that influence the amount of drugs transfer into human breast milk. J Pharm Biomed Anal 29:103–119, 2002

Alexander FW: Sodium valproate and pregnancy. Arch Dis Child 54:240, 1979

Allen S: A quantitative analysis of the process, mediating variables, and impact of traumatic childbirth. J Reprod Infant Psychol 16:107–131, 1998

Altshuler LL, Burt VK, McMullen M, et al: Breastfeeding and sertraline: a 24-hour analysis. J Clin Psychiatry 56:243–245, 1995

Altshuler LL, Cohen LS, Szuba MP, et al: Pharmacologic management of psychiatric illness in pregnancy: dilemmas and guidelines. Am J Psychiatry 153:592–606, 1996

Alwan S, Reefhuis J, Rasmussen SA, et al: Use of selective serotonin-reuptake inhibitors in pregnancy and the risk of birth defects. N Engl J Med 356:2684–2692, 2007

Ambresin G, Berney P, Schulz P, et al: Olanzapine excretion into breast milk: a case report. J Clin Psychopharmacol 24:93–95, 2004

American Academy of Pediatrics, Committee on Drugs: The transfer of drugs and other chemicals into human milk. Pediatrics 108:776–789, 2001

Andrade SE, McPhillips H, Loren D, et al: Antidepressant medication use and risk of persistent pulmonary hypertension of the newborn. Pharmacoepidemiol Drug Safety 18:246–252, 2009

Ardinger H, Atkin J, Blackston RD, et al: Verification of the fetal valproate syndrome phenotype. Am J Med Genet 29:171–185, 1988

Assencio-Ferreira VJ, Abraham R, Veiga JC, et al: Metopic suture craniosynostosis: sodium valproate teratogenic effect: case report [Portuguese]. Arquivos de Neuro-Psiquiatria 59:417–420, 2001

Athinarayanan P, Peirog SH, Nigam SK, et al: Chlordiazepoxide withdrawal in the neonate. Am J Obstet Gynecol 124:212–213, 1976

Audus KL: Controlling drug delivery across the placenta. Eur J Pharmacol Sci 8:161–165, 1999

Backes CR, Cordero L: Withdrawal symptoms in the neonate from presumptive intrauterine exposure to diazepam: report of case. J Am Osteopath Assoc 79:584–585, 1980

Bardy AH, Granström ML, Hiilesmaa VK: Valproic acid and breast feeding, in Epilepsy, Pregnancy, and the Child. Edited by Janz D, Dam M, Richens A. New York, Raven Press 1982a, pp 359–360

Bardy AH, Teramo K, Hiilesmaa VK: Apparent plasma clearances of phenytoin, phenobarbitone, primidone, and carbamazepine during pregnancy: results of the prospective Helsinki study, in Epilepsy, Pregnancy, and the Child. Edited by Janz D, Dam M, Richens A, et al. New York, Raven Press, 1982b, pp 141–145

Barnas C, Bergant A, Hummer A, et al: Clozapine concentrations in maternal and fetal plasma, amniotic fluid, and breast milk (abstract). Am J Psychiatry 151:945, 1994

Barry WS, St. Clair SM: Exposure to benzodiazepines in utero. Lancet 1(8547):1436–1437, 1987

Barson AJ: Malformed infant (letter). BMJ 2:45, 1972

Battino D, Avanzini G, Bossi L, et al: Monitoring of antiepileptic drug plasma levels during pregnancy and puerperium, in Epilepsy, Pregnancy, and the Child. Edited by Janz D, Dam M, Richens A, et al. New York, Raven Press, 1982, pp 147–154

Bennedsen BE, Mortensen PB, Olesen AV, et al: Obstetric complications in women with schizophrenia. Schizophr Res 47:167–175, 2001

Berard A, Ramos E, Rey E, et al: First trimester exposure to paroxetine and risk of cardiac malformations in infants: the importance of dosage. Birth Defects Res Part B: Dev Reprod Toxicol 80:18–27, 2007

Bergman U, Rosa FW, Baum C, et al: Effects of exposure to benzodiazepine during fetal life. Lancet 340:694–696, 1992

Bertossi M, Virgintino D, Errede M, et al: Immunohistochemical and ultrastructural characterization of cortical plate microvasculature in the human fetus telencephalon. Microvasc Res 58:49–61, 1999

Bescoby-Chambers N, Forster P, Bates G: Foetal valproate syndrome and autism: additional evidence of an association. Dev Med Child Neurol 43:847, 2001

Birnbaum C, Cohen LS, Bailey JW, et al: Serum concentrations of antidepressants and benzodiazepines in nursing infants: a case series. Pediatrics 104:1–6, 1999

Bitnum S: Possible effects of chlordiazepoxide on the foetus. Can Med Assoc J 100:351, 1969

Bjerkedal T, Czeizel A, Goujard J, et al: Valproic acid and spina bifida. Lancet 2(8307):1096, 1982

Black MM, Matula K: Essentials of Bayley Scales of Infant Development—II Assessment. New York, Wiley, 2000

Bologa M, Tang B, Klein J, et al: Pregnancy-induced changes in drug metabolism in epileptic women. J Pharmacol Exp Ther 267:735–740, 1991

Boobis AR, Lewis PJ: Pharmacokinetics in pregnancy, in Clinical Pharmacology in Obstetrics. Edited by Lewis P. Boston, MA, Wright-PSG, 1983, pp 6–54

Boshier A, Wilton LV, Shakir SA: Evaluation of the safety of bupropion (Zyban) for smoking cessation from experience gained in general practice use in England in 2000. Eur J Clin Pharmacol 59:767–773, 2003

Brent NB, Wisner KL: Fluoxetine and carbamazepine concentrations in a nursing mother/infant pair. Clin Pediatr 37:41–44, 1998

Briggs GG, Samson JH, Ambrose PJ, et al: Excretion of bupropion in breast milk. Ann Pharmacother 27:431–433, 1993

Briggs GG, Freeman RK, Yaffe SJ: Drugs in Pregnancy and Lactation, 4th Edition. Philadelphia, PA, Lippincott Williams & Wilkins, 1994

Briggs GG, Freeman RK, Yaffe SJ: Drugs in Pregnancy and Lactation, 7th Edition. Philadelphia, PA, Lippincott Williams & Wilkins, 2005

Brockington IF, Winokur G, Dean C: Puerperal psychosis, in Motherhood and Mental Illness. Edited by Brockington IF, Kumar R. London, Academic Press, 1982, pp 37–69

Buesching DP, Glasser ML, Frate DA: Progression of depression in the prenatal and postpartum periods. Women Health 11:61–78, 1988

Buist A, Norman TR, Dennerstein L: Breastfeeding and the use of psychotropic medication: a review. J Affect Disord 19:197–206, 1990

Burch K, Wells B: Fluoxetine/norfluoxetine concentrations in human milk. Pediatrics 89:676–677, 1992

Canger R, Battino D, Canevini MP, et al: Malformations in offspring of women with epilepsy: a prospective study. Epilepsia 40:1231–1236, 1999

Capello CF, Bourke CH, Ritchie JC, et al: Serotonin transporter occupancy in rats exposed to serotonin reuptake inhibitors in utero or via breast milk. J Pharmacol Exp Ther J Pharmacol Exp Ther 339:275–285, 2011

Casper RC, Fleisher BE, Lee-Ancajas JC, et al: Follow-up of children of depressed mothers exposed or not exposed to antidepressant drugs during pregnancy. J Pediatr 142:402–408, 2003

Centers for Disease Control: Spina bifida incidence at birth—United States, 1983–1990. MMWR Morb Mortal Wkly Rep 41:497–500, 1992

Chambers CD, Johnson KA, Dick LM, et al: Birth outcomes in pregnant women taking fluoxetine. N Engl J Med 335:1010–1015, 1996

Chambers CD, Hernandez-Diaz S, Van Marter LJ, et al: Selective serotonin-reuptake inhibitors and risk of persistent pulmonary hypertension of the newborn. N Engl J Med 354:579–587, 2006

Chun-Fai-Chan B, Koren G, Fayez I, et al: Pregnancy outcome of women exposed to bupropion during pregnancy: a prospective comparative study. Am J Obstet Gynecol 192:932–936, 2005

Cleary MF: Fluphenazine decanoate during pregnancy. Am J Psychiatry 134:815–816, 1977

Cohen LS, Friedman JM, Jefferson JW, et al: A reevaluation of risk of in utero exposures to lithium. JAMA 271:146–150, 1994

Cohen LS, Altshuler LL, Harlow BL, et al: Relapse of major depression during pregnancy in women who maintain or discontinue antidepressant treatment. JAMA 295:499–507, 2006 (Erratum appears in JAMA 296:170, 2006)

Cole JA, Ephross SA, Cosmatos IS, et al: Paroxetine in the first trimester and the prevalence of congenital malformations. Pharmacoepidemiol Drug Saf 16:1075–1085, 2007

Coppola D, Russo LJ, Kwarta RF, et al: Evaluating the postmarketing experience of risperidone use during pregnancy: pregnancy and neonatal outcomes. Drug Saf 30:247–264, 2007

Costei AM, Kozer E, Ho T, et al: Perinatal outcome following third trimester exposure to paroxetine. Arch Pediatr Adolesc Med 156:1129–1132, 2002

Croke S, Buist A, Hackett LP, et al: Olanzapine excretion in human breast milk: estimation of infant exposure. Int J Neuropsychopharmacol 5:243–247, 2002

Cutrona CE: Causal attributions and perinatal depression. J Abnorm Psychol 92:161–172, 1986

Dalens B, Raynaud EJ, Gaulme J: Teratogenicity of valproic acid. J Pediatr 97:332–333, 1980

Dallemagne G, Weiss B: Altered behavior of mice following postnatal treatment with haloperidol. Pharmacol Biochem Behav 16:761–767, 1982

Dam J, Christiansen J, Munck O, et al: Antiepileptic drugs: metabolism in pregnancy. Clin Pharmacokinet 4:53–62, 1979

Dean JC, Moore SJ, Osborne A, et al: Fetal anticonvulsant syndrome and mutation in the maternal MTHFR gene. Clin Genet 56:216–220, 1999

de Haan GJ, Edelbroek P, Segers J, et al: Gestation-induced changes in lamotrigine pharmacokinetics: a monotherapy study. Neurology 63:571–573, 2004

Dev V, Krupp P: The side-effects and safety of clozapine. Rev Contemp Pharmacother 6:197–208, 1995

Di Liberti JH, Farndon PA, Dennis NR, et al: The fetal valproate syndrome. Am J Med Genet 19:473–481, 1984

Di Michele V, Ramenghi LA, Sabatino G: Clozapine and lorazepam administration in pregnancy. Eur Psychiatry 11:214, 1996

Dickinson RG, Harland RC, Lynn RK, et al: Transmission of valproic acid (Depakene) across the placenta: half-life of the drug in mother and baby. J Pediatr 94:832–835, 1979

Dickson RA, Hogg L: Pregnancy of a patient treated with clozapine. Psychiatr Serv 49:1081–1083, 1998

Djulus J, Koren G, Einarson TR, et al: Exposure to mirtazapine during pregnancy: a prospective, comparative study of birth outcomes. J Clin Psychiatry 67:1280–1284, 2006

Dodd S, Stocky A, Buist A, et al: Sertraline in paired blood plasma and breast-milk samples from nursing mothers. Hum Psychopharmacol 15:261–264, 2000

Dolk H, Jentink J, Loane M, et al: Does Lamotrigine use in pregnancy increase orofacial cleft risk relative to other malformations? Neurology 71:714–722, 2008

Dominguez-Salgado M, Morales A, Santiago Gomez R, et al: Gestational lamotrigine monotherapy: congenital malformations and psychomotor development (abstract). Epilepsia 45 (suppl 7):229–230, 2004

Downey G, Coyne JC: Children of depressed parents: an integrative review. Psychol Bull 108:50–76, 1990

Duffy CL: Postpartum depression: identifying women at risk. Genesis 11:21, 1983

Ebbesen F, Joergensen AM, Hoseth E, et al: Neonatal hypoglycaemia and withdrawal symptoms after exposure in utero to valproate. Arch Dis Child Fetal Neonatal Ed 83:F124–F129, 2000

Edlund MJ, Craig TJ: Antipsychotic drug use and birth defects: an epidemiologic reassessment. Compr Psychiatry 25:244–248, 1976

Eggermont E: Withdrawal symptoms in neonates associated with maternal imipramine therapy. Lancet 2(7830):680, 1973

Einarson A, Fatoye B, Sarkar M, et al: Pregnancy outcome following gestational exposure to venlafaxine: a multicenter prospective controlled study. Am J Psychiatry 158:1728–1730, 2001

Einarson A, Bonari L, Voyer-Lavigne S, et al: A multicentre prospective controlled study to determine the safety of trazodone and nefazodone use during pregnancy. Can J Psychiatry 48:106–110, 2003

Elia J, Katz IR, Simpson GM: Teratogenicity of psychotherapeutic medications. Psychopharmacol Bull 23:531–586, 1987

Engelhard IM, van den Hout MA, Arntz A. Posttraumatic stress disorder after pregnancy loss. Gen Hosp Psychiatry 23:62–66, 2001

Entman SS, Vaughn WK: Lack of relation of oral clefts to diazepam use in pregnancy. N Engl J Med 310:1121–1122, 1984

Epperson C, Anderson G, McDougle C: Sertraline and breast-feeding. N Engl J Med 336:1189–1190, 1997

Epperson N, Czarkowski KA, Ward-O'Brien D, et al: Maternal sertraline treatment and serotonin transport in breast-feeding mother-infant pairs. Am J Psychiatry 158:1631–1637, 2001

Ericson A, Källén B, Wiholm BE: Delivery outcome after the use of antidepressants in early pregnancy. Eur J Clin Pharmacol 55:503–508, 1999

Erkkola R, Kanto J, Sellman R: Diazepam in early human pregnancy. Acta Obstet Gynecol Scand 53:135–138, 1974

Erkkola R, Kero P, Kanto J, et al: Severe abuse of psychotropic drugs during pregnancy with good perinatal outcome. Ann Clin Res 15:88–91, 1983

Eros E, Czeizel AE, Rockenbauer M, et al: A population-based case-control teratologic study of nitrazepam, medazepam, tofisopam, alprazolam, and clonazepam treatment during pregnancy. Eur J Obstet Gynecol Reprod Biol 101:147–154, 2002

Falterman CG, Richardson CJ: Small left colon syndrome associated with maternal ingestion of psychotropic drugs. J Pediatr 97:308–310, 1980

Fisher JN, Edgren BE, Mammel MC, et al: Neonatal apnea associated with clonazepam therapy: a case report. Obstet Gynecol 66:348–358, 1985

Fones C: Posttraumatic stress disorder occurring after painful childbirth. J Nerv Ment Dis 184:195–196, 1996

Fotopoulou C, Kretz R, Bauer S, et al: Prospectively assessed changes in lamotrigine-concentration in women with epilepsy during pregnancy, lactation and the neonatal period. Epilepsy Res 85:60–64, 2009

Franco V, Mazzucchelli I, Gatti G, et al: Changes in lamotrigine pharmacokinetics during pregnancy and the puerperium. Ther Drug Monit 30:544–547, 2008

Frederiksen MC: Physiologic changes in pregnancy and their effect on drug disposition. Semin Perinatol 25:120–123, 2001

Frey B, Schubiger G, Musy JP: Transient cholestatic hepatitis in a neonate associated with carbamazepine exposure during pregnancy and breast-feeding. Eur J Pediatr 150:136–138, 1990

Frey B, Braegger CP, Ghelfi D: Neonatal cholestatic hepatitis from carbamazepine exposure during pregnancy and breast feeding. Ann Pharmacother 36:644–647, 2002

Frieder B, Epstein S, Grimm VE: The effects of exposure to diazepam during various stages of gestation or during lactation on the development and behavior of rat pups. Psychopharmacology 83:51–55, 1984

Friedman JM, Polifka JE: Teratogenic Effects of Drugs: A Resource for Clinicians (TERIS), 2nd Edition. Baltimore, MD, Johns Hopkins University Press, 2000, pp ix–x

Friedman SH, Rosenthal MB: Treatment of perinatal delusional disorder: a case report. Int J Psychiatry Med 33:391–394, 2003

Fries H: Lithium in pregnancy. Lancet 1(7658): 1233, 1970

Froescher W, Eichelbaum M, Nieson M, et al: Antiepileptic therapy with carbamazepine and valproic acid during pregnancy and the lactation period, in Advances in Epileptology: The 12th Epilepsy International Symposium. Edited by Dam M, Gram L, Penry JK. New York, Raven Press, 1981, pp 581–588

Froescher W, Eichelbaum M, Niesen M, et al: Carbamazepine levels in breast milk. Ther Drug Monit 6:266–271, 1984a

Froescher W, Gugler R, Niesen M, et al: Protein binding of valproic acid in maternal and umbilical cord serum. Epilepsia 25:244–249, 1984b

Gaily E, Kantola-Sorsa E, Granstrom ML: Specific cognitive dysfunction in children with epileptic mothers. Dev Med Child Neurol 32:403–414, 1990

Galler JR, Harrison RH, Ramsey F, et al: Maternal depressive symptoms affect infant cognitive development in Barbados. J Child Psychol Psychiatry 41:747–757, 2000

Gardiner SJ, Kristensen JH, Begg EJ, et al: Transfer of olanzapine into breast milk, calculation of infant drug dose, and effect on breast-fed infants. Am J Psychiatry 160:1428–1431, 2003

Gerhardsson M, Alfredsson L: In-utero exposure to benzodiazepines. Lancet 1(8533):628, 1987

GlaxoSmithKline: Epidemiology study: Updated preliminary report on bupropion and other antidepressants, including paroxetine in pregnancy and the occurrence of cardiovascular and major congenital malformations (study EPIP083). 2005. Available at: http://ctr,gsk.co.uk/summary/paroxetine/epip083part2.pdf. Accessed January 2008.

GlaxoSmithKline Corp: International Pregnancy Registry: interim report (1 September 1992 through 31 March 2007). Wilmington, NC, Inveresk, 2007

Glaze R, Chapman G, Murray D: Recurrence of puerperal psychosis during late pregnancy. Br J Psychiatry 159:567–569, 1991

Goldberg HL, DiMascio A: Psychotropic drugs in pregnancy, in Psychopharmacology: A Generation of Progress. Edited by Lipton HL, DiMascio A, Killam KF. New York, Raven, 1978, pp 1047–1055

Goldstein DJ, Sundell KL, Corbin LA: Birth outcomes in pregnant women taking fluoxetine. N Engl J Med 336:872–873, 1997

Goldstein DJ, Corbin LA, Fung MC: Olanzapine-exposed pregnancies and lactation: early experience. J Clin Psychopharmacol 20:399–403, 2000

Hallberg P, Sjöblom V: The use of selective serotonin reuptake inhibitors during pregnancy and breastfeeding: a review and clinical aspects. J Clin Psychopharmacol 25:59–73, 2005

Haram K: "Floppy infant syndrome" and maternal diazepam. Lancet 2(8038):612–613, 1977

Hartz SC, Heinonen OP, Shapiro S, et al: Antenatal exposure to meprobamate and chlordiazepoxide in relation to malformations, mental development, and childhood mortality. N Engl J Med 292:726–728, 1975

Hassmannova J, Myslivecek J: Inhibitory and excitatory adult learning after prenatal diazepam application. Studia Psychologica 36:323–326, 1994

Hedegaard M, Henriksen T, Sabroe S, et al: The relationship between psychological distress during pregnancy and birth weight for gestational age. Acta Obstet Gynecol Scand 75:32–39, 1996

Heikkinen T, Ekblad U, Kero P, et al: Citalopram in pregnancy and lactation. Clin Pharmacol Ther 72:184–191, 2002

Hendrick V, Fukuchi A, Altshuler LL, et al: Use of sertraline, paroxetine, and fluvoxamine by nursing women. Br J Psychiatry 179:163–166, 2001a

Hendrick V, Stowe ZN, Altshuler LL, et al: Fluoxetine in nursing infants and breast milk. Biol Psychiatry 50:775–782, 2001b

Hendrick V, Smith LM, Suri R, et al: Birth outcomes after prenatal exposure to antidepressant medication. Am J Obstet Gynecol 188:812–815, 2003a

Hendrick V, Stowe ZN, Altshuler LL, et al: Placental passage of antidepressant medication. Am J Psychiatry 160:993–996, 2003b

Hernandez-Diaz S, Werler MM, Walker AM, et al: Neural tube defects in relation to use of folic acid antagonists during pregnancy. Am J Epidemiol 153:961–968, 2001

Hertzberg T, Wahlbeck K: The impact of pregnancy and puerperium on panic disorder: a review. J Psychosom Obstet Gynecol 20:59–64, 1999

Hill RC, McIvor RJ, Wojnar-Horton RE, et al: Risperidone distribution and excretion into human milk: case report and estimated infant exposure during breast-feeding. J Clin Psychopharmacol 20:285–286, 2000

Hill RM, Stern L: Drugs in pregnancy: effects on the fetus and newborn. Curr Ther 20:131–150, 1979

Hill RM, Desmond MM, Kay JL: Extrapyramidal dysfunction in an infant of a schizophrenic mother. J Pediatr 69:589–595, 1966

Hirsch MS, Swartz MN: Antiviral agents. N Engl J Med 302:903–907, 1980

Hoffeld DR, McNew J, Webster RL: Effect of tranquilizing drugs during pregnancy on activity of offspring. Nature 218:357–358, 1968

Holmes LB, Wyszynski DF, Baldwin EJ, et al: Increased risk for non-syndromic cleft palate among infants exposed to lamotrigine during pregnancy (abstract). Birth Defects Res Part A Clin Mol Teratol 76:318, 2006

Hostetter A, Stowe ZN, McLaughlin E, et al: The dose of selective serotonin reuptake inhibitors across pregnancy: clinical implications. Depress Anx 11:51–57, 2000

Ilett K, Hackett L, Dusci L, et al: Distribution and excretion of venlafaxine and O-desmethylvenlafaxine in human milk. Br J Clin Pharmacol 45:459–462, 1998

Ilett KF, Hackett LP, Kristensen JH, et al: Transfer of risperidone and 9-hydroxyrisperidone into human milk. Ann Pharmacother 38:273–276, 2004

Jacobsen SJ, Jones K, Johnson K, et al: Prospective multicentre study of pregnancy outcome after lithium exposure during first trimester. Lancet 339:530–533, 1992

Jager-Roman E, Deichl A, Jakob S, et al: Fetal growth, major malformations, and minor anomalies in infants born to women receiving valproic acid. J Pediatr 108:997–1004, 1986

Jaiswal A, Bhattacharya S: Effects of gestational undernutrition, stress and diazepam treatment on spatial discrimination learning and retention in young rats. Indian J Exp Biol 31:353–359, 1993

James ME: Neuroleptic malignant syndrome in pregnancy. Psychosomatics 29:112–119, 1988

Jameson PB, Gelfand DM, Kulcsar E, et al: Mother-toddler interaction patterns associated with maternal depression. Dev Psychopathol 9:537–550, 1997

Jenike MA, Hyman S, Baer L, et al: A controlled trial of fluvoxamine in obsessive-compulsive disorder: implications for a serotonergic theory. Am J Psychiatry 147:1209–1215, 1990

Jensen P, Olesen O, Bertelsen A, et al: Citalopram and desmethylcitalopram concentrations in breast milk and in serum of mother and infant. Ther Drug Monit 19:236–239, 1997

Jentink J, Dolk H, Loane MA, et al: Intrauterine exposure to carbamazepine and specific congenital malformations: systematic review and case-control study. BMJ 341:c6581, 2010

Jones KL, Lacro RV, Johnson KA, et al: Pattern of malformations in the children of women treated with carbamazepine during pregnancy. N Engl J Med 320:1661–1666, 1989

Källén B: Neonate characteristics after maternal use of antidepressants in late pregnancy. Arch Pediatr Adolesc Med 158:312–316, 2004

Källén B, Tandberg A: Lithium and pregnancy: a cohort of manic-depressive women. Acta Psychiatr Scand 68:134–139, 1983

Källén B, Olausson PO: Maternal use of selective serotonin re-uptake inhibitors and persistent pulmonary hypertension of the newborn. Pharmacoepidemiol Drug Safety 17:801–806, 2008

Kaneko S, Suzuki K, Sato T, et al: The problems of antiepileptic medication in the neonatal period: is breast-feeding advisable? in Epilepsy, Pregnancy and the Child. Edited by Janz D, Dam M, Richens A. New York, Raven Press, 1982, pp 343–348

Kaneko S, Battino D, Andermann E, et al: Congenital malformations due to antiepileptic drugs. Epilepsy Res 33:145–158, 1999

Kaplan HI, Sadock BJ: Pocket Handbook of Psychiatric Drug Treatment. Baltimore, MD, Williams & Wilkins, 1993

Karlsson K, Lindstedt G, Lundberg PA, et al: Letter: Transplacental lithium poisoning: reversible inhibition of fetal thyroid. Lancet 1(7919):1295, 1975

Kendell R, Chalmers J, Platz C: Epidemiology of puerperal psychosis. Br J Psychiatry 150:662–673, 1987

Kendler KS, Kessler RC, Neale MC, et al: The prediction of major depression in women: toward an integrated etiologic model. Am J Psychiatry 150:1139–1148, 1993

Kennedy D, Koren G: Valproic acid use in psychiatry: issues in treating women of reproductive age. J Psychiatry Neurosci 23:223–228, 1998

Kirchheiner J, Berghofer A, Bolk-Weischedel D: Healthy outcome under olanzapine treatment in a pregnant woman. Pharmacopsychiatry 33:78–80, 2000

Kirksey A, Groziak SM: Maternal drug use: evaluation of risks to breast-fed infants. World Rev Nutr Diet 43:60–79, 1984

Koch S, Jager-Roman E, Rating D, et al: Possible teratogenic effect of valproate during pregnancy. J Pediatr 103:1007–1008, 1983

Kok TH, Taitz LS, Bennett MJ, et al: Drowsiness due to clemastine transmitted in breast milk. Lancet 1(8277):914–915, 1982

Korebrits C, Ramirez M, Watson L, et al: Maternal corticotropin-releasing hormone is increased with impending preterm birth. J Clin Endocrinol Metab 83:1585–1591, 1998

Kornhuber J, Weller M: Postpartum psychosis and mastitis: a new indication for clozapine? Am J Psychiatry 148:1751–1752, 1991

Kozma C: Valproic acid embryopathy: report of two siblings with further expansion of the phenotypic abnormalities and a review of the literature. Am J Med Genet 98:168–175, 2001

Kriel RL, Cloyd J: Clonazepam and pregnancy. Ann Neurol 11:544, 1982

Kris EB: Children of mothers maintained on pharmacotherapy during pregnancy and postpartum. Curr Ther Res 7:785–789, 1965

Kris EB, Carmichael D: Chlorpromazine maintenance therapy during pregnancy and confinement. Psychiatr Q 31:690–695, 1957

Kristensen J, Ilett K, Dusci L, et al: Distribution and excretion of sertraline and N-desmethylsertraline in human milk. Br J Clin Pharmacol 45:453–457, 1998

Kristensen J, Ilett K, Hackett L, et al: Distribution and excretion of fluoxetine and norfluoxetine in human milk. Br J Clin Pharmacol 48:521–527, 1999

Kuhnz W, Jager-Roman E, Rating D, et al: Carbamazepine and carbamazepine-10,11-epoxide during pregnancy and postnatal period in epileptic mothers and their nursed infants: pharmacokinetics and clinical effects. Pediatr Pharmacol 3:199–208, 1983

Kulin N, Pastuszak A, Sage S, et al: Pregnancy outcome following maternal use of the new selective serotonin reuptake inhibitors: a prospective controlled multicenter study. JAMA 279:609–610, 1998

Kumar R, Robson KM: A prospective study of emotional disorders in childbearing women. Br J Psychiatry 144:35–47, 1984

Laegreid L, Olegard R, Wahlstrom J, et al: Abnormalities in children exposed to benzodiazepines in utero. Lancet 1(8524):108–109, 1987

Laine K, Heikkinen T, Ekblad U, et al: Effects of exposure to selective serotonin reuptake inhibitors during pregnancy on serotonergic symptoms in newborns and cord blood monoamine and prolactin concentrations. Arch Gen Psychiatry 60:720–726, 2003

Lajeunie E, Le Merrer M, Marchac D, et al: Syndromal and nonsyndromal primary trigonocephaly: analysis of 237 patients. Am J Med Genet 75:211–215, 1998

Lajeunie E, Barcik U, Thorne JA, et al: Craniosynostosis and fetal exposure to sodium valproate. J Neurosurg 95:778–782, 2001

Lander CM, Livingstone I, Tyrer JH, et al: The clearance of anticonvulsant drugs in pregnancy. Clin Exp Neurol 17:71–78, 1980

Lee A, Giesbrecht E, Dunn E, et al: Excretion of quetiapine in breast milk. Am J Psychiatry 161:1715–1716, 2004

Lester B, Cucca J, Andreozzi L, et al: Possible association between fluoxetine hydrochloride and colic in an infant. J Am Acad Child Adolesc Psychiatry 32:1253–1255, 1993

Lindhout D, Schmidt D: In-utero exposure to valproate and neural tube defects. Lancet 1(8494): 329–333, 1986

Liporace J, Kao A, D'Abreu A: Concerns regarding lamotrigine and breast-feeding. Epilepsy Behav 5:102–105, 2004

Little BB: Pharmacokinetics during pregnancy: evidence-based maternal dose formulation. Obstet Gynecol 93:858–868, 1999

Llewellyn AM, Stowe ZN, Strader JR: The use of lithium and management of women with bipolar disorder during pregnancy and lactation. J Clin Psychiatry 59 (suppl 6):57–64, 1998

Lobo ED, Loghin C, Knadler MP, et al: Pharmacokinetics of duloxetine in breast milk and plasma of healthy postpartum women. Clin Pharmacokinetics 47:103–109, 2008

Louik C, Lin AE, Werler MM, et al: First-trimester use of selective serotonin-reuptake inhibitors and the risk of birth defects. N Engl J Med 356:2675–2683, 2007

Luoma I, Tamminen T, Kaukonen P, et al: Longitudinal study of maternal depressive symptoms and child well-being. J Am Acad Child Adolesc Psychiatry 40:1367–1374, 2001

Luoma I, Kaukonen P, Mäntymaa M, et al: A longitudinal study of maternal depressive symptoms, negative expectations and perceptions of child problems. Child Psychiatry Hum Dev 35:37–53, 2004

Lutz UC, Hiemke, Wiatr G, et al: Aripiprazole in pregnancy and lactation: a case report. J Clin Psychopharmacol 30:204–205, 2010

Lyons-Ruth K, Wolfe R, Lyubchik A: Depression and the parenting of young children: making the case for early preventive mental health services. Harv Rev Psychiatry 8:148–153, 2000

Mammen O, Perel JM, Rudolph G, et al: Sertraline and norsertraline levels in three breastfed infants. J Clin Psychiatry 58:100–103, 1997

Mandelli M, Morselli PL, Nordio S, et al: Placental transfer of diazepam and its disposition in the newborn. Clin Pharmacol Ther 17:564–572, 1975

Manly PC, McMahon RJ, Bradley CF, et al: Depressive attributional style and depression following childbirth. J Abnorm Psychol 91:245–254, 1982

Marcus SM, Flynn HA, Blow FC, et al: Depressive symptoms among pregnant women screened in obstetrics settings. J Womens Health (Larchmt) 12:373–380, 2003

Martinez A, Malphurs J, Field T, et al: Depressed mothers' and their infants' interactions with nondepressed partners. Infant Ment Health J 17:74–80, 1996

Martinez-Frias ML: Clinical manifestation of prenatal exposure to valproic acid using case reports and epidemiologic information. Am J Med Genet 37:277–282, 1990

Martins C, Gaffan EA: Effects of early maternal depression on patterns of infant-mother attachment: a meta-analytic investigation. J Child Psychol Psychiatry 41:737–746, 2000

Maschi S, Clavenna A, Campi R, et al: Neonatal outcome following pregnancy exposure to antidepressants: a prospective controlled cohort study. BJOG 115:283–289, 2008

Matalon S, Schechtman S, Goldzweig G, et al: The teratogenic effect of carbamazepine: a meta-analysis of 1255 exposures. Reprod Toxicol 16:9–17, 2002

Matheson I, Pande H, Alertson AR: Respiratory depression caused by N-desmethyldoxepine in breast milk. Lancet 2(8464):1124, 1985

Matheson I, Skjaeraasen J: Milk concentrations of flupenthixol, nortriptyline and zuclopenthixol and between-breast differences in two patients. Eur J Clin Pharmacol 35:217–220, 1988

Mazzi E: Possible neonatal diazepam withdrawal: a case report. Am J Obstet Gynecol 129:586–587, 1977

McAuley DM, O'Neill MP, Moore J, et al: Lorazepam premedication for labour. Br J Obstet Gynecol 89:149–154, 1982

McBride WG: Limb deformities associated with iminodibenzyl hydrochloride. Med J Aust 1:175–178, 1972

McElhatton PR, Garbis HM, Elefant E, et al: The outcome of pregnancy in 689 women exposed to therapeutic doses of antidepressants: a collaborative study of the European Network of Teratology Information Services (ENTIS). Reprod Toxicol 10:285–294, 1996

McEvoy JP, Hatcher A, Appelbaum PS, et al: Chronic schizophrenic women's attitudes toward sex, pregnancy, birth control, and childrearing. Hosp Community Psychiatry 34:536–539, 1983

McKenna K, Koren G, Tetelbaum M, et al: Pregnancy outcome of women using atypical antipsychotic drugs: a prospective comparison study. J Clin Psychiatry 66:444–449, 2005

McMahon CL, Braddock SR: Septo-optic dysplasia as a manifestation of valproic acid embryopathy. Teratology 64:83–86, 2001

McNeil TF, Kaij L, Malmquist-Larson A: Women with nonorganic psychosis: mental disturbance during pregnancy. Acta Psychiatr Scand 70:127–139, 1984a

McNeil TF, Kaij L, Malmquist-Larson A: Women with nonorganic psychosis: pregnancy's effect on mental health during pregnancy. Acta Psychiatr Scand 70:140–148, 1984b

McVearry KM, Gaillard WD, VanMeter J, et al: A prospective study of cognitive fluency and originality in children exposed in utero to carbamazepine, lamotrigine, or valproate monotherapy. Epilepsy Behav 16:609–616, 2009

Meador KJ, Baker GA, Finnell RH, et al: In utero antiepileptic drug exposure: fetal death and malformations. Neurology 67:407–412, 2006

Meador KJ, Baker GA, Browning N, et al: Cognitive function at 3 years of age after fetal exposure to antiepileptic drugs. N Engl J Med 360:1597–1605, 2009

Meador JK, Baker GA, Browning N, et al: Foetal antiepileptic drug exposure and verbal versus non-verbal abilities at three years of age. Brain 134 (pt 2):396–404, 2011

Meijer A: Child psychiatric sequelae of maternal war stress. Acta Psychiatr Scand 72:505–511, 1985

Merlob P, Mor N, Litwin A: Transient hepatic dysfunction in an infant of an epileptic mother treated with carbamazepine during pregnancy and breastfeeding. Ann Pharmacother 26:1563–1565, 1992

Milkovich L, Van den Berg BJ: An evaluation of the teratogenicity of certain antinauseant drugs. Am J Obstet Gynecol 125:244–248, 1976

Miller LJ: Clinical strategies for the use of psychotropic drugs during pregnancy. Psychiatr Med 9:275–298, 1991

Miller LJ, Finnerty M: Sexuality, pregnancy, and childrearing among women with schizophrenia-spectrum disorders. Psychiatr Serv 47:502–506, 1996

Misri S, Sivertz K: Tricyclic drugs in pregnancy and lactation: a preliminary report. Int J Psychiatry Med 21:157–171, 1991

Misri S, Oberlander TF, Fairbrother N, et al: Relation between prenatal maternal mood and anxiety and neonatal health. Can J Psychiatry 49:684–689, 2004

Mizrahi EM, Hobbs JF, Goldsmith DI: Nephrogenic diabetes insipidus in transplacental lithium intoxication. J Pediatr 94:493–495, 1979

Molgaard-Nielsen D, Hviid A: Newer-generation antiepileptic drugs and the risk of major birth defects. JAMA 305:1996–2002, 2011

Moore SJ, Turnpenny P, Quinn A, et al: A clinical study of 57 children with fetal anticonvulsant syndromes. J Med Genet 37:489–497, 2000

Moore WM, Hellegers AE, Battaglia FC: In vitro permeability of different layers of human placenta to carbohydrates and urea. Am J Obstet Gynecol 96:951–955, 1966

Morgan DJ: Drug disposition in mother and foetus. Clin Exp Pharmacol Physiol 24:869–873, 1997

Moriarty AJ, Nance NR: Trifluoperazine and pregnancy. Can Med Assoc J 88:375–376, 1963

Morrow J, Russell A, Guthrie E, et al: Malformation risks of antiepileptic drugs in pregnancy: a prospective study from the UK Epilepsy and Pregnancy Register. J Neurol Neurosurg Psychiatry 77:193–198, 2006

Moses-Kolko EL, Bogen D, Perel J, et al: Neonatal signs after late in utero exposure to serotonin reuptake inhibitors: literature review and implications for clinical applications. JAMA 293:2372–2383, 2005

Mountain KR, Hirsh J, Gallus AS: Neonatal coagulation defect due to anticonvulsant drug treatment in pregnancy. Lancet 1(7641):265–268, 1970

Myllynen PK, Pienimaki PK, Vahakangas KH: Transplacental passage of lamotrigine in a human placental perfusion system in vitro and in maternal and cord blood in vivo. Eur J Clin Pharmacol 58:677–682, 2003

Myslivecek J, Hassmannova J, Josifko M: Impact of prenatal low-dose diazepam or chlorpromazine on reflex and motor development and inhibitory-learning. Homeost Health Dis 33:77–88, 1991

Nadebaum C, Anderson V, Vajda F, et al: The Australian brain and cognition and antiepileptic drugs study: IQ in school-aged children exposed to sodium valproate and polytherapy. J Intl Neuropsychol Soc 17:133–142, 2011a

Nadebaum C, Anderson V, Vajda F, et al: Language skills of school-aged children prenatally exposed to antiepileptic drugs. Neurology 76:719–726, 2011b

Nau H, Rating D, Koch S, et al: Valproic acid and its metabolites: placental transfer, neonatal pharmacokinetics, transfer via mother's milk and clinical status in neonates of epileptic mothers. J Pharmacol Exp Ther 219:768–777, 1981

Nau H, Kuhnz W, Egger HJ, et al: Anticonvulsants during pregnancy and lactation: transplacental, maternal and neonatal pharmacokinetics. Clin Pharmacokinet 7:508–543, 1982a

Nau H, Wittfoht W, Rating D, et al: Pharmacokinetics of valproic acid and its metabolites in a pregnant patient: stable isotope methodology, in Epilepsy, Pregnancy, and the Child. Edited by Janz D, Bossi L, Dam M, et al: New York, Raven Press, 1982b, pp 131–139

Newport DJ, Stowe ZN, Nemeroff CB: Parental depression: animal models of an adverse life event. Am J Psychiatry 159:1265–1283, 2002

Newport DJ, Viguera AC, Beach AJ, et al: Lithium placental passage and obstetrical outcome: implications for clinical management during late pregnancy. Am J Psychiatry 162:2162–2170, 2005

Newport DJ, Calamaras MR, DeVane CL, et al: Atypical antipsychotic administration during late pregnancy: placental passage and obstetrical outcomes. Am J Psychiatry 164:1214–1220, 2007a

Newport DJ, Levey LC, Ragan K, et al: Suicidal ideation in pregnancy: assessment and clinical implications. Arch Womens Ment Health 10:181–187, 2007b

Newport DJ, Brennan PA, Green P, et al: Maternal depression and medication exposure during pregnancy: comparison of retrospective recall to prospective documentation. Br J Obstet Gynaecol 115:681–688, 2008a

Newport DJ, Pennell PB, Calamaras MR, et al: Lamotrigine in breast milk and nursing infants: determination of exposure. Pediatrics 122:e223–e231, 2008b

Newport DJ, Stowe ZN, Viguera AC, et al: Lamotrigine in bipolar disorder: efficacy during pregnancy. Bipolar Disord 10:432–436, 2008c

Newport DJ, Ritchie JC, Knight BT, et al: Venlafaxine in human breast milk and nursing infant plasma: determination of exposure. J Clin Psychiatry 70:1304–1310, 2009

Newport DJ, Ji S, Long Q, et al: Maternal depression and anxiety differentially impact fetal exposures during pregnancy. J Clin Psychiatry 73:247–251, 2012

New York State Department of Health: Congenital Malformations Registry Summary Report: Statistical Summary of Children Born in 1998–2001 and Diagnosed Through 2003. Troy, NY, Congenital Malformations Registry, New York State Department of Health, 2005. Available at: http://www.health.state. ny.us/nysdoh/cmr/docs/98report.pdf. Accessed November 2007.

Niebyl JR, Blake DA, Freeman JM, et al: Carbamazepine levels in pregnancy and lactation. Obstet Gynecol 53:139–140, 1979

Nora JJ, Nora AH, Toews WH: Letter: Lithium, Ebstein's anomaly, and other congenital heart defects. Lancet 2(7880):594–595, 1974

Nordmo E, Aronsen L, Wasland K, et al: Severe apnea in an infant exposed to lamotrigine in breast milk. Ann Pharmacother 43:1893–1897, 2009

Nulman I, Rovet J, Stewart DE, et al: Neurodevelopment of children exposed in utero to antidepressant drugs. N Engl J Med 336:258–262, 1997a

Nulman I, Scolnick D, Chitayat D, et al: Findings in children exposed in utero to phenytoin and carbamazepine monotherapy: independent effects of epilepsy and medications. Am J Med Genet 68:18–24, 1997b

Nulman I, Rovet J, Stewart DE, et al: Child development following exposure to tricyclic antidepressants or fluoxetine throughout fetal life: a prospective, controlled study. Am J Psychiatry 159:1889–1895, 2002

Nurnberg HG, Prudic J: Guidelines for treatment of psychosis during pregnancy. Hosp Community Psychiatry 35:67–71, 1984

Oberlander TF, Misri S, Fitzgerald CE, et al: Pharmacologic factors associated with transient neonatal symptoms following prenatal psychotropic medication exposure. J Clin Psychiatry 65:230–237, 2004

Oberlander TF, Warburton W, Misri S, et al: Neonatal outcomes after prenatal exposure to selective serotonin reuptake inhibitor antidepressants and maternal depression using population-based linked health data. Arch Gen Psychiatry 63:898–906, 2006

Oberlander TF, Reebye P, Misri S, et al: Externalizing and attentional behaviors in children of depressed mothers treated with a selective serotonin reuptake inhibitor antidepressant during pregnancy. Arch Pediatr Adolesc Med 161:22–29, 2007

O'Connor MO, Johnson GH, James DI: Intrauterine effect of phenothiazines. Med J Aust 1:416–417, 1981

O'Connor TG, Heron J, Golding J, et al: Maternal antenatal anxiety and behavioural/emotional problems in children: a test of a programming hypothesis. J Child Psychol Psychiatry 44:1025–1036, 2003

Oesterheld JR: A review of developmental aspects of cytochrome P450. J Child Adolesc Psychopharmacol 8:161–174, 1998

O'Hara MW, Rehm LP, Campbell SB: Predicting depressive symptomatology: cognitive-behavioural models and postpartum depression. J Abnorm Psychol 91:457–461, 1982

Ohman I, Vitols S, Tomson T: Lamotrigine in pregnancy: pharmacokinetics during delivery, in the neonate, and during lactation. Epilepsia 41:709–713, 2000

Ohman R, Hagg S, Carleborg L, et al: Excretion of paroxetine into breast milk. J Clin Psychiatry 60:519–523, 1999

Omtzigt JG, Nau H, Los FJ, et al: The disposition of valproate and its metabolites in the late first trimester and early second trimester of pregnancy in maternal serum, urine, and amniotic fluid: effect of dose, co-medication, and the presence of spina bifida. Eur J Clin Pharmacol 43:381–388, 1992

Omtzigt JG, Los FJ, Meijer JW, et al: The 10,11-epoxide-10,11-diol pathway of carbamazepine in early pregnancy in maternal serum, urine, and amniotic fluid: effect of dose, comedication, and relation to outcome of pregnancy. Ther Drug Monit 15:1–10, 1993

Ordy JM, Samorajski T, Collins RL: Prenatal chlorpromazine effects on liver survival and behavior of mice offspring. J Pharmacol Exp Ther 151:110–125, 1966

Ornoy A, Cohen E: Outcome of children born to epileptic mothers treated with carbamazepine during pregnancy. Arch Dis Child 75:517–520, 1996

Orr S, Miller C: Maternal depressive symptoms and the risk of poor pregnancy outcome. Epidemiol Rev 17:165–170, 1995

Orr ST, James SA, Blackmore Prince C: Maternal prenatal depressive symptoms and spontaneous preterm births among African-American women in Baltimore, Maryland. Am J Epidemiol 156:797–802, 2002

Otani K: Risk factors for the increased seizure frequency during pregnancy and puerperium. Folia Psychiatr Neurol Jpn 39:33–41, 1985

Pacifici GM, Nottoli R: Placental transfer of drugs administered to the mother. Clin Pharmacokinet 28:235–269, 1995

Page-Sharp M, Kristensen JH, Hackett LP, et al: Transfer of lamotrigine into breast milk. Ann Pharmacother 40:1470–1471, 2006

Parkin DE: Probable Benadryl withdrawal manifestations in a newborn infant. J Pediatr 85:580, 1974

Pastuszak A, Schick-Boschetto B, Zuber C, et al: Pregnancy outcome following first trimester exposure to fluoxetine (Prozac). JAMA 269:2246–2248, 1993

Paulson GW, Paulson RB: Teratogenic effects of anticonvulsants. Arch Neurol 38:140–143, 1981

Pennell PB, Newport DJ, Stowe ZN, et al: The impact of pregnancy and childbirth on the metabolism of lamotrigine. Neurology 62:292–295, 2004

Pennell PB, Peng L, Newport DJ, et al: Lamotrigine in pregnancy: clearance, therapeutic drug monitoring, and seizure frequency. Neurology 70 (22 pt 2):2130–2136, 2008

Perkin R, Bland J, Peacock J, et al: The effect of anxiety and depression during pregnancy on obstetric complications. Br J Obstet Gynaecol 100:629–634, 1993

Petrenaite V, Sabers A, Hansen-Schwartz J: Individual changes in lamotrigine plasma concentrations during pregnancy. Epilepsy Res 65:185–188, 2005

Philbert A, Pederson B, Dam M: Concentration of valproate during pregnancy in the newborn and in breast milk. Acta Neurol Scand 72:460–463, 1985

Piontek CM, Baab S, Peindl KS, et al: Serum valproate levels in 6 breast-feeding mother-infant pairs. J Clin Psychiatry 61:170–172, 2000

Piontek CM, Wisner KL, Perel JM, et al: Serum fluvoxamine levels in breastfed infants. J Clin Psychiatry 52:111–113, 2001

Pynnonen S, Sillanpaa M: Letter: carbamazepine and mother's milk. Lancet 2(7934):563, 1975

Pynnonen S, Kanto J, Sillanpaa M, et al: Carbamazepine: placental transport, tissue concentrations in foetus and newborn, and level in milk. Acta Pharmacol Toxicol 41:244–253, 1977

Rambeck B, Kurlemann G, Stodieck SR, et al: Concentrations of lamotrigine in a mother on lamotrigine treatment and her newborn child. Eur J Clin Pharmacol 51:481–484, 1997

Rampono J, Hackett LP, Kristensen JH, et al: Transfer of escitalopram and its metabolite desmethylescitalopram into breastmilk. Br J Clin Pharmacol 62:316–322, 2006

Rampono J, Simmer K, Ilett KF, et al: Placental transfer of SSRI and SNRI antidepressants and effects on the neonate. Pharmacopsychiatry 42:95–100, 2009

Rampono J, Teoh S, Hackett LP, et al: Estimation of desvenlafaxine transfer into milk and infant exposure during its use in lactating women with postnatal depression. Arch Womens Mental Health 14:49–53, 2011

Rawlings WJ, Ferguson R, Maddison TG: Phenmetrazine and trifluoperazine. Med J Aust 1:370, 1963

Rieder RO, Rosenthal D, Wender P, et al: The offspring of schizophrenics: fetal and neonatal deaths. Arch Gen Psychiatry 32:200–211, 1975

Rimm AA, Katayama AC, Diaz M, et al: A meta-analysis of controlled studies comparing major malformation rates in IVF and ICSI infants with naturally conceived children. J Assist Reprod Genet 21:437–443, 2004

Riordan D, Appleby L, Faragher B: Mother-infant interaction in post-partum women with schizophrenia and affective disorders. Psychol Med 29:991–995, 1999

Robertson RT, Majka JA, Peter CP, et al: Effects of prenatal exposure to chlorpromazine on postnatal development and behavior of rats. Toxicol Appl Pharmacol 53:541–549, 1980

Rodriguez-Pinilla E, Arroyo I, Fondevilla J, et al: Prenatal exposure to valproic acid during pregnancy and limb deficiencies: a case-control study. Am J Med Genet 90:376–381, 2000

Rosa FW: Spina bifida in infants of women treated with carbamazepine during pregnancy. N Engl J Med 324:674–677, 1991

Rosenberg L, Mitchell AA, Parsells JL, et al: Lack of relation of oral clefts to diazepam use during pregnancy. N Engl J Med 309:1281–1285, 1984

Rumeau-Rouquette C, Goujard J, Huel G: Possible teratogenic effect of phenothiazines in human beings. Teratology 15:57–64, 1977

Sabers A, Dam M, A-Rogvi-Hansen B, et al: Epilepsy and pregnancy: lamotrigine as main drug used. Acta Neurol Scand 109:9–13, 2004

Samrén E, van Duijn C, Koch S, et al: Maternal use of antiepileptic drugs and the risk of major congenital malformations: a joint European prospective study of human teratogenesis associated with maternal epilepsy. Epilepsia 38:981–990, 1997

Samrén E, van Duijn C, Christiaens G, et al: Antiepileptic drug regimens and major congenital abnormalities in the offspring. Ann Neurol 46:739–746, 1999

Sanchis A, Rosique D, Catala J: Adverse effects of maternal lorazepam on neonates. Ann Pharmacother 25:1137–1138, 1991

Sathanandar S, Blesi K, Tran T, et al: Lamotrigine clearance increases markedly during pregnancy. Epilepsia 41:246, 2000

Saxén I: Cleft palate and maternal diphenhydramine intake. Lancet 1(7854):407–408, 1974

Saxén I: Association between oral clefts and drugs taken during pregnancy. Int J Epidemiol 4:37–44, 1975

Saxén I, Saxén L: Letter: Association between maternal intake of diazepam and oral clefts. Lancet 2(7933):498, 1974

Schatzberg AF, Cole JO: Manual of Clinical Psychopharmacology, 2nd Edition. Washington, DC, American Psychiatric Press, 1991

Schell L: Environmental noise and human prenatal growth. Am J Physiol Anthropol 56:63–70, 1981

Schick-Boschetto B, Zuber C: Alprazolam exposure during early human pregnancy. Teratology 45: 460, 1992

Schlotterbeck P, Leube D, Kircher T, et al: Aripiprazole in human milk. Int J Neuropsychopharmacol 10:433, 2007

Schlotterbeck P, Saur R, Hiemke C, et al: Low concentration of ziprasidone in human milk: a case report. Int J Neuropsychopharmacol 12:437–438, 2009

Schmidt K, Olesen O, Jensen P: Citalopram and breast-feeding: serum concentration and side effects in the infant. Biol Psychiatry 47:164–165, 2000

Schou M: What happened later to the lithium babies? Follow-up study of children born without malformations. Acta Psychiatr Scand 54:193–197, 1976

Schou M, Amdisen A: Lithium and pregnancy, III: lithium ingestion by children breast-fed by women on lithium treatment. BMJ 2:138, 1973

Scokel PW, Jones WD: Infant jaundice after phenothiazine drugs for labor: an enigma. Obstet Gynecol 20:124–127, 1962

Scolnick D, Nulman I, Rovet J, et al: Neurodevelopment of children exposed in utero to phenytoin and carbamazepine monotherapy. JAMA 271:767–770, 1994

Shallcross R, Bromley RL, Irwin B, et al: Child development following in utero exposure: levetiracetam vs sodium valproate. Neurology 76:383–389, 2011

Shannon RW, Fraser GP, Aitken RG, et al: Diazepam in preeclamptic toxaemia with special reference to its effect on the newborn infant. Br J Clin Pract 26:271–275, 1972

Shiono PH, Mills JL: Oral clefts and diazepam use during pregnancy. N Engl J Med 311:919–920, 1984

Simon GE, Cunningham ML, Davis RL: Outcomes of prenatal antidepressant exposure. Am J Psychiatry 159:2055–2061, 2002

Sivojelezova A, Shuhaiber S, Sarkissian L, et al: Citalopram use in pregnancy: prospective comparative evaluation of pregnancy and fetal outcome. Am J Obstet Gynecol 193:2004–2009, 2005

Skausig OB, Schou M: Breast feeding during lithium therapy [Danish]. Ugeskrift for Laeger 139:400–401, 1977

Slone D, Siskind V, Heinonen OP, et al: Antenatal exposure to the phenothiazines in relation to congenital malformations, perinatal mortality rate, birth weight, and intelligence quotient score. Am J Obstet Gynecol 128:468–486, 1977

Smith MV, Poschman K, Cavaleri MA, et al: Symptoms of posttraumatic stress disorder in a community sample of low-income pregnant women. Am J Psychiatry 163:881–884, 2006

Sodhi P, Poddar B, Parmar V: Fatal cardiac malformation in fetal valproate syndrome. Indian J Pediatr 68:989–990, 2001

Sondergaard C, Olsen J, Friis-Hasche E, et al: Psychosocial distress during pregnancy and the risk of infantile colic: a follow-up study. Acta Paediatr 92:811–816, 2003

Speight AN: Floppy-infant syndrome and maternal diazepam and/or nitrazepam. Lancet 2(8043): 878, 1977

Spigset O, Carleborg L, Norstrom A, et al: Paroxetine level in breast milk. J Clin Psychiatry 57: 39, 1996

Spigset O, Carleborg L, Ohman R, et al: Excretion of citalopram in breast milk. Br J Clin Pharmacol 44:295–298, 1997

St. Clair SM, Schirmer RG: First trimester exposure to alprazolam. Obstet Gynecol 80:843–846, 1992

Stahl MM, Neiderud J, Vinge E: Thrombocytopenic purpura and anemia in a breast-fed infant whose mother was treated with valproic acid. J Pediatr 130:1001–1003, 1997

Steer R, Scholl T, Hediger M, et al: Self-reported depression and negative pregnancy outcomes. Epidemiology 45:1093–1099, 1992

Stewart R, Karas B, Springer P: Haloperidol excretion in human milk. Am J Psychiatry 137:849–850, 1980

Stirrat GM, Edington P, Berry DJ: Transplacental passage of chlordiazepoxide. BMJ 2:729, 1974

Stoner SC, Sommi RW, Marken PA, et al: Clozapine use in two full-term pregnancies. J Clin Psychiatry 58:364–365, 1997

Stott D: Follow-up study from birth of the effects of prenatal stresses. Dev Med Child Neurol 15: 770–787, 1973

Stowe ZN, Nemeroff CB: Women at risk for postpartum-onset major depression. Am J Obstet Gynecol 173:639–645, 1995

Stowe ZN, Owens MJ, Landry JC, et al: Sertraline and desmethylsertraline in human breast milk and nursing infants. Am J Psychiatry 154:1255–1260, 1997

Stowe ZN, Cohen LS, Hostetter A, et al: Paroxetine in breast milk and nursing infants. Am J Psychiatry 157:185–189, 2000

Stowe ZN, Hostetter A, Owens MJ, et al: The pharmacokinetics of sertraline excretion into human breast milk: determinants of infant serum concentrations. J Clin Psychiatry 64:73–80, 2003

Stowe Z, Hostetter A, Newport D: The onset of postpartum depression: implications for clinical screening in obstetrical and primary care. Am J Obstet Gynecol 192:522–526, 2005

Sullivan FM, McElhatton PR: A comparison of the teratogenic activity of the antiepileptic drugs carbamazepine, clonazepam, ethosuximide, phenobarbital, phenytoin, and pyrimidone in mice. Toxicol Appl Pharmacol 40:365–378, 1977

Summerfield RJ, Nielsen MS: Excretion of lorazepam into breast milk. Br J Anaesth 57:1042–1043, 1985

Suri R, Stowe ZN, Hendrick V, et al: Estimates of nursing infant daily dose of fluoxetine through breast milk. Biol Psychiatry 52:446–451, 2002

Swedish Centre for Epidemiology: Registration of congenital malformations in the Swedish Health Registers. Stockholm, Sweden, National Board of Health and Welfare, Centre for Epidemiology, June 18, 2004. Available at: http://www.socialstyrelsen.se/Publicerat/2004/5120/2004-112-1.htm. Accessed December 2007.

Sykes PA, Quarrie J, Alexander FW: Lithium carbonate and breast-feeding. BMJ 2:1299, 1976

Taddio A, Ito S, Koren G: Excretion of fluoxetine and its metabolite norfluoxetine in human breast milk. J Clin Pharmacol 36:42–47, 1996

Targum S, Davenport Y, Webster M: Postpartum mania in bipolar manic-depressive patients withdrawn from lithium carbonate. J Nerv Ment Dis 167:572–574, 1979

Tenyi T, Tixler M: Clozapine in the treatment of pregnant schizophrenic women. Psychiatria Danubina 10:15–18, 1998

Thisted E, Ebbesen F: Malformations, withdrawal manifestations, and hypoglycaemia after exposure to valproate in utero. Arch Dis Child 69:288–291, 1993

Tomson T, Lindborn U, Ekqvist B, et al: Disposition of carbamazepine and phenytoin in pregnancy. Epilepsia 35:131–135, 1994

Tomson T, Ohman I, Vitols S: Lamotrigine in pregnancy and lactation: a case report. Epilepsia 38:1039–1041, 1997

Tran TA, Leppik IE, Blesi K, et al: Lamotrigine clearance during pregnancy. Neurology 59:251–255, 2002

Troutman B, Cutrona C: Nonpsychotic postpartum depression among adolescent mothers. J Abnorm Psychol 99:69–78, 1990

Tsuru N, Maeda T, Tsuruoka M: Three cases of delivery under sodium valproate—placental transfer, milk transfer and probable teratogenicity of sodium valproate. Jpn J Psychiatry Neurol 42:89–96, 1988

Tunnessen WW, Hertz CG: Toxic effects of lithium in newborn infants: a commentary. J Pediatr 81:804–807, 1972

Turton P, Hughes P, Evans CD, et al: Incidence, correlates and predictors of post-traumatic stress disorder in the pregnancy after stillbirth. Br J Psychiatry 178:556–560, 2001

U.S. Food and Drug Administration: 21 CFR Part 201—Content and format of labeling for human prescription drug and biological products; requirements for pregnancy and lactation labeling. Federal Register 73:30831–30868, 2008

Vajda FJ, O'Brien TJ, Hitchcock A, et al: The Australian registry of anti-epileptic drugs in pregnancy: experience after 30 months. J Clin Neurosci 10:543–549, 2003

Van den Bergh BR, Marcoen A: High antenatal maternal anxiety is related to ADHD symptoms, externalizing problems, and anxiety in 8- and 9-year-olds. Child Dev 75:1085–1097, 2004

Van der Pol MC, Hadders-Algra M, Huisjes MJ, et al: Antiepileptic medication in pregnancy: late effects on the children's nervous system development. Am J Obstet Gynecol 164:121–128, 1991

Van Waes A, Van de Velde EJ: Safety evaluation of haloperidol in the treatment of hyperemesis gravidarum. J Clin Pharmacol 9:224–227, 1969

Viguera AC, Newport DJ, Ritchie JC, et al: Lithium from breast milk in nursing infants: clinical implications. Am J Psychiatry 164:342–345, 2007a

Viguera AC, Whitfield T, Baldessarini RJ, et al: Risk of recurrence in women with bipolar disorder during pregnancy: prospective study of mood stabilizer discontinuation. Am J Psychiatry 164:1817–1824, 2007b

von Unruh GE, Froescher W, Hoffmann F, et al: Valproic acid in breast milk: how much is really there? Ther Drug Monit 6:272–276, 1984

Waldman MD, Safferman AZ: Pregnancy and clozapine. Am J Psychiatry 150:168–169, 1993

Wang JS, Newport DJ, Stowe ZN, et al: The emerging importance of transporter proteins in the psychopharmacological treatment of the pregnant patient. Drug Metab Rev 39:723–746, 2007

Warner A: Drug use in the neonate: inter-relationships of pharmacokinetics, toxicity and biochemical maturity. Clin Chem 32:721–727, 1986

Watson JP, Elliott SA, Rugg AJ, et al: Psychiatric disorder in pregnancy and the first postnatal year. Br J Psychiatry 144:453–462, 1984

Weinstein MR, Goldfield M: Lithium carbonate treatment during pregnancy: report of a case. Dis Nerv System 30:828–832, 1969

Weinstein MR, Goldfield MD: Cardiovascular malformations with lithium use during pregnancy. Am J Psychiatry 132:529–531, 1975

Weissman MM, Prusoff BA, Gammon GD, et al: Psychopathology in the children (ages 6–18) of depressed and normal parents. J Am Acad Child Adolesc Psychiatry 23:78–84, 1984

Welch R, Findlay J: Excretion of drugs in human breast milk. Drug Metab Rev 12:261–277, 1981

Wesson DR, Camber S, Harkey M, et al: Diazepam and desmethyldiazepam in breast milk. J Psychoactive Drugs 17:55–56, 1985

Whalley LJ, Blain PG, Prime JK: Haloperidol secreted in breast milk. BMJ 282:1746–1747, 1981

Whitelaw AG, Cummings AJ, McFadyen IR: Effect of maternal lorazepam on the neonate. BMJ 282:1106–1108, 1981

Whitworth A, Stuppaeck C, Yazdi K, et al: Olanzapine and breast-feeding: changes of plasma concentrations of olanzapine in a breast-fed infant over a period of 5 months. J Psychopharmacol 24:121–123, 2010

Wide K, Winbladh B, Tomson BWT, et al: Psychomotor development and minor anomalies in children exposed to antiepileptic drugs in utero: a prospective population based study. Dev Med Child Neurol 42:87–92, 2000

Williams G, King J, Cunningham M, et al: Fetal valproate syndrome and autism: additional evidence of an association. Dev Med Child Neurol 43:202–206, 2001

Williams KE, Koran L: Obsessive-compulsive disorder in pregnancy, the puerperium, and the premenstruum. J Clin Psychiatry 58:330–334, 1997

Williams PG, Hersh JH: A male with fetal valproate syndrome and autism. Dev Med Child Neurol 39:632–634, 1997

Wilson KL, Zelig CM, Harvey JP, et al: Persistent pulmonary hypertension of the newborn is associated with mode of delivery and not with maternal use of selective serotonin reuptake inhibitors. Am J Perinatol 28:19–24, 2011

Wilson JT, Brown RD, Cherek DR, et al: Drug excretion in human breast milk: principles, pharmacokinetics and projected consequences. Clin Pharmacokinet 5:1–66, 1980

Wilson N, Forfar JC, Godman MJ: Atrial flutter in the newborn resulting from maternal lithium ingestion. Arch Dis Child 58:538–549, 1983

Wilton LV, Pearce GL, Martin RM, et al: The outcomes of pregnancy in women exposed to newly marketed drugs in general practice in England. Br J Obstet Gynaecol 105:882–889, 1998

Winter RM: In utero exposure to benzodiazepines. Lancet 1(8533):627, 1987

Winter RM, Donnai D, Burn J, et al: Fetal valproate syndrome: is there a recognizable phenotype? J Med Genet 24:692–695, 1987

Wisner KL, Perel JM: Psychopharmacologic agents and electroconvulsive therapy during pregnancy and the puerperium, in Psychiatric Consultation in Childbirth Settings: Parent- and Child-Oriented Approaches. Edited by Cohen RL. New York, Plenum, 1988, pp 165–206

Wisner KL, Perel JM: Serum levels of valproate and carbamazepine in breastfeeding mother-infant pairs. J Clin Psychopharmacol 18:167–169, 1998

Wisner KL, Perel JM, Wheeler SB: Tricyclic dose requirements across pregnancy. Am J Psychiatry 150:1541–1542, 1993

Wisner KL, Peindl KS, Hanusa BH: Effect of childbearing on the natural history of panic disorder with comorbid mood disorder. J Affect Disord 41:173–180, 1996a

Wisner KL, Perel JM, Findling RL: Antidepressant treatment during breast-feeding. Am J Psychiatry 153:1132–1137, 1996b

Wisner K, Perel J, Blumer J: Serum sertraline and N-desmethylsertraline levels in breast-feeding mother-infant pairs. Am J Psychiatry 155:690–692, 1998

Woods DL, Malan AF: Side effects of maternal diazepam on the newborn infant. S Afr Med J 54:636, 1978

Woody JN, London WL, Wilbanks GD: Lithium toxicity in a newborn. Pediatrics 47:94–96, 1971

Wreitland MA: Excretion of oxazepam in breast milk. Eur J Clin Pharmacol 33:209–210, 1987

Wright S, Dawling S, Ashford J: Excretion of fluvoxamine in breast milk. Br J Clin Pharmacol 31:209, 1991

Wyska E, Jusko WJ: Approaches to pharmacokinetic/pharmacodynamic modeling during pregnancy. Semin Perinatol 25:124–132, 2001

Yerby MS, Friel PN, Miller DQ: Carbamazepine protein binding and disposition in pregnancy. Ther Drug Monit 7:269–273, 1985

Yerby MS, Friel PN, McCormick K, et al: Pharmacokinetics of anticonvulsants in pregnancy: alterations in plasma protein binding. Epilepsy Res 5:223–228, 1990

Yerby MS, Friel PN, McCormick K: Antiepileptic drug disposition during pregnancy. Neurology 42:12–16, 1992

Yoshida K, Smith B, Craggs M, et al: Fluoxetine in breast-milk and developmental outcome of breast-fed infants. Br J Psychiatry 172:175–178, 1998a

Yoshida K, Smith B, Craggs M, et al: Neuroleptic drugs in breast-milk: a study of pharmacokinetics and of possible adverse effects in breast-fed infants. Psychol Med 28:81–91, 1998b

Zambaldi CF, Cantilino A, Montenegro AC, et al: Postpartum obsessive-compulsive disorder: prevalence and clinical characteristics. Compr Psychiatry 50:503–509, 2009

Zeskind PS, Stephens LE: Maternal selective serotonin reuptake inhibitor use during pregnancy and newborn neurobehavior. Pediatrics 113:368–375, 2004

Zuckerman B, Amaro H, Bauchner H, et al: Depressive symptoms during pregnancy: relationship to poor health behaviors. Am J Obstet Gynecol 160:1107–1111, 1989

INDEX

*Page numbers printed in **boldface** type refer to tables or figures.*